The ASCRS Textbook of Colon and Rectal Surgery

The ASCRS Textbook of Colon and Rectal Surgery

Third Edition

Volume 1

Editors

Scott R. Steele, MD
Tracy L. Hull, MD
Thomas E. Read, MD
Theodore J. Saclarides, MD
Anthony J. Senagore, MD
Charles B. Whitlow, MD

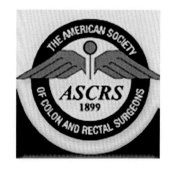

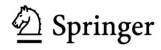

Editors
Scott R. Steele, M.D
Chief, Division of Colorectal Surgery
University Hospitals Case Medical Center
Professor of Surgery
Case Western Reserve University
Cleveland, OH, USA

Thomas E. Read, MD
Professor of Surgery
Tufts University School of Medicine
Lahey Hospital & Medical Center
Burlington, MA, USA

Anthony J. Senagore, MD
Professor, Chief of Gastrointestinal Surgery
University of Texas Medical Branch at Galveston
Galveston, TX, USA

Tracy L. Hull, MD
Professor of Surgery
Cleveland Clinic
Cleveland, OH, USA

Theodore J. Saclarides, MD
Ambrose and Gladys Bowyer
Professor of Surgery
Loyola University
Chicago, IL, USA

Charles B. Whitlow, MD
Chief, Colorectal Surgery
Ochsner Medical Center
New Orleans, LA, USA

Videos to this book can be accessed at http://link.springer.com/book/10.1007/978-3-319-25970-3

ISBN 978-3-319-25968-0   ISBN 978-3-319-25970-3   (eBook)
DOI 10.1007/978-3-319-25970-3

Library of Congress Control Number: 2016936561

Springer Cham Heidelberg New York Dordrecht London

Jointly published with The American Society of Colon and Rectal Surgeons, Arlington Heights, IL, USA

Printed on acid-free paper

Springer International Publishing AG Switzerland is part of Springer Science+Business Media (www.springer.com)

Foreword

One given definition of the word *textbook* is "a book used as *a standard* work for the study of a particular subject." Our collective goal for the third edition of the American Society of Colon and Rectal Surgeons' *ASCRS Textbook of Colon and Rectal Surgery* was to make this volume *the standard* for the study of colon and rectal surgery, providing a valuable resource for surgeons and healthcare providers at all stages of their career caring for patients with colorectal disease. In line with previous editions, we aimed to build upon the collective experience and expertise from national and international experts in the field, providing a completely revamped, up-to-date tome covering the wide breadth of colorectal disease. In addition to providing all newly written chapters, we have reorganized the text around the "pillars" of colorectal disease: perioperative (including endoscopy), anorectal disease, benign disease (including inflammatory bowel disease), malignancy, pelvic floor disorders, and a "miscellaneous" section that covers aspects both inside and beyond the operating room that are pertinent to providers at every level. This restructuring coincides effectively with the ASCRS Online Education Portal (www.fascrs.org) and mirrors the configuration of the Society's collection of educational and CME-accredited programs including CREST and CARSEP. In addition, each chapter contains several **Key Concepts** that succinctly depict the major learning objectives for individual sections and are in line with the Core Curriculum for Colon and Rectal Surgery provided by the Association of Program Directors in Colon and Rectal Surgery and the key topics used by the American Board of Colon and Rectal Surgery.

In addition, we have expanded beyond the initial print-only edition to encompass a multimedia platform with the availability of an electronic version of the text along with online videos depicting procedures, tips and tricks, and complications—all easily accessible through desktops, tablets, and smartphones to accommodate the mobile healthcare world in which we live.

While this textbook was originally conceived as a means of providing state of the art information to residents in training and fully trained surgeons, our hope, more than anything, is that this volume continues to support the mission of the American Society of Colon and Rectal Surgeons as the world's most established authority on colon and rectal disease. We are honored to have been a part of this project and wish to thank the leaders of the ASCRS for their continued support of the textbook. We especially would like to recognize the editors of the first and second editions for having the vision and purpose to produce such high-quality, evidence-based texts that have made the *ASCRS Textbook of Colon and Rectal Surgery* the success and reference it remains today. Lastly, we would like to thank our Developmental Editor Elektra McDermott for her extraordinary efforts and thoroughness in overseeing and ensuring its timely completion, and each chapter author and coauthor(s) for their devotion to this task and to the mission of the ASCRS. Since inception, it has been our privilege and pleasure to work with this tremendous gathering of authors and editors, as their unique contributions have come together to make this textbook a reality.

Cleveland, OH	Scott R. Steele, MD
Cleveland, OH	Tracy Hull, MD
Burlington, MA	Thomas Read, MD
Chicago, IL	Theodore Saclarides, MD
Galveston, TX	Anthony Senagore, MD
New Orleans, LA	Charles Whitlow, MD

Preface

The field of Colon and Rectal Surgery has a long and respected tradition of patient service, knowledge expansion, and education. The American Society of Colon and Rectal Surgeons (ASCRS) is the premier professional organization of this specialty. The leaders of our Society (ASCRS) recognized that there were several textbooks in the field of Colorectal Surgery, but none of which could be deemed as truly representative of the collective objective views of the ASCRS. At the inaugural meeting of the senior and associate editors, prior to the 2007 publication of the *ASCRS Textbook of Colon and Rectal Surgery* 1st edition, the group made several fundamental decisions. One of those decisions was to have chapters extensively referenced, authoritatively written, appropriately illustrated, and as unbiased as possible. This very important latter point was strictly enforced by adherence by the chapter authors to ASCRS materials including the evidence-based ASCRS clinical practice guidelines, core subjects, presentations at our annual meeting, questions in the colon and rectal self-assessment program (CARSEP), and material otherwise presented through official society vehicles. In addition, first edition chapters were, in general, written by a "junior" and a "senior" coauthor. A second decision was a rotation schedule for the editors: two to three of the editors would rotate off after each edition. This would provide wider participation and ensure that the text would represent the specialty as a whole and not a select group of individuals.

The overwhelming success of the first edition led to the publication of a second edition in 2011. The second edition expanded upon the first edition, added new authors, supplemented a significant number of color plates, and increased the text itself from 810 to 946 pages. The vision provided by the leaders of our Society was certainly correct, as attested to by the tremendous interest in both editions of the ASCRS textbooks. We are proud that the standardized reference for evidence-based material in Colorectal Surgery is the work product of our Society members, owned by our Society, and has become a source of financial support to our Society. In addition, a corresponding manual (the *ASCRS Manual of Colon and Rectal Surgery*), designed more towards residents in training and physicians desiring a focused reference, has been released for each edition and has also been exceptionally popular.

The continued rapid expansion of knowledge, in part attested by the increased number of pages in each subsequent edition, as well as the new technologies and new techniques has ensured the longevity of our work and has necessitated this third edition. We congratulate the current editors Drs. Scott Steele, Tracy Hull, Thomas Read, Anthony Senagore, Theodore Sacclarides, and Charles Whitlow on their tremendous accomplishment. We also thank all of the chapter authors and coauthors whose dedication, devotion, energy, and expertise have enabled the editors to produce this volume. The third edition has been reorganized and completely rewritten to reflect advances in our specialty and the evolution of our practice. In addition, the current grouping of topics serves as a framework for the ongoing educational efforts of the Society and certification process by the American Board of Colon and Rectal Surgery.

New developments in the management of colorectal diseases and our colleagues' continued search for answers have produced the need for this and future editions of the *ASCRS Textbook of Colon and Rectal Surgery.* We are gratified that this significant educational endeavor continues to flourish. We commend this work to every practitioner of colorectal surgery throughout the world and eagerly await reports of its success.

New Orleans, LA   Dave Beck, MD
Weston, FL   Steven Wexner, MD

Contents

Volume 1

Part I   Perioperative/Endoscopy

Part II   Anorectal Disease

Part III   Malignant Disease

Volume 2

Contributors

Editors

Tracy Hull, MD
Department of Surgery, Cleveland Clinic, Cleveland, OH, USA

Thomas Read, MD
Tufts University School of Medicine, Lahey Hospital & Medical Center,
Burlington, MA, USA

Theodore Saclarides, MD
Loyola University, Chicago, IL, USA

Anthony Senagore, MD
University of Texas Medical Branch at Galveston,
Galveston, TX, USA

Scott R. Steele, MD
Division of Colorectal Surgery, University Hospitals Case Medical Center,
Case Western Reserve University, Cleveland, OH, USA

Charles Whitlow, MD
Colorectal Surgery, Ochsner Medical Center, New Orleans, LA, USA

Authors

Cary B. Aarons, MD
Division of Colon and Rectal Surgery, Hospital of the University of Pennsylvania,
Philadelphia, PA, USA

Maher A. Abbas, MD, FACS, FASCRS
Digestive Disease Institute, Cleveland Clinic Abu Dhabi Hospital, Abu Dhabi, UAE

Karim Alavi, MD, MPH
Colon and Rectal Surgery Fellowship Program, Department of Surgery,
University of Massachusetts Medical School, Worcester, MA, USA

Dennis K. Ames, JD
La Follette, Johnson, Dehaas, Fesler, and Ames, Santa Ana, CA, USA

Glenn T. Ault, MD, MSEd
Division of Colorectal Surgery, Department of Surgery, University of Southern California,
Los Angeles, CA, USA

Jennifer M. Ayscue, MD, FACS, FASCRS
Section of Colon & Rectal Surgery, Department of Surgery,
MedStar Washington Hospital Center, Washington, DC, USA

Amir L. Bastawrous, MD, MBA
Swedish Colon and Rectal Clinic, Swedish Cancer Institute, Seattle, WA, USA

Joshua I.S. Bleier, MD, FACS, FASCRS
Perelman School of Medicine, University of Pennsylvania Health System, Philadelphia, PA, USA

Liliana Bordeianou, MD
Department of Surgery, Massachusetts General Hospital, Boston, MA, USA

Raul Martin Bosio, MD, MSBS
Division of Colon and Rectal Surgery, Department of Surgery,
University Hospitals Case Medical Center, Case Western Reserve University,
Cleveland, OH, USA

W. Donald Buie, MD, MSc, FRCSC, FACS
Department of Surgery, Foothills Hospital, University of Calgary, Calgary, AB, Canada

Jamie Cannon, MD
Division of Gastrointestinal Surgery, Department of Surgery, University of Alabama-
Birmingham, Birmingham, AL, USA

Evie Carchman, MD
Department of General Surgery, University of Wisconsin, Madison, WI, USA

Joseph C. Carmichael, MD
Department of Surgery, University of California, Irvine, Irvine, CA, USA

Peter A. Cataldo, MD, FACS, FASCRS
Department of Surgery, University of Vermont Medical Center,
University of Vermont College of Medicine, Burlington, VT, USA

Thomas E. Cataldo, MD, FACS, FASCRS
Division of Colon and Rectal Surgery, Department of Surgery,
Beth Israel Deaconess Medical Center, Harvard Medical School, Boston, MA, USA

Andrea Cercek, MD
Department of Medicine, Memorial Sloan Kettering Cancer Center, New York, NY, USA

Bradley J. Champagne, MD, FACS, FASCRS
Department of Surgery, University Hospital Case Medical Center, Cleveland, OH, USA

George J Chang, MD, MS
New Technologies in Oncologic Surgery Program, Department of Surgical Oncology,
The University of MD Anderson Cancer Center, Houston, TX, USA

Dorin T. Colibaseanu, MD
Department of General Surgery, Mayo Clinic, Rochester, MN, USA

Kyle G. Cologne, MD
Division of Colorectal Surgery, University of Southern California Keck School of Medicine,
Los Angeles, CA, USA

Tara M. Connelly, MD, MB, BCh, MSc
Division of Colon and Rectal Surgery, Milton S. Hershey Medical Center, Hershey, PA, USA

Jennifer S. Davids, MD
Department of Surgery, Division of Colon and Rectal Surgery, University of Massachusetts
Memorial Medical Center, Worcester, MA, USA

Bradley R. Davis, MD, FACS, FASCRS
Department of Surgery, Charlotte Hospitals Medical Center, Charlotte, NC, USA

Kurt Davis, MD
Department of Surgery, William Beaumont Army Medical Center, El Paso, TX, USA

Conor P. Delaney, MD, MCh, PhD, FRCSI, FACS, FASCRS
Department of Colorectal Surgery, Digestive Disease Institute, Cleveland Clinic, Cleveland,
OH, USA

Eric J. Dozois, MD
Department of Surgery, Mayo Clinic, Rochester, MN, USA

Jonathan Efron, MD
Department of Surgery, Johns Hopkins Hospital, Johns Hopkins University, Baltimore, MD, USA

Peter F. Ehrlich, MD, MSc
Section of Pediatric Surgery, C.S. Mott Children's Hospital, University of Michigan,
Ann Arbor, MI, USA

Marwan Fakih, MD
Department of Medical Oncology and Therapeutic Diagnostics, City of Hope Medical
Center, Duarte, CA, USA

Daniel Feingold, MD
Columbia University, New York, NY, USA

Alessandro Fichera, MD, FACS, FASCRS
Section of Gastrointestinal Surgery, Department of Surgery, University of Washington,
Seattle, WA, USA

Todd D. Francone, MD, MPH
Department of Colon and Rectal Surgery, Lahey Hospital & Medical Center,
Tufts University Medical Center, Burlington, MA, USA

Charles M. Friel, MD
Department of Surgery, University of Virginia Medical Center, Charlottesville, VA, USA

Wolfgang B. Gaertner, MSc, MD
Department of Colon and Rectal Surgery, University of Minnesota Medical Center,
Minneapolis, MN, USA

Julio Garcia-Aguilar, MD, PhD
Department of Surgery, Memorial Sloan Kettering Cancer Center, New York, NY, USA

Kelly A. Garrett, MD, FACS, FASCRS
Section of Colon and Rectal Surgery, Department of General Surgery, New York Presbyterian
Hospital, Weill Cornell Medical College, New York, NY, USA

Stephen R. Gorfine, MD
Division of Colorectal Surgery, Department of Surgery, The Mount Sinai Hospital,
New York, NY, USA

Brooke Gurland, MD
Department of Colorectal Surgery, Cleveland Clinic Lerner College of Medicine, Cleveland,
OH, USA

Eric M Haas, MD, FACS, FASCRS
Division of Colon and Rectal Surgery, Houston Methodist Hospital, Houston, TX, USA;
Minimally Invasive Colon and Rectal Surgery Fellowship, The University of Texas Medical
School, Houston, TX, USA; Colorectal Surgical Associates, LLP LTD, Houston, TX, USA

Karin E. Hardiman, MD, PhD
Division of Colorectal Surgery, University of Michigan, Ann Arbor, MI, USA

Dana M Hayden, MD, MPH
Department of General Surgery, Loyola University Medical Center, Maywood, IL, USA

Charles P. Heise, MD, FACS, FASCRS
Department of Surgery, University of WI School of Medicine and Public Health, Madison,
WI, USA

Alan J. Herline, MD
Department of Surgery, Georgia Regents University, Augusta, GA, USA

Daniel O. Herzig, MD, FACS, FASCRS
Division of Gastroenterology and General Surgery, Department of Surgery, Oregon Health
and Science University, Portland, OR, USA

Rebecca E. Hoedema, MS, MD, FACS, FASCRS
Department of Colon and Rectal Surgery, Spectrum Health/Ferguson Clinic, Grand Rapids,
MI, USA

Stefan D. Holubar, MD, MS, FACS, FASCRS
Department of Surgery, Dartmouth-Hitchcock Medical Center, Lebanon, NH, USA

Steven R. Hunt, MD
Section of Colon and Rectal Surgery, Division of General Surgery, Barnes Jewish Hospital,
St. Louis, MO, USA; Department of Surgery, Section of Colon and Rectal Surgery,
Washington University School of Medicine, St. Louis, MO, USA

Neil Hyman, MD, FACS, FASCRS
Section of Colon and Rectal Surgery, University of Chicago Medicine, Chicago, IL, USA

Eric K. Johnson, MD
Uniformed Services University of the Health Sciences, Bethesda MD, USA;
Department of Surgery, Madigan Army Medical Center, Joint Base Lewis-McChord, WA, USA

Andreas M. Kaiser, MD, FACS, FASCRS
Keck Medical Center of the University of Southern California, Los Angeles, CA, USA

Matthew F. Kalady, MD
Comprehensive Colorectal Cancer Program, Department of Colorectal Surgery, Cleveland
Clinic, Cleveland, OH, USA

Brian R. Kann, MD, FACS, FASCRS
Department of Colon & Rectal Surgery, Ochsner Medical Center, New Orleans, LA, USA

Muneera R Kapadia, MD, MME
Department of Surgery, University of Iowa Hospitals and Clinics, Iowa City, IA, USA

Kevin R. Kasten, MD
Department of Surgery, Vidant Medical Center, Brody School of Medicine at East Carolina University, Greenville, NC, USA

Gregory D. Kennedy, MD, PhD
Department of Surgery, University of Wisconsin Hospital and Clinics, Madison, WI, USA

Jason D. Keune, MD, MBA
Department of Surgery, St. Louis University School of Medicine, St. Louis, MO, USA

Cindy Kin, MD
Department of Surgery, Stanford University Medical Center, Stanford, CA, USA

P. Ravi Kiran, MBBS, MS (Gen Surgery), FRCS (Eng), FRCS (Glas), FACS, MSc (EBM) Oxford
Center for Innovation and Outcomes Research, Columbia University Medical Center, New York, NY, USA; Mailman School of Public Health, New York, NY, USA; Division of Colorectal Surgery, Department of Colorectal Surgery, New York Presbyterian Hospital, New York, NY, USA

Walter A. Koltun, MD, FACS, FASCRS
Department of Surgery, Division of Colon and Rectal Surgery, Penn State Milton S. Hershey Medical Center, Hershey, PA, USA

Mukta Katdare Krane, MD, FACS
Department of Surgery, University of Washington, Seattle, WA, USA

Anjali S. Kumar, MD, MPH, FACS, FASCRS
Director, Colon & Rectal Surgery Program, Department of Surgery, Virginia Mason Medical Center, Seattle, WA, USA

Alex Jenny Ky, MD
Department of Surgery, Mount Sinai School of Medicine, New York, NY, USA

Frederick R. Lane, MD
Kendrick Colon and Rectal Center, Franciscan St. Francis Health Indianapolis, Indianapolis, IN, USA

Erin O. Lange, MD, MSPH
Department of Surgery, University of Washington Medical Center, Seattle, WA, USA

Sang W. Lee, MD, FACS, FASCRS
Department of General Surgery, Section of Colon and Rectal Surgery, Weill Cornell Medical College, New York Presbyterian Hospital, New York, NY, USA
Keck School of Medicine, University of Southern California, Los Angeles, CA, USA

Kim C. Lu, MD, FACS, FASCRS
Division of Gastrointestinal and General Surgery, Department of Surgery, Oregon Health and Science University, Portland, OR, USA

Martin Luchtefeld, MD, FACS, FASCRS
Department of Colon and Rectal Surgery, Spectrum Health/Ferguson Clinic, Grand Rapids, MI, USA

Anthony R. MacLean, MD, FRCSC, FACS
Department of Surgery, Foothills Medical Centre, University of Calgary, Calgary, AB, Canada

Helen M. MacRae, MD, MA, FRCSC, FACS
Department of Surgery, Mount Sinai Hospital, Toronto, ON, Canada

Najjia N. Mahmoud, MD
Division of Colon and Rectal Surgery, Department of Surgery, University of Philadelphia, Philadelphia, PA, USA

Christopher R. Mantyh, MD
Department of Surgery, Duke University Medical Center, Durham, NC, USA

Jorge Marcet, MD
Department of Surgery, Tampa General Hospital, Tampa, FL, USA

David J. Maron, MD, MBA
Colorectal Surgery Residency Program, Department of Colorectal Surgery, Cleveland Clinic Florida, Weston, FL, USA

Dipen C. Maun, MD
Kendrick Colon and Rectal Center, Franciscan St. Francis Health Indianapolis, Indianapolis, IN, USA

Justin A. Maykel, MD
Division of Colon and Rectal Surgery, Department of Surgery, University of Massachusetts Memorial Medical Center, Worcester, MA, USA

Michael F. McGee, MD, FACS, FASCRS
Division of Gastrointestinal and Oncologic Surgery, Northwestern University Feinberg School of Medicine, Chicago, IL, USA

M. Shane McNevin, MD, FASCRS
Sacred Heart Hospital, Spokane, WA, USA

Genevieve B. Melton, MD, PhD
Department of Surgery, University of Minnesota Medical Center, Minneapolis, MN, USA

John Migaly, MD, FACS, FASCRS
Department of Surgery/Advanced Oncologic and GI Surgery, Duke University Hospital, Durham, NC, USA

Steven Mills, MD
Department of Surgery, University of California, Irvine, Orange, CA, USA

Husein Moloo, MD, MSc, FRCS
Department of Surgery, Ottawa Hospital Research Institute, University of Ottawa, Ottawa, ON, Canada

Roberta Muldoon, MD
Department of Surgery, Vanderbilt University Hospital, Nashville, TN, USA

Matthew Mutch, MD, FACS, FASCRS
Section of Colon and Rectal Surgery, Department of Surgery, Washington University School of Medicine, St. Louis, MO, USA

Garrett M. Nash, MD, MPH
Department of Surgery, Memorial Sloan Kettering Cancer Center, New York, NY, USA

Guy R. Orangio, MD, FACS, FASCRS
Division of Colon and Rectal Surgery, Department of Surgery, University Hospital, Louisiana State University, New Orleans, LA, USA

Emmanouil P. Pappou, MD, PhD
Department of Colorectal Surgery, Columbia University, New York, NY, USA

Ian M. Paquette, MD
Department of Surgery, University of Cincinnati Medical Center, Cincinnati, OH, USA

Marie Fidela R. Paraiso, MD
Department of Obstetrics and Gynecology, Cleveland Clinic, Cleveland, OH, USA

W. Brian Perry, MD, FASCRS
Audie L. Murphy VA Medical Center, San Antonio, TX, USA

Matthew M. Philp, MD, FACS, FASCRS
Division of Colon and Rectal Surgery, Temple University Hospital, Philadelphia, PA, USA

Vitaly Y. Poylin, MD, FACS, FASCRS
Division of Colon and Rectal Surgery, Department of Surgery, Beth Israel Deaconess Medical Center, Harvard Medical School, Boston, MA, USA

Isabelle Raîche, MD, FRCS
Department of Surgery, The Ottawa Hospital, University of Ottawa, Ottawa, ON, Canada

Jan Rakinic, MD
Section of Colorectal Surgery, Department of Surgery, Southern Illinois University, Springfield, IL, USA

Scott E. Regenbogen, MD, MPH
Division of Colorectal Surgery, University of Michigan, Ann Arbor, MI, USA

Rocco Ricciardi, MD, MPH
Lahey Hospital and Medical Center, Burlington, MA, USA

Howard M. Ross, MD
Department of Surgery, Temple University Health System, Philadelphia, PA, USA

Andrew Russ, MD
Department of Surgery, University Colon and Rectal Surgery, University of Tennessee Medical Center, Knoxville, TX, USA

Tushar Samdani, MD, MS, DNB(Surg)
Department of Colorectal Surgery, Medstar Saint Mary's Hospital, Leonardo Town, MD, USA

Dana R. Sands, MD, FACS, FASCRS
Department of Colorectal Surgery, Cleveland Clinic Florida, Weston, FL, USA

Giulano A. Santoro, MD, PhD
Department of Colorectal Surgery, Digestive Disease Institute, Cleveland Clinic Abu Dhabi, Abu Dhabi, UAE

Stephen M. Sentovich, MD, MBA
Department of Surgical Oncology, City of Hope, Duarte, CA, USA

Matthew L. Silviera, MD
Section of Colon and Rectal Surgery, Department of Surgery, Barnes Jewish Hospital, Washington University School of Medicine, St. Louis, MO, USA

Michael J. Snyder, MD, FACS
Colon and Rectal Surgery Residency Program, The University of Texas Medical School at Houston, Houston, TX, USA; Department of Surgery, Houston Methodist TMC, Houston, TX, USA

Mattias Soop, MD, PhD
Department of Surgery, Salford Royal NHS Foundation Trust, Manchester Academic Health Science Center, The University of Manchester, Manchester, UK

Constantine P. Spanos, MD, FACS, FASCRS
Department of Surgery, Aristotelian University of Thessaloniki, Panorama-Thessaloniki, Greece

David B. Stewart Sr. , MD, FACS, FASCRS
Division of Colorectal Surgery, Department of Surgery, M. S. Hershey Medical Center, The Pennsylvania State University, Hershey, PA, USA

Scott A. Strong, MD
Division of GI and Oncologic Surgery, Northwestern Medicine, Chicago, IL, USA

Daniel Teitelbaum, MD
Section of Pediatric Surgery, University of Michigan C.S. Mott Children's Hospital, Ann Arbor, MI, USA

Amy J. Thorsen, MD
Department of Colon and Rectal Surgery, University of Minnesota, Minneapolis, MN, USA

Konstantin Umanskiy, MD, FACS, FASCRS
Section of Colon and Rectal Surgery, University of Chicago Medicine, Chicago, IL, USA

Cecile A. Unger, MD, MPH
Department of Obstetrics and Gynecology, Cleveland Clinic, Cleveland, OH, USA

Michael A. Valente, DO, FACS, FASCRS
Department of Colorectal Surgery, Digestive Disease Institute, Cleveland Clinic, Cleveland, OH, USA

H. David Vargas, MD, FACS, FASCRS
Department of Colon and Rectal Surgery, Ochsner Medical Center, New Orleans, LA, USA

Madhulika K. Varma, MD
Division of Colon and Rectal Surgery, University of California-San Francisco, San Francisco, CA, USA

Martin R Weiser, MD
Department of Surgery, Memorial Sloan Kettering Cancer Center, New York, NY, USA

Mark Welton, MD, MHCM
Department of Surgery, Stanford Health Care, Stanford, CA, USA

Elizabeth C. Wick, MD
Department of Surgery, Johns Hopkins Hospital, Johns Hopkins University, Baltimore, MD, USA

Kirsten Bass Wilkins, MD, FACS, FASCRS
UMDNJ Robert Wood Johnson University Hospital, Edison, NJ, USA

Y. Nancy You, MD, MHSc
Department of Surgical Oncology, University of Texas MD Anderson Cancer Center, Houston, TX, USA

Massarat Zutshi, MD
Department of Colorectal Surgery, Lerner College of Medicine, Cleveland Clinic, Cleveland, OH, USA

Part I
Perioperative/Endoscopy

1
Anatomy and Embryology of the Colon, Rectum, and Anus

Joseph C. Carmichael and Steven Mills

Key Concepts

- The dentate line represents a true division between embryonic endoderm and ectoderm.
- The location of the anterior peritoneal reflection is highly variable and can be significantly altered by disease such as rectal prolapse.
- The right and left ischioanal space communicate posteriorly through the deep postanal space between the levator ani muscle and anococcygeal ligament.
- The junction between the midgut (superior mesenteric artery) and the hindgut (inferior mesenteric artery) leads to a potential watershed area in the area of the splenic flexure.
- There is a normal, three-stage process by which the intestinal tract rotates during development beginning with herniation of the midgut followed by return of the midgut to the abdominal cavity and ending with its fixation.

Anatomy of the Anal Canal and Pelvic Floor

Textbooks of anatomy would define the "anatomic" anal canal as beginning at the dentate line and extending to the anal verge. This definition is one defined truly by the embryology and mucosal histology. However, the "surgical" anal canal, as first defined by Milligan and Morgan, [1] extends from the anorectal ring to the anal verge. The surgical definition of the anal canal takes in to account the surrounding musculature that is critical to consider during the conduct of operations from low anterior resection to anal fistulotomy. The surgical anal canal is formed by the internal anal sphincter, external anal sphincter, and puborectalis (Figure 1-1) and is easily identified on digital examination and ultrasound imaging. On average, the surgical anal canal is longer in males than in females. Intraoperative measurements of the posterior anal canal have estimated the surgical anal canal to

be 4.4 cm in men compared with 4.0 cm in women [2]. In addition, the anal canal was shown to be a unique muscular unit in that its length did not change with age.

The anatomy of the anal canal has also been characterized using magnetic resonance imaging. MR imaging does not show a difference in the length of the posterior anal canal in men and women, but does show that the anterior and posterior external anal sphincter length (not including the puborectalis) is significantly shorter in women [3].

The anal canal forms proximally where the rectum passes through the pelvic hiatus and joins with the puborectalis muscle. Starting at this location, the muscular anal canal can be thought of as a "tube within a tube." The inner tube is the visceral smooth muscle of the internal anal sphincter and longitudinal layer that is innervated by the autonomic nervous system. The outer muscular tube consists of somatic muscles including the components of the puborectalis and external anal sphincter [4]. It is the outer muscular tube that provides conscious control over continence and is strengthened during Kegal exercises. The external anal sphincter extends distal to the internal anal sphincter and the anal canal terminates at the anal verge where the superficial and subcutaneous portions of the external anal sphincter join the dermis.

Anal Canal Epithelium

The proximal anal canal has a pink appearance and is lined by the columnar epithelium of the rectal mucosa. Six to twelve millimeters proximal to the dentate line, the anal transition zone (ATZ) begins. The ATZ appears purple in color and represents an area of gradual transition of columnar epithelium to squamous epithelium. The columns of Morgagni are noted in this area were redundant columns of tissue are noted with anal crypts at their base. This forms the rippled dentate line (or pectinate line) which may be most easily identified by locating the anal crypts at the base of the Columns of Morgagni. Anal crypts are connected to

© Springer International Publishing 2016
S.R. Steele et al. (eds.), *The ASCRS Textbook of Colon and Rectal Surgery*, DOI 10.1007/978-3-319-25970-3_1

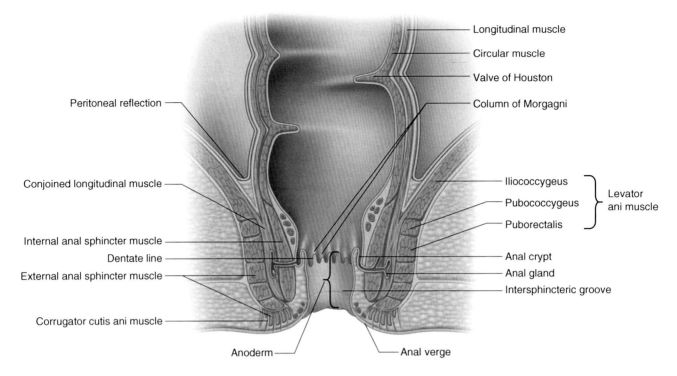

Peritoneal reflection

Conjoined longitudinal muscle

Internal anal sphincter muscle
Dentate line
External anal sphincter muscle

Corrugator cutis ani muscle

Anoderm

Longitudinal muscle

Circular muscle

Valve of Houston

Column of Morgagni

Iliococcygeus
Pubococcygeus   Levator
                       ani muscle
Puborectalis

Anal crypt
Anal gland
Intersphincteric groove

Anal verge

FIGURE 1-1. Anal canal.

underlying anal glands which are the presumed source of sepsis in the majority of anorectal abscesses and fistula. On average, there are six anal glands surrounding the anal canal (range 3–12) [4–6] and they tend to be more concentrated in the posterior quadrants. More than one gland may open into the same crypt and some crypts may not be connected to anal glands. The anal gland ducts proceed inferior and lateral from the anal canal and enter the submucosa where two-thirds enter the internal anal sphincter and half terminate in the intersphincteric plane [5]. It is theorized that obstruction of these ducts leads to anal fistula and abscess [4]. Knowledge of the anatomy also explains why the internal opening of a "cryptoglandular" anal fistula should typically be at the dentate line.

Distal to the dentate line, the anoderm begins and extends for approximately 1.5 cm. Anoderm has squamous histology and is devoid of hair, sebaceous glands, and sweat glands. At the anal verge, the anal canal lining becomes, thickened, pigmented and contains hair follicles—this represents normal skin.

The dentate line represents a true division between embryonic endoderm and ectoderm. Proximal to the dentate line, the innervation is via the sympathetic and parasympathetic systems, with venous, arterial, and lymphatic drainage associated with the hypogastric vessels. Distal to the dentate line, the innervation is via somatic nerves with blood supply and drainage from the inferior hemorrhoidal system.

Internal Anal Sphincter

The internal anal sphincter (IAS) is the downward continuation of the circular smooth muscle of the rectum and terminates with a rounded edge approximately 1 cm proximal to the distal aspect of the external anal sphincter. 3D imaging studies of this muscle demonstrate the overall volume does not vary according to gender, but the distribution is different with women tending to have a thicker medial/distal internal anal sphincter [7]. Overall, the IAS was found to be approximately 2 mm in thickness and 35 mm in length. The authors note that on any study, it is difficult to identify the proximal portion of the IAS as it is a continuation of the wall of the lower rectum.

Conjoined Longitudinal Muscle

The anatomy and function of the perianal connective tissue is often overlooked, but plays a significant role in normal anorectal function. Measuring approximately 0.5–2.0 mm in thickness, the conjoined longitudinal muscle (or conjoined longitudinal coat) lies in between the internal and external anal sphincters. It begins at the anorectal ring as an extension of the longitudinal rectal muscle fibers and descends caudally joined by fibers of the puborectalis muscle [8]. At its most caudal aspect, some of the conjoined longitudinal muscle fibers (referred to as *corrugator cutis ani muscle*) traverse the distal external anal sphincter and insert into the perianal skin and some enter the fat of the ischiorectal fossa. Fibers of the conjoined longitudinal muscle also pass obliquely and caudally through the internal anal sphincter to interlace in a network within the subepithelial space. These subepithelial smooth muscle fibers were originally described by Treitz in 1853 [9] and have been referred to as Treitz's muscle. They have also been referred to *corrugator cutis ani*, *musculus submucosae ani*, *mucosal suspensory ligament*, and *musculus canalis ani* [10] It has been hypothesized by Thomson that disruption of Treitz's muscles results in anal cushion prolapse, vascular outflow obstruction, and hemorrhoidal bleeding and thrombosis [11]. Haas and Fox have hypothesized that the conjoined longitudinal muscle, along with the network of connective tissue that it supports, plays a role in minimizing anal incontinence after sphincterotomy.

External Anal Sphincter

The external anal sphincter (EAS) is composed of striated muscle that forms an elliptical tube around the internal anal sphincter and conjoined longitudinal muscle. As it extends beyond the distal most aspect of the internal anal sphincter the intersphincteric groove is formed. At its distal most aspect, *corrugator cutis ani muscle* fibers from the conjoined longitudinal muscle traverse the external anal sphincter and insert into the perianal skin. Milligan and Morgan described the external anal sphincter as having three distinct divisions from proximal to distal that were termed: sphincter ani externus profundus, superficialis, and subcutaneus [1]. With time, this theory of three distinct divisions was proven invalid by Goligher who demonstrated that the external anal sphincter was truly a continuous sheet of skeletal muscle extending up to the puborectalis and levator ani muscles [12]. While the external anal sphincter does not have three distinct anatomic layers, it is not uncommon to see the proximal portion of the EAS referred to as deep EAS, the mid-portion referred to as the superficial EAS and the most distal aspect as the subcutaneous EAS. The mid EAS has posterior attachment to the coccyx via the anococcygeal ligament and the proximal EAS becomes continuous with the puborectalis muscle. Anteriorly, the proximal EAS forms a portion of the perineal body with the transverse perineal muscle. There are clear differences in the morphology of the anterior external anal sphincter that have been demonstrated on both MRI and three dimensional endoanal ultrasound studies in normal male and female volunteers [13, 14]. The normal female external anal sphincter has a variable natural defect occurring along its proximal anterior length below the level of the puborectalis sling that was demonstrated in 75% of nulliparous volunteers. This defect correlated with findings on anal manometry and the authors noted that it can make interpretation of an isolated endoanal ultrasound difficult resulting in over-reporting of obstetric sphincter defects [13]. This natural defect of the anterior anal sphincter provides some justification as to why anterior anal sphincterotomy is not routinely recommended in women.

The external anal sphincter is innervated on each side by the inferior rectal branch of the pudendal nerve (S2 and S3) and by the perineal branch of S4. There is substantial overlap in the pudendal innervation of the external anal sphincter muscle on the two sides which enables re-innervation to be partially accomplished from the contralateral side following nerve injury [15].

Perineal Body

The perineal body represents the intersection of the external anal sphincter, superficial transverse perinei, deep transverse perinei, and bulbospongiosus (also referred to as bulbocavernosus) muscles (Figure 1-2). Recent research, based on advanced magnetic resonance and ultrasound imaging, has suggested that the transverse perinei (TP) and bulbospongiosus (BS) muscles contribute significantly to anal continence [16]. It has been proposed that the EAS, TP and BS muscles be collectively referred to as the "EAS complex muscles." In this theory, the EAS complex morphology is "purse string" shaped rather than the typical "donut" shape previously considered. When these muscles are considered as a functional unit, it lends further support to the idea that it is critical to attempt to repair the perineal body during overlapping sphincter reconstructions.

Pelvic Floor Muscles

In addition to the anal sphincter and perineal body, the levator ani (LA) muscles contribute to pelvic organ support. For example, injury to the LA is seen in 55% of women with pelvic organ prolapse, but in only 16% without prolapse [17]. The LA has three subdivisions including the pubococcygeus (aka pubovisceral), puborectalis, and iliococcygeus. Some authors had previously suggested that the puborectalis was part of the deep portion of the EAS [18]; however, a significant amount of evidence has been presented to the contrary. In vivo MRI measurements in women have shown distinct, visible muscle fascicle directions for each of the three LA component muscles [19]. Embryology studies have also demonstrated that the puborectalis muscle is a portion of the LA muscle and shares a common primordium with the iliococcygeus and pubococcygeus muscles [20].

Innervation of the levator ani muscles has been described in detailed cadaveric studies [21]. The contemporary cadaveric studies suggest that the LA muscles are innervated by the pudendal nerve branches: perineal nerve and inferior rectal nerve as well as direct sacral nerves S3 and/or S4 (i.e., levator ani nerve) [22]. The pubococcygeus muscle and

Female Pelvic Floor

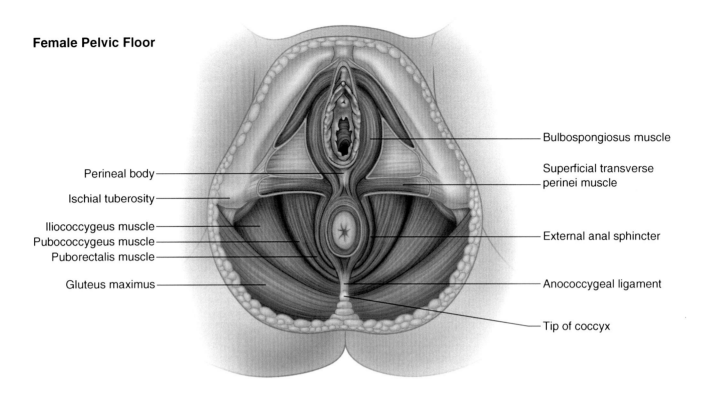

Bulbospongiosus muscle

Superficial transverse
perinei muscle

Perineal body

Ischial tuberosity

External anal sphincter

Iliococcygeus muscle
Pubococcygeus muscle
Puborectalis muscle

Gluteus maximus

Anococcygeal ligament

Tip of coccyx

Male Pelvic Floor

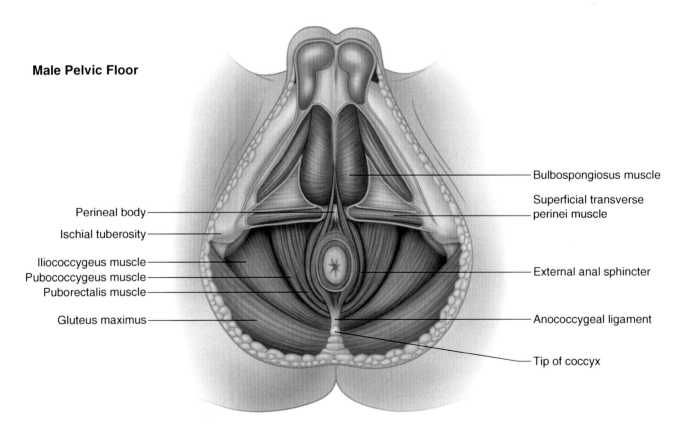

Bulbospongiosus muscle

Superficial transverse
perinei muscle

Perineal body

Ischial tuberosity

Iliococcygeus muscle
Pubococcygeus muscle
Puborectalis muscle

External anal sphincter

Gluteus maximus

Anococcygeal ligament

Tip of coccyx

FIGURE 1-2. Pelvic floor muscles.

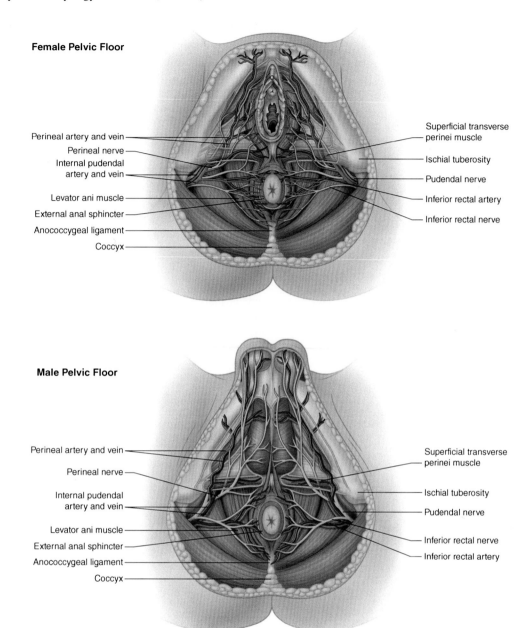

FIGURE 1-3. Pelvic floor nerves and blood supply.

puborectalis muscle are primarily innervated by the pudendal nerve branches while the iliococcygeus muscle is primarily innervated by the direct sacral nerves S3 and/or S4 (Figure 1-3).

Puborectalis Muscle

The puborectalis muscle (PRM) fibers arise from the lower part of the symphysis pubis and from the superior fascia of the urogenital diaphragm and run alongside the anorectal junction. Posterior to the rectum, the fibers join forming a sling. The "anorectal ring" is composed of the upper borders of the internal anal sphincter and puborectalis

muscle [1]. Contraction of the PRM sling causes a horizontal force [19] that closes the pelvic diaphragm and decreases the anorectal angle during squeeze. This is widely considered the most important contributing factor to gross fecal continence.

Iliococcygeus Muscle

Iliococcygeus muscle (ICM) fibers arise from the ischial spines and posterior obturator fascia, pass inferior/posterior and medially, and insert into the distal sacrum, coccyx, and anococcygeal raphe. The ICM, along with the pubococcygeus muscle, contributes to "lifting" of the pelvic floor [19].

Pubococcygeus Muscle

The pubococcygeus (PCM) muscle lies medial to the PRM. PCM fibers arise from the anterior half of the obturator fascia and the high posterior pubis. The PCM fibers are directed posterior/inferior and medially, where they intersect with fibers from the opposite side and form the anococcygeal raphe (or anococcygeal ligament). PCM muscle fibers insert in the distal sacrum and tip of the coccyx. Portions of the PCM contribute to the conjoined longitudinal muscle. The PCM forms the "levator hiatus" as it ellipses the lower rectum, urethra, and either the vagina in women or the dorsal vein of the penis in men. The levator hiatus is connected to the intrahiatal organs by a fascial condensation called the "hiatal ligament" (Figure 1-4). The hiatal ligament arises circumferentially around the hiatal margin as a continuation of the fascia on the pelvic surface of the levator muscle [23]. Enlargement of the levator hiatus has been implicated as a cause of female pelvic organ prolapse [24]. The PCM is the portion of the levator ani that is typically injured during traumatic vaginal delivery [25].

Anatomy of the Rectum

The rectum is arbitrarily considered to have three distinct parts: the upper, middle, and lower rectum. Although not anatomically distinct, the upper, mid, and lower rectal divisions are important when considering surgical treatment of rectal cancer. From the anal verge, the lower rectum is 0–7 cm; middle rectum, 7–12 cm; and upper rectum 12–15 cm [26]. However, the rectum is actually variable in length and may extend beyond 15 cm from the anal verge. The upper rectum can be distinguished from the sigmoid colon by the absence of taenia coli and epiploic appendages.

The majority of the rectum lies outside of the peritoneal cavity, although anteriorly and laterally the upper rectum is covered by a layer of visceral peritoneum down to the peritoneal reflection. The location of the anterior peritoneal reflection is highly variable and can be significantly altered by disease such as rectal prolapse. One study sought to identify the location of the anterior peritoneal reflection in 50 patients

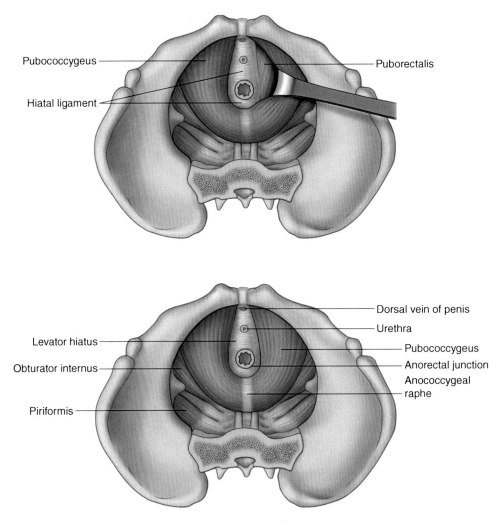

FIGURE 1-4. Pelvic floor anatomy, abdominal view.

who were undergoing laparotomy [27]. It was found that the anterior peritoneal reflection was located on average 9 cm from the anal verge in females and 9.7 cm from the anal verge in males—there was no statistically significant difference based on gender.

Mesorectum

The origin of the word "mesorectum" is difficult to identify and may be attributed to Maunsell in 1892 [28], but was certainly later popularized by Heald [29]. Unfortunately, the term mesorectum is a misnomer that is not generally acknowledged in classic texts of anatomy such as the *Nomina Anatomica* [30]. In anatomic terms, the prefix "meso" refers to two layers of peritoneum that suspend an organ and the suffix applied indicates the target organ (e.g., mesocolon). The term "meso" cannot be assigned to the rectum, as it implies a mobile, suspended rectum, which may only be the case in patients with rectal prolapse.

The mesorectum is a term employed by surgeons to describe the fascial envelope of the rectum that is excised during surgical treatment of rectal cancer. Indeed, failure to completely excise this envelope intact has been associated with an increased incidence of local recurrence of rectal cancer [31]. The mesorectum is contained within the fascia propria. The fascia propria is an upward projection of the parietal endopelvic fascia that lines the walls and floor of the pelvis. The fascia propria encloses the perirectal fat, lymphatics, blood vessels, and nerves and is not considered a barrier strong enough to prevent the spread of infection or malignancy [32].

Presacral Fascia

The presacral fascia is a thickened portion of the parietal endopelvic fascia overlying the sacrum that covers the presacral veins and hypogastric nerves (Figure 1-5). It extends laterally to cover the piriformis and upper coccyx. As the presacral fascia extends laterally, it becomes continuous with the fascia propria and contributes to the lateral ligaments of the rectum. Caudally, this fascia extends to the anorectal junction covering the anococcygeal ligament. During total mesorectal excision, the fascia propria is elevated sharply off the presacral fascia. Leaving the presacral fascia intact eliminates the possibility of causing presacral bleeding.

Retrosacral Fascia

The retrosacral fascia originates at the third and fourth portion [33] of the sacrum and extends anteriorly to the posterior layer of the fascia propria 3–5 cm proximal to the anorectal junction [34]. This tough fascia layer is surgically relevant as it must be sharply incised during total mesorectal excision [32]. The space posterior to the retrosacral fascia is referred to as the supralevator or retrorectal space.

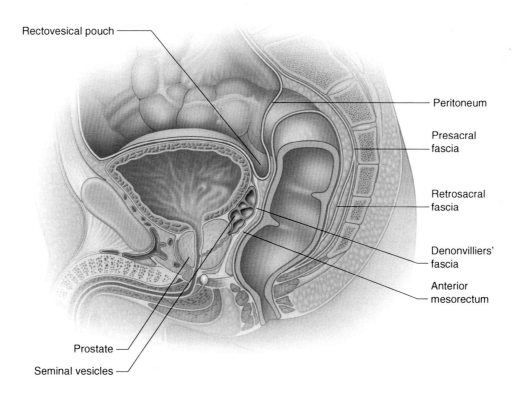

Figure 1-5. Fascial relationships of the rectum.

Waldeyer's Fascia

There is significant confusion about what Waldeyer's fascia represents as the eponym has been used to describe the presacral fascia, the retrosacral fascia or all fascia posterior to the rectum. In Waldeyer's original description of pelvic fascia, there was no particular emphasis on the presacral component [32, 34]. While the debate continues regarding "Waldeyer's fascia," it is important to simply understand that the phrase can have the potential to mean presacral fascia, rectosacral, or retrorectal fascia [35].

Denonvilliers' Fascia

Denonvilliers' fascia arises from the fusion of the two walls of the embryological peritoneal cul-de-sac and extends from the deepest point of the rectovesical pouch to the pelvic floor [36]. Originally described by Denonvilliers in 1836 as a "prostato-peritoneal" membranous layer between the rectum and seminal vesicles, Denonvilliers' fascia is also present in females as part of the rectovaginal septum and is sometimes referred to as rectovaginal fascia. It is found immediately beneath the vaginal epithelium and is clearly what most would consider as part of the vaginal wall. It merges superiorly with the cardinal/uterosacral complex in females or the rectovesical pouch in males. It merges laterally with the endopelvic fascia overlying the levator muscle and distally with the perineal body. It contains collagen, some strands of smooth muscle and heavy elastin fibers. Rectoceles represent a defect in this layer that allows the rectum to bulge anteriorly [37].

Microscopically, the Denonvilliers' fascia has two layers; however, it is not possible to discern two layers during pelvic dissection [36]. In the anterior rectal plane, the mesorectum is contained by the fascia propria which lies dorsal to Denonvilliers' fascia. The cavernous nerves run in neurovascular bundles at the anterolateral border of Denonvilliers' fascia.

Lateral Ligaments

While frequently referred to by surgeons, there are two controversial points regarding the lateral ligaments of the rectum. First, do the lateral ligaments exist? Second, what do they contain? Miles refers to division of the lateral ligaments of the rectum in his seminal description of abdominoperineal resection in 1908. Specifically, he notes "In these structures the middle hemorrhoidal arteries are found but seldom require a ligature" [38]. It is interesting to note that at least one modern cadaveric dissection study identified the presence of a middle rectal artery in only 22% of specimens [33] which could be a contributing factor as to why Miles saw no significant bleeding in this area.

Total mesorectal excision, as popularized and described by Heald involves sharp dissection along the fascia propria circumferentially to the pelvic floor. While acknowledging that the middle rectal vessels are "divided as far from the carcinoma as possible," Heald does not mention "lateral ligaments" of the rectum at all [39].

In an extensive review of the anatomy of the lateral ligament, Church notes that it is a common misconception that the lateral ligaments contain the middle rectal artery at all. It appears that the lateral ligaments comprise "primarily nerves and connective tissue" and their division without bleeding attests to the absence of a "significant accessory rectal artery in this location in the majority of patients" [32].

In a separate cadaveric study, the lateral ligaments of the rectum were identified as trapezoid structures originating from mesorectum and anchored to the endopelvic fascia at the level of the midrectum. It was recommended that, as lateral extensions of the mesorectum, the ligaments must be cut and included in the total mesorectal excision (TME) specimen. It was further noted that the lateral ligaments did not contain middle rectal arteries or nerve structures of importance. The urogenital bundle runs just above the lateral ligament at its point of insertion on the endopelvic fascia, the middle rectal artery (if present) runs posterior to the lateral ligament and the nervi recti fibers (which originate from the inferior hypogastric plexus) course transversely under the lateral ligament to the rectal wall [40]. Other modern cadaveric investigations note the rarity of middle rectal arteries and the absence of clinically relevant neurovascular structures in the lateral ligaments [41].

Valves of Houston

The rectum has been classically described to have three distinct, semicircular, inner folds called valves of Houston (Figure 1-1) with the superior and inferior valves located on the left side of the rectum and the more prominent middle rectal valve on the right; however, this is not uniformly the case [42]. Only 45.5% of patients will have the classic three valve rectal anatomy; 32.5% will have only two valves; and, 10.25% may have four valves.

Anorectal Spaces

It is important to acknowledge and understand the anorectal spaces created by the various myofascial relationships in the pelvis as these spaces help us understand how anorectal sepsis can spread throughout the pelvis.

Perianal Space

The perianal space contains external hemorrhoid cushions, the subcutaneous external anal sphincter and the distal internal anal sphincter. The perianal space is in communication with the intersphincteric space (Figure 1-6). The perianal space has its cephalad boundary at the dentate line and laterally to the subcutaneous fat of the buttocks or is contained by fibers

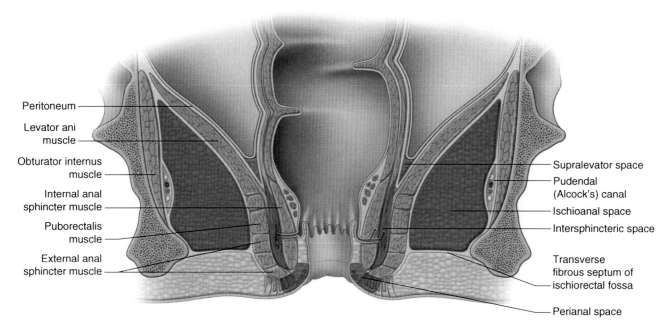

FIGURE 1-6. Perianal and perirectal spaces, coronal view.

extending from the conjoined longitudinal muscle often referred to as *corrugator cutis ani* muscle fibers. Otherwise, the perianal space is contained by anoderm.

Intersphincteric Space

The intersphincteric space is the potential space that lies between the internal and external anal sphincter and is continuous with the perianal space. It is of clinical importance as cryptoglandular infections tend to begin in this area and expand elsewhere to create anal fistula [4].

Submucous Space

This space lies between the medial boarder of the internal anal sphincter and the anal mucosa proximal to the dentate line. It is continuous with the submucosa of the rectum. This area contains internal hemorrhoid vascular cushions.

Ischioanal/Ischiorectal Space

The ischioanal (also referred to as ischiorectal) space is the largest anorectal space. It has been described as a pyramid shape with its apex at the levator muscle insertion into the obturator fascia. The medial boarder is thus the levator ani muscle and external anal sphincter. The obturator internus muscle and obturator fascia make up the lateral boarder of the ischioanal space. The posterior boundary is formed by the lower border of the gluteus maximus muscle and the sacrotuberous ligament. The space is has an anterior boundary formed by the superficial and deep transverse perineal muscles. The caudal boundary is skin of the perineum. The ischioanal fossa contains adipose tissue, pudendal nerve branches and superficial branches of the internal pudendal vessels. The right and left ischioanal space communicate posteriorly through the deep postanal space between the levator ani muscle and anococcygeal ligament (Figure 1-7) [43]. When the ischioanal and perianal spaces are regarded as a single space, it is referred to as the ischioanal fossa [35].

Supralevator Space

The upper boundary of the supralevator space is the peritoneum, the lateral boundary is the pelvic wall, the medial boundary is the rectum and the inferior boarder is the levator ani muscle (Figure 1-8).

Superficial and Deep Postanal Spaces

These spaces are located posterior to the anus and inferior to the levator muscle. The superficial postanal space is more caudal and is located between the anococcygeal ligament and the skin. The superficial postanal space allows communication of perianal space sepsis.

The deep postanal space (retrosphincteric space of Courtney) [44] is located between the levator ani muscle and the anococcygeal raphe. This space allows ischioanal sepsis to track from one side to the other resulting in the so called "horseshoe" abscess.

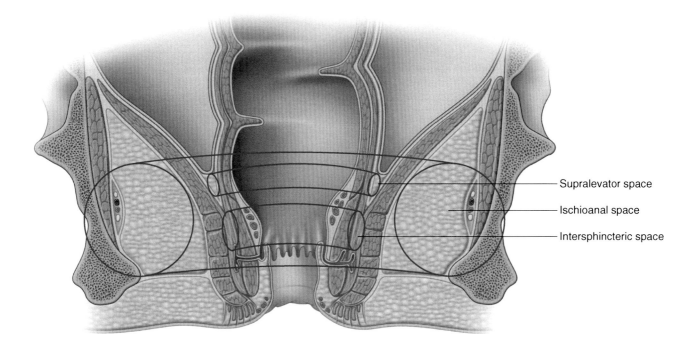

FIGURE 1-7. Communication of the anorectal spaces.

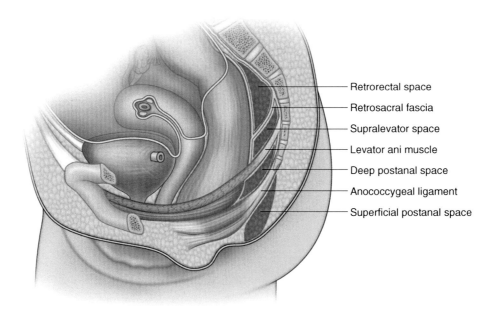

FIGURE 1-8. Perianal and perirectal spaces, lateral view.

Retrorectal Space

The retrorectal space is found between the presacral fascia and fascia propria. It contains no major blood vessels or nerves. It is limited laterally by the lateral ligaments of the piriformis fascia and inferiorly by the retrosacral fascia. The fascia propria and presacral fascia come together at the apex of this space [32].

Rectal Blood Supply

The rectum is supplied by the superior, middle, and inferior rectal (hemorrhoidal) arteries (Figure 1-9). Both the middle and inferior hemorrhoidal vessels are paired arteries and the superior rectal artery is not.

Superior Rectal Artery

The superior rectal artery (SRA) is the continuation of the inferior mesenteric artery and is so named after the inferior mesentcric artery crosses the left iliac vessels. The SRA gives off a rectosigmoid branch, an upper rectal branch, and then bifurcates into right and left terminal branches in 80%

[45] of cases as it descends caudally in the mesorectum. On average, eight terminal branches of the SRA have been identified in the distal rectal wall [46].

Middle Rectal Artery

The middle rectal artery (MRA) has been variably noted in many studies. It may be found on one or both sides of the rectum and has been noted to be present 12–28% of the time [41, 47]. At least one study reported the presence of the middle rectal artery in at least 91% of cadaveric specimens [40]. The MRA originates from the anterior division of the internal iliac or pudendal arteries. Please see the "Lateral Ligament" discussion above for more review on the anatomic course of the middle rectal artery.

Inferior Rectal Artery

The inferior rectal arteries (IRA) are paired vessels that originate as branches of the internal pudendal artery which receives its blood supply from the internal iliac artery. The artery originates in the pudendal canal and is entirely extra-pelvic (caudal to the levator ani) in its distribution. The IRA

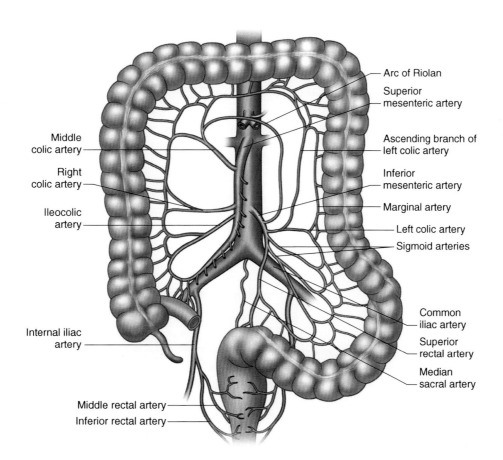

Figure 1-9. Arterial anatomy of the colon and rectum.

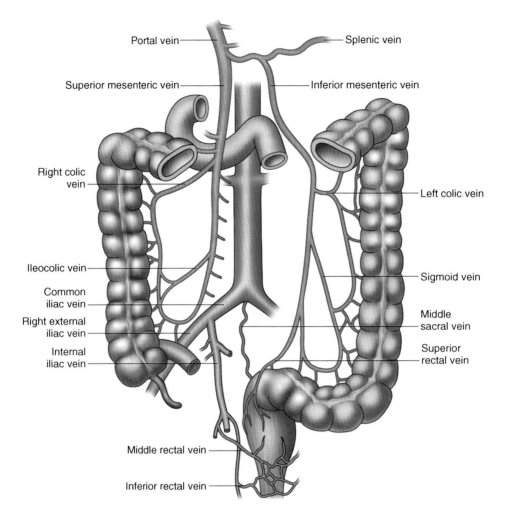

Portal vein

Splenic vein

Superior mesenteric vein

Inferior mesenteric vein

Right colic vein

Left colic vein

Ileocolic vein

Sigmoid vein

Common iliac vein

Middle sacral vein

Right external iliac vein

Superior rectal vein

Internal iliac vein

Middle rectal vein

Inferior rectal vein

FIGURE 1-10. Venous anatomy of the colon and rectum.

traverses the obturator fascia, the ischiorectal fossa and pierces the wall of the anal canal in the region of the external anal sphincter [32].

Venous and Lymphatic Drainage of the Rectum and Anus

Venous drainage from the rectum and anus occurs via both the portal and systemic systems. Middle and inferior rectal veins drain to the systemic systems via the internal iliac vein while the superior rectal vein drains the rectum and upper anal canal into the portal system via the inferior mesenteric vein (Figure 1-10).

Lymphatics from the upper two-thirds of the rectum drain to the inferior mesenteric lymph nodes and then to the para-aortic lymph nodes. Lymphatic drainage from the lower third of the rectum occurs along the superior rectal artery and laterally along the middle rectal artery to the internal iliac lymph nodes. In the anal canal, lymphatic above the dentate drain to the inferior mesenteric and internal iliac lymph nodes. Below the dentate line lymphatics drain along the inferior rectal lymphatics to the superficial inguinal nodes.

Innervation of the Rectum and Anus

Sympathetic fibers arise from L1, L2, and L3 and pass through the sympathetic chains and join the pre-aortic plexus (Figure 1-11). From there, they run adjacent and dorsal to the inferior mesenteric artery as the mesenteric plexus and inner-vate the upper rectum. The lower rectum is innervated by the presacral nerves from the hypogastric plexus. Two main hypogastric nerves, on either side of the rectum, carry sympa-thetic information form the hypogastric plexus to the pelvic plexus. The pelvic plexus lies on the lateral side of the pelvis at the level of the lower third of the rectum adjacent to the lateral stalks (please see discussion of lateral stalks above).

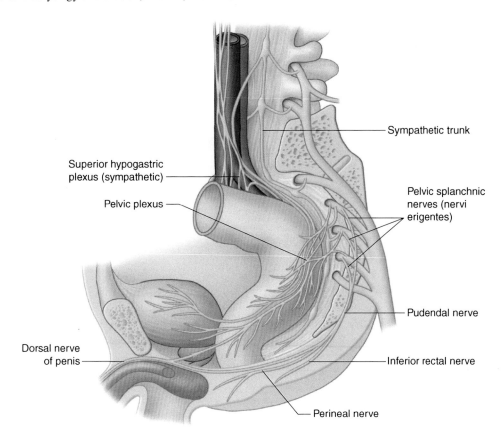

Superior hypogastric
plexus (sympathetic)

Pelvic plexus

Dorsal nerve
of penis

Sympathetic trunk

Pelvic splanchnic
nerves (nervi
erigentes)

Pudendal nerve

Inferior rectal nerve

Perineal nerve

FIGURE 1-11. Nerves of the rectum.

Parasympathetic fibers to the rectum and anal canal originate from S2, S3, and S4 to penetrate through the sacral foramen and are called the nervi erigentes. These nerves course laterally and anterior to join the sympathetic hypogastric nerves and form the pelvic plexus on the pelvic sidewall. From here, postganglionic mixed parasympathetic and sympathetic nerve fibers supply the rectum, genital organs, and anal canal. The periprostatic plexus is considered a subdivision of the pelvic plexus and supplies the prostate, seminal vesicles, corpora cavernosa, vas deferens, urethra, ejaculatory ducts, and bulbourethral glands.

The internal anal sphincter is innervated by sympathetic (L5) and parasympathetic (S2, S3, and S4) nerves following the same route as the nerves to the rectum as noted above. The external anal sphincter is innervated on each side by the inferior rectal branch of the internal pudendal nerve (S2 and S3) and by the perineal branch of S4. Anal sensation is mediated by the inferior rectal branch of the pudendal nerve.

Anatomy of the Colon

The colon is a long tubular organ consisting of muscle and connective tissue with an inner mucosal layer. The diameter of the colon differs depending upon which segment is evaluated, and generally decreases in diameter as one travels proximal to distal (cecum about 7 cm and sigmoid colon about 2.5 cm in diameter). The overall length is variable with an average length approximating 150 cm. The right and left sides of the colon are fused to the posterior retroperitoneum (secondarily retroperitonealized) while the transverse colon and sigmoid colon are relatively free within the peritoneum. The transverse colon is held in position via its attachments to the right/left colon at the flexures (hepatic and splenic, respectively) and is further fused to the omentum. Generally speaking the colon is located peripherally within the abdomen with the small bowel located centrally.

There are three important anatomic points of differentiation between the colon and the small intestine: the appendices epiploicae, the taeniae coli, and the haustra. The appendices epiploicae are non-mesenteric fat protruding from the serosal surface of the colon. They are likely residual from the anti-mesenteric fat of the embryologic intestine which dissipates (unlike the omentum on the stomach). The taenia coli are three thickened bands of outer, longitudinal muscle of the colon. This outer layer of muscle is indeed circumferentially complete [48], but is considerably thicker in three areas represented by the taenia. The three taeniae have been given separate names by some: *taenia libera* to represent the anterior band, *taenia mesocolica* for the posteromedial band, and *taenia omentalis* for posterolateral band. The bands are continuous from their origin at the base of the appendix until the rectosigmoid junction where they converge (marking an anatomically identifiable differentiation between the sigmoid colon and rectum). Though they run along the full length of the colon, they are not as long as the bowel wall. This difference in length results in outpouchings of the bowel wall between the taenia referred to as haustra. The haustra are further septated by the plicae semilunares.

Cecum

The proximal most portion of the colon is termed the cecum, a sac-like segment of colon below (proximal to) the ileocecal valve. The cecum is variable in size, but generally is about 8 cm in length and 7 cm in diameter. At its base is the appendix. Terminating in the posteromedial area of the cecum is the terminal ileum (ileocecal valve). The cecum is generally covered by visceral peritoneum, with more variability near the transition to the ascending colon (upper or distal cecum). The ileocecal valve is a circular muscular sphincter which appears as a slit-like ("fish-mouth") opening noted on an endoscopic evaluation of the cecum. The valve is not competent in all patients, but when present, its competence leads to the urgency of a colon obstruction as it develops into a closed-loop obstruction. Regulation of ileal emptying into the colon appears to be the prime task in ileocecal valve function [49].

The Appendix

The appendix is an elongated, true diverticulum arising from the base of the cecum. The appendiceal orifice is generally about 3–4 cm from the ileocecal valve. The appendix itself is of variable length (2–20 cm) and is about 5 mm in diameter in the non-inflamed state. Blood is supplied to the appendix via the appendiceal vessels contained within the mesoappendix. This results in the most common location of the appendix being medially on the cecum toward the ileum, but the appendix does have great variability in its location including pelvic, retrocecal, preileal, retroileal, and subcecal.

Ascending Colon

From its beginning at the ileocecal valve to its terminus at the hepatic flexure where it turns sharply medially to become the transverse colon, the ascending colon measures on average, about 15–18 cm. Its anterior surface is covered in visceral peritoneum while its posterior surface is fused with the retroperitoneum. The lateral peritoneal reflection can be seen as a thickened line termed the white line of Toldt, which can serve as a surgeon's guide for mobilization of the ascending colon off of its attachments to the retroperitoneum, most

notably the right kidney (Gerotta's fascia) and the loop of the duodenum located posterior and superior to the ileocolic vessels. The right ureter and the right gonadal vessels pass posteriorly to the ascending mesocolon within the retroperitoneum.

Transverse Colon

The transverse colon traverses the upper abdomen from the hepatic flexure on the right to the splenic flexure on the left. It is generally the longest section of colon (averaging 45–50 cm) and swoops inferiorly as it crosses the abdomen. The entire transverse colon is covered by visceral peritoneum, but the greater omentum is fused to the anterosuperior surface of the transverse colon. Superior to the transverse mesocolon, inferior to the stomach, and posterior to the omentum is the pocket of the peritoneal cavity termed the lesser sac, with the pancreas forming the posterior most aspect. The splenic flexure is the sharp turn from the transversely oriented transverse colon to the longitudinally oriented descending colon. It can be adherent to the spleen and to the diaphragm via the phrenocolic ligament.

Descending Colon

The descending colon travels inferiorly from the splenic flexure for the course of about 25 cm. It is fused to the retroperitoneum (similarly to the ascending colon) and overlies the left kidney as well as the back/retroperitoneal musculature. Its anterior and lateral surfaces are covered with visceral peritoneum and the lateral peritoneal reflection (white line of Toldt) is again present.

Sigmoid Colon

The sigmoid colon is the most variable of the colon segments. It is generally 35–45 cm in length. It is covered by visceral peritoneum, thereby making it mobile. Its shape is considered "omega-shaped" but its configuration and attachments are variable. Its mesentery is of variable length, but is fused to the pelvic walls in an inverted-V shape creating a recess termed the intersigmoid fossa. Through this recess travel the left ureter, gonadal vessels, and often the left colic vessels.

Rectosigmoid Junction

The end of the sigmoid colon and the beginning of the rectum is termed the rectosigmoid junction. It is noted by the confluence of the taeniae coli and the end of epiploicae appendices. While some surgeons have historically considered the rectosigmoid junction to be a general area (comprising about 5 cm of distal sigmoid and about 5 cm of proximal rectum), others have described a distinct and clearly defined segment. It is the narrowest portion of the large intestine, measuring 2–2.5 cm in diameter. Endoscopically, it is noted as a narrow and often sharply angulated area above the relatively capacious rectum, and above the three rectal valves.

In the early nineteenth century, it was proposed that the sigmoid acts as a reservoir for stool, thus aiding in continence [50]. Subsequently, an area of thickened circular muscle within the wall of the rectosigmoid was described and felt to function as a sphincter of sorts. Historically, it has been variably named the *sphincter ani tertius, rectosigmoid sphincter*, and *pylorus sigmoidorectalis* [51–55]. A more recent evaluation of the rectosigmoid junction utilizing anatomic and histologic studies as well as radiographic evaluation concluded that there was an anatomic sphincter at the rectosigmoid junction [56]. Microscopic evaluation of the area does reveal thickening of the circular muscle layer as it progresses toward the rectum. Though not identifiable externally, radiologic evaluation can identify the area as a narrow, contractile segment [56].

Blood Supply

The colon receives blood supply from two main sources, branches of the Superior Mesenteric Artery (SMA) (cecum, ascending, and transverse colon) and branches of the Inferior Mesenteric Artery (IMA) (descending and sigmoid colon) (Figure 1-9). There is a watershed area between these two main sources located just proximal to the splenic flexure where branches of the left branch of the middle colic artery anastomose with those of the left colic artery. This area represents the border of the embryologic midgut and hindgut. Though the blood supply to the colon is somewhat variable, there are some general common arteries. The cecum and right colon are supplied by the terminus of the SMA, the ileocolic artery. The right colic artery is less consistent and, when present, can arise directly from the SMA, from the ileocolic, or from other sources. The transverse colon is supplied via the middle colic artery, which branches early to form right and left branches. The middle colic artery originates directly from the SMA. The left colon and sigmoid colon are supplied by branches of the IMA, namely the left colic and a variable number of sigmoid branches. After the final branches to the sigmoid colon, the IMA continues inferiorly as the superior hemorrhoidal (rectal) artery.

Superior Mesenteric Artery

The superior mesenteric artery (SMA) is the second, unpaired anterior branch off of the aorta (Figure 1-9). It arises posterior to the upper edge of the pancreas (near the L1 vertebrae), courses posterior to the pancreas, and then crosses over the third portion of the duodenum to continue within the base of the mesentery. From its left side, the SMA gives rise to up to 20 small intestinal branches while the colic branches originate from its ride side. The most constant of the colic branches is the ileocolic vessel which courses through the ascending mesocolon where it divides into a superior (ascending) branch and an inferior (descending) branch [57]. A true right colic artery is absent up to 20% of the time and, when present, typically arises from the SMA. Alternatively, the right colic artery can arise from the ileocolic vessels or from the middle colic vessels [45, 57, 58]. The middle colic artery arises from the SMA near the inferior border of the pancreas. It branches early to give off right and left branches. The right branch supplies the hepatic flexure and right half of the transverse colon. The left branch supplies the left half of the transverse colon to the splenic flexure. In up to 33% of patients, the left branch of the middle colic artery can be the sole supplier of the splenic flexure [57, 59].

Inferior Mesenteric Artery

The inferior mesenteric artery (IMA) (Figure 1-9) is the third unpaired, anterior branch off of the aorta, originating 3–4 cm above the aortic bifurcation at the level of the L2 to L3 vertebrae. As the IMA travels inferiorly and to the left, it gives off the left colic artery and several sigmoidal branches. After these branches, the IMA becomes the superior hemorrhoidal (rectal) artery as it crosses over the left common iliac artery. The left colic artery divides into an ascending branch (splenic flexure) and a descending branch (the descending colon). The sigmoidal branches form a fairly rich arcade within the sigmoid mesocolon (similar to that seen within the small bowel mesentery). The superior hemorrhoidal artery carries into the mesorectum and into the rectum. The superior hemorrhoidal artery bifurcates in about 80% of patients.

The Marginal Artery and Other Mesenteric Collaterals

The major arteries noted above account for the main source of blood within the mesentery. However, the anatomy of the mesenteric circulation and the collaterals within the mesentery remain less clear. Haller first described a central artery anastomosing all mesenteric branches in 1786 [60]. When Drummond demonstrated its surgical significance in the early twentieth century, it became known as the marginal artery of Drummond [61, 62]. The marginal artery (Figure 1-9) has been shown to be discontinuous or even absent in some patients, most notably at the splenic flexure (Griffiths' critical point), where it may be absent in up to 50% of patients [63]. This area of potential ischemia is the embryologic connection between the midgut and hindgut. Inadequacy of the marginal artery likely accounts for this area being most severely affected in cases of colonic ischemia. Another potential (though controversial) site of ischemia is at a discontinuous area of marginal artery located at the rectosigmoid junction termed Sudeck's critical point. Surgical experience would question whether this potential area of ischemia exists; a recent fluorescence study indicates that it does [64], though its clinical importance remains in doubt.

Venous Drainage

Venous drainage of the colon largely follows the arterial supply with superior and inferior mesenteric veins draining both the right and left halves of the colon (Figure 1-10). They ultimately meet at the portal vein to reach the intrahepatic system. The superior mesenteric vein (SMV) travels parallel and to the right of the artery. The inferior mesenteric vein (IMV) does not travel with the artery, but rather takes a longer path superiorly to join the splenic vein. It separates from the artery within the left colon mesentery and runs along the base of the mesentery where it can be found just lateral to the ligament of Treitz and the duodenum before joining the splenic vein on the opposite (superior) side of the transverse mesocolon. Dissecting posterior to the IMV can allow for separation of the mesenteric structures from the retroperitoneal structures during a medial-to-lateral dissection.

Lymphatic Drainage

The colon wall has a dense network of lymphatic plexuses. These lymphatics drain into extramural lymphatic channels which follow the vascular supply of the colon. Lymph nodes are plentiful and are typically divided into four main groups. The *epiploic* group lies adjacent to the bowel wall just below the peritoneum and in the epiploicae. The *paracolic* nodes are along the marginal artery and the vascular arcades. They are most filtering of the nodes. The *intermediate* nodes are situated on the primary colic vessels. The *main* or *principal* nodes are on the superior and inferior mesenteric vessels. Once the lymph leaves the main nodes, it drains into the cisterna chili via the para-aortic chain.

Nervous Innervation

The colon is innervated by the sympathetic and parasympathetic nervous systems and closely follows the arterial blood supply. The sympathetic innervation of the right half of the colon originates from the lower six thoracic splanchnic nerves which synapse within the celiac, pre-aortic, and superior mesenteric ganglia. The post-ganglionic fibers then follow the SMA to the right colon. The sympathetic innervation for the left half originates from L1, L2, and L3.

Parasympathetic fibers to the right colon come from the posterior (right) branch of the Vagus Nerve and celiac plexus. They travel along the SMA to synapse with the nerves within the intrinsic autonomic plexuses of the bowel wall. On the left side, the parasympathetic innervation comes from S2, S3, and S4 via splanchnic nerves.

Embryology

The embryologic development of the GI system is complex. That said, however, a working knowledge of the development of the small bowel, colon, and anorectum is critical for a colorectal surgeon as it can aid in understanding pathophysiology and is essential for recognizing surgical planes.

Anus and Rectum

The colon distal to the splenic flexure, including the rectum and the anal canal (proximal to the dentate line), are derived from the hindgut and therefore have vascular supply from the inferior mesenteric vessels (Figure 1-9). The dentate line (Figure 1-1) is the fusion plane between the endodermal and ectodermal tubes. The cloacal portion of the anal canal has both endodermal and ectodermal components which develop into the anal transitional zone [65]. The terminal portion of the hindgut or cloaca fuses with the proctodeum (an ingrowth from the anal pit).

The cloaca originates at the portion of the rectum below the pubococcygeal line while the hindgut originates above it. Before the fifth week of development, the intestinal and urogenital tracts are joined at the level of the cloaca. By the eighth week, the urorectal septum migrates caudally to divide the cloacal closing plate into an anterior urogenital plate and a posterior anal plate. Anorectal rings result from a posterior displacement in the septum and the resultant smaller anal opening. By the tenth week, the anal tubercles fuse into a horseshoe shaped structure dorsally and into the perineal body anteriorly. The external anal sphincter forms from the posterior aspects of the cloacal sphincter earlier than the development of the internal sphincter. The internal sphincter develops from enlarging fibers of the circular muscle layer of the rectum [66]. The sphincters migrate during their development with the internal sphincter moving caudally while the external sphincter enlarges cephalad. Meanwhile, the longitudinal muscle descends into the intersphincteric plane [6]. In females, the female genital organs form from the Müllerian ducts and join the urogenital sinus by the 16th week of development. In contrast, in males, the urogenital membrane obliterates with fusion of the genital folds while the sinus develops into the urethra.

Normal inestinal rotation

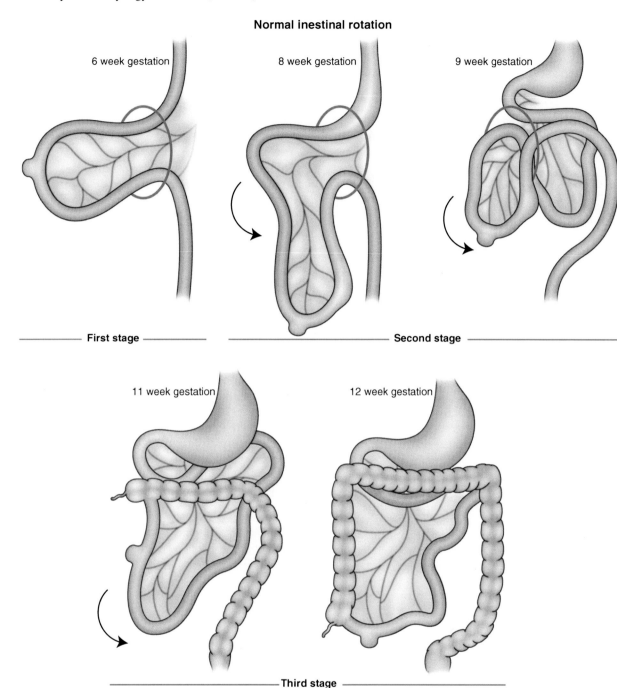

6 week gestation

8 week gestation

9 week gestation

——————— First stage ——————— ——————— Second stage ———————

11 week gestation

12 week gestation

——————— Third stage ———————

FIGURE 1-12. Summary of normal intestinal rotation during development.

Colon and Small Intestine

The endodermal roof of the yolk sac develops into the primitive gut tube. This initially straight tube is suspended upon a common mesentery. By week 3 of development, it has three discernible segments; namely the foregut, midgut, and hindgut. The midgut starts below the pancreatic papilla to form the small intestine and the first half of the colon (all supplied by the superior mesenteric artery). The distal colon and rectum, as well as the anal canal develop from the hindgut and are therefore supplied by the inferior mesenteric artery.

There is a normal process by which the intestinal tract rotates (Figure 1-12). The first stage is the physiologic herniation of the midgut, the second stage is its return to the abdomen, and the third stage is the fixation of the midgut. Abnormalities in this normal process lead to various malformations (see below). The physiologic herniation (first stage) occurs between weeks 6 and 8 of development. The primitive gut tube elongates over the superior mesenteric artery and bulges out through the umbilical cord (Figure 1-13). During the eighth week, these contents move in a counterclockwise fashion, turning 90° from the sagittal to the horizontal plane (Figure 1-14). Anomalies at this stage are rare, but include situs inversus, duodenal inversion, and extroversion of the cloaca. During the second stage (tenth week of gestation),

the midgut loops return to the peritoneal cavity and simultaneously rotate an additional 180° in the counterclockwise direction (Figure 1-15). The pre-arterial portion of the duodenum returns to the abdomen first, followed by the counterclockwise rotation around the superior mesenteric vessels, resulting in the duodenum lying behind them. The colon returns after the rotation, resulting in their anterior location. Anomalies in this stage are more common and result in nonrotation, malrotation, reversed rotation, internal hernia, and omphalocele. The third stage (fixation of the midgut) begins once the intestines have returned to the peritoneal cavity and end at birth. The cecum migrates to the right lower quadrant from its initial position in the upper abdomen (Figure 1-16). After the completion of this 270° counterclockwise rotation, fusion begins, typically at week 12–13. This results in fusion of the duodenum as well as the ascending and descending colon (Figure 1-17).

Major Anomalies of Rotation

Non-rotation

The midgut returns to the peritoneum without any of the normal rotation. This results in the small intestine being on the right side of the abdomen and the colon on the left side (Figure 1-18). This condition can remain asymptomatic (a finding noted at laparoscopy or laparotomy) or result in volvulus affecting the entirety of the small intestine. The twist generally occurs at the duodenojejunal junction as well as the midtransverse colon.

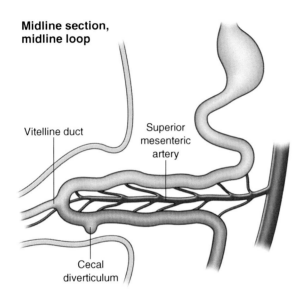

FIGURE 1-13. Elongation of the midgut loop.

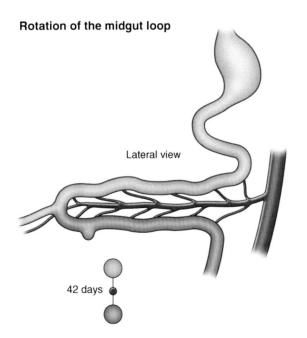
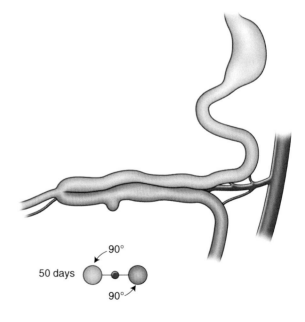

FIGURE 1-14. Rotation of the midgut loop.

FIGURE 1-15. Return of the
intestinal loop to the abdomen.

Return to the abdomen

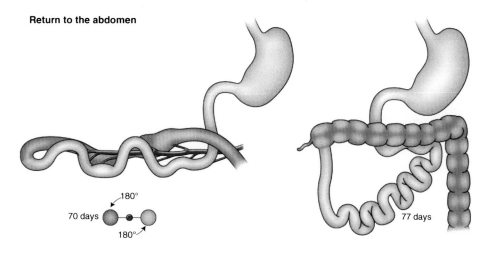

Later fetal period

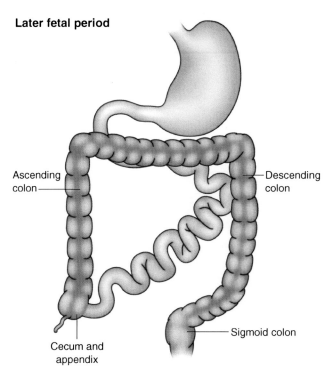

FIGURE 1-16. Later fetal development.

Malrotation

There is normal initial rotation, but the cecum fails to complete the normal 270° rotation around the mesentery. This results in the cecum being located in the mid-upper abdomen with lateral bands (Ladd's bands) fixating it to the right abdominal wall (Figure 1-19). These bands can result in extrinsic compression of the duodenum.

Reversed Rotation

Clockwise (rather than counterclockwise) rotation of the midgut results in the transverse colon being posterior to the superior mesenteric artery while the duodenum lies anterior to it.

Omphalocele

An omphalocele is, basically, the retention of the midgut within the umbilical sac and its failure to return to the peritoneal cavity.

Internal Hernias

Internal hernias, as well as congenital obstructive bands, can cause congenital bowel obstructions. These are considered failures of the process of fixation (the third stage of rotation). This can be the result of an incomplete fusion of the mesothelium or when structures are abnormally rotated. Retroperitoneal hernias can occur in various positions, most notably paraduodenal, paracecal, and intersigmoid.

Other Congenital Malformations of the Colon and Small Intestine

Proximal Colon Duplication

There are three general types of colonic duplication: mesenteric cysts, diverticula, and long colon duplication [67]. Mesenteric cysts are lined with intestinal epithelium and variable amounts of smooth muscle. They are found within the colonic mesentery or posterior to the rectum (within the mesorectum). They may be closely adherent to the bowel

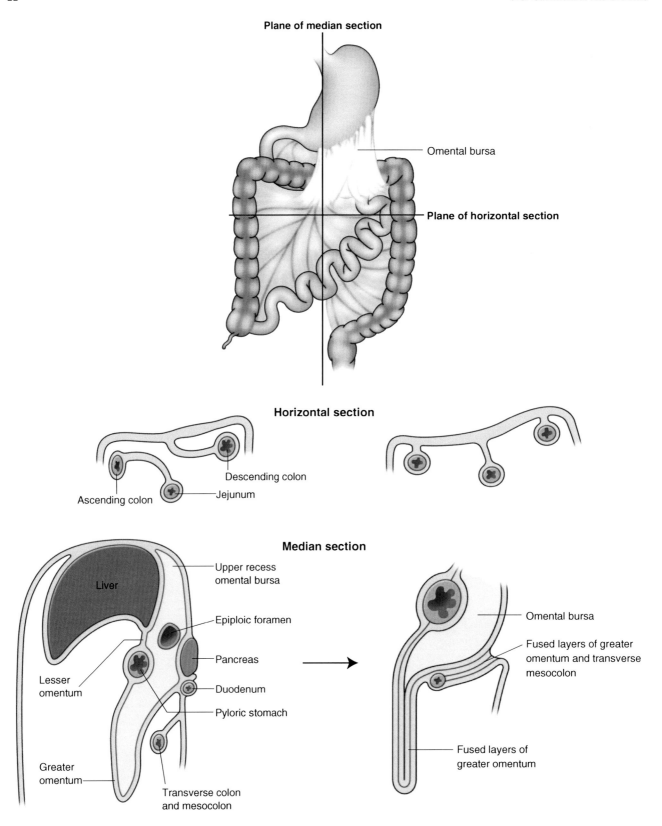

FIGURE 1-17. Development of the mesentery and omental fusion.

Nonrotation

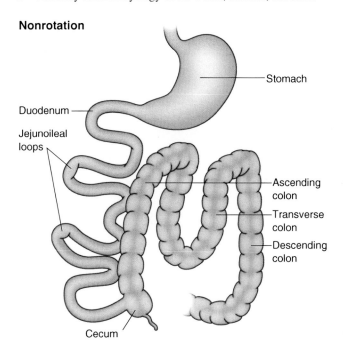

FIGURE 1-18. Intestinal non-rotation.

Intestinal Malrotation

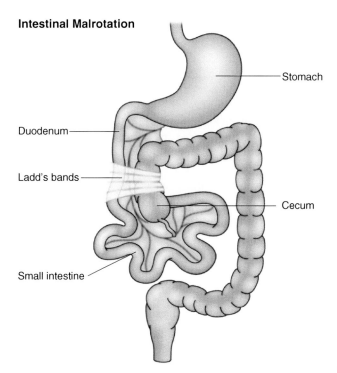

FIGURE 1-19. Intestinal malrotation.

wall or separate from it. They generally present as a mass or with intestinal obstruction as they enlarge. Diverticula can be found on the mesenteric or antimesenteric sides of the colon and are outpouchings of the bowel wall. They often contain heterotopic gastric or pancreatic tissue. Long colonic duplications of the colon are the rarest form of duplication. They

parallel the functional colon and often share a common wall throughout most of their length. They usually run the entire length of the colon and rectum and there is an association with other genitourinary abnormalities.

Meckel's Diverticulum

A Meckel's diverticulum is the remnant of the vitelline or omphalomesenteric duct (Figure 1-13). It arises from the antimesenteric aspect of the terminal ileum, most commonly within 50 cm of the ileocecal valve. They can be associated with a fibrous band connecting the diverticulum to the umbilicus (leading to obstruction) or it may contain ectopic gastric mucosa or pancreatic tissue (leading to bleeding or perforation) (Figure 1-20). An indirect hernia containing a Meckel's diverticulum is termed a Littre's hernia. Meckel's diverticulum is generally asymptomatic and, per autopsy series, is found in up to 3% of the population [68]. Surgical complications, which are more common in children than adults, include hemorrhage, obstruction, diverticulitis, perforation, and umbilical discharge. Generally, there is no hard indication for excision of an incidentally discovered Meckel's diverticulum, though its removal is generally safe [69, 70].

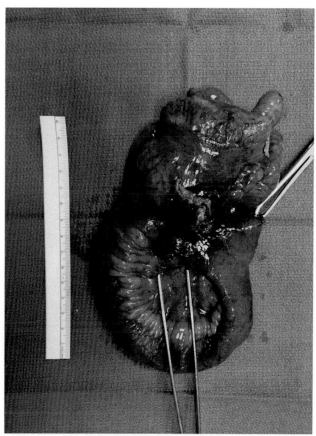

FIGURE 1-20. Perforated Meckel's diverticulum with fistula to ileum.

Atresia of the Colon

Colonic atresia, representing only 5% of all gastrointestinal atresias, is a rare cause of congenital obstruction. They are likely the result of vascular compromise during development [71]. They vary in severity from a membranous diaphragm blocking the lumen to a fibrous cord-like remnant, on to a complete absence of a segment [72].

Hirschsprung's Disease

This nonlethal anomaly, which is more common in males, results from the absence of ganglion cells within the myenteric plexus of the colon. It is caused by interruption of the normal migration of the neuroenteric cells from the neural crest before they reach the rectum. This results in dilation and hypertonicity of the proximal colon. The extent of the aganglionosis is variable, though the internal sphincter is always involved. Its severity is dependent upon the length of the involved segment. It is discussed fully in Chap. 64.

Anorectal Malformations

Abnormalities in the normal development of the anorectum can be attributed to "developmental arrest" at various stages of normal development. These abnormalities are often noted in concert with spinal, sacral, and lower limb defects, as noted by Duhamel and theorized to be related to a "syndrome of caudal regression" [73]. Indeed, skeletal and urinary anomalies are associated in up to 70% [74], while digestive tract anomalies (e.g., tracheoesophageal fistula or esophageal stenosis), cardiac, and abdominal wall abnormalities are also noted in patients with anorectal anomalies. While these are discussed in detail in Chap. 64, a few notable traits are worth pointing out.

Anal Stenosis

While anal stenosis in a newborn is relatively common, noted in 25–39% of infants, symptomatic stenosis is only noted in 25% of these children [75]. The majority of these children undergo spontaneous dilation in the first 3–6 months of life.

Membranous Atresia

This very rare condition is characterized by the presence of a thin membrane of skin between the blind end of the anal canal and the surface. It is also termed the covered anus. It is more common in males.

Anal Agenesis

The rectum develops to below the puborectalis where it either ends in an ectopic opening (fistula) in the perineum, vulva, or urethra, or it ends blindly (less commonly). The sphincter is present at its normal site.

Anorectal Agenesis

Anorectal agenesis is the most common type of "imperforate anus." More common in males, the rectum ends well caudal to the surface and the anus is represented by a dimple with the anal sphincter usually being normal in location. In most cases, there is a fistula to the urethra or vagina. High fistulae (to the vagina or urethra) with anorectal agenesis develop as early as the sixth or seventh week of gestation while the low fistulae (perineal) or anal ectopia develop later, in the eighth or ninth week of development.

Rectal Atresia or "High Atresia"

In rectal atresia, the rectum and the anal canal are separated from one another by an atretic portion. It is embryologically the distal most type of colon atresia, but is still considered an anorectal disorder clinically.

Persistent Cloaca

This rare condition, which only occurs in female infants, is the result of total failure of descent of the urorectal septum. It occurs at a very early stage of development.

Conclusion

It is said that to understand abnormal, you must first understand the normal. No where is that more of a true statement than with human anatomy. Further, to understand the pathophysiology of colorectal and anorectal disease mandates a wide-ranging knowledge base of the underlying anatomy and embryology. To properly care for these patients, one must first have a strong foundation and understanding the anatomical "building blocks" of the human body.

Acknowledgment This chapter was written by José Marcio Neves Jorge and Angelita Habr-Gama in the first and second editions of this textbook.

References

1. Milligan ETC, Morgan CN. Surgical anatomy of the anal canal: with special reference to anorectal fistulae. Lancet. 1934;2(5804):1150–6.
2. Nivatvongs S, Stern HS, Fryd DS. The length of the anal canal. Dis Colon Rectum. 1981;24(8):600–1.
3. Morren GL, Beets-Tan RG, van Engelshoven JM. Anatomy of the anal canal and perianal structures as defined by phased-array magnetic resonance imaging. Br J Surg. 2001;88(11):1506–12.
4. Parks AG. Pathogenesis and treatment of fistuila-in-ano. Br Med J. 1961;1(5224):463–9.
5. Lilius HG. Fistula-in-ano, an investigation of human foetal anal ducts and intramuscular glands and a clinical study of 150 patients. Acta Chir Scand Suppl. 1968;383:7–88.

6. Barleben A, Mills S. Anorectal anatomy and physiology. Surg Clin North Am. 2010;90(1):1–15. Table of Contents.

7. Sboarina A, et al. Shape and volume of internal anal sphincter showed by three-dimensional anorectal ultrasonography. Eur J Radiol. 2012;81(7):1479–82.

8. Haas PA, Fox Jr TA. The importance of the perianal connective tissue in the surgical anatomy and function of the anus. Dis Colon Rectum. 1977;20(4):303–13.

9. Treitz W. Ueber einen neuen Muskel am Duodenum des Menschen, uber elsatische Sehnen, und einige andere anatomische Verhaltnisse. Vierteljahrschrift Praktische Heilkunde (Prager). 1853;37:133–44.

10. Chang SC, Shih JJM, Shih JYM, Lee HHC. Review of Treitz's muscles and their implications in a hemorrhoidectomy and hemorrhoidopexy. Fu-Jen J Med. 2006;4(1):1–6.

11. Thomson WH. The nature of haemorrhoids. Br J Surg. 1975;62(7):542–52.

12. Goligher JC, Leacock AG, Brossy JJ. The surgical anatomy of the anal canal. Br J Surg. 1955;43(177):51–61.

13. Bollard RC, et al. Normal female anal sphincter: difficulties in interpretation explained. Dis Colon Rectum. 2002;45(2): 171–5.

14. Hussain SM, Stoker J, Lameris JS. Anal sphincter complex: endoanal MR imaging of normal anatomy. Radiology. 1995;197(3):671–7.

15. Wunderlich M, Swash M. The overlapping innervation of the two sides of the external anal sphincter by the pudendal nerves. J Neurol Sci. 1983;59(1):97–109.

16. Mittal RK, et al. Purse-string morphology of external anal sphincter revealed by novel imaging techniques. Am J Physiol Gastrointest Liver Physiol. 2014;306(6):G505–14.

17. DeLancey JO, et al. Comparison of levator ani muscle defects and function in women with and without pelvic organ prolapse. Obstet Gynecol. 2007;109(2 Pt 1):295–302.

18. Shafik A. New concept of the anatomy of the anal sphincter mechanism and the physiology of defecation. II. Anatomy of the levator ani muscle with special reference to puborectalis. Invest Urol. 1975;13(3):175–82.

19. Betschart C, et al. Comparison of muscle fiber directions between different levator ani muscle subdivisions: in vivo MRI measurements in women. Int Urogynecol J. 2014;25(9): 1263–8.

20. Levi AC, Borghi F, Garavoglia M. Development of the anal canal muscles. Dis Colon Rectum. 1991;34(3):262–6.

21. Grigorescu BA, et al. Innervation of the levator ani muscles: description of the nerve branches to the pubococcygeus, iliococcygeus, and puborectalis muscles. Int Urogynecol J Pelvic Floor Dysfunct. 2008;19(1):107–16.

22. Wallner C, et al. Evidence for the innervation of the puborectalis muscle by the levator ani nerve. Neurogastroenterol Motil. 2006;18(12):1121–2.

23. Shafik A. A new concept of the anatomy of the anal sphincter mechanism and the physiology of defecation. VIII. Levator hiatus and tunnel: anatomy and function. Dis Colon Rectum. 1979;22(8):539–49.

24. Andrew BP, et al. Enlargement of the levator hiatus in female pelvic organ prolapse: cause or effect? Aust N Z J Obstet Gynaecol. 2013;53(1):74–8.

25. DeLancey JO, et al. Comparison of the puborectal muscle on MRI in women with POP and levator ani defects with those with normal support and no defect. Int Urogynecol J. 2012;23(1):73–7.

26. Heald RJ, Moran BJ. Embryology and anatomy of the rectum. Semin Surg Oncol. 1998;15(2):66–71.

27. Najarian MM, et al. Determination of the peritoneal reflection using intraoperative proctoscopy. Dis Colon Rectum. 2004;47(12):2080–5.

28. Chapuis P, et al. Mobilization of the rectum: anatomic concepts and the bookshelf revisited. Dis Colon Rectum. 2002;45(1):1–8. discussion 8–9.

29. Heald RJ, Husband EM, Ryall RD. The mesorectum in rectal cancer surgery—the clue to pelvic recurrence? Br J Surg. 1982;69(10):613–6.

30. Nomina Anatomica. 6th ed. Singapore: Churchill Livingstone; 1989.

31. Quirke P, et al. Effect of the plane of surgery achieved on local recurrence in patients with operable rectal cancer: a prospective study using data from the MRC CR07 and NCIC-CTG CO16 randomised clinical trial. Lancet. 2009;373(9666):821–8.

32. Church JM, Raudkivi PJ, Hill GL. The surgical anatomy of the rectum—a review with particular relevance to the hazards of rectal mobilisation. Int J Colorectal Dis. 1987;2(3):158–66.

33. Sato K, Sato T. The vascular and neuronal composition of the lateral ligament of the rectum and the rectosacral fascia. Surg Radiol Anat. 1991;13(1):17–22.

34. Crapp AR, Cuthbertson AM. William Waldeyer and the rectosacral fascia. Surg Gynecol Obstet. 1974;138(2):252–6.

35. Gordon PH, Nivatvongs S. Principles and practice of surgery for the colon, rectum, and anus. 3rd ed. New York, NY: Informa Healthcare USA, Inc.; 2007.

36. Lindsey I, et al. Anatomy of Denonvilliers' fascia and pelvic nerves, impotence, and implications for the colorectal surgeon. Br J Surg. 2000;87(10):1288–99.

37. Richardson AC. The rectovaginal septum revisited: its relationship to rectocele and its importance in rectocele repair. Clin Obstet Gynecol. 1993;36(4):976–83.

38. Corman ML. Classic articles in colonic and rectal surgery. A method of performing abdominoperineal excision for carcinoma of the rectum and of the terminal portion of the pelvic colon: by W. Ernest Miles, 1869–1947. Dis Colon Rectum. 1980;23(3):202–5.

39. Heald RJ, Ryall RD. Recurrence and survival after total mesorectal excision for rectal cancer. Lancet. 1986;1(8496):1479–82.

40. Nano M, et al. Contribution to the surgical anatomy of the ligaments of the rectum. Dis Colon Rectum. 2000;43(11):1592–7. discussion 1597–8.

41. Lin M, et al. The anatomy of lateral ligament of the rectum and its role in total mesorectal excision. World J Surg. 2010;34(3):594–8.

42. Abramson DJ. The valves of Houston in adults. Am J Surg. 1978;136(3):334–6.

43. Llauger J, et al. The normal and pathologic ischiorectal fossa at CT and MR imaging. Radiographics. 1998;18(1):61–82. quiz 146.

44. Courtney H. The posterior subsphincteric space; its relation to posterior horseshoe fistula. Surg Gynecol Obstet. 1949;89(2): 222–6.

45. Michaels NA, Siddharth P, Kornblith PL, Park WW. The variant blood supply to the small and large intestines: its importance in regional resections. A new anatomic study based on four hundred dissections with a complete review of the literature. J Int Coll Surg. 1963;39:127–70.

46. Schuurman JP, Go PM, Bleys RL. Anatomical branches of the superior rectal artery in the distal rectum. Colorectal Dis. 2009;11(9):967–71.

47. Ayoub SF. Arterial supply to the human rectum. Acta Anat (Basel). 1978;100(3):317–27.

48. Fraser ID, et al. Longitudinal muscle of muscularis externa in human and nonhuman primate colon. Arch Surg. 1981;116(1):61–3.

49. Guyton AC. Textbook of medical physiology. Philadelphia, PA: WB Saunders; 1986.

50. O'Beirne J, editor. New views of the process of defecation and their application to the pathology and treatment of diseases of the stomach, bowels and other organs. Dublin: Hodges and Smith; 1833.

51. Hyrtl J. Handbuch der topographischen anatomie und ihrer praktisch medicinisch-chirurgischen anwendungen. II. Band. 4th ed. Wien: Braumüller; 1860.

52. Mayo WJ. A study of the rectosigmoid. Surg Gynecol Obstet. 1917;25:616–21.

53. Cantlie J. The sigmoid flexure in health and disease. J Trop Med Hyg. 1915;18:1–7.

54. Otis WJ. Some observations on the structure of the rectum. J Anat Physiol. 1898;32:59–63.

55. Balli R. The sphincters of the colon. Radiology. 1939;33:372–6.

56. Shafik A, et al. Rectosigmoid junction: anatomical, histological, and radiological studies with special reference to a sphincteric function. Int J Colorectal Dis. 1999;14(4–5):237–44.

57. Sonneland J, Anson BJ, Beaton LE. Surgical anatomy of the arterial supply to the colon from the superior mesenteric artery based upon a study of 600 specimens. Surg Gynecol Obstet. 1958;106(4):385–98.

58. Steward JA, Rankin FW. Blood supply of the large intestine. Its surgical considerations. Arch Surg. 1933;26:843–91.

59. Griffiths JD. Surgical anatomy of the blood supply of the distal colon. Ann R Coll Surg Engl. 1956;19(4):241–56.

60. Haller A. The large intestine. In: Cullen W, editor. First lines of physiology. A reprint of the 1786 edition, Sources of science, vol. 32. New York, NY: Johnson; 1966. p. 139–40.

61. Drummond H. Some points relating to the surgical anatomy of the arterial supply of the large intestine. Proc R Soc Med. 1913;7:185–93.

62. Drummond H. The arterial supply of the rectum and pelvic colon. Br J Surg. 1914;1:677–85.

63. Meyers CB. Griffiths' point: critical anastomosis at the splenic flexure. Am J Roentgenol. 1976;126:77.

64. Watanabe J, et al. Evaluation of the intestinal blood flow near the rectosigmoid junction using the indocyanine green fluorescence method in a colorectal cancer surgery. Int J Colorectal Dis. 2015;30(3):329–35.

65. Skandalakis JE, Gray SW, Ricketts R. The colon and rectum. In: Skadalakis JE, Gray SW, editors. Embryology for surgeons. The embryological basis for the treatment of congenital anomalies. Baltimore, MD: Williams & Wilkins; 1994. p. 242–81.

66. Nobles VP. The development of the human anal canal. J Anat. 1984;138:575.

67. McPherson AG, Trapnell JE, Airth GR. Duplication of the colon. Br J Surg. 1969;56(2):138–42.

68. Benson CD. Surgical implications of Meckel's diverticulum. In: Ravitch MM, Welch KJ, Benson CD, editors. Pediatric surgery. Chicago, IL: Year Book Medical Publishers; 1979. p. 955.

69. Zani A, et al. Incidentally detected Meckel diverticulum: to resect or not to resect? Ann Surg. 2008;247(2):276–81.

70. Park JJ, et al. Meckel diverticulum: the Mayo Clinic experience with 1476 patients (1950–2002). Ann Surg. 2005;241(3):529–33.

71. Fomolo JL. Congenital lesions: intussusception and volvulus. In: Zuidema GD, editor. Shackelford's surgery of the alimentary tract. Philadelphia, PA: WB Saunders; 1991. p. 45–51.

72. Louw JH. Investigations into the etiology of congenital atresia of the colon. Dis Colon Rectum. 1964;7:471–8.

73. Duhamel B. From the mermaid to anal imperforation: The syndrome of caudal regression. Arch Dis Child. 1961;36(186):152–5.

74. Moore TC, Lawrence EA. Congenital malformations of the rectum and anus. II. Associated anomalies encountered in a series of 120 cases. Surg Gynecol Obstet. 1952;95(3):281–8.

75. Brown SS, Schoen AH. Congenital anorectal stricture. J Pediatr. 1950;36(6):746–51.

2

Colonic Physiology

Joshua I.S. Bleier and Kirsten Bass Wilkins

Key Concepts

- Colonic innervation is supplied by both extrinsic and intrinsic pathways. The extrinsic pathways are derived from the autonomic nervous system including parasympathetic and sympathetic routes. Parasympathetic input is excitatory while sympathetic input is inhibitory to colonic motor function. The intrinsic colonic nervous system consists of the myenteric plexus.
- Short chain fatty acids are produced by the colon as a result of the fermentation of complex carbohydrates by colonic flora. The SCFA, butyrate, is the primary energy source of the colon.
- The colon absorbs sodium and water and secretes bicarbonate and potassium. Aldosterone mediates the process of active sodium absorption in the colon.
- Colonic contractile events are divided into (1) segmental contractions and (2) propagated contractions (including low-amplitude and high-amplitude propagating contractions, LAPC and HAPC, respectively). The main function of HAPC is to propagate colonic contents towards the anus.
- The Interstitial cells of Cajal (ICC) are the primary pacemaker cells governing the function of the enteric nervous system.

Introduction

The colon plays a central role in gastrointestinal (GI) physiology. There are multiple functions that the colon and rectum serve. The primary role of the colon is one of absorption of excess water and electrolytes, serving to salvage valuable fluid and unabsorbed nutrients as well as to create solid stool. It also plays a central role in bacterial homeostasis, serving as a home to billions of commensal bacteria whose role is symbiotic in maintaining the health of the colonic epithelium. The rectum has evolved complicated and elegant mechanisms to store feces and accommodate it while allowing for the selective egress of stool or gas. Understanding the physiologic and histologic components of the colon and rectum are critical to understanding normal and pathologic states.

Embryology

Understanding the embryology of the colon and rectum provides essential information for understanding its function. During the third and fourth weeks of gestation, the primitive gut arises from the cephalic caudal and lateral foldings of the dorsal endoderm lined yolk sac. The mucosa arises from the endodermal layer, however the muscular wall, connective tissue and outer serosal surface arises from the mesodermal layer. By the fourth week of gestation, three distinct regions have differentiated based on their blood supply. The midgut, supplied by the superior mesenteric artery, begins distal to the confluence of the common bile duct in the third portion of the duodenum and includes the proximal two-thirds of the transverse colon. This portion of the intestine maintains a connection to the yolk sac via the vitelline duct. Absence of its obliteration results in a Meckel's diverticulum. The hindgut, which comprises the rest of the distal GI tract, includes the distal transverse colon, descending colon, sigmoid colon, and rectum. This is supplied by the inferior mesenteric artery (IMA). During the fifth week of gestation, the midgut undergoes a rapid elongation which exceeds the capacity of the abdominal cavity. This results in a physiologic herniation through the abdominal wall at the umbilicus. Through the sixth week, continued elongation results in a 90° counterclockwise rotation around the superior mesenteric artery (SMA). The small intestine continues its significant growth, forming loops, while the caudal end enlarges into the cecal bud. During the tenth week, herniated bowel returns to the abdominal cavity, completing an additional 180° counterclockwise loop which leaves the proximal small bowel on the left, and the colon on the right. The dorsal mesentery of

© Springer International Publishing 2016

S.R. Steele et al. (eds.), *The ASCRS Textbook of Colon and Rectal Surgery*, DOI 10.1007/978-3-319-25970-3_2

the ascending and descending colon shortens and involutes resulting in secondary retroperitoneal fixation [1]. The embryology of the distal rectum is more complex. It initially begins as the cloaca which is a specialized area comprising endodermal and ectodermally derived tissue. The cloaca exists as a continuation between the urogenital and GI tracts, however, during the sixth week it begins to divide and differentiate into the anterior urogenital and posterior anorectal and sphincter components. At the same time, the urogenital and GI tracts become separated by caudal migration of the urogenital septum. During the tenth week, while the majority of the midgut is returning to the abdomen, the external anal sphincter is formed in the posterior cloaca as the descent of the urogenital septum becomes complete. The internal anal sphincter is formed during the 12th week by enlargement and specialization of the circular muscle layer of the rectum [1].

Colonic Anatomy

Introduction

The colonic epithelium has both absorptive and secretory functions. The colon is highly efficient at absorbing sodium chloride, water, and short chain fatty acids. In addition, the colonic epithelium secretes bicarbonate, potassium chloride, and mucus. The colonic epithelium is a typical electrolyte-transporting layer that is capable of moving large quantities of water and salt from the lumen towards the blood. Under normal circumstances, the colon is presented with between 1 and 2 l of electrolyte-rich fluid per day. Under normal physiologic conditions, nearly 90% of this fluid is absorbed. The end result is the excretion of feces that has a sodium concentration that approximates 30 mmol/l and a potassium concentration of approximately 75 mmol/l. Under normal circumstances, fecal and plasma osmolality are similar. Colonic epithelial cells are polarized and equipped with numerous ion channels, carriers, and pumps that are localized on both the luminal and basolateral membranes. Many transport proteins have been identified and their functions elucidated. While an in-depth discussion of these mechanisms is beyond the scope of this chapter, important aspects are highlighted below.

Colonic Wall Anatomy

The luminal surface of the colon is lined by epithelium. Deep to this is the submucosal layer, rich in vascular and lymphatic supply. This is surrounded by the continuous inner circular muscle layer and the outer longitudinal muscle layer which has three condensations known as taenia coli. The serosa, or outer layer of the colon, is surrounded by visceral peritoneum.

Colonic Epithelial Cell Types

Three main cell types are present in the colonic epithelium including columnar epithelial cells, goblet cells, and enterochromaffin cells. Columnar epithelial and goblet cells comprise nearly 95% of the cells in the colonic epithelium. The surface and crypt epithelial cells can be differentiated from one another based on proliferative activity, degree of differentiation, and function. Crypt epithelium is highly proliferative, relatively undifferentiated, and secretes chloride. The surface epithelium in contrast has low proliferative activity, is well-differentiated, and is highly absorptive. In general, epithelial cells become increasingly differentiated the farther they are from the crypt base. Thus, the base of the crypts forms the source of continually regenerating epithelial cells. This polarization provides distinct histologic characteristics, which are easily identified on standard H and E staining (Figures 2-1 and 2-2). Recent evidence, however, indicates that ion absorption and secretion occurs at both the surface and crypt levels [2]. The role of the enterochromaffin cells is discussed below.

The cells responsible for the enteric nervous system, the enteric ganglia, are located in the submucosa, otherwise known as Meissner's plexus. An additional layer of ganglia are located between the inner circular and outer longitudinal muscle layers known as Auerbach's plexus. The interstitial cells of Cajal (ICC), are specialized, c-kit positive cells that are thought to primarily serve as the pacemaker cell of the enteric nervous system, linking the colonic submucosa electrochemically with the myenteric plexi. These are the cells of origin of GI stromal tumors (GISTs) which arise from the colonic wall rather than the mucosa [3].

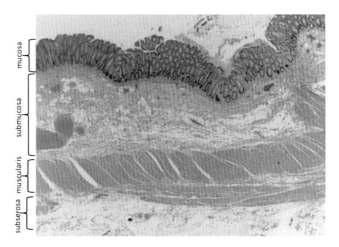

FIGURE 2-1. Normal colonic mucosa. H and E, 250×. The layers of the normal colonic wall are indicated by the *brackets. Courtesy of Julieta E. Barroeta, MD.*

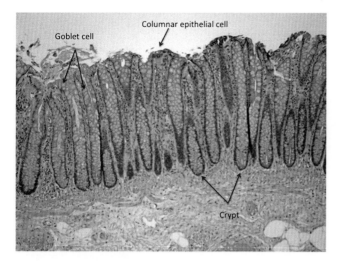

FIGURE 2-2. Normal colonic mucosa. H and E, 1000×. Epithelial cells types are clearly visible including goblet cells and columnar epithelial cells. The crypts are the source of the continually regenerating mucosal cells. *Courtesy of Julieta E. Barroeta, MD.*

Colonic Flora

By the time enteric contents reach the colon, the majority of nutrients have been digested and absorbed by the small intestine. This leaves a fluid rich in electrolytes, bile salts, and undigested starches. These are the primary substrates upon which the colon functions. The colon is home to an enormous quantity of autochthonous flora consisting of more than 400 species of bacteria. Feces contains as many as $10^{11}-10^{12}$ bacteria/gram of stool, and these bacteria contribute to approximately 50% of fecal mass. The majority of these bacteria are anaerobes which feed on residual proteins and undigested carbohydrates. This microflora contributes several important functions to the host including metabolic support of the colonocyte and gut-associated lymphoid tissue (GALT), which contributes significantly to both innate and adaptive immunity. *Bacteroides* species compose the predominant bacterial type throughout the colon, and they are responsible for almost 2/3 of the bacteria within the proximal colon and 70% of the bacteria in the rectum. The other predominant species are facultative aerobes and comprise *Escherichia*, *Klebsiella*, *Proteus*, *lactobacillus*, and *enterococci*. Unlike the majority of the proximal GI tract, the colonic mucosa does not receive its primary nutrition from blood-borne nutrients. In the colon and rectum, luminal contents provide the primary substrate. The main source of the substrate is undigested dietary fiber. This is metabolized by colonic bacteria through the process of *fermentation*. Cellulose is a partially fermented starch, which leaves behind bulk, whereas fruit pectins are completely metabolized (clarify). The primary end products of this process include short chain fatty acids, including butyrate, and gas. Several of the common dietary complex carbohydrates, including lignin and psyllium, are not metabolized at all, but remain as hydrophilic molecules in stool. These lead to water retention and stool bulking. Butyrate is the main source of energy for the colonocyte. This provides the substrate necessary to maintain epithelial integrity and developmental functions that stimulate epithelial cell differentiation and immune function. Protein fermentation, or *putrefaction*, may result in the formation of potentially toxic metabolites including phenols, indoles, and amines. These toxic end products of bacterial metabolism can lead to mucosal injury, reactive hyperproliferation, and possible promotion of carcinogenesis. Increased stool bulk is felt to provide enhanced colonic transit resulting in decreased time of exposure of the colonic lumen to these toxins, as well as a decreased need for higher intracolonic pressures necessary for segmental motility, a process which may retard the development of diverticular disease. Taken together, these aspects are the reason for many of the recommendations for dietary supplementation with indigestible fiber [4].

Electrolyte Regulation and Water Absorption

Sodium chloride absorption occurs by both electroneutral and electrogenic active transport mechanisms. While electroneutral absorption takes place in both the surface and crypt epithelium, electrogenic absorption appears to be confined to the surface epithelium. A majority of sodium chloride absorption occurs in the proximal colon and is driven primarily through electroneutral absorption by tightly coupled luminal Na^+/H^+ and Cl^-/HCO_3^- exchange. This process is driven by the basolateral Na^+-K^+-ATPase resulting in 1 mol of ATP being hydrolyzed for every 3 mol of NaCl absorbed. Three types of Na^+/H^+ exchangers (NHE) have been identified in colonic epithelium. Similarly, several Cl^- exchange mechanisms have been identified. The luminal Cl^-/HCO_3^- exchange is represented by the anion exchanger type 1 (AE1). A separate Cl^-/OH^- exchange is represented by a protein called DRA (downregulated in colonic adenomas). Human DRA mutations are responsible for congenital chloride diarrhea [2].

Epithelial cells in the distal colon participate in electrogenic absorption of sodium. The epithelial sodium channel (ENaC) mediates this absorption and is located on the luminal surface. Sodium is taken up by the ENaC on the luminal surface and is excreted on the basolateral side by the Na^+-K^+-ATPase. Potassium is secreted on the luminal side and is driven by the electrogenic uptake of sodium. Chloride is absorbed through luminal cystic fibrosis conductance regulator (CFTR) and other chloride channels. Chloride is then excreted on the basolateral side via multiple mechanisms including KCL cotransporter (KCC1), Cl^- channels, and Cl^-/HCO_3^- anion exchangers [2]. The net result is tight regulation of electrolyte secretion in excreted stool (Figure 2-3).

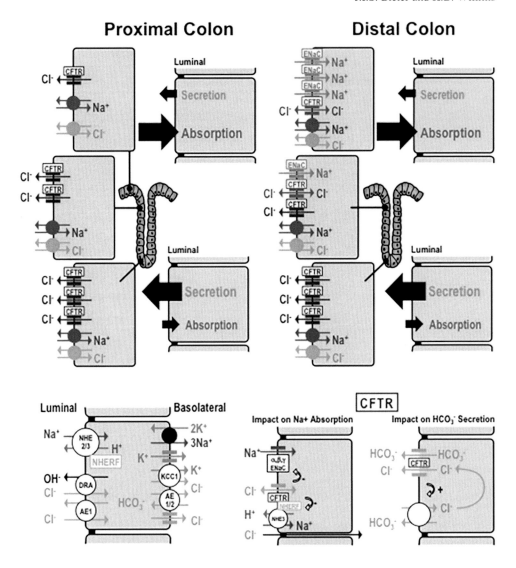

Regulation of sodium absorption is complex and multiple mechanisms are involved. One mechanism of sodium absorption regulation is by feedback inhibition. Namely, changes in intracellular sodium concentration during sodium chloride absorption downregulate ENaC activity. Blood pressure and potassium levels also regulate sodium absorption via angiotensin II. Aldosterone, a mineralocorticoid, is the final endocrine signal in the renin–angiotensin–aldosterone pathway that targets renal and colonic epithelium. Aldosterone is a steroid hormone that is synthesized in the *zona glomerulosa* of the adrenal cortex. Previously, it was thought that aldosterone regulated sodium absorption solely via luminal ENaC. However, aldosterone also increases activity of NHE3. Therefore, aldosterone plays a role in both electrogenic and electroneutral active sodium absorption. Early and late phase aldosterone genomic actions have been identified. In the first 1–6 h, aldosterone-induced proteins including serum and glucocorticoid-inducible kinase (Sgk), corticosteroid hormone-induced factor (CHIF), and K-Ras (KRAS) increase the posttranslational activation of existing ion channels and other proteins involved in ion transport such as ENAc. In the late phase (>6 h), aldosterone acts via the upregulation of nuclear transcription of these receptors. In addition, electroneutral absorption is known to be regulated in response to some G protein-linked receptors, tyrosine kinase-coupled receptors, and protein kinases. For example, activation of protein kinase C, Ca^{2+}/calmodulin-dependent kinase, and increases in cAMP inhibit NHE3 [2, 5].

Evidence also points towards the regulation of sodium absorption by CFTR. ENaC, NHE3, and CFTR are coexpressed in colonic epithelial cells and thus CFTR plays a role in both the electrogenic and electroneutral absorption of electrolytes. CFTR inhibits both electroneutral NaCl absorption as well as electrogenic Na^+ absorption. In the crypts, CFTR is a cAMP-mediated chloride channel that is essential for chloride secretion. In patients with cystic fibrosis, mutations in CFTR result in both impaired chloride secretion and enhanced sodium absorption [2, 6].

Along with the kidneys, the colon assists with potassium homeostasis through the absorption and secretion of potassium. Active potassium absorption is restricted to the distal colon and is mediated by H^+-K^+-ATPase [2].

Water is passively absorbed and can be transported by various pathways including through paracellular shunts and through transcellular flux potentially through aquaporin channels located on luminal and basolateral membrane surfaces [2].

Short Chain Fatty Acid Absorption

As indicated earlier, short chain fatty acids (SCFA) are produced during fermentation of dietary fibers by luminal bacteria. The most common short chain fatty acids include acetate, proprionate, and butyrate. Short chain fatty acids are absorbed by nonionic diffusion and paracellular absorption in the proximal colon. Butyrate is the main energy source for the colonocyte. Butyrate also plays a major role in the stimulation of sodium chloride absorption and inhibition of chloride secretion. Absorption of SCFA plays a significant role in NaCl absorption presumably by the acidification of colonocytes and activation of luminal Na^+/H^+ exchangers. Chloride absorption is also upregulated by increased HCO_3^- production and stimulation of the luminal Cl^-/HCO_3^- exchanger. This HCO_3^- luminal secretion is paramount in regulating luminal intestinal pH. It has been proposed that antibiotic associated diarrhea is secondary to decreased butyrate production resulting in net secretion of fluid [2, 7].

In addition to its role in ionic absorption, butyrate has several other important functions. Butyrate has a trophic effect and stimulates cell proliferation in the crypts. It also reduces the number and size of aberrant crypt foci. This is important as aberrant crypt foci are the earliest precursors of colonic neoplasms. In colon cancer cell lines, butyrate induces apoptosis and cell cycle arrest via inhibition of histone deacetylase. Butyrate also has an anti-inflammatory role primarily by inhibition of nuclear factor kB (NF-kB) in colonic epithelial cells. Some studies have implicated impaired butyrate metabolism in patients with ulcerative colitis. Butyrate stimulates the production of MUC2 mucin and thus may play a role in maintaining the colonic defense barrier. In addition, butyrate may play a role in intestinal motility by regulating gene expression in the enteric nervous system. Finally, butyrate may decrease visceral sensitivity [7, 8].

Despite, the benefits of butyrate discussed above, commercially available butyrate available for oral administration is limited by its short half-life, poor palatability, and side effects such as nausea and anorexia. Rectal formulations are most commonly utilized at this time. Prebiotics and probiotics which produce butyrate are alternative methods of delivery. Prebiotics are nutrients (typically carbohydrates) that support the growth of probiotics bacteria. Probiotics are live bacteria that when consumed in sufficient quantities confer positive health benefits [7, 8].

Secretory Role of the Colonic Epithelium

Another major function of the colonic epithelium is electrolyte secretion. Electrolyte secretion may help transport mucus from the crypts and mucus secretion may be activated by an increase in intracellular cAMP that parallels electrolyte secretion. Chloride secretion occurs predominantly in the crypt cells, but can occur from the surface epithelium as well. Chloride secretion is activated by cAMP-dependent stimulation of CFTR chloride channels. CFTR is the gene product that is affected by any of a number of mutations that cause cystic fibrosis. CFTR is the predominant Cl^- channel in the colon and is responsible for both cAMP- and Ca^{2+}-mediated chloride secretion. CFTR is primarily activated by protein kinase A; however, other second messenger pathways are involved including protein kinase C, cGMP, and calmodulin-dependent kinase [2, 6].

Additional Cl^- channels have been identified in the colonic mucosa that belong to a family of ClC Cl^- channels. The ClC-2 channel is found in colonic epithelium and is regulated by changes in intracellular pH as well as cell volume. They have been localized at tight junction complexes in the crypts [2]. Lubiprostone accelerates colonic transport through the activation of ClC-2 channels on the apical membrane of epithelial cells [9, 10].

As mentioned above, bicarbonate is also secreted to the luminal side of the epithelium and is responsible for the slightly alkaline pH of the colonic lumen [2].

Secretion of electrolytes is often accompanied by secretion of macromolecules. Mucus is probably the most important of these macromolecules and this mucus creates a barrier between the colonic luminal contents and the epithelium [2]. Secreted mucus in the colon forms two distinct layers. The outer loose layer contains bacteria and lubricates feces and protects epithelial cells from abrasion and chemical insult. An inner layer is essentially sterile and is a dense gel that contains antimicrobial peptides, enzymes, and secretory immunoglobulin A (IgA) amongst other substances [3]. Mucus is secreted from goblet cells as well as crypt epithelial cells. Cholinergic stimulation releases preformed mucus. Increased intracellular cAMP induces mucus synthesis. Prostaglandins stimulate mucus secretion from columnar epithelial cells [2].

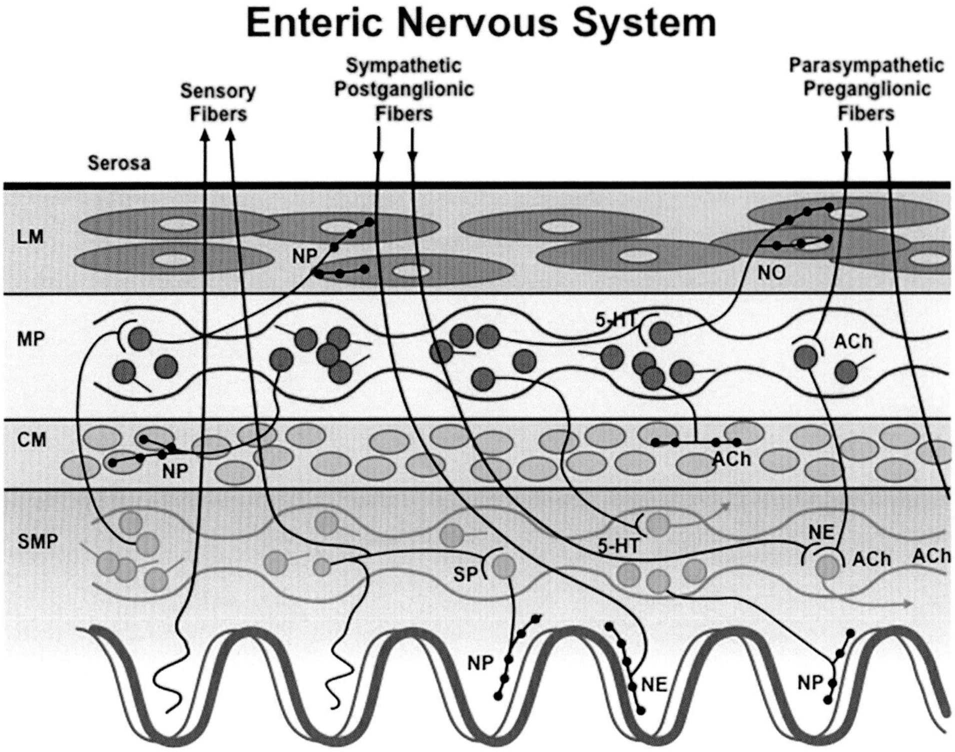

FIGURE 2-4. Schematic representation of the components of the enteric nervous system. *Courtesy of Robin Noel.*

Enteric Nervous System

Regulation of Electrolyte and Water Absorption and Secretion

Under normal physiologic conditions, there is a net absorption of sodium chloride and water. Under pathologic conditions, active Cl⁻ secretion predisposes to the development of diarrhea. Secretion and absorption are mediated by endocrine, paracrine, autocrine, immunologic, and neuronal input [2, 6]. The major neuronal input is via the myenteric (Auerbach's) plexus and the submucosal (Meissner's) plexus. These plexi innervate epithelial as well as vascular smooth muscle cells and regulate colonic blood flow, absorption, and secretion. Food substances, bile acids, and bacterial or viral toxins may act as secretagogues. Secretory hormones and neurotransmitters include vasoactive intestinal polypeptide (VIP), acetylcholine (ACh), histamine, secretin, and serotonin. Substances that inhibit secretion include growth hormone, neuropeptide Y, somatostatin, opiates, and norepinephrine [2]. There is also evidence to suggest that small gaseous molecules, gasotransmitters, also play a role in regulating colonic ion transport. Examples of gasotransmitters include nitric oxide, carbon monoxide, and hydrogen sulfide [6].

Colonic Innervation

Nerves supplying the colon serve to control and modulate colonic motor function. These nerves have a multitude of functions including the following: (1) afferent input via chemoreceptors and mechanoreceptors, (2) efferent output to smooth muscles cells that either stimulate or inhibit

contraction by the release of neurotransmitters, (3) modulate the release of neurotransmitters through the release of neuromodulators, (4) control colonic sphincter activity for functions including defecation, and (5) generate signals for the initiation of propagating and nonpropagating motor complexes (see below) [11].

The nerves that control these functions are of both extrinsic and intrinsic origin. The extrinsic pathways originate from the central and autonomic (sympathetic and parasympathetic) nervous systems. Intrinsic innervation consists of the enteric nervous system [11, 12].

It is speculated that central control contributes minimally to baseline colonic tone except as it relates to defecation when voluntary relaxation of the external anal sphincter and contraction of abdominal musculature is required. It is unknown whether the central nervous system provides continuous input to colonic motor control [11].

Autonomic pathways run along parasympathetic and sympathetic chains. Each of these pathways include afferent (sensory) and efferent (motor) innervation. Vagal and pelvic nerves provide parasympathetic input to the colon. Vagal fibers reach the proximal colon along the posterior vagal trunk that follows the arterial blood supply along superior mesenteric arterial branches. The rectum and distal colon receives parasympathetic input from the sacral nerves (S2–S4) through the pelvic plexus. Parasympathetic stimulation stimulates motor activity of the circular and longitudinal muscle throughout the colon. Unlike vagal afferents, the pelvic afferents contain pain fibers and thus convey visceral sensory input (Figure 2-4). Acetylcholine is the major cholinergic parasympathetic neurotransmitter. Noncholinergic neurotransmitters may also play a role [11, 12].

Sympathetic fibers originate from several sources including the lumbar ventral roots (L2–L5), postganglionic hypogastric nerves, and the splanchnic nerves (T5–T12). The lumbar ventral nerve roots provide the main sympathetic supply to the colon. These nerves synapse on the inferior mesenteric ganglia. From there, the post-ganglionic nerves course along the inferior mesenteric artery to synapse on the enteric ganglia. The postganglionic hypogastric nerves also originate from the inferior mesenteric ganglia and then join the pelvic plexus. The hypogastric nerves primarily innervate the anal sphincters. The splanchnic nerves reach the proximal colon as they course along the blood supply. It is speculated that the lumbar nerves innervate the entire colon while the splanchnic nerves likely only innervate the proximal colon. The primary targets of the sympathetic efferent pathways include myenteric ganglia, submucosal ganglia, blood vessels, and sphincters. Sympathetic innervation is inhibitory to the myenteric ganglia and thus inhibits colonic contractions. However, sympathetic input to sphincter muscle is excitatory. Taken together, sympathetic input decreases peristalsis. Amongst numerous other substances, norepinephrine is a neurotransmitter that is known to exert inhibitory effects via a-2 adrenergic receptors in the myenteric plexus [13, 14].

While central and autonomic innervation is important, the intrinsic (enteric) nervous system is unique in that colon can continue to function even when these circuits have been interrupted. Specifically, the colon exhibits reflexes in the absence of extrinsic neural input. This is due to the complex system of 200–600 million ganglia that comprise the enteric nervous system. These ganglia arise from neural crest cells that colonize the gut during embryological development. The enteric nervous system consists of full reflex circuits comprising sensory neurons, interneurons, and motor neurons. This complex system is regulated by a multitude of neurotransmitters and neuromodulators and is responsible not only for controlling colonic motor activity, but also mucosal ion absorption and secretion and intestinal blood flow [3, 11, 12, 15].

Two major sets of ganglia are found in the colon. The myenteric or Auerbach's plexus is located between the longitudinal and circular smooth muscle layers and plays a crucial role in colonic smooth muscle function. The submucosal or Meissner's plexus regulates ion transport [3, 13–15]. The extreme importance of these two plexuses is clear in children with Hirschsprung's disease in which the ganglia of the myenteric and submucosal plexuses are congenitally absent. The aganglionic segments do not relax and peristalsis is disturbed resulting in severe constipation [14]. There is also a mucosal abnormality predisposing to enterocolitis. Nearly 20 types of enteric neurons have been identified and every class of CNS neurotransmitters has been identified in the enteric nervous system. Besides neurotransmitters, other chemicals act in an endocrine or paracrine function to influence the enteric nervous system. While not totally inclusive, substances identified as playing a role in the enteric nervous system include acetylcholine, norepinephrine, 5-hydroxy-tryptamine (serotonin), dopamine, substance P, neurotensin, vasoactive intestinal peptide, somatostatin, prostaglandins, and neuropeptide Y [11, 12, 16].

Intrinsic primary afferent neurons (IPANs) are the neurons through which enteric reflexes are initiated. These were initially described as Type II neurons with long axonal processes extending to the mucosa and other neurons. However, it has become clear that other non-Type II neurons also play a crucial role in enteric sensation. Nonetheless, these IPANs function to sense changes in luminal chemistry and pressure as well as colonic muscular tone. IPANs are present in the myenteric and submucosal plexi [12, 14, 15]. While the IPANs monitor luminal stimuli, they need to do this transepithelially, since nerve fibers do not directly have contact with the colonic lumen. Therefore, sensory transducer cells in the epithelium are present to respond to mucosal changes. Enterochromaffin (EC) cells represent a type of this sensory transducer cell. EC cells contain large quantities of serotonin. Nearly 95% of serotonin is found in the gut and most of that is stored in the EC cells. When EC cells are stimulated, serotonin is secreted from the basolateral surface of the EC cells of the lamina propria. This is where the serotonin has access to nerve fibers. Serotonin can be excitatory or inhibitory depending on which type of serotonin receptor with which it interacts. Serotonin is not catabolized by enzymes, but is taken up by specific serotonin reuptake transporters (SERT) present in serotonergic neurons. While beyond the scope of this chapter, it is worth mentioning that in patients with irritable bowel syndrome, mucosal expression of SERT is reduced. The importance of serotonin in the enteric nervous system and the role it plays in irritable bowel syndrome has allowed the development of medications to reduce the symptoms of IBS [3, 12, 15]. The 5-HT3 antagonist, alosetron, has been approved for treatment of IBS-associated diarrhea in women [10, 15]. On the other hand, the 5-HT4 agonist, tegaserod, was initially approved for the treatment of IBS-associated constipation. Tegaserod was withdrawn from the market by the FDA in 2007 because of concerns of potential adverse cardiac events [9, 12, 15].

Colonic Motility

Basic colonic motility requirements include slow net caudal propulsion, extensive mixing of semisolid stool, and uniform exposure of luminal contents to the mucosal surface. The colon also needs to rapidly move stool caudally during mass movements. In addition, the colon must be able to store fecal material in the colon until defecation. As reviewed above, most colonic motility is involuntary and is primarily mediated by the enteric nervous system in association with autonomic parasympathetic and sympathetic input.

Cellular Basis of Motility

The muscular apparatus of the colon consists of two distinctive layers of smooth muscle cells including the circular and longitudinal layers. These smooth muscle cells are interconnected by gap junctions that allow electrical signals to spread in coordinated fashion. Very important to this function are the colonic pacemaker cells, also called the interstitial cells of Cajal. The ICC are cells of mesenchymal origin. The ICC generates electrical pacemaker activity that provides the smooth muscle with the mechanism to produce propulsive rhythmic activity. They also appear to serve as conduits for muscle innervation and may transmit sensory information. In colon biopsy specimens, ICC density is able to be measured by c-Kit immunohistochemistry. ICC occur in the submucosa and myenteric borders [3, 17–20]. ICC of the submucosa (ICC-SM) generate electrical stimuli with an oscillatory pattern of 2–4 Hz. Coupling of the ICC-SM to smooth muscle cells triggers large, slow repetitive depolarizations of the smooth muscle referred to as slow waves. Higher frequency oscillations (17–18 Hz) are generated in the ICC of the myenteric border (ICC-MP), but the slow waves from the ICC-SM seem to predominate [17–19].

Motility Patterns and Measurement

Intraluminal colonic motility measurements (manometry and barostat studies) have provided an understanding of colonic motility patterns. Colonic motor activity is not rhythmic, but is characterized by brief (phasic) and sustained (tonic) contractions. At least seven different patterns of human colonic phasic pressure activity have been identified. These include non-propagating and propagating pressure waves and contractions. Non-propagating pressure waves occur randomly for at least 30 s. Simultaneous pressure waves occur simultaneously at least 10 cm apart with an onset time of <1 s. Periodic colonic motor activity also manifests as discrete random bursts of phasic and tonic pressure waves with a frequency of ≥ 3 per minute and a cycle duration of ≥ 3 per minute. Similar discrete bursts of phasic and tonic pressure waves also occur in the rectosigmoid and occur predominantly at night and are referred to as periodic rectal motor activity (PRMA). The function of these non-propagating waves is not well delineated, but they may serve as a means for local mixing of luminal contents and may allow for adequate mucosal sampling [19–22].

Propagating pressure waves and contractions serve to propel the colonic contents in aborad and orad directions. Aborad pressure waves include propagating pressure waves that migrate aborad across ≥ 10 cm at a velocity of 0.5 cm/s and high amplitude propagated contractions (HAPC) of pressures ≥ 75 mmHg and that migrate aborad ≥ 15 cm. HAPCs occur approximately six times a day and serve to move stool *en masse* across the colon. Frequently, but not always, these occur prior to defecation. There are also retrograde waves that migrate orad ≥ 15 cm with a velocity of >0.5 cm/s [19, 21, 22].

Clear physiologic patterns of colonic motor activity are recognized. Phasic activity demonstrates diurnal variation with activity decreasing during sleep and increasing upon awakening. Phasic activity also increases within a few minutes after a meal and continues for up to 2.5 h depending on the nutrient composition and caloric content of the meal. High fat meals elicit more of a response than carbohydrate rich meals. At least 500 kcal needs to be ingested to predictably cause a colonic response to the meal. Finally, colonic instillation of bisacodyl or intravenous neostigmine induces HAPCs. Colonic tone can be measured with a barostat. In physiologic states, colonic tone increases in response to a meal [17, 21–23].

Altered colonic motility may be manifest as constipation. Patients with constipation can be evaluated with several modalities including radiopaque marker studies, radionuclide scintigraphy, magnetic resonance imaging, dynamic defecography, wireless motility capsule (smart pill®, Given Imaging) evaluation, and colonic manometry/barostat studies [17, 18, 22, 23]. While the details of these modalities are discussed in subsequent chapters, it is worth mentioning several common findings in patients with slow transit constipation. Patients with slow transit constipation have a reduced frequency of HAPCs. These patients also lack the normal phasic response that is elicited by the intake of a meal. The diurnal variation of colonic motor activity also may be abnormal in patients with slow transit constipation. Colonic bisacodyl administration also produces a blunted HAPC response in patients with slow transit constipation. A diminished increase in colonic tone following a meal has also been observed in slow transit constipation [21–24]. Loss and injury to the ICC has also been observed in patients with constipation [20]. Taken together, slow transit constipation may be associated with both myopathic and neuropathic etiologies.

Clinical Aspects of Colon Physiology

Ultimately, the main goal of understanding the concepts behind colonic physiology is to be able to translate these into effective therapy for the problems that plague our patients. Subsequent chapters in the text deal more specifically with these issues, but to illustrate this concept, we can consider the use of sacral neuromodulation (SNM). This is not a new therapy; however, its FDA approval for the treatment of fecal incontinence has brought it into the spotlight more recently. In addition to its efficacy for fecal incontinence and its complex interaction with the pelvic floor, European data has also shown its efficacy for the treatment of colonic motility disorders, specifically chronic constipation as well as low anterior resection syndrome. The postulated effectors for its success are based on the known principles of colonic motility illustrated in this chapter. Dinning et al. performed an elegant study in which patients with slow-transit constipation were treated with SNM. A manometry catheter was positioned colonoscopically, with its tip fixed in the cecum. Electrodes were then placed in both the S2 and S3 foramina and stimulated. They found that stimulation to the S3 nerve root significantly increased pan-colonic antegrade propagating sequences (PS), while stimulation at S2 significantly increased retrograde PSs. During a 3-week trial 75% of patients reported increase frequency of bowel movements and decreased laxative use [25]. The true mechanism of SNM on the enteric nervous system is not known; however, it is hypothesized to affect autonomic innervation, largely through CNS-mediated effects.

The colorectum is a complex organ with multiple roles in human homeostasis. By increasing understanding of its anatomy and complex physiologic components, the colorectal surgeon can gain not only a better understanding of its normal role, but the etiology of derangement in pathophysiologic conditions, as well as an opportunity to develop new therapies based on its known functions. These examples are demonstrated with much greater detail throughout other sections of the text.

References

1. Szmulowicz U, Hull T. Colonic physiology. In: Beck DE, Roberts P, Saclarides T, Senagore A, Stamos M, Wexner SD, editors. The ASCRS textbook of colon and rectal surgery. 2nd ed. New York: Springer Science+Business media LLC; 2011. p. 23.
2. Kunzelmann K, Mall M. Electrolyte transport in the mammalian colon: mechanisms and implications for disease. Physiol Rev. 2002;82(1):245–89.
3. Sellers RS, Morton D. The colon: from banal to brilliant. Toxicol Pathol. 2014;42(1):67–81.
4. Fry R, Mahmoud N, Maron D, Bleier J. Chapter 52: Colon and rectum. In: Townsend C, Beauchamp R, Evers B, Mattox K, editors. Sabiston textbook of surgery. 19th ed. Philadelphia: Elsevier Saunders; 2012. p. 1294.
5. Booth RE, Johnson JP, Stockand JD. Aldosterone. Adv Physiol Educ. 2002;26(1–4):8–20.
6. Pouokam E, Steidle J, Diener M. Regulation of colonic ion transport by gasotransmitters. Biol Pharm Bull. 2011;34(6):789–93.
7. Canani RB, Costanzo MD, Leone L, Pedata M, Meli R, Calignano A. Potential beneficial effects of butyrate in intestinal and extraintestinal diseases. World J Gastroenterol. 2011;17(12):1519–28.
8. Leonel AJ, Alvarez-Leite JI. Butyrate: implications for intestinal function. Curr Opin Clin Nutr Metab Care. 2012;15(5):474–9.
9. Hussain ZH, Everhart K, Lacy BE. Treatment of chronic constipation: prescription medications and surgical therapies. Gastroenterol Hepatol. 2015;11(2):104.
10. Chey WD, Kurlander J, Eswaran S. Irritable bowel syndrome: a clinical review. JAMA. 2015;313(9):949–58.
11. Sarna SK. Colonic motor activity. Surg Clin North Am. 1993;73(6):1201–23.
12. Furness JB, Callaghan BP, Rivera LR, Cho HJ. The enteric nervous system and gastrointestinal innervation: integrated local and central control. Adv Exp Med Biol. 2014;817:39–71.
13. Sarna SK. Physiology and pathophysiology of colonic motor activity (2). Dig Dis Sci. 1991;36(7):998–1018.
14. Furness JB. The enteric nervous system: normal functions and enteric neuropathies. Neurogastroenterol Motil. 2008;20 Suppl 1:32–8.
15. Gershon MD. Nerves, reflexes, and the enteric nervous system: pathogenesis of the irritable bowel syndrome. J Clin Gastroenterol. 2005;39(5 Suppl 3):S184–93.
16. Straub RH, Wiest R, Strauch UG, Harle P, Scholmerich J. The role of the sympathetic nervous system in intestinal inflammation. Gut. 2006;55(11):1640–9.
17. Gudsoorkar VS, Quigley EM. Colorectal sensation and motility. Curr Opin Gastroenterol. 2014;30(1):75–83.
18. Quigley EM. What we have learned about colonic motility: normal and disturbed. Curr Opin Gastroenterol. 2010;26(1):53–60.
19. Brookes SJ, Dinning PG, Gladman MA. Neuroanatomy and physiology of colorectal function and defaecation: from basic science to human clinical studies. Neurogastroenterol Motil. 2009;21 Suppl 2:9–19.
20. Huizinga JD, Chen JH. Interstitial cells of Cajal: update on basic and clinical science. Curr Gastroenterol Rep. 2014;16(1):363.
21. Bassotti G, de Roberto G, Castellani D, Sediari L, Morelli A. Normal aspects of colorectal motility and abnormalities in slow transit constipation. World J Gastroenterol. 2005;11(18):2691–6.
22. Camilleri M, Bharucha AE, di Lorenzo C, Hasler WL, Prather CM, Rao SS, et al. American Neurogastroenterology and Motility Society consensus statement on intraluminal measurement of gastrointestinal and colonic motility in clinical practice. Neurogastroenterol Motil. 2008;20(12):1269–82.
23. Dinning PG, Smith TK, Scott SM. Pathophysiology of colonic causes of chronic constipation. Neurogastroenterol Motil. 2009;21 Suppl 2:20–30.
24. Bassotti G, Crowell MD, Whitehead WE. Contractile activity of the human colon: lessons from 24 hour studies. Gut. 1993;34(1):129–33.
25. Dinning PG, Fuentealba SE, Kennedy ML, Lubowski DZ, Cook IJ. Sacral nerve stimulation induces pan-colonic propagating pressure waves and increases defecation frequency in patients with slow-transit constipation. Colorectal Dis. 2007;9(2):123–32.

3

Anal Physiology: The Physiology of Continence and Defecation

Vitaliy Poylin and Thomas E. Cataldo

Abbreviations

RAIR   Rectoanal inhibitory reflex
SNS   Sacral nerve stimulation
FI   Fecal incontinence
MR   Magnetic resonance

Key Concepts

- The innervation of the anal sphincter complex is a mixed sympathetic and parasympathetic crossed over system that provides redundant safeguards to continence.
- Normal continence and defecation require intact sensation and motor control and reflexes to sense, retain, and voluntarily expect the rectal contents at a socially appropriate time and place.
- The normal physiology of the anus can be disturbed in a variety of ways resulting in lack of control, inability to expel, or chronic pelvic pain.
- The process of childbirth can contribute significantly to alteration in anorectal anatomy and physiology resulting in a variety of disorders of defecation and/or incontinence.

Introduction

The physiology of the anus and its surrounding structures is in essence the physiology of continence and controlled defecation. This is a physiology of balance and continuous feedback and complex reflexes. Normal continence requires a balance between the pressure inside the rectum and the combined tone of the internal and external sphincters. Defecation and the controlled passage of gas or stool at socially

appropriate circumstances required very fine sensation and ability to discern the rectal contents. Defecation requires the balance to tip in favor of the rectal pressure and contraction with simultaneous coordinated relaxation of the pelvic floor and internal and external sphincters. Disturbance in any part of this complex balance can result in incontinence either through reduced anal tone, excess rectal contraction, reduced sensation, or the inability to differentiate the consistency of the rectal contents. Alternatively, disorders tipping in the opposite direction may result in inability to properly or completely empty the rectum. Additionally, more proximal conditions resulting in chronic diarrhea or constipation may tip the balance. And forces even higher can contribute to the behavioral and psychosocial aspects of ordered and disordered function of the rectum and anal canal.

It is the patient and skilled practitioner who listens to what the patient can teach and tell about how and what they are doing combined with a good working knowledge of anorectal physiology that can effectively intervene in disorders of defecation.

Normal Anatomy and Physiology

For a detailed discussion on the anal anatomy, see Chap. 1. Briefly, the musculature of the anus is made up of three concentric cylindrical structures. The internal sphincter is derived as an extension of the involuntary circular smooth muscle of the rectum. The longitudinal muscle is derived from the outer longitudinal smooth muscle of the rectum, and ultimately does extend into the anus and turns medially through the internal sphincter to comprise the muscles of Treitz that support the internal hemorrhoids. Lastly, the external sphincter is derived from the voluntary striated muscle of the pelvic floor.

The internal sphincter begins as a condensation of the inner circular involuntary smooth muscle of the GI tract at the top of the surgical anal canal, as the top of the anorectal ring.

Electronic supplementary material: The online version of this chapter (doi:10.1007/978-3-319-25970-3_3) contains supplementary material, which is available to authorized users.

S.R. Steele et al. (eds.), *The ASCRS Textbook of Colon and Rectal Surgery*, DOI 10.1007/978-3-319-25970-3_3

It extends downward to just proximal to the end of the external sphincter in the non-retracted or effaced state. The length of the normal internal sphincter can vary from under 2 to over 4 cm. In the unstimulated state, the internal sphincter is chronically contracting and contributes approximately 50–75 % of the resting tone of the anus. It appears as a 2–3-mm hypoechoic band on transanal ultrasound imaging [1]. The internal sphincter may not represent a perfect cylinder in all patients. Proximal anterior defects have been demonstrated in nulliparous women [2]. Length and bulk of the sphincter can be reduced if deprived of innervation or hormones in postmenopausal women (progesterone).

The external sphincter is a cylinder of striated muscle that extends downward from the levator ani muscle to the distal anoderm. Like the internal sphincter, it exists in a chronically contracting state, but has the potential when stimulated under voluntary control, to more than double the tone of the anus above the resting state. It was initially considered to be divided into three separate segments, deep, superficial, and subcutaneous; this is no longer thought to be a meaningful distinction [3].

Between the internal and external sphincters is a layer of mixed smooth and striated muscle that is made up of an extension of the longitudinal outer muscle of the bowel and some striated extensions of the levator ani muscle. As it extends downward, some aspects of the muscle cross medially through the internal sphincter to contribute to the suspensory muscles that hold the hemorrhoid complex in place (Trietz's muscle). Distally, the conjoined muscle extends to the anoderm and through the external sphincter radially to form the corrugator cutis ani [1, 4, 5].

Innervation of the Anus and Pelvic Floor

The parasympathetic fibers to the rectum and anal canal emerge from the sacral foramina at the S2, 3, 4 levels. They join the sympathetic hypogastric nerves in the pelvic plexus. From there mixed postganglionic fibers extend to the lower rectum and anal canal. Thereby internal sphincter is innervated by L5–S4 mixed autonomic function in crossed fashion so that unilateral injury still results in preserved function. The external sphincter is similarly innervated from branches of S2–3 via the inferior rectal branch of the pudendal nerve and the perineal branch of S4. This nervous distribution also carries the nerves of sensation and contributes to the functional aspects of continence. The upper anal canal contains a high density of free and organized sensory nerve endings [1, 6, 7]. Organized nerve endings include Meisner's corpuscles (touch), Krause's bulbs (cold), Golgi-Mazzoni bodies (pressure), and genital corpuscles (friction).

Normal Continence

Rectal Capacity

Normal continence first requires a location to temporarily hold and assess the contents and expel them under control. The rectum therefore needs both a baseline capacity and the compliance to expand and the force to expel. The empty rectum is a low pressure vessel with the capacity to receive stool from the sigmoid. It must have the capacity to expand significantly to accommodate stool under pressure. Patients with diminished rectal capacity will suffer from fecal frequency, urgency and frequently may contribute to incontinence.

Pressure and Motility

Baseline pressure in the rectum is low, about 5 mmHg with frequent low amplitude contractions every 6–12 s. Occasional high pressure waves up to 100 mmHg have been demonstrated. The anal canal shows overlapping of resting tone with small oscillations of pressure and frequency of 15 cycles/min and cm H_2O. Pressure in the anal canal ranges 10–14 times that of the rectum. Motor activity is more frequent, and contractile waves are of higher amplitude in the rectum than in the sigmoid [6]. This reverse gradient provides a pressure barrier resisting forward motion of stool and may propel stool back into the sigmoid as part of delaying bowel movements when it is not convenient [7]. Slow waves are observed in the anal canal with increasing frequency distally. This gradient is thought to help maintain continence by propelling the contents back into the rectum and helps keep the canal empty.

Rectoanal Sensation and Sampling

The rectum does not itself have receptors for proprioception. The conscious sensation of the need to defecate lives in the levators and the anal canal, hence the preserved sensation in patients who have had complete proctectomies and anal anastomoses. Distention of the rectum triggers contraction of the external anal sphincter and significant internal anal sphincter contraction. As first described by Gowers in 1877 [8] the rectoanal inhibitory reflex (RAIR) is thought to allow the highly innervated sensitive epithelial lining of the upper anal canal to sample the contents of the distal rectum to determine its quality and consistency. This allows the patient to accurately discern flatus from stool, and liquid stool from firm. Alterations in this mechanism, either through reduced sensation, or impaired sampling can result in incontinence either through overflow or inability to discern that defecation is occurring. Impaired anal sensation has been associated with childbirth, perineal descent, and mucosectomy [9–11].

Structural Considerations

In addition to the baseline resultant tone provided by the anal sphincter complex and the puborectalis sling, the entire structure is held closed by the angulation created by the puborectalis in its chronically contracted unstimulated state. This angle between the axis of the anus and the axis of the rectum is between 80° and 90° and is responsible for the majority of gross fecal continence. It may increase normally above 90 while sitting and will extend beyond 110° during normal defecation. In cases of dysfunctional defecation where the puborectalis does not sufficiently relax the angle can be enhanced by squatting and flexing the hips to an angle of less than 90°. The flap valve theory advocated by Parks suggests the anterior rectal mucosa constitutes a flap that lies over the upper end of the anal canal. Increased inter abdominal pressure not associated with defecation increased the angulation and closes flap more firmly over the upper anal canal. The flap is opened when the perineum descends and the anorectal angle is straightened. The anterior mucosal flap certainly seems to be a component of the issue when patients suffer from obstructed defecation and have evidence of internal rectal prolapse.

Role of Hemorrhoids in Normal Continence

It has also been postulated that the normal function of the hemorrhoids, in a non-pathologic state serve as an additional important component of normal continence. Stelzner referred to the hemorrhoids as the corpora cavernosum of the anus [12]. These vascular cushions have the ability to expand as needed to create a seal above the anus creating the fine tuning of continence. This concept is supported by the observation that after formal hemorrhoidectomy some patients experience minor alterations in continence.

Sensation and Innervation

Within the pelvis, the innervation of the proximal anal canal descends from the rectum. The rectum has a mixed sympathetic and parasympathetic innervation derived from the hypogastric nerves and the sacral parasympathetic nerves through the pelvic plexi. Extrapelvic innervation comes to the anus from the pudendal nerve derived from S2 to S4 via the inferior rectal nerve and ultimately spreads around the anus from both sides entering at lateral to slightly anterior positions. There is known to be significant crossover innervation around the anus as a complete disruption of either pudendal nerve does not result in asymmetric sphincter atrophy or fecal incontinence.

Sensory innervation within the rectum is sensitive only to stretch, resulting in vague sensation to visceral pelvic pain. Distal rectal stretch or distention can result in significant parasympathetic stimulation of the vagus nerve, thereby resulting in bradycardia and hypotension. The lack of pain-sensitive innervation proximal to a short distance from the dentate line is what allows some hemorrhoid treatments to be performed with relatively limited discomfort, e.g., elastic band ligation, injection sclerotherapy, and stapled hemorrhoidopexy. Somatic sensory innervation begins in the anal transitional zone proximal to the dentate line for a short variable distance 0.3–1.5 cm [13]. Within this zone, there is a dense collection of nerve endings for pain, touch, pressure, and temperature. As such they are theorized to be an integral part of the sampling aspect of the continence mechanism [14]. These fibers are derived from the pudendal branches, and complete anesthesia to this area can be provided by bilateral anal nerve blockade.

Normal Defecation

Normal defecation is a complicated mechanism that relies on a close interaction between the somatic and autonomic nervous system, which includes the conscious and unconscious control of both sensory input and muscle contraction. The process starts with stool arriving into the rectum and sampling as described above. If it is not an appropriate time for defecation, the anal sphincter will contract and rectum will start to distend [7]. This process continues with progressive distention of the rectum without a person's full awareness; patients are often unaware that they have stool in the vault during rectal exam. Conscious sampling, however, is also present during this process (one can differentiate between gas and stool and allow gas to pass, even with full rectum). As the rectum continues to expand, a person becomes aware (with continuous sampling) There is an urge defecate that usually lasts for a few seconds and can be controlled by further contraction of external anal sphincter (efferent nerve endings end in lumbosacral spine which is under higher control, that allows conscious suppression of the urge) [15, 16].

When it becomes socially appropriate to proceed, the defecation process again relies on both conscious and unconscious response. The process starts with contraction of abdominal musculature (Valsalva), which is also associated with contraction of the sigmoid colon to move stool forward. Pelvic floor musculature on the other hand relaxes, which is a combination of relaxation of puborectalis (releases sling around anorectal junction) and relaxation of remaining levator muscle. This allows the pelvic floor to descend slightly and straighten the anorectal angle. The rectum itself starts to contract and both internal and external sphincters relax. Even if the sphincters are not completely relaxed, at this point pressure in the rectum exceeds pressure in the anal canal and defecation will occur. This process can also be aided by assuming the squatting position, which increases the intra-abdominal pressure and straightens the rectum further. If the conscious decision to defecate is made during sampling (rectum is contracting, internal sphincters already partially relaxed) allowing the external sphincters to relax, then defecation will occur [17–19]. Once begun a number of patterns can occur. There may be a single evacuation of the rectal contents accompanied by mass peristalsis of the left and sigmoid colon clearing the bowel in one continuous movement, or the passage of smaller volumes of stool individually over a short time requiring recurrent efforts and straining [20]. These two patterns and variations thereof are dictated by the habits of the patient and other factors including the overall consistency of the stool.

If a large volume of stool is delivered quickly to the rectum, normal rectal compliance and accommodation may be insufficient. In this case the patient with normal sensation and function will have a sense of acute urgency and can forestall defecation for 40–60 s with the use of voluntary contraction of the external sphincter to allow accommodation or move to a socially appropriate location to evacuate.

For obvious reasons, studying this process can be difficult, and thus our understanding of it relies on what is observed during testing (e.g., defecography—Video 3.1; and anal manometric studies) [2, 6], patients with neurologic deficits (specifically spinal injuries) [21] and animal studies. Animal studies revealed the presence of different, more sensitive mechanoreceptors in the rectum, when compared to the colon that are most responsive to tension and rapid distention [22–24]. These tension mechanoreceptors respond to both rectal distension and muscle contraction consistent with the observation that rectal filling sensation coincides with the period of raised rectal pressure during rectal distension [3–6].

Physiology of Tibial Nerve and Sacral Nerve Root Stimulation in Fecal Continence

For many years it has been recognized that chronic electrical stimulation of nerves entering the pelvis has had effects of visceral function and activity. Unilateral stimulation of the S3 or S4 nerve as it exits the foramen has been used for urinary incontinence for over 30 years; meanwhile benefits for fecal incontinence have been recognized as well. Most recently, sacral nerve stimulation has shown encouraging results for idiopathic constipation as well [25–27].

The exact mechanism of how sacral nerve stimulation creates its effect remains unclear. The physiological control of defecation relies on the coordinated sensory and motor efforts of the colon, rectum, and anus. Current opinion is that disordered defecation is secondary to several disturbances of anorectal and colonic physiology and not purely a sphincter disturbance in patients with FI or colonic transit failure in constipation. It is therefore likely that the therapeutic effects of SNS are due not only to peripheral motor stimulation of the anal sphincter complex in patients with FI as was initially proposed, but instead due to changes in the motor and/or sensory function of the combined functional anorectal unit. Such a hypothesis would explain the "paradox" of SNS effectiveness in both FI and chronic constipation, i.e., it is likely that SNS is effective in both conditions not due to paradoxical actions in each, but instead by improvement of common pathophysiologies. This hypothesis also explains why FI and disordered defecation so frequently coexist [28]. Similarly, intermittent stimulation of the posterior tibial nerve has a beneficial effect on fecal incontinence through a mechanism that is not fully understood [29].

In 2014, Carrington et al. performed an exhaustive review of the scientific literature regarding sacral and peripheral nerve stimulation for fecal incontinence and constipation [15]. To summarize their findings, SNS had no demonstrable effect of rectal compliance or motility. It did seem to reduce hypersensitivity in those with reduced capacity and hypersensitivity, while increasing sensitivity in those patients with reduced sensitivity. Additionally sacral nerve stimulation increases mucosal blood flow when on and returns to baseline when off. There are higher levels of the neuropeptide substance P identified in rectal biopsies of those undergoing stimulation, which reverses after it is discontinued. The exact importance or impact of these two phenomena has not been identified as yet. Forty studies have examined changes in anal sphincter function through the use of anorectal manometry. Direct comparison between studies is difficult, as equipment specifications, study protocol, and method of results reporting is extremely variable between centers. Fourteen studies reported a significant increase in voluntary anal squeeze, with eight of these also reporting an increase in resting pressure.

Spinal Cord Injuries and Defecation

The most interesting and informative studies in normal and abnormal defecation are provided by patients with spinal cord injuries. However, it is important to remember that this is a very heterogeneous group of patients with degrees of injury that can vary significantly from patient to patient [7]. High spinal cord injuries (above T7) interrupt higher control and sensation of the abdominal and pelvic floor musculature as well as colon in rectum [12, 29, 30]. This combination allows for lower tone in the colon and rectum. The decrease in propulsive ability of the colon, the decrease in tone resulting in distention and slower transit through the colon explains the constipation that often accompanies high spinal cord injuries. These patients are often unable to generate adequate intra-abdominal pressure or take squatting position to aid defecation [11, 13, 31]. At the same time, there is an unopposed stimulation of the lower neurons that increase contraction and spasticity of the pelvic floor and external anal sphincters.

Sensation is often also impaired which can eliminate the normal urge to defecate. Interestingly, this often does not affect mechanoreceptors and some patients will report vague sensation of pressure that is then interpreted as a need to defecate [31–33]. As a result, these patients often have chronic constipation caused by both diminished sensation and inability to move stool forward [12, 13]. This is combined with pelvic floor dysfunction and the inability to identify the urge to defecate and an inability to relax the pelvic floor. They often rely on a strict bowel program, which is a combination of laxatives, rectal stimulation and manual disimpaction [11–13]. Rectal stimulation can allow some patents to have decreased anal sphincter pressure. They can also experience fecal incontinence as a result of overflow and overfill of the rectum and well as damage to sphincters from manual disimpaction [12–14, 34].

Patients with low spinal cord injuries such as Cauda Equina Syndrome often have impaired afferent fibers that results in loss of tone in the internal and external sphincter muscle as well as impaired sensation. This can result in significant incontinence since any generation of intra-abdominal pressure may result in bowel movement [11–13].

Obstructed Defecation

Obstructed defecation is a poorly understood group of disorders resulted from an alteration in sensation, muscle relaxation or both. In many patients with these problems, the exact cause is multifactorial and/or the inciting event is not easily identifiable [35]. It is possible that an abnormality in the sensory mechanism is the primary insult in a number of patients [36]. Normal sensation is an integral part of normal defecation. It allows for appropriate reflexes, mostly importantly the anal sampling RAIR. Some causes of abnormal sensation can be fairly evident in patients such as those with significant proctitis (infectious or inflammatory) or those after anorectal injury/surgery. In the absence of above, the etiology is less clear. Dysfunction may be associated with conscious/subconscious inhibition of the need to defecate during childhood [15, 16, 37, 38]. According to this theory, repeated delays in defecation result in altered sensation that eventually leads to dyscoordination between the anorectal and pelvic floor musculature. As this process continues, even though patient may continue to experience "normal" urge to defecate, changes in sensation cause an increase in stimulation of lower (lumbosacral) neuronal loop; the relaxing effects of the upper parts of the nervous system are insufficient to overpower the abnormal stimulation. Once this occurs, and pelvic floor musculature such as puborectalis and sphincter complex fail to relax appropriately, increasingly higher intra-abdominal pressure is needed to overpower the rectal/anal pressure to evacuate [39]. This failure can be associated with pain and a feeling of incomplete evacuation.

Independent of what part of normal defecation was affected first, over time there is probably significant damage to the sensory pathways including receptors, efferent nerves and muscles. With time, this process will also start affecting the structural integrity of the pelvic floor. Obstructed defecation disorders include intussusception, rectocele, non-relaxing puborectalis/levator muscle spasm, dyssynergic puborectalis, as well as enterocele and rectal prolapse. Although causes of enterocele and rectal prolapse may be complex, these disorders in their pure form are mechanical obstructions to defecation and thus beyond the scope of this chapter. Here we describe a few pathological conditions that are more directly affected abnormalities in sensory-muscular neurological loop.

Intussusception is mucosal descent causing blockage of the lower rectum/anal canal. It is possible that it is a primary process in some patients arising from redundancy of mucosa, possibly poor tone, and pelvic floor descent (either primary structural problems or as a result of childbirth and muscle/nerve damage in women). In most patients it is likely a secondary process resulting from increased pushing and decreased relaxation. Once developed, intussusception itself generates mechanical blockage to defecation and further attempts to generate more pressure to evacuate stool [17–19, 40].

Rectocele likely develops by a similar process. It is defined as greater than 2 cm of rectal wall out pouching or bowing anteriorly while straining. It can be accompanied by intussusception. Rectoceles are caused by abnormal relaxation of the pelvic floor/sphincter complex or structural defects in the rectal wall created during childbirth. As a result, when a patient attempts to evacuate, generated pressure delivers stool anteriorly towards the weakened portion of the wall that is not contracting appropriately. This generates a sensation of bulge and incomplete evacuation and can be at least in part relieved in women by pushing on the vagina in the initial stages of the disease (Figure 3-1; Video 3.2). However, a rectocele itself is a very common finding on the exam and only a small proportion of patients who have it will ever have symptoms. Most symptomatic patients likely have a combination of a weaker rectal wall as well as dyssynergy of the sphincters or puburectalis [15, 41].

Pelvic floor dyssynergy (pelvic outlet obstruction) results from a failure of the puborectalis and/or sphincter complex to relax. It can also be caused by an abnormal contraction during evacuation. As a result, when a patient tries to evacuate the anorectal angle may not increase or may even become sharper. A patient's natural response is to generate higher pressures in which only further worsens the symptoms. Over time, these changes likely cause more damage to the musculature and nerves. Similar to the rest of the disorders in this group, rectal sensation is also impaired, but whether it is a result of long-term damage or from an inciting event is unclear [15, 16, 18].

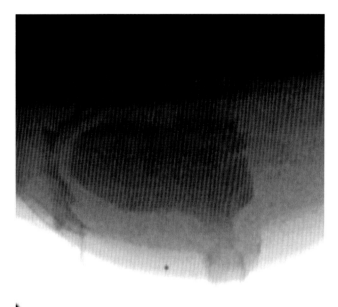

FIGURE 3-1. Defecography still image of a rectocele.

Functional Anorectal Pain

Most causes of anorectal pain can be routinely ascribed to such common conditions as anal fissures, hemorrhoidal disease, or inflammatory bowel diseases (see Chap. 11). There is a small group of disorders, however, that seem to be related to more functional, rather than structural problems [42].

Levator ani syndrome (levator spasm, puborectalis syndrome) is often described as dull pain, high in the rectum that is often made worse with sitting. By definition, it should last more than 20 min at the time and other causes are excluded [43]. Etiology of this condition is unclear. Interestingly, even though episodes may be triggered by difficult defecation (along with emotional stress among other things) it is not always associated with difficulty evacuating. Similar to other functional disorders, it is possible that alternations in sensation, and perhaps behaviors (deferring defecation, damage with hard stool) could contribute to the development and propagation of this problem. In addition, it is thought that prolonged muscle contraction may result in compression of vasculature, which then leads to relative ischemia and an increase in anaerobic consumptions. That in turn can cause activation of nociceptors in the muscle (bradykinin, Substance P), and further decrease in relaxation with spasm and pain [15, 16, 22].

Proctalgia fugax is a sudden severe anal pain, lasting seconds to minutes, that disappears completely. The etiology is unknown, but it seems to be related to stress. It is associated in some patients with a thickened internal sphincter muscle. Some studies suggest smooth muscle contraction is responsible for this pain [15, 16, 44].

Pathophysiology of Obstetric-Related Problems

One of the worrisome potential sequelae of pregnancy and delivery is fecal incontinence. It can develop as a result of direct disruption of the anal sphincter, muscle, connective tissue or pudendal nerve injury [45]. During pregnancy, there is direct pressure on the pelvic floor as well as hormonal changes. Progesterone, released during pregnancy, acts by suppressing contraction of smooth muscle and prevents premature uterine contraction. This leads to decreased gut motility (that can contribute to constipation) and diminished tonic contraction of anal sphincters [25, 46]. Androgen, progesterone, and estrogen receptors are found in squamous epithelium of the anal canal, indirectly supporting possible effects of this hormone on the sphincters [47]. In addition, progesterone causes ligamentous laxity [48]. When combined with increased intra-abdominal pressure, these changes contribute to stretching of the pelvic floor musculature, widening of the levator hiatus, and potentially pudendal nerve injury. The pudendal nerve can be affected during pregnancy by stretching as well as traction injury during delivery as described below [49]. Pudendal nerve injury can affect both external sphincters by de-innervating them and causing muscle atrophy as well as by affecting sensory components and altering RAIR. Evidence of neuropathy in pelvic floor musculature has been found after delivery as well as in idiopathic FI and constipation.

Labor further complicates issues of continence. Pushing during labor can significantly exacerbate the above problem [50]. It can be associated with further muscle stretching or even evulsion and pudendal nerve injury [25]. This explains why a longer second stage of labor (pushing) is associated with higher rates later in life. In addition, there is likely effects of traction injury (increased baby weight is associated with higher chances of immediate and long-term problems). Use of additional devices to aid labor such as forceps and vacuum is associated with increased incidence of FI [25, 51]. This is likely related to direct damage to the sphincters as well as traction injury. Tearing and episiotomy are additional risk factors for FI and related to direct damage to the sphincter complex. Cesarean section is associated with lower incidences of flatus and stool incontinence, but this difference is smaller when comparing emergent Cesarean sections and vaginal deliveries. Emergent cesarean are often initiated after failure of labor to progress following significant pushing [52]. Although many women experience immediate mild problems with incontinence to flatus or stool, most have enough reserves to compensate. Presence of symptoms after delivery is an additional risk factor for developing significant incontinence in the future when age further weakens already damages muscles and nerves.

Urogynecological Considerations and Pelvic Pain

With all its complexity, the pelvic floor is anatomically very small area. It includes pelvic musculature and their corresponding nerves responsible not only for maintenance of continence and normal defecation, but also normal urinary gynecologic function. Not surprisingly, although dysfunction in any single system is common, more than one system is frequently affected. For example, physiologic and muscular changes associated with pregnancy and labor which effects the posterior compartment often has similar effects on middle and anterior compartment structures as well. Uterine prolapse is more common in multiparous women, especially in complicated deliveries. Urinary problems including incontinence are also common [16, 25]. The mechanism for urinary issues is likely the same as in posterior compartment problems, which is a combination of hormonal effects as well as direct damage to the pelvic floor muscle, nerves, and sphincters. Widening of the levator hiatus has been shown to affect middle and anterior compartments as well as posterior one. This can result in uterine and bladder prolapse in addition to rectal prolapse, intussusception, and rectocele [21]. Pregnancy and delivery effects on anal sphincters can affect urinary sphincters as well. It is common for women presenting with urinary incontinence to report fecal incontinence as well [16, 25]. As a result, urogynecologists see and treat a number of patients with anorectal problems, especially since the treatments available are similar between specialties (e.g., pelvic floor physical therapy, sacral nerve stimulation). Pelvic floor prolapse problems, especially of the middle compartment, may contribute to obstructed defecation. For this reason care should be taken to obtain full history of pelvic floor problems. Otherwise one risks missing significant contributors to patients' symptoms and may compromise success of treatment.

Another common problem is pelvic pain, and women with these symptoms are often referred directly to gynecologists, although underlying cause could be levator spasm or pelvic floor dyssynergy [23]. These problems are also commonly treated by our urogynecology colleagues utilizing similar techniques including physical therapy and other pelvic floor relaxation techniques. Diagnostic techniques employed by urogynecologists to diagnose anterior pelvic problems are often the same (MR defecography and conventional cine defecography, anal manometry). As a result, when patients present with anorectal problems related to pelvic floor issues, one has to maintain vigilance in identifying related problems with anterior and middle compartment since they can affect overall symptom control as well as how these problems are ultimately addressed.

References

1. Jorge JMN, Habr-Gama A. Anatomy and embryology of the colon rectum and anus. In: Wolff BG, Fleshman JW, Beck DE, Pemberton JH, Wexner SD, editors. The ASCRS textbook of colon and rectal surgery. New York, NY: Springer; 2007. p. 1–11.
2. Bollard RC, Gardiner A, Lindow S, Phillips K, Duthie GS. Normal female anal sphincter: difficulties in interpretation explained. Dis Colon Rectum. 2002;45:171–5.
3. Gordon PH. Anatomy and physiology of the anorectum. In: Fazio VW, Church JM, Delaney CP, editors. Current therapy in colon and rectal surgery. 2nd ed. Philadelphia, PA: Elsevier Mosby; 2005. p. 1–4.
4. Milligan ETC, Morgan CN, Jones LE, Officer R. Surgical anatomy of the anal canal and the operative treatment of haemorrhoids. Dis Colon Rectum. 1985;28:620–8.
5. Morgan CN. The surgical anatomy of the anal canal and rectum. Postgrad Med J. 1936;12:287–314.
6. Taylor I, Duthie HL, Amallwwod R, et al. Large bowel myoelectrical activity in man. Gut. 1975;16:808–14.
7. Gordon PH. Anorectal anatomy and physiology. Gastroenterol Clin North Am. 2001;30:1–13.
8. Gowers WR. The automatic action of the sphincter ani. Proc R Soc Lond. 1877;26:77–84.
9. Cornes H, Bartolo DCC, Stirra T. Changes in anal canal sensation after childbirth. Br J Surg. 1991;78:74–7.
10. Miller R, Bartolo DCC, Cervero F, Mortenson NJ. Differences in anal sensation in continent and incontinent patients with perineal descent. Int J Colorectal Dis. 1989;4:45–9.
11. Keighley MRB. Abdominal mucosectomy reduces the incidence of soiling and sphincter damage after restorative proctocolectomy and J-pouch. Dis Colon Rectum. 1987;39:386–90.
12. Stelzner F. The morphological principles of anorectal continence. In: Rickham PP, Hecker WSH, Prevot J, editors. Anorectal malformations and associated diseases, Progress in pediatric surgery series, vol. 9. Munich: Urban & Schwarzberg; 1976. p. 1–6.
13. Kaiser AM, Ortega AE. Anorectal anatomy. Surg Clin North Am. 2002;82:1125–38.
14. Duthie HL, Gairns FW. Sensory nerve-endings and sensation in the anal region of man. Br J Surg. 1960;206:585–95.
15. Sangwan YP, Solla JA. Internal anal sphincter: advances and insights. Dis Colon Rectum. 1998;41:1297–311.
16. Palit S, Lunniss PJ, Scott SM. The physiology of human defecation. Dig Dis Sci. 2012;57:1445–64.
17. Bajwa A, Emmanuel A. The physiology of continence and evacuation. Best Pract Res Clin Gastroenterol. 2009;23:477–85.
18. Brookes SJ, Dinning PG, Gladman MA. Neuroanatomy and physiology of colorectal function and defaecation: from basic science to human clinical studies. Neurogastroenterol Motil. 2009;21 Suppl 2:9–19.
19. Gurjar SV, Jones OM. Physiology: evacuation, pelvic floor and continence mechanisms. Surgery. 2011;29(8):358–61.
20. Lubowski DZ, Meagher AP, Smart AC, et al. Scintigraphic assessment of colonic function during defecation. Int J Colorectal Dis. 1995;10:91–3.

21. Brading AF, Ramalingam T. Mechanisms controlling normal defecation and the potential effects of spinal cord injury. In: Weaver LC, Polosa C, editors. Progress in brain research 2006; vol 152:p. 345-358 (Chapter 23).

22. Broens PMA, Penninckx FM, Ochoa JB. Fecal continence revisited: the anal external sphincter continence reflex. Dis Colon Rectum. 2013;56:1273–81.

23. Lynn PA, Olsson C, Zagorodnyuk V, et al. Rectal intraganglionic laminar endings are transduction sites of extrinsic mechanoreceptors in the guinea pig rectum. Gastroenterology. 2003; 125:589–601.

24. Lynn PA, Blackshaw LA. In vitro recordings of afferent fibres with receptive fields in the serosa, muscle and mucosa of rat colon. J Physiol. 1999;518(Pt 1):271–82.

25. Tanagho EA, Schmidt RA. Electrical stimulation in the clinical management of the neurogenic bladder. J Urol. 1988;140: 1331–9.

26. Ganio E, Luc AR, Clerico G, Trompetto M. Sacral nerve stimulation for treatment of fecal incontinence: a novel approach for intractable fecal incontinence. Dis Colon Rectum. 2001;44:619–29.

27. Malouf AJ, Wiesel PH, Nicholls T, Nicholls RJ, Kamm MA. Sacral nerve stimulation for idiopathic slow transit constipation. Gastroenterol Clin North Am. 2001;118:4448–9.

28. Carrington EV et al. A systematic review of sacral nerve stimulation mechanisms in the treatment of fecal incontinence and constipation. Neurogastroenterol Motil. 2014;26(9):1222–37.

29. Thumas TO, Dudding TC, et al. A systemic review of posterior tibial nerve stimulation for faecal incontinence. Colorectal Dis. 2012;15:519–26.

30. Ebert E. Gastrointestinal involvement in spinal cord injury: a clinical perspective. J Gastrointestin Liver Dis. 2012;21(1): 75–82.

31. Lynch AC, Frizelle FA. Colorectal motility and defecation after spinal cord injury in humans. In: Weaver LC, Polosa C, editors. Progress in brain research 2006;vol 152:193–203 (Chapter 23).

32. Nout YS, Leedy GM, Beattie MS, Bresnahan JS. Alterations in eliminative and sexual reflexes after spinal cord injury: defecatory function and development of spasticity in pelvic floor musculature. In: Weaver LC, Polosa C, editors. Progress in brain research 2006;vol 152:359–273 (Chapter 23).

33. Preziosi G, Raptis DA, Raeburn A, Panicker J, Emmanuel A. Autonomic rectal dysfunction in patients with multiple sclerosis and bowel symptoms is secondary to spinal cord disease. Dis Colon Rectum. 2014;57:514–21.

34. Valle's M, Mearin F. Pathophysiology of bowel dysfunction in patients with motor incomplete spinal cord injury: comparison with patients with motor complete spinal cord injury. Dis Colon Rectum. 2009;52:1589–97.

35. Bharucha AE, Rao SSC. An update on anorectal disorders for gastroenterologists. Gastroenterology. 2014;146:37–45.

36. Bharucha AE, Wald A, Enck P, Rao S. Functional anorectal disorders. Gastroenterology. 2006;130:1510–8.

37. van Ginkel R, Reitsma JB, Buller HA, et al. Childhood constipation: longitudinal follow-up beyond puberty. Gastroenterology. 2003;125:67–72.

38. Rao SSC, Tuteja AK, Vellema T, et al. Dyssynergic defecation: demographics, symptoms, stool patterns and quality of life. J Clin Gastroenterol. 2004;38:680–5.

39. Rao SS, Welcher KD, Leistikow JS. Obstructive defecation: a failure of rectoanal coordination. Am J Gastroenterol. 1998;93: 1042–50.

40. Andromanakos N, Skandalakis P, Troupis T, Filippou D. Constipation of anorectal outlet obstruction: pathophysiology, evaluation and management. J Gastroenterol Hepatol. 2006;21: 638–46.

41. Felt-Bersma RJ, Tiersma ES, Cuesta MA. Rectal prolapse, rectal intussusception, rectocele, solitary rectal ulcer syndrome, and enterocele. Gastroenterol Clin North Am. 2008;37: 645–68.

42. Atkin GK, Suliman A, Vaizey CJ. Patient characteristics and treatment outcome in functional anorectal pain. Dis Colon Rectum. 2011;54:870–5.

43. Hull M, Cort MM. Evaluation of the levator ani and pelvic wall muscles in levator ani syndrome. Urol Nus. 2009; 29(4):225.

44. Eckardt VF, Dodt O, Kanzler G, Bernhard G. Anorectal function and morphology in patients with sporadic proctalgia fugax. Dis Colon Rectum. 2004;39:755–62.

45. Shin GH, Toto EL, Schey R. Pregnancy and postpartum bowel changes: constipation and fecal incontinence. Am J Gastroenterol. 2015;110:521–9.

46. Chiloiro M, Darconza G, Piccioli E, et al. Gastric emptying and orocecal transit time in pregnancy. J Gastroenterol. 2001;36: 538–43.

47. Oettling G, Franz HB. Mapping of androgen, estrogen and progesterone receptors in the anal continence organ. Eur J Obstet Gynecol Reprod Biol. 1998;77:785–95.

48. Shultz SJ, Wideman L, Montgomery MM, et al. Changes in serum collagen markers, IGF-I, and knee joint laxity across the menstrual cycle. J Orthop Res. 2012;30:1405–12.

49. Parks AG, Swash M. Denervation of the anal sphincter causing idiopathic anorectal incontinence. J R Coll Surg Edinb. 1979; 24:94–6.

50. Bharucha AE, Fletcher JG, Melton III LJ, et al. Obstetric trauma, pelvic floor injury and fecal incontinence: a population-based case–control study. Am J Gastroenterol. 2012;107: 902–11.

51. Dudding TC, Vaizey CJ, Kamm MJ. Obstetric anal sphincter injury incidence, risk factors, and management. Ann Surg. 2008;247(2):224–37.

52. Pretlove SJ, Thompson PJ, Toozs-Hobson PM, et al. Does the mode of delivery predispose women to anal incontinence in the first year postpartum? A comparative systematic review. BJOG. 2008;115:421–34.

4

Endoscopy

Kurt Davis and Michael A. Valente

Key Concepts

- The endoscopic examination is critical for patients with colorectal complaints and is a key component of the complete colorectal examination.
- The anoscopic examination is the best way to adequately evaluate the anoderm, dentate line and evaluate for internal and external hemorrhoids, and anal masses.
- Multiple bowel preparation regimens exist, but regardless of which prep is chosen, splitting the timing into the half the day prior to and half the day of the procedure results in a better prep.
- There is no ideal sedation medication, but the endoscopist must be familiar with the side effect profile of any medications being used and be prepared and comfortable with any reversal agents.
- Adjunctive maneuvers employed with endoscopy serve as the markers between seasoned experts and novices: these include abdominal pressure, adjusting position, torqueing, and dithering.
- PillCam endoscopy allows the clinician to evaluate the small bowel for occult gastrointestinal bleeding, insipient tumors, polyposis syndromes, or Crohn's disease.

Introduction

The endoscopic evaluation of the patient with colorectal complaints forms the keystone of the physical examination. It allows the physician to visually assess the entirety of the intestinal tract from the mouth to the anus and allows for the diagnosis, treatment, and monitoring of the effectiveness of any therapy. It is imperative for all physicians treating patients with colorectal diseases to be facile in the more common endoscopic diagnostic and therapeutic techniques.

The Complete Anorectal Examination

While performing any anorectal or endoscopic examination, an anxiety-free and modest environment must be created. Most patients will exhibit nervousness, and apprehension, which can cause anal or gluteal spasm that will preclude an accurate assessment. The examiner must reassure the patient and keep anxiety and embarrassment to a minimum. This can be accomplished by effective communication, keeping the patient covered as much as possible, keeping ancillary personnel in the room to a minimum and not rushing through the examination. Physicians should strive to actively communicate with the patient as the examination is progressing.

Before a discussion on endoscopic techniques, a thorough understanding of the initial steps of the anorectal examination is compulsory for success and patient well-being and satisfaction. Before any instrument is inserted, a focused history must be obtained coupled with a local examination. The local examination is an important precursor to any endoscopic examination and consists of: proper patient positioning, visual inspection, and manual palpation of the anorectal region followed by the digital rectal examination. Once this stepwise examination is complete, then inspection of the colon, rectum, and anus can commence.

Patient Position

There are two positions that may be used for effective anorectal examination. The choice of position may depend on several variables including available equipment, patient age and comorbid status, and physician preference. Regardless of the position chosen, both the patient and the examiner must be comfortable in order to carry out an effective anorectal and endoscopic evaluation.

© Springer International Publishing 2016
S.R. Steele et al. (eds.), *The ASCRS Textbook of Colon and Rectal Surgery*, DOI 10.1007/978-3-319-25970-3_4

FIGURE 4-1. Prone jackknife
position. Reprinted with
permission, Cleveland Clinic
Center for Medical Art &
Photography ©2015. All
Rights Reserved.

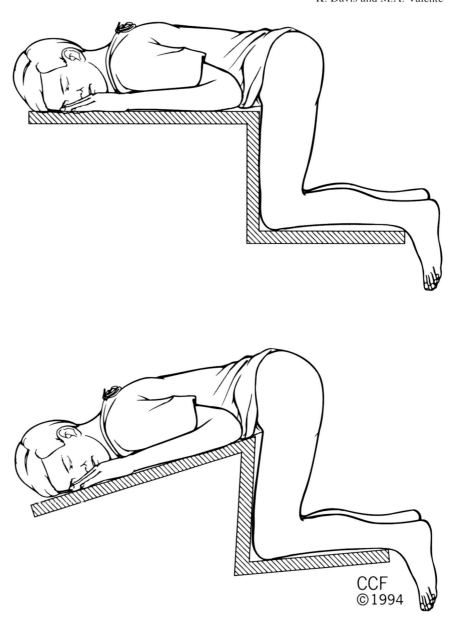

Prone Jackknife

The prone jackknife position (knee-chest), performed with
the aid of a specialized proctoscopic table is commonly
employed and allows for excellent visualization of the
entire anus and perianal and perineal region, as well as the
sacrococcygeal region. The patient kneels on the padded
portion of the table and leans forward with their trunk and
arms extended forward (Figure 4-1). The table is angled
forward gradually so that the patient's buttocks and
perineum are superior, while the head and feet are inferior.
This is a comfortable position for the examiner and also
allows for easy insertion of the anoscope, proctoscope, or
flexible sigmoidoscope. This position is well tolerated by
most patients, but should be avoided in various situations,
such as debilitated patients, recent abdominal surgery,
cardiopulmonary issues, various arthritic/rheumatologic
conditions, or late pregnancy.

Left Lateral

The left lateral recumbent (Sims') position is also widely used,
especially if a specialty bed is not readily available (Figure 4-2).
This position is very well tolerated and is well suited for
elderly or debilitated patients. The patient lies on their left side
and the thighs are flexed as to form a 90° angle with the trunk.
It is imperative that the buttocks project slightly beyond the
edge of the examining table. This position will allow for excellent visualization of the perianal and sacral regions, but the
anterior perineum is often obscured and requires the retraction
of the buttock by an assistant. Anoscopic or endoscopic evaluation is easily performed in this position.

Inspection and Palpation

Proper stepwise visual inspection of the perineum, anal canal,
rectum, and vagina should precede any other examination.

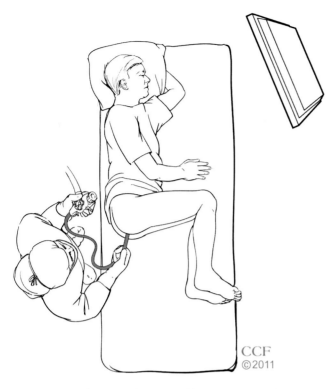

FIGURE 4-2. Left lateral (Sims') position. Reprinted with permission, Cleveland Clinic Center for Medical Art & Photography ©2015. All Rights Reserved.

Proper lighting is essential, and various light sources are commercially available, including overhead lights, gooseneck lamps, or headlamps. It should be noted that the "clock-face" nomenclature is not recommended for localizing anorectal findings. This nomenclature is dependent upon the position of the patient, and hence different interpretations of the true location may differ from examiner to examiner. It is more proper to delineate anatomical location using the cardinal quadrants (i.e., left lateral, right anterior, right posterior). This is the practice most commonly employed by colorectal surgeons.

An overall assessment of the shape of the buttock and inspection of the lower sacrococcygeal area is undertaken. This is followed by the gentle spreading of the buttocks to gain proper exposure. A great deal of information can be gained from visualization. The physician should examine for and document any scarring, fecal soiling, purulence, blood or mucous drainage, excoriations, erythema, anal sphincter shape, perineal body bulk, hemorrhoidal disease, skin tags, overt signs of inflammatory bowel disease, external fistulous openings, rectal prolapse, neoplasm, and any evidence of previous anorectal surgery. Next, the patient is asked to strain (Valsalva maneuver) to help determine and assess for perineal descent, uterine, vaginal, or bladder prolapse, or rectal prolapse. It should be noted that the best position to evaluate rectal prolapse is in the sitting position on the toilet or commode after an enema has been administered. Gentle and directed palpation of the anorectal region also gives the examiner a great detail of information. Gently touching the anal verge

will elicit the anocutaneous reflex (anal wink), which is indicative of an intact pudendal nerve. Additionally, gentle spreading of the anus will help elicit an anal fissure or ulceration. Palpation of the gluteal region can help identify an abscess, external opening of a fistulous tract, or possibly a mass.

Digital Rectal Examination

The digital rectal examination (DRE) is simple and is typically well tolerated and should be performed before all endoscopy of the rectum and colon. A well-performed DRE will provide information regarding the contents and potential pathology of the anal canal, distal rectum, and adjacent organs. The DRE may also permit an assessment of the neurological function of the muscles of fecal continence. While the medical school maxim of the only patient not receiving a DRE is the one that lacks an anus is obviously excessive—there are relative contraindications to performing this portion of the exam. These include painful lesions such as an anal fissure, thrombosed external hemorrhoids, grade IV internal hemorrhoids, and neutropenic patients. The keys to a successful DRE can be summarized by simple rules: adequate lubrication, gentleness, and attention to detail [1]. It is important to minimize pain during DRE as this may affect patient cooperation during endoscopy.

After proper communication with the patient, a well-lubricated index finger is placed across the anus to lubricate the general area. The fingertip is then gently inserted into the anal opening. Lubrication should be warmed if possible, and lidocaine jelly should also be available. If the patient's response is an involuntary spasm of the internal sphincter, the examiner should withdraw their fingertip and gently try again. Ask the patient to bear down as to pass a stool. This maneuver will cause relaxation of the entire sphincter complex and should facilitate an easy digital insertion [2]. The finger should be gradually and slowly advanced. The distal rectum and anal canal along with surrounding structures should be investigated in an organized and stepwise fashion. Resting anal tone followed by squeeze tone should be assessed. Assessment should be made of the entire circumference of the lumen by gently sweeping around the entire anus and distal rectum. Anteriorly in a male, the prostate should be palpated and assessed for nodularity, hypertrophy and firmness. In the female, anteriorly palpate for a rectocele. The cervix and uterus can also be palpated. Posteriorly, the presence of a presacral (retrorectal) mass may be palpated. Bimanual examination may be necessary when examining a female patient in order to adequately examine the rectovaginal septum and associated adnexal structures. Redundant rectal mucosa may be palpated as well as a stricture or narrowing. Induration or a fibrous cord, representing an internal fistulous opening, may also be felt on DRE. Exclusion of any masses should be carefully performed. The patient should be asked to perform a Valsalva maneuver to potentially bring any lesions of the upper rectum or the rectosigmoid into the examiners reach. If a mass is palpated, its size, position,

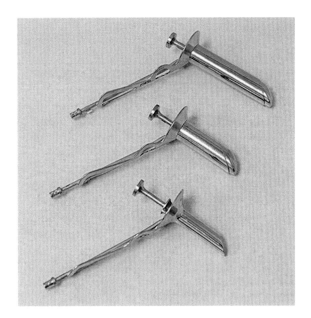

FIGURE 4-3. Various beveled anoscopes. From *top* to *bottom*: Large Hirschmann (short bevel); Buie-Hirschmann anoscope (long bevel); small (pediatric) Hirschmann anoscope.

characteristics (sessile, polypoid, ulcerated), mobility (mobile, tethered, fixed), and relationship to other structures (distance from the anal verge, distance for the anorectal ring) must be accurately recorded.

The levator ani/puborectalis muscles can also be assessed on DRE with evaluation of both the strength and function of these muscles, along with any tenderness on direct palpation, indicating a possible pelvic pain disorder. When a patient with good sphincter function is asked to squeeze these muscles, the examiner's finger will feel the muscle tighten and will have his finger pulled up into the rectum. Additionally, when the examiner pulls posteriorly on these muscles, the anal opening should gape and then return to normal, representing an intact reflex pathway to the thoracolumbar spinal cord.

Anoscopy/Proctoscopy

The anorectal examination in most cases should be followed with some component of an endoscopic investigation to complete the workup. This may include anoscopy, proctoscopy, or flexible endoscopy. Anoscopy and proctoscopy are typically performed in the clinic setting without sedation or mechanical bowel preparation and are tolerated quite well by the patient.

It should be noted that the term proctoscopy will be used as to describe the rigid scope implemented to evaluate the rectum and the distal sigmoid colon. Therefore, "rigid proctosigmoioscope" or "proctosigmoidoscopy" will be referred to as "rigid proctoscopy" or "proctoscopy." Sigmoidoscopy refers to the use of the flexible sigmoidoscope.

Anoscopy

Anoscopy is the examination of the anal canal and the distal rectum. Anoscopy offers the best way to adequately evaluate the anoderm, dentate line, internal and external hemorrhoids, papillae, fissures, anal masses, and distal rectal mucosa.

The anoscope is a relatively simple instrument consisting of an obturator, the scope itself, and a light source. There exist several variations in type, size, and length of anoscopes available. Additionally, commercially available anoscopes include slotted or beveled styles, reusable or disposable, and lighted or unlighted. The particular type of instrument and light source used are based on individual preference, expense, and prior training (Figure 4-3).

Regardless of the choice of instrument used, the examination is initiated only after a DRE has been performed (if a DRE is unable to be performed secondary to pain, spasm, or stenosis, an anoscopic exam should not be attempted). For most instances, cleansing of the anorectum with an enema is not warranted. The anoscope (with obturator in place) is liberally lubricated and gently and gradually advanced until the instrument is fully inserted. It is important to align the anoscope along the anterior–posterior axis of the anus. If unsuccessful due to patient intolerance, remove the scope, reapply lubrication and try again. After successful insertion, the obturator is removed and examination of the anorectum undertaken. The obturator should then be reinserted while the scope still in the anus, and the anoscope is gently rotated to examine a new area.

The prone jackknife position offers good visualization and ease of insertion as well does the lateral position, however, an assistant must retract the buttock if the lateral position is utilized. During the examination, the patient is asked to strain while the anoscope is withdrawn to visualize any prolapsing anorectal mucosa or hemorrhoidal tissue. During the anoscopic examination, hemorrhoids may be banded or sclerosing agents injected and biopsies of any suspicious lesions may be obtained. Complications are rare, but may include occasional bleeding from hemorrhoids or inadvertently tearing the anoderm.

Proctoscopy

Rigid proctoscopy is suitable to examine the rectum, and in some patients, the distal sigmoid colon may also be evaluated. Similar to the anoscope, the proctoscope consists of an obturator, the scope itself, and a light source. Illumination is supplied by a built-in light source and a lens is attached to the external orifice of the scope after the obturator is removed. The main difference between an anoscope is that a proctoscope needs to hold air so the rectum can be distended. This is achieved by having a bellows attached to the scope, which allows for insufflation of air to gain better visualization and negotiation of the scope proximally through the rectum. A suction device or cotton tipped swabs can be used to remove any endoluminal debris or fluid or to enhance visualization (Figure 4-4). Ideally, the patient should receive an enema preparation within 2 h of

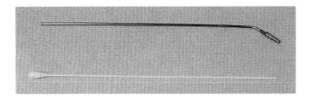

FIGURE 4-4. Proctoscopy suction catheter and long cotton-tipped applicators for clearing small amounts of fecal debris. The cotton-tipped swaps are also used for manipulating the rectal and anal mucosa during anoscopy and proctoscopy.

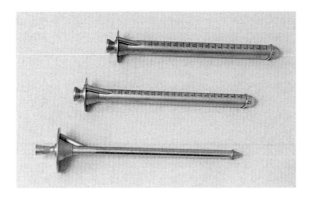

FIGURE 4-5. Proctoscopes. From *top* to *bottom*: large proctoscope, length 25 cm, diameter 19 mm; standard proctoscope, length 25 cm, diameter 15 mm; pediatric proctoscope, length 25 cm, diameter 11 mm.

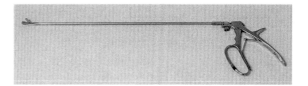

FIGURE 4-6. Turell angulated biopsy forceps. A curved upper jaw allows for 360° rotation. A variety of jaw sizes and types are available.

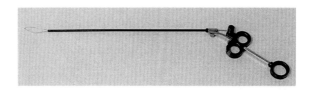

FIGURE 4-7. Rigid-wire (Frankfelt) snare. This snare allows for polypectomy or tumor debulking via the anoscope or proctoscope.

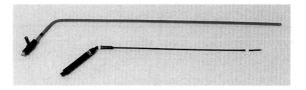

FIGURE 4-8. Suction catheter/electrocoagulation catheter. From *top* to *bottom*: an insulated catheter for combining suction and electrocautery, and an electrocoagulation catheter.

the procedure in order to clear any stool, which may make passage of the scope and visualization difficult.

Proctoscopes are available in three sizes, all 25 cm in length. Different luminal diameters include 11, 15, and 19 mm (Figure 4-5). The largest scope is suited best for polypectomy or biopsies in which electrocoagulation may be needed. In most patients, the 15 mm × 25 cm scope is ideal for a general inspection. There is also a disposable plastic, self-lighted proctoscope which is available for use.

The procedure can be performed in either the prone jackknife or left lateral position as previously described. When properly performed, the patient feels little to no discomfort. Pain may occur with stretching of the rectosigmoid mesentery due to over insufflation of air or the scope hitting the rectal wall. An overzealous examiner trying to advance the scope too quickly or too proximal is the main cause of patient discomfort. Unfortunately, the art of using the rigid proctoscope has declined in recent years due to the ubiquity of flexible endoscopy. The proctoscope however, still has important indications, especially in the identification and precise localization of rectal lesions or in the evaluation of rectal bleeding. Contraindications are similar to anoscopy and include painful anorectal condition such as acute fissure, incarcerated hemorrhoids, recent anorectal surgery (<1 month), or anal stenosis.

After adequate lubrication, while the obturator is held in place with the right thumb, the instrument is gently inserted into the anal canal and advanced approximately 4–5 cm in the general direction of the umbilicus. The scope is then aimed toward the sacrum and advanced for an additional 4–5 cm. The obturator is then removed and the viewing lens is placed. Minimal air insufflation is used in order to open the bowel lumen and gently withdrawing and advancing the scope to straighten out angulations proximally aids in achieving successful navigation. It should be noted that the distal extent reached on proctoscopic examinations averages approximately 17–20 cm and very rarely can the scope be inserted to its full length [3]. If at any time the insertion becomes difficult or painful to the patient, the procedure should be terminated and the farthest extend reached should be recorded.

As the proctoscope is withdrawn from the farthest extent reached, careful examination is performed of the entire circumference of the rectal wall with minimal air insufflation and rotation of the scope. The valves of Houston are flattened out with the tip of the scope to reveal areas just proximal to the folds. If any lesions are found, accurate measurements and descriptions are necessary. These include: size of the lesion, the exact distance from the anal verge, appearance, and location on the bowel wall. Several different types of biopsy forceps are available (Figure 4-6) and biopsies can be done in the office setting with or without the use of electrocautery. Additionally, polyps or small lesions can be snared (Figure 4-7) or fulgurated. Proper suction, electrocautery and irrigation devices should be readily available in the examining room for these purposes (Figure 4-8).

Serious complications during rigid proctoscopy are rare, with bleeding the most common, especially after biopsy or polypectomy. Perforation is a very rare occurrence and should not happen with proper technique. Before the introduction of flexible endoscopy, rigid proctoscopy was the standard technique to evaluate the distal sigmoid and rectum and large series of patients have shown minimal to no complications [4, 5]. Perforation of a normal rectum or sigmoid colon is a rare occurrence, but passing a scope or excess insufflation in a diseased or inflamed rectosigmoid may prove hazardous and caution must be undertaken in patients with inflammatory bowel disease, radiation proctitis, diverticulosis/diverticulitis, volvulus, or malignancy.

Anal and Rectal Ultrasound

Endoanal ultrasonography (EUS) is a highly reliable and reproducible imaging modality that provides information on the anatomy and function of pelvic floor structures, anorectal disease processes, and anorectal tumors. In experienced hands, EUS is accurate, with high sensitivity and specificity for detecting anal sphincter injuries. Advantages of EUS include the relatively inexpensive cost to perform and its widespread availability. One obvious disadvantage of EUS is that like all ultrasound examinations, it is an operator-dependent test, with varied published results for the same disease process.

Circumferential assessment of the anal canal and distal rectum is made possible by a 360° rotating transducer that is either a 7 or 10 megaHertz (MHz) probe for two-dimensional (2D) units or a 13 MHz probe for three-dimensional (3D) (Figure 4-9). In recent years, the use of 3D units has increased, with a similar sensitivity in detecting both external and internal sphincter defects, but it has been demonstrated that with the 3D units, intra-observer variation is decreased and thereby the diagnosis of pathology has been increased [6].

Prior to testing, patients receive an enema to clear the anorectum of any stool that may interfere with images due to artifact. Additionally, as with rigid proctoscopy above, EUS should not be performed on patients diagnosed with anal stenosis or fissure-in-ano, as this will undoubtedly render the test uncomfortable for the patient and difficult for the examiner to perform. EUS is most commonly performed with the patient in the left lateral recumbent position. After a gentle DRE, the well-lubricated ultrasound probe is inserted and slowly advanced and then withdrawn to view the entire area of the anal canal/rectum (in modern systems, a crystal moves up and down along the transducer to acquire images while the probe is held stationary).

The anal canal is divided into three levels on EUS: upper, middle, and lower based on anatomic landmarks. The upper anal canal is defined by the U-shaped puborectalis muscle; the middle canal has both EAS and IAS muscles visible (this is also where the IAS is at maximum width); and in the lower anal canal, only the most distal external sphincter fibers are visualized (Figures 4-10, 4-11, and 4-12). Highly reflective tissue on EUS reveals a hyperechoic (white) image, while poorly reflective tissues are hypoechoic (black). Thus, the smooth muscle-based IAS, which has higher water content, shows up black on EUS. In postobstetrical sphincter injuries, the defect is usually located anteriorly and encompasses the EAS and may involve the IAS as well. In cases of postsurgical or posttraumatic injuries of the anal sphincters, defects can involve either or both muscles and may be unifocal or multifocal in nature (Figure 4-13). The accuracy of EUS compared to surgical findings has been reported to be as high as 90–100% by some authors and additionally, EUS has been used after operative sphincter repair to show the overlap of the muscles and to confirm a proper repair has been performed.

Flexible Endoscopy

Flexible Endoscopic Insertion Techniques

Due to the fact that no two colons are the same, the techniques described here are generalizations and guidelines to help navigate the flexible endoscope to its completion. The technique of performing an endoscopic examination, like any invasive procedure, is best learned under the watchful eye of a seasoned mentor, rather than reading a text; however, there are some points that can be generalized.

The keys to a comfortable and efficient endoscopic examination include a mastery of the insertion techniques described here to maintain a straight scope while keeping pain and trauma to the patient at a minimum. The skilled endoscopist must be able to use torque, tip deflection, dithering/jiggle, and push and pullback techniques as second nature in order to successfully achieve these goals. The techniques described here apply to both sigmoidoscopy and colonoscopy.

Torque

The twisting motion applied to the shaft of the scope by the endoscopist's right hand is called torque (Figure 4-14). Torque is an essential technique that allows for a stiffening of the scope and alters the direction in which the tip deflection controls work. Torque also has the ability to increase the scopes resistance to avoid troublesome loops. Torque can be to the right (clockwise) or left (counterclockwise) based on whichever direction seems to work best for the task at hand. Gentle torque is used while keeping the scope straight and a more forceful torque is used when removing or following a loop.

Tip Deflection

The tip of the endoscope should always be kept in the middle of the bowel lumen. The techniques of torque, pull/push, and

Figure 4-9. B-K Medical (Herlev, Denmark) three-dimensional anorectal ultrasound equipment.

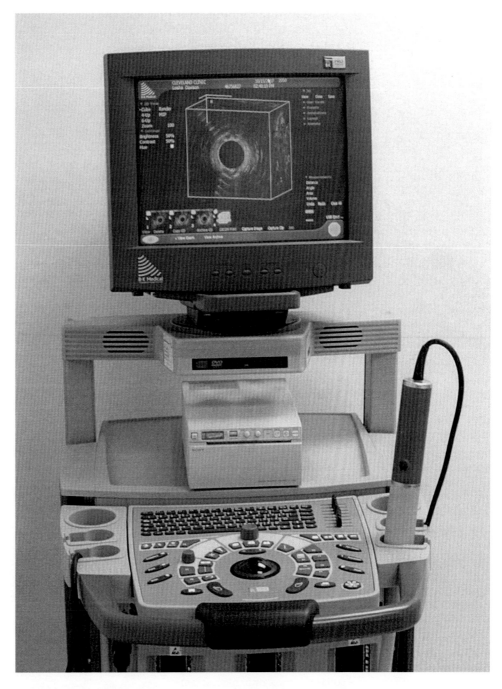

dithering-jiggle will tend to move the tip in several directions. The endoscopist should bring the tip back by controlling both the outer and inner controls with their left hand. With practice, the endoscopist should be able to control and use both tip deflection control knobs in different directions with only the thumb of the left hand. The preference of locking one or both of the knobs is operator dependent. It should be noted, however, that the endoscopist should strive to keep their right hand on the shaft and their left hand on the tip deflection controls throughout the examination in order to maintain proper feel of the scope and to not miss opportunities for advancement and also to avoid "losing ground" by having the scope slide retrograde.

Dithering/Jiggle

The rapid up-and-down, side-to-side, and to-and-fro movements of the shaft of the scope are referred to as dithering or jiggle (Figure 4-15). This technique can be combined with rapid torqueing and rapid in-and-out movements of the scope. The object of this important maneuver is to pleat the colon onto the shaft of the endoscope in order to shorten the colon and to keep the scope straight. Every endoscopist should employ this technique throughout the entire insertion, even when scope advancement appears easy in a straight portion of the colon, especially the descending and transverse colon.

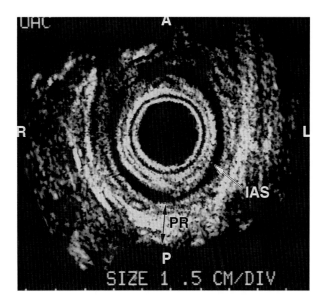

FIGURE 4-10. Two-dimensional endoanal ultrasound view of the U-shaped puborectalis muscle (PR). *IAS* internal anal sphincter.

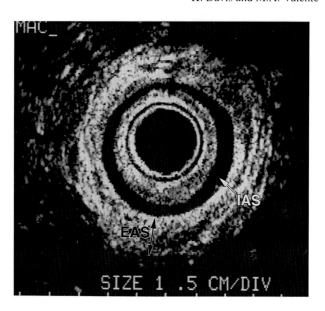

FIGURE 4-11. Two-dimensional ultrasound from the mid-anal canal. This ultrasound image represents normal, intact internal anal sphincter (IAS) (hypoechoic) and external anal sphincter (EAS), (hyperechoic).

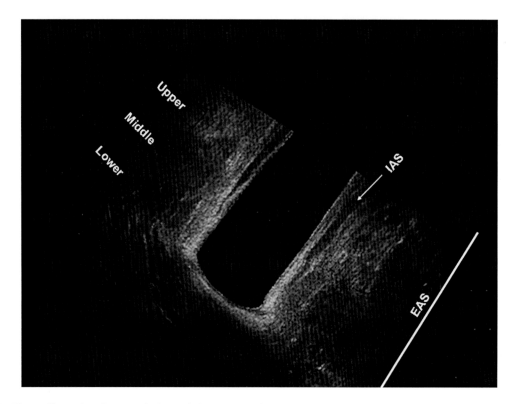

FIGURE 4-12. Three-dimensional coronal view of the upper, middle, and lower anal canal. *EAS* external anal sphincter, *IAS* internal anal sphincter.

Aspiration of Air and Breath Holding

As insufflation of air accumulates during the procedure, the colon becomes distended and elongates, thereby making the goal of reaching the cecum farther away and often causing discomfort to the patient. The judicious and cautious use of air is important during the examination, but thoughtful and calculated aspiration/suction of air is an important adjunct insertion technique. Aspiration of air can allow the scope to

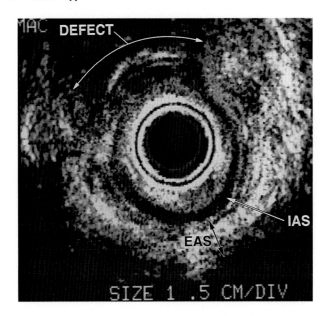

Figure 4-13. Anteriorly located defect of both the EAS and IAS in the mid anal canal.

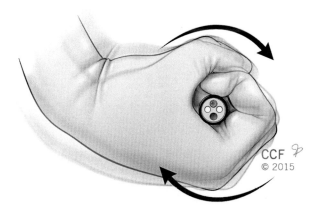

Figure 4-14. Torque—a twisting motion of the endoscopist's right hand to the left (counterclockwise) or right (clockwise). Reprinted with permission, Cleveland Clinic Center for Medical Art & Photography ©2015. All Rights Reserved.

advance the tip past a turn (especially at the hepatic flexure) without needed to push the scope forward and likely forming a loop. Once the tip of the scope is past the turn, advancement is much easier due to the straightness of the scope.

Another technique to help the scope around the flexure is the "breath-hold" maneuver. While negotiating difficult turns and bends (especially the hepatic and splenic flexure), have the patient take a deep breath in and hold it. This causes the diaphragm to drop and pushes the flexures over the scope and thereby allows the scope to pass [7]. Aspiration of air and breath holding can be used in conjunction along with precise abdominal pressure techniques.

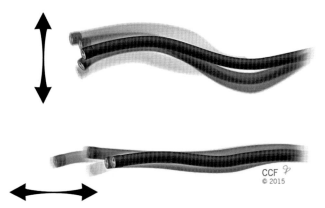

Figure 4-15. Jiggle (Dithering)—rapid side-to-side, up-and-down, and to-and-fro movements of the endoscope in order to pleat or "accordion" the colon onto the scope's shaft. Reprinted with permission, Cleveland Clinic Center for Medical Art & Photography ©2015. All Rights Reserved.

Slide-By

The technique of pushing blindly into a turn or bend with maximum tip deflection and without full visualization of the colon lumen to guide the scope along the curvature of the bowel wall to advance the scope past the turn is termed a slide-by technique. Slide-by is a controversial technique that should never be used by unsupervised trainees or novice endoscopists due to the potential dangers and complications that may occur, namely perforation. Slide-by should be terminated if there is any resistance to forward advancement or the mucosa becomes blanched at the tip of the scope. Slide-by can be very painful to the patient because it causes tension on the bowel mesentery and will need to be terminated if not tolerated by the patient. Once the slide-by is successful, the scope needs to be straightened and any loops need to be reduced. Modern endoscopes have a great deal of tip deflection and thus, slide-by is not as commonly employed as when endoscopy was in its infancy (Fig. 4.16).

Adjunctive Maneuvers for More Difficult Examinations

The adjunctive maneuvers employed with endoscopy often serve as the markers between seasoned experts and novices. There are several different maneuvers including abdominal pressure and other external manipulation provided by an assistant under the direct supervision of the endoscopist. In addition it is possible to adjust the position of the patient to either the supine or prone positions. There are also commercially produced overtubes, which are seldom required now with the advent of adjustable stiffness endoscopes. All of these adjunctive maneuvers are designed to reduce the loop formation of the endoscope or to prevent it from reforming

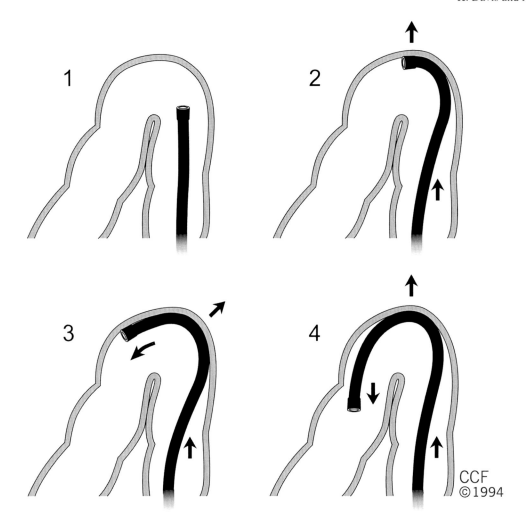

FIGURE 4-16. Slide-by technique. The colonoscope is blindly pushed around a bend, guided by the curve of the scope and the curvature of the bowel wall. Slide-by should be terminated with excessive patient pain or blanching of the mucosa occurs. This technique should be avoided in diseased bowel or in the presence of diverticuli. Reprinted with permission, Cleveland Clinic Center for Medical Art & Photography ©2015. All Rights Reserved.

once it has been reduced. In one study evaluating the use of ancillary techniques, directed abdominal pressure was used in 56% of colonoscopies, while turning to the left and right was performed in 17% and 23% of exams respectively [7]. Like all techniques, however, they are best learned under the supervision of a seasoned endoscopist.

The most likely cause of a difficult examination is the formation of a loop, which makes further advancement of the scope impossible, painful, and potentially harmful. It should be remembered that when facing a difficult-to-negotiate area of the colon, a different technique must be employed to facilitate success. It is the authors' opinion that once a technique has failed twice, a new technique should be employed. The technique of withdrawing the scope all the back to the rectosigmoid and starting the procedure over is a valuable maneuver and again should not be overlooked. It may be necessary during a difficult examination to "take a few steps backwards in order to move forward."

Patient Position

While the procedure starts with the patient on their left side, transitioning to a supine position may ease the navigation of the sigmoid, sigmoid/descending, splenic flexure, and hepatic flexure. Alternatively, if the patient begins supine, turning to the left lateral will help achieve the same goal. While the patient is being moved with the assistance of the endoscopy team, the endoscopist should keep their eye on the screen and attempt to maintain the scope in the middle of the lumen, as it is common for the scope to lose its position during patient movement. Turning the patient to their right side is a technique that is especially useful when the examination has reached the ascending colon and it cannot be advanced into the cecum. Placing the patient into a prone position can also be performed, but this position is often difficult and cumbersome for the staff and the patient. Patient safety must be maintained during this maneuver. The authors finds this technique useful very occasionally to help the scope navigate in more obese individuals, as the act of having their abdomen on the bed supplies abdominal pressure.

Abdominal Pressure

The technique of splinting certain redundant areas of the colon with external pressure via the abdominal wall may help reduction in loop formation. However, this technique is most effective when a known loop is present and the endoscopist can guide the staff to apply pressure in the correct location. The most common areas of looping are the sigmoid and transverse colon, but simply pressing on different areas of the abdomen will often clue the examiner where the problem exists. Initial attempts at "blind pressure" should be from superior and right of the umbilicus directed toward the left lower quadrant. This has the effect of stabilizing the sigmoid colon and giving counter-pressure to the scope. However, pressure may need to be applied to different areas of the abdomen in order to successfully reduce the loop. The scope should be in the middle of the lumen and as straight as possible before pressure is asserted. This technique should be performed gently and it should not cause the patient any discomfort.

Turning the Scope

During the navigation of a very difficult or acute turn, it may help to change the entire angle of approach of the scope. This is accomplished by torqueing the shaft 180°, while keeping the tip of the scope stabilized in the middle with the help of the deflection knobs (Figure 4-17).

Sigmoidoscopy

The use of the flexible sigmoidoscopy (FS) in the office setting has increased in popularity due to its many applications, ease of use and high yield of findings over conventional rigid proctoscopy. In approximately 50–85% of patients, the entire sigmoid colon can be evaluated and in some patients, the splenic flexure can be reached as well. The flexible sigmoidoscope is easier to handle and the technique is easier to learn than colonoscopy, but nonetheless, supervised training is compulsory. In terms of selective screening purposes, the flexible sigmoidoscope offers a three to sixfold increase in the yield of findings, especially neoplasms, in the rectum and sigmoid colon compared to rigid proctoscopy. It should be noted, however, that FS is not an adequate substitute to colonoscopy for detection of colonic polyps and neoplasms.

The flexible sigmoidoscope is available from various companies with minor variations between them. In general, the channel size ranges between 2.6 and 3.8 mm, the diameter of the scope ranges between 12 and 14 mm and the length varies from 60 to 71 cm (Figure 4-18). As with most instruments in a surgeon's armamentarium, the exact instrument selected is based on surgeon preference in regards to availability, cost and surgeon experience.

The indications for FS in the office setting are broad. FS is an excellent tool to evaluate the patient with bright red rectal bleeding as well as a myriad of other conditions such as in radiation proctitis, nonspecific proctitis, rectal ulcer, anorectal Crohn's disease, or suspected distal neoplasms. FS also

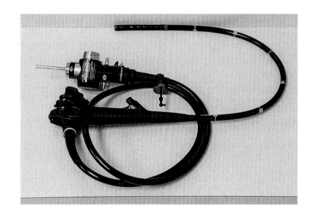

Figure 4-18. Flexible sigmoidoscope.

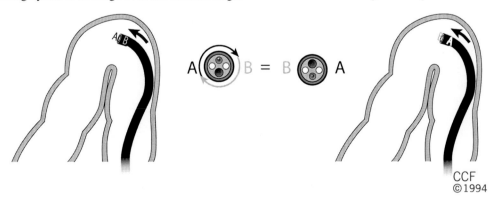

Figure 4-17. Turning the scope. This maneuver allows the examiner to change the angle of approach to a turn. Scope torque of 180° is accomplished while the deflection controls keep the tip centered in the lumen. Reprinted with permission, Cleveland Clinic Center for Medical Art & Photography ©2015. All Rights Reserved.

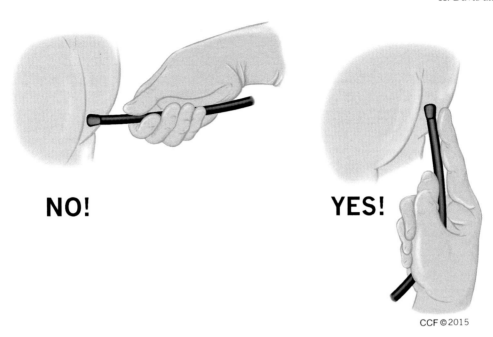

NO!   YES!

FIGURE 4-19. The flexible endoscope should be inserted "side first" for less painful passage through the anal canal. Reprinted with permission, Cleveland Clinic Center for Medical Art & Photography ©2015. All Rights Reserved.

has utility in examining and acquiring cultures or biopsies of the distal colorectum in diarrheal states, ruling out *Clostridium difficile*, infectious and ischemic colitis. Radiographical abnormalities can be confirmed with the use FS as well as diagnosing or for the follow-up of inflammatory bowel disease. Additionally, postoperative evaluation of distal anastomoses can rapidly be performed, evaluating for stricture or recurrence of cancer as well as recurrences after local excision.

Patients are typically given one to two enemas prior to the procedure and generally do not require oral laxatives or dietary restrictions. The position that offers the easiest approach is the left lateral recumbent but the prone jackknife position can also be used. Sedation is not typically necessary in the vast majority of patients.

The well lubricated scope is inserted "side first" rather than "end on" which allows for the edge of the endoscope to act as a leading point and avoids pushing the blunt end "*en face*" against the anal sphincter with subsequent trauma and pain (Figure 4-19) [2]. After proper insertion of the scope, gentle air insufflation is achieved and the scope is advanced under direct visualization to approximately 10–12 cm. The instrument is then passed into the sigmoid colon by a combination of torqueing in either the clockwise or counterclockwise direction and short advancement and withdrawal (dithering). These maneuvers are used to advance the scope as far as the splenic flexure, if amendable. The endoscopist should use a combination of these techniques along with air insufflation, suction and irrigation to successfully advance the scope. After the scope has been advanced to its extent, careful and thoughtful withdrawal is achieved slowly, in order to evaluate the entire mucosal surface. Any lesions that are detected can be biopsied or have brush cytology performed to establish a diagnosis. Additionally, small polyps can be removed with cold or hot biopsy forceps. Larger polyp removal may be best suited during a subsequent colonoscopy when a full bowel preparation has been achieved. It is important to remember that FS is excellent at examining the proximal and mid rectum as well as the left and sigmoid colon, but is suboptimal for the most distal anorectal disorders, and therefore, another method such as anoscopy should be employed to visualize this area.

Complications of FS are uncommon but may be serious or life threatening when they do occur. Over distention of air will cause abdominal pain and patient discomfort or possibly perforation due to barotrauma. Perforation is most common at the distal sigmoid where it angulates from the relatively fixed rectum at the sacral promontory. It is critical for the endoscopist to be aware of any patient discomfort during the procedure, to use as little insufflation as necessary and abort the procedure if necessary. Electrocoagulation should be avoided or used very judiciously in biopsies or snare techniques unless the patient has received a full mechanical bowel preparation to reduce the risk of explosion due to the presence of hydrogen and methane gas present within the bowel lumen.

Colonoscopy

The colonoscopic examination is often at the center of the evaluation and treatment of many patients with intestinal complaints. A thorough colonoscopy allows the physician to completely evaluate the mucosa of the terminal ileum, colon, and rectum as well as to obtain biopsies or photodocumentation of any abnormalities identified. The colonoscopy also remains at the forefront of the screening for colorectal carcinoma. The procedure also plays a central part of the clinical practice of most colon and rectal surgeons. Over 90% of colon and rectal surgeons reported performing colonoscopies as part of their regular practice, with these surgeons reporting an average of over 40 endoscopic procedures a month. Clearly the performance of colonoscopy plays a central role in the training and practice of colorectal surgeons across the world [8].

Indications and Contraindications

The specific indications for performing a colonoscopy are multiple and the endoscopic evaluation and management of these conditions is covered in the appropriate sections elsewhere in this text. There does exist some debate regarding the appropriateness of performing the procedure in varying clinical scenarios and an attempt to ensure the appropriateness of the procedure has been sought. In 2000, the American Society for Gastrointestinal Endoscopy and in 2008 the European Panel on the Appropriateness of Gastrointestinal Endoscopy was revised to EPAGE II [9]. Each published their respective appropriateness guidelines regarding when to perform a colonoscopy. The EPAGE II guidelines are intended to serve as a guide for referring physicians and is available to the clinician online at: http://www.epage.ch/, allowing the consulting physician to ensure the procedure is indicated prior to making the referral to an endoscopist. Despite the existence of these guidelines, they have not been widely accepted [10].

Using either of these two sets of guidelines, there are numerous publications demonstrating that many colonoscopies are indeed inappropriate. Using the ASGE guidelines there have been reports ranging from a 13% inappropriate procedure rate [11] to 18% [12]. These are even higher when the European criteria are utilized. Inappropriate procedure rates of 30% are reported [13], and these percentages have been confirmed in several multi-institutional studies [14, 15]. One reason for these high numbers is that an open access practice pattern is common among many physicians who perform endoscopy [16]. Indeed, these guidelines are designed primarily for the open access endoscopy scenario, where the endoscopist serves more as a technician: performing and interpreting the procedure for the physician ordering the procedure. These studies show that it is often surgeons that fall outside the ordering guidelines. Since colon and rectal surgeons seldom perform endoscopy in these open access systems, there are no studies evaluating the appropriateness of colonoscopies performed by these subspecialty surgeons.

The only absolute contraindication for performing a colonoscopy is in a patient who requires immediate operative intervention. All other contraindications are relative and are at the discretion of the endoscopist. Patients with active colitis or those with a recent intestinal anastomosis are at higher risk for complications but a careful endoscopic examination can be safely conducted in these patients [17]. As with any procedure being performed, the benefits must outweigh the risks.

Bowel Preparation

Unlike in elective colon surgery there is no controversy surrounding the necessity of mechanical bowel preparation prior to a colonoscopy. The bowel prep is of critical importance in order to be able to adequately examine the entire colon, with inadequate cleaning reported in up to 27% of patients [18]. It is often considered the most unpleasant part of the procedure on the part of the patient and a great deal of research has gone into making it more effective and the process more palatable for the patient. Despite this, the optimal regimen has yet to be determined [19]. While many practitioners add additional dietary restrictions such as protein restriction or a low residue diet for 2–3 days prior to the procedure but there are no studies that validate these practices.

There remain numerous options for bowel preparation prior to the procedure with three broad categories of agents in use: osmotic agents, polyethylene glycol (PEG) solutions and stimulants. The choice is somewhat practice-dependent, although more practitioners use PEG-based preparations in their practices than the osmotic agents. Osmotic agents such as Sodium Phosphate and Magnesium Citrate work by increasing the passage of extracellular fluid across the bowel wall. Following the FDA alert regarding renal damage associated with oral sodium phosphate with bowel cleansing prior to colonoscopy in 2008, its use declined precipitously in the USA [20, 21], yet it remains a viable option [22]. The potential side effects associated with its use include nephropathy and renal insufficiency resulting from the tubular deposition of phosphate [23]. These side effects are uncommon; yet, with many and potentially better options, most practitioners including the authors forgo using it in clinical practice. Stimulants such as Senna and Bisacodyl increase bowel wall smooth muscle activity, and are primarily used as adjuncts to one of the other preps rather than as a stand-alone prep [24].

There is also good evidence to suggest that regardless which agent is chosen, splitting the timing into the half-day prior to and half-day of the procedure results in an overall better cleansing [25]. The majority of patients seem willing to comply with this split preparation and this results in an improvement in the number of satisfactory bowel preparations [26]. At least one meta-analysis demonstrates that a 4-L split-dose PEG is superior to other preparation strategies [27]. It is also critical that the instructions that are given to the patient are understood. It is beneficial if the language is tailored to the individual and instructions should include commonly asked questions, as this will increase patient understanding and compliance with whichever agent(s) is chosen [28].

The reporting of the quality of the bowel prep is both an important part of documentation of the procedure as well as a standard of quality. An adequate bowel preparation should be achieved and documented in greater than 85% of procedures [29]. There are numerous scales for grading the adequacy of the bowel prep, yet none is proven superior. The Aronchick scale grades the overall quality on a scale of 5 (excellent) to 0 (inadequate) [30]. The Ottawa [31], Boston [32] and Chicago [33] scales grade the preparation quality in different anatomic areas of the colon adding them together to form a total score. These scores range up to 9 for the Boston, 14 for the Ottawa and 36 for the Chicago. The easiest and therefore the most commonly employed is the 4-point scale of excellent, good, fair, and poor. Regardless of which scale is chosen, they are all subjective and therefore subject to bias.

Special Considerations

The Difficult-to-Prep Patient

With the high number of patients with an inadequate bowel prep, as above, it is not uncommon to encounter patients with a prior history of a poor bowel prep presenting for a repeat evaluation. It is recommend that patients undergo early repeat colonoscopy when the bowel preparation quality is deemed inadequate, defined as the inability to detect polyps smaller than 5 mm [34]. Adenomas and high-risk lesions are frequently detected on repeat colonoscopy in these inadequate prep patients, suggesting that these lesions were likely missed at the time of the initial evaluation [35].

There are no prospective studies dealing with this patient population and the practices are individualized. Some practitioners either increase the amount of liquid diet by 1 day or add an osmotic or cathartic agent to the existing regimen. In addition antiemetics or anxiolytics may be added in an attempt to make the prep more palatable to the patient. It has also been demonstrated that patients tolerate a larger volume PEG prep solution [36]. In hospitalized patients it has also been demonstrated that the prep can be administered via a gastroscope the day prior to colonoscopy, improving patient tolerance and the subsequent quality of bowel preparation for colonoscopy [37]. Ultimately the clinician is left to their best clinical judgment.

The Patient Requiring Antibiotics

The data regarding the need for prophylactic antibiotics for patients undergoing a colonoscopy is lacking. While there are case reports of endocarditis following colonoscopy, the need for antibiotic prophylaxis for patients undergoing elective endoscopy is rare. Antibiotic prophylaxis against infective endocarditis is not routinely recommended for colonoscopy although there is some evidence suggesting that infective endocarditis due to *Streptococcus* and *Enterococcus* species may indeed warrant prophylaxis in these patients [38] Based upon current guidelines antibiotic prophylaxis is reserved for individuals with cardiac valvular disease at high risk of infective endocarditis. There has been a small but significant increase in the incidence of infective endocarditis since 2008, when the more restrictive guidelines regarding the lack of need for prophylaxis were issued [39], but the clinical significance remains unclear at this time [40, 41].

The ASGE guidelines published in 2003 and revised in 2008 (Table 4-1) divide the patients into high, moderate, and low risk based upon the cardiac risk factors [42]. However, even high-risk patients are not required to have antimicrobial prophylaxis prior to endoscopic procedures. In patients who fall into the high-risk category, a frank discussion with the patient's cardiologist or infectious disease specialist is warranted.

TABLE 4-1. Antibiotic prophylaxis for elective colonoscopy ± biopsy

Conditions	Patient risk	Antibiotics
Prosthetic heart valves	High-risk patients	Prophylaxis is optional
History of endocarditis		
Systemic-pulmonary shunt		
Complex cyanotic congenital heart disease		
Cardiac Transplant with valvulopathy		
Other congenital cardiac abnormalities	Moderate-risk patients	Prophylaxis is not recommended
Mitral valve prolapse with regurgitation		
Rheumatic heart disease		
Hypertrophic cardiomyopathy		
CABG	Low-risk patients	Prophylaxis is not recommended
Defibrillators		
Pacemakers		
Repaired septal defect or PDA		
Physiologic heart murmurs		
Mitral valve prolapse without regurgitation		
Prosthetic joints <6 months	Patients to consider prophylaxis	Consider prophylaxis
Peritoneal dialysis		
Vascular grafts	Insufficient data	Consider prophylaxis

The Anticoagulated Patient

The anticoagulated patient poses an even larger dilemma for the endoscopist. As the number of anticoagulation medications and the number of patients receiving these medications increase coupled with the rising number of colonoscopies performed, this clinical scenario is frequently encountered, and can be expected to increase. While a diagnostic colonoscopy itself poses little bleeding risk, the possibility of biopsies or polypectomy must be considered. It is imperative that the endoscopist weighs the risk of possible thrombotic events if any medication is withdrawn against those of bleeding. This must often be done prior to the procedure, when knowledge of any pathology or whether any biopsy or polypectomy does not exist.

According to the 2005 ASGE guidelines [43], a diagnostic colonoscopy or a colonoscopy with biopsy is considered a low-risk procedure for causing hemorrhage. A polypectomy however is considered to be a high-risk procedure and any anticoagulant medications should be adjusted according to the medication that is being taken (Table 4-2) [44–47]. These decisions will often need to be coordinated with the physician monitoring the anticoagulant, as it is often not within the purview of the endoscopist to evaluate the thrombotic risk. When to reinitiate anticoagulation is another difficult issue that must take into account what was performed at the time of the endoscopy, with the recommendation being to reinitiate the therapy as soon as hemostasis has been confirmed, which is obviously difficult [48]. The incidence of post-polypectomy hemorrhage peaks at 4–6 days and this risk extends to at least 14 days. In general, the morbidity of a thromboembolic event is greater than that of hemorrhage—therefore, resuming anticoagulation as soon as possible and treating hemorrhagic complications as they occur seems to be the most prudent management strategy.

Incomplete Colonoscopy

A complete colonoscopy examination to the cecum should be achieved in >95% for screening cases and is considered a major benchmark of quality. The slight decrease in colorectal cancer incidence over the past several decades is attributed in part to early detection and removal of colorectal polyps before they progress to invasive malignancy [49]. This decrease is attributed mostly to left sided lesions versus right sided lesions due to potential genetic factors, missed lesions, poor bowel preparation, and incomplete examinations [50]. Right-sided colon lesions tend to more flat and depressed which undoubtedly contributes to missing these lesions.

Rates of incomplete colonoscopy range from 5 to 25% and reasons are varied [49, 51]. Whatever the reason for incompletion, a secondary examination must be offered to the patient. The dilemma of what to do after an incomplete colonoscopy is best approached by delineating what was the specific reason for the incomplete exam.

TABLE 4-2. Management of anticoagulation medications for elective lower GI endoscopy

↑ Risk procedures			↓ Risk procedures
Polypectomy >1 cm			Diagnostic endoscopy
Endoscopic dilatation			Flexible sigmoidoscopy/colonoscopy ±biopsy
			Stent placement without dilation
Medications			
Medication	Risk	Medication instructions	Medication restart
Warfarin		Hold 3–5 days prior	
A-fib		Hold warfarin and start UFH or LMWH when INR ≤2.0	
A-fib w h/o embolic event		Hold warfarin and start UFH or LMWH when INR ≤2.0	
Mechanical valvular heart disease			
Low molecular weight heparin (LMWH)	↓	No medication adjustment necessary	
	↑	D/C 8 h prior to procedure	Restarting medication Individualized
Bridging LMWH: to replace Heparin Window		Consider 1 mg/kg q 12 h	D/C as above
D/C Warfarin 3–5 days prior to procedure			
Thienopyridines: clopidogrel/ticlopidine	↓	No change necessary	
	↑	D/C 7–10 days prior to procedure, consider continuing aspirin if on dual therapy	Restarting individualized
Dipridamole	↓	If no preexisting bleeding disorder, no change necessary	
	↑	Unknown	
GIIb/IIIa inhibitor		Medication not usually used in patients undergoing elective procedures. Consult with Prescribing Physician or Cardiology	

Patients who had an incomplete colonoscopy due to an unsatisfactory or poor prep must be re-educated on the preparation process, as above. A repeat colonoscopy in this situation is the most logical and effective approach [52, 53]. In patients whom the procedure was terminated secondary to tortuosity or pain, a repeat colonoscopy under alternate analgesia or a repeat colonoscopy with a more experienced endoscopist may be appropriate [49, 53]. Alternatively, CT colonoscopy (virtual colonoscopy) may also be performed with good success. It should be noted that any lesion >6 mm found on CT colonoscopy will require a standard colonoscopy as follow-up. As a final option, a double (air and ingested contrast) barium enema can be considered. Even though barium enema has been available for decades and is an accepted screening tool for colorectal carcinoma, a recent large population-based study showed a cancer miss rate of 22%, which makes this a very poor second test to either standard or CT colonoscopy [54].

In patients in whom the colonoscopy was incomplete secondary to stricture or an obstructing lesion, options include on-table colonoscopy at the time of resection, preoperative CT colonoscopy, or postoperative colonoscopy [49].

Procedure

The Endoscopy Suite

Unlike the flexible sigmoidoscopic examination that can be adequately performed in the office, a full colonoscopy typically requires a larger space with more equipment. The endoscopy suite should provide an adequate amount of space for the necessary endoscopic equipment and patient stretcher as well as allow adequate egress of staff and equipment. It is important that clear and unobstructed sight lines are maintained for all of the personnel in the endoscopy suite such that adequate visualization on the patient as well as any monitoring equipment is maintained at all times. It is dark in the endoscopy suite and the endoscopist is concentrating on the procedure therefore it is imperative to have a designated person, who's primary responsibility is for monitoring the patient throughout the procedure.

If sedation is to be used, as is most commonly performed in the USA, it is important that oxygen and routine EKG monitoring are performed. A consensus statement states that patients who are having their procedure performed under moderate or deep sedation "must have continuous monitoring before, during, and after the administration of sedatives." Monitoring may detect early signs of patient distress, such as changes in cardiovascular or pulmonary parameters prior to any clinically significant compromise. Standard monitoring of sedated patients undergoing GI endoscopic procedures includes recording the heart rate, blood pressure, respiratory rate, and oxygen saturation. Although electronic monitoring equipment often facilitates assessment of patient status, it does not replace a well-trained and vigilant assistant [55].

Instruments

As with flexible sigmoidoscopes above, there are numerous manufacturers of colonoscopes that typically vary from 130 to 168 cm in length. There are also pediatric colonoscopes that are smaller in diameter than the typical adult endoscope: 11.3 mm versus 12.8 mm. The basic colonoscope consists of a suction channel, an air/water channel, and fiber-optic bundles for light transmission, along with a biopsy port, which is connected into the suction channel (Figure 4-20a, b). Modern colonoscopes commonly possess variable stiffness controls that allow the endoscopist to vary the rigidity of the endoscope dependent on the clinical situation. It is hypothesized that this ability decreases the need for external over the tube stiffeners, and they have been proven to decrease procedure-related pain and the doses of sedative medications during colonoscopy [56].

Sedation

There are numerous studies evaluating the optimal method in which to sedate the patient for colonoscopy procedures and there is ample dogma employed as well. As with a bowel prep, there is no perfect sedation regimen but the endoscopist must be familiar with the side effect profile of medications being used and be prepared and comfortable with any reversal agents. While there is literature demonstrating that colonoscopy can be performed adequately and safely on the un-sedated patient, the practice in the USA is rare. In one study, less than half of the endoscopists polled practiced unsedated colonoscopy, listing a lack of patient acceptance as the most common reason for not offering it [57]. In an evaluation of Canadian gastroenterologists and colon and rectal surgeons, the endoscopists reported using sedation for more than 90% of colonoscopies they performed. The most common sedation regimen was a combination of midazolam and fentanyl [58]. While the combination of a narcotic with a benzodiazepine remains popular for providing colonoscopy sedation, several alternate medications have been evaluated.

Nitrous Oxide

Nitrous oxide is one medication that has been found effective in several studies to be effective for colonoscopic sedation. While some studies show that it is not an effective substitution for intravenous sedation and analgesics [59], there are several studies that show it to work well in that setting. In a review of seven randomized trials using nitrous oxide for colonoscopy, four showed that nitrous oxide is as good at controlling pain as conventional methods, while another showed that sedation was actually improved [60]. Despite this it is unlikely that Nitrous Oxide will become widely used in clinical practice.

FIGURE 4-20. (a) End-on view of the endoscopic tip, showing suction/biopsy channel, air/water channel, lens, and light source. (b) Basic endoscope design. Reprinted with permission, Cleveland Clinic Center for Medical Art & Photography ©2015. All Rights Reserved.

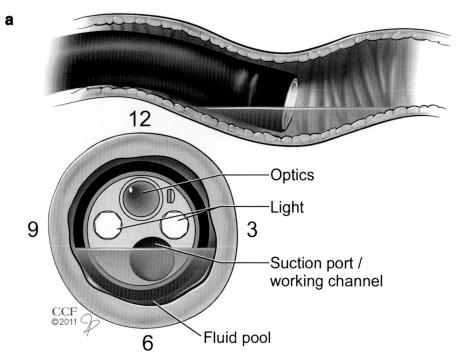

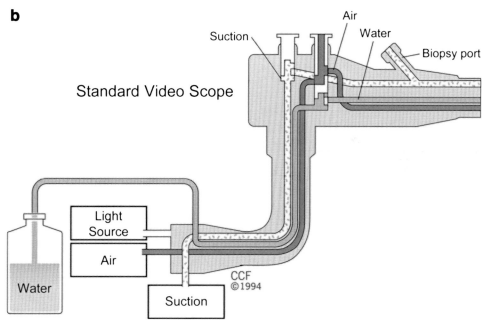

Ketamine

Ketamine is another medication that has demonstrated beneficial in colonoscopy. In one study, the addition of low-dose ketamine to a standard sedation regimen resulted in more rapid and better quality of sedation with stable hemodynamic status, and similar recovery times [61]. Due to a lack of familiarity with the medication and concerns regarding central nervous system alteration this medication is also unlikely to receive widespread use for endoscopic sedation.

Propofol

By far, the preponderance of the recent literature involving sedation for endoscopy involves the use of propofol, which has increased substantially among endoscopists [62]. In a Cochrane Review of the randomized controlled studies comparing propofol with standard sedation of a narcotic and benzodiazepine, the findings were that recovery and discharge times were shorter with the use of propofol. In addition, there was higher patient satisfaction with use of propofol. No difference in the procedure time, the cecal intubation rate or the incidence of complications was noted [63]. A later meta-analysis confirmed these findings [64].

One criticism of the use of propofol is that an anesthesia provider is typically required to administer the agent—thereby increasing the cost associated with the procedure. It has been demonstrated that the medication can be delivered in a patient controlled setting [65] or by a nurse under the supervision of the endoscopist [66]. These methods are likely to remain in the minority, however, and the question remains unanswered in an era of cost containment whether the benefits listed above justify its use.

Colonoscopy Technique

Colonoscopy is the most challenging endoscopic examination, and appropriate training, practice, attention to detail, and patience is needed in order to successfully complete this examination. The act of negotiating a 5–6 ft flexible tube through a tortuous colon painlessly and efficiently while performing detailed surveillance and therapeutic maneuvers is a difficult task. This section will describe successful navigation to the full extent of the colonoscopy relying on the principles mentioned prior.

Anal Intubation

The well-lubricated colonoscope is inserted as previously described for sigmoidoscopy. The examiner must make sure that the scope is brought over to the patient straight without any twists or loops from the endoscopy tower.

The Rectum and Rectosigmoid

Once the endoscope is placed into the anus, it is advanced into the rectum while insufflating an appropriate amount of air to distend the rectum. The distensibility of the rectum is an easy way to evaluate rectal compliance based on how easily and how much the rectum distends. Negotiating through the rectum is usually not difficult, but if difficulty is encountered going through the three valves of Houston (Figure 4-21), torque can be employed to reach the rectosigmoid.

The rectosigmoid can pose extreme difficulty and is often one of the more challenging areas of the colonoscopy. There is often an acute angle at this junction from a redundant and floppy sigmoid colon. If the patient has undergone prior pelvic surgery, especially hysterectomy, the sigmoid may become fixed and adherent which makes negotiation of the turn difficult and often painful. In other patients (usually males) this turn is obtuse and very easy to advance. In situations where the turn is difficult, a combination of all the basic maneuvers discussed should be employed. The scope should be kept as straight as possible as a combination of short advancements—withdrawals with jiggle and a slight clockwise

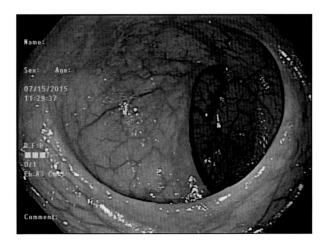

FIGURE 4-21. The first and second rectal valves of Houston. Note the large submucosal venous plexus.

torque (this torque may be considerable in certain individuals) should be employed to advance the scope into the sigmoid colon. This portion of the exam requires adequate patient sedation and relaxation. For the most acute angles, multiple small advancing steps toward getting the tip of the scope past the angle with tip deflection and torque are needed. Slide-by maneuvers should not be routinely performed.

Once the scope advances into the sigmoid, tip deflection and some torque will help reduce any loops. If this is not possible, the scope can be carefully inserted farther into the sigmoid with the loop still in place as long as this does not cause too much patient discomfort. Once the descending colon comes into view, any loops should be reduced with withdrawal and torqueing maneuvers. This may require a substantial torque with the right hand and usually the endoscopist can feel the scope reduce and any patient discomfort or pain will usually abate at this time. It should be noted that successful completion of the procedure is quite low if the rectosigmoid loop is not reduced [67].

Sigmoid Colon

The sigmoid colon is the most tortuous segment of the colon with associated high muscular tone, spasm, and a higher incidence of diverticulosis (Figure 4-22). The sigmoid colon is not fixed and can be very redundant and elongated. The sigmoid readily accepts the endoscope and a considerable length of scope can be inserted. All of these factors contribute to making this a difficult-to-navigate segment requiring insertion-pull back, jiggle, and a variable amount of torque (usually clockwise). These maneuvers will allow the sigmoid to "accordion" over the scope, which allows for efficient advancement and the prevention of loop formation.

Diverticula, when present, can be of various sizes and the larger ones can be dangerous as they can be mistaken for the true bowel lumen. Careful navigation around a diverticula

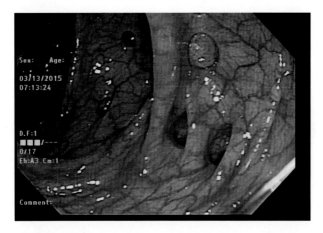

FIGURE 4-22. The sigmoid colon has variable degrees of tortuosity, spasm, diverticular disease, and muscular tone.

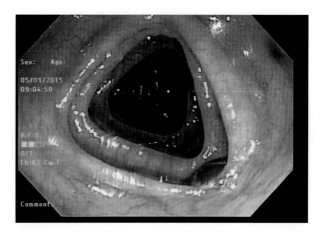

FIGURE 4-23. Transverse colon: note the common triangular appearance of the lumen.

laden sigmoid requires patience and the pull back techniques in order to gain a broader view of the colon. Perforation of a diverticulum can occur if too forceful or blind advancement (slide-by) is incorporated.

Sigmoid-Descending Junction

The junction of the sigmoid and descending colon can be difficult if a sigmoid loop is present or has only been partially reduced. Keeping the scope straight and gently advancing and withdrawing 1–2 cm at a time usually works, as opposed to pushing through the loop which will undoubtedly cause pain. One can also attempt to apply abdominal pressure at this point or turn the patient position to supine (or lateral) in attempts to advance into the descending colon.

Descending Colon

The descending colon is usually straighter and less muscular than the sigmoid colon. It should be noted that even though this segment of the colon is easier to advance, jiggle, torque, air suction, and push and pullback techniques should still be employed to pleat the colon over the scope.

Splenic Flexure

After advancing through the descending colon, the splenic flexure is the next obstacle. The splenic flexure is identified by the strong cardiac pulsations often seen and occasionally the blue shadow from the spleen itself. Often, this is a simple 90° turn that can be easily negotiated with some tip deflection and torque and other times, the splenic flexure may be a series of turns and twists in multiple planes. A difficult splenic flexure should be treated as already described using tip deflection, torque and push and pull techniques. Often,

changing patient position or externally splinting the sigmoid with abdominal pressure can achieve flexure passage as well. It should be noted that the straighter the sigmoid colon is, the easier the splenic flexure will be. A sigmoid loop can form during this portion of the exam if forward push is used to get past the flexure.

Transverse Colon

The transverse colon is characterized by the triangular appearance formed by the taenia coli (Figure 4-23). If no proximal loop has been formed, the scope will advance readily through this segment. If a loop is formed in the splenic flexure or the sigmoid, application of abdominal pressure at the sigmoid coupled with a strong torque (left or right) will usually reduce the loop and allow for a one-to-one advancement rather than a paradoxical advance. It should be remembered that torque, jiggle, and push-pull should be employed even when this segment is straight.

One area of difficulty may be in the mid-transverse colon. The mid transverse colon may exhibit ptosis and descend down into the pelvis and could be fixed with adhesions, especially following pelvic surgery. Loops are commonly created during this part of the exam, and external pressure and changing the patient position to either right lateral or supine will help with advancement.

Hepatic Flexure

The hepatic flexure is often recognized by the large blue shadow from the liver (especially in thin patients) (Figure 4-24). As one advances through the transverse colon, the hepatic flexure comes into view, often with a variable amount of pooling liquid stool. If the flexure turn is very acute, the novice endoscopist often mistakes this "fools cecum" for the true one, believing that they are at the end of

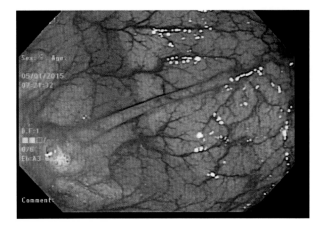

FIGURE 4-24. Hepatic flexure: note the *blue shadow* from the liver. There is usually a sharp turn which can be quite difficult to negotiate.

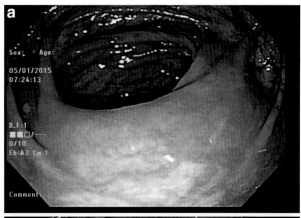

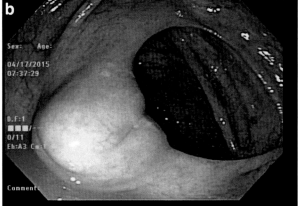

FIGURE 4-25. Different appearance of the ileocecal valve. (**a**) Flat and subtle. (**b**) Polypoid and obvious.

the colon. As with any other turn or flexure, if the scope is straight, advancement will be easier than if a loop is formed proximally. Often, one can gently push through a loop and get into the ascending colon and then reduce the loop. At other times, the examiner may find it useful to use air suction and abdominal pressure techniques to negotiate this turn. Another technique previously mentioned, involves having the patient take a deep breath of air to push the diaphragm down, and thus, the scope down into the ascending colon.

Ascending Colon and Ileocecal Valve

As the scope advances past the hepatic flexure into the ascending colon, prevention of a new loop is critical, as any proximal loop at this point will make further advancement of the scope extremely difficult. Pushing through a loop in the ascending colon is not as successful as it is on the left side of the colon since there are many bowel loops to accommodate before push pressure is transmitted to the end of the scope [67]. It can be very common to have the entire length of the scope inserted and there is still additional colon to traverse, due to inappropriate or minimal pleating techniques and the presence of loops. A change in patient position to either supine, right lateral, or prone coupled with the basic inser-tion techniques will prove to be extremely important in these situations and help advance the scope to the cecum.

The ileocecal valve is a fold at the base of the ascending colon that may appear as an obvious polypoid-like yellowish mass or can be totally hidden (Figure 4-25a, b). When the valve is not easily recognizable, the presence of gas, stool, or bile flowing from it is helpful to aid in its identification.

Cecum

The complete colonoscopic examination is ensured when the cecum has been reached. This blind sac is characterized by the "crow's foot" which is made up of the muscular arrange-ment of the colonic wall and the crescent or circular shaped appendicle orifice (Figure 4-26a, b). These landmarks are extremely important in quality assurance of a complete examination and photodocumentation is mandatory. Relying on trans-illumination of the scope through the abdominal wall in the right lower quadrant can be deceptive and is inad-equate evidence of a complete examination. Careful and detailed examination of the entire cecum is important due to the fact that many cecal lesions, including serrated adenomas are flat or recessed and can be quite deceptive and easily missed with a casual examination.

Ileocecal Valve Intubation

It is common for some endoscopists to routinely advance the endoscope into the terminal ileum. While it is considered a critical assessment when performing either an initial evaluation or follow-up for Crohn's disease, or in a search for obscure bleeding, it is unclear the precise role of routine visu-alization of the terminal ileum on colonoscopy. It is a skill, and the ability of the endoscopist to perform the maneuver improves with practice. The technique involves first remov-ing any loops from the colonoscope, as significant looping of the instrument make entering the ileum much more techni-cally challenging. The edge of the ileocecal valve is hooked with the curved endoscope and the scope is then gently inserted into the ileum when the lumen is visualized (Figure 4-27). The intubation of the ileum confirms a complete colonoscopic evaluation and this confirmation can often be a frustrating endeavor for beginning endoscopist [68].

In an assessment of the ileal intubation learning curve, 50 procedures was the benchmark, but once learned could

be accomplished in most patients in less than 1 min [69]. The addition of routine ileoscopy to screening colonoscopy has been demonstrated to detect asymptomatic small bowel carcinoid tumors and has led some to argue that this should be considered part of the endoscopic examination [70]. A large study at the Mayo Clinic involving over 6000 patients however did not validate this. Terminal ileum intubation showed gross abnormalities in only 1% of the patients, and pathologic abnormalities were identified for only 0.3% of the patients. These authors concluded that intubation of the terminal ileum should not be a required part of screening colonoscopy [71].

Terminal Ileum

If the endoscopist chooses to intubate the ileum, it is easily recognizable by its granular appearance and its increased motility (Figure 4-28). Quite often in younger patients, there will be innumerable lymphoid follicles that may resemble small polyps. The scope should be advanced as far as it is

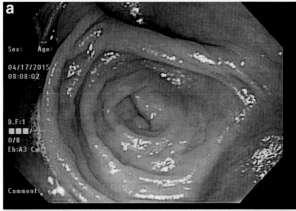

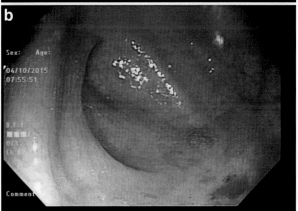

FIGURE 4-26. Reaching and proper identification of the cecum is compulsory for a complete examination. (**a**) Round appendiceal orifice with associated crow's foot. (**b**) Crescent shaped appendiceal orifice.

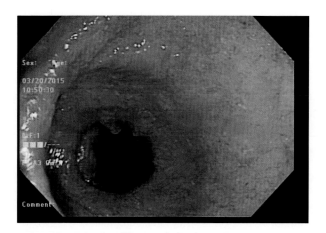

FIGURE 4-28. Terminal ileum: note the granular mucosa and the fine muscular folds.

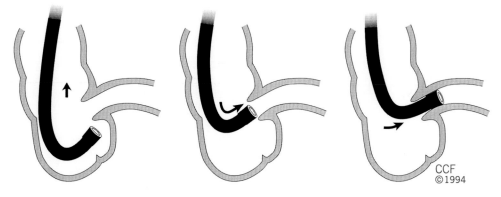

FIGURE 4-27. Intubation of the ileocecal valve: identification of the orifice, impacting the scope while giving air insufflation and then waiting for the bowel to relax before advancement into the terminal ileum. Reprinted with permission, Cleveland Clinic Center for Medical Art & Photography ©2015. All Rights Reserved.

comfortable and appropriate biopsies taken when needed. One should try to keep air insufflation to a minimum during this portion of the examination.

Alternate Techniques

CO₂ Insufflation

Two alternatives to traditional air infusion colonoscopy are water-assisted colonoscopy and insufflation with Carbon Dioxide. Due to the fact that CO_2 is more rapidly expelled from the colon than air, the hypothesis is that due to this rapid diffusion, there will be decreased pain associated with CO_2 infusion compared to air. Some evaluations have been consistent with this [72] hypothesis, while others have not shared these findings [73]. Due to the paucity of literature documenting efficacy, the technique must be considered experimental at this point.

Water Insufflation

The second method shows more promise. It involves the infusion of water without air and subsequent suctioning either during the insertion or withdrawal of the endoscope [74]. It has been demonstrated in limited studies that the use of water-assisted colonoscopy has a positive effect on patients, predominantly with lower levels of pain during the procedure [75, 76]. In addition, one study demonstrated that water immersion colonoscopy prevented loop formation in the sigmoid colon [77]. In a meta-analysis of nine studies, warm water infusion was demonstrated to be less painful than standard air insufflation, while reducing the need for sedation or analgesia during the procedure. There is a higher incomplete colonoscopy rate with this technique, however, and the endoscopist must consider this if considering employing this technique [78]. Interestingly when the methods of water insufflation and CO_2 insufflation are compared to each other, there is no significant reduction in either moderate or severe pain with either technique, compared with patients receiving no sedation [79].

Chromocolonoscopy (Chromoendoscopy)

Chromocolonoscopy involves the use of dye with spray catheters to spray coat the colonic mucosa in an attempt to increase the visualization of the mucosa. The dye enhances delineation, thereby aiding the endoscopist in differentiating between small structures, especially small and flat neoplastic lesions that are hard to recognize with traditional endoscopy. There has been some demonstrated benefit with this technology in high-risk populations such as those with inflammatory bowel disease or those with known genetic disorders [80, 81], due to the difficulty in differentiating abnormal from normal mucosa in some of these patients. The technology

has primarily demonstrated an increase in the yield of small polyps in the general population, however. Due to this lack of clinical significance in the population as a whole, there is a questioning of the necessity for widespread application of the technique [82].

High Definition/NBI Endoscopy

High definition endoscopes with wider angle viewing capability have the ability to increase the magnification and the visualization in endoscopy. High definition endoscopy has not proven superior in the ability to detect additional colon neoplasms, however [83]. Narrow Bandwidth Imaging (NBI) uses a filter to narrow the blue and green wave light and eliminates the red wavelength from standard white light. This leads to an accentuation of the microvasculature and improved visualization of pathology. The endoscopist is able to rapidly switch between white light and NBI views with the use of a foot pedal [84]. It has been noted in small studies that using NBI technology there is an increase in the number of adenomatous polyps detected [85]. In addition surface patterns differentiation between hyperplastic and adenomatous polyps is enhanced [86]. Due to this ability to better predict histology, NBI technology may play a role in the future resection and discarding of diminutive polyps, but it has not received widespread acceptance.

Full Spectrum Endoscopy

Full spectrum endoscopy uses three cameras, with the two additional cameras located adjacent to the scope's tip. This allows simultaneous viewing of all three cameras, which the endoscopist has from three adjacently located monitors. This colonoscopy platform has been demonstrated to be feasible, usable, and safe [87]. Despite the impressive visualization that is gained from the additional cameras, at this point, there is no proven benefit regarding increased adenoma detection, making it only a viable alternative to traditional endoscope technology [88].

Retroflexion

Many endoscopists routinely perform retroflexion, or the turning of the endoscope back upon itself in a U shape, in order to obtain a better view than with straight viewing. There is sparse data on either the benefits or the risks associated with the routine use of retroflexion of the endoscope in the rectum. There is one study that using the retroflexion technique with sigmoidoscopy increases adenoma detection [89]. Other studies cast some doubt on this. In one study of over 450 patients, in only 9 cases did the retroflex view identifiable pathology—predominantly hyperplastic polyps [90]. In another study of over 1500 patients, only 7 polyps were visualized solely by retroflexion. Six of these were hyperplastic and one was a

4 mm sessile tubular adenoma [91]. More concerning than a low yield is a higher rectal perforation rate reported associated with the technique [92]. The procedure can undoubtedly be performed safely, and some experts tout that it provides valuable information and photodocumentation of benign disease at the rectal outlet such as hemorrhoids [93]. It is unclear if the limited data is worth any added risk.

There is some data that retroflexion performed in the ascending colon, may offer benefit, however. One study evaluating routine retroflexion in the right colon showed that it could be safely achieved in the majority of patients undergoing screening colonoscopy [94]. In addition retroflexion identified additional polyps, predominantly adenomas, increasing the polyp yield as well as the adenoma detection rate in one study [95]. Due to the concerns regarding missed lesions in the right colon, retroflexion in patients with polyps identified on initial forward viewing should be considered.

Complications

While the performance of colonoscopy is very safe with several million procedures performed every year with no untoward events—it is an invasive procedure and complications are possible. These should be discussed with the patient frankly and documented prior to the procedure. The complications can be broadly grouped into those relating directly form the procedure such as bleeding and perforation and those relating to the sedation involved with the procedure—primarily cardiac and pulmonary complications. The exact incidence of complications varies widely in the literature, from 4.0 for 10,000 colonoscopies [96] to 17.8 per 1000 procedures [97]. The incidence varies somewhat depending on what exactly is considered a complication, and looking only at serious complications, defined as those resulting in hospital admission within 30 days of the procedure occur with a rate of 1 per 1000 [98–100] to 5.0 per 1000 exams [101, 102].

Sedation Complications

There are obviously risks associated with the administration of any medication, particularly sedative medications. The reason for the monitoring guidelines outlined above is to monitor for just these risks [103]. The primary concerns regarding the administration of sedation revolve around the cardiac and pulmonary complications associated with these medicines.

Vasovagal/Cardiac Arrhythmia

A vasovagal reaction is a slowing of the heart rate, often accompanied by a drop in blood pressure. This is believed to reflect the stimulation of the vagus nerve. It is common during colonoscopy and has been reported to occur in up to 16% of cases [104]. It is most likely not related to sedation, however, as the occurrence is unrelated to sedative medication administration and [105] it more likely results from the distension of the bowel or from a relative hypovolemic state resulting from the bowel prep. A vasovagal reaction is typically self-limited, but should be addressed by colonoscopic aspiration of air and/or reduction of loops. It typically requires no medical intervention other than monitoring and IV fluid administration. True cardiac arrhythmias are uncommon in association with colonoscopy. While there are reports of life threatening cardiac dysrhythmias during the procedure, these are primarily from case reports [106, 107]. Cardiac arrhythmias occur in approximately 2% of patients while undergoing endoscopic procedures [108] but the vast majority of these require no medical intervention [109].

The administration of sedative medications, particularly midazolam does cause transient hypotension in 20% of patients, with ST-segment depression in 7% of them [110]. It has also been noted in patients undergoing endoscopy that there is evidence of cardiac arrhythmias in 16%, with ischemic changes noted in 4% of those [108]. The clinical significance of these changes is unclear, however, as these are only electrocardiographic abnormalities. When comparing patients not having a colonoscopy, the incidence of myocardial infarction or stroke is similar to patients undergoing colonoscopy [111], implying that the procedure does not place the patient at increased risk for a cardiac event. In addition, it has been demonstrated that endoscopic procedures are safe and beneficial in patients after recent MI and should be performed if necessary in this patient population [112]. Colonoscopy in patients with a recent myocardial infarction is associated with a higher rate of minor, transient, and primarily cardiovascular complications compared with control patients but is infrequently associated with major complications [113].

Pulmonary

The incidence of pulmonary complications is even less common than for cardiac events, and any evidence of pulmonary issues following a colonoscopy should prompt the endoscopist to consider the abdomen as the ultimate source. The majority of patients that are undergoing colonoscopy are older and patients over 80 have not surprisingly demonstrated higher rates of pulmonary complications [111]. There are reports of aspiration following the administration of sedative medications for colonoscopy [114], but this is a very uncommon event. In addition, there are also numerous reports of pneumothorax or pneumomediastinum, following a colonoscopy [115]. These events are most commonly related to an intra-abdominal perforation, however, and should prompt a quick investigation for that possibility [116].

Procedural Complications

Procedural complications such as bleeding, perforation, and post-polypectomy syndrome serve as the other broad classification of complications. There are reports of unusual occurrences such as colonoscopes becoming incarcerated in either inguinal or ventral hernias [117, 118], but these are extremely uncommon events and serve primarily to warn the practitioner that there is always something else that can go wrong with any procedure. All endoscopists should be aware of the more common risks associated with the endoscopy and attempt to mitigate them.

Splenic Injury

The incidence of splenic injury in association with a colonoscopy is uncommon but is something that many endoscopists will encounter. A comprehensive literature search identified just over 100 patients worldwide with this complication [119]. It is likely that it is a much more common occurrence, however, as most of the cases in the literature are severe and the patients reported typically are managed with splenectomy [120]. There are likely many more cases that are not reported that are managed nonoperatively or even go unrecognized. It is believed that the etiology of this injury is from traction and subsequent tearing of the splenocolic ligament during the procedure, with subcapsular hematoma the most common injury pattern seen [121]. Splenic rupture at colonoscopy usually presents with abdominal pain developing within the first 24 h [122], although patients can present anywhere from a few hours to several days following the procedure [123]. Selection criteria for operative management may be extrapolated from those used for the management of traumatic splenic injury, but while there are reports of using splenic embolization [124], as mentioned above, the majority of patients in the literature have required splenectomy.

Perforation

A perforation of the colon during a colonoscopy can be a devastating complication that can result in serious morbidity or mortality. While it is uncommon, endoscopists will likely encounter it at some point in their career. The exact incidence of perforation is difficult to precisely define, but it is much less than 1/1000 procedures, with rates of 0.012% [125] to 0.016% reported in large studies [126]. It is believed to be more common when the procedure is performed in a diseased colon such as in inflammatory bowel disease patients, but a large study of IBD patients showed a low perforation rate of 0.16% [127]. In most series attempting to examine the etiology of the complication, the incidence is as common when a biopsy is performed as from a diagnostic endoscopy alone [99, 128, 129].

There are three mechanisms believed to be responsible for colonoscopic perforation. The first is believed to be a mechanical perforation resulting from direct trauma from the colonoscope itself [130]. The most common anatomic site for perforation is the sigmoid colon, occurring in up to [131] 74% in some series [132]. This would be consistent with direct trauma, as the sigmoid is the narrowest and most tortuous section of the colon. The second mechanism is believed to be a result of barotrauma from air insufflation, and the ascending colon or cecum, which would be the most susceptible to this mechanism, is the second most common location for a perforation. However, one series that examined specifically patients that had a cecal perforation found that cecal pathology such as inflammation or ulceration contributed to the perforation in most of these patients [133]. The final etiology of perforation is believed to be from therapeutic procedures such as polypectomy or the dilation of strictures.

The management depends not only on the condition of the patient, but on what the etiology of the perforation is felt to be. If the patient presents acutely and has peritonitis, the management is relatively clear and the patient warrants an emergent celiotomy. If the patient had a therapeutic endoscopy, and is clinically stable, then an attempt at nonoperative management is acceptable. The management with bowel rest and IV antibiotics has been demonstrated to be successful in 13/21 patients in one series of patients, all of whom had a perforation resulting from a therapeutic colonoscopy [134]. Perforations from a diagnostic colonoscopy are likely larger and are less successfully managed with nonoperative treatment [135]. The operative management of colonoscopic perforations has evolved as well. As in the trauma literature, if the patient requires surgical intervention, primary repair or resection with a primary anastomosis has proven to be an effective management strategy [132].

One emerging technology is the use of clips to manage a perforation that is either identified endoscopically or as prophylaxis when the endoscopist feels that the tissue has been thinned to the point that a perforation is likely. There are several case series reported in the literature with good results. A literature review of perforations managed with this technology show that if the clips were placed for a perforation during therapeutic colonoscopy it is successful in 69–93% of cases [136]. In one cohort of 27 patients with perforation from a therapeutic colonoscopy, the placement of clips resulted in successful nonoperative management in 25 of these patients [137]. In another review of 28 visible or suspected perforations, 13/19 evident and 8/9 suspected perforations underwent successful endoscopic closure with clips [138]. Clearly this technology has a place in the endoscopist's armamentarium, but should also be employed with surgical consultation, so that early decisions regarding operative management can be made.

Post-polypectomy Syndrome

Post-polypectomy syndrome is a spectrum of symptoms including abdominal pain, fever, leukocytosis, peritoneal tenderness, and guarding, following a colonoscopic polypectomy.

It is believed to be the result of an electrocoagulation injury to the colonic wall, thereby creating a transmural burn with localized peritoneal inflammation, but without evidence of perforation. It has carried several other monikers as well, including post-polypectomy coagulation syndrome and transmural burn syndrome. Typically patients present several days following a colonoscopy with fever, localized abdominal pain, and leukocytosis and may have localized peritoneal signs on physical examination. The majority of these patients do not require surgical treatment and are usually adequately managed with bowel rest, intravenous hydration, broad-spectrum parenteral antibiotics until symptoms resolution [139]. In one series, all patients were successfully managed medically without the need for surgery, with a median hospitalization of 5 days [140]. In an attempt to identify risk factors, one study found that polyp size greater than 2 cm and the presence of hypertension were the largest risk factors [141], but any patient who undergoes a polypectomy with cautery is at risk.

Bleeding

Bleeding following a polypectomy is the most common serious complication following a colonoscopy and patients should be given specific written instructions regarding the actions they should take if it should occur. It is estimated that significant bleeding, requiring a patient to seek medical care, occurs in over [142] 3% of all colonoscopic polypectomies, with significant bleeding in over 1% [143–146]. While bleeding can happen immediately when the polyp is removed, this is typically dealt with by the endoscopist at the time of the procedure [147]. Clinically significant hemorrhage typically manifests itself 4–6 days following the procedure when there is clot dissolution [145].

There have been several studies attempting to elucidate those patients at higher risk for this complication. A difficult colonoscopy with procedural bleeding is one group of patients at higher risk [148]. Hypertension has also been noted to be not only a risk for bleeding, but for increasing the interval between the polypectomy and hemorrhage [149] In addition, patients on anticoagulation medications are not surprisingly at higher risk, with 34% of patients in one series having been recently restarted on their anticoagulant medications [145]. While there is an increased risk with anticoagulants, surprisingly, this risk is not seen with aspirin, NSAIDS, or other antiplatelet medications [150]. The size of the polyps excised is the most consistent predictor of delayed hemorrhage after a polypectomy [151]. It is much more common with larger polyps. Polyps greater than 2.0 cm diameter were noted to experience bleeding 3.8% of the time, compared to 0.3% when the polyps removed were smaller than 2 cm in one study [148]. In addition to the absolute size, the risk is noted to increase by 13% for every 1 mm increase in polyp diameter. While polyp size correlates with bleeding, the type of polyp either sessile or pedunculated has not been demonstrated to be a risk factor [152]. The location

of the polyp has, however, with polyps located in the right colon more susceptible to bleeding [153]. Microscopic examination of the vascular supply of resected polyps reveal that sessile and thick-stalked pedunculated polyps are supplied with more vessels than other polyps. Patients with polyps larger than 17 mm, pedunculated polyps with a stalk diameter >5 mm obviously place the patient at higher risk [154]. The endoscopist should obviously recognize those patients that are at highest risk for post-procedural bleeding and counsel them appropriately.

The initial management of a patient with post-polypectomy bleeding is identical to any other patient with intestinal bleeding. The patient should have coagulation parameters measured and resuscitation should be based upon hemodynamic parameters. There are no specific transfusion triggers with post-polypectomy bleeding, but advanced age is predictive of a patient receiving a transfusion [155]. Almost all patients can be managed with a repeat endoscopy and rarely are operative or other interventions necessary, although angiographic embolization has been demonstrated to be effective in the management of post-polypectomy bleeding [156]. The endoscopist should be familiar with advanced endoscopic hemostatic techniques for these procedures, or consult an experienced colleague.

As with the management of perforation above, endoscopic clipping has been demonstrated beneficial in patients at increased risk for post-polypectomy hemorrhage. In one evaluation of polyps 2 cm or larger, there was a significantly decreased rate of post-procedure bleeding when the site was prophylactically clipped [157]. In addition, clipping has been shown to be beneficial in anticoagulated patients with lesions larger than 1 cm who were able to undergo successful polypectomy without interrupting the anticoagulation or antiplatelet medications [158].

Infectious Complications

A word of caution should be made regarding the extremely rare infectious complications associated with endoscopy. Although it is uncommon, it is associated with sensationalistic press coverage when it does occur. The endoscopist should have a basic understanding of the process involved in the cleaning of the endoscopes and endoscopic equipment, as the majority of infectious complications result from breaches in cleaning procedures. In one survey of endoscopy centers, it was found that a significant number of centers did not conform to guidelines regarding the cleaning, processing and care of endoscopes [159]. A separate study found that several of the guidelines are inconsistent with one another, making it difficult to determine which guideline to follow [160]. *Salmonella*, *Pseudomonas*, and *Mycobacterium* species are the most commonly transmitted organisms associated with endoscopic equipment [161] and the ability of these bacteria to form biofilms on the inner channel surfaces is believed to contribute to their ability to survive the decontamination process [162]. There have recently been reports of Carbapenem-resistant organisms associated with endoscopy as well [163]. The endoscopist should always be vigilant regarding the equipment used and ensure that proper protocols are in place and are being followed.

Training and the Use of Simulation

The training of medical personnel to safely and adequately perform colonoscopy is obviously critical. The criteria of what constitutes adequate training is controversial, however. Gastroenterologists perform the vast majority of colonoscopies and there are understandably differences in the manner in which different specialists, either gastroenterologists or surgeons educate and evaluate their trainees in performing procedures. Most of the literature on the topic involves gastroenterology fellows, and tends to focus on the number of procedures necessary in order to achieve competency. Surgical trainees obviously spend more time throughout their education learning procedural skills and it is doubtful that the two groups can be adequately compared regarding the speed or alacrity with which they learn procedures. It is unlikely that there will ever be a consensus on what constitutes adequate training. What is clear is that colonoscopy is a critical element in the treatment of the patient with colorectal disease and the colorectal surgeon must continue to be involved and have a voice in the education of the next generation of endoscopists.

The ability to perform a colonoscopy is undoubtedly a skill and as with any skill, the ability to perform it improves with repetition. It is a point of contention exactly how many of these repetitions a trainee must perform. In evaluating first year gastroenterology fellows, it was found that the ability to intubate the cecum successfully improved and reached the requisite standard of competence—defined as completing the task greater than 90% of the time and within 20 min after 150 procedures had been performed [164]. When comparing first and third year gastroenterology fellows, it was found that competence improved throughout training but an independent completion rate of 90% was not obtained until after 500 colonoscopies were performed [165]. As with the ability to technically perform the procedure, quality metrics improve with experience as well. In one study, the adenoma detection rate (ADR) increased by year of training [166]. Another study however showed that from the beginning of their education, trainees were able to provide high-quality investigations, again using ADR as the quality indicator benchmark [167]. In one of the few comparisons between gastroenterology and surgery trainees, there was a disparity in endoscopic performance between trainees favoring the gastroenterology trainees [168]. A different study showed that following the use of endoscopy simulation surgery residents were capable of performing colonoscopy equivalent to their gastroenterology counterparts using quality metrics as the benchmark [169].

Simulation

The practice of endoscopy lends itself well to simulation, yet it has not been fully embraced. While surgical simulation is difficult to portray, basic endoscopy skills are well illustrated. Due to the myriad of surgical procedures that are performed and the manner in which they are performed, it is difficult to incorporate surgical simulation into the educational curriculum. Endoscopy, lends itself much better to simulation. The improvement of trainees using simulation is most noticeable during the beginning of their endoscopic experience [170]. Following a 6-h colonoscopy simulation, trainees were noted to significantly outperform those who did not have the training but these advantages are negligible after approximately 30 procedures on patients [171].

Despite this reported advantage, the technology has not received widespread adoption in gastroenterology training. In a survey of active gastroenterology fellows, they noted that while half of the programs have endoscopic simulators, only 15% are required to use them prior to performing endoscopy on patients [172]. In a review of program directors, this was confirmed with 15% requiring their fellows to use simulation prior to clinical cases, with only one program having a minimum number of hours required in simulation training. The majority of the program directors felt that there is a need for endoscopic simulator training [173]. The reasons for a lack of embracing simulation are unclear. An attractive method to increase the quality of colonoscopy performance and to increase the skill levels of trainees without excessive numbers of procedures is the incorporation of endoscopy simulation into the curriculum of training programs that train endoscopists.

Documentation and Quality

Documentation

After completion of the procedure it is important to adequately document any findings as well as any adjunctive procedures that were performed at the time. It is imperative to photodocument any lesions or areas that were biopsied, as well as the endoscopists interpretation of these lesions. An attempt to place the location anatomically should be made, as the distance of the inserted colonoscopy can vary greatly depending upon looping and can vary depending on whether the measurement was taken on insertion or while the endoscope was being withdrawn. In addition, if any lesion was biopsied, or if a polyp was excised, the note should document whether the excision was complete or whether there was grossly abnormal tissue remaining.

A Multi-Society Task Force on Colorectal Cancer developed a consensus-based set of data points that reflected what should be included in any colonoscopy report (Table 4-3) [174].

TABLE 4-3. Recommended elements in standard colonoscopy report

---

Documentation of informed consent

Facility where endoscopy performed

Patient demographics and history

Age/sex

Receiving anticoagulation: if yes, document management plan

Need for antibiotic prophylaxis: if yes, document reason and management plan

Assessment of patient risk and comorbidity

ASA classification

Indication(s) for procedure

   Procedure: technical description

      Procedure date and time

      Procedure performed with additional qualifiers (CPT codes, polypectomy, etc.)

      Sedation: medications given and by the type of provider responsible

      Level of sedation (conscious, deep, general anesthesia)

      Extent of examination by anatomic segment: cecum, ascending colon, etc.

      If cecum is not reached, provide reason

      Method of documentation: i.e., photo of ileocecal valve and/or appendiceal orifice

      Time of examination: scope was inserted, withdrawal started, when withdrawn from patient

      Retroflexion in rectum (yes/no)

      Bowel prep: type of preparation, quality, adequate or inadequate to detect polyps >5 mm

      Technical performance: not technically difficult or examination difficult

      Patient discomfort/looping/need for special maneuvers including turning patient

      Type of instrument used: model and instrument number

Colonoscopic findings

   Colonic masses or polyp(s)

      Anatomic location: length/size (mm)

      Descriptors: pedunculated/sessile/flat/obstructive (% of lumen reduced)/ulcerated

      Biopsy obtained: hot/cold or snare/tattoo (if performed)

      Fulguration or ablation with cautery

      Completely removed (yes/no)/retrieved (yes/no)/sent to pathology (yes/no)

   Mucosal abnormality

      Suspected diagnosis: ulcerative colitis, Crohn's, ischemia, infection

      Anatomic location/extent/pathology obtained (yes/no)

   Other findings

Diverticulosis/arteriovenous malformations/hemorrhoids

Assessment

   Follow-up plan

      Immediate follow-up/further tests, referrals/medication changes

      Follow-up appointments and recommendation for follow-up colonoscopy and tests

      Documentation of communication directly to the patient and referring physician

   Pathology

      Pathology results reviewed, communicated with referring provider with recommendation for follow-up and communicated with patient

---

Adapted from Lieberman D, Nadel M et al. Standardized colonoscopy reporting and data system: report of the Quality Assurance Task Group of the National Colorectal Cancer Roundtable. Gastrointest Endosc 2007 May;65(6):757–66 (17)

There are numerous commercially available software programs that allow rapid and accurate documentation and these guidelines will look familiar to any provider who has utilized these systems. Unfortunately, the very ease of these programs and their check-box design allow trainees or busy professionals to perform documentation that is inadequate. In one study involving both community hospitals and academic centers several deficiencies in reporting were identified. For example, bowel preparation quality was reported in only 20%, but more concerning, the description of polyp appearance was present in only in 34% of notes [175]. In another study, photodocumentation was often missing and the size and morphology of polyps was present in only slightly more than 60% of cases [176]. Other studies show a consistent lack of documenting the quality of the bowel preparation, lack of documentation of the cecal landmarks as well as poor procedural interpretation [177, 178]. Clearly physicians who perform these procedures must not only ensure that the procedure is done well and safely, but that it is properly documented and these findings are relayed to the patient and any other treating physicians.

Quality

There is increasing attention to quantifiable measures of quality in medicine, and colonoscopy lends itself well to metric analysis and therefore there has been a great deal of attention paid to these performance measures [179]. Almost 14 million colonoscopies are performed annually in the USA and there is understandably a great deal of attention paid to quality associated with the procedure. The five most frequently cited quality measures are cecal intubation rate, adherence to recommended screening and surveillance interval, adenoma detection rate, quality of bowel preparation, and colonoscopy withdrawal time [180]. While some of these elements are addressed elsewhere in this text, is imperative that surgeons remain involved in these discussions and the continuing quest for quality improvement for our profession and for our patients.

PillCam Endoscopy

The advent of PillCam endoscopy (PCE) has revolutionized the evaluation of the small intestine. It allows the clinician to evaluate this portion of the intestine that was previously relegated to inaccurate or uncomfortable studies such as small bowel radiographic series or enteroclysis. The procedure is most commonly used in patients with occult gastrointestinal bleeding or in the search for other small bowel pathology, such as insipient tumors, polyposis syndromes, or Crohn's disease [181]. It typically is performed after an upper and lower endoscopic examination has already been completed; however, it can complement the latter as well, as in at least one study 28% of abnormalities identified on PCE were within the area normally covered by an endoscopic exam [182]. The use of PillCam endoscopy is easy to perform and learn and is a natural adjunct in the endoscopists' armamentarium. Capsule endoscopy does not require a bowel preparation, but most patients are instructed to remain either NPO or on a clear liquid diet for 10–12 h prior to the procedure. The patient swallows the disposable capsule, which then transmits images wirelessly to a recorder, and the clinician can review the images at a time when it is convenient to spend the 15–60 min, on average, for image viewing and documentation [183].

PillCam endoscopy has been demonstrated to play a significant role in Crohn's disease, where the small intestine is difficult to visualize radiographically. While there are concerns for evaluating patients with stricturing Crohn's disease, as the capsule can be retained at the location of a stricture [184, 185], this is typically less of a concern for a surgeon contemplating operative management and can serve as a

marker of stricture location enabling the procedure to be performed with minimally invasive techniques. PCE has resulted in medication changes in up to 60% of patients in some studies and [186] has proven superior to other imaging modalities in identifying obscure sources of intestinal bleeding and is beneficial in the localization of small bowel neoplasms [187, 188]. In addition, there is data that PCE may play a role in screening for colonic neoplasm, or in the evaluation of large intestinal inflammatory bowel disease. It is clear that the uses for this technology will only expand and physicians who treat intestinal disease will have to be familiar with the technology [189].

Summary

The endoscopic evaluation of the patient with colorectal complaints is essential in both the diagnosis and management of the patient. It allows the physician to visually assess the entirety of the intestinal tract and should not be thought of as a separate entity, but as an adjunct in the examination of the colorectal patient. These techniques should be familiar to the colorectal surgeon, and surgeons should continue to play a role in the testing, training, and advancement of endoscopic techniques and technology.

References

1. Ashburn J, Church J. Open sesame revisited. Am J Gastroenterol. 2013;108(1):143. doi:10.1038/ajg.2012.382.
2. Farmer KC, Church JM. Open sesame: tips for traversing the anal canal. Dis Colon Rectum. 1992;35(11):1092–3.
3. Nivatvongs S, Fryd DS. How far does the proctosigmoidoscope reach? A prospective study of 1000 patients. N Engl J Med. 1980;303(7):380–2.
4. Gibertson VA. Proctosigmoidoscopy and polypectomy in reducing the incidence of rectal cancer. Cancer. 1974;34(3 suppl):936–9.
5. Nelson RL, Abcarian H, Prasad ML. Iatrogenic perforation of the colon and rectum. Dis Colon Rectum. 1982;25(4):305–8.
6. Christensen AF, Nyhuus B, Nielsen MB, Christensen H. Three-dimensional anal endosonography may improve diagnostic confidence of detecting damage to the anal sphincter complex. Br J Radiol. 2005;78(928):308–11.
7. Xhaja X, Church J. The use of ancillary techniques to aid colonoscope insertion. Surg Endosc. 2014;28(6):1936–9.
8. Kann BR, Margolin DA, Brill SA, et al. The importance of colonoscopy in colorectal surgeons' practices: results of a survey. Dis Colon Rectum. 2006;49(11):1763–7.
9. Juillerat P, et al. EPAGE II. Presentation of methodology, general results and analysis of complications. Endoscopy. 2009;41:240–6.
10. Gimeno-García AZ, Quintero E. Colonoscopy appropriateness: really needed or a waste of time? World J Gastrointest Endosc. 2015;7(2):94–101.
11. Chan TH, Goh KL. Appropriateness of colonoscopy using the ASGE guidelines: experience in a large Asian hospital. Chin J Dig Dis. 2006;7(1):24–32.

12. Suriani R, Rizzetto M, Mazzucco D, et al. Appropriateness of colonoscopy in a digestive endoscopy unit: a prospective study using ASGE guidelines. J Eval Clin Pract. 2009;15(1):41–5.

13. Gimeno García AZ, González Y, Quintero E, et al. Clinical validation of the European Panel on the Appropriateness of Gastrointestinal Endoscopy (EPAGE) II criteria in an open-access unit: a prospective study. Endoscopy. 2012;44(1):32–7.

14. Petruzziello L, Hassan C, Alvaro D, et al. Appropriateness of the indication for colonoscopy: is the endoscopist the 'gold standard'? J Clin Gastroenterol. 2012;46(7):590–4.

15. Eskeland SL, Dalén E, Sponheim J, et al. European panel on the appropriateness of gastrointestinal endoscopy II guidelines help in selecting and prioritizing patients referred to colonoscopy—a quality control study. Scand J Gastroenterol. 2014;49(4):492–500.

16. Zuccaro G. Treatment and referral guidelines in gastroenterology. Gastroenterol Clin North Am. 1997;26:845–57.

17. Cappell MS, Ghandi D, Huh C. A study of the safety and clinical efficacy of flexible sigmoidoscopy and colonoscopy after recent colonic surgery in 52 patients. Am J Gastroenterol. 1995;90:1130–4.

18. Froelich F, Wietlisbach V, Gonvers JJ, et al. Impact of colonic cleansing on quality and diagnostic yield of colonoscopy: the European Panel of Appropriateness of Gastrointestinal Endoscopy European multicenter study. Gastrointest Endosc. 2005;61(3):378–84.

19. Kao D, Lalor E, Sandha G, et al. A randomized controlled trial of four precolonoscopy bowel cleansing regimens. Can J Gastroenterol. 2011;25(12):657–62.

20. Markowitz GS, Stokes MB, Radhakrishnan J, et al. Acute phosphate nephropathy following oral sodium phosphate bowel purgative: an underrecognized cause of chronic renal failure. J Am Soc Nephrol. 2005;16:3389–96.

21. Markowitz GS, Perazella MA. Acute phosphate nephropathy. Kidney Int. 2009;76:1027–34.

22. Cohen LB. Advances in bowel preparation for colonoscopy. Gastrointest Endosc Clin N Am. 2015;25(2):183–97.

23. Brunelli SM, Lewis JD, Gupta M, et al. Risk of kidney injury following oral phosphosoda bowel preparations. J Am Soc Nephrol. 2007;18:3199–205.

24. Hookey LC, Depew WT, Vanner SJ. A prospective randomized trial comparing low-dose oral sodium phosphate plus stimulant laxatives with large volume polyethylene glycol solution for colon cleansing. Am J Gastroenterol. 2004;99(11):2217–22.

25. Gurudu SR, Ramirez FC, Harrison ME, et al. Increased adenoma detection rate with system-wide implementation of a split-dose preparation for colonoscopy. Gastrointest Endosc. 2012;76(3):603–8.e1.

26. Kilgore TW, Abdinoor AA, Szary NM, et al. Bowel preparation with split-dose polyethylene glycol before colonoscopy: a meta-analysis of randomized controlled trials. Gastrointest Endosc. 2011;73(6):1240–5.

27. Enestvedt BK, Tofani C, Laine LA, et al. 4-Liter split-dose polyethylene glycol is superior to other bowel preparations, based on systematic review and meta-analysis. Clin Gastroenterol Hepatol. 2012;10(11):1225–31.

28. Abuksis G, Mor M, Segal N, et al. A patient education program is cost-effective for preventing failure of endoscopic procedures in a gastroenterology department. Am J Gastroenterol. 2001;96(6):1786–90.

29. Johnson DA, Barkun AN, Cohen LB, et al. Optimizing adequacy of bowel cleansing for colonoscopy: recommendations from the US multi-society task force on colorectal cancer. Gastroenterology. 2014;147(4):903–24.

30. Aronchick CA, Lipshutz WH, Wright SH, et al. A novel tableted purgative for colonoscopic preparation: efficacy and safety comparisons with Colyte and Fleet Phospho-Soda. Gastrointest Endosc. 2000;52:346–52.

31. Rostom A, Jolicoeur E. Validation of a new scale for the assessment of bowel preparation quality. Gastrointest Endosc. 2004;59(4):482–6.

32. Calderwood AH, Schroy PC, Lieberman DA, et al. Boston Bowel Preparation Scale scores provide a standardized definition of adequate for describing bowel cleanliness. Gastrointest Endosc. 2014;80(2):269–76.

33. Gerard DP, Foster DB, Raiser MW, et al. Validation of a new bowel preparation scale for measuring colon cleansing for colonoscopy: the Chicago bowel preparation scale. Clin Transl Gastroenterol. 2013;4:e43.

34. Clark BT, Rustagi T, Laine L. What level of bowel prep quality requires early repeat colonoscopy: systematic review and meta-analysis of the impact of preparation quality on adenoma detection rate. Am J Gastroenterol. 2014;109(11):1714–23.

35. Chokshi RV, Hovis CE, Hollander T, et al. Prevalence of missed adenomas in patients with inadequate bowel preparation on screening colonoscopy. Gastrointest Endosc. 2012;75(6):1197–203.

36. Poon CM, Lee DW, Mak SK, et al. Two liters of polyethylene glycol-electrolyte lavage solution versus sodium phosphate as bowel cleansing regimen for colonoscopy: a prospective randomized controlled trial. Endoscopy. 2002;34(7):560–3.

37. Barclay RL. Esophagogastroduodenoscopy-assisted bowel preparation for colonoscopy. World J Gastrointest Endosc. 2013;5(3):95–101.

38. Patanè S. Is there a need for bacterial endocarditis prophylaxis in patients undergoing gastrointestinal endoscopy? J Cardiovasc Transl Res. 2014;7(3):372–4.

39. Wilson W, Taubert KA, Gewitz M, et al. Prevention of infective endocarditis: guidelines from the American Heart Association: a guideline from the American Heart Association Rheumatic Fever, Endocarditis, and Kawasaki Disease Committee, Council on Cardiovascular Disease in the Young, and the Council on Clinical Cardiology, Council on Cardiovascular Surgery and Anesthesia, and the Quality of Care and Outcomes Research Interdisciplinary Working Group. Circulation. 2007;116:1736–54.

40. Duval X, Delahaye F, Alla F, et al. Temporal trends in infective endocarditis in the context of prophylaxis guideline modifications: three successive population-based surveys. J Am Coll Cardiol. 2012;59(22):1968–76.

41. Dayer MJ, Jones S, Prendergast B, et al. Incidence of infective endocarditis in England, 2000–13: a secular trend, interrupted time-series analysis. Lancet. 2014. doi:10.1016/S0140-6736(14)62007-9.

42. Banerjee S, Shen B, Baron TH, et al. Antibiotic prophylaxis for GI endoscopy. Gastrointest Endosc. 2008;67:791–8.

43. Zuckerman MJ, Hirota WK, Adler DG, et al. ASGE guideline: the management of low-molecular-weight heparin and non-aspirin antiplatelet agents for endoscopic procedures. Gastrointest Endosc. 2005;61:189–94.

44. Khashab MA, Chithadi KV, Acosta RD, et al. Antibiotic prophylaxis for GI endoscopy. Gastrointest Endosc. 2015;81(1):
81–9.

45. Piraino B, Bernardini J, Brown E, et al. ISPD position statement on reducing the risks of peritoneal dialysis-related infections. Perit Dial Int. 2011;31:614–30.

46. Meyer GW, Artis AL. Antibiotic prophylaxis for orthopedic
prostheses and GI procedures: report of a survey. Am
J Gastroenterol. 1997;92:989–91.

47. Anderson MA, Ben-Menachem T, Gan SI, et al. Management
of antithrombotic agents for endoscopic procedures.
Gastrointest Endosc. 2009;70:1060.

48. Fujimoto K, Fujishiro M, Kato M, et al. Guidelines for gastroenterological endoscopy in patients undergoing antithrombotic treatment. Dig Endosc. 2014;26:1–14.

49. Ridolfi TJ, Valente MA, Church JM. Achieving a complete
colonic evaluation with incomplete colonospcy is worth the
effort. Dis Colon Rectum. 2014;57:383–7.

50. Baxter NN, Goldwasser MA, Paszat LF, Saskin R, Urbach
DR, Rabeneck L. Association of colonoscopy and death from
colorectal cancer. Ann Intern Med. 2009;150:1–8.

51. Church JM. Complete colonoscopy: how often? And if not,
why not? Am J Gastroenterol. 1994;89:556–60.

52. Rizek R, Paszat LF, Stukel TA, Saskin R, Li C, Rabeneck
L. Rates of complete colonic evaluation after incomplete colo-
noscopy and their associated factors: a population-based study.
Med Care. 2009;47:48–52.

53. Kao KT, Tam M, Sekhon H, Wijeratne R, Haigh PI, Abbas MA.
Should barium enema be the next step following an incomplete
colonoscopy? Int J Colorectal Dis. 2010;25:1353–7.

54. Toma J, Paszat LF, Gunraj N, Rabeneck L. Rates of new or
missed colorectal cancer after barium enema and their risk factors: a population-based study. Am J Gastroenterol. 2008;
103:3142–8.

55. Baron JP, Hirota TH, Waring WK, et al. Guidelines for conscious sedation and monitoring during gastrointestinal endoscopy. Gastrointest Endosc. 2003;58(3):317.

56. Lee DW, Li AC, Ko CW, et al. Use of a variable-stiffness colonoscope decreases the dose of patient-controlled sedation during colonoscopy: a randomized comparison of 3 colonoscopes.
Gastrointest Endosc. 2007;65(3):424–9.

57. Faulx AL, Vela S, Das A, et al. The changing landscape of
practice patterns regarding unsedated endoscopy and propofol
use: a national Web survey. Gastrointest Endosc. 2005;62(1):
9–15.

58. Porostocky P, Chiba N, Colacino P, et al. A survey of sedation
practices for colonoscopy in Canada. Can J Gastroenterol.
2011;25(5):255–60.

59. Loberg M, Furholm S, Hoff I, et al. Nitrous oxide for analgesia
in colonoscopy without sedation. Gastrointest Endosc.
2011;74(6):1347–53.

60. Aboumarzouk OM, Agarwal T, Syed Nong Chek SA et al.
Nitrous oxide for colonoscopy. Cochrane Database Syst Rev
2011;(8):CD008506.

61. Tuncali B, Pekcan YO, Celebi A, et al. Addition of low-dose
ketamine to midazolam-fentanyl-propofol-based sedation for
colonoscopy: a randomized, double-blind, controlled trial.
J Clin Anesth. 2015;27:301–6.

62. Childers RE, Williams JL, Sonnenberg A. Practice patterns of
sedation for colonoscopy. Gastrointest Endosc. 2015;82(3):
503–11.

63. Singh H, Poluha W, Cheung M et al. Propofol for sedation during colonoscopy. Cochrane Database Syst Rev 2008;(4):
CD006268.

64. Wang D, Chen C, Chen J, et al. The use of propofol as a sedative agent in gastrointestinal endoscopy: a meta-analysis.
PLoS One. 2013;8(1):e53311.

65. Bright E, Roseveare C, Dalgleish D, et al. Patient-controlled
sedation for colonoscopy: a randomized trial comparing
patient-controlled administration of propofol and alfentanil
with physician-administered midazolam and pethidine.
Endoscopy. 2003;35(8):683–7.

66. Ulmer BJ, Hansen JJ, Overley CA, et al. Propofol versus mid-
azolam/fentanyl for outpatient colonoscopy: administration by
nurses supervised by endoscopists. Clin Gastroenterol Hepatol.
2003;1(6):425–32.

67. Church JM. Colonoscopy. In: Church JM, editor. Endoscopy
of the colon, rectum, and anus. New York: Igaku-Shoin; 1995.
p. 99–135.

68. Cirocco WC, Rusin LC. The reliability of cecal landmarks
during colonoscopy. Surg Endosc. 1993;7(1):33–6.

69. Iacopini G, Frontespezi S, Vitale MA, et al. Routine ileoscopy
at colonoscopy: a prospective evaluation of learning curve and
skill-keeping line. Gastrointest Endosc. 2006;63(2):250–6.

70. Ten Cate EM, Wong LA, Groff WL, et al. Post-surgical surveillance of locally advanced ileal carcinoids found by routine
ileal intubation during screening colonoscopy: a case series.
J Med Case Rep. 2014;8:444.

71. Kennedy G, Larson D, Wolff B, et al. Routine ileal intubation
during screening colonoscopy: a useful maneuver? Surg
Endosc. 2008;22(12):2606–8.

72. Uraoka T, Kato J, Kuriyama M, et al. CO(2) insufflation for
potentially difficult colonoscopies: efficacy when used by less
experienced colonoscopists. World J Gastroenterol. 2009;
15(41):5186–92.

73. Chen PJ, Li CH, Huang TY, et al. Carbon dioxide insufflation
does not reduce pain scores during colonoscope insertion in
unsedated patients: a randomized, controlled trial. Gastrointest
Endosc. 2013;77(1):79–89.

74. Leung FW. Water-aided colonoscopy. Gastroenterol Clin
North Am. 2013;42(3):507–19.

75. Church JM. Warm water irrigation for dealing with spasm during colonoscopy: simple, inexpensive, and effective.
Gastrointest Endosc. 2002;56(5):672–4.

76. Miroslav V, Klemen M. Warm water immersion vs. standard
air insufflation for colonoscopy: comparison of two techniques. Hepatogastroenterology. 2014;61(136):2209–11.

77. Asai S, Fujimoto N, Tanoue K, et al. Water immersion colonoscopy facilitates straight passage of the colonoscope through
the sigmoid colon without loop formation: randomized
controlled trial. Dig Endosc. 2015;27(3):345–53.

78. Rabenstein T, Radaelli F, Zolk O. Warm water infusion
colonoscopy: a review and meta-analysis. Endoscopy. 2012;
44(10):940–51.

79. Garborg K, Kaminski MF, Lindenburger W, et al. Water
exchange versus carbon dioxide insufflation in unsedated
colonoscopy: a multicenter randomized controlled trial.
Endoscopy. 2015;47(3):192–9.

80. Bartel MJ, Picco MF, Wallace MB. Chromocolonoscopy.
Gastrointest Endosc Clin N Am. 2015;25(2):243–60.

81. Huneburg R, Lammert F, Rabe C, et al. Chromocolonoscopy
detects more adenomas than white light colonoscopy or

narrow band imaging colonoscopy in hereditary nonpolyposis colorectal cancer screening. Endoscopy. 2009;41(4): 316–22.

82. Kahi CJ, Anderson JC, Waxman I, et al. High-definition chromocolonoscopy vs. high-definition white light colonoscopy for average-risk colorectal cancer screening. Am J Gastroenterol. 2010;105(6):1301–7.

83. Pellise M, Fernandez-Esparrach G, Cardenas A, et al. Impact of wide-angle, high-definition endoscopy in the diagnosis of colorectal neoplasia: a randomized controlled trial. Gastroenterology. 2008;135(4):1062–8.

84. Singh R, Mei SC, Sethi S. Advanced endoscopic imaging in Barrett's oesophagus: a review on current practice. World J Gastroenterol. 2011;17(38):4271–6.

85. Rastogi A, Early DS, Gupta N, et al. Randomized, controlled trial of standard-definition white-light, high-definition white-light, and narrow-band imaging colonoscopy for the detection of colon polyps and prediction of polyp histology. Gastrointest Endosc. 2011;74(3):593–602.

86. Rastogi A, Keighley J, Singh V, et al. High accuracy of narrow band imaging without magnification for the real-time characterization of polyp histology and its comparison with high-definition white light colonoscopy: a prospective study. Am J Gastroenterol. 2009;104(10):2422–30.

87. Gralnek IM, Segol O, Suissa A, et al. A prospective cohort study evaluating a novel colonoscopy platform featuring full-spectrum endoscopy. Endoscopy. 2013;45(9):697–702.

88. Gralnek IM, Siersema PD, Halpern Z, et al. Standard forward-viewing colonoscopy versus full-spectrum endoscopy: an international, multicentre, randomised, tandem colonoscopy trial. Lancet Oncol. 2014;15(3):353–60.

89. Hanson JM, Atkin WS, Cunliffe WJ, et al. Rectal retroflexion: an essential part of lower gastrointestinal endoscopic examination. Dis Colon Rectum. 2001;44(11):1706–8.

90. Cutler AF, Pop A. Fifteen years later: colonoscopic retroflexion revisited. Am J Gastroenterol. 1999;94(6):1537–8.

91. Saad A, Rex DK. Routine rectal retroflexion during colonoscopy has a low yield for neoplasia. World J Gastroenterol. 2008;14(42):6503–5.

92. Quallick MR, Brown WR. Rectal perforation during colonoscopic retroflexion: a large, prospective experience in an academic center. Gastrointest Endosc. 2009;69(4):960–3.

93. Rex DK, Vemulapalli KC. Retroflexion in colonoscopy: why? where? when? how? what value? Gastroenterology. 2013; 144(5):882–3.

94. Kushnir VM, Oh YS, Hollander T, et al. Impact of retroflexion vs. second forward view examination of the right colon on adenoma detection: a comparison study. Am J Gastroenterol. 2015;110(3):415–22.

95. Chandran S, Parker F, Vaughan R, et al. Right-sided adenoma detection with retroflexion versus forward-view colonoscopy. Gastrointest Endosc. 2015;81(3):608–13.

96. Niv Y, Gershtansky Y, Kenett RS, et al. Complications in colonoscopy: analysis of 7-year physician-reported adverse events. Eur J Gastroenterol Hepatol. 2011;23(6):492–8.

97. Chan AO, Lee LN, Chan AC, Ho WN, Chan QW, Lau S, Chan JW. Predictive factors for colonoscopy complications. Hong Kong Med J. 2015;21(1):23–9.

98. Stock C, Ihle P, Sieg A, et al. Adverse events requiring hospitalization within 30 days after outpatient screening and nonscreening colonoscopies. Gastrointest Endosc. 2013;77(3):419–29.

99. Ko CW, Riffle S, Michaels L, et al. Serious complications within 30 days of screening and surveillance colonoscopy are uncommon. Clin Gastroenterol Hepatol. 2010;8(2):166–73.

100. Castro G, Azrak MF, Seeff LC, Royalty J. Outpatient colonoscopy complications in the CDC's Colorectal Cancer Screening Demonstration Program: a prospective analysis. Cancer. 2013;119 Suppl 15:2849–54.

101. Levin TR, Zhao W, Conell C, et al. Complications of colonoscopy in an integrated health care delivery system. Ann Intern Med. 2006;145(12):880–6.

102. Nelson DB, McQuaid KR, Bond JH, et al. Procedural success and complications of large-scale screening colonoscopy. Gastrointest Endosc. 2002;55(3):307–14.

103. Alam M, Schuman BM, Duvernoy WF, et al. Continuous electrocardiographic monitoring during colonoscopy. Gastrointest Endosc. 1976;22:203.

104. Herman LL, Kurtz RC, McKee KJ, et al. Risk factors associated with vasovagal reactions during colonoscopy. Gastrointest Endosc. 1993;39(3):388–91.

105. Da Silva RM. Syncope: epidemiology, etiology, and prognosis. Front Physiol. 2014;5:471.

106. Davison ET, Levine M, Meyerowitz R. Ventricular fibrillation during colonoscopy: case report and review of the literature. Am J Gastroenterol. 1985;80:690–3.

107. Ugajin T, Miyatani H, Momomura S, et al. Ventricular fibrillation during colonoscopy: a case report—colonoscopy in high-risk patients should be performed with ECG monitoring. Intern Med. 2008;47(7):609–12.

108. Gupta SC, Gopalswamy N, Sarkar A, et al. Cardiac arrhythmias and electrocardiographic changes during upper and lower gastrointestinal endoscopy. Mil Med. 1990;155(1):9–11.

109. Eckardt VF, Kanzler G, Schmitt T, Eckardt AJ, Bernhard G. Complications and adverse effects of colonoscopy with selective sedation. Gastrointest Endosc. 1999;49(5):560–5.

110. Ristikankare M, Julkunen R, Mattila M, et al. Conscious sedation and cardiorespiratory safety during colonoscopy. Gastrointest Endosc. 2000;52(1):48–54.

111. Day LW, Kwon A, Inadomi JM, Walter LC, Somsouk M. Adverse events in older patients undergoing colonoscopy: a systematic review and meta-analysis. Gastrointest Endosc. 2011;74(4):885–96.

112. Cena M, Gomez J, Alyousef T, et al. Safety of endoscopic procedures after acute myocardial infarction: a systematic review. Cardiol J. 2012;19(5):447–52.

113. Cappell MS. Safety and efficacy of colonoscopy after myocardial infarction: an analysis of 100 study patients and 100 control patients at two tertiary cardiac referral hospitals. Gastrointest Endosc. 2004;60(6):901–9.

114. Lois F. An unusual cause of regurgitation during colonoscopy. Acta Anaesthesiol Belg. 2009;60(3):195–7.

115. Webb T. Pneumothorax and pneumomediatinum during colonoscopy. Anaesth Intensive Care. 1998;26:302–4.

116. Marwan K, Farmer KC, Varley C, Chapple KS. Pneumothorax, pneumomediastinum, pneumoperitoneum, pneumoretroperitoneum and subcutaneous emphysema following diagnostic colonoscopy. Ann R Coll Surg Engl. 2007;89(5):W20–1.

117. Koltun WA, Coller JA. Incarceration of colonoscope in an inguinal hernia. "Pulley" technique of removal. Dis Colon Rectum. 1991;3:191–3.

118. Leisser A, Delpre G, Kadish U. Colonoscope incarceration: an avoidable event. Gastrointest Endosc. 1990;36(6):637–8.

119. Singla S, Keller D, Thirunavukarasu P, et al. Splenic injury during colonoscopy—a complication that warrants urgent attention. J Gastrointest Surg. 2012;16(6):1225–34.

120. Kamath AS, Iqbal CW, Sarr MG, et al. Colonoscopic splenic injuries: incidence and management. J Gastrointest Surg. 2009;13(12):2136–40.

121. Michetti CP, Smeltzer E, Fakhry SM. Splenic injury due to colonoscopy: analysis of the world literature, a new case report, and recommendations for management. Am Surg. 2010;76(11):1198–204.

122. Ahmed A, Eller PM, Schiffman FJ. Splenic rupture: an unusual complication of colonoscopy. Am J Gastroenterol. 1997;92: 2101–4.

123. Petersen CR, Adamsen S, Gocht-Jensen P, et al. Splenic injury after colonoscopy. Endoscopy. 2008;40(1):76–9.

124. Stein DF, Myaing M, Guillaume C. Splenic rupture after colonoscopy treated by splenic artery embolization. Gastrointest Endosc. 2002;55:946–89.

125. Shi X, Shan Y, Yu E, et al. Lower rate of colonoscopic perforation: 110,785 patients of colonoscopy performed by colorectal surgeons in a large teaching hospital in China. Surg Endosc. 2014;28(8):2309–16.

126. Rathgaber SW, Wick TM. Colonoscopy completion and complication rates in a community gastroenterology practice. Gastrointest Endosc. 2006;64(4):556–62.

127. Buisson A, Chevaux JB, Hudziak H, et al. Colonoscopic perforations in inflammatory bowel disease: a retrospective study in a French referral centre. Dig Liver Dis. 2013;45(7):569–72.

128. Araujo SE, Seid VE, Caravatto PP, Dumarco R. Incidence and management of colonoscopic colon perforations: 10 years' experience. Hepatogastroenterology. 2009;56(96):1633–6.

129. Polter DE. Risk of colon perforation during colonoscopy at Baylor University Medical Center. Proc (Bayl Univ Med Cent). 2015;28(1):3–6.

130. Damore LJ, Rantis PC, Vernava AM, Longo WE. Colonoscopic perforations. Etiology, diagnosis, and management. Dis Colon Rectum. 1996;39(11):1308–14.

131. Korman LY, Overholt BF, Box T, Winker CK. Perforation during colonoscopy in endoscopic ambulatory surgical centers. Gastrointest Endosc. 2003;58(4):554–7.

132. Luning TH, Keemers-Gels ME, Barendregt WB, et al. Colonoscopic perforations: a review of 30,366 patients. Surg Endosc. 2007;21(6):994–7.

133. Foliente RL, Chang AC, Youssef AI, et al. Endoscopic cecal perforation: mechanisms of injury. Am J Gastroenterol. 1996;91:705–8.

134. Orsoni P, Berdah S, Verrier C, et al. Colonic perforation due to colonoscopy: a retrospective study of 48 cases. Endoscopy. 1997;29(3):160–4.

135. Avgerinos DV, Llaguna OH, Lo AY, Leitman IM. Evolving management of colonoscopic perforations. J Gastrointest Surg. 2008;12(10):1783–9.

136. Trecca A, Gaj F, Gagliardi G. Our experience with endoscopic repair of large colonoscopic perforations and review of the literature. Tech Coloproctol. 2008;12(4):315–21.

137. Magdeburg R, Collet P, Post S, et al. Endoclipping of iatrogenic colonic perforation to avoid surgery. Surg Endosc. 2008;22: 1500–4.

138. Yang DH, Byeon JS, Lee KH, et al. Is endoscopic closure with clips effective for both diagnostic and therapeutic colonoscopy-associated bowel perforation? Surg Endosc. 2010;24(5): 1177–85.

139. Kim HW. What is different between postpolypectomy fever and postpolypectomy coagulation syndrome? Clin Endosc. 2014;47(3):205–6.

140. Cha JM, Lim KS, Lee SH, et al. Clinical outcomes and risk factors of post-polypectomy coagulation syndrome: a multi-center, retrospective, case-control study. Endoscopy. 2013; 45(3):202–7.

141. Lee SH, Kim KJ, Yang DH, et al. Postpolypectomy fever, a rare adverse event of polypectomy: nested case-control study. Clin Endosc. 2014;47(3):236–41.

142. Rabeneck L, Paszat LF, Hilsden RJ, et al. Bleeding and perforation after outpatient colonoscopy and their risk factors in usual clinical practice. Gastroenterology. 2008;135:1899–906.

143. Waye JD. Management of complications of colonoscopic polypectomy. Gastroenterologist. 1993;1(2):158–64.

144. Rosen L, Bub DS, Reed JF, Nastasee SA. Hemorrhage following colonoscopic polypectomy. Dis Colon Rectum. 1993; 36(12):1126–31.

145. Sawhney MS, Salfiti N, Nelson DB, et al. Risk factors for severe delayed postpolypectomy bleeding. Endoscopy. 2008;40(2):115–9.

146. Heldwein W, Dollhopf M, Rösch T, et al. The Munich Polypectomy Study (MUPS): prospective analysis of complications and risk factors in 4000 colonic snare polypectomies. Endoscopy. 2005;37:1116–22.

147. Kim HS, Kim TI, Kim WH, et al. Risk factors for immediate postpolypectomy bleeding of the colon: a multicenter study. Am J Gastroenterol. 2006;101(6):1333–41.

148. Wu XR, Church JM, Jarrar A, et al. Risk factors for delayed postpolypectomy bleeding: how to minimize your patients' risk. Int J Colorectal Dis. 2013;28(8):1127–34.

149. Watabe H, Yamaji Y, Okamoto M, et al. Risk assessment for delayed hemorrhagic complication of colonic polypectomy: polyp-related factors and patient related factors. Gastrointest Endosc. 2006;64:73–8.

150. Hui AJ, Wong RM, Ching JY, et al. Risk of colonoscopic polypectomy bleeding with anticoagulants and antiplatelet agents: analysis of 1657 cases. Gastrointest Endosc. 2004;59:44–8.

151. Moon HS, Park SW, Kim DH, et al. Only the size of resected polyps is an independent risk factor for delayed postpolypectomy hemorrhage: a 10-year single-center case-control study. Ann Coloproctol. 2014;30(4):182–5.

152. Buddingh KT, Herngreen T, Haringsma J, et al. Location in the right hemi-colon is an independent risk factor for delayed post-polypectomy hemorrhage: a multi-center case-control study. Am J Gastroenterol. 2011;106(6):1119–24.

153. Choung BS, Kim SH, Ahn DS, et al. Incidence and risk factors of delayed postpolypectomy bleeding: a retrospective cohort study. J Clin Gastroenterol. 2014;48(9):784–9.

154. Dobrowolski S, Dobosz M, Babicki A, et al. Blood supply of colorectal polyps correlates with risk of bleeding after colonoscopic polypectomy. Gastrointest Endosc. 2006;63(7):1004–9.

155. Sorbi D, Norton I, Conio M, et al. Postpolypectomy lower GI bleeding: descriptive analysis. Gastrointest Endosc. 2000;51: 690–6.

156. Rossetti A, Buchs NC, Breguet R, et al. Transarterial embolization in acute colonic bleeding: review of 11 years of experience and long-term results. Int J Colorectal Dis. 2012;28:777–82.

157. Liaquat H, Rohn E, Rex DK. Prophylactic clip closure reduced the risk of delayed postpolypectomy hemorrhage: experience in 277 clipped large sessile or flat colorectal lesions and 247 control lesions. Gastrointest Endosc. 2013;77(3):401–7.

158. Katsinelos P, Fasoulas K, Chatzimavroudis G, et al. Prophylactic clip application before endoscopic resection of large pedunculated colorectal polyps in patients receiving anticoagulation or antiplatelet medications. Surg Laparosc Endosc Percutan Tech. 2012;22(5):e254–8.

159. Cheung RJ, Ortiz D, DiMarino AJ. GI endoscopic reprocessing practices in the United States. Gastrointest Endosc. 1999;50(3):362–8.

160. Muscarella LF. Inconsistencies in endoscope-reprocessing and infection-control guidelines: the importance of endoscope drying. Am J Gastroenterol. 2006;101(9):2147–54.

161. Spach DH, Silverstein FE, Stamm WE. Transmission of infection by gastrointestinal endoscopy and bronchoscopy. Ann Intern Med. 1993;118(2):117–28.

162. Kovaleva J, Peters FT, van der Mei HC, Degener JE. Transmission of infection by flexible gastrointestinal endoscopy and bronchoscopy. Clin Microbiol Rev. 2013;26(2):231–54.

163. Kola A, Piening B, Pape UF, et al. An outbreak of carbapenem-resistant OXA-48–producing Klebsiella pneumonia associated to duodenoscopy. Antimicrob Resist Infect Control. 2015;4:8.

164. Lee SH, Chung IK, Kim SJ, et al. An adequate level of training for technical competence in screening and diagnostic colonoscopy: a prospective multicenter evaluation of the learning curve. Gastrointest Endosc. 2008;67(4):683–9.

165. Spier BJ, Benson M, Pfau PR, et al. Colonoscopy training in gastroenterology fellowships: determining competence. Gastrointest Endosc. 2010;71(2):319–24.

166. Peters SL, Hasan AG, Jacobson NB, Austin GL. Level of fellowship training increases adenoma detection rates. Clin Gastroenterol Hepatol. 2010;8(5):439–42.

167. Klare P, Ascher S, Wagenpfeil S, et al. Trainee colonoscopists fulfil quality standards for the detection of adenomatous polyps. BMC Med Educ. 2015;15(1):312.

168. Leyden JE, Doherty GA, Hanley A, et al. Quality of colonoscopy performance among gastroenterology and surgical trainees: a need for common training standards for all trainees? Endoscopy. 2011;43(11):935–40.

169. Williams MR, Crossett JR, Cleveland EM, et al. Equivalence in colonoscopy results between gastroenterologists and general surgery residents following an endoscopy simulation curriculum. J Surg Educ. 2015;72(4):654–7.

170. Cohen J, Cohen SA, Vora KC, et al. Multicenter, randomized, controlled trial of virtual-reality simulator training in acquisition of competency in colonoscopy. Gastrointest Endosc. 2006;64:361–8.

171. Sedlack RE, Kolars JC. Computer simulator training enhances the competency of gastroenterology fellows at colonoscopy: results of a pilot study. Am J Gastroenterol. 2004;99:33–7.

172. Jirapinyo P, Imaeda AB, Thompson CC. Endoscopic training in gastroenterology fellowship: adherence to core curriculum guidelines. Surg Endosc. 2015;24:4110–4.

173. Jirapinyo P, Thompson CC. Current status of endoscopic simulation in gastroenterology fellowship training programs. Surg Endosc. 2015;29(7):1913–9.

174. Lieberman D, Nadel M, Smith RA, et al. Standardized colonoscopy reporting and data system: report of the Quality Assurance Task Group of the National Colorectal Cancer Roundtable. Gastrointest Endosc. 2007;65(6):757–66.

175. Singh H, Kaita L, Taylor G, et al. Practice and documentation of performance of colonoscopy in a central Canadian health region. Can J Gastroenterol Hepatol. 2014;28(4):185–90.

176. Beaulieu D, Barkun A, Martel M. Quality audit of colonoscopy reports amongst patients screened or surveilled for colorectal neoplasia. World J Gastroenterol. 2012;18(27):3551–7.

177. Robertson DJ, Lawrence LB, Shaheen NJ, et al. Quality of colonoscopy reporting: a process of care study. Am J Gastroenterol. 2002;97(10):2651–6.

178. De Jonge V, Sint Nicolaas J, Cahen DL, et al. Quality evaluation of colonoscopy reporting and colonoscopy performance in daily clinical practice. Gastrointest Endosc. 2012;75(1):98–106.

179. Bourikas LA, Tsiamoulos ZP, Haycock A, et al. How we can measure quality in colonoscopy? World J Gastrointest Endosc. 2013;5(10):468–75.

180. Ketwaroo GA, Sawhney MS. Quality measures and quality improvements in colonoscopy. Curr Opin Gastroenterol. 2015;31(1):56–61.

181. Hale MF, Sidhu R, McAlindon ME. Capsule endoscopy: current practice and future directions. World J Gastroenterol. 2014;20(24):7752–9.

182. Hoedemaker RA, Westerhof J, Weersma RK, et al. Non-small-bowel abnormalities identified during small bowel capsule endoscopy. World J Gastroenterol. 2014;20(14):4025–9.

183. Goenka MK, Majumder S, Goenka U. Capsule endoscopy: present status and future expectation. World J Gastroenterol. 2014;20(29):10024–37.

184. O'Donnell S, Qasim A, Ryan BM, et al. The role of capsule endoscopy in small bowel Crohn's disease. J Crohns Colitis. 2009;3(4):282–6.

185. Long MD, Barnes E, Isaacs K, et al. Impact of capsule endoscopy on management of inflammatory bowel disease: a single tertiary care center experience. Inflamm Bowel Dis. 2011;17(9):1855–62.

186. Dionisio PM, Gurudu SR, Leighton JA, et al. Capsule endoscopy has a significantly higher diagnostic yield in patients with suspected and established small-bowel Crohn's disease: a meta-analysis. Am J Gastroenterol. 2010;105(6):1240–8.

187. Triester SL, Leighton JA, Leontiadis GI, et al. A meta-analysis of the yield of capsule endoscopy compared to other diagnostic modalities in patients with obscure gastrointestinal bleeding. Am J Gastroenterol. 2005;100(11):2407–18.

188. Zagorowicz ES, Pietrzak AM, Wronska E, et al. Small bowel tumors detected and missed during capsule endoscopy: single center experience. World J Gastroenterol. 2013;19(47):9043–8.

189. Van Gossum A. Wireless capsule endoscopy of the large intestine: a review with future projections. Curr Opin Gastroenterol. 2014;30(5):472–6.

5

Endoscopic Management of Polyps, Polypectomy, and Combined Endoscopic and Laparoscopic Surgery

Kelly A. Garrett and Sang W. Lee

Key Concepts

- Colonoscopic polypectomy is the treatment of choice for diagnosing and removing most colon polyps.
- Operator variability influences the quality of colonoscopy for both detection and resection.
- Multiple questions remain about best practice techniques for colonoscopic polypectomy.
- EMR of colorectal lesions is safe and effective but results in piecemeal resection that may prevent accurate histological diagnosis. Colonoscopy surveillance is required to assess for and manage local recurrence of neoplasia.
- ESD is able to resect superficial lesions en bloc regardless of tumor size, location, and fibrosis. These advantages come at a cost of an increased risk of perforation, bleeding, and a longer procedure time as compared with EMR.
- Combined endo-laparoscopic surgery is an adjunct to endoscopic polypectomy that may help to avoid colectomy.

Introduction

It is estimated that 93,090 new cases of colon cancer will be diagnosed in the year 2015 with almost 50,000 estimated deaths due to colon cancer [1]. Although colon cancer is still the third most common cause of cancer related mortality in the USA, there has been a steady decline in the colorectal cancer incidence since the mid-1980s which is partially attributed to the introduction of colorectal cancer screening [2]. There has even been a more rapid decline in recent years (4% or greater per year from 2008 to 2011) which may be multifactorial but likely reflects the increased use of screening colonoscopy. Among adults aged 50–75 years, colonoscopy use increased from 19.1% in 2000 to 54.5% in 2013 [3].

Electronic supplementary material: The online version of this chapter (doi:10.1007/978-3-319-25970-3_5) contains supplementary material, which is available to authorized users.

Recently published data of the long-term follow-up from patients enrolled in the National Polyp Study provides evidence that colonoscopic removal of adenomatous polyps reduces colon cancer incidence and related mortality [4].

Colonoscopic polypectomy is the treatment of choice for diagnosing and removing most colon polyps. In the past decade, polypectomy technique, instrumentation, and evolution of endoscopy skills have improved polyp detection rates and the ability to remove polyps. Even so, large polyps or polyps in an anatomically difficult location can be challenging to remove endoscopically. Traditionally the most common recommendation for these patients has been to undergo a colon resection. Although the laparoscopic approach has reduced the morbidity of an abdominal operation, it still poses potential morbidities related to bowel resection. A combined approach using both laparoscopy and colonoscopy has more recently been described as an alternative to bowel resection in select patients with polyps that cannot be removed endoscopically. This chapter addresses endoscopic polypectomy—basic and advanced techniques and combined endoscopic endo-laparoscopic techniques.

Identification of Polyps

Although there is little dispute about the impact of colonoscopy, there remains marked variability in the quality of colonoscopy. Indicators of quality colonoscopy include cecal intubation, withdrawal time, and polyp detection rate [5]. The need for cecal intubation is based on the persistent finding that a substantial fraction of colorectal neoplasms are located in the proximal colon including the cecum. Low cecal intubation rates have been associated with higher rates of interval proximal colon cancers [6]. Colonoscopy studies in screening patients in the USA have reported cecal intubation rates of 97% or higher [7, 8]. As the detection of neoplastic lesions is the primary goal of most colonoscopic examinations, careful inspection of the mucosa is essential.

In 2002, the US Multi-Society Task Force on Colorectal Cancer recommended a withdrawal time (defined as the time from cecal intubation to the time the colonoscope is withdrawn out of the anus) of at least 6 min as an indicator of quality colonoscopy [9]. In 2006, Barclay et al. found a correlation between longer withdrawal time and an increased rate in the detection of adenomas [10]. There have been variations in the adenoma detection rates (ADR) and for this reason, targets for ADR have been recommended. The American Society for Gastrointestinal Endoscopy (ASGE) and the American College of Gastroenterology (ACG) recommends a minimum target for overall ADR of at least 25% based on the observation that higher ADRs were associated with a reduced risk of both proximal and distal cancer [11, 12].

Criteria for Polypectomy

Polyps occur in all parts of the colon. It is the current practice, that when polyps are detected that they should be removed as any adenomatous tissue visualized should be assumed to carry some malignant potential [13, 14]. It is widely accepted that more than 95% of colorectal cancers arise from adenomatous polyps [15, 16]. This adenoma-carcinoma sequence is well described and is often an indolent process that takes many years. Polyps are characterized by their size and morphology (pedunculated or sessile), which are two important features that may predict underlying malignancy and should guide how polyps are managed. As defined by the US National Polyp Study, an advanced adenoma is one that is ≥1 cm in size or contains high grade dysplasia or appreciable villous tissue. When screening colonoscopy is performed in average-risk, asymptomatic individuals over the age of 50, the prevalence of advanced adenomas ranges from 6 to 9% [7]. It is accepted that removal of large adenomas is advisable to prevent progression to colorectal cancer. The malignant potential of adenomas <0.5 cm is not as well studied. In order to determine the clinical significance of polyps <0.5 cm, a retrospective study from Vienna, 7590 adenomatous polyps from 4216 patients between 1978 and 1996 were analyzed. Size was the strongest predictor of advanced pathologic features. Advanced pathologic features were defined as high grade dysplasia or invasive cancer. The percentages of adenomas with advanced pathologic features were 3.4%, 13.5% and 38.5% for adenomas <0.5 cm, 0.5–1.0 cm and >1 cm respectively. Villous change, left sided location and age ≥60 were also associated with advanced pathologic features. No invasive cancer was found in any polyp ≤0.5 cm, but since 3.4% of these contained high-grade dysplasia, the authors recommended removal whenever possible [17]. Another study found that a small (≤0.5 cm) right sided polyp in a young patient (≤60 years of age) has only a 3.8% risk for containing advanced pathologic features whereas polyps in patients over age 60, in the presence of anemia, polyp size >1 cm, or left sided location as single or

combined parameters had a maximum predictive value of 75.4% for advanced adenomas [18].

There are several reasons why a polyp should not be removed during colonoscopy. If there are characteristics suspicious for malignancy and if its endoscopic appearance suggests penetration deeper than the submucosa, a polypectomy should not be performed. The characteristics of a polyp that may be indicative of malignancy are firmness or hardness, mucosal irregularity, vascular pattern on narrow band imaging, ulceration or central umbilication, large size, and if the polyp does not lift with submucosal injection [19, 20]. In these cases, one would consider biopsy of the polyp instead of removal. Large polyp size may be another reason to defer polypectomy. Large polyps in the cecum have a higher risk of perforation during resection, and therefore, one may consider doing a combined endo-laparoscopic approach. Finally, a polypectomy should not be performed if the risks outweigh the benefits. Examples of this would be any polyp in an asymptomatic patient whose life expectancy is less than 2 years (patients with terminal cancer), polyps discovered during unfavorable circumstances (patients undergoing workup for bleeding), patients with comorbidities or on medications that would make polypectomy too risky (anticoagulation) [19].

Polypectomy Techniques

Polypectomy is fundamental to the practice of colonoscopy. The principles of polypectomy are to remove all visible adenomatous tissue. There are many different techniques that are used in creating a wide variability in practice. Reasons for variability likely reflect the lack of standardized polypectomy protocols, difference in training and experience, mis-sizing of polyps, and concern regarding adverse events and time constraints [21].

Polypectomy is best performed with the polyp in the 5–7 o'clock position. Cold forceps biopsy is the simplest method of polypectomy. This is frequently used for diminutive lesions (polyps <5 mm). In a survey of 187 gastroenterologists, forceps removal was the resection technique of choice for lesions 1–3 mm in size [22]. The technique for polypectomy using cold biopsy forceps is simple. The biopsy forceps is passed through the biopsy channel of the colonoscope and the jaws are positioned over the polyp. The polyp tissue is grasped and removed. The forceps is removed for tissue retrieval [23]. This technique requires minimal manipulation, uses no electrocautery, and has an insignificant risk of perforation [24]. Frequently however, more than one bite is needed to remove all polypoid tissue. In addition, after the initial bite, minor bleeding can obscure the field, increasing the risk of leaving residual polyp behind. Biopsy and histologic evaluation of polypectomy sites after what was considered a complete cold forceps polypectomy can show residual polypoid tissue in 29–38% of specimens [25–27]. In addition, if two bites are taken in one pass, the tissue obtained with the first bite can become dislodged and get lost. Therefore, a single-bite polypectomy may be more efficient and decrease the risk of incomplete polypectomy. In comparing jumbo forceps (jaw volume 12.44 mm) to standard forceps (jaw volume 7.22 mm) in a randomized controlled trial, a trend toward a higher complete histologic eradication was noted with the jumbo forceps but this did not reach statistical significance [28].

Another method of removing small polyps is with the application of electrocautery to the forceps during tissue removal. The application of thermal energy fulgurates the base of the polyp while the specimen is protected in the jaws of the forceps [29]. There are several drawbacks to this technique, which have caused it to fall out of favor. There may be architectural distortion from thermal energy resulting in impaired histologic evaluation of the specimen [30]. This technique has also been associated with an increased risk of delayed bleeding and perforation in the right colon [31, 32]. It has also been suggested that the use of hot biopsy forceps is unreliable in completely removing all adenomatous tissue with 17% of polypectomy sites revealing persistent viable polyp remnants [33]. National societies recommend avoidance of hot biopsy forceps for polyps >5 mm and those in the right colon [34, 35].

Snare polypectomy is the preferred method for polypectomy among clinical gastroenterologists [22]. Once the instrument is passed through the working channel of the scope, the snare is extended from a plastic sheath and then passed around the base of the polyp. Once it is in proper position, the snare is closed transecting the base of the polyp. Advancing the catheter tip or sheath to the base of the polyp will avoid the snare from slipping back over the head of the polyp [23]. Snare polypectomy can be done with a cold technique or combined with electrocautery. It has been suggested that cold snaring is the preferred technique for all small (<10 mm) and most diminutive polyps but this has not been well studied [36, 37]. The technique of cold snaring allows for a resection of a 1–2 mm margin of normal tissue around the polyp. Bleeding is typically minor and not significant [38]. Several randomized controlled trials have shown that the risk of bleeding is similar between cold and hot snare polypectomy in lesions up to 8 mm and use of the cold snare may actually shorten procedure times [38–40]. The application of electrocautery with snare polypectomy is more common for larger polyps (>7–8 mm) and pedunculated polyps [21, 22, 41]. As previously stated, the polyp should optimally be in the 5–7 o'clock position and if it is a pedunculated polyp, one may consider repositioning the patient so the base of the polyp is not in a dependent position to make post-polypectomy bleeding easier to control. When using electrocautery, the polyp should be tented toward the center of the lumen to stretch the submucosa away from the muscularis propria and serosa. The duration of energy delivery should be minimized to prevent injury to the wall of the colon. For pedunculated polyps, the snare should be closed at a third or

halfway from the base of the polyp to ensure a sufficient stump to regrasp if there is immediate bleeding. Energy should be applied early and the snare should be closed slowly [23]. There are many different snare devices available and there are no trials to establish the advantage of one device over another. In a study looking at 147,174 subcentimeter polyps from the English Bowel Cancer Screening Program, pedunculated polyps were most commonly removed using hot snare (84.7%) although this technique was used somewhat less frequently in the right side of the colon than in the left side for all polyps sizes (69.6% vs. 88.3%, $p<0.001$). For non-pedunculated polyps, hot snare was also the most commonly used technique overall (29.2%) [21].

Endoscopic Mucosal Resection

Large polyps, those involving more than one third of the circumference of the colon or two haustral folds, or those with a flat or depressed morphology are more challenging to remove with the standard polypectomy technique. [42] Endoscopic mucosal resection (EMR) can assist in removal of these lesions that may otherwise require surgical intervention. EMR allows removal of superficial tumors of the gastrointestinal tract. This technique was originally described and popularized in Japan for the treatment of gastric and esophageal tumors. It was further described for removal of colorectal polyps that were not amenable to traditional endoscopic polypectomy techniques. Because the plane of resection of EMR is typically the middle to deep submucosal layer, compared with standard polypectomy, which normally provides resection at the mucosal layer, EMR offers the potential advantage of providing en bloc resection specimens for histopathologic analysis. Unfortunately however, EMR tends to result in piecemeal excision of polyps which can cause difficulty with histologic diagnosis, staging and evaluation of margins. In addition, in contrast to the stomach, the colon wall is much thinner which can lead to higher rates of complications, i.e., perforation. Indications for EMR include adenomas or small well differentiated carcinomas that are confined to the mucosa or with superficial invasion of the submucosa, polyps less than 1/3 the circumference of the lumen and flat or depressed polyps [42].

EMR is a modification of conventional snare polypectomy. A solution is injected into the submucosa beneath the lesion. This serves to elevate the mucosal layer that contains the lesion on a submucosal fluid cushion providing a safety zone for snare resection. Many different solutions have been used for injection including normal saline, hypertonic saline, 50% dextrose, glycerol solutions, hyaluronic acid, and diluted epinephrine solution. The ideal agent prolongs the "pillow effect" which decreases the risk of bleeding and perforation [42]. Once the lesion is raised, snare polypectomy is performed. For large lesions, piecemeal polypectomy is invariably required. The cap-assisted technique (EMRC) is

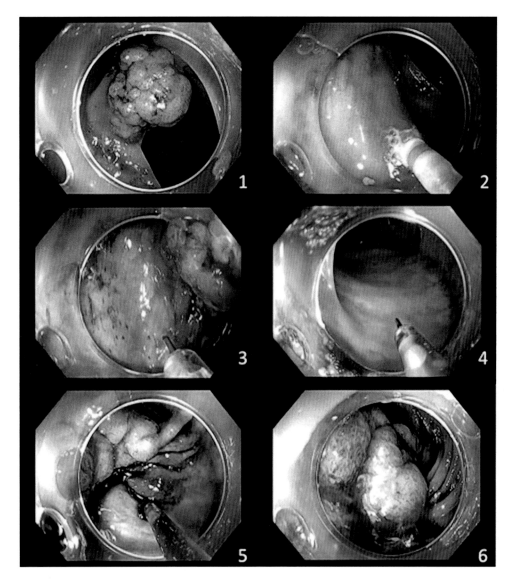

FIGURE 5-1. Illustration of piecemeal endoscopic mucosal resection. 1–6: mucosal lift by submucosal injection of indigo carmine.

another method used which involves a cap with a lip on the distal end. A snare is positioned around the lip of the cap and then the target mucosa is suctioned into the cap. Once the tissue is aspirated, the snare is then closed around the tissue (Figures 5-1 and 5-2). The benefits of this technique are reported better visualization and the possibility of resecting lesions in variable positions. The pressure of the cap on the wall of the colon allows flattening of the folds maximizing the view of interhaustral lesions. This technique is frequently performed in the stomach in Japan. EMRC is not as popular for colorectal polyps for fear of entrapping the muscularis propria into the snare, therefore increasing the risk of perforation [43].

EMR is limited by the difficulty in determining which lesions are likely to be confined to the mucosa. In a prospective, multicenter cohort, risk factors for submucosal invasion and

failure of successful EMR were identified. In their experience, risk factors for submucosal invasion were Paris classification 0-IIa+c morphology, non-granular surface morphology, or Kudo pit pattern type V (Tables 5-1 and 5-2). The presence of multiple risks factors magnified the risk of submucosal invasion [44]. In this study, EMR was attempted on 464 patients and successful in 89% of patients. Risk factors for failure included a prior attempt at EMR (OR=3.8; 95% CI: 1.77–7.94), difficult position (OR=2.17; 95%CI: 1.14–4.12) and ileocecal valve involvement (OR=3.38; 95%CI: 1.20–9.52).

EMR is effective and practical with good outcomes (Table 5-3). When performed by experts, anywhere from 3 to 7% of patients are referred for surgical resection because of inability to remove the polyp endoscopically [45, 46]. Approximately 44% of lesions are removed en bloc and the remaining are removed piecemeal [45]. Complication rates

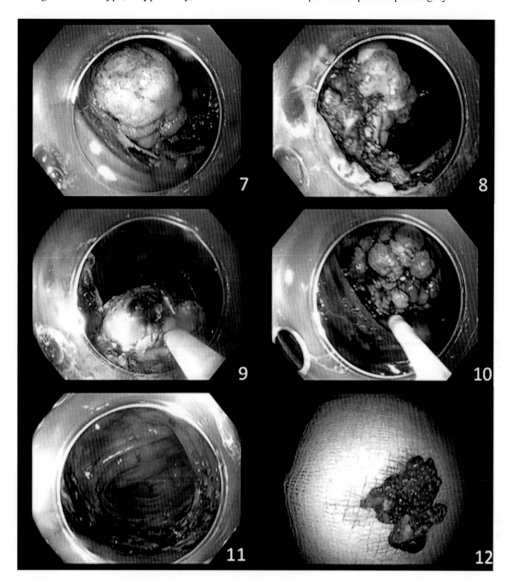

FIGURE 5-2. Illustration of piecemeal endoscopic mucosal resection. 7–10: Piecemeal hot snare polypectomy. 11: intact muscularis. 12: Removed specimen.

TABLE 5-1. Paris classification

Pedunculated	Ip
Subpedunculated	Isp
Sessile, higher than height of closed forceps (2.5 mm)	Is
Slightly elevated, below height of closed forceps (2.5 mm)	IIa
Completely flat lesion, does not protrude above mucosal surface	IIb
Slightly depressed, lower than mucosa but depth < 1.2 mm	IIc
Excavated/ulcerated, deep ulcer below mucosa below 1.2 mm	III

TABLE 5-2. Kudo pit pattern

Pit pattern type	Characteristics
I	Round pits
II	Stellar or papillary pits
III S	Small tubular or round pits (smaller than type I pits)
III L	Large tubular or round pits (larger than type I pits)
IV	Branch-like or gyrus-like pits
V	Irregular or non-structured pits (absence of pit pattern)

are low. Intraprocedural bleeding occurs in about 8% of patients, post-procedural bleeding in 0–1%, and perforation 1–2% [45, 46]. Local recurrence after EMR is variable and reported in up to 27% of cases [47]. In a multicenter, prospective study of 1000 consecutive patients treated with

EMR where the lesion was thought to have been completely treated, early recurrent/residual adenoma (4 months following EMR) was present in 16% and late recurrent/residual adenoma (16 months following EMR) was uncommon (4%). On multivariate analysis, risk factors for recurrence were

Table 5-3. Endoscopic mucosal resection

Author	Year	Polyps	Polyp size (cm)	Macroscopic classification	Operating time (min)	En bloc resection (%)	LOS (day)	Leakage/ fistula (%)	Postoperative bleeding (%)	Cancer (%)	Depth	Recurrence (%)
Gomez	2014	131	3.3	NA	NA	27	NA	3	2.3	7.6	Unknown	17
Maguire	2014	269	2.8	NA	NA	0	NA	1.3	3	16	Tis: 6.3%; T1: 9.3%	24
Knabe	2013	252	>2.0	Paris	NA	12	NA	1.6	1.6	3.2	Unknown	22
Buchner	2012	315	2.3	Paris	NA	54	<1	0.4	7.2	4.4	Unknown	27
Conio	2004	139	2.0	NA	NA	0	NA	0	0	12.2	Tis: 6; T1: 3; T2: 21.9 1	
Stergiou	2002	68	>3.0	Sessile/pedunculated	NA	38	NA	0	4	10	Unknown	29

LOS length of stay, Tis carcinoma in situ, NA not available

lesion size >4 cm, use of argon plasma coagulation to ablate adenomatous tissue and intraprocedural bleeding. The recurrent adenoma was usually unifocal and diminutive, and was managed endoscopically in 93% of cases [45]. Further reported risk factors for recurrence include granular appearance of the lesion and distal rectal lesions. Incomplete resection and resections with deep positive margins should be considered for surgery [48].

Endoscopic Submucosal Dissection

The technique of endoscopic submucosal dissection (ESD) developed for en bloc resection for large and ulcerative lesions in the stomach has been widely accepted in Japan for the treatment of early gastric cancer [49]. Compared with EMR, ESD has the advantage of definitively permitting an en bloc and therefore histologically complete resection. With this technique, one is able to resect superficial lesions regardless of tumor size, location, and fibrosis [50–52]. These advantages come at the cost of an increased risk of perforation, bleeding, and a longer procedure time as compared with EMR. [53]

As the major difference between surgical resection and endoscopic resection is the absence of lymph node dissection, endoscopic resection should only be considered in lesions that have an insignificant risk of lymph node metastasis. The risk of lymphatic disease is largely based on a tumor's depth of invasion, and hence, a large part of the evaluation is determining this. Therefore, the use of ESD for colorectal lesions has been limited to patients who have undergone accurate preoperative diagnosis. This technique is indicated when an en bloc resection cannot be done with EMR. It is also indicated for polyps with intramucosal to shallow submucosal invasion as well as lesions with submucosal fibrosis that cannot be lifted with submucosal injection during conventional EMR. It may also be indicated in sporadic localized tumors in conditions of chronic inflammation such as ulcerative colitis or local residual or recurrent early carcinomas after endoscopic resection [54]. Experience with ESD outside of Japan is still limited. In a consensus statement by a panel of experts, the goals of ESD remain: treating mucosal cancer, achieving an R0 resection, meeting quality standards, ensuring the procedure is performed by endoscopists trained in this technique and under institutional review board approval [55].

The technique of ESD is similar to EMR in that it involves a single channel scope and submucosal injection. The border of the lesion may first be marked out by injecting indigo carmine or using indigo carmine dye spray. A variety of solutions have been used for submucosal injection but the most common are normal saline, glycerol or hyaluronic acid. Normal saline is safe and widely available but the lift that it

creates is of short duration, which may come at a disadvantage. For safety in the thin walls of the colon, longer lasting solutions such as glycerol or hyaluronic acid are needed [56]. The optimal injection solution should achieve and maintain the necessary submucosal lifting height and duration, not influence the histological evaluation, not have tissue toxicity and be easily prepared and administrated [57]. Once the lesion is lifted, specialized endoscopic knives help to dissect out the lesion (Figure 5-3). There are a variety of knives available but the two traditional types of needle knives and insulted tip knives. Both types of knives are used in combination with electrocautery to dissect and separate the mucosal and submucosal layers. Bleeding is common during ESD, and therefore, management of bleeding is important for the procedure to be successful. Hemostasis is maintained using either monopolar or bipolar coagulation forceps, which can increase the risk of perforation or hemoclips, which can obstruct the plane of dissection [56].

Similar to new techniques elsewhere, ESD has a high learning curve. Compared with gastric lesions, ESD in the colon and rectum is more difficult due to anatomic features (thin wall, peristalsis, folds) and the position of the endoscopic is less stable especially outside of the rectum. Probst and colleagues divided their experience with ESD into three periods and demonstrated a clear learning curve over time with resection rates increasing and procedure times decreasing as expected. They suggest a learning curve of 25–50 cases [58]. Others have suggested 40 procedures are necessary to acquire skill in avoiding perforation and 80 cases to be proficient in resecting large colorectal lesions [59]. Successful en bloc resection may be as low as 60% in initial cases but increases up to 88–97% with experience [58–60]. Similarly, R0 resection rate improves with experience and is reported as high as 96% [58]. Procedural complications are higher than with EMR and consist of bleeding in 1.5–7.9% and perforation in up to 10.7% of cases (Table 5-4) [58, 60, 61]. Frequently, complications are successfully treated with endoscopic clipping. Follow up and surveillance after ESD should be case dependent. The aim of surveillance is to detect residual disease or recurrent disease early. The follow up plan should be based on whether resection was en bloc or piecemeal, the pathology of the lesion, risk factors for multiple lesions and underlying disease [54].

Combined Endo-Laparoscopic Surgery (CELS)

As previously discussed, large polyps or polyps within or behind a haustral fold can be very challenging to remove endoscopically. Although EMR and ESD are performed for

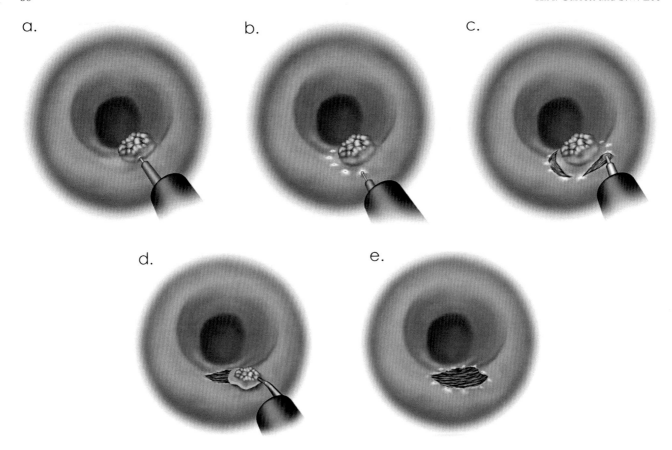

FIGURE 5-3. Steps of endoscopic submucosal dissection. (**a**) submucosal injection. (**b**) marking of the resection margin. (**c**) submucosal dissection using a needle knife. (**d**) extraction of specimen. (**e**) intact muscularis.

these polyps, these techniques are not widely available and require a high level of technical skill. Traditionally, the most common recommendation for these patients has been segmental colectomy—an oncologic resection. Although the laparoscopic approach can minimize the morbidity associated with colectomy, only a minority of the colon resections performed in the USA are being done laparoscopically [62]. Furthermore, even if a minimally invasive approach is used, it still entails a major abdominal operation with associated morbidities. Combined endo-laparoscopic surgery (CELS) has been described as an alternative to bowel resection in select patients.

Laparoscopic assisted polypectomy was first described in 1993 as a means to avoid bowel resection [63]. Larger retrospective studies have since been published indicating that the technique is safe and effective [64–69]. There are several ways in which laparoscopic assistance during colonoscopic polypectomy can be helpful: (1) the underlying colon can be invaginated to assist in snaring of a flat polyp, (2) laparoscopic mobilization of flexures and angulated colon can provide better access and exposure, and (3) full-thickness injury to the colon can be detected and repaired laparoscopically. Simultaneous performance of laparoscopy and colonoscopy can often present technical challenges. Insufflation using room air during colonoscopy can significantly obscure the laparoscopic view and compromise exposure. A technique of laparoscopically clamping the terminal ileum to minimize bowel distention has been described, but colonic distension is still a major impediment with this method [63, 64]. The use of carbon dioxide (CO_2) for insufflation during

TABLE 5-4. Endoscopic submucosal dissection

Author	Year	Polyps	Polyp size (cm)	Macroscopic classification	Operating time (min)	En bloc resection	LOS (day)	Perforation (%)	Postoperative bleeding (%)	R0 resection rate (%)	Cancer (%)	Depth	Recurrence (%)
Saito	2014	900	3.7	Paris	60	91	NA	2.7	1.7	87	74	Unknown	NA
Toyonaga	2014	468	3	NA	60	99	NA	1.5	1.5	NA	66	Tis: 49%; T1: 17%; T2: 0.4%	NA
Lee	2013	874	2.7	sessile/pedunculated	54	97	3.5	5.3	0.5	91.2	43	Tis: 28%; T1: 15%; T2: 0.2%	0.4
Yoshida	2013	530	3.1	protruding/superficial	93	91	NA	4.1	2.3	NA	54	Tis: 41%; T1: 12%	NA
Nakamura	2014	300	3.0	LST/ non-LST	90	91.7	5	1.7	5	91	99	M-SM-s: 92%; SM-d: 7%	NA

LOS length of stay, NA not available, Tis carcinoma in situ, M-SM-s mucosal or shallow submucosal invasion <1000 mcm from the muscularis mucosae, SM-d >1000 mcm of submucosal invasion

TABLE 5-5. Combined endo-laparoscopic surgery

Author	Year	Patients	Polyps	Polyp size, (cm)	Frozen section	Operating time (min)	Intraoperative complications (%)	Postoperative complications,%	Mortality (%)	LOS (days)	Tis (%)	Submucosal cancer (%)	Successful endoscopic resection (%)	Conversion to open surgery (%)	Prognosis (m=months)
Goh	2014	30	30	1.4	–	105 (75–125)	0	13.3	0	2.0	HGD 26.7	6.7	73	0	no recurrence at 20m
SW Lee	2013	75	75	3 (1–7)	if needed	145 (50–249)	0	9.2	0	1	HGD 9.3	6.7	74	3	10% recurrence at 65m
Wood	2011	13	16	3 (2–5)	all	NA	0	15	0	2	7.7		77	0	NA
Grunhagen	2011	11	12	2 (0.6–4.5)	–	45 (15–80)	0	18.1	0	1	9	0	82	0	no recurrences at 11m
Cruz	2011	25	25	2.4 (1–4)	–	92.7 (60–145)	0	8	0	1.5	8	4	76	0	NA
Agrawal	2010	19	19	0.6–6	all	35.3–37	0	5.6	0	0–14	5.3		58	NA	no recurrences at 3m
Wilhelm	2009	146	154	NA	–	100 (40–272)	1	25	0.7	8	11		73	5	Local recurrence of adenoma 0.9% at 35m
Franklin	2009	176	251	3.7 (2–6)	all	96.5	0	10	0	1.1	10.2		91	0	no recurrences at 65m

NA not available, HGD high grade dysplasia, Tis carcinoma in situ, LOS length of stay colonoscopy has been shown to be safe and can remedy this issue. CO_2 gas is absorbed approximately 150-times faster than room air so there is minimal unwanted distention of the colon providing excellent simultaneous endoscopic and laparoscopic visualization [70].

Consideration for CELS starts by reviewing the initial procedure report and photographs looking for any concerning signs of malignancy, such as ulceration and hypervascularity. Presence of high-grade dysplasia is concerning for malignancy but is not necessarily a contraindication to performing CELS. In our practice, prior to obtaining laparoscopic access to the abdomen, colonoscopy is performed and at that point, decision is made whether the polyp is resectable using colonoscopy alone or if laparoscopic assistance is needed (Video 5.1). If laparoscopic assistance is needed, then abdominal access is performed. The exact location of the polyp is determined by visualizing the tattoo mark and manipulating the polyp laparoscopically while visualizing the polyp endoscopically. For laterally and retroperitoneally located polyps, the colon needs to be mobilized. Polyps located on the mesenteric side may be difficult to visualize and laparoscopically repair in case of perforation. Once the polyp is identified intraluminally, using laparoscopic manipulation, the base of the polyp is exposed. The lesion can then be elevated further with submucosal injection. Malignancy is suspected with specific morphology (ulceration, central umbilication, or a vascular pattern on narrow-band imaging) or if the polyp does not lift up with injection. If there is no suspicion of malignancy, polypectomy is performed using snare and electrocautery. The wall of the colon can be invaginated laparoscopically to aid in optimal snaring of the polyp. While polypectomy is performed, the serosal aspect of the colon can be monitored for thermal related changes. If a full-thickness burn of perforation is even suspected, repair can be done intracorporeally. An air leak test can also be performed using insufflation with the colonoscope. If the polyp feels firm on palpation or seems in any way suspicious for malignancy after excision, an intraoperative frozen section can be performed. In select patients with cecal or right colon polyps, if the polyp is located on the anti-mesenteric side of the colon, a colonoscopic assisted laparoscopic wall excision can be performed using a laparoscopic stapler. When the stapler is placed across the bowel wall, colonoscopy can be used to monitor the margins of excision and the ileocecal valve when in the cecum.

Several published studies have similarly addressed this combined technique, considering it a safe and effective method to avoid colectomy and remove difficult polyps in many cases (Table 5-5). A large study describing a 10-year experience with the technique of combined laparoscopic endoscopic resection reported results on 146 patients with 156 lesions. The authors performed four separate techniques combining endoscopy and laparoscopy but only eight patients (5.4%) had laparoscopic-assisted endoscopic resection. Most of the patients (76.7%) underwent either an endoscopic-assisted transluminal resection, which was done through a colotomy. In addition, the mean length of stay was 8 days, which is long compared with other studies. This may have been due to the nature of the resections. There was also a 25% complication rate, which may have contributed to the prolonged length of stay. Although there was only a 0.9% local recurrence rate, with a follow up of 2.9 years [65]. One of the largest studies to date was reported by Franklin and Portillo describing the technique of laparoscopic-monitored colonoscopic polypectomy in 176 patients with excision of 251 polyps. The procedure was performed successfully in all but four patients (97.8%). This study was an update of two previous publications from their group in 2000 and 2007. In their practice, all specimens were sent for frozen section and ultimately, 18 (10.2%) patients required colectomy for cancer [71].

Overall, technical success rates for CELS are consistently reported between 74 and 97%. Postoperative complications are typically minor and less than 5%. Recurrence rates are low, reported in 10–15% and can typically be approached endoscopically or with CELS [65, 69, 70].

Conclusion

Polypectomy is fundamental to the practice of colonoscopy. A range of techniques is available and the choice of technique should be tailored to the size, site, and morphology of the polyp. There is a wide variation in practice. Advanced endoscopic techniques such as EMR, ESD, and combined endo-laparoscopic techniques provide options for patients with benign polyps not amenable to traditional endoscopic removal that would have otherwise undergone colon resection. Although polyp removal using these advanced techniques may be an effective alternative in select patients, they require both experience and expertise to become an available option in a surgeon's armamentarium [66, 70, 71].

References

1. Siegel RL, Miller KD, Jemal A. Cancer statistics, 2015. CA Cancer J Clin. 2015;65(1):5–29.
2. Edwards BK, Ward E, Kohler BA, et al. Annual report to the nation on the status of cancer, 1975–2006, featuring colorectal cancer trends and impact of interventions (risk factors, screening, and treatment) to reduce future rates. Cancer. 2010;116(3):544–73.
3. Centers for Disease Control and Prevention. National Center for Health Statistics. National heath interview surveys 2000, 2013. public use data files. Updated 2014.
4. Zauber AG, Winawer SJ, O'Brien MJ, et al. Colonoscopic polypectomy and long-term prevention of colorectal-cancer deaths. N Engl J Med. 2012;366(8):687–96.
5. Baker SL, Miller RA, Creighton A, Aguilar PS. Effect of 6-minute colonoscopy withdrawal time policy on polyp detection rate in a community hospital. Gastroenterol Nurs. 2015;38(2): 96–9.

6. Baxter NN, Sutradhar R, Forbes SS, Paszat LF, Saskin R, Rabeneck L. Analysis of administrative data finds endoscopist quality measures associated with postcolonoscopy colorectal cancer. Gastroenterology. 2011;140(1):65–72.

7. Lieberman DA, Weiss DG, Bond JH, Ahnen DJ, Garewal H, Chejfec G. Use of colonoscopy to screen asymptomatic adults for colorectal cancer. veterans affairs cooperative study group 380. N Engl J Med. 2000;343(3):162–8.

8. Rathgaber SW, Wick TM. Colonoscopy completion and complication rates in a community gastroenterology practice. Gastrointest Endosc. 2006;64(4):556–62.

9. Rex DK, Bond JH, Winawer S, et al. Quality in the technical performance of colonoscopy and the continuous quality improvement process for colonoscopy: recommendations of the U.S. multi-society task force on colorectal cancer. Am J Gastroenterol. 2002;97(6):1296–308.

10. Barclay RL, Vicari JJ, Doughty AS, Johanson JF, Greenlaw RL. Colonoscopic withdrawal times and adenoma detection during screening colonoscopy. N Engl J Med. 2006;355(24): 2533–41.

11. Corley DA, Jensen CD, Marks AR, et al. Adenoma detection rate and risk of colorectal cancer and death. N Engl J Med. 2014;370(14):1298–306.

12. Rex DK, Schoenfeld PS, Cohen J, et al. Quality indicators for colonoscopy. Gastrointest Endosc. 2015;81(1):31–53.

13. Chapuis PH, Dent OF, Goulston KJ. Clinical accuracy in the diagnosis of small polyps using the flexible fiberoptic sigmoidoscope. Dis Colon Rectum. 1982;25(7):669–72.

14. Neale AV, Demers RY, Budev H, Scott RO. Physician accuracy in diagnosing colorectal polyps. Dis Colon Rectum. 1987; 30(4):247–50.

15. Bujanda L, Cosme A, Gil I, Arenas-Mirave JI. Malignant colorectal polyps. World J Gastroenterol. 2010;16(25): 3103–11.

16. Molatore S, Ranzani GN. Genetics of colorectal polyps. Tech Coloproctol. 2004;8 Suppl 2:s240–2.

17. Gschwantler M, Kriwanek S, Langner E, et al. High-grade dysplasia and invasive carcinoma in colorectal adenomas: a multivariate analysis of the impact of adenoma and patient characteristics. Eur J Gastroenterol Hepatol. 2002;14(2):183–8.

18. Kulling D, Christ AD, Karaaslan N, Fried M, Bauerfeind P. Is histological investigation of polyps always necessary? Endoscopy. 2001;33(5):428–32.

19. Church J. Polyp treatment. In: Endoscopy of the colon, rectum and anus. 1st ed. Japan: Igaku-Shoin; 1995. p. 156–78.

20. Lee SW, Garrett KA, Shin JH, Trencheva K, Sonoda T, Milsom JW. Dynamic article: long-term outcomes of patients undergoing combined endolaparoscopic surgery for benign colon polyps. Dis Colon Rectum. 2013;56(7):869–73.

21. Din S, Ball AJ, Taylor E, Rutter M, Riley SA, Johal S. Polypectomy practices of sub-centimeter polyps in the English Bowel Cancer Screening Programme. Surg Endosc. 2015; 29(11): 3224-3230.

22. Singh N, Harrison M, Rex DK. A survey of colonoscopic polypectomy practices among clinical gastroenterologists. Gastrointest Endosc. 2004;60(3):414–8.

23. Kedia P, Waye JD. Colon polypectomy: a review of routine and advanced techniques. J Clin Gastroenterol. 2013;47(8): 657–65.

24. Rex DK. Preventing colorectal cancer and cancer mortality with colonoscopy: What we know and what we don't know. Endoscopy. 2010;42(4):320–3.

25. Woods A, Sanowski RA, Wadas DD, Manne RK, Friess SW. Eradication of diminutive polyps: a prospective evaluation of bipolar coagulation versus conventional biopsy removal. Gastrointest Endosc. 1989;35(6):536–40.

26. Efthymiou M, Taylor AC, Desmond PV, Allen PB, Chen RY. Biopsy forceps is inadequate for the resection of diminutive polyps. Endoscopy. 2011;43(4):312–6.

27. Liu S, Ho SB, Krinsky ML. Quality of polyp resection during colonoscopy: are we achieving polyp clearance? Dig Dis Sci. 2012;57(7):1786–91.

28. Draganov PV, Chang MN, Alkhasawneh A, et al. Randomized, controlled trial of standard, large-capacity versus jumbo biopsy forceps for polypectomy of small, sessile, colorectal polyps. Gastrointest Endosc. 2012;75(1):118–26.

29. Williams CB. Small polyps: the virtues and the dangers of hot biopsy. Gastrointest Endosc. 1991;37(3):394–5.

30. Monkemuller KE, Fry LC, Jones BH, Wells C, Mikolaenko I, Eloubeidi M. Histological quality of polyps resected using the cold versus hot biopsy technique. Endoscopy. 2004;36(5):432–6.

31. Vanagunas A, Jacob P, Vakil N. Adequacy of "hot biopsy" for the treatment of diminutive polyps: a prospective randomized trial. Am J Gastroenterol. 1989;84(4):383–5.

32. Savides TJ, See JA, Jensen DM, Jutabha R, Machicado GA, Hirabayashi K. Randomized controlled study of injury in the canine right colon from simultaneous biopsy and coagulation with different hot biopsy forceps. Gastrointest Endosc. 1995; 42(6):573–8.

33. Peluso F, Goldner F. Follow-up of hot biopsy forceps treatment of diminutive colonic polyps. Gastrointest Endosc. 1991;37(6): 604–6.

34. Gilbert DA, DiMarino AJ, Jensen DM, et al. Status evaluation: hot biopsy forceps. American society for gastrointestinal endoscopy. technology assessment committee. Gastrointest Endosc. 1992;38(6):753–6.

35. Riley S. Colonoscopic polypectomy and endoscopic mucosal resection: A practical guide. http://www.bsg.org.uk/clinical-guidance/endoscopy/colonoscopic-polypectomy-and-endoscopic-mucosal-resection-a-practical-guide.html. Updated 2008. Accessed 5 June 2015.

36. Kim JS, Lee BI, Choi H, et al. Cold snare polypectomy versus cold forceps polypectomy for diminutive and small colorectal polyps: A randomized controlled trial. Gastrointest Endosc. 2015;81(3):741–7.

37. Hewett DG. Colonoscopic polypectomy: current techniques and controversies. Gastroenterol Clin North Am. 2013;42(3): 443–58.

38. Paspatis GA, Tribonias G, Konstantinidis K, et al. A prospective randomized comparison of cold vs hot snare polypectomy in the occurrence of postpolypectomy bleeding in small colonic polyps. Colorectal Dis. 2011;13(10):e345–8.

39. Lee CK, Shim JJ, Jang JY. Cold snare polypectomy vs. cold forceps polypectomy using double-biopsy technique for removal of diminutive colorectal polyps: a prospective randomized study. Am J Gastroenterol. 2013;108(10):1593–600.

40. Ichise Y, Horiuchi A, Nakayama Y, Tanaka N. Prospective randomized comparison of cold snare polypectomy and

conventional polypectomy for small colorectal polyps. Digestion. 2011;84(1):78–81.

41. Van Gossum A, Cozzoli A, Adler M, Taton G, Cremer M. Colonoscopic snare polypectomy: Analysis of 1485 resections comparing two types of current. Gastrointest Endosc. 1992;38(4):472–5.

42. Repici A, Pellicano R, Strangio G, Danese S, Fagoonee S, Malesci A. Endoscopic mucosal resection for early colorectal neoplasia: pathologic basis, procedures, and outcomes. Dis Colon Rectum. 2009;52(8):1502–15.

43. Conio M, Blanchi S, Repici A, Ruggeri C, Fisher DA, Filiberti R. Cap-assisted endoscopic mucosal resection for colorectal polyps. Dis Colon Rectum. 2010;53(6):919–27.

44. Moss A, Bourke MJ, Williams SJ, et al. Endoscopic mucosal resection outcomes and prediction of submucosal cancer from advanced colonic mucosal neoplasia. Gastroenterology. 2011;140(7):1909–18.

45. Moss A, Williams SJ, Hourigan LF, et al. Long-term adenoma recurrence following wide-field endoscopic mucosal resection (WF-EMR) for advanced colonic mucosal neoplasia is infrequent: results and risk factors in 1000 cases from the australian colonic EMR (ACE) study. Gut. 2015;64(1):57–65.

46. Luigiano C, Consolo P, Scaffidi MG, et al. Endoscopic mucosal resection for large and giant sessile and flat colorectal polyps: a single-center experience with long-term follow-up. Endoscopy. 2009;41(10):829–35.

47. Buchner AM, Guarner-Argente C, Ginsberg GG. Outcomes of EMR of defiant colorectal lesions directed to an endoscopy referral center. Gastrointest Endosc. 2012;76(2):255–63.

48. Steele SR, Johnson EK, Champagne B, et al. Endoscopy and polyps-diagnostic and therapeutic advances in management. World J Gastroenterol. 2013;19(27):4277–88.

49. Japanese Gastric Cancer Association. Japanese gastric cancer treatment guidelines 2010 (ver.3). Gastric Cancer. 2011;14:113–23.

50. Gotoda T, Ho KY, Soetikno R, Kaltenbach T, Draganov P. Gastric ESD: current status and future directions of devices and training. Gastrointest Endosc Clin N Am. 2014;24(2):213–33.

51. Draganov PV, Gotoda T, Chavalitdhamrong D, Wallace MB. Techniques of endoscopic submucosal dissection: application for the western endoscopist? Gastrointest Endosc. 2013;78(5):677–88.

52. Ono S, Fujishiro M, Koike K. Endoscopic submucosal dissection for superficial esophageal neoplasms. World J Gastrointest Endosc. 2012;4(5):162–6.

53. Oda I, Suzuki H, Nonaka S, Yoshinaga S. Complications of gastric endoscopic submucosal dissection. Dig Endosc. 2013;25 Suppl 1:71–8.

54. Tanaka S, Kashida H, Saito Y, et al. JGES guidelines for colorectal endoscopic submucosal dissection/endoscopic mucosal resection. Dig Endosc. 2015;27(4):417–34.

55. Deprez PH, Bergman JJ, Meisner S, et al. Current practice with endoscopic submucosal dissection in Europe: position statement from a panel of experts. Endoscopy. 2010;42(10):853–8.

56. Bhatt A, Abe S, Kumaravel A, Vargo J, Saito Y. Indications and techniques for endoscopic submucosal dissection. Am J Gastroenterol. 2015.

57. Huai ZY, Feng Xian W, Chang Jiang L, Xi Chen W. Submucosal injection solution for endoscopic resection in gastrointestinal tract: a traditional and network meta-analysis. Gastroenterol Res Pract. 2015;2015:702768.

58. Probst A, Golger D, Anthuber M, Markl B, Messmann H. Endoscopic submucosal dissection in large sessile lesions of the rectosigmoid: learning curve in a european center. Endoscopy. 2012;44(7):660–7.

59. Hotta K, Oyama T, Shinohara T, et al. Learning curve for endoscopic submucosal dissection of large colorectal tumors. Dig Endosc. 2010;22(4):302–6.

60. Saito Y, Uraoka T, Yamaguchi Y, et al. A prospective, multicenter study of 1111 colorectal endoscopic submucosal dissections (with video). Gastrointest Endosc. 2010;72(6):1217–25.

61. Kobayashi N, Yoshitake N, Hirahara Y, et al. Matched case–control study comparing endoscopic submucosal dissection and endoscopic mucosal resection for colorectal tumors. J Gastroenterol Hepatol. 2012;27(4):728–33.

62. Steele SR, Brown TA, Rush RM, Martin MJ. Laparoscopic vs open colectomy for colon cancer: results from a large nationwide population-based analysis. J Gastrointest Surg. 2008;12(3):583–91.

63. Beck DE, Karulf RE. Laparoscopic-assisted full-thickness endoscopic polypectomy. Dis Colon Rectum. 1993;36(7):693–5.

64. Franklin Jr ME, Diaz-E JA, Abrego D, Parra-Davila E, Glass JL. Laparoscopic-assisted colonoscopic polypectomy: the Texas Endosurgery Institute experience. Dis Colon Rectum. 2000;43(9):1246–9.

65. Wilhelm D, von Delius S, Weber L, et al. Combined laparoscopic-endoscopic resections of colorectal polyps: 10-year experience and follow-up. Surg Endosc. 2009;23(4):688–93.

66. Ommer A, Limmer J, Mollenberg H, Peitgen K, Albrecht KH, Walz MK. Laparoscopic-assisted colonoscopic polypectomy—indications and results. Zentralbl Chir. 2003;128(3):195–8.

67. Franklin Jr ME, Leyva-Alvizo A, Abrego-Medina D, et al. Laparoscopically monitored colonoscopic polypectomy: an established form of endoluminal therapy for colorectal polyps. Surg Endosc. 2007;21(9):1650–3.

68. Winter H, Lang RA, Spelsberg FW, Jauch KW, Huttl TP. Laparoscopic colonoscopic rendezvous procedures for the treatment of polyps and early stage carcinomas of the colon. Int J Colorectal Dis. 2007;22(11):1377–81.

69. Lee SW, Garrett KA, Shin JH, Trencheva K, Sonoda T, Milsom JW. Dynamic article: long-term outcomes of patients undergoing combined endolaparoscopic surgery for benign colon polyps. Dis Colon Rectum. 2013;56(7):869–73.

70. Yan J, Trencheva K, Lee SW, Sonoda T, Shukla P, Milsom JW. Treatment for right colon polyps not removable using standard colonoscopy: combined laparoscopic-colonoscopic approach. Dis Colon Rectum. 2011;54(6):753–8.

71. Franklin Jr ME, Portillo G. Laparoscopic monitored colonoscopic polypectomy: long-term follow-up. World J Surg. 2009;33(6):1306–9.

6
Preoperative Assessment of Colorectal Patients

Jennifer S. Davids and Justin A. Maykel

Key Concepts

- A thorough history and physical exam performed by the surgeon is the single best preoperative "test."
- Complex surgical patients with multiple comorbidities need careful preoperative assessment in order to minimize risk of perioperative complications.
- Preoperative laboratory studies should be ordered on a selective basis, as "routine" preoperative labs on otherwise asymptomatic, healthy patients have low diagnostic yield.
- Depending on patient's risk factors, a preoperative cardiac risk assessment should be made and appropriate testing obtained. Cardiac medications should be continued, although beta blockers should not be initiated in the preoperative setting. Cardiac interventions should be performed for standard indications, independent of the need for abdominal surgery.
- Smoking cessation should be strongly encouraged prior to elective surgery.
- The surgeon should carefully review the patient's medication list, paying particular attention to anticoagulants, immunosuppressants, and chemotherapy agents.

Evaluation of the Routine Colorectal Patient

In Office by Surgeon

The in-office surgical consultation, including a detailed history and physical exam performed by the surgeon, is the single most important part of the preoperative evaluation. This also includes a thorough review of the patient's medical record, which often will uncover additional relevant medical and surgical history, as well as medications. Particularly for complex patients with known cardiopulmonary disease or other major comorbidities (as well as patients with surgical diseases involving multidisciplinary care teams such as inflammatory

bowel disease (IBD) and rectal cancer), it is essential to obtain the names, phone numbers, and e-mail addresses of the patients' specialists for further communication and coordination of care. Many patients shuttle between different hospital systems and despite advances in information technologies, fluid communication between specialists remains challenging. The task of coordinating these patients' preoperative care can be enormously time-consuming for the busy surgeon; however, it is incredibly important to communicate and exchange vital information prior to elective surgery, in order to minimize risk of perioperative complications.

Major Abdominal Surgery

It goes without saying that the surgeon should personally perform a detailed history and physical examination of every patient undergoing elective abdominal surgery. The history should make sure to include a detailed list of active medications, including blood thinners and over-the-counter drugs or topical agents. The history should include complementary or alternative medicine practices and substances. Personal and/or family history of clotting or bleeding disorders (or bleeding complications from prior surgery) should be obtained. Additionally, the surgeon should ask about activity level, in order to estimate exercise capacity. Poor baseline exercise capacity has been shown to correlate with increased risk of perioperative cardiac complications [1]. Can the patient walk up a flight of stairs, do heavy housework, or walk up a hill? "Yes" to these questions indicates that the patient can perform at least four METs (metabolic equivalents) and if otherwise healthy, the patient does not need a preoperative cardiac workup [2].

Anorectal Surgery

Anorectal surgical procedures are considered low acuity and do not trigger the major physiologic changes associated with major abdominal surgery. Accordingly it is not necessary to obtain any additional preoperative workup for healthy patients undergoing

© Springer International Publishing 2016
S.R. Steele et al. (eds.), *The ASCRS Textbook of Colon and Rectal Surgery*, DOI 10.1007/978-3-319-25970-3_6

elective anorectal procedures. This includes patients who are over 50 years old, with comorbidities such as hypertension, hyperlipidemia, and diabetes that are well-compensated and properly managed by their PCP or specialists.

Preoperative Testing

Laboratory Studies

Multiple studies have demonstrated that routine preoperative labs are very low-yield in identifying abnormalities that require a change in management in healthy, asymptomatic patients. A selective approach to preoperative laboratory studies should be taken, based on the evidence outlined in this section. A landmark retrospective study of 2000 patients undergoing elective surgery demonstrated that approximately 60% of all preoperative laboratory studies were not indicated, and only 0.2% of these non-indicated tests (which occurred in ten patients) revealed abnormalities that could potentially result in a change in management [3]. Further analysis of these ten individual patient charts was performed and it was determined that no further actions were taken in any instance. When laboratory tests are indicated, lab values from the 4 month timeframe prior to surgery may be used, unless there has been a change in clinical status (uptodate. com, preoperative evaluation of the healthy patient).

Hemoglobin is recommended for all patients age 65 or older who are undergoing abdominal surgery. Younger patients should be tested if there is potential for major blood loss, or if the history is suggestive of anemia. *White blood cell count* as a screening test is of limited utility, but is certainly relevant in cases where recent infection has been treated or in the setting of immunosuppression. *Platelet counts* should be checked if the patient will undergo spinal or epidural anesthesia. *Coagulation studies and bleeding time* are not needed in patients with no personal or family history of bleeding disorders. Further, abnormal prothrombin time and bleeding time have not been shown in large studies to correlate with increased risk of intraoperative or postoperative bleeding complications [4, 5]. Pre-transfusion testing consisting of *ABO and Rh typing* ("type and screen") should be performed preoperatively in all patients undergoing major abdominal surgery, including bowel resection. This is particularly important for patients who have a significant transfusion history, who may have multiple alloantibodies.

Serum *creatinine* should be checked in patients 50 years or older, as elevated creatinine is an independent predictor of increased postoperative cardiac complications [6], as well as mortality [7] in elective noncardiac surgery. Further, some anesthetics require dose adjustments for patients with impaired renal function, so this information is vital to our anesthesia colleagues. Routine *electrolytes* are not required unless the patient has a history of prior electrolyte abnormalities, chronic kidney disease, or diuretic use. Routine blood **glucose** measurements are not indicated in nondiabetic patients, as the incidence of asymptomatic hyperglyce-

mia is low [8]. The same logic also applies to *liver function tests*, which also should not be routinely ordered in a healthy, asymptomatic patient [4]. Routine *urinalysis* does not need to be performed in healthy, asymptomatic patients, and should be only performed on a more selective basis, in patients with history of frequent urinary tract infections or other relevant urinary symptoms. In most instances, asymptomatic patients with positive urinalyses may be treated empirically for urinary tract infection, and may proceed with elective abdominal surgery as scheduled. Most studies of the utility of preoperative urinalysis are from the orthopedic surgery literature, and they do not demonstrate a correlation between preoperative positive urinalysis or bacteriuria and postoperative infectious complications [9].

Pregnancy tests should be performed on all women of childbearing age, if the results would alter management [10]. While serum human chorionic gonadotropin (HCG) assays are the most sensitive in detecting very early pregnancy, most urine pregnancy tests are positive within a week of a missed period, and can be processed quickly in the preoperative setting.

Electrocardiogram

Electrocardiograms (ECGs) are quick, noninvasive, and inexpensive; consequently, they are overutilized in the routine preoperative workup of most patients. In asymptomatic patients undergoing low-risk surgery, ECG is unlikely to identify abnormalities that result in a change in management. Further, the incidence of abnormal ECGs is very low in patients under 45 years old. According to the ACC/AHA guidelines, preoperative ECG should be performed on patients with known heart disease, peripheral arterial disease, or cerebrovascular disease [11].

Chest X-Ray

The American College of Physicians recommends obtaining chest X-ray (CXR) for patients with known cardiopulmonary disease, as well as all patients 50 years or older who require major abdominal surgery [12]. The American Heart Association also recommends CXR (posterior–anterior and lateral views) on obese patients with BMI $\geq$ 40 [13]. Despite these recommendations, CXR are low yield in identifying clinically significant abnormalities that alter management [14].

Patients with Specific Comorbidities

Assessment of Cardiac Risk

The overall risk of perioperative cardiac events is low in patients undergoing elective noncardiac surgery; however, it is essential to identify patients who may be at increased risk, in order to optimize them preoperatively and thereby minimize their potential for adverse perioperative cardiac events. A large study of over 8000 high-risk patients undergoing noncardiac surgery demonstrated that postoperative myocardial infarction is associated with high 30-day mortality (11.6%), and the majority (65%) was not associated with ischemic symptoms [15]. It is therefore important to ensure that these risks are identified preoperatively and patients are optimized, as these adverse events can range from subtle to fatal.

Initial Workup

The most common postoperative cardiac events include myocardial infarction, heart failure, arrhythmia, and cardiac arrest. The first step is to obtain a detailed history and physical during the office consultation. Patients should be asked whether they can climb two flights of stairs, and/or walk four city blocks (noting that some may have orthopedic issues limiting these tasks) [16]. They should also be asked about the following symptoms: palpitations, chest pain, syncope, dyspnea, orthopnea. Not only is history of cardiac disease important (including valvular or ischemic heart disease, cardiomyopathy, and arrhythmia), but history of diabetes, renal impairment, peripheral artery disease, and cerebrovascular disease is also highly relevant in assessing risk due to their association with coronary artery disease.

There are several validated models that can be used by the clinician to predict risk of perioperative cardiac adverse events. The simplest of these models is the Revised Goldman Cardiac Risk Index (RCRI) (Table 6-1) [6]. Other user-friendly models include the American College of Surgeons' National Surgical Quality Improvement Program (ACS-NSQIP) risk calculator, which requires more input variables, but also will provide quantification of other, noncardiac risks [17]. The calculator is online, and accessible at http://riskcalculator.facs.org.

Who Needs Additional Testing?

The extent of preoperative workup is based on the patient's estimated risk according to these models. Patients with less than 1% risk of perioperative death from cardiac disease do not require additional workup. Patients whose risk is 1% or more are likely to have a known history of recent myocardial infarction, unstable angina, heart failure, valvular disease, or arrhythmias. These patients should be evaluated preoperatively by their cardiologist, as the decisions regarding which additional testing to pursue, if any, is rarely simple. The American College of Cardiology/American Heart Association (ACC/AHA) guidelines suggest that functional performance status is an important indicator of whether additional testing is necessary in higher risk patients [11]. Further testing may include echocardiography, stress test (exercise or pharmacologic), 24-h ambulatory monitoring and cardiac catheterization. Generally, additional testing is not usually performed beyond what is ordinarily needed if the patient were not undergoing surgery, as this has not been shown to improve perioperative outcomes in noncardiac, nonvascular surgery.

Preoperative "Optimization"

Once the preoperative cardiac assessment has been completed and risk estimated, the primary care physician or cardiologist may institute treatment that optimally limits the risk of a perioperative cardiac adverse event. While long-standing beta-blockers should be continued, beta-blockers should NOT be initiated in the preoperative setting. While there may be a benefit with regard to non fatal MI, multiple studies and meta-analyses have documented a significantly increased risk of non fatal stroke and mortality when beta-blockers are started as soon as 24 h before surgery [18, 19]. Antihypertensive medications can be adjusted to avoid perioperative hypotension, targeting a systolic blood pressure of 116–130 mmHg and heart rate of 60–70 beats per minute [18, 20]. When diagnosed, new dysrhythmias can be controlled with antiarrhythmic agents. Decompensated heart failure increases perioperative risk and this risk may be mitigated by treatment with ACE inhibitors, aldosterone antagonists, and digoxin for at least 1 week preoperatively [21]. While cardiac catheterization should be reserved for patients with high-risk features on noninvasive testing (including

TABLE 6-1. Revised Goldman Cardiac Risk Index (RCRI) [6]

Six Independent Predictors of Major Cardiac Complications [1, 85]
• High-risk type of surgery (examples include vascular surgery and any open intraperitoneal or intrathoracic procedures)
• History of ischemic heart disease (history of myocardial infarction (MI) or a positive exercise test, current complaint of chest pain considered to be secondary to myocardial ischemia, use of nitrate therapy, or ECG with pathological Q waves; do not count prior coronary revascularization procedure unless one of the other criteria for ischemic heart disease is present)
• History of heat failure (HF)
• History of cerebrovascular disease
• Diabetes mellitus requiring treatment with insulin
• Preoperative serum creatinine <2.0 mg/dL (177 μmol/L)
Rate of cardiac death, nonfatal myocardial infarction, and nonfatal cardiac arrest according to the number of predictors [2]
• No risk factors—0.4% (95% CI: 0.1–0.8)
• One risk factor—1.0% (95% CI: 0.5–1-4)
• Two risk factors—2.4% (95% CI: 1.3–3.5)
• Three or more risk factors—5.4% (95% CI: 2.8–7.9)

reversible large anterior wall defect, multiple reversible defects, ischemia occurring at a low heart rate, extensive stress-induced wall motion abnormalities, transient ischemic dilatation) the role for percutaneous coronary intervention (PCI) or operative revascularization remains controversial. While the discussion is beyond the scope of this chapter, revascularization should be reserved for those patients who meet criteria for cardiac intervention regardless of the need for non cardiac surgery and the timing should be chosen based on the indication for and urgency associated with the colorectal resection.

Coronary Stent Management

For patients with either a bare-metal stent (BMS) or drug-eluting stent (DES), the current recommendation is to continue dual antiplatelet therapy (aspirin plus an oral antiplatelet agent such as clopidogrel) for at least 12 months. For patients who need to undergo nonemergent noncardiac surgery, the recommendation is to complete at least 1 month dual antiplatelet therapy preoperatively for BMS, and at least 6 months for DES [22, 23].

These recommendations are based on existing data that quantifies risk of postoperative coronary and cerebrovascular thrombotic events in this patient population. The RECO study is a prospective multicenter observational cohort study of 1134 consecutive patients with coronary stents undergoing noncardiac surgery from 2007 to 2009. The goal of the study was to quantify risk of adverse cardiac and cerebrovascular events (MACCEs) and major bleeding, and to risk stratify patients according to preoperative characteristics. Of the study group, 54.9% had bare-metal stents (BMS) only, and 32.4% had drug-eluting stents (DES) (± BMS); in 12.7% the stent type was unknown. Overall, there was a 10.9% rate of MACCEs, and a 9.5% rate of hemorrhagic complications. Multivariable logistic regression was used to determine preoperative characteristics that were risk factors for MACCEs, which included the following: complete cessation of oral antiplatelet agent >5 days preoperatively, preoperative hemoglobin <10 g/dl, creatinine clearance <30 ml/min, and emergency or high-risk surgery. Risk factors for major bleeding included hemoglobin <10 g/dl, creatinine clearance 30–60 ml/min, duration from stent implantation to surgery <3 months, and high-risk surgery. This study highlights the importance of delaying elective surgery >3 months after stent placement if possible, as well as the need to maintain oral antiplatelet agents through the perioperative period in order to minimize risk for major adverse cardiac and cerebrovascular events.

Not infrequently colon and rectal surgeons are presented with patients who require urgent abdominal surgery, who also have recently implanted DES. A common scenario is the patient who has a lower gastrointestinal bleed while on oral antiplatelet therapy after DES implantation, who is found on colonoscopy to have a bleeding colon cancer. Patients on oral antiplatelet agents for recently implanted drug-eluting coronary stents can be safely "bridged" with IV infusions of shorter-acting antiplatelet agents. A pilot study of 30 patients with recently implanted DES (median 4 months; range 1–12 months) undergoing major (ten had abdominal surgery) or eye surgery had clopidogrel withheld 5 days preoperatively and were bridged with tirofiban (started 24 h later, discontinued 4 h preoperatively and restarted 2 h postoperatively until clopidogrel is resumed) [24]. Fourteen of the patients (47%) were maintained on aspirin throughout the perioperative course. There were no adverse cardiac events during the index hospitalization, and 28 patients (93%) did not experience significant postoperative bleeding. One of the two patients had an anastomotic bleed after partial colectomy that occurred 4 days after restarting clopidogrel; this was controlled with endoscopic clip placement. This study demonstrates the importance of careful coordination with the inpatient cardiologist in order to optimize outcomes for these complex patients who require urgent abdominal surgery while on antiplatelet therapy for a recently placed coronary stent.

AICD/Management

For nonemergent procedures, it is essential that these high-risk and complex cardiac patients are evaluated by a cardiologist, preferably the patient's own electrophysiologist. The importance of communication between the cardiologist and anesthesiologist cannot be overstated; above all, it is the obligation of the colon and rectal surgeon to ensure that this occurs. Patients with automatic implantable cardioverter-defibrillators (AICD) often have underlying ischemic heart disease, which should not be overlooked during the preoperative assessment. It is important for the anesthesiologist to find out from the cardiologist whether the patient is pacemaker-dependent, which means that the patient has atrial, ventricular, or both chambers paced 100% of the time. For patients who are not pacemaker-dependent, the anesthesiologist should place a magnet over the device, which will prevent inappropriate delivery of shocks [2]. For patients who are pacemaker-dependent, the device may need to be reprogrammed intraoperatively. All AICD patients should have an external defibrillator and transcutaneous pacer immediately available, and the pads should be affixed to the patient at the start of the case. In emergent settings, in which a formal cardiology consultation is not feasible, a 12-lead EKG can be used to determine pacemaker-dependence.

It is important for the surgeon to understand that AICD activity can be affected by monopolar cautery, causing electromagnetic interference [2]. This can result in delivery of inappropriate shocks to the patient, or inadequate pacing. Intent to use monopolar cautery should be clearly communicated to the anesthesia team prior to the case. Use of bipolar whenever possible can help decrease risk of electromagnetic interference but is not feasible for most colorectal procedures.

Assessment of Pulmonary Risk

COPD

Patients with chronic obstructive pulmonary disorder (COPD) are at high risk of perioperative pulmonary complications. Preoperative optimization of pulmonary function is the best way to minimize risk. These patients should be evaluated by their primary care physician, or pulmonologist, if they see a specialist. Bronchodilators should be continued perioperatively. Glucocorticoid use must be balanced against potential for increased risk of surgical complications such as anastomotic leak (see below section on steroids); tapering down or off is advantageous if at all possible, and should be discussed with the specialist. A randomized controlled trial of 48 high-risk pulmonary patients demonstrated significant decrease in postoperative pulmonary complications, 60% versus 22% ($p < .01$), in the group receiving aggressive pulmonary care, which included bronchodilators, antibiotics, chest physical therapy, nebulizers, and smoking cessation, compared to a group who did not receive these therapies [25].

Obstructive Sleep Apnea (OSA)

Obstructive sleep apnea (OSA) is the most common sleep disorder, and is characterized by upper airway obstruction, causing apneic episodes. Rates of OSA are on the rise, partially due to increased incidence of obesity, a major risk factor. A study of almost 1000 patients revealed that 60% of surgical patients with moderate-to-severe OSA are undiagnosed by the anesthetist, and 92% were undiagnosed by the surgeon [26]. OSA is important to recognize preoperatively, as it is a risk factor for perioperative cardiopulmonary complications, and is associated with unplanned ICU admission [27]. One reason why OSA is under diagnosed is that it can present with a wide range of symptoms, beyond the more classically described loud snoring, daytime sleepiness, and witnessed apnea by a sleep partner. Other symptoms include morning headaches, poor concentration, altered mood, vivid or disturbing dreams, restless sleep, GERD, and nocturia [28].

Patients undergoing major abdominal surgery should be screened for OSA, particularly those with high BMI and multiple comorbidities. There are several simple and efficient clinical screening tools available, including the STOP-Bang questionnaire (Table 6-2) [29]. Patients with high scores who are undergoing major abdominal surgery should be referred to a pulmonologist for a formal workup. A randomized controlled trial of 177 patients with documented OSA demonstrated that patients who used auto-titrated continuous positive airway pressure (APAP) perioperatively ($N = 87$) had significantly decreased rates of hypoxia and apnea compared to the untreated group ($N = 90$); the APAP group had three events/hour postoperatively, decreased from their preoperative baseline of 30 events/hour ($P < 0.001$), and the control group had 31.9 events/hour, increased from preoperative baseline of 30.4 events/hour ($P = 0.302$). Importantly, the investigators noted compliance rates (defined as wearing the device nightly) of only 45%, which was most commonly attributed to generalized discomfort, nausea, or vomiting [30]. Patients with a known diagnosis of OSA should provide the anesthesiologist with documentation of their sleep study results and recent pulmonary consultations, and should bring their CPAP machine to the hospital for perioperative use.

Diabetes

Diabetic patients represent a complex subset of surgical patients, who often have long-term complications of their disease (neuropathy, visual impairment), as well as other

TABLE 6-2. STOP-bang questionnaire [29, 84]

○ Yes	○ No	*Snoring?* Do you *Snore Loudly* (loud enough to be heard through closed doors or your bed-partner elbows you for snoring at night)?
○ Yes	○ No	*Tired?* Do you often feel *Tired, Fatigued, or Sleepy* during the daytime (such as falling asleep during driving)?
○ Yes	○ No	*Observed?* Has anyone *Observed* you *Stop Breathing* or *Choking/Gasping* during your sleep?
○ Yes	○ No	*Pressure?* Do you have or are being treated for *High Blood Pressure*
○ Yes	○ No	*Body Mass Index more than 35 kg/m2?*
○ Yes	○ No	*Age older than 50 years old?*
○ Yes	○ No	*Neck size large? (Measured around Adams apple)* For male, is your shirt collar 17 in. or larger? For female, is your shirt collar 16 in. or larger?
○ Yes	○ No	*Gender = Male?*

Scoring criteria*:

Low risk of OSA: Yes to 0–2 questions

Intermediate risk of OSA: Yes to 3–4 questions

High risk of OSA: Yes to 5–8 questions

OSA obstructive sleep apnea

related comorbidities, such as chronic renal insufficiency and cardiovascular disease [6, 31]. The initial office consultation with the surgeon should include a detailed history, focusing on the type and duration of diabetes, symptoms, how glucose is monitored at home, baseline glucose range, glycated hemoglobin (A1C) levels, related symptoms, as well as the contact information of their primary care physician and/or endocrinologist. Diabetic patients undergoing major abdominal surgery should have the following as part of their preoperative workup: ECG, CXR, serum creatinine, serum glucose, and an AIC level (within 4–6 weeks preoperatively). In particular, elevated A1C levels have been shown in cardiac surgery to be associated with increased risk of surgical complications, including infections, myocardial infarction, and death [32]. Close perioperative involvement of the anesthesiologist is also critical, as some patients undergoing major operations will require preoperative intravenous insulin infusion to attain euglycemia prior to initiation of surgery [33].

Obesity

More than one-thirds of adults in the USA are obese, which is defined as having body-mass index (BMI) of 30 or more. One in 20 adults is considered super-obese (BMI of 40 or more) [34]. BMI is considered a screening tool to identify obesity, and is calculated as the patient's weight (in kilograms) divided by square of the height (in meters). An online BMI calculator is available at on the CDC website (http://www.cdc.gov/healthyweight/assessing/bmi/adult_BMI/english_bmi_calculator/bmi_calculator.html).

Despite the fact that the obese patient creates substantial technical challenges for the surgeon, they do not have significantly greater risk of perioperative mortality. A prospective multicenter study of over 100,000 patients undergoing nonbariatric surgery demonstrated that overweight and obese patients actually had a statistically significantly lower postoperative mortality, compared to nonobese patients (overweight patients: OR 0.85, 95% CI 0.75–0.99; moderately obese OR 0.73, CI 0.57–0.94). This unexpected result was termed the "obesity paradox" and can potentially be explained by increased nutritional stores, as well as the chronic inflammatory state of obesity that may prime these patients for the inflammatory surge of surgery [35].

In terms of postoperative morbidity, obese patients undergoing nonbariatric abdominal surgery have been shown to have increased risk of perioperative venous thromboembolism and superficial site infection. A prospective study of over 6000 patients found that the risk of superficial site infection after open abdominal surgery was 4% for obese versus 3% for nonobese patients, $P=0.03$ [36].

Obese patients pose significant intraoperative challenges, some of which can be mitigated with appropriate preoperative planning. For example, if a stoma may be needed, a visit from the enterostomal therapist is extremely important, as marking on the thinner upper abdomen will be helpful. It is especially important to ensure that these patients are able to reach the stoma so they can care for it independently. Both laparoscopic and open surgery is technically demanding in obese patients; however, if feasible, laparoscopic surgery has the advantage to the patient of smaller incisions and improved visualization for the surgeon. Avoiding lower midline and Pfannenstiel incisions is helpful in minimizing superficial site infections and other wound-related complications in the obese patient with a large pannus. Clear communication with the operating room staff prior to the case is essential, to ensure availability of long instruments, deep retractors, appropriate beds and equipment such as blood pressure cuffs and large pneumatic compression boots.

Malnutrition

Colorectal surgeons are commonly faced with challenging patients who are malnourished due to advanced malignancies or inflammatory bowel disease that result in intestinal blockages, intestinal fistulas, poor absorptive capacity, and large volume losses from the GI tract. Nutritional risk tends to be a reflection of the patient's overall health, and in oncology has correlated with the Eastern Cooperative Oncology Group score and the presence of anorexia or fatigue [37]. Such nutritional risk is associated with increased postoperative complications, longer length of stay, and higher mortality following elective surgery [38, 39], and is particularly pronounced in patient with colorectal cancer [40]. Incidence remains under recognized and malnutrition continues to negatively impact postoperative recovery and patient outcomes, as well as mortality [41]. Although logistically challenging, nutritional support can be delivered in the preoperative or postoperative setting and can be administered via the enteral and parenteral routes. Most studies are limited by heterogeneous patient populations, variable study designs, different feeding protocols that often result in parenteral overfeeding, and outdated methodologies. When delivered appropriately, the malnourished colorectal patient realizes several benefits from perioperative nutritional support including fewer postoperative complications, shorter hospital length of stay, and lower mortality [42].

The evaluation of the potentially malnourished patient begins with the history and physical examination. Most patients will complain of some degree of intolerance of oral intake as a result of poor appetite, nausea, abdominal bloating, abdominal pain, and weakness. Patients will relate a recent weight loss, typically over a 1–3 month time period. On physical examination, the patient appears thin, pale, and weak with muscle wasting and loose skin. These variables can be objectified using grading systems such as the relatively intuitive Subjective Global Assessment (SGA) to classify patients as well nourished, moderately malnourished, or severely malnourished [43]. The SGA utilizes five features of the history (weight loss over 6 months, dietary intake change, gastrointestinal symptoms, functional capacity, and the impact of disease on nutritional requirements) and four features of the clinical exam (loss of subcutaneous fat, muscle wasting, ankle edema, sacral edema, ascites) to elicit a SGA rank based on subjective weighting.

Serum albumin level has been considered the "classic" test reflecting overall nutritional status, with serum concentration of <3.0 g/dL defining the "malnourished state." However, in real practice its utility and reliability is limited as levels fluctuate for many reasons, including production alterations in the catabolic or anabolic states, external losses, or redistribution between the various fluid compartments of the body [44]. Other short turnover proteins such as prealbumin, transferrin, and retinol binding protein have similar limitations as nutritional markers as a result of variable half-lives and response to dietary intake and renal/liver dysfunction, although all of these proteins can be useful when followed as trends over time.

Inflammatory bowel disease, intestinal obstruction, large tumors, fistulizing diseases, and patients with diarrhea are often unable to sustain themselves orally due to a poor appetite or resultant abdominal bloating and pain. This limits the ability to intervene preoperatively, particularly when considering utilizing the enteral route. Options include oral nutritional supplements (standard or immunonutrition) or feeding via nasoenteric feeding tubes. Total parenteral nutrition (TPN) can be uses as long as central intravenous access is obtained, an appropriate formula is prescribed (1.5 g per kilogram and 25 kcal per kilogram) and tight glycemic control is maintained (serum blood sugars <150 g/dL). Unfortunately, the use of preoperative nutrition has not been well studied in the malnourished GI surgery patient populations. A recent Cochrane review [45] highlights this paucity of evidence and the reality that many of the studies are outdated, with only two trials evaluating the administration of enteral nutrition (years 1992 and 2009) including only 120 participants and a high risk of bias. Neither study showed any difference in primary outcomes. The three studies that evaluated preoperative parenteral nutrition (years 1982, 1988, and 1992) showed a significant reduction in postoperative complications, predominantly in malnourished patients.

Solid Organ Transplant Recipients

The introduction of novel, more effective immunosuppression regimens has resulted in improved long-term survival after solid organ transplant. Over 150,000 patients in the USA are living with functional kidney transplants, and this number is on the rise. It is increasingly common for surgeons to encounter transplant patients in their practice, in both the elective and emergency settings. The vast majority of these patients are maintained on chronic immunosuppressive regimens. These agents are generally continued throughout the perioperative and early postoperative period in order to minimize risk of rejection. It is therefore essential that surgeons

familiarize themselves with the more commonly used immunosuppressive agents and their potential to impact perioperative outcomes. Communication with the transplant team of physicians is necessary prior to elective surgery.

The newer immunosuppressive agents, sirolimus and everolimus, which belong to the drug class known as inhibitors of the mammalian target of rapamycin (mTOR), have been shown to negatively impact healing of surgical wounds. mTOR is a cytoplasmic kinase that is essential for cell growth and proliferation [46]. Inhibition of lymphocyte proliferation despite stimulation results in immunosuppression. This same mechanism is also responsible for inhibition of the wound healing process. In a prospective trial of 123 patients randomized to receive either sirolimus or tacrolimus on postoperative day 4 after kidney transplant, Dean et al. found a significantly higher rate of wound-related complications (including superficial site infection and incisional hernias) in the sirolimus cohort, compared those receiving tacrolimus (47% vs. 8%, $P < 0.0001$) [47]. This data has prompted clinicians to replace mTOR inhibitors with tacrolimus for 6 weeks prior to elective surgery.

Substance Abuse

All surgical patients should be asked about their use of tobacco, alcohol, and street drugs. A large database study from 2002 determined that 7.6% of Americans had a substance abuse disorder within the prior year (95% CI 6.6–8.6%) [48]. The surgeon must also recognize narcotic dependency and use of prescription opioids that are not medically indicated. It is important for surgeons to make patients feel comfortable in answering these questions honestly and accurately. It is never safe to simply assume that a particular patient does not fit the expected profile of an "alcoholic" or "drug addict." Substance abuse has been shown to affect the elderly [49], as well as highly functional individuals with families and careers [50]. It is therefore critical to screen *all* patients preoperatively in order to minimize perioperative risk.

Alcohol

Alcoholism has been shown to be associated with a number of different perioperative complications, in a dose-dependent manner. Large studies have demonstrated that alcoholism is associated with surgical site and other infections, cardiopulmonary complications, and also correlates with longer hospital stay, increased rates of ICU stay, and increased rates of reoperation [51, 52]. The AUDIT-C questionnaire is a validated screening tool that can be used by the clinician to identify patients at high risk for perioperative complications (Table 6-3) [53]. A randomized controlled trial of 41 patients with alcoholism (defined as consumption >60 g ethanol per day) undergoing elective colorectal surgery demonstrated that abstinence 1 month preoperatively was associated with fewer cardiac complications, including myocardial ischemia

TABLE 6-3. AUDIT—C questionnaire

Question # 1: How often did you have a drink containing alcohol in the past year?	
Never	(0 points)
Monthly or less	(1 point)
Two to four times a month	(2 points)
Two to three times per week	(3 points)
Four or more times a week	(4 points)
Question # 2: How many drinks did you have on a typical day when you were drinking in the past year?	
1 or 2	(0 points)
3 or 4	(1 point)
5 or 6	(2 points)
7 to 9	(3 points)
10 or more	(4 points)
Question # 3: How often did you have six or more drinks on one occasion in the past year?	
Never	(0 points)
Less than monthly	(1 point)
Monthly	(2 points)
Weekly	(3 points)
Daily or almost daily	(4 points)

The AUDIT-C score on a scale of 0–12 (scores of 0 reflect no alcohol use). In men, a score of 4 or more is considered positive; in women, a score of 3 or more is considered positive

(23% vs. 85%, $P<0.05$) and arrhythmias (33% vs. 86%, $P<0.05$), as well as overall decreased complication rate (31% vs. 74%, $P=0.02$) [54]. It is unknown what the optimal alcohol-free interval is prior to elective surgery, in terms of maximizing risk reduction, although the trial investigators recommend 3–8 weeks, highlighting the importance of intensive counseling and monitoring of these patients during this interval [55].

Tobacco

Smoking has been shown in multiple studies to increase perioperative pulmonary risk, as well as risk of wound infections, neurologic complications, and ICU admission [56]. The best way to minimize this risk is to encourage patients to quit smoking prior to elective surgery. Previously it was felt that smoking cessation less than 8 weeks preoperatively was associated with a paradoxical increase in pulmonary complications, possibly due to a compensatory increase in secretions. This has now been disproven in multiple large studies. A large trial of 522 smokers undergoing gastric cancer surgery compared risk of postoperative pulmonary complications between three groups: (1) active smokers or those who quit less than 2 weeks prior to surgery, (2) those who quit 4–8 weeks prior, and (3) those who quit 8 or more weeks prior to surgery. The odds ratio for postoperative pulmonary complications were 2.92 for group 1 (95% CI 1.45–5.90), 0.98 for group 2 (0.28–3.45), and 1.42 for group 3 (0.66–3.05) [57]. Therefore, the recommendation is to encourage smoking cessation, regardless of the timing of surgery, although ideally surgery can be planned for at least 4 weeks from the "quit date."

Opioids

There are many different types of patients with chronic opioid dependence, including: abusers of street drugs such as heroin; abusers of prescription-only opioids; patients with prior history of opioid abuse, maintained on long-acting agents such as methadone; and patients on long-term narcotics prescribed for a chronic medical condition. Overall, prescription opioid use is on the rise in the USA and therefore this is being encountered by the surgeon with increasing frequency [58]. For all patients on narcotics, the surgeon should always ask preoperatively what the indication is, how long they have been taking it, side-effects (such as constipation), if there is a plan to wean off the drug, as well as who has been prescribing it. The patient's responses should be corroborated with the prescribing physician and/or medical record. Regardless of whether it is warranted for an underlying condition, opioid dependency will result in increased narcotic requirements perioperatively. Whenever possible, it is helpful to involve the acute pain management service preoperatively, in anticipation of these issues, in order to provide the best perioperative pain management. Non-narcotic adjunct therapies can be considered, including thoracic epidural catheters, transversus abdominus plane (TAP) blocks, as well as drugs such as ketorolac (Toradol), acetaminophen and gabapentin (Neurontin). Preoperatively, a clear plan should be made with the patient and the clinician who has been prescribing chronic opioids regarding postoperative pain management following hospital discharge, particularly who will be prescribing, and for how long. This is instrumental in avoiding concerns in the outpatient setting with over-prescribing and relapse.

Other Illicit Drugs

All patients undergoing elective surgery should be screened for the use of illicit drugs— not just "street drugs," but also other prescription-only drugs, such as benzodiazepines, that are not medically indicated. For patients requiring elective surgery, intensive efforts should be made to encourage cessation prior to planned surgery. This requires clear communication with the patient's primary care physician and/or psychiatrist. Discussion of individual drugs is beyond the scope of this chapter; however, additional information is well-summarized in this 2014 reference from the anesthesia literature [59].

Medications

In the era of polypharmacy, it is essential for the colorectal surgeon to carefully assess the patient's current medication list. Novel anticoagulants, chemotherapy, and immunosuppressants may be disguised by long, difficult to pronounce names. It is therefore critical for surgeons to be familiar with these newer agents. In many instances, patients are maintained indefinitely on medications that may pose significant perioperative risk. Discussing these situations preoperatively with the prescribing physician is essential, as the need for surgery may provide the necessary impetus to discontinue chronic medications that are no longer necessary or applicable.

Anticoagulation

In recent years, several novel oral anticoagulants have become commercially available and are widely used in patients with atrial fibrillation or history of stroke, as well as in patients with coronary or endovascular stents. When determining how to manage anticoagulation perioperatively, risk of bleeding must be balanced against the risk of thromboembolic complications. Additionally, it should be determined whether "bridging" with a short-acting anticoagulant is necessary. Although there are evidence-based guidelines, these decisions should be made on a case-by-case basis, and should closely involve the patient's cardiologist and/or hematologist. The patient should be educated upfront about the potential risks involved and to recognize that the ability to restart the medication postoperatively relates to the extent of surgery and associated bleeding risk.

Clopidogrel (Plavix) is a member of the platelet receptor PY12 blocker drug class, and is used in patients with history of myocardial infarction or stroke, as well as recent coronary or peripheral vascular stent placement. For most patients, the maintenance dose is 75 mg orally per day. If the decision has been made to discontinue clopidogrel prior to elective surgery, it should be discontinued 5–7 days preoperatively [23]. Clopidogrel should be restarted as soon as possible after surgery. A more extensive discussion of clopidogrel earlier in the chapter—refer to the section on "Coronary Stent Management."

Warfarin (Coumadin) is an inhibitor of vitamin-K-dependent clotting factor synthesis (factors II, VII, IX, and X). The half-life of warfarin is 36–42 h. Therapeutic dose range is measured by the prothrombin time (PT), which is generally maintained at a goal of INR (international normalized ratio) 2.0–3.0 for most conditions. Patients with cardiac valves may be maintained at higher doses, with a goal INR 2.5–3.5. For elective surgery, warfarin should be discontinued 5 days preoperatively. Most abdominal surgery is safe to perform when INR is ≤1.4 [60]. Ideally, INR should be checked the day prior to surgery, if possible. For urgent surgery (within 1–2 days), warfarin can be reversed with vitamin K (2.5–5 mg oral or intravenous). For emergency surgery, warfarin can be rapidly reversed with fresh frozen plasma (FFP), which contains the necessary clotting factors [61]. Provided that there was adequate hemostasis during surgery, warfarin may be restarted (at the preoperative dose) as early as 12–24 h postoperatively, although the timing depends on indication for anticoagulation (for example short term thromboembolic risk is higher with a mechanical mitral valve compared to atrial fibrillation).

Heparin binds to and inactivates antithrombin III and has a half-life of 45 min. Unfractionated heparin is administered as an IV infusion, using a weight-based nomogram to titrate the dose [62, 63]. Compared to low molecular weight heparin, unfractionated heparin is less costly, is easier and faster to reverse, and is preferable in patients with renal insufficiency (the dose is not affected by creatinine clearance). Unfractionated heparin should be held 6 h prior to surgery. *Enoxaparin (Lovenox)* is a low molecular weight heparin that has comparable efficacy to unfractionated heparin, but has many advantages. It is easier to use, is administered as a subcutaneous injection (and therefore can be given in the outpatient setting) and does not require monitoring. Its half-life is 3–5 h. It can be given at prophylactic dose for venous thromboembolism, as well as therapeutic, weight-based dose. In preparation for surgery, if twice-daily dosing is used, the evening dose should be held on the night prior to surgery; if once daily dosing is being used, a half-dose should be given the morning prior to surgery [60]. Other low molecular weight heparin products available in the USA include dalteparin (Fragmin) and tinzaparin (Innohep). Patients on any heparin derivative need to be monitored for heparin-induced thrombocytopenia (HIT), although this risk is less significant with low molecular weight heparin. Heparin products can be reversed with protamine sulfate.

Apixaban (Eliquis) is an oral factor Xa inhibitor that is commonly used in patients with atrial fibrillation, as well as for both prophylaxis and treatment of venous thromboembolism. Additionally, apixaban has been used as postoperative DVT prophylaxis after hip surgery [64]. The major advantage of apixaban over coumadin is that drug levels do not need to be checked routinely (although the drug does prolong PT/PTT/INR). The drug is dosed twice daily, is unaffected by dietary intake, and can be crushed and administered via nasogastric tube. The dose must be decreased for Cr ≥ 1.5, as well as for age >80 and body weight ≤60 kg. The drug is generally well-tolerated with a favorable side-effect profile. Apixaban should be discontinued a minimum of 48 h prior to abdominal or anorectal surgery, although depending on the indication for anticoagulation, it would be acceptable to discontinue it 24 h preoperatively for anorectal surgery, if necessary from a risk standpoint. There is a boxed warning regarding the use of neuraxial anesthesia and risk of spinal or epidural hematoma (which could result in temporary or permanent paralysis), as the optimal interval from drug discontinuation to intervention is not well-defined. Therefore we recommend not using this drug for perioperative anticoagulation if an epidural catheter or spinal anesthesia is planned. Although not routinely used to assess drug levels, anti-Factor 10a (Anti-FXa) levels can help guide management. There are currently no specific reversal agents for this drug.

Aspirin impairs platelet function primarily by downstream effects of irreversibly inhibiting cyclooxygenase-1 (COX-1). Its antiplatelet effects start as soon as 30 min after ingestion, and last throughout the platelet life span, which ranges from 8 to 10 days.

Despite the fact that there is no clear consensus among surgeons regarding perioperative aspirin use in noncardiac surgery, the risk of aspirin on postoperative bleeding is actually well studied in the literature. Perioperative continuation of low-dose (81 mg) aspirin in low-risk patients (for primary prevention of thrombotic cardiovascular events) undergoing abdominal surgery has not been shown in randomized controlled trials to be associated with an increase in major postoperative bleeding complications [65] . Other larger randomized controlled studies have demonstrated comparable results in patients at higher risk for adverse cardiovascular thromboembolic events, who are on chronic low-dose aspirin for secondary prevention of myocardial infarction or stroke. The STRATAGEM trial randomized 291 patients undergoing elective intermediate- or high-risk noncardiac surgery (of which 20% was abdominal surgery) to receive low-dose (75 mg) aspirin versus placebo starting 10 days preoperatively; these patients were all on long-term aspirin or another antiplatelet agent for secondary prevention of cardiovascular thromboembolic events [66]. Although the study was underpowered due to difficulty with recruitment, the investigators found no statistically significant difference in the rate of major bleeding complications within 30 days postoperatively between the aspirin and placebo groups, 6.2% versus 5.5%, respectively; $P=0.81$. Importantly, they also found no difference in the rate of cardiovascular thrombotic events, 3.4% versus 2.7%, $P=0.75$. Surprisingly, very few studies specifically evaluate the perioperative risk of high-dose (325 mg) aspirin; many of the larger studies on antiplatelet agents do not even take the aspirin dose into account [67]. A retrospective analysis of 1017 patients undergoing elective pancreatic resection compared patients on aspirin (55 patients on 325 mg aspirin, 234 patients on 81 mg aspirin) to no-aspirin ($n=728$), and found no significant dif-

ference in rate of blood transfusion within 30 days postoperatively between groups (29% versus 26% $P=.37$) [68]. The higher dose aspirin group was too small to stratify risk according to aspirin dose.

In our practice, we do not discontinue low-dose "baby" aspirin perioperatively for anorectal or abdominal cases, regardless of the indication for its use. For patients on high-dose (325 mg) aspirin, the decision is more individualized and requires input of the patient's cardiologist and/or vascular surgeon. If the decision is made to discontinue aspirin preoperatively, it should be held for 7 days prior to surgery.

Immunosuppressive Agents

Corticosteroids have been shown to impair wound healing in both animal models as well as clinical studies. In animal models, corticosteroids have been shown to alter multiple independent signaling pathways, impairing all three phases of wound healing: inflammatory, proliferative, and remodeling. Clinical studies have also demonstrated a higher rate of anastomotic complications in patients on chronic steroids [69]. A prospective study performed in the 1980s specifically evaluated the risk of steroids in Crohn's patients, and demonstrated in multivariate analysis that corticosteroids were associated with an increased overall postoperative complication rate in Crohn's patients undergoing surgery involving bowel anastomosis (15.4% vs. 6.7%; $p=.03$) [70]. One of the largest studies looking at anastomotic leak in colorectal patients included 250 left sided resections with anastomosis. The overall anastomotic leak rate was 7.5%. When patients were administered corticosteroids, either perioperatively or long term, the multivariate model concluded that corticosteroid use increased the risk for AL by more than seven times (OR, 7.52; standard error, 4.47; $P=0.001$; 95% CI, 2.35–24.08 [71]. A meta-analysis evaluating the risk of corticosteroids on colorectal anastomotic integrity is included 9564 patients from 12 studies demonstrated an overall leak rate of 6.77% (95% CI 5.48–9.06) compared to 3.26% (95% CI 2.94–3.58) in the non-corticosteroid group [72]. In addition, corticosteroids impact wound healing and are a risk factor for the development of superficial and deep surgical site infections and have even been shown to impact postoperative mortality [73]. Ultimately, this understanding allows the surgeon to better counsel the patient regarding possible postoperative complications, wean steroids during the preoperative period when possible, and make decisions in the operating room (such as the decision to create diverting stoma and wounds closure) to optimize patient outcomes.

Immunomodulators, including azathioprine and 6-mercaptopurine, are used in both Crohn's disease and ulcerative colitis to maintain steroid-induced remission. These drugs often take 3–4 months until clinical benefit is apparent, and have infrequent but serious side-effects such as leucopenia, liver function abnormalities, pancreatitis, and lymphoma.

A retrospective study of 417 operations involving bowel anastomoses for Crohn's disease demonstrated no difference in the rate of anastomotic complications for patients on immunomodulators (10% vs. 14%; $p=0.263$) [74]. Similar to the studies above, they also found that in multivariate analysis, corticosteroids (preoperative prednisolone 20 mg or more) was a predictor of anastomotic complication (OR 0.355, 95% CI 0.167–0.756; $p=0.007$). Accordingly these medications are often continued until surgery.

Biologic agents include infliximab (Remicade), a chimeric monoclonal antibody that targets tumor necrosis factor, a proinflammatory cytokine that has been shown to be elevated in inflamed tissue of IBD patients. Biologics including infliximab have been demonstrated to induce remission and control symptoms in patients with moderate-to-severe Crohn's and ulcerative colitis. With more widespread use of biologic agents such in other inflammatory conditions such as rheumatoid arthritis and psoriasis, surgeons are seeing a larger percentage of patients on these agents perioperatively. Krane et al. performed a retrospective analysis of 518 patients with IBD undergoing elective laparoscopic bowel resection, of which 142 patients were on preoperative infliximab [75]. There was no difference in the rate of anastomotic leak, which was overall low in both groups (2.1% with infliximab versus 1.3% without; $p=0.81$). A significantly higher percentage of the patients on infliximab were also on steroids, 73.9% vs. 58.8%, $p=0.006$, and still this did not impact anastomotic leak rate. Overall the existing literature is limited and controversial but biologic agents are thought to impact wound healing and most surgeons prefer to hold these agents for 4–6 weeks if possible prior to major abdominal surgery [76].

Chemotherapy

Through a myriad of mechanisms, the final common pathway of cytotoxic chemotherapy is induction of cell death. Ideally this effect is minimized in nontumor cells, including healing anastomoses. Large studies have attempted to evaluate the overall effect of neoadjuvant and adjuvant chemotherapy on the rate of anastomotic leak, and there have been conflicting results. In a recent single-center study of 797 patients with a single anastomosis, Lucan et al. determined in multivariate analysis that preoperative chemotherapy was one of the strongest independent risk factors for anastomotic leak, with an odds ratio of 2.85 (95% CI 1.21–6.73, $P=0.017$) [77]. Morse et al. performed a similar study of 682 patients with intestinal anastomoses over a 5 year period, and determined in bivariate analysis that chemotherapy (administered within 6 weeks of the operation) was not a risk factor for anastomotic leak.

Bevacizumab (Avastin) is a humanized monoclonal antibody, which targets vascular endothelial growth factor A (VEGF-A), and is thought to work in solid tumors by restricting neoangiogenesis, which is necessary for tumor growth. It is the first of the antiangiogenic drugs to be approved for first-line treatment of metastatic colorectal cancer, and is also used for other solid tumors including breast, kidney, ovarian, and lung cancer. Bevacizumab is associated with increased incidence of postoperative complications, including impaired wound healing and anastomotic leak. Consequently, phase II and III studies of bevacizumab for colorectal cancer excluded patients who underwent major surgery within the previous 28 days [78–80]. Yoshioka et al. retrospectively evaluated 78 patients with resectable advanced or metastatic colorectal cancer who received neoadjuvant bevacizumab prior to surgical resection (this included 46 rectal resections and 4 colectomies) [81]. Overall median interval from last bevacizumab dose to surgery was 9 weeks; anastomotic leaks occurred in six patients, four of which required re-laparotomy. The mean interval from surgery to diagnosis of anastomotic leak was 15.8 days (range 4–34 days). Although the authors did not document mean in-hospital length of stay, presumably most of the leaks occurred after discharge. In multivariate analysis, primary colorectal anastomosis was the only independent predictive risk factor for major postoperative complications (OR 8.285; $P=0.013$). Interestingly, the interval from last bevacizumab dose to surgery was not an independent risk factor for postoperative complications. Bevacizumab has also been associated with late anastomotic complications [82]. Unsurprisingly, other newer antiangiogenic drugs have also been implicated in the development of anastomotic leak, including pazopanib and aflibercept in small series and case reports [83]. As with most chemotherapy agents, these agents are held for 6 weeks before major surgery, when possible.

Conclusion

The preoperative assessment of colorectal surgery patients should be comprehensive and often requires involvement of physicians from multiple specialties. The assessment of cardiopulmonary risk has been well studied and tends to be the focus of most surgeons. Attention to other organ systems as well as comorbidities such as substance abuse, malnutrition, and obesity deserve specific attention. Medications including anticoagulation and immunosuppressive agents are commonly encountered and their optimal management (or cessation) demands a balance between the treatment of conditions and the risk of bleeding and wound healing. With a thorough preoperative patient evaluation, patient outcomes can be optimized, by minimizing the risk of perioperative complications.

References

1. Reilly DF, McNeely MJ, Doerner D, Greenberg DL, Staiger TO, Geist MJ, et al. Self-reported exercise tolerance and the risk of serious perioperative complications. Arch Intern Med. 1999;159(18):2185–92.
2. American Society of Anesthesiologists. Practice advisory for the perioperative management of patients with cardiac implantable

electronic devices: pacemakers and implantable cardioverter-defibrillators: an updated report by the american society of anesthesiologists task force on perioperative management of patients with cardiac implantable electronic devices. Anesthesiology. 2011;114(2):247–61.

3. Kaplan EB, Sheiner LB, Boeckmann AJ, Roizen MF, Beal SL, Cohen SN, et al. The usefulness of preoperative laboratory screening. JAMA. 1985;253(24):3576–81.

4. Smetana GW, Macpherson DS. The case against routine preoperative laboratory testing. Med Clin North Am. 2003;87(1):7–40.

5. Peterson P, Hayes TE, Arkin CF, Bovill EG, Fairweather RB, Rock Jr WA, et al. The preoperative bleeding time test lacks clinical benefit: College of American Pathologists' and American Society of Clinical Pathologists' position article. Arch Surg. 1998;133(2):134–9.

6. Lee TH, Marcantonio ER, Mangione CM, Thomas EJ, Polanczyk CA, Cook EF, et al. Derivation and prospective validation of a simple index for prediction of cardiac risk of major noncardiac surgery. Circulation. 1999;100(10):1043–9.

7. Mathew A, Devereaux PJ, O'Hare A, Tonelli M, Thiessen-Philbrook H, Nevis IF, et al. Chronic kidney disease and postoperative mortality: a systematic review and meta-analysis. Kidney Int. 2008;73(9):1069–81.

8. Grek S, Gravenstein N, Morey TE, Rice MJ. A cost-effective screening method for preoperative hyperglycemia. Anesth Analg. 2009;109(5):1622–4.

9. Bouvet C, Lubbeke A, Bandi C, Pagani L, Stern R, Hoffmeyer P, et al. Is there any benefit in pre-operative urinary analysis before elective total joint replacement? Bone Joint J. 2014;96-b(3):390–4.

10. Apfelbaum JL, Connis RT, Nickinovich DG, Pasternak LR, Arens JF, Caplan RA, et al. Practice advisory for preanesthesia evaluation: an updated report by the American Society of Anesthesiologists Task Force on Preanesthesia Evaluation. Anesthesiology. 2012;116(3):522–38.

11. Fleisher LA, Fleischmann KE, Auerbach AD, Barnason SA, Beckman JA, Bozkurt B, et al. 2014 ACC/AHA guideline on perioperative cardiovascular evaluation and management of patients undergoing noncardiac surgery: executive summary: a report of the American College of Cardiology/American Heart Association Task Force on practice guidelines. Developed in collaboration with the American College of Surgeons, American Society of Anesthesiologists, American Society of Echocardiography, American Society of Nuclear Cardiology, Heart Rhythm Society, Society for Cardiovascular Angiography and Interventions, Society of Cardiovascular Anesthesiologists, and Society of Vascular Medicine Endorsed by the Society of Hospital Medicine. Journal of nuclear cardiology : official publication of the American Society of Nuclear Cardiology. 2015;22(1):162–215

12. Smetana GW, Lawrence VA, Cornell JE. Preoperative pulmonary risk stratification for noncardiothoracic surgery: systematic review for the American College of Physicians. Ann Intern Med. 2006;144(8):581–95.

13. Poirier P, Alpert MA, Fleisher LA, Thompson PD, Sugerman HJ, Burke LE, et al. Cardiovascular evaluation and management of severely obese patients undergoing surgery: a science advisory from the American Heart Association. Circulation. 2009;120(1):86–95.

14. Archer C, Levy AR, McGregor M. Value of routine preoperative chest x-rays: a meta-analysis. Can J Anaesth. 1993;40(11):1022–7.

15. Devereaux PJ, Xavier D, Pogue J, Guyatt G, Sigamani A, Garutti I, et al. Characteristics and short-term prognosis of perioperative myocardial infarction in patients undergoing noncardiac surgery: a cohort study. Ann Intern Med. 2011;154(8):523–8.

16. Girish M, Trayner Jr E, Dammann O, Pinto-Plata V, Celli B. Symptom-limited stair climbing as a predictor of postoperative cardiopulmonary complications after high-risk surgery. Chest. 2001;120(4):1147–51.

17. Bilimoria KY, Liu Y, Paruch JL, Zhou L, Kmiecik TE, Ko CY, et al. Development and evaluation of the universal ACS NSQIP surgical risk calculator: a decision aid and informed consent tool for patients and surgeons. J Am Coll Surg. 2013;217(5):833–42.e1-3.

18. Devereaux PJ, Yang H, Yusuf S, Guyatt G, Leslie K, Villar JC, et al. Effects of extended-release metoprolol succinate in patients undergoing non-cardiac surgery (POISE trial): a randomised controlled trial. Lancet. 2008;371(9627):1839–47.

19. Wijeysundera DN, Duncan D, Nkonde-Price C, Virani SS, Washam JB, Fleischmann KE, et al. Perioperative beta blockade in noncardiac surgery: a systematic review for the 2014 ACC/AHA guideline on perioperative cardiovascular evaluation and management of patients undergoing noncardiac surgery: a report of the American College of Cardiology/American Heart Association Task Force on Practice Guidelines. Circulation. 2014;130(24):2246–64.

20. Bouri S, Shun-Shin MJ, Cole GD, Mayet J, Francis DP. Meta-analysis of secure randomised controlled trials of beta-blockade to prevent perioperative death in non-cardiac surgery. Heart. 2014;100(6):456–64.

21. Kumar R, McKinney WP, Raj G, Heudebert GR, Heller HJ, Koetting M, et al. Adverse cardiac events after surgery: assessing risk in a veteran population. J Gen Intern Med. 2001;16(8):507–18.

22. Singla S, Sachdeva R, Uretsky BF. The risk of adverse cardiac and bleeding events following noncardiac surgery relative to antiplatelet therapy in patients with prior percutaneous coronary intervention. J Am Coll Cardiol. 2012;60(20):2005–16.

23. Dweck MR, Cruden NL. Noncardiac surgery in patients with coronary artery stents. Arch Intern Med. 2012;172(14):1054–5.

24. Savonitto S, D'Urbano M, Caracciolo M, Barlocco F, Mariani G, Nichelatti M, et al. Urgent surgery in patients with a recently implanted coronary drug-eluting stent: a phase II study of "bridging" antiplatelet therapy with tirofiban during temporary withdrawal of clopidogrel. Br J Anaesth. 2010;104(3):285–91.

25. Stein M, Cassara EL. Preoperative pulmonary evaluation and therapy for surgery patients. JAMA. 1970;211(5):787–90.

26. Singh M, Liao P, Kobah S, Wijeysundera DN, Shapiro C, Chung F. Proportion of surgical patients with undiagnosed obstructive sleep apnoea. Br J Anaesth. 2013;110(4):629–36.

27. Kaw R, Chung F, Pasupuleti V, Mehta J, Gay PC, Hernandez AV. Meta-analysis of the association between obstructive sleep apnoea and postoperative outcome. Br J Anaesth. 2012;109(6):897–906.

28. Chung F, Elsaid H. Screening for obstructive sleep apnea before surgery: why is it important? Curr Opin Anaesthesiol. 2009;22(3):405–11.

29. Chung F, Subramanyam R, Liao P, Sasaki E, Shapiro C, Sun Y. High STOP-Bang score indicates a high probability of obstructive sleep apnoea. Br J Anaesth. 2012;108(5):768–75.

30. Liao P, Luo Q, Elsaid H, Kang W, Shapiro CM, Chung F. Perioperative auto-titrated continuous positive airway pressure treatment in surgical patients with obstructive sleep apnea: a randomized controlled trial. Anesthesiology. 2013;119(4):837–47.

31. Kannel WB, McGee DL. Diabetes and cardiovascular risk factors: the Framingham study. Circulation. 1979;59(1):8–13.

32. Halkos ME, Puskas JD, Lattouf OM, Kilgo P, Kerendi F, Song HK, et al. Elevated preoperative hemoglobin A1c level is predictive of adverse events after coronary artery bypass surgery. J Thorac Cardiovasc Surg. 2008;136(3):631–40.

33. Pezzarossa A, Taddei F, Cimicchi MC, Rossini E, Contini S, Bonora E, et al. Perioperative management of diabetic subjects. Subcutaneous versus intravenous insulin administration during glucose-potassium infusion. Diabetes Care. 1988;11(1):52–8.

34. Flegal KM, Carroll MD, Kit BK, Ogden CL. Prevalence of obesity and trends in the distribution of body mass index among US adults, 1999–2010. JAMA. 2012;307(5):491–7.

35. Mullen JT, Moorman DW, Davenport DL. The obesity paradox: body mass index and outcomes in patients undergoing nonbariatric general surgery. Ann Surg. 2009;250(1):166–72.

36. Dindo D, Muller MK, Weber M, Clavien PA. Obesity in general elective surgery. Lancet. 2003;361(9374):2032–5.

37. Mariani L, Lo Vullo S, Bozzetti F. Weight loss in cancer patients: a plea for a better awareness of the issue. Support Care Cancer. 2012;20(2):301–9.

38. Mullen JL, Gertner MH, Buzby GP, Goodhart GL, Rosato EF. Implications of malnutrition in the surgical patient. Arch Surg. 1979;114(2):121–5.

39. Sorensen J, Kondrup J, Prokopowicz J, Schiesser M, Krahenbuhl L, Meier R, et al. EuroOOPS: an international, multicentre study to implement nutritional risk screening and evaluate clinical outcome. Clin Nutr. 2008;27(3):340–9.

40. Schwegler I, von Holzen A, Gutzwiller JP, Schlumpf R, Muhlebach S, Stanga Z. Nutritional risk is a clinical predictor of postoperative mortality and morbidity in surgery for colorectal cancer. Br J Surg. 2010;97(1):92–7.

41. Panis Y, Maggiori L, Caranhac G, Bretagnol F, Vicaut E. Mortality after colorectal cancer surgery: a French survey of more than 84,000 patients. Ann Surg. 2011;254(5):738–43. discussion 43–4.

42. Wu GH, Liu ZH, Wu ZH, Wu ZG. Perioperative artificial nutrition in malnourished gastrointestinal cancer patients. World J Gastroenterol. 2006;12(15):2441–4.

43. Baker JP, Detsky AS, Wesson DE, Wolman SL, Stewart S, Whitewell J, et al. Nutritional assessment: a comparison of clinical judgement and objective measurements. N Engl J Med. 1982;306(16):969–72.

44. Doweiko JP, Nompleggi DJ. The role of albumin in human physiology and pathophysiology, Part III: Albumin and disease states. JPEN J Parenter Enteral Nutr. 1991;15(4):476–83.

45. Burden S, Todd C, Hill J, Lal S. Pre-operative nutrition support in patients undergoing gastrointestinal surgery. Cochrane Database Syst Rev. 2012;11:Cd008879.

46. Bootun R. Effects of immunosuppressive therapy on wound healing. Int Wound J. 2013;10(1):98–104.

47. Dean PG, Lund WJ, Larson TS, Prieto M, Nyberg SL, Ishitani MB, et al. Wound-healing complications after kidney transplan-

tation: a prospective, randomized comparison of sirolimus and tacrolimus. Transplantation. 2004;77(10):1555–61.

48. Narrow WE, Rae DS, Robins LN, Regier DA. Revised prevalence estimates of mental disorders in the United States: using a clinical significance criterion to reconcile 2 surveys' estimates. Arch Gen Psychiatry. 2002;59(2):115–23.

49. Kraemer KL, Conigliaro J, Saitz R. Managing alcohol withdrawal in the elderly. Drugs Aging. 1999;14(6):409–25.

50. Pihkala H, Sandlund M. Parenthood and opioid dependence. Subst Abuse Rehabil. 2015;6:33–40.

51. Bradley KA, Rubinsky AD, Sun H, Bryson CL, Bishop MJ, Blough DK, et al. Alcohol screening and risk of postoperative complications in male VA patients undergoing major non-cardiac surgery. J Gen Intern Med. 2011;26(2):162–9.

52. Rubinsky AD, Sun H, Blough DK, Maynard C, Bryson CL, Harris AH, et al. AUDIT-C alcohol screening results and postoperative inpatient health care use. J Am Coll Surg. 2012; 214(3):296–305.e1.

53. Bush K, Kivlahan DR, McDonell MB, Fihn SD, Bradley KA. The AUDIT alcohol consumption questions (AUDIT-C): an effective brief screening test for problem drinking. Ambulatory Care Quality Improvement Project (ACQUIP). Alcohol Use Disorders Identification Test. Arch Intern Med. 1998;158(16):1789–95.

54. Tonnesen H, Rosenberg J, Nielsen HJ, Rasmussen V, Hauge C, Pedersen IK, et al. Effect of preoperative abstinence on poor postoperative outcome in alcohol misusers: randomised controlled trial. BMJ. 1999;318(7194):1311–6.

55. Tonnesen H, Nielsen PR, Lauritzen JB, Moller AM. Smoking and alcohol intervention before surgery: evidence for best practice. Br J Anaesth. 2009;102(3):297–306.

56. Gronkjaer M, Eliasen M, Skov-Ettrup LS, Tolstrup JS, Christiansen AH, Mikkelsen SS, et al. Preoperative smoking status and postoperative complications: a systematic review and meta-analysis. Ann Surg. 2014;259(1):52–71.

57. Jung KH, Kim SM, Choi MG, Lee JH, Noh JH, Sohn TS, et al. Preoperative smoking cessation can reduce postoperative complications in gastric cancer surgery. Gastric Cancer. 2015;18:683–90.

58. Frenk SM, Porter KS, Paulozzi LJ. Prescription opioid analgesic use among adults: United States, 1999–2012. NCHS data brief. 2015;189:1–8.

59. Vadivelu N, Mitra S, Kaye AD, Urman RD. Perioperative analgesia and challenges in the drug-addicted and drug-dependent patient. Best Pract Res Clin Anaesthesiol. 2014;28(1):91–101.

60. Douketis JD, Spyropoulos AC, Spencer FA, Mayr M, Jaffer AK, Eckman MH, et al. Perioperative management of antithrombotic therapy: Antithrombotic Therapy and Prevention of Thrombosis, 9th ed: American College of Chest Physicians Evidence-Based Clinical Practice Guidelines. Chest. 2012;141(2 Suppl):e326S–50S.

61. Levy JH, Tanaka KA, Dietrich W. Perioperative hemostatic management of patients treated with vitamin K antagonists. Anesthesiology. 2008;109(5):918–26.

62. Colvin BT, Barrowcliffe TW. The British Society for Haematology Guidelines on the use and monitoring of heparin 1992: second revision. BCSH Haemostasis and Thrombosis Task Force. J Clin Pathol. 1993;46(2):97–103.

63. Bernardi E, Piccioli A, Oliboni G, Zuin R, Girolami A, Prandoni P. Nomograms for the administration of unfractionated heparin

in the initial treatment of acute thromboembolism--an over-view. Thromb Haemost. 2000;84(1):22–6.

64. Maniscalco P, Caforio M, Imberti D, Porcellini G, Benedetti R. Apixaban versus enoxaparin in elective major orthopedic surgery: a clinical review. Clin Appl Thromb Hemost. 2015; 21(2):115–9.

65. Antolovic D, Reissfelder C, Rakow A, Contin P, Rahbari NN, Buchler MW, et al. A randomised controlled trial to evaluate and optimize the use of antiplatelet agents in the perioperative management in patients undergoing general and abdominal surgery--the APAP trial (ISRCTN45810007). BMC Surg. 2011;11:7.

66. Mantz J, Samama CM, Tubach F, Devereaux PJ, Collet JP, Albaladejo P, et al. Impact of preoperative maintenance or inter-ruption of aspirin on thrombotic and bleeding events after elec-tive non-cardiac surgery: the multicentre, randomized, blinded, placebo-controlled, STRATAGEM trial. Br J Anaesth. 2011;107(6):899–910.

67. Sahebally SM, Healy D, Coffey JC, Walsh SR. Should patients taking aspirin for secondary prevention continue or discontinue the medication prior to elective, abdominal surgery? Best evi-dence topic (BET). Int J Surg. 2014;12(5):16–21.

68. Wolf AM, Pucci MJ, Gabale SD, McIntyre CA, Irizarry AM, Kennedy EP, et al. Safety of perioperative aspirin therapy in pancreatic operations. Surgery. 2014;155(1):39–46.

69. Wang AS, Armstrong EJ, Armstrong AW. Corticosteroids and wound healing: clinical considerations in the perioperative period. Am J Surg. 2013;206(3):410–7.

70. Post S, Betzler M, von Ditfurth B, Schurmann G, Kuppers P, Herfarth C. Risks of intestinal anastomoses in Crohn's disease. Ann Surg. 1991;213(1):37–42.

71. Slieker JC, Komen N, Mannaerts GH, Karsten TM, Willemsen P, Murawska M, et al. Long-term and perioperative corticoste-roids in anastomotic leakage: a prospective study of 259 left-sided colorectal anastomoses. Arch Surg. 2012;147(5):447–52.

72. Eriksen TF, Lassen CB, Gogenur I. Treatment with corticoste-roids and the risk of anastomotic leakage following lower gas-trointestinal surgery: a literature survey. Colorectal Dis. 2014;16(5):O154–60.

73. Ismael H, Horst M, Farooq M, Jordon J, Patton JH, Rubinfeld IS. Adverse effects of preoperative steroid use on surgical out-comes. Am J Surg. 2011;201(3):305–8. discussion 8–9.

74. El-Hussuna A, Andersen J, Bisgaard T, Jess P, Henriksen M, Oehlenschlager J, et al. Biologic treatment or immunomodula-tion is not associated with postoperative anastomotic complica-tions in abdominal surgery for Crohn's disease. Scand J Gastroenterol. 2012;47(6):662–8.

75. Krane MK, Allaix ME, Zoccali M, Umanskiy K, Rubin MA, Villa A, et al. Preoperative infliximab therapy does not increase morbidity and mortality after laparoscopic resection for inflam-matory bowel disease. Dis Colon Rectum. 2013;56(4):449–57.

76. Ali T, Yun L, Rubin DT. Risk of post-operative complications associated with anti-TNF therapy in inflammatory bowel dis-ease. World J Gastroenterol. 2012;18(3):197–204.

77. Lujan JJ, Nemeth ZH, Barratt-Stopper PA, Bustami R, Koshenkov VP, Rolandelli RH. Factors influencing the outcome of intestinal anastomosis. Am Surg. 2011;77(9):1169–75.

78. Kabbinavar F, Hurwitz HI, Fehrenbacher L, Meropol NJ, Novotny WF, Lieberman G, et al. Phase II, randomized trial comparing bevacizumab plus fluorouracil (FU)/leucovorin (LV) with FU/LV alone in patients with metastatic colorectal cancer. J Clin Oncol. 2003;21(1):60–5.

79. Kabbinavar FF, Schulz J, McCleod M, Patel T, Hamm JT, Hecht JR, et al. Addition of bevacizumab to bolus fluorouracil and leu-covorin in first-line metastatic colorectal cancer: results of a ran-domized phase II trial. J Clin Oncol. 2005;23(16):3697–705.

80. Hurwitz H, Fehrenbacher L, Novotny W, Cartwright T, Hainsworth J, Heim W, et al. Bevacizumab plus irinotecan, fluorouracil, and leucovorin for metastatic colorectal cancer. N Engl J Med. 2004;350(23):2335–42.

81. Yoshioka Y, Uehara K, Ebata T, Yokoyama Y, Mitsuma A, Ando Y, et al. Postoperative complications following neoadjuvant bevacizumab treatment for advanced colorectal cancer. Surg Today. 2014;44(7):1300–6.

82. Deshaies I, Malka D, Soria JC, Massard C, Bahleda R, Elias D. Antiangiogenic agents and late anastomotic complications. J Surg Oncol. 2010;101(2):180–3.

83. Eveno C, le Maignan C, Soyer P, Camus M, Barranger E, Pocard M. Late anastomotic colonic dehiscence due to antian-giogenic treatment, a specific drug-class complication requiring specific treatment: an example of pazopanib complication. Clin Res Hepatol Gastroenterol. 2011;35(2):135–9.

84. Chung F, Yegneswaran B, Liao P, et al. STOP questionnaire: a tool to screen patients for obstructive sleep apnea. Anesthesiology. 2008;108:812–21.

85. Devereaux PJ, Goldman L, Cook DJ, Gilbert K, Leslie K, Guyatt GH. Perioperative cardiac events in patients undergoing noncardiac surgery: a review of the magnitude of the problem, the pathophysiology of the events and methods to estimate and communicate risk. CMAJ. 2005;173(6):627–34.

7

Optimizing Outcomes with Enhanced Recovery

Conor P. Delaney and Raul Martin Bosio

Key Concepts

- Enhanced recovery pathways (ERPs) include measures for preoperative management, intraoperative care, postoperative recovery, and pathway quality evaluation.
- ERP improves the quality of patient care by establishing standardized care paths based on evidence-based literature and current practice guidelines.
- A modified frailty index (MFI) allows for preoperative risk stratification and identifies patients that will require extra healthcare resources.
- A combination of oral antibiotics administered during the preoperative phase combined with intravenous antibiotics administered within 1 h of surgery appears to be the most efficacious strategy to decrease SSI.
- Measurement of ERP compliance is necessary to make sure the individual stated pathway items are being accomplished.

Introduction

Among the goals of a successful surgical practice, delivering high-quality patient-centered care while maintaining a low procedure-specific morbidity and readmission rate is of paramount importance. Facilitating a patient's recovery and assisting them to return to their usual activities safely, but also as soon as possible, should be viewed as part of these goals [1]. Accomplishing these goals benefits not only patients, but by decreasing length of hospital stay (LOS) and costs associated with diagnosis and treatments of complications, they also help to improve the efficiency with which healthcare is provided [2–5].

In the era of bundled payment, "pay for performance," and ongoing cuts in healthcare reimbursement, decreasing hospital operating expenses may contribute to increasing or at least maintaining hospitals' financial viability [6]. Cost-analysis data demonstrating that a specific healthcare system is able to deliver comparable patient care at a lower cost may also influence insurance preference to established contracts with a specific healthcare system over another.

Minimally invasive techniques have had a major impact on postoperative recovery, contributing to a reduction in LOS and cost [6]. In many subspecialties, these techniques have now substituted open operations and become the standard of care. However, optimizing patient recovery goes far beyond a particular technical approach. It requires a multidisciplinary approach that includes not only surgeons, anesthesiologists, and nurses, among others but also the patient himself. Enhanced recovery protocols (ERPs) start at the surgeon's office by engaging the patients in this process, managing expectations, and converting them from a passive recipient of care into an active member of this recovery team. Standardization of perioperative care measures combined with minimally invasive colorectal surgery has decreased, in our hands, LOS to an average of 2.6 days, without a significant impact on readmission rate [7–12].

What Is an ERP?

Traditionally, pre-, intra-, and postoperative management had varied depending on individuals' practice preferences of the various members of the healthcare team involved. This approach creates significant variability throughout the healthcare process, since surgeons, anesthesiologists, hospitalists, and ancillary support to name some managed patients based on past experiences, usually gained during residency or school training. This variability increases complications and healthcare cost as patients are not necessarily managed according to current recommendations [2, 4, 5, 10–33].

In an effort to reduce postoperative complication rates and decrease or contain healthcare costs, the concept of creating specific evidence-based protocols or pathways where the various components of pre-, intra-, and postoperative care are outlined and could, therefore, be followed by all the

© Springer International Publishing 2016
S.R. Steele et al. (eds.), *The ASCRS Textbook of Colon and Rectal Surgery*, DOI 10.1007/978-3-319-25970-3_7

members that participate in any given healthcare episode was developed [2, 3, 10, 16, 17, 23].

Initially called fast-track pathways, these care paths are now most commonly called enhanced recovery pathways (ERPs), which refer to the multimodality patients' care approach where patients' orders are clearly established based on evidence-based literature and current practice guidelines. These orders are then routinely followed, minimizing variability among providers with the goals of decreasing morbidity and mortality rates and increasing quality of care as a result. The decrease in healthcare resource utilization achieved as a result of decreased complications, and LOS contribute to decrease costs [10, 15, 21, 23, 25]. As patients progress through a healthcare intervention, specialty-specific order sets clearly outline patients' management at any given point in time, from the preoperative encounter until care is completed, generally at the time of hospital discharge.

The direct consequences of the application of specialty-specific pathways are well documented and include a reduction in morbidity, mortality, and length of hospital stay (LOS). This reduction in LOS is seen both after open and laparoscopic operations when compared to patients that are managed outside a pathway. An even greater reduction in LOS is seen when open versus laparoscopic colorectal procedures coupled to a perioperative pathway are compared. This difference persists even when readmission rates are included into the overall LOS for any given patient [7, 10, 12, 16–18, 21, 22, 27, 30–32, 34–42].

Components of an ERP

From a practical standpoint, ERP can be divided in four parts: (a) preoperative management, (b) intraoperative care, (c) postoperative recovery, and (d) quality pathway evaluation measures.

Each part includes a series of measures or steps as follows:

(a) *Preoperative management*: (1) preoperative evaluation (i.e., frailty score and pre-habilitation); (2) fasting prior to surgery, mechanical bowel preparation, and preoperative antibiotics usage; (3) patient education; and (4) analgesia (*for practical purposes, as it overlaps with pre-, intra-, and postoperative management, analgesia is addressed as a whole in the intraoperative section*).

(b) *Intraoperative care*: (1) minimally invasive colorectal surgery when possible, (2) standardized intraoperative fluid resuscitation, (3) analgesia, and (4) venous thromboembolism prophylaxis (VTE).

(c) *Postoperative recovery*: (1) analgesia; (2) intravenous fluid management; (3) early oral feeding and ambulation; (4) prevention of postoperative nausea and vomiting (PONV) and postoperative ileus (POI), role of nasogastric tube and motility agents; (5) venous thromboembolism prophylaxis (VTE); and (6) discharge planning, follow-up, and coordination of care.

(d) *Quality pathway evaluation measures*: (1) electronic order sets creation and updates to comply with best practice parameter guidelines and evidence-based literature, (2) implementation and monitoring of pathway application, and (3) quality improvement measures.

Enhanced Recovery Pathways (ERPs) After Surgery: Challenging "Traditional" Patients' Care Management

Traditionally, postoperative care varies depending on surgeon's preferences and his understanding of patients' clinical condition. In general, perioperative management practices learned during training tend to be maintained once in practice despite evidence that would suggest that new available pathways may help decrease postoperative complications, length of stay, and the associated healthcare cost. Furthermore, compliance with ERP application has been associated with improved outcomes, decreased LOS, and cost reduction [19, 43].

Multiple factors may impact the application of new models of care. Limited time to interact with patients both in the preoperative setting and during the inpatient stay leads to a feeling of lack of control when attempting to implement changes. As surgeons adjust to the demands of current practice styles, and the implementation of electronic medical records, providing coverage to multiple hospitals and to increase productivity, modifying patient care patterns learned through personal experience during training in favor of new care pathways described on medical literature, but without any clinical experience is difficult [44–46].

However, as teaching hospitals expose trainees to these new models of care, a new generation of surgeons is entering the working force with the knowledge and experience to implement and lead these changes.

Electronic medical records, with the capability of creating order sets, also play an important role in eliminating variability in patients' management as they provide a blue print that is easily reproduced from patient to patient.

Successful implementation of these new models of care depends not only on the surgeon; on the contrary, they required significant institutional support as multiple teams across the healthcare spectrum are necessary in order to improve patients' care and reduce costs [47, 48]. As pathways are developed and implemented, full potential can be achieved with active participation from anesthesiologists, nursing staff, physical therapists, and ostomy teams. This increase in resource utilization may contribute to a perception of increased cost and healthcare expenditure and lead to a lack of support from hospitals' administration. Although there is an initial increase in cost, the increased healthcare expenditure is offset through a reduction in patients' morbidity and length of hospital stay [49–51].

TABLE 7-1. Quality measures between patients managed within and outside an established enhanced recovery pathway (ERP)

Author	Within ERP	Outside ERP	Morbidity (ERP vs. non-ERP)	LOS (days) (ERP vs. non-ERP)	Readmission rates (ERPs vs. non-ERP)
Bradshaw et al. [155]	36	36	8% vs. 11%	4.9 vs. 6	3% vs. 3%
Basse et al. [157]	130	130	25% vs. 55%	3.3 vs. 10	21% vs. 12%
Anderson et al. [158]	14	11	28% vs. 45%	3.9 vs. 6.9[a]	0% vs. 0%
Raue et al. [156]	23	29	17% vs. 24%	4 vs. 7	4 % vs. 7 %
Delaney et al. [15]	33	31	22% vs. 30%	5.2 vs. 5.8[a]	9.7% vs. 18.2%
Gatt et al. [159]	19	20	47% vs. 75%	6.6 vs. 9[a]	5.3% vs. 20%
Khoo et al. [59]	35	35	25% vs. 51%	5 vs. 7[a]	9% vs. 3%
Serclova et al. [160]	52	51	21% vs. 48%	7.4 vs. 10.4[a]	0% vs. 0%
Muller et al. 2009 [161]	75	76	21% vs. 49%	6.7 vs. 10.3[a]	3.9% vs. 2.6%
LAFA 2011 laparoscopic [153]	100	109	34% vs. 37%	5 vs. 6	6% vs. 6.4%
LAFA 2011 open [154]	93	98	43% vs. 41%	6 vs. 7	7.4 % vs. 7.1 %

[a]Mean length of stay (LOS)
Data obtained and combined into current table from Wind et al. [153], Vlug et al. [154], and Adamina et al. [1]

The concept of "team" is key to the success of these changes in patients care practices, as surgeons alone without the appropriate supportive environment may encounter difficulties in improving patient experience. Monitoring adherence to a given pathway allows for quality control measures to be periodically evaluated, ensuring participation of the various teams involved and allows for modifications to the pathway to be implemented as necessary [52–54].

At the end, incorporating an enhanced recovery pathway (ERP) into a practice or hospital system should lead to improve patient care, decreased morbidity and mortality, reduced length of hospital stay (LOS) and healthcare cost, while maintaining or even decreasing readmission rates (Table 7-1) [1].

Where Does the Pathway Start?

The answer to this question needs to be considered both from the surgeon and from an institutional viewpoint.

From a surgeons' perspective, in its simplest form, an ERP starts with a surgeon implementing a specialty-specific order set. As the use of ERP is applicable to most specialties across the board and affects hospitals' expenditure and therefore profit margins, more advanced setups require the participation of multiple teams (surgery, anesthesia, nursing, etc.) [55].

As specialty-specific ERPs are created, institutional support facilitates their introduction and use. Creation of specialty-/department-specific committees allows for input from these teams to be incorporated into the ERP. There is no point in modifying preoperative fasting time to 2 h for liquids, to cite an example, if the individual anesthesiologist will not accept and be willing to anesthetize a patient due to his own practice preferences, despite the fact that guidelines indicate that such practice is safe [56–58]. Multiple examples like this one can be described, and consensus is necessary among healthcare providers and ancillary teams as the

institution moves forward in the development of these pathways. Teams usually involved include, but are not limited to, surgeons, nursing staff, physical therapist, information technology personnel, residents, respiratory therapist, and ostomy team members. The configuration of these committees may vary, as pathways have been successfully implemented across multiple specialties and specialty-specific needs are targeted [59].

Preoperative Management

Preoperative Evaluation: Frailty Score and Pre-habilitation

Several patient factors can negatively affect the outcome after elective colorectal surgery. Among them, nutritional status has been directly associated with outcomes and should be viewed as part of the preoperative assessment of patients within an ERP program [60]. Several tools can be used to evaluate nutritional status. The subjective global assessment (SGA) tool allows patients to be stratified in well, moderate, and severe malnutrition (SGA-A, SGA-B, and SGA-C, respectively). Postoperative complications after colorectal surgery, as well as LOS, have both increased as patients' nutritional status worsens. Morbidity increases from 11% for SGA-A to 31% and 41% for SGA-B and SGA-C. Length of stay increases as well, with hospital days increasing from 4 to 5 and 7, respectively, for SGA-A, SGA-B, and SGA-C [61]. Prolonged preoperative nutrition, either enteral (whenever use of the gastrointestinal tract is possible) or parenteral, may improve nutrition within 2–3 weeks and decrease complications. Therefore, preoperative nutritional assessment and optimization should be part of an ERP, as both morbidity and LOS improve when appropriate steps are implemented [62, 63].

Frailty, defined as a decrease in physiologic reserve and multisystem impairment independently of the normal aging process, where patients show a combination of decreased muscle mass and functionality, signs of chronic inflammation, and altered metabolism, is also a marker of increased postoperative morbidity and mortality as well as prolonged LOS [64, 65].

A modified frailty index (MFI) allows for preoperative risk stratification and may allow to identify patients that will require extra healthcare resources early on and to plan in accordance. Eleven variables are considered, and some of them can be optimized preoperatively, such as chronic obstructive pulmonary disease or congestive heart failure [66]. Published data has demonstrated a correlation with LOS, and utilization of MFI may allow surgeons to identify patients early on that may require additional healthcare resource utilization. Data suggest that approximately 61% of patients with a MFI of 1 or less had a LOS between 1 and 3 days, while more than 50% of patients with a MFI of 3 or more are hospitalized between 4 and 8 days [61].

Preoperative optimization is recommended when possible, and certain measures such as stopping alcohol or smoking 4 weeks prior to surgery are associated with improved outcomes [60, 61, 64]. Pre-habilitation, a term that refers to a structured process, aims to improve patients' capacity to respond to surgical stress, and decreased postoperative complications are currently an area of research within ERP protocols. Although creation of a structured program that combines preoperative exercise training, nutritional support, and optimization of chronic disease processes appears as a logical progression of preoperative management, there is not sufficient data at this time to support the allocation of resources to the creation of such programs. They represent, however, an avenue for active research with potential to positively impact patients' outcomes and could be considered at the time of creation of an ERP.

Fasting Prior to Surgery, Mechanical Bowel Preparation, and Preoperative Antibiotics Usage

Classic preoperative management teaching had focus on limitation of oral intake prior to surgery, the role of mechanical bowel preparation, and antibiotics usage [60].

Traditionally, patients are asked to fast from midnight onwards prior to surgery. Published literature has evaluated the role of carbohydrate loading prior to elective surgery. Solid intake is then limited to 6 h prior to surgery and carbohydrate-rich fluids to 2 h. It appears to be of some benefit in terms of decreasing postoperative insulin resistance, LOS, and patient satisfaction (i.e., decreased in thirst); however, the level of evidence is low, and further studies are required to determine how it may affect patient recovery. Some literature suggests that preoperative carbohydrate

loading improves PONV and decreases loss of muscle mass. However, further studies are needed, as patient benefits may not be superior when preoperative oral glucose is compared to intravenous glucose infusion during surgery. Independent of potential benefits, reducing fasting times and the usage of preoperative carbohydrate drinks up to 2 h prior to surgery is safe as there is no increased risk of anesthesia complications [67–70].

Mechanical bowel preparation prior to colorectal surgery has also been a topic of debate, with a large body of literature showing that there is no difference in outcomes whether mechanical preparation is used or not [71–74]. A Cochrane review that included 5805 patients demonstrated no difference in wound infection, anastomotic leakage, intra-abdominal infectious complications, or need for reoperation independently of whether a mechanical bowel preparation was used or not [75]. However, colonic manipulation during laparoscopic surgery is easier when a mechanical bowel preparation is used. Jung et al. randomized 1343 patients to mechanical bowel preparation versus no preparation and found similar results. This study, published in 2007, evaluated patients enrolled between 1999 and 2005 [76]. Recently, long-term follow-up data from this study found a change in cancer-specific survival when a mechanical bowel preparation was used. The 10-year cancer-specific survival was 84.1% versus 78% for patient who underwent mechanical bowel preparation versus those who did not [77]. However, Van't Sant et al. reviewed data from 382 patients (median follow-up 7.6 years) and found no difference in survival among groups (bowel preparation vs. none) [78]. Although further studies are now needed in order to evaluate the relationship of mechanical bowel preparation and long-term specific survival, as the authors themselves point out, surgeons should consider reviewing their current practices, as mechanical bowel preparation may not change early postoperative outcomes, but it may impact long-term survival.

It is our practice to use mechanical bowel preparation when a patient will be diverted, for left colon and rectal resections, when an intracorporeal anastomosis is planned, and in those cases that may require an intraoperative colonoscopy. As a result of the data mentioned above, mechanical bowel preparation for right colectomies is being used by part of our team.

The third component of the preoperative management includes the usage of antibiotics prior to surgery. Adequate coverage should include both aerobic and anaerobic flora. Meta-analyses have shown that there is a decrease in surgical wound infection (SSI) when antibiotics usage is compared to placebo. A risk reduction of at least 75% has been found with a decrease in wound infection from 40% to 14–6% [79–82]. As surgeons currently administer antibiotics routinely within 1 h of the surgical starting time as part of compliance with Surgical Care Improvement Project guidelines (SCIP), the decision-making process currently centers in what the ideal regimen is. The ideal regimen should not only control SSI but also consider cost and adverse effects of a selected regimen. A combination of oral antibiotics administered during the preoperative phase (usually while the patient undergoes mechanical bowel preparation) combined with intravenous antibiotics administered within 1 h of surgery appears to be the most efficacious strategy to decrease SSI (6.5%). Continuation of antibiotics beyond 24 h after elective surgery offers no benefit, and it is not recommended under current guidelines [79, 83]. It is our practice to give antibiotics the day prior to surgery during the bowel preparation, followed by one dose in the operating room. Re-dosing varies depending on the antibiotic used half live and the length of the case.

Patient Education

From a surgeon-patient interaction perspective, an ERP starts in the first office visit. The concept of early hospital discharge is not new. The first reports are from the 1990s. Although successful implementation was demonstrated back then, they also showed that managing patients' expectations is important, as a significant number of patients felt they were discharged home too early despite meeting discharge criteria, based mainly in their perception of inpatient postoperative recovery times.

Patient education is a key component of an ERP. The concept or view of patients being passive recipients of care should be changed. Patients should be actively engaged in the recovery process and understand that they play a significant role in decreasing complications. A motivated patient, with clear goals to meet in mind, is more likely to comply with perioperative tasks such as ambulating, incentive spirometry usage, and reduction of narcotics intake to name a few [1, 3, 60].

These goals and expectations can be discussed during the preoperative encounter and reinforced by written educational material, preoperative meeting with the ostomy team when necessary, and encouraging the patient to communicate their questions or concerns as needed. Easy patient accessibility to the care team, in many cases through a nurse practitioner or a medical assistant, plays an important role in the development of the patient-physician-healthcare team relationship. From a patient's perspective, being discharged home in postoperative day 2 or 3 after a major abdominal surgery may be perceived as a daunting scenario. Easy accessibility to the healthcare team through healthcare extenders helps develop trust in the system and contributes to improve patient satisfaction. Institutional support plays an important role in this process, as resources need to be available to incorporate, for example, nurse practitioner into the teams. However, having someone available within the team to address patients' questions once discharged, either through phone or email communication, can contribute to decrease readmission rates and should be seen as part of the efforts to improve care and patient satisfaction.

Intraoperative Pathway

Minimally Invasive Colorectal Surgery

Current data shows that only 50–70% of colorectal resections in the United States are performed in a minimally invasive fashion. The national average LOS after colorectal surgery reported by Medicare is approximately 9 days; a substantial variability in the quality of care that has been delivered can be seen when LOS of 2–3 days is common after laparoscopic colorectal resections [1, 6, 14, 18, 23, 30, 42, 84]. From an economic point of view, the average cost per inpatient day in the United States varies between $1625 and $2025 (2010 data). This difference in LOS represents gross savings of approximately $9750 per patient per hospital stay.

Minimally invasive colorectal surgery combined with enhanced recovery protocols has shown to decrease LOS to an average as low as 2.6 days, with some patients being safely discharged home within 24 h. At the same time, early hospital discharge has been associated to readmission rates comparable to patients being managed outside an ERP [4, 7–10, 12, 38, 40, 41, 85].

ERP can be successfully applied for patients undergoing open colorectal procedures, with data supporting a decrease in morbidity and LOS compared to non-pathway patients. However, LOS is invariably longer when compared to patients undergoing a minimally invasive procedure. Therefore, procedures performed open, laparoscopic, and in an emergent basis should be managed within the established ERP, with minimally invasive surgery preferred over open when possible [5, 8, 10–12, 17, 24, 26, 31, 38, 40, 41, 43, 86, 87].

Intraoperative Fluid Administration

Fluid administration during surgery is an area of ongoing debate. As fluid homeostasis is affected by changes in several hormones during the postoperative period, the amount of fluid given during the surgery itself varies significantly based on individual practices. Historically, fluid resuscitation tends to overestimate requirements which translate into early postoperative weight gain secondary to fluid retention and third spacing [55]. Studies using restrictive fluid resuscitation strategies have shown a decrease in cardiopulmonary complications and LOS without an adverse effect in anastomotic leakage or surgical-specific complications. However, the data is not clear regarding the optimal strategy, as different studies had used different regimens, with variations in the type of fluid used (colloid vs. crystalloid) and the option of increasing fluid administration based on intraoperative clinical parameter interpretation by the individual anesthesiologist [88]. These situations make comparison difficult; therefore, there are no clear guidelines as to what the ideal regimen is. By measuring intraoperative "real-time" volume status using transesophageal Doppler to determine stroke volume and vasopressor medication once normovolemia is achieved, a LOS as low as 2.7 days has been reported, with a subgroup of patients being discharged home within 23 h [55]. This approach, described as a goal-directed therapy, as patients' fluid resuscitation is tailored based on individual needs, has shown similar results to data published by Delaney et al., who has reported a similar LOS without the need of additional intraoperative equipment (i.e., transesophageal Doppler probe) and the need of anesthesiologists with that particular skill set. Both these factors may increase cost without a clear change in outcomes in elective cases or in patients with minimal comorbidities [88–97]. These results are further validated by Senagore et al., who randomized patients undergoing a minimally invasive procedure within an ERP pathway and compared standard versus goal-directed fluid resuscitation. The standard group has a shorter LOS (64.9 h vs. 75.5 h, respectively) [98].

Currently, intraoperative restrictive fluid administration appears to be superior to traditional intraoperative fluid resuscitation protocols, and a standardized anesthesia protocol should be established as part of an ERP. However, further studies are necessary to determine the role of goal-directed therapy, independent of whether intraoperative transesophageal Doppler monitoring or finger-probe monitoring is used, as there may be a subset of patients that could benefit from this technology [55].

Analgesia

From our standpoint, pain control starts prior to surgery, continues during the procedure and the hospital stay, and adequately maintains based on specific patients' needs after discharge. Pain management is described in this part of the chapter; however, the ERP should address pre-, intra-, and postoperative pain control.

Adequate pain control is of paramount importance after surgery, as patients are more likely to ambulate and resume some routine daily activities sooner when postoperative pain is well managed. The opposite is also true, as patients with inadequate pain control are most likely to remain in bed, to avoid deep breathing and actively engaging in their recovery, as they perceive pain as a limiting factor to what they can do. At the same time, it is considered a patient's right and patients' satisfaction can be negatively affected when pain management is not adequate. It is not only indicative of poor patient management in most cases, but it may also affect hospital reimbursement as patients' satisfaction becomes tied to it [55, 60].

There is no ideal pain regimen, as analgesia requirements vary from patient to patient and type of analgesic used is influenced by patients' history of chronic narcotics usage, liver and kidney function's profiles, and age to name some. Ideally, the selected analgesia regimen will control patients' pain while minimizing the development of adverse effects, such as PONV, POI hypotension, or kidney injury, among others.

Blocking nociceptor activation prior to a painful stimulus, a term described as "preemptive" analgesia, has been extensively discussed in the medical literature. However, high-quality data to support its usage is scarce. Preemptive analgesia includes multiple interventions, from oral analgesic administration starting the day prior to surgery to placement of epidural catheters or spinal analgesia prior to the beginning of the procedure or local infiltration of the surgical sites in the case of laparoscopy. Data supporting these different strategies varies; however, simple measures such as preoperative intake of oral medication should be considered as part of an ERP. Nonsteroidal anti-inflammatory drugs (NSAIDs) such as ibuprofen or diclofenac are usually incorporated into the ERP and administered starting 24 h prior or the day of surgery [99–101]. Gabapentin, a central acting agent, can also be started in the preoperative stage, and it is part of the ERP protocol used by the authors. Data regarding the use of short- and long-acting anxiolytic medication has been reported; however, these drugs are currently not recommended by the ERAS society [60, 102–106].

Intraoperatively, local infiltration of the surgical port sites has not shown to decrease postoperative pain requirements. Liposomal bupivacaine may be used; however, there is yet no evidence to support its use. On the contrary, peripheral nerve blocks such as a transverse abdominis muscle pain (TAP) block have shown to decrease postoperative opioid usage. It is a technically simple, low-cost procedure that can easily be performed under laparoscopic or ultrasound guidance [107–109].

Postoperative analgesia has also been subject to extensive debate. The use of epidural analgesia versus a combination of intravenous opioids delivered using patient controlled analgesia (PCA) equipment and scheduled intravenous NSAIDs such as ketorolac and/or paracetamol appears to be similar in controlling pain in most cases. Although the use of epidural catheters may improve pain scores initially, overall pain control, LOS, and patient satisfaction appear to favor the latter [33, 110–115].

The combination of an opioid PCA and intravenous ketorolac or acetaminophen in the initial postoperative phase (postoperative day zero or 1) followed by a combination of these medications by mouth as soon as patients start oral intake is favored by the author and is part of the standard ERP protocol and the electronic order sets.

A combination of epidural analgesia administered and intravenous opioids and NSAIDs is an alternative that should be considered in chronic opioids users. Epidurals analgesia may be limited to the administration of a local anesthetic or to a combination of a local anesthetic and opioids. Although there is extensive data regarding the use of thoracic epidural analgesia documenting its safety, it is an invasive procedure with associated complications such as pruritus, urinary retention, and postoperative hypotension. Postoperative hypotension secondary to an inhibition of the sympathetic tone is of particular importance when using an epidural catheter. In these cases, patients may benefit from a decrease in the amount of medication being delivered rather than from the administration of intravenous fluids boluses [115, 116].

A one-time intrathecal administration of an opioid and local anesthetic (0.5% bupivacaine) followed by a combination of a narcotics PCA and NSAIDs appears to be superior than both of the abovementioned options; however, it is an invasive procedure, and further data is required to determine its real impact on LOS [116]. It is not currently part of our standard ERP.

Venous Thromboembolism Prophylaxis (VTE)

Venous thromboembolism prophylaxis is currently part of the SCIP guidelines and commonly built in as part of the mandatory electronic admission order sets. SCIP guidelines require starting of prophylaxis within 24 h of surgery. This allows for variability in the usage of the medication, as surgeons may opt to administer it prior to the surgical procedure itself or within the 24 h period. Data supporting the use of either unfractionated heparin versus low molecular weight heparin shows very little difference between these prophylactic agents. However, data regarding the length of prophylaxis after surgery is still controversial [60, 117]. A Cochrane meta-analysis that included four randomized trials demonstrated a reduction in VTE from 1.7 to 0.2% when prophylaxis was maintained for 4 weeks [118]. However, a database review of more than 52,000 patients found that the prevalence of postoperative symptomatic VTE after only inpatient prophylaxis was 0.67% [119, 120]. A recently published randomized controlled trial of 1 versus 4 weeks of pharmacological VTE prophylaxis specifically after colorectal laparoscopic surgery showed that VTE occurred in 9.7% versus 0.9%, respectively [121]. Symptoms of VTE were present in only two and one patient respectively. No episodes of pulmonary embolism occurred in either group. Guidelines indicated that prophylaxis should be continued for 4 weeks, especially in oncologic patients [60].

In our practice, patients with limited mobility, being discharged to a skill nursing facility, morbid obese, with advanced malignancies, with coagulation disorders, or with prior history of VTE or PE, are usually discharged on a 4-week course.

Postoperative Recovery

Analgesia

Pain control should continue during the inpatient stay as well as after discharge. Pain management strategies have been described earlier in the chapter. From an outpatient pain management standpoint, a gradual decrease in medication usage is expected. Medication (both opioids and NSAIDs) should be prescribed, keeping this in mind and considering the potential for abuse associated with narcotics usage. The amount of narcotics usage in the United States is significantly higher when compared to the rest of the world, and efforts are being implemented at a government level to monitor opioids usage. A fine line is required to maintain adequate pain control and patients' satisfaction while preventing abuse.

It is our practice to start a combination of acetaminophen and NSAIDs the day after surgery unless a specific contraindication exists. These medications are scheduled, while opioids are used for breakthrough pain control. Opioid PCA is usually discontinued in postoperative day 1 after a laparoscopic resection.

Intravenous Fluid Management

ERP have demonstrated the safety of initiating early oral intake, thus being able to decrease intravenous fluid requirements. At the same time, published data indicated that restricting intravenous fluids to less than <2 l/day versus >3 l/day are associated with increase gastric emptying, faster recovery of gastrointestinal function, and overall decrease morbidity and LOS [55]. It is our practice to limit or stop intravenous fluids within 24–48 h of surgery.

Early Oral Feeding, Ambulation, and Role of Nasogastric Tube

A large body of literature has shown that early introduction of oral intake within 24 h of surgery is safely tolerated in 70–90% of patients. Even though a Cochrane review and a meta-analysis fail to show a reduction in LOS when early feeding is introduced, numerous single institution reports over the last 10 years or more have reported average LOS of just over 2 days, and restarting oral intake within the first day of surgery has been an integral part of their ERPs [122]. Although early feeding increases the risk of vomiting [123], the risk of aspiration pneumonia remains the same whether feeding is started early on or after return of bowel function (absolute risk of 0–6.3% vs. 0–7.1%, respectively) [122–126]. Early feeding has also been associated with a decrease in insulin resistance, hyperglycemia, and wound infection.

Encouraging and facilitating early ambulation through the aid of ancillary staff while the patient is still in the hospital is key to achieve the goal of a short LOS. Early ambulation helps decrease muscle waste and helps prevent a reduction in gastrointestinal motility associated with an increased time in bed [125, 126].

Prevention of Postoperative Nausea and Vomiting (PONV) and Postoperative Ileus (POI): Role of Nasogastric Tube and Motility Agents

ERP routinely includes medications that try to decrease PONV and prevent the development of POI. Several classes of antiemetics are available, and each class has been shown to be superior to placebo in the management of PONV. A combination of two or more drugs decreases even further the incidence of PONV [127–133].

A single dose of intravenous dexamethasone during surgery combined with ondansetron (serotonergic 5-HT3 receptor antagonists) appears to be the most adequate strategy to prevent PONV. Ondansetron is continued during the postoperative period at a dose of 4 mg every 6–8 h as needed. Studies have demonstrated a decreased incidence in PONV with ondansetron compared to metoclopramide. For patients at increased risk of developing PONV, a combination of a transdermal scopolamine patch and ondansetron can be used with studies suggesting increased efficacy when compared to ondansetron alone [131, 132].

Postoperative ileus (POI) refers to a transient impairment in gastrointestinal motility that prevents oral intake. Various definitions of POI have been proposed. Classically, it has been described as a delay to restart oral intake for more than 3 days after laparoscopic surgery or to more than 5 days after open procedures. Senagore et al. proposed an alternative classification by describing POI as any situation that requires a return to "nil per os" or the insertion of a nasogastric tube (NG). He further defines ileus as primary or secondary based on whether it is associated (secondary) or not to any other complication (i.e., anastomotic leakage) [9, 128, 129].

Primary POI causes not only patient discomfort and delays hospital discharge; it is a significant cause of healthcare expenditure, accounting for approximately $750 million per year [55, 132].

Alvimopan, a peripheral-acting mu-opioid receptor antagonist, has been shown to decrease the time required for return of gastrointestinal function and decrease POI and LOS after open and laparoscopic colorectal surgery. However, its role after laparoscopic colorectal surgery and an established ERP is less clear; Delaney et al. described a reduction in POI from 4 to 12% when comparing two matched laparoscopic colectomy groups when alvimopan was used. However, LOS (3.6 vs. 3.7 days) and hospital readmission rates (4% vs. 4.2%) were the same in both groups [134–141].

Oral magnesium oxide was described to facilitate return of bowel function after colonic surgery and as part of an ERP protocol. However, the data available is small and have not been validated in further studies.

Bisacodyl, either orally or as a suppository, facilitates return of bowel function; however, LOS is unchanged, and the amount of data available is limited [142, 143].

Chewing sugarless gum postoperatively has also been associated with a decreased time to return of bowel function and decreased LOS. The level of evidence is very robust, and its associated cost and reported adverse effects (i.e., bloating) are minimal [144–147].

Nasogastric tube decompression has been shown to have no role as a preemptive measure to prevent PONV or POI. Furthermore, it delays return of bowel function and hospital discharge. Therapeutic NG decompression still has a role in the treatment of POI; however, its usage is required in less than 10% of patients [148–150].

Venous Thromboembolism Prophylaxis (VTE)

VTE prophylaxis should be initiated within 24 h per SCIP guidelines. This topic has been addressed earlier on the chapter while discussing intraoperative management; however, addressing VTE prophylaxis is mandatory during the postoperative period under current practice parameters.

Discharge Planning, Follow-Up, and Coordination of Care

Discharge planning, follow-up, and coordination of care with other healthcare teams (i.e., predischarge appointments coordination with the different healthcare provider such as oncology, as needed) should be initiated early on during hospital stay. This process is facilitated by the electronic medical records system and electronic orders/appointments scheduling. Incorporation of ancillary support staff such as nurse practitioners, stoma therapists, social workers, and physical therapists as members of the ERP team allows for active education, planning, early identification of patients that may need home care or to be discharged to physical rehabilitation or extended care facilities, and decreased unnecessary hospital stay secondary to poor planning or administrative delays such as insurance approval [2, 9, 15, 21, 29, 31, 151, 152].

Quality Pathway Evaluation Measures

Electronic Order Set Creation and Updates to Comply with Best Practice Parameters Guidelines and Evidence-Based Literature

Creation of specialty-specific order sets requires the participation of the various members that contribute on a daily basis to patient care and application of the ERP. This includes surgeons, anesthesiologists, information technology personnel, nurses, ostomy/wound care team members, physical therapist, residents, and social workers to name a few. Data have shown that the initial cost of implementing an ERP is offset by the reduction in morbidity and LOS achieved with the subsequent pathway implementation. Regular meetings are required to ensure that the ERP and the associated order sets remain in compliance with changes in practice parameters, evidence-based guidelines, and government and insurance policies [1, 43, 60].

Implementation and Monitoring of Pathway Application

Compliance and application of the numerous components of an ERP have been shown to vary within members of any given colorectal group. Changes in members of the ERP can impact the way ERPs are implemented, and morbidity and LOS may change accordingly. Mobile Internet-based applications currently exist and are being used in high-volume centers to monitor in real-time ERP compliance and to identify variables that can affect its application, such as individual surgeon's preferences or a lack of support personnel. As information technology progresses and variables that affect patient care are identified, an opportunity for further improvement of ERP may occur. There is no data at the present time to evaluate its effect in overall patients' experience, quality of care, and healthcare cost [153–156].

Quality Improvement Measures

Since the beginning of the century and secondary to high morbidity and mortality rates and a constant increase in healthcare cost, numerous programs have been developed to try to standardize care. With the objective of improving quality by decreasing variability among healthcare providers and contain cost, programs such as SCIP and National Surgical Quality Improvement Program (NSQIP) were developed. Over time, regional initiatives supported by private funding also developed as the opportunity to change individuals' practice styles toward an evidence-based, and best practice guidance model was seen as a way to achieve those goals.

Compliance with SCIP measures is becoming part of everyday practice. However, some of the standardized measures have failed to significantly improve quality. Internal practice monitoring and benchmarking them to national standards, as long as confounding variables can be included (i.e., tertiary center patients' complexity and postoperative morbidity), may allow physicians and hospitals to modify practice parameters and improve outcomes [1, 36–38, 45, 48, 64]. An easy-to-apply metric to evaluate for quality in colorectal surgery was described by the senior author of this chapter. The HARM score takes into consideration hospital stay, readmission, and mortality rates. The score is calculated by giving each patient discharge a value from 1 to 10. As the hospital mean HARM score increases from <2, to 2–3, to 3–4 and more than 4, an increase in complication rates after elective

colorectal surgery is seen, changing from 15.2% to 18.2%, to 24.0%, and to 35.6%, respectively. This metric provides surgeons a low-cost tool to compare quality and may allow for identification of true outlier performers [152].

Conclusion

The combination of ERPs and minimally invasive colorectal techniques has demonstrated a reduction in morbidity and mortality and overall length of hospital stay and is associated with a low readmission rate. This multimodal approach, based on interdisciplinary work, contributes to the standardization of patients' care and, as a result, contributes to increase quality of care. Its implementation through specialty-specific order sets covers the whole episode of care, from preoperative management until completion of care is achieved. Continuous pathway monitoring allows for updates in the order sets to be made to adjust to changes in best practice parameters and pathway compliance. Overall, the decrease in complications associated with the implementation of an ERP and minimally invasive colorectal surgery achieves the goals of improving quality of patients' care while simultaneously reducing healthcare-related cost when compared to patients managed outside a specific pathway [1–3, 6–9, 13–16, 18, 21, 35–38, 45, 47, 48, 62, 64, 84, 86].

References

1. Adamina M, Kehlet H, Tomlinson GA, Senagore AJ, Delaney CP. Enhanced recovery pathways optimize health outcomes and resource utilization: a meta-analysis of randomized controlled trials in colorectal surgery. Surgery. 2011;149(6):830–40.
2. Asgeirsson T, Jrebi N, Feo L, Kerwel T, Luchtefeld M, Senagore AJ. Incremental cost of complications in colectomy: a warranty guided approach to surgical quality improvement. Am J Surg. 2014;207(3):422–6. discussion 5–6.
3. Chestovich PJ, Lin AY, Yoo J. Fast-track pathways in colorectal surgery. Surg Clin North Am. 2013;93(1):21–32.
4. Senagore AJ, Delaney CP. A critical analysis of laparoscopic colectomy at a single institution: lessons learned after 1000 cases. Am J Surg. 2006;191(3):377–80.
5. Senagore AJ, Stulberg JJ, Byrnes J, Delaney CP. A national comparison of laparoscopic vs. open colectomy using the National Surgical Quality Improvement Project data. Dis Colon Rectum. 2009;52(2):183–6.
6. Bosio RM, Smith BM, Aybar PS, Senagore AJ. Implementation of laparoscopic colectomy with fast-track care in an academic medical center: benefits of a fully ascended learning curve and specialty expertise. Am J Surg. 2007;193(3):413–5. discussion 5–6.
7. Delaney CP, Chang E, Senagore AJ, Broder M. Clinical outcomes and resource utilization associated with laparoscopic and open colectomy using a large national database. Ann Surg. 2008;247(5):819–24.
8. Delaney CP, Kiran RP, Senagore AJ, Brady K, Fazio VW. Case-matched comparison of clinical and financial outcome after

laparoscopic or open colorectal surgery. Ann Surg. 2003;238(1):67–72.

9. Delaney CP, Senagore AJ, Gerkin TM, Beard TL, Zingaro WM, Tomaszewski KJ, et al. Association of surgical care practices with length of stay and use of clinical protocols after elective bowel resection: results of a national survey. Am J Surg. 2010;199(3):299–304. discussion 304.

10. Keller DS, Lawrence JK, Nobel T, Delaney CP. Optimizing cost and short-term outcomes for elderly patients in laparoscopic colonic surgery. Surg Endosc. 2013;27(12):4463–8.

11. Lawrence JK, Keller DS, Samia H, Ermlich B, Brady KM, Nobel T, et al. Discharge within 24 to 72 hours of colorectal surgery is associated with low readmission rates when using enhanced recovery pathways. J Am Coll Surg. 2013;216(3):390–4.

12. Rossi G, Vaccarezza H, Vaccaro CA, Mentz RE, Im V, Alvarez A, et al. Two-day hospital stay after laparoscopic colorectal surgery under an enhanced recovery after surgery (ERAS) pathway. World J Surg. 2013;37(10):2483–9.

13. Bloomstone JA, Loftus T, Hutchison R. ERAS: enhancing recovery one evidence-based step at a time. Anesth Analg. 2015;120(1):256.

14. Bona S, Molteni M, Rosati R, Elmore U, Bagnoli P, Monzani R, et al. Introducing an enhanced recovery after surgery program in colorectal surgery: a single center experience. World J Gastroenterol. 2014;20(46):17578–87.

15. Delaney CP, Zutshi M, Senagore AJ, Remzi FH, Hammel J, Fazio VW. Prospective, randomized, controlled trial between a pathway of controlled rehabilitation with early ambulation and diet and traditional postoperative care after laparotomy and intestinal resection. Dis Colon Rectum. 2003;46(7):851–9.

16. Eglinton TW. The era of ERAS: a new standard of perioperative care. N Z Med J. 2013;126(1369):6–7.

17. Feldman LS, Delaney CP. Laparoscopy plus enhanced recovery: optimizing the benefits of MIS through SAGES 'SMART' program. Surg Endosc. 2014;28(5):1403–6.

18. Gignoux B, Pasquer A, Vulliez A, Lanz T. Outpatient colectomy within an enhanced recovery program. J Visc Surg. 2015;152(1):11–5.

19. ERAS Compliance Group. The impact of enhanced recovery protocol compliance on elective colorectal cancer resection: results from an international registry. Ann Surg. 2015;261(6):1153–9.

20. Kariv Y, Delaney CP, Casillas S, Hammel J, Nocero J, Bast J, et al. Long-term outcome after laparoscopic and open surgery for rectal prolapse: a case-control study. Surg Endosc. 2006;20(1):35–42.

21. Kariv Y, Delaney CP, Senagore AJ, Manilich EA, Hammel JP, Church JM, et al. Clinical outcomes and cost analysis of a "fast track" postoperative care pathway for ileal pouch-anal anastomosis: a case control study. Dis Colon Rectum. 2007;50(2):137–46.

22. Ljungqvist O. ERAS—enhanced recovery after surgery: moving evidence-based perioperative care to practice. JPEN J Parenter Enteral Nutr. 2014;38(5):559–66.

23. Lohsiriwat V. Enhanced recovery after surgery vs conventional care in emergency colorectal surgery. World J Gastroenterol. 2014;20(38):13950–5.

24. Noel JK, Fahrbach K, Estok R, Cella C, Frame D, Linz H, et al. Minimally invasive colorectal resection outcomes: short-term comparison with open procedures. J Am Coll Surg. 2007;204(2):291–307.

25. Oda Y, Kakinohana M. Introduction of ERAS((R)) program into clinical practice: from preoperative management to postoperative evaluation: opening remarks. J Anesth. 2014;28(1):141–2.

26. Patel SS, Patel MS, Mahanti S, Ortega A, Ault GT, Kaiser AM, et al. Laparoscopic versus open colon resections in California: a cross-sectional analysis. Am Surg. 2012;78(10):1063–5.

27. Pokala N, Delaney CP, Senagore AJ, Brady KM, Fazio VW. Laparoscopic vs open total colectomy: a case-matched comparative study. Surg Endosc. 2005;19(4):531–5.

28. Rona K, Choi J, Sigle G, Kidd S, Ault G, Senagore AJ. Enhanced recovery protocol: implementation at a county institution with limited resources. Am Surg. 2012;78(10):1041–4.

29. Senagore AJ, Madbouly KM, Fazio VW, Duepree HJ, Brady KM, Delaney CP. Advantages of laparoscopic colectomy in older patients. Arch Surg. 2003;138(3):252–6.

30. Spanjersberg WR, van Sambeeck JD, Bremers A, Rosman C, van Laarhoven CJ. Systematic review and meta-analysis for laparoscopic versus open colon surgery with or without an ERAS programme. Surg Endosc. 2015;29:3443–53.

31. Steele SR, Bleier J, Champagne B, Hassan I, Russ A, Senagore AJ, et al. Improving outcomes and cost-effectiveness of colorectal surgery. J Gastrointest Surg. 2014;18(11):1944–56.

32. Zutshi M, Delaney CP, Senagore AJ, Fazio VW. Shorter hospital stay associated with fastrack postoperative care pathways and laparoscopic intestinal resection are not associated with increased physical activity. Colorectal Dis. 2004;6(6):477–80.

33. Zutshi M, Delaney CP, Senagore AJ, Mekhail N, Lewis B, Connor JT, et al. Randomized controlled trial comparing the controlled rehabilitation with early ambulation and diet pathway versus the controlled rehabilitation with early ambulation and diet with preemptive epidural anesthesia/analgesia after laparotomy and intestinal resection. Am J Surg. 2005;189(3):268–72.

34. Delaney CP, Fazio VW, Remzi FH, Hammel J, Church JM, Hull TL, et al. Prospective, age-related analysis of surgical results, functional outcome, and quality of life after ileal pouch-anal anastomosis. Ann Surg. 2003;238(2):221–8.

35. Gillissen F, Ament SM, Maessen JM, Dejong CH, Dirksen CD, van der Weijden T, et al. Sustainability of an enhanced recovery after surgery program (ERAS) in colonic surgery. World J Surg. 2015;39(2):526–33.

36. Hoffman RL, Bartlett EK, Ko C, Mahmoud N, Karakousis GC, Kelz RR. Early discharge and readmission after colorectal resection. J Surg Res. 2014;190(2):579–86.

37. Kehlet H. Enhanced Recovery After Surgery (ERAS): good for now, but what about the future? Can J Anaesth. 2015;62(2):99–104.

38. Keller DS, Bankwitz B, Woconish D, Champagne BJ, Reynolds Jr HL, Stein SL, et al. Predicting who will fail early discharge after laparoscopic colorectal surgery with an established enhanced recovery pathway. Surg Endosc. 2014;28(1):74–9.

39. Keller DS, Delaney CP. Current evidence in gastrointestinal surgery: natural orifice translumenal endoscopic surgery (NOTES). J Gastrointest Surg. 2013;17(10):1857–62.

40. Keller DS, Khorgami Z, Swendseid B, Khan S, Delaney CP. Identifying causes for high readmission rates after stoma reversal. Surg Endosc. 2014;28(4):1263–8.

41. Kiran RP, Delaney CP, Senagore AJ, Steel M, Garafalo T, Fazio VW. Outcomes and prediction of hospital readmission after intestinal surgery. J Am Coll Surg. 2004;198(6):877–83.

42. Zhuang CL, Ye XZ, Zhang XD, Chen BC, Yu Z. Enhanced recovery after surgery programs versus traditional care for colorectal surgery: a meta-analysis of randomized controlled trials. Dis Colon Rectum. 2013;56(5):667–78.

43. Thiele RH, Rea KM, Turrentine FE, Friel CM, Hassinger TE, Goudreau BJ, et al. Standardization of care: impact of an enhanced recovery protocol on length of stay, complications, and direct costs after colorectal surgery. J Am Coll Surg. 2015;220(4):430–43.

44. Fearon KC, Ljungqvist O, Von Meyenfeldt M, Revhaug A, Dejong CH, Lassen K, et al. Enhanced recovery after surgery: a consensus review of clinical care for patients undergoing colonic resection. Clin Nutr. 2005;24(3):466–77.

45. Kehlet H, Buchler MW, Beart Jr RW, Billingham RP, Williamson R. Care after colonic operation—is it evidence-based? Results from a multinational survey in Europe and the United States. J Am Coll Surg. 2006;202(1):45–54.

46. Lassen K, Hannemann P, Ljungqvist O, Fearon K, Dejong CH, von Meyenfeldt MF, et al. Patterns in current perioperative practice: survey of colorectal surgeons in five northern European countries. BMJ. 2005;330(7505):1420–1.

47. Cabana MD, Rand CS, Powe NR, Wu AW, Wilson MH, Abboud PA, et al. Why don't physicians follow clinical practice guidelines? A framework for improvement. JAMA. 1999;282(15):1458–65.

48. Kehlet H, Wilmore DW. Evidence-based surgical care and the evolution of fast-track surgery. Ann Surg. 2008;248(2):189–98.

49. Kahokehr A, Sammour T, Zargar-Shoshtari K, Thompson L, Hill AG. Implementation of ERAS and how to overcome the barriers. Int J Surg. 2009;7(1):16–9.

50. Sammour T, Zargar-Shoshtari K, Bhat A, Kahokehr A, Hill AG. A programme of Enhanced Recovery After Surgery (ERAS) is a cost-effective intervention in elective colonic surgery. N Z Med J. 2010;123(1319):61–70.

51. Srinivasa S, Sammour T, Kahokehr A, Hill AG. Enhanced Recovery After Surgery (ERAS) protocols must be considered when determining optimal perioperative care in colorectal surgery. Ann Surg. 2010;252(2):409. author reply 409–10.

52. Henry A, Stopfkuchen-Evans M, Wolf L, Bader A, Goldberg J, Kelley R, et al. Implementation of an Eras pathway in an Academic Medical Center: measurement of compliance and results. Dis Colon Rectum. 2015;58(5), E220.

53. Miller T, Ernst FR, Krukas MR, Gan T. Level of compliance with the Enhanced Recovery after Surgery (Eras) protocol and postoperative outcomes. Anesth Analg. 2013;116:100.

54. Patel A, Marimuthu K, Mathew G. Enhanced recovery after surgery (ERAS) card: a simple intervention to improve junior doctor compliance. Br J Surg. 2011;98:131–2.

55. Stein SL. Perioperative management. Clin Colon Rectal Surg. 2013;26(3):137–8.

56. Eriksson LI, Sandin R. Fasting guidelines in different countries. Acta Anaesthesiol Scand. 1996;40(8 Pt 2):971–4.

57. Smith I, Kranke P, Murat I, Smith A, O'Sullivan G, Soreide E, et al. Perioperative fasting in adults and children: guidelines from the European Society of Anaesthesiology. Eur J Anaesthesiol. 2011;28(8):556–69.

58. Soreide E, Eriksson LI, Hirlekar G, Eriksson H, Henneberg SW, Sandin R, et al. Pre-operative fasting guidelines: an update. Acta Anaesthesiol Scand. 2005;49(8):1041–7.

59. Khoo CK, Vickery CJ, Forsyth N, Vinall NS, Eyre-Brook IA. A prospective randomized controlled trial of multimodal perioperative management protocol in patients undergoing elective colorectal resection for cancer. Ann Surg. 2007; 245(6):867–72.

60. Gustafsson UO, Scott MJ, Schwenk W, Demartines N, Roulin D, Francis N, et al. Guidelines for perioperative care in elective colonic surgery: Enhanced Recovery After Surgery (ERAS((R))) Society recommendations. World J Surg. 2013;37(2):259–84.

61. Lohsiriwat V. The influence of preoperative nutritional status on the outcomes of an enhanced recovery after surgery (ERAS) programme for colorectal cancer surgery. Tech Coloproctol. 2014;18(11):1075–80.

62. Kehlet H. Multimodal approach to control postoperative pathophysiology and rehabilitation. Br J Anaesth. 1997;78(5):606–17.

63. Waitzberg DL, Saito H, Plank LD, Jamieson GG, Jagannath P, Hwang TL, et al. Postsurgical infections are reduced with specialized nutrition support. World J Surg. 2006;30(8):1592–604.

64. Keller DS, Bankwitz B, Nobel T, Delaney CP. Using frailty to predict who will fail early discharge after laparoscopic colorectal surgery with an established recovery pathway. Dis Colon Rectum. 2014;57(3):337–42.

65. Kulminski AM, Ukraintseva SV, Culminskaya IV, Arbeev KG, Land KC, Akushevich L, et al. Cumulative deficits and physiological indices as predictors of mortality and long life. J Gerontol A Biol Sci Med Sci. 2008;63(10):1053–9.

66. Farhat JS, Velanovich V, Falvo AJ, Horst HM, Swartz A, Patton Jr JH, et al. Are the frail destined to fail? Frailty index as predictor of surgical morbidity and mortality in the elderly. J Trauma Acute Care Surg. 2012;72(6):1526–30. discussion 30–1.

67. Hausel J, Nygren J, Lagerkranser M, Hellstrom PM, Hammarqvist F, Almstrom C, et al. A carbohydrate-rich drink reduces preoperative discomfort in elective surgery patients. Anesth Analg. 2001;93(5):1344–50.

68. Svanfeldt M, Thorell A, Hausel J, Soop M, Nygren J, Ljungqvist O. Effect of "preoperative" oral carbohydrate treatment on insulin action—a randomised cross-over unblinded study in healthy subjects. Clin Nutr. 2005;24(5):815–21.

69. Svanfeldt M, Thorell A, Hausel J, Soop M, Rooyackers O, Nygren J, et al. Randomized clinical trial of the effect of preoperative oral carbohydrate treatment on postoperative whole-body protein and glucose kinetics. Br J Surg. 2007;94(11): 1342–50.

70. Noblett SE, Watson DS, Huong H, Davison B, Hainsworth PJ, Horgan AF. Pre-operative oral carbohydrate loading in colorectal surgery: a randomized controlled trial. Colorectal Dis. 2006;8(7):563–9.

71. Contant CM, Hop WC, van't Sant HP, Oostvogel HJ, Smeets HJ, Stassen LP, et al. Mechanical bowel preparation for elective colorectal surgery: a multicentre randomised trial. Lancet. 2007;370(9605):2112–7.

72. Slim K, Vicaut E, Launay-Savary MV, Contant C, Chipponi J. Updated systematic review and meta-analysis of randomized clinical trials on the role of mechanical bowel preparation before colorectal surgery. Ann Surg. 2009;249(2):203–9.

73. van't Sant HP, Weidema WF, Hop WC, Lange JF, Contant CM. Evaluation of morbidity and mortality after anastomotic leakage following elective colorectal surgery in patients treated with or without mechanical bowel preparation. Am J Surg. 2011;202(3):321–4.

74. Van't Sant HP, Weidema WF, Hop WC, Oostvogel HJ, Contant CM. The influence of mechanical bowel preparation in elective lower colorectal surgery. Ann Surg. 2010;251(1):59–63.

75. Guenaga KF, Matos D, Wille-Jorgensen P. Mechanical bowel preparation for elective colorectal surgery. Cochrane Database Syst Rev. 2011;9, CD001544.

76. Jung B, Pahlman L, Nystrom PO, Nilsson E, Mechanical Bowel Preparation Study Group. Multicentre randomized clinical trial of mechanical bowel preparation in elective colonic resection. Br J Surg. 2007;94(6):689–95.

77. Collin A, Jung B, Nilsson E, Pahlman L, Folkesson J. Impact of mechanical bowel preparation on survival after colonic cancer resection. Br J Surg. 2014;101(12):1594–600.

78. Van't Sant HP, Kamman A, Hop WC, van der Heijden M, Lange JF, Contant CM. The influence of mechanical bowel preparation on long-term survival in patients surgically treated for colorectal cancer. Am J Surg. 2015;210(1):106–10.

79. Morris MS, Graham LA, Chu DI, Cannon JA, Hawn MT. Oral antibiotic bowel preparation significantly reduces surgical site infection rates and readmission rates in elective colorectal surgery. Ann Surg. 2015;261(6):1034–40.

80. Nelson RL, Gladman E, Barbateskovic M. Antimicrobial prophylaxis for colorectal surgery. Cochrane Database Syst Rev. 2014;5, CD001181.

81. Nelson RL, Glenny AM, Song F. Antimicrobial prophylaxis for colorectal surgery. Cochrane Database Syst Rev. 2009;1, CD001181.

82. Roos D, Dijksman LM, Tijssen JG, Gouma DJ, Gerhards MF, Oudemans-van Straaten HM. Systematic review of perioperative selective decontamination of the digestive tract in elective gastrointestinal surgery. Br J Surg. 2013;100(12):1579–88.

83. Song F, Glenny AM. Antimicrobial prophylaxis in colorectal surgery: a systematic review of randomized controlled trials. Br J Surg. 1998;85(9):1232–41.

84. Bakker N, Cakir H, Doodeman HJ, Houdijk AP. Eight years of experience with Enhanced Recovery After Surgery in patients with colon cancer: impact of measures to improve adherence. Surgery. 2015;157(6):1130–6.

85. Senagore AJ, Brannigan A, Kiran RP, Brady K, Delaney CP. Diagnosis-related group assignment in laparoscopic and open colectomy: financial implications for payer and provider. Dis Colon Rectum. 2005;48(5):1016–20.

86. Delaney CP, Fazio VW, Senagore AJ, Robinson B, Halverson AL, Remzi FH. 'Fast track' postoperative management protocol for patients with high co-morbidity undergoing complex abdominal and pelvic colorectal surgery. Br J Surg. 2001;88(11):1533–8.

87. Tekkis PP, Senagore AJ, Delaney CP. Conversion rates in laparoscopic colorectal surgery: a predictive model with, 1253 patients. Surg Endosc. 2005;19(1):47–54.

88. Bleier JI, Aarons CB. Perioperative fluid restriction. Clin Colon Rectal Surg. 2013;26(3):197–202.

89. Abraham-Nordling M, Hjern F, Pollack J, Prytz M, Borg T, Kressner U. Randomized clinical trial of fluid restriction in colorectal surgery. Br J Surg. 2012;99(2):186–91.

90. Boersema GS, van der Laan L, Wijsman JH. A close look at postoperative fluid management and electrolyte disorders after gastrointestinal surgery in a teaching hospital where patients are treated according to the ERAS protocol. Surg Today. 2014;44(11):2052–7.

91. Boland MR, Noorani A, Varty K, Coffey JC, Agha R, Walsh SR. Perioperative fluid restriction in major abdominal surgery: systematic review and meta-analysis of randomized, clinical trials. World J Surg. 2013;37(6):1193–202.

92. MacKay G. Randomized clinical trial of the effect of postoperative intravenous fluid restriction on recovery after elective colorectal surgery (Br J Surg 2006;93:1469–1474). Br J Surg. 2007;94(3):383.

93. MacKay G, Ihedioha U, McConnachie A, Serpell M, Molloy RG, Fearon KC, et al. Intravenous fluid and sodium restriction has no effect on recovery from colorectal surgery: an observer blinded randomized clinical trial. Br J Surg. 2006;93(7):901–2.

94. Miller TE, Roche AM, Mythen M. Fluid management and goal-directed therapy as an adjunct to Enhanced Recovery After Surgery (ERAS). Can J Anaesth. 2015;62(2):158–68.

95. Morera FJ. Randomized clinical trial of the effect of postoperative intravenous fluid restriction on recovery after elective colorectal surgery (Br J Surg 2006;93:1469–1474). Br J Surg. 2007;94(3):382–3.

96. Phan TD, An V, D'Souza B, Rattray MJ, Johnston MJ, Cowie BS. A randomised controlled trial of fluid restriction compared to oesophageal Doppler-guided goal-directed fluid therapy in elective major colorectal surgery within an Enhanced Recovery After Surgery program. Anaesth Intensive Care. 2014;42(6):752–60.

97. Tornero-Campello G. Randomized clinical trial of the effect of postoperative intravenous fluid restriction on recovery after elective colorectal surgery (Br J Surg 2006;93:1469–1474). Br J Surg. 2007;94(3):382.

98. Senagore AJ, Emery T, Luchtefeld M, Kim D, Dujovny N, Hoedema R. Fluid management for laparoscopic colectomy: a prospective, randomized assessment of goal-directed administration of balanced salt solution or hetastarch coupled with an enhanced recovery program. Dis Colon Rectum. 2009;52(12):1935–40.

99. American Society of Anesthesiologists Task Force on Acute Pain Management. Practice guidelines for acute pain management in the perioperative setting: an updated report by the American Society of Anesthesiologists Task Force on Acute Pain Management. Anesthesiology. 2012;116(2):248–73.

100. Garimella V, Cellini C. Postoperative pain control. Clin Colon Rectal Surg. 2013;26(3):191–6.

101. Ong CK, Lirk P, Seymour RA, Jenkins BJ. The efficacy of preemptive analgesia for acute postoperative pain management: a meta-analysis. Anesth Analg. 2005;100(3):757–73. table of contents.

102. Parikh HG, Dash SK, Upasani CB. Study of the effect of oral gabapentin used as preemptive analgesia to attenuate postoperative pain in patients undergoing abdominal surgery under general anesthesia. Saudi J Anaesth. 2010;4(3):137–41.

103. Siddiqui NT, Fischer H, Guerina L, Friedman Z. Effect of a preoperative gabapentin on postoperative analgesia in patients with inflammatory bowel disease following major bowel surgery: a randomized, placebo-controlled trial. Pain Pract. 2014;14(2):132–9.

104. Tirault M, Foucan L, Debaene B, Frasca D, Lebrun T, Bernard JC, et al. Gabapentin premedication: assessment of preoperative anxiolysis and postoperative patient satisfaction. Acta Anaesthesiol Belg. 2010;61(4):203–9.

105. Adachi YU, Nishino J, Suzuki K, Obata Y, Doi M, Sato S. Preemptive analgesia by preoperative administration of nonsteroidal anti-inflammatory drugs. J Anesth. 2007;21(2):294.

106. Mezei M, Hahn O, Penzes I. Preemptive analgesia—preoperative diclofenac sodium for postoperative analgesia in general surgery. Magy Seb. 2002;55(5):313–7.

107. Favuzza J, Brady K, Delaney CP. Transversus abdominis plane blocks and enhanced recovery pathways: making the 23-h hospital stay a realistic goal after laparoscopic colorectal surgery. Surg Endosc. 2013;27(7):2481–6.

108. Keller DS, Ermlich BO, Delaney CP. Demonstrating the benefits of transversus abdominis plane blocks on patient outcomes in laparoscopic colorectal surgery: review of 200 consecutive cases. J Am Coll Surg. 2014;219(6):1143–8.

109. Keller DS, Ermlich BO, Schiltz N, Champagne BJ, Reynolds Jr HL, Stein SL, et al. The effect of transversus abdominis plane blocks on postoperative pain in laparoscopic colorectal surgery: a prospective, randomized, double-blind trial. Dis Colon Rectum. 2014;57(11):1290–7.

110. Hubner M, Blanc C, Roulin D, Winiker M, Gander S, Demartines N. Randomized clinical trial on epidural versus patient-controlled analgesia for laparoscopic colorectal surgery within an enhanced recovery pathway. Ann Surg. 2015;261(4):648–53.

111. Hubner M, Schafer M, Demartines N, Muller S, Maurer K, Baulig W, et al. Impact of restrictive intravenous fluid replacement and combined epidural analgesia on perioperative volume balance and renal function within a Fast Track program. J Surg Res. 2012;173(1):68–74.

112. Kaminski JP, Pai A, Ailabouni L, Park JJ, Marecik SJ, Prasad LM, et al. Role of epidural and patient-controlled analgesia in site-specific laparoscopic colorectal surgery. JSLS. 2014;18(4).

113. Khan SA, Khokhar HA, Nasr AR, Carton E, El-Masry S. Effect of epidural analgesia on bowel function in laparoscopic colorectal surgery: a systematic review and meta-analysis. Surg Endosc. 2013;27(7):2581–91.

114. Marret E, Remy C, Bonnet F, Postoperative Pain Forum Group. Meta-analysis of epidural analgesia versus parenteral opioid analgesia after colorectal surgery. Br J Surg. 2007; 94(6):665–73.

115. Zingg U, Miskovic D, Hamel CT, Erni L, Oertli D, Metzger U. Influence of thoracic epidural analgesia on postoperative pain relief and ileus after laparoscopic colorectal resection: benefit with epidural analgesia. Surg Endosc. 2009;23(2): 276–82.

116. Levy BF, Scott MJ, Fawcett W, Fry C, Rockall TA. Randomized clinical trial of epidural, spinal or patient-controlled analgesia for patients undergoing laparoscopic colorectal surgery. Br J Surg. 2011;98(8):1068–78.

117. Douketis JD. Perioperative management of antithrombotic therapy: antithrombotic therapy and prevention of thrombosis, 9th ed: American College of Chest Physicians evidence-based clinical practice guidelines. Chest. 2012;141, e326S. Erratum in Chest. 2012;141(4):1129.

118. Rasmussen MS, Jorgensen LN, Wille-Jorgensen P. Prolonged thromboprophylaxis with low molecular weight heparin for abdominal or pelvic surgery. Cochrane Database Syst Rev. 2009;1, CD004318.

119. Fleming FJ. Operative approach and venous thromboembolism in colorectal surgery: casual or causal association? Dis Colon Rectum. 2011;54(12):1463–4.

120. Fleming FJ, Kim MJ, Salloum RM, Young KC, Monson JR. How much do we need to worry about venous thromboembolism after hospital discharge? A study of colorectal surgery patients using the National Surgical Quality Improvement Program database. Dis Colon Rectum. 2010;53(10):1355–60.

121. Pai A, Hurtuk MG, Park JJ, Marecik SJ, Prasad LM. A randomized study on 1-week versus 4-week prophylaxis for venous thromboembolism after laparoscopic surgery for colorectal cancer. Ann Surg. 2014 Sep 10. [Epub ahead of print].

122. Ng WQ, Neill J. Evidence for early oral feeding of patients after elective open colorectal surgery: a literature review. J Clin Nurs. 2006;15(6):696–709.

123. Lewis SJ, Andersen HK, Thomas S. Early enteral nutrition within 24 h of intestinal surgery versus later commencement of feeding: a systematic review and meta-analysis. J Gastrointest Surg. 2009;13(3):569–75.

124. Henriksen MG, Hansen HV, Hessov I. Early oral nutrition after elective colorectal surgery: influence of balanced analgesia and enforced mobilization. Nutrition. 2002;18(3):263–7.

125. Henriksen MG, Jensen MB, Hansen HV, Jespersen TW, Hessov I. Enforced mobilization, early oral feeding, and balanced analgesia improve convalescence after colorectal surgery. Nutrition. 2002;18(2):147–52.

126. Zhuang CL, Ye XZ, Zhang CJ, Dong QT, Chen BC, Yu Z. Early versus traditional postoperative oral feeding in patients undergoing elective colorectal surgery: a meta-analysis of randomized clinical trials. Digest Surg. 2013;30(3):225–32.

127. Asgeirsson T, El-Badawi KI, Mahmood A, Barletta J, Luchtefeld M, Senagore AJ. Postoperative ileus: it costs more than you expect. J Am Coll Surg. 2010;210(2):228–31.

128. Barletta JF, Asgeirsson T, Senagore AJ. Influence of intravenous opioid dose on postoperative ileus. Ann Pharmacother. 2011;45(7–8):916–23.

129. Barletta JF, Senagore AJ. Reducing the burden of postoperative ileus: evaluating and implementing an evidence-based strategy. World J Surg. 2014;38(8):1966–77.

130. Bungard TJ, Kale-Pradhan PB. Prokinetic agents for the treatment of postoperative ileus in adults: a review of the literature. Pharmacotherapy. 1999;19(4):416–23.

131. Harms BA, Heise CP. Pharmacologic management of postoperative ileus: the next chapter in GI surgery. Ann Surg. 2007;245(3):364–5.

132. Person B, Wexner SD. The management of postoperative ileus. Curr Probl Surg. 2006;43(1):6–65.

133. Stewart D, Waxman K. Management of postoperative ileus. Am J Ther. 2007;14(6):561–6.

134. Barletta JF, Asgeirsson T, El-Badawi KI, Senagore AJ. Introduction of alvimopan into an enhanced recovery protocol for colectomy offers benefit in open but not laparoscopic colectomy. J Laparoendosc Adv Surg Tech A. 2011;21(10): 887–91.

135. Bell TJ, Poston SA, Kraft MD, Senagore AJ, Delaney CP, Techner L. Economic analysis of alvimopan in North American phase III efficacy trials. Am J Health Syst Pharm. 2009; 66(15):1362–8.

136. Bell TJ, Poston SA, Kraft MD, Senagore AJ, Techner L. Economic analysis of alvimopan—a clarification and commentary. Pharmacotherapy. 2013;33(5):e81–2.

137. Delaney CP, Wolff BG, Viscusi ER, Senagore AJ, Fort JG, Du W, et al. Alvimopan, for postoperative ileus following bowel resection: a pooled analysis of phase III studies. Ann Surg. 2007;245(3):355–63.

138. Leslie JB. Alvimopan for the management of postoperative ileus. Ann Pharmacother. 2005;39(9):1502–10.

139. Ludwig K, Viscusi ER, Wolff BG, Delaney CP, Senagore A, Techner L. Alvimopan for the management of postoperative ileus after bowel resection: characterization of clinical benefit by pooled responder analysis. World J Surg. 2010;34(9):2185–90.

140. Senagore AJ, Bauer JJ, Du W, Techner L. Alvimopan accelerates gastrointestinal recovery after bowel resection regardless of age, gender, race, or concomitant medication use. Surgery. 2007;142(4):478–86.

141. Simorov A, Thompson J, Oleynikov D. Alvimopan reduces length of stay and costs in patients undergoing segmental colonic resections: results from multicenter national administrative database. Am J Surg. 2014;208(6):919–25.

142. Wiriyakosol S, Kongdan Y, Euanorasetr C, Wacharachaisurapol N, Lertsithichai P. Randomized controlled trial of bisacodyl suppository versus placebo for postoperative ileus after elective colectomy for colon cancer. Asian J Surg. 2007;30(3):167–72.

143. Zingg U, Miskovic D, Pasternak I, Meyer P, Hamel CT, Metzger U. Effect of bisacodyl on postoperative bowel motility in elective colorectal surgery: a prospective, randomized trial. Int J Colorectal Dis. 2008;23(12):1175–83.

144. Keller D, Stein SL. Facilitating return of bowel function after colorectal surgery: alvimopan and gum chewing. Clin Colon Rectal Surg. 2013;26(3):186–90.

145. Purkayastha S, Tilney HS, Darzi AW, Tekkis PP. Meta-analysis of randomized studies evaluating chewing gum to enhance postoperative recovery following colectomy. Arch Surg. 2008;143(8):788–93.

146. Hocevar BJ, Robinson B, Gray M. Does chewing gum shorten the duration of postoperative ileus in patients undergoing abdominal surgery and creation of a stoma? J Wound Ostomy Continence Nurs. 2010;37(2):140–6.

147. Chan MK, Law WL. Use of chewing gum in reducing postoperative ileus after elective colorectal resection: a systematic review. Dis Colon Rectum. 2007;50(12):2149–57.

148. Nelson RL. A systematic review of prophylactic nasogastric suction after abdominal surgery. Dis Colon Rectum. 2004;47(4):640.

149. Nelson R, Tse B, Edwards S. Systematic review of prophylactic nasogastric decompression after abdominal operations. Br J Surg. 2005;92(6):673–80.

150. Rao W, Zhang X, Zhang J, Yan R, Hu Z, Wang Q. The role of nasogastric tube in decompression after elective colon and rectum surgery: a meta-analysis. Int J Colorectal Dis. 2011;26(4):423–9.

151. O'Brien DP, Senagore A, Merlino J, Brady K, Delaney C. Predictors and outcome of readmission after laparoscopic intestinal surgery. World J Surg. 2007;31(12):2430–5.

152. Keller DS, Chien HL, Hashemi L, Senagore AJ, Delaney CP. The HARM score: a novel, easy measure to evaluate quality and outcomes in colorectal surgery. Ann Surg. 2014;259(6):1119–25.

153. Wind J, Polle SW, Fung Kon Jin PH, Dejong CH, von Meyenfeldt MF, Ubbink DT, Gouma DJ, Bemelman WA, Laparoscopy and/or Fast Track Multimodal Management Versus Standard Care (LAFA) Study Group; Enhanced Recovery after Surgery (ERAS) Group. Systematic review of enhanced recovery programmes in colonic surgery. Br J Surg. 2006;93(7):800–9.

154. Vlug MS, Wind J, van der Zaag E, Ubbink DT, Cense HA, Bemelman WA. Systematic review of laparoscopic vs open colonic surgery within an enhanced recovery programme. Colorectal Dis. 2009;11(4):335–43.

155. Bradshaw BG, Liu SS, Thirlby RC. Standardized perioperative care protocols and reduced length of stay after colon surgery. J Am Coll Surg. 1998;186(5):501–6.

156. Raue W, Haase O, Junghans T, et al. 'Fast-track' multimodal rehabilitation program improves outcome after laparoscopic sigmoidectomy: a controlled prospective evaluation. Surg Endosc. 2004;18(10):1463–8.

157. Basse L, Raskov HH, Hjort Jakobsen D, Sonne E, Billesbolle P, Hendel HW, et al. Accelerated postoperative recovery programme after colonic resection improves physical performance, pulmonary function and body composition. Br J Surg. 2002;89:446–53.

158. Anderson AD, McNaught CE, MacFie J, Tring I, Barker P, Mitchell CJ. Randomized clinical trial of multimodal optimization and standard perioperative surgical care. Br J Surg. 2003;90:1497–504.

159. Gatt M, Anderson AD, Reddy BS, Hayward-Sampson P, Tring IC, MacFie J. Randomized clinical trial of multimodal optimization of surgical care in patients undergoing major colonic resection. Br J Surg. 2005;92:1354–62.

160. Serclová Z, Dytrych P, Marvan J, Nová K, Hankeová Z, Ryska O, Slégrová Z, Buresová L, Trávníková L, Antos F. Fast-track in open intestinal surgery: prospective randomized study (Clinical Trials Gov Identifier no. NCT00123456). Clin Nutr. 2009;28(6):618–24.

161. Muller S, Zalunardo MP, et al. A fast-track program reduces complications and length of hospital stay after open colonic surgery. Gastroenterology. 2009;136:842–7.

8

Postoperative Complications

Andrew Russ and Gregory D. Kennedy

Key Concepts

- Thorough preoperative evaluation including assessment of social situation, cognitive status, and comorbidities contribute to safe postoperative recovery.
- Laparoscopic approach to colorectal surgery is associated with a decreased risk for postoperative complications.
- Risk for mortality after major postoperative complications is a reflection of surgeon as well as the system in which the surgeon operates.
- Meticulous operative technique with particular attention to hemostasis will lead to improved postoperative outcomes.
- Postoperative management with an enhanced recovery after surgery protocol leads to decreased postoperative complications.
- Bowel preparation with oral antibiotics correlates with a decreased risk of superficial surgical site infection.

Introduction

Postoperative complications are common in colorectal surgery with an incidence as high as 40 % depending upon the study. Many studies have been reported which characterize the complications and their frequency. The overarching goal of this chapter is to highlight some of this literature in an attempt to give the reader a broad overview of some of the issues surrounding postoperative complications.

Preoperative Considerations and Prediction of Postoperative Complications

Given the frequency of postoperative complications and their implications on quality of life, much current work focuses on prevention of complications. To that end, many authors have used the database that has come out of the American College of Surgeons National Surgical Quality Improvement Program (NSQIP) to characterize postoperative complications [1–6]. Perhaps one of the most significant developments is that of the ACS NSQIP surgical risk calculator [7, 8]. This tool uses procedure-specific information to provide an accurate prediction both of risk for various complications as well as hospital length of stay. Importantly, the ACS NSQIP calculator provides risk stratification that allows the patient to see their risk in the context of other more average-risk patients. Figure. 8-1a, b is an example of a report obtained from the ACS NSQIP risk calculator. These types of tools allow surgeons to not only anticipate various complications but to guide patient counseling on expected outcomes. This type of informed consent allows surgeons to consider the outcomes that are most important to patients so they can make decisions that align with their goals of life [9, 10].

While this risk calculator seems to accurately predict postoperative complications [8], risk prediction is dependent upon the accuracy of the data entered into the model. Furthermore, factors exist that impact the outcomes that cannot be measured by any specific model. For example, Dr. Senagore's group investigated the accuracy of the ACS NSQIP risk calculator in predicting outcomes in a high-volume minimally invasive colorectal surgery practice [11]. The authors of this study found that the risk calculator generally overestimated the rate of complications [11]. The authors proposed that the discrepancy in the observed to expected rate of complications was related to the inability of the calculator to account for surgeon-specific experience, volume, and prior outcomes. However, the authors did not report how well the results of the calculator correlated with the actual patient outcomes on a per-patient basis, which is a major limitation to their conclusions. Nonetheless, it is clear that any prediction calculator developed will always be able to be improved with more accurate data input.

Patient comorbidity clearly impacts risk for postoperative complications [1]. The NSQIP risk calculator, as well

S.R. Steele et al. (eds.), *The ASCRS Textbook of Colon and Rectal Surgery*, DOI 10.1007/978-3-319-25970-3_8

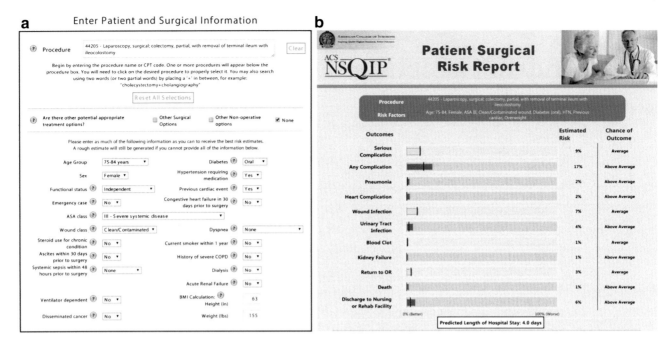

FIGURE 8-1. A sample of the American College of Surgeons risk calculator is shown. The calculator was found at http://riskcalculator.facs.org/ and details of a made-up patient were inserted according to the instructions. (**a**) In this example, a 77-year-old female patient will undergo a laparoscopic right hemicolectomy. Her made-up comorbidities were inserted and the risk calculator was run. (**b**) Results of the risk calculation were obtained and shown here. This sample patient was found to be of average risk for serious complication and slightly higher than average risk for any complication. Risks for specific complications are shown. © American College of Surgeons, used with permission.

as many other investigators, has clearly shown the impact of these comorbidities on risk for postoperative complications. However, as patients with surgical problems age, surgeons must be able to address issues that are specific to the older adult population. In particular, it is important to begin to understand how frailty, cognitive impairment, and social support impact patient outcomes. These variables are largely neglected by any current predictive nomogram, but it is clear that these factors contribute to postoperative outcomes. For example, cognitive impairment has been shown to correlate with discharge to a higher level of care in the older adult population [12]. In this study, 41 % of patients with a score ≤14 on the mini-mental status examination (MMSE) were discharged to a higher-level care facility compared to only 11 % of patients who scored >14 (OR 4.76, CI 1.72–13.17, $P=0.003$) [12]. These findings indicate that preoperative cognitive impairment is an important predictor of discharge destination. Others have also found that preoperative cognitive impairment correlated with a higher risk for postoperative complications (42 % rate of complications in the impaired group compared to 24 % in the intact group, $P=0.011$) [13]. Cognitive impairment also correlated with longer length of stay and higher 6-month mortality. Taken together, the data indicate that cognitive impairment should be considered an important predictor of outcome when dealing with the older adult population.

Another commonly forgotten consideration in the high-risk older adult population is frailty. Frailty is a syndrome characterized by age-related declines in functional reserves across an array of physiologic systems. The syndrome is highly prevalent in older adults and confers a high risk for falls, disability, hospitalization, and institutionalization. Despite the prevalence of this syndrome in older adults and the wide recognition of the importance of frailty on postoperative outcomes, it has not been well defined in the literature until recently. Many different strategies have been used to measure frailty [14]. Perhaps the best measurement is termed the frailty phenotype that is characterized by unintentional weight loss, decreased energy, and decrease in activity and strength [15]. It is clear that frailty directly impacts postoperative outcomes in the older adult population [16, 17]. In fact, given all of the issues associated with surgical care of the older adult patient, the American College of Surgeons assembled a task force of experts to put together a best practice guideline for the optimal preoperative assessment of this group of patients [18].

Finally, as a patient is assessed in clinic for an operation, another important factor likely to impact the recovery course is the social structure of the patient. Many authors have investigated how social structure impacts postoperative recovery and results have been mixed [19]. In general, it is thought that social structure contributes to postoperative recovery either in alleviating anxiety, pain, or response to pain [20, 21]. One group from Michigan recently examined the concept of social connectedness as it relates to postoperative recovery [22]. They found that patients with more social connectedness, as measured by number of friends and family as well as by interaction within the network, experienced less subjective pain and less perceived unpleasantness from the pain as compared to patients who had less social connectedness [22]. While it is clear that a patient's social structure is related to their perception of the recovery, it is not understood if connectedness contributes to recovery after suffering a major complication or if the concept of connectedness contributes to a patient's underlying risk for suffering a postoperative complication. It is likely that social connectedness does contribute to risk, as patients who are alone may have poor overall health and malnutrition [23].

As we consider the future, we must begin to consider how to properly counsel patients prior to surgical intervention. Quality measures, including outcomes related to safety, effectiveness, and patient centeredness, are already included in many facets of clinical practice such as credentialing and reimbursement. Therefore, it is imperative that all surgeons embrace these measures, become more comfortable with the details, and strive to improve outcomes. Risk stratification systems such as the ACS NSQIP risk calculator will be important in preoperative assessment. How these assessments will be used to change management and outcomes remains to be determined. Future work will focus on enhancing the scoring systems as well as understanding how a surgeon can modify the approach to improve surgical outcomes.

Intraoperative Factors that Contribute to Postoperative Outcomes

Operative Approach and Postoperative Impact

Laparoscopy for colon surgery was first reported in a small case series in the early 1990s [24]. Shortly after these reports, Dr. Wexner and his group published results from their earliest prospective studies, which found no difference in outcomes between open and laparoscopic-assisted colectomy [25, 26]. These studies began the debate on the role of laparoscopy in the treatment of colorectal diseases. Multiple subsequent publications have highlighted the benefit of a laparoscopic approach to colorectal surgery. Nonetheless, it is interesting to note that in many circles this debate continues in spite of the multiple published studies highlighting the benefits of a laparoscopic approach to colorectal surgery. However, it is important to consider those endpoints that are affected by surgical approach in order to fully appreciate the benefit of laparoscopy in improving outcomes.

Postoperative bowel obstruction is a common complication of many abdominal and pelvic surgical procedures. Given the unpredictable timing and potentially quite delayed presentation of postoperative bowel obstruction, it is difficult to know the exact incidence of this complication. A landmark paper published in 1999 by Beck et al. used the Health Care Financing Administration dataset from 1993 to address this question. They found that between 12.4 and 17 % of Medicare beneficiaries undergoing either pelvic or abdominal operations suffered a bowel obstruction sometime within 2 years of the primary operation [27]. Importantly, this study found the incidence of bowel obstruction to be quite a bit higher than previous reports. Since this paper, others have found the incidence of bowel obstruction due to adhesive disease to be less than 3 % and to be dependent upon the cavity in which the operation was performed [28]. For example, in one study, an operation on the lower GI tract carried a higher risk for bowel obstruction than did an operation on the abdominal wall only (3.8 % versus 0.5 %) [28]. The evidence regarding the impact of laparoscopy on the development of postoperative bowel obstruction is somewhat mixed [28, 29]. A retrospective study of nearly 300 patients undergoing restorative proctocolectomy at a single institution found no difference in incidence of postoperative small bowel obstruction between open and laparoscopic approaches [30]. In summary, the use of laparoscopy may decrease adhesion formation, which likely will result in lower rates of adhesive postoperative bowel obstruction.

The impact of laparoscopy on other complications and outcomes is more clear. The prospective randomized controlled trial reported by the Clinical Outcomes of Surgical Therapy Study Group found that perioperative recovery was faster in subjects randomized to laparoscopy compared to those undergoing open procedures, as reflected by a shorter hospital length of stay [31]. Rates of intraoperative complications, 30-day mortality, complications at discharge and at 60 days, hospital readmission, and reoperation were similar between groups [31]. Similarly, results from the MRC CLASICC trial demonstrated shorter length of stay for patients treated with a laparoscopic approach, with no difference in 30-day or 3-month complications [32]. While these randomized controlled trials failed to show differences in some short-term outcomes between operative approaches, it should be noted that they were not designed to detect these differences. Furthermore, randomized controlled trials are inherently biased and nonrepresentative of the daily practice of medicine and surgery, which highlights the importance of observational and comparative effectiveness studies [33].

A review of the literature reveals several comparative effectiveness studies looking at the issue of laparoscopic versus open approach to colon surgery. In general, all have found that minimally invasive techniques are correlated with improved short-term outcomes. Specifically, these studies report at least a 50 % reduction in superficial surgical site infections, a 50 % reduction in deep wound infection, and a significant reduction in postoperative length of stay in patients who have a laparoscopic operation [5, 34–42]. However, these studies have generally reported similar mortality associated with the two approaches, suggesting that while surgical approach may decrease some types of postoperative complications, other outcomes such as mortality are more complex and multifactorial. In fact, when examining the so-called "failure to rescue" phenomenon first published by Silber in 1992 [43], it is clear that the surgeon, surgical volume, and the system in which the surgeon operates contribute to the rate of postoperative mortality following major complications [44–46].

In summary, operative approach clearly relates to the development of postoperative complications. The exact mechanism of protection provided by the minimally invasive approach is unknown and is not reflected in every outcome. Therefore, future research should address the complication phenotype, and surgeons should strive to reduce variability in operative approach.

Luminal Organ Injuries and Postoperative Impact

In 2003, the Agency for Healthcare Research and Quality (AHRQ) proposed a set of patient safety indicators (PSIs) intended to reflect the quality of care delivered in hospitals. Several PSIs are included in the current CMS pay for performance plan, directly affecting reimbursement. These PSIs are presumed to be preventable by provider or system changes and include iatrogenic events such as accidental puncture or laceration (APL) during a procedure. Accidental puncture or laceration is defined as an accidental perforation of a blood vessel, nerve, or organ occurring during a procedure [47]. When applying this definition to over two million Veterans Health Administration admissions, 7023 were flagged for APL. These included serosal tears, enterotomy, and injury to the ureter, bladder, spleen, and blood vessels. Of true APLs, 27 % were minor injuries such as small serosal tears with no clinically significant impact [48]. The clinical significance of serosal tears is also found to be minimal in other large-volume studies [49]. In fact, further evidence from the Cleveland Clinic group found that accidental puncture laceration was more correlated with complexity of the operation and largely had no impact on postoperative recovery [49]. Since the rate of APL is publicly available and used in pay for performance models, it is important that we fully understand the limitations of this PSI. These data suggest that the utility of APL is limited and better measures of safety are necessary if we are to compare organizations in a fair and non-biased fashion.

Vascular Injury and Failure of Hemostatic Devices

Blood loss has been shown in many studies to correlate with outcomes across various different types of operations [50–52]. Using the NSQIP PUF database, Greenblatt et al. found intraoperative blood transfusion to be significantly associated with postoperative complications in patients undergoing surgery for rectal cancer [53]. These results are consistent with those found in the single-institution study published by Gu and others examining outcomes in patients undergoing ileal pouch-anal anastomosis [50]. Halabi et al. demonstrated a dose-dependent effect of blood transfusion, with worse outcomes in patients receiving more than 3 or more units of blood compared to those receiving only 1–2 units of blood [54]. All of these data together indicate that careful attention to hemostasis is not only consistent with good operative technique but also contributes to decreased postoperative morbidity.

The exact incidence of major vascular injury during colorectal surgery is unclear. However, examination of the surgical literature indicates that major vascular injury is relatively rare. For example, in a series of 404 patients undergoing retroperitoneal laparoscopic nephrectomy, Meraney and colleagues reported seven patients who had major vascular injuries. Conversion to open or repair of the injury through the extraction site was necessary in three of the seven patients. Overall postoperative complication rate in the group sustaining an injury was 25 % [55]. Others have examined the rate of trocar injuries to the vasculature at the time of laparoscopy [56, 57]. One series examined the number of trocar injuries reported to the FDA through the Center of Devices and Radiological Health [56]. In this study, the authors found 408 cases of vascular injury reported to the FDA as a result of trocar insertion. It is impossible to know the actual incidence from this study without a denominator; however, they did note that 26 of the 408 patients died as a result of the injury for a mortality rate of around 6 % [56]. The actual incidence of trocar injury was reported by Larobina and Nottle in a case series report as well as a literature review [57]. Here they found no major vascular injuries in their case series of 5900 patients and a rate of 0.04 % in a literature review which included over 760,000 patients [57]. They concluded that vascular injuries at the time of trocar insertion are rare and can be eliminated by an open, Hasson access technique [57].

While it is difficult to know the exact impact of vascular injuries and blood loss on postoperative outcomes, there is enough data to warrant meticulous attention to hemostasis. There are a myriad of minimally invasive and open instruments available for hemostasis during colorectal procedures. These devices can be used for adhesiolysis, dividing embryological attachments, ligating mesentery, and even ligating named vascular pedicles. The technology continues to evolve at a rapid pace. A recent Cochrane review looked at various commercially available instruments used for laparoscopic colectomy. It evaluated six separate randomized controlled trials including a total of 446 patients [58]. These trials evaluated laparoscopic staplers and clips, as well as electrothermal bipolar vessel sealers (EBVS), monopolar electrocautery scissors (MES), and ultrasonic coagulating shears (UCS) [58]. This review found significantly less blood loss in studies using UCS compared to MES. Overall, hemostatic control was found to be improved in UCS and EBVS over

MES. No definite conclusion on the cost difference between these three instruments was made in this review. This review also found that laparoscopic staples/clips used for pedicle ligation in colectomy were associated with more failures in vessel ligation and cost more when compared to EBVS [58]. Additionally, a randomized clinical trial comparing the cost and effectiveness of bipolar sealers versus clip and vascular staples for laparoscopic colorectal resection found that bipolar sealers reduced both the time spent and the cost of disposable instruments for achieving vascular control [59]. Another prospective randomized trial by Marcello and colleagues found increased failure rates in cases where vascular staplers and clips were used for pedicle ligation [60]. However, the amount of blood loss associated with device failure was higher in those using EBVS for pedicle ligation [60].

The choice of ideal device remains largely up to surgeon preference. There are now multiple instruments capable of 7 mm vessel sealing with various other capabilities. Based on the current available literature, electrothermal bipolar vessel sealing allows for faster operating times, less blood loss, and less sealing failure [58]. However, sealing failure with an energy device often leads to more blood loss than sealing failure with the use of clips and vascular staplers [60]. It is our practice to take vascular pedicles with an electrothermal bipolar vessel sealing device. For device failure or inadequate seal, we favor the use of clips or alternatively an endo-loop, as blindly sealing vessels in a crimson field is often fraught with complication. In the setting of a known atherosclerotic vessel, the application of a vascular stapler should be considered.

Urologic Injuries and Their Management

Ureteral Injury

One of the most dreaded complications related to colorectal surgery is ureteral injury, which thankfully remains an exceedingly rare occurrence. Iatrogenic ureteral injury has a documented incidence of 0.3–1.5 % in most studies. A retrospective analysis of over two million colorectal surgical procedures found an incidence of 0.28 %; however, a significantly higher incidence was found in the latter time period of this analysis, suggesting a trend toward increasing rate of this complication [61]. Risk factors for ureteral injury in this study included the presence of rectal cancer, adhesions, metastatic cancer, weight loss/malnutrition, and teaching hospitals. A study by Palaniappa et al. examined their series of over 5000 patients undergoing colectomy for various indications [62]. They found a significantly higher rate of ureteral injury associated with laparoscopic colectomy compared to open (0.66 % versus 0.15 %, $P < 0.05$) [62]. They also found that female sex, increased operative blood loss, and reoperation conferred an increased risk of iatrogenic injury [62]. Ureteral injuries were associated with higher morbidity and mortality, longer length of stay, and higher hospital charges by over $30,000 [61]. It does appear

that experience and working through the learning curve lead to a decrease in these types of iatrogenic injuries [63].

Preoperative or intraoperative ureteral catheterization is sometimes used to aid in identification of the ureters and subsequent injury. Most data suggest that placement of ureteral stents neither reduces the incidence of injury nor ensures intraoperative identification of injury [64]. In an NSQIP analysis, there was an increasing trend of ureteral stent use over time from 1.1 to 4.4 % from 2005 to 2011 [65]. Independent predictors of stent utilization included diverticular disease, LAR and APR, recent radiation therapy, and more recent year of operation [65]. After adjustment for baseline patient and operative characteristics, there were no statistically significant differences in any primary or secondary endpoints, including overall renal complications. There was, however, a statistically significant increase in length of stay associated with stent utilization, which was also observed by Halabi and colleagues [61, 65].

Early identification of injury is paramount in minimizing morbidity and preserving renal function. Diagnosis of a suspected injury can be confirmed with an on-table intravenous pyelogram (IVP), retrograde injection of methylene blue, intravenous administration of methylene blue or indigo carmine, or ureteral catheter contrast administration. Injuries can be classified as a laceration, ligation, devascularization, or energy related. Transection and laceration are repaired based on location of injury. General principles include use of absorbable suture (to prevent stone formation), tension-free spatulated anastomosis over an indwelling stent, and placement of a closed suction drain. For those injuries in the proximal one-third (2 % of injuries), repair depends on length of the damaged segment. Simple spatulated ureteroureterostomy (UU) is the preferred method of repair. For additional mobilization, a nephropexy can be performed with fixation to the psoas tendon. Bowel interposition can be utilized for long-segment damage. Additionally, a psoas hitch or Boari flap can be used to reach the upper ureter; however, these procedures are more commonly used for injuries of the middle or distal third. Injuries to the middle third account for 7 % of ureteral injuries, and the preferred method of repair is via ureteroureterostomy for short-segment injury. A psoas hitch or Boari flap should be used if a tension-free anastomosis is not possible, with the Boari flap preferred for injuries spanning longer and more proximal distances. Lastly, a transureteroureterostomy (TUU) can be performed with anastomosis to the contralateral uninjured ureter. Injuries to the distal one-third of the ureter are preferentially repaired with ureteroneocystostomy. A Foley catheter should be left in place for 7–14 days with stent removal 4–6 weeks after surgery [64].

Bladder Injury

Bladder injury also presents a significant management challenge for the colorectal surgeon. These injuries can present in a delayed fashion or at the time of initial surgery. Risk factors include previous operations, radiation treatment, malignant infiltration, chronic infection, and inflammatory conditions. Radiographic diagnosis can be obtained with CT cystogram or fluoroscopic cystogram. Untoward complications of missed bladder injury can include development of a colovesical or enterovesical fistula. Abdominopelvic CT scan with oral and rectal contrast may be performed for accurate diagnosis [64].

Primary repair (cystorrhaphy) with placement of closed suction drains is the preferred approach when injury is immediately recognized. Small extraperitoneal injuries can be effectively treated with 7–14 days of Foley catheter decompression. Larger or intraperitoneal bladder injuries require operative repair. For injuries to the ventral bladder, dome, or posterior bladder away from ureteral orifices, the bladder can be repaired primarily with two-layer mucosal and seromuscular closure using absorbable suture. A third layer, in the fashion of Lembert, can be added for high-risk cases. Permanent suture must be avoided to prevent the long-term development of bladder stones. For injuries involving the posterior bladder or trigone, near the ureteral orifices, inspection for ureteral injury is mandatory via mobilization of the space of Retzius and subsequent anterior cystotomy, allowing for full exposure of the trigone and interior of the bladder. Indigo carmine can then be administered intravenously to aid in identification of ureteral orifices. Posterior repair is then performed through this anterior cystotomy [66]. Delayed diagnosis of urine leak from the bladder is often managed with percutaneous drainage of a urinoma and continued Foley catheter decompression. Finally, it is always prudent to at least consider consultation with specialized services when faced with difficult scenarios and specific complications. This allows for the obvious support with the repair as well as additional advice in difficult scenarios.

Urethral Injury

Perhaps the least frequent intraoperative urologic injury involves those to the urethra. The most common urethral injury during colon and rectal surgery is related to traumatic Foley catheter placement. The exact rate of this injury in the colorectal patient population is difficult to ascertain. Kashefi and others prospectively studied men in their institution over 1 year and found the rate to be 3.2/1000 catheter insertions [67]. After the implementation of an educational program teaching the inserter to investigate for the presence of risk factors such as benign prostatic hypertrophy, the incidence decreased to 0.7/1000 catheter insertions [67]. Direct injuries also occur during extirpative surgery. Many of these patients have a history of radiation therapy and are prone to fistula formation. Intraoperatively, retrograde injection of methylene blue-tinted saline can aid in diagnosis. The most common presentation of a urethral injury is postoperatively by virtue of fistula formation. Cystoscopy, retrograde urethrogram, exam under anesthesia, and CT scan with both oral and rectal contrast help to delineate the location of injury, which has significant impact on reparative options [64].

Primary repair at the time of injury in two layers with absorbable suture is of course the preferred method. In the setting of poor tissue or neoadjuvant radiation, utilization of an omental flap or local tissue flap can reduce the risk of postoperative fistula formation. In the case of extensive urethral loss recognized at the time of surgery, local tissue flaps may be used to aid in reconstruction. If repair is not feasible, a suprapubic catheter should be placed and repair can be performed after several months [64].

Injuries recognized postoperatively with resultant fistula formation must be staged according to location, size, and history of radiation treatment. Spontaneous closure of recto-urethral fistula is extremely rare [68]:

Stage 1—low (<4 cm from anal verge, nonirradiated)
Stage 2—high (>4 cm from anal verge, nonirradiated)
Stage 3—small (<2 cm diameter, irradiated)
Stage 4—large (>2 cm diameter, irradiated)
Stage 5—large (ischial decubitus fistula)

Principles of repair include transection and closure of fistulas and placement of interposed local or regional tissue flaps or grafts [69]. Fecal diversion is recommended for stages 3 through 5, usually in advance. Reparative choices depend on local tissue integrity and staging. A suprapubic catheter is recommended in addition to a Foley catheter for adequate decompression and drainage [70]. Transanal advancement flap alone can be performed for stage 1 fistulas or in combination with other techniques for higher-stage fistulas [71]. Perineal approaches and transanal or transsphincteric approaches have also been described [72, 73]. Other operative approaches include harvest and interposition of regional myofascial flaps [74, 75]. Muscle interposition repairs can be used alone or in combination with abdominoperineal pull-through with resection of the fistula and hand-sewn colo-anal anastomosis [76].

Postoperative Management Decisions that Contribute to Postoperative Complications

IV Fluid Management

There is little doubt that the administration of intravenous fluids contributes to postoperative complications. In a study published by Lobo et al., 20 patients were randomly allocated to either standard fluid management or a restricted fluid protocol [77]. Patients randomized to a restricted protocol had earlier return of bowel function as measured using radioscintigraphic studies, as well as shorter length of stay and lower rates of complications [77]. While this was a small study, other larger trials examining fluid restriction as part of an enhanced recovery after surgery (ERAS) pathway have clearly shown that fluid restriction is an essential component of these protocols [78–81]. In a meta-analysis of randomized controlled trials, Adamina et al. found that length of stay was reduced by an average of 2.5 days and postoperative morbidity was 50 % lower in patients managed on an ERAS protocol compared to those receiving standard postoperative care [80]. The authors of this study estimated that one complication was avoided for every 4.5 patients managed on the ERAS protocol [80]. Of course, outside of an ERAS protocol, the management of fluids should be tailored to each individual patient [82]. In support of this principle, a trial of liberal fluid management versus fluid restriction in patients not being managed in an ERAS fashion was published by Mackay and others [83]. In this study, fluid restriction had no impact on early return of bowel function [83]. In contrast, patients in the restricted arm had a slight increase in their postoperative levels of serum BUN and creatinine, which did not reach statistical significance. In general, the data indicate that fluid restriction is a critical part of an ERAS protocol and that patients have improved outcomes when managed on these types of regimented pathways.

Wound Management

While there are no clear guidelines for the postoperative management of wounds, there are some general recommendations that may lead to lower rates of postoperative superficial surgical site infections (SSIs). Dressings are considered a standard of care in the management of surgical wounds, but there has been no standardization [84]. A recent Cochrane review on the topic of wound dressings and their effect on wound infection was published by Dumville and colleagues [84]. In this manuscript, the authors identified 20 randomized controlled trials, all of which had significant methodological problems. Despite the limitations of the studies, the authors performed a thorough review and found no evidence that one type of wound dressing decreased incidence of SSI over any other type [84]. In short, dressing selection should be left up to the operating surgeon and should probably reflect cost and convenience. Table 8-1 lists features of an ideal wound dressing [84].

Some have recently been interested in using new technology to manage wounds. For example, the utility of a negative pressure wound dressing on primarily closed wounds for the prevention of wound infections has been examined [85–87]. In general, the work with negative pressure units is filled with bias, and the role for this technology for the prevention of wound infections remains to be seen.

The etiology of a wound infection is largely unknown. While contamination at the time of surgery contributes to risk for infection, it has been thought that a wound hematoma or seroma may be the inciting event that leads to the postoperative infection in those cases where contamination did not occur. In an attempt to eliminate this fluid collection from the wound, Towfigh and others randomized 76 patients with high-risk wounds to either daily wound probing or standard wound management [88]. Patients treated with daily

TABLE 8-1 Features of an ideal wound dressing

1. The ability of the dressing to absorb and contain exudate without leakage or strike-through
2. Lack of particulate contaminants left in the wound by the dressing
3. Thermal insulation
4. Impermeability to water and bacteria
5. Suitability of the dressing for use with different skin closures (sutures, staples)
6. Avoidance of wound trauma on dressing removal
7. Frequency with which the dressing needs to be changed
8. Provision of pain relief
9. Cosmesis and comfort
10. Effect on formation of scar tissue

wound probing had lower rates of SSI (3 % versus 19 %) and shorter postoperative stay by 2 days [88]. While these results were promising, they have unfortunately never been reproduced or expanded to a larger population in general or colorectal surgery. In summary, there is no good evidence that any one wound management strategy is better than another. The choice of management strategies should be based on institutional experience and buy-in of the surgeons involved and should ultimately be incorporated into an institutional SSI reduction bundle which packages all care around the episode of surgery in order to reduce wound infection risk [89–93].

Bladder Management

Urinary tract infection (UTI) and catheter-associated UTI (CAUTI) are frequently encountered postoperative complications related to colorectal surgery procedures. A study from the NSQIP PUF found the rate of UTI after colorectal resection to be 4.1 % compared to 1.8 % after other general surgery operations [94]. The authors concluded that the actual rate of UTI in colorectal surgery patients is higher than expected by predictive models. Factors that correlated with an increased risk for developing a postoperative UTI included female sex; ASA class >2; procedure of a total colectomy, proctocolectomy, or APR; functional status of partially or totally dependent; and age greater than 75 [94]. Other significant factors such as presence of indwelling catheter, number of catheter days, and incidence of postoperative urinary retention are known to strongly associate with risk for UTI but are unfortunately not included in the NSQIP database. Therefore, while NSQIP database studies indicate that colorectal procedures are high risk, they offer little insight into the modifiable source of this risk.

In 2008, the Centers for Medicare and Medicaid Services (CMS) implemented a policy whereby they would reduce payment for hospitalizations that included a preventable complication [95–97]. Effective for discharges beginning October 1, 2014, CMS instituted a 1 % payment reduction for those hospitals whose ranking falls in the bottom quartile of conditions acquired during the hospital stay [97]. Included among these hospital-acquired conditions is the surveillance measure of catheter-associated urinary tract infection (CAUTI). Best practices and care bundles have been widely published in attempts to decrease the rates of CAUTI [98, 99]. While CMS has emphasized CAUTI, many in the hospital-acquired infection community point to the limitations of these surveillance definitions. For example, it is clear that a CAUTI is often not relevant to the care of the patient diagnosed after an unindicated urinalysis has revealed the presence of asymptomatic bacteriuria [100, 101]. However, the unintended negative consequences of such a urinalysis cannot be ignored [100, 101]. The unnecessary antibiotic use that often results from this type of test result leads to increased risk exposure to the patient and increased antibiotic pressure on the patient's microbial environment and ultimately contributes to the selection of multidrug-resistant organisms.

Given all of these implications of CAUTI, it makes sense that surgeons pay attention to these measures and contribute our efforts to the improvement of patient safety and reduction of hospital-acquired conditions. The question facing surgeons is how to effectively do this while still managing the patient according to a standard of care. For example, if all catheters are discontinued upon completion of an operation, we will certainly reduce the rate of CAUTI in our patient population. However, Kwaan et al. have found that early removal of the urinary catheter increases rates of urinary retention in patients undergoing pelvic surgery [102]. These high rates of urinary retention lead to increased catheter reinsertion, which likely contributes to an increased rate of urinary tract infection in patients who suffer postoperative urinary retention (POUR) [103]. However, a randomized controlled trial of early catheter removal in patients with an epidural was performed by Coyle and colleagues [104]. Here the authors found no difference in rates of POUR in epidural patients who had their catheter removed on postoperative day number 2 compared to those patients who had their catheters removed after the epidural was removed [104]. The conclusions drawn from these studies must be tempered given the clear limitations of both data and study design. Therefore, before a policy of early catheter removal can be instituted for all patients undergoing colorectal surgery, we must better understand the problem of POUR and implement effective methods to deal with this complex problem.

Pain Management

Perioperative pain is a potent trigger for the stress response that can activate the autonomic nervous system and may contribute to adverse postoperative outcomes. While there is very little evidence that poor pain control itself contributes to worse postoperative outcomes, one study found that hospitals with low patient satisfaction scores related to pain control had higher rates of postoperative mortality compared to similar hospitals [105]. Others have found that poor postoperative pain control after thoracotomy was associated with the

development of chronic long-term pain [106]. While it is not clear if poor pain control contributes to those complications colorectal surgeons commonly worry about (anastomotic leak, wound infection, etc.), Lynch and colleagues did find a correlation between high postoperative pain scores and the development of postoperative delirium [107]. In addition, high pain is often treated with high doses of opioids, which increases risk for respiratory depression and other complications related to oversedation [108]. Irrespective of the lack of high-quality data showing a clear relationship between poor pain control and postoperative complications, very few surgeons will argue against the principle of good pain control in order to ensure humane, high-quality postoperative care of all patients.

Because of the many obvious negative implications of poor pain control, many studies have assessed the best route of analgesic delivery. Specifically, many studies have examined intravenous versus epidural delivery of pain medications and have, in general, found that epidural delivery results in improved postoperative pain control [109–113]. Randomized controlled trials of laparoscopic versus open colectomy have found pain scores to be generally decreased in patients undergoing laparoscopic colectomy [114]. Therefore, as laparoscopy becomes more widespread in colorectal surgery, the use of postoperative epidural must be reexamined. In fact, a meta-analysis recently published found that although pain control was improved by the use of an epidural in patients undergoing laparoscopic colectomy, there was no difference in return of bowel function and no impact on length of stay [115]. Other studies have found no real differences between epidural and patient-controlled intravenously delivered analgesia [115–118]. Enhanced recovery after surgery protocols have largely adopted non-opioid-based pain regimens, and more work is focusing on local blocks, such as the transversus abdominis plane (TAP) block, to enhance pain control [119, 120]. Further studies are needed to identify the ideal pain control regimen for patients undergoing laparoscopic and open colorectal surgery. Regardless, it is clear that adequate pain control improves the overall patient experience.

Impact of Hospital Structure on Postoperative Complications

Academic Medical Center

The impact of resident training on patient outcome has long been debated in both the academic and lay press. In fact, Kiran et al. found a correlation between increased rates of complications and resident involvement in patient care [121]. While these results must be interpreted in the light of the limitations within the NSQIP participant use file, they do suggest that resident participation may be potentially detrimental to patient care. However, they also found that resident participation was associated with a lower rate of failure to rescue, indicating that even though patients treated at an academic medical center may have a slightly higher rate of complications, they have a lower mortality rate as a result of these complications [121]. This is likely related to resident hospital presence at all hours allowing rapidity of assessment and implementation of rescue measures. Others have similarly queried the NSQIP dataset from various years and similarly found that resident participation increases rates of postoperative complications [122–124]. While the NSQIP database controls for many factors of patient morbidity that increase risk for postoperative complications, there are many limitations of the dataset that must be considered prior to drawing hard and fast conclusions. First, missing data fields is a common problem of this database, which limits risk stratification. In addition, there is no control for the attending surgeon's gestalt assessment of risk, which also contributes to operative approach and ultimately to the operation performed.

While the above studies have examined the question of resident impact on outcomes from the binary, yes-no perspective, others have examined this question from the seasonal perspective. In particular, Englesbe et al. examined the rate of complications according to the time of year using the NSQIP dataset [125]. They found that patients treated later in the academic year had lower rates of mortality and morbidity [125]. While these results are intriguing, they still fail to control for confounding variables including differences in the environment that may contribute to complications. In fact, one study of over one million patients undergoing coronary artery bypass grafting examined outcomes by time of year in both academic and nonacademic medical centers [126]. The authors of this study found that rates of complications were higher in the first part of the year, independent of teaching status. However, they found that the rate of mortality following complication, or failure to rescue, was higher in patients treated at nonacademic medical centers. They concluded that a seasonal variation to complications and mortality exists in medical centers and cannot be explained by the presence of trainees alone [126]. In summary, it is not entirely clear that trainee presence is independently associated with postoperative complications. Furthermore, mortality rates after major complications seem to be lower in hospitals that have training programs. These findings suggest that more studies are necessary to clearly define the relationship between resident training and patient outcomes, as well as the source of the seasonal variability in postoperative morbidity and mortality.

Surgical Volume and Postoperative Complications

Much has been written on the effect of surgical volume on complications. On the surface, these papers seem to be largely self-serving works that conclude low-volume surgeons have higher rates of mortality and complications, which would necessitate referral to higher-volume surgeons. While this may be true on some level, a more critical evaluation of the literature reveals that there is a very complex interplay between the volume of the surgeon and the volume of the institution. This interplay can be seen quite nicely in two papers written by Dr. Birkemeyer and colleagues [127, 128]. In these papers, he first described a relationship between hospital volume and postoperative mortality for specific complicated operations—pancreatectomy, esophagectomy, etc. [128]. In general, they found that the rate of mortality after all resections, including proctectomy, decreased as the volume of the procedure increased at the hospital. The group then expanded this work and looked at the impact of provider volume on these mortality rates [127]. They found that provider volume could mitigate some of the effect of the institutional volume for some operations. However, not all of the effect on mortality could be explained by provider volume. The end result is a complex relationship between provider and institutional volume, suggesting that the system in which a patient undergoes an operation contributes to outcomes. This type of work has been demonstrated multiple times using many different datasets over the years [129–136]. While most of this work has indicated that higher volume is associated with improved outcomes, little work has been accomplished in understanding the mechanism behind this complex observation. Specifically, it would be interesting to truly understand the impact of the hospital system on outcomes. In recent work, Ghaferi et al. examined the features of hospital systems that correlate with low rates of mortality after major complications [44]. In this study from the Nationwide Inpatient Sample database, the authors found that teaching hospitals with more than 200 beds, increased nurse-to-patient ratio, and with a high level of technology had lower rates of failure to rescue [44]. While the results were not completely surprising, this study lays the groundwork for future investigations into how systems of care directly impact patient outcomes.

Prevention and Management of Specific Complications

Wound Complications

Wound complications and, specifically, surgical site infections (SSIs) are among the most common source of nosocomial morbidity for patients undergoing surgical procedures. SSIs are associated with increased hospital length of stay, increased risk of mortality, and decreased health-related quality of life [137, 138]. This risk is significantly increased in those patients undergoing colorectal surgery [139]. This of course is related to the clean-contaminated nature of many colorectal procedures and exteriorization of the bowel. Wound infections are commonly thought of as occurring in the superficial tissues, deep tissues, or organ space. The bulk of this discussion will focus on the prevention and treatment of superficial surgical site infection. However, all principles are applicable to deep surgical site infections and many are also applicable to organ-space infections.

It has been estimated that an SSI adds between $10,000 and $25,000 to the care of a patient depending on extent of infection [140, 141]. Given the implications of SSI on both patient outcomes and healthcare costs, much effort has been directed toward the prevention of these complications. Preoperative, perioperative, and postoperative interventions have been implemented in an attempt to decrease the rates of wound infections in all patients.

Preoperative Considerations

There are a myriad of patient-specific factors that predispose to an increased risk of perioperative complications. The number of people classified as overweight [body mass index (BMI)=25 to <30 kg/m^2] or obese (BMI ≥ 30 kg/m^2) is at pandemic proportions. The prevalence of obesity is increasing and significantly influences overall survival of the general population. The most recent data from the United States show that 40 % of adult men and 30 % of women fall within the overweight category [142]. Elevated BMI has been a validated risk factor for SSIs, with some reporting SSI rate as high as 60 % among obese patients [143–148]. However, BMI does not account for all risks associated with wound infection. In an attempt to better quantify the impact of BMI on both medical and surgical complications, there has been recent interest in the role of waist circumference (WC) and waist-to-hip ratio (WHR) on the development of cardiovascular events, as well as specifically the relationship between these measurements and perioperative outcomes of colorectal surgery. Waist circumference is thought to better reflect abdominal adiposity, including the subcutaneous fat layer, and intra-abdominal visceral adiposity. The INTERHEART study found that increased WC and WHR was predictive of myocardial infarction. To evaluate the effect of WC and WHR on surgical complications, a prospective, multicenter, international study of 1349 patients undergoing elective colorectal surgery was performed. Increased WHR was identified as an independent predictor of intraoperative complications, conversion, medical complications, and re-interventions, whereas increased BMI was a risk factor only for abdominal wall complications [149].

Another well-established risk factor for SSI is administration of allogeneic blood transfusion [139, 150, 151]. It is hypothesized that the underlying mechanism is related to transfusion-induced immunosuppression [150]. In addition to the deleterious effect that transfusion may have on disease-free survival in colorectal cancer patients, reduction in SSI risk is another compelling reason to use blood judiciously in colorectal surgery patients [152].

Perioperative Interventions

The role of mechanical bowel preparation in the prevention of SSIs has been extensively studied and debated. The data are conflicting, and oftentimes the arguments for or against bowel preparation relate more to personal preference than to evidence. That being said, much has been written on this topic. For example, there have been three recent meta-analyses of RCTs evaluating the need for mechanical bowel prep prior to surgery. One study evaluating nine RCTs demonstrated a significant increase in the percentage of anastomotic leak in prepared patients (6.2 % versus 3.2 % [OR 2.03]) [153]. An update of this analysis failed to detect significant differences in anastomotic leakage or SSI between those patients receiving and not receiving bowel preps [154]. A second meta-analysis similarly found no difference in anastomotic leakage rates; however, analysis of secondary outcomes yielded a significant difference in SSI, favoring no MBP [155]. Despite these results, the majority of colorectal surgeons still favor the use of mechanical bowel prep. Reasons for this include improved handling of a prepared colon and reduction of stool burden proximal to a fresh anastomosis. Interestingly, recently, a large retrospective review of nearly 10,000 patients did not find any difference in SSI between those with and without MBP. However, the use of oral antibiotics alone was associated with a 67 % decrease in SSI, and oral antibiotics plus mechanical bowel prep were associated with a 57 % decrease in SSI. Additionally, hospitals with higher rates of oral antibiotics had lower SSI rates [156].

Skin preparation has also been extensively examined in relation to wound infection risk. Various skin prep techniques and products are available for colorectal procedures, but clear evidence supporting one over another is lacking. In one randomized controlled trial, the use of chlorhexidine-alcohol rather than povidone-iodine was shown to significantly reduce both superficial surgical site infections and deep incisional infections but had no demonstrable effect on organ-space infections [157]. Another group performed a sequential implementation study in which different skin preparation agents were serially used over the course of a defined time period [158]. The authors of this study found the lowest rates of SSI in the time frame that used iodine povacrylex in isopropyl alcohol, which subsequently led to institutional adoption of this skin prep agent [158]. This is a perfect example of classic quality improvement work characterized by the FOCUS-PDCA process (Figure 8-2) [159–161]. This quality improvement model facilitates concrete steps toward a defined goal and ultimately implementation of change to enhance patient care. However, it is important to note that quality improvement is an iterative process. As implied in Figure 8-2, the FOCUS-PDCA process is a cycle that repeats itself. This cycle allows us to always search for a better "best practice."

Another relatively straightforward intervention at the time of operation that may prevent superficial SSI is the use of a wound protector. While there are conflicting data regarding the utility of these devices in preventing wound infections in abdominal surgery, a recent randomized study of 130 consecutive patients undergoing elective, open, colorectal surgery found that the use of a wound protector was significantly

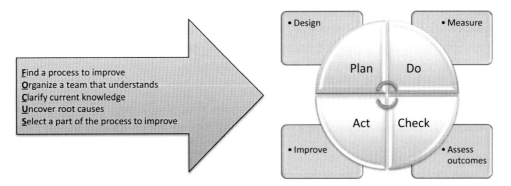

FIGURE 8-2. FOCUS-PDCA cycle is shown. The key to a successful quality improvement process is the continuous assessment and process improvement implied by the cycle.

associated with reduced incidence of incisional SSI [162]. A recent meta-analysis supported these results, concluding that the use of a dual-ring wound protector is associated with decreased risk for SSI [163].

In addition to interventions aimed directly at reducing microbial burden, treatments that improve oxygen delivery to the wound have also been examined in the context of SSI prevention. Murray et al. [164] performed a review of level 1 evidence looking at non-pharmacologic modalities for decreasing the incidence of SSI. These include easily implemented, cost-effective interventions with a low-risk profile such as administration of supranormal oxygen, active rewarming strategies, and adjustment in wound closure techniques. Several prospective randomized trials have attempted to define the impact of supranormal levels of oxygen during anesthesia on SSI [165–168]. A meta-analysis of such trials demonstrated a significant decrease in SSI with the use of 80 % FIO2 in the perioperative setting, favoring the use of perioperative hyperoxia. In contrast, a recent multicenter study [PROXI] that randomized patients to receive 80 % FIO2 intraoperatively and 2 h postoperatively versus 30 % FIO2 in a similar fashion found no difference in outcomes [168]. Of note, none of these studies reported any adverse events attributable to the administration of supranormal levels of oxygen [164]. Another readily available intervention that has been shown to reduce SSI in colorectal surgery patients involves the application of an active warming strategy perioperatively [169, 170].

Multiple reports have demonstrated the utility of closing the midline wound with a suture length-to-wound length ratio of at least 4 [171]. This technique mandates taking either >10 mm fascial bites at greater intervals than previously recommended or alternatively smaller bites of the fascial edge (5–8 mm) in closer intervals. These techniques were compared in a randomized controlled trial which demonstrated a significant increase in SSI and incisional hernia when utilizing the former approach [172]. Specific to colorectal surgery, ileostomy closure poses a unique challenge with regard to infection. In this setting, purse-string closure of ileostomy wounds has been significantly associated with reduced SSI rate in a meta-analysis of three RCTs [173, 174].

In summary, multiple low-risk perioperative interventions can be taken that likely improve short-term outcomes. This phase of care should not be neglected when implementing a bundle of care designed to decrease risk for surgical site infection. Such a bundle might include bowel preparation with oral antibiotics, skin preparation with a chlorhexidine-based agent, hyperoxygenation, active warming, and meticulous closure with careful attention to tension and hemostasis, all of which together may contribute to improved outcomes.

Management of Superficial Surgical Site Infection

Given the enormity of the problem of surgical site infections, it is clear that the best management strategy is one of prevention. Regardless of the interventions taken to prevent these hospital-acquired infections, it seems that the most efficient method involves standardizing the practice to include a bundle of care that is included for every operation. Dr. Cima and others have recently published their experience on a surgical site infection reduction bundle at their institution in Rochester, MN. They have found a reduction of surgical site infections from 9.8 % pre-bundle to 4.0 % after the bundle implementation [92]. Monitoring of compliance with the care bundle is also critically important. As shown by Waits et al., compliance with all parts of a bundle correlates with a lower risk of wound infection (2.5 % in those hospitals with 100 % compliance compared to 17.5 % in those hospitals that were the most noncompliant) [175]. We have similarly implemented a surgical site infection reduction bundle in our hospital and have seen our rate of SSI as monitored by NSQIP to drop into the "as expected" range with the most recent site report showing our rate of SSI in colorectal surgery to be in the second decile (data not shown). The adoption of bundled care ensures all members of the surgical team are focused on the safety of the patient and gives the team a template from which to work.

Despite all attempts to prevent surgical site infections in colorectal surgery, the average institution will continue to see rates of infections near 10 %. Therefore, understanding the principles of treatment is critical. For an uncomplicated superficial surgical site infection, the standard treatment is drainage of the infection and local wound care without the routine use of antibiotics [176–178]. If patients exhibit signs and symptoms of shock, one must suspect the presence of a deeper infection. This type of infection may involve the deeper layers of the wound (muscle and fascia) or may even involve the organ space. Aggressive interventional therapy is often required to adequately treat a deep surgical site infection and organ-space infections may require reoperation as well. It is critical that the surgeon stay intimately involved in all aspects of the patient's care and also remain vigilant as the best treatment of these infections is often through early identification and infection control.

Cardiovascular and Respiratory Complications

Additional postoperative complications befall those undergoing colorectal surgery. These include cardiovascular complications, which as mentioned have an increased incidence in those patients with an elevated BMI, as well as more recently found, elevated waist-to-hip ratio. In the previously mentioned study of 1349 patients, which identified elevated waist-to-hip ratio (WHR) as a predictor for postoperative complications, the incidences of stroke, deep venous thrombosis, myocardial infarction, congestive heart failure, and pulmonary embolism were all less than 1 %. All complications, to include cardiovascular and respiratory complications, as well as sepsis and septic shock, were previously shown to be decreased in those patients undergoing laparoscopic colorectal procedures compared to those patients undergoing similar procedures in an open fashion [34, 179].

Postoperative venous thromboembolism carries a current prevalence of 1.4–2.4 % in colorectal surgery patients and is one of the most important potentially preventable conditions leading to increases in morbidity, mortality, hospitalization length, and hospital charges [180–182]. A recent study of 116,029 patients utilizing the ACS NSQIP database analyzed the incidence, risk factors, and 30-day outcomes of VTE in patients undergoing colorectal procedures [183]. Risk-adjusted analysis for preoperative factors associated with DVT included age greater than 70, African American race, ASA score >2, hypoalbuminemia, disseminated cancer, steroid use, and obesity. Additionally, open colorectal procedures had a higher risk of postoperative DVT compared to laparoscopic procedures, as did emergently admitted patients, ulcerative colitis on pathology, and anesthesia length greater than 150 min. Similarly, with regard to PE, risk-adjusted analysis found that age greater than 70, emergency admission, open surgery, hypoalbuminemia, steroid use, and obesity all conferred a significantly increased risk of postoperative PE. Additionally, as expected, mortality risk is

significantly increased among those patients diagnosed with PE. This analysis also found that the majority of VTE and PE events occurred during the first week after surgery; however, interestingly, they also found that 34.6 % and 29.3 % of patients diagnosed with VTE and PE, respectively, were diagnosed after discharge [183].

These data underscore the importance of VTE and PE prophylaxis in the perioperative setting and also suggest a possible role for anticoagulating after discharge. It is our practice to administer 5000 units of unfractionated heparin (UFH) prior to skin incision and to immediately implement additional prophylaxis to include UFH or LWMH, on postoperative day 1, provided there are no contraindications. We do not routinely anticoagulate after discharge; however, this practice should be considered as we evaluate the most recent literature. Specifically, a recent randomized prospective analysis evaluating 1-week versus 4-week prophylaxis in patients undergoing laparoscopic colorectal surgery for colorectal cancer found a significant reduction in rates of VTE among those undergoing 4-week prophylaxis with LMWH with similar rates of bleeding between the two groups [184].

Mortality and Failure to Rescue

While postoperative mortality is uncommon after elective colorectal surgery [34, 35], it would be remiss to not address this particular outcome as the patient population ages and becomes higher risk. Fortunately, even in the oldest patient populations undergoing elective colectomy for colon cancer, the rate of mortality is at most 4 % in hospitals participating in the NSQIP program [185]. Given this relatively low rate of postoperative mortality, it is worth considering what leads to death after surgery. In general, mortality after elective surgery does not occur in isolation but rather follows another major complication. In fact, the Agency for Healthcare Research and Quality (AHRQ) has defined death rate among surgical inpatients with serious treatable complications as a patient safety indicator in order to track this metric across institutions. Failure to rescue is defined as death per 1000 surgical discharges among patients aged 18–89 with serious treatable complications such as deep vein thrombosis/pulmonary embolism, pneumonia, sepsis, shock/cardiac arrest, or gastrointestinal hemorrhage/acute ulcer [186]. Failure to rescue is considered a measure of the system of care in which a patient is treated and was discussed previously in relation to the impact of resident involvement on postoperative outcomes at academic medical centers. Sheetz and colleagues examined failure to rescue rates across the state of Michigan using the Michigan Surgical Quality Collaborative [187]. Failure to rescue rates varied by hospital even when controlling for differences in patient characteristics, and rates of complications were highest in the hospitals with the highest mortality [187]. These results suggest that failure to rescue is more related to the system of care than to the patient population. Ghaferi et al. similarly found that systems-related factors such as number of hospital beds, teaching status, nurse-to-patient ratio, and high technology utilization correlated with low failure to rescue rates [44]. More research is necessary to further delineate both risk and mitigating factors for failure to rescue after major complications.

Long-Term Complications

Many colorectal surgery interventions result in long-term physiological changes for patients. Effective management and patient counseling require a thorough understanding of potential long-term complications and their natural history.

Genitourinary Complications

Bladder dysfunction following colorectal surgery is most commonly related to extirpative procedures in the region of the autonomic pelvic plexus. Abdominoperineal resection and low anterior resection have incidences of postoperative bladder dysfunction of nearly 50 % and 15–25 %, respectively [188]. The most common sequel of autonomic nerve damage during colorectal surgery is parasympathetic detrusor denervation, resulting in impaired contractility of the bladder. A majority of patients will regain the ability to empty the bladder; however, this can take up to 6 months. In the interim, the bladder is managed with clean intermittent catheterization. If careful bladder care is neglected, deleterious effects such as hydronephrosis, urinary reflux, pyelonephritis, and declining renal function may ensue [189]. The use of urodynamics allows for objective measurements to identify those patients at risk, and treatment must be highly individualized [189].

Fertility Complications

Female patients undergoing pelvic procedures should be engaged in a thoughtful discussion preoperatively of the potential risk for fertility problems. A meta-analysis found a postoperative infertility rate of 48 % after restorative proctocolectomy for ulcerative colitis, compared to 15 % preoperatively [190]. Additionally, a systematic literature review was undertaken to evaluate the impact of restorative proctocolectomy on sexual function, urinary function, fertility, pregnancy, and delivery in patients with ulcerative colitis. Infertility rates of 12 % before surgery and 26 % after surgery were reported among 945 patients in seven studies [191]. However, some authors contend that this is more likely related to the disease process itself, rather than the type of surgery performed. A cross-sectional study of FAP patients found no association between fertility problems and

type of surgery but did report an increased risk of fertility difficulty in women undergoing surgical procedures earlier in life [192].

Bowel Dysfunction

Pelvic surgery that includes restoration of bowel continuity is not only technically complicated but introduces new physiology to the life of the patients. For example, low anterior resection syndrome includes a variety of symptoms, including fecal incontinence, urgency, frequent bowel movements, and clustering of bowel movements [193]. When undergoing a procedure for rectal cancer, it is often assumed that restorative and sphincter-sparing techniques afford patients a quality of life, which is superior to that of a permanent stoma, with equivalent oncological outcome. This has been challenged by recent inquiries comparing patients' quality of life postoperatively following low anterior resection and abdominoperineal resection for rectal cancer. Certain prospective studies found better cognitive and social function, as well as less symptomatology with respect to pain, sleep disturbance, diarrhea, and constipation in those undergoing abdominoperineal resection. Those undergoing low anterior resection reported better sexual function; however, 72 % reported some degree of fecal incontinence [194]. A recent Cochrane review further calls into question that the quality of life (QoL) with a permanent stoma is inferior to the QoL of those with restored bowel continuity. This review did not find evidence that the QoL after anterior resection is superior to that of patients who had undergone abdominoperineal resection or Hartmann's procedure [195]. This lack of significance led some authors to surmise that this was in direct relation to bowel function postoperatively. Indeed, 50–90 % of patients undergoing sphincter-sparing low anterior resection have some degree of bowel dysfunction postoperatively [196, 197]. Using a validated LARS score [198], Juul et al. found that the quality of life after rectal cancer surgery is closely associated with the severity of the low anterior resection syndrome [193].

The etiology of the symptoms constituting LAR syndrome is unknown; however, it is often manifest by some degree of fecal or gas incontinence, clustering of bowel movements, frequency, and urgency. The severity of symptoms also seems to correlate with tumor height more than 5 cm, total mesorectal excision, and patient treatment with radiotherapy [199]. In fact, Marijnen et al. found that short-term preoperative radiotherapy led to significantly slower recovery from defecation problems, a negative effect on sexual functioning in males and females, as well as more ejaculation disorders and erectile functioning in males, when compared to those patients who did not undergo preoperative radiotherapy [200]. This did not, however, affect health-related quality of life in their study. Interestingly, when patients who underwent low anterior resection versus abdominoperineal resection were compared, those who underwent APR scored better on physical and psychologic dimensions of quality of life [200]. An additional randomized controlled trial found that a short course of preoperative radiotherapy increased male sexual dysfunction, as well as an increased level of fecal incontinence [201]. Taken together, the risk of bowel dysfunction after surgery can be directly attributed to difficulties with symptoms related to the low anterior resection syndrome. While previous reports have assumed that the quality of life with restorative and sphincter-sparing procedures is greater than the quality of life with a permanent stoma, this is not always the case. When evaluating a patient with rectal cancer, specifically one who qualifies for neoadjuvant treatment, an earnest conversation must be had regarding postoperative functional outcomes.

Impact of Postoperative Complications on Oncologic Outcomes

It is clear that postoperative complications carry implications for short-term quality of life and negatively impact the cost of care. In addition, there is evidence that postoperative complications impact long-term oncologic outcomes [202, 203]. While the exact mechanism of the impact on long-term survival is unclear, it seems likely that postoperative complications result in either delay in receiving or complete omission of chemotherapy in patients with clear indications for systemic treatment. Hendren and colleagues used the SEER-Medicare database from 1993 to 2005 to examine risk for chemotherapy omission [203]. Patients who suffered postoperative complications were more likely to have chemotherapy omitted, but this was unable to be correlated with long-term survival [203]. Tevis and colleagues looked at this question in patients undergoing surgery for rectal cancer [202]. In this cohort, patients with postoperative complications had worse long-term survival than did those with no complications. Postoperative complications independently correlated with decreased overall survival even in patients who received chemotherapy, suggesting that in addition to omission of chemotherapy, complications may otherwise lead to poor long-term survival [202]. While no single study has definitively answered the question, most have found similar negative correlations between postoperative complications and long-term survival, suggesting that there is a relationship between the two. Further work is required to fully understand this relationship.

Conclusion

Postoperative complications after colorectal surgery are common. While we should strive to make postoperative complications, so-called never events, given the imprecise and uncontrollable nature of our profession, it is unlikely that we will achieve such a status. Therefore, we must have a good understanding of the issues related to these complica-

tions and be able to work through the implications of these complications. Research to better understand risk factors and preoperative risk mitigation may continue to lead to improved outcomes. How risk modulation can be achieved with surgical approach and intraoperative management must also be examined if we want to continue to improve outcomes. While quality improvement efforts are difficult and not always rewarding, it is clear that continued focus on preventing postoperative complications is beneficial not only to the patient's short-term health and quality of life but will also deliver downstream benefits such as improved long-term physiologic and oncologic outcomes. Finally, it is self-evident that improvements in short-term outcomes will have a positive impact on the healthcare delivery system by decreasing costs associated with postoperative complications.

References

1. Dahlke AR, Merkow RP, Chung JW, et al. Comparison of postoperative complication risk prediction approaches based on factors known preoperatively to surgeons versus patients. Surgery. 2014;156(1):39–45.
2. Sherman SK, Hrabe JE, Charlton ME, Cromwell JW, Byrn JC. Development of an improved risk calculator for complications in proctectomy. J Gastrointest Surg. 2014;18(5):986–94.
3. Fischer JP, Wes AM, Tuggle CT, Serletti JM, Wu LC. Risk analysis and stratification of surgical morbidity after immediate breast reconstruction. J Am Coll Surg. 2013;217(5): 780–7.
4. Nelson MT, Greenblatt DY, Soma G, Rajimanickam V, Greenberg CC, Kent KC. Preoperative factors predict mortality after major lower-extremity amputation. Surgery. 2012;152(4):685–94. discussion 694–6.
5. Greenblatt DY, Kelly KJ, Rajamanickam V, et al. Preoperative factors predict perioperative morbidity and mortality after pancreaticoduodenectomy. Ann Surg Oncol. 2011;18(8): 2126–35.
6. Davenport DL, Henderson WG, Khuri SF, Mentzer Jr RM. Preoperative risk factors and surgical complexity are more predictive of costs than postoperative complications: a case study using the National Surgical Quality Improvement Program (NSQIP) database. Ann Surg. 2005;242(4):463–8. discussion 468–71.
7. New ACS NSQIP Surgical Risk Calculator offers personalized estimates of surgical complications. Bull Am Coll Surg. 2013;98(10):72–3.
8. Bilimoria KY, Liu Y, Paruch JL, et al. Development and evaluation of the universal ACS NSQIP surgical risk calculator: a decision aid and informed consent tool for patients and surgeons. J Am Coll Surg. 2013;217(5):833–42 e831–33.
9. Schwarze ML, Brasel KJ, Mosenthal AC. Beyond 30-day mortality: aligning surgical quality with outcomes that patients value. JAMA Surg. 2014;149(7):631–2.
10. Paruch JL, Ko CY, Bilimoria KY. An opportunity to improve informed consent and shared decision making: the role of the ACS NSQIP Surgical Risk Calculator in oncology. Ann Surg Oncol. 2014;21(1):5–7.
11. Cologne KG, Keller DS, Liwanag L, Devaraj B, Senagore AJ. Use of the American College of Surgeons NSQIP Surgical Risk Calculator for laparoscopic colectomy: how good is it

and how can we improve it? J Am Coll Surg. 2015;220(3):281–6.

12. Ehlenbach CC, Tevis SE, Kennedy GD, Oltmann SC. Preoperative impairment is associated with a higher post-discharge level of care. J Surg Res. 2015;193(1):1–6.

13. Robinson TN, Wu DS, Pointer LF, Dunn CL, Moss M. Preoperative cognitive dysfunction is related to adverse postoperative outcomes in the elderly. J Am Coll Surg. 2012;215(1):12–7. discussion 17–8.

14. Bouillon K, Kivimaki M, Hamer M, et al. Measures of frailty in population-based studies: an overview. BMC Geriatr. 2013;13:64.

15. Fried LP, Tangen CM, Walston J, et al. Frailty in older adults: evidence for a phenotype. J Gerontol A Biol Sci Med Sci. 2001;56(3):M146–56.

16. Robinson TN, Wallace JI, Wu DS, et al. Accumulated frailty characteristics predict postoperative discharge institutionalization in the geriatric patient. J Am Coll Surg. 2011;213(1):37–42. discussion 42–4.

17. Robinson TN, Wu DS, Pointer L, Dunn CL, Cleveland Jr JC, Moss M. Simple frailty score predicts postoperative complications across surgical specialties. Am J Surg. 2013;206(4):544–50.

18. Chow WB, Rosenthal RA, Merkow RP, Ko CY, Esnaola NF. Optimal preoperative assessment of the geriatric surgical patient: a best practices guideline from the American College of Surgeons National Surgical Quality Improvement Program and the American Geriatrics Society. J Am Coll Surg. 2012;215(4):453–66.

19. Mavros MN, Athanasiou S, Gkegkes ID, Polyzos KA, Peppas G, Falagas ME. Do psychological variables affect early surgical recovery? PLoS One. 2011;6(5):e20306.

20. Okkonen E, Vanhanen H. Family support, living alone, and subjective health of a patient in connection with a coronary artery bypass surgery. Heart Lung. 2006;35(4):234–44.

21. Kulik JA, Mahler HI. Social support and recovery from surgery. Health Psychol. 1989;8(2):221–38.

22. Mitchinson AR, Kim HM, Geisser M, Rosenberg JM, Hinshaw DB. Social connectedness and patient recovery after major operations. J Am Coll Surg. 2008;206(2):292–300.

23. Ferry M, Sidobre B, Lambertin A, Barberger-Gateau P. The SOLINUT study: analysis of the interaction between nutrition and loneliness in persons aged over 70 years. J Nutr Health Aging. 2005;9(4):261–8.

24. Jacobs M, Verdeja JC, Goldstein HS. Minimally invasive colon resection (laparoscopic colectomy). Surg Laparosc Endosc. 1991;1(3):144–50.

25. Wexner SD, Cohen SM, Johansen OB, Nogueras JJ, Jagelman DG. Laparoscopic colorectal surgery: a prospective assessment and current perspective. Br J Surg. 1993;80(12):1602–5.

26. Wexner SD, Johansen OB, Nogueras JJ, Jagelman DG. Laparoscopic total abdominal colectomy. A prospective trial. Dis Colon Rectum. 1992;35(7):651–5.

27. Beck DE, Opelka FG, Bailey HR, Rauh SM, Pashos CL. Incidence of small-bowel obstruction and adhesiolysis after open colorectal and general surgery. Dis Colon Rectum. 1999;42(2):241–8.

28. ten Broek RP, Issa Y, van Santbrink EJ, et al. Burden of adhesions in abdominal and pelvic surgery: systematic review and met-analysis. BMJ. 2013;347:f5588.

29. Duepree HJ, Senagore AJ, Delaney CP, Fazio VW. Does means of access affect the incidence of small bowel obstruction and ventral hernia after bowel resection? Laparoscopy versus laparotomy. J Am Coll Surg. 2003;197(2):177–81.

30. Dolejs S, Kennedy G, Heise CP. Small bowel obstruction following restorative proctocolectomy: affected by a laparoscopic approach? J Surg Res. 2011;170(2):202–8.

31. Clinical Outcomes of Surgical Therapy Study Group. A comparison of laparoscopically assisted and open colectomy for colon cancer. N Engl J Med. 2004;350(20):2050–9.

32. Guillou PJ, Quirke P, Thorpe H, et al. Short-term endpoints of conventional versus laparoscopic-assisted surgery in patients with colorectal cancer (MRC CLASICC trial): multicentre, randomised controlled trial. Lancet. 2005;365(9472):1718–26.

33. Yang W, Zilov A, Soewondo P, Bech OM, Sekkal F, Home PD. Observational studies: going beyond the boundaries of randomized controlled trials. Diabetes Res Clin Pract. 2010;88 Suppl 1:S3–9.

34. Kennedy GD, Heise C, Rajamanickam V, Harms B, Foley EF. Laparoscopy decreases postoperative complication rates after abdominal colectomy: results from the national surgical quality improvement program. Ann Surg. 2009;249(4):596–601.

35. Bilimoria KY, Bentrem DJ, Merkow RP, et al. Laparoscopic-assisted vs. open colectomy for cancer: comparison of short-term outcomes from 121 hospitals. J Gastrointest Surg. 2008;12(11):2001–9.

36. Bilimoria KY, Bentrem DJ, Nelson H, et al. Use and outcomes of laparoscopic-assisted colectomy for cancer in the United States. Arch Surg. 2008;143(9):832–9. discussion 839–40.

37. Wilson MZ, Hollenbeak CS, Stewart DB. Laparoscopic colectomy is associated with a lower incidence of postoperative complications than open colectomy: a propensity score-matched cohort analysis. Colorectal Dis. 2014;16(5):382–9.

38. Speicher PJ, Englum BR, Jiang B, Pietrobon R, Mantyh CR, Migaly J. The impact of laparoscopic versus open approach on reoperation rate after segmental colectomy: a propensity analysis. J Gastrointest Surg. 2014;18(2):378–84.

39. Causey MW, Stoddard D, Johnson EK, et al. Laparoscopy impacts outcomes favorably following colectomy for ulcerative colitis: a critical analysis of the ACS-NSQIP database. Surg Endosc. 2013;27(2):603–9.

40. Aimaq R, Akopian G, Kaufman HS. Surgical site infection rates in laparoscopic versus open colorectal surgery. Am Surg. 2011;77(10):1290–4.

41. Stefanou AJ, Reickert CA, Velanovich V, Falvo A, Rubinfeld I. Laparoscopic colectomy significantly decreases length of stay compared with open operation. Surg Endosc. 2012;26(1):144–8.

42. Kiran RP, El-Gazzaz GH, Vogel JD, Remzi FH. Laparoscopic approach significantly reduces surgical site infections after colorectal surgery: data from national surgical quality improvement program. J Am Coll Surg. 2010;211(2):232–8.

43. Silber JH, Williams SV, Krakauer H, Schwartz JS. Hospital and patient characteristics associated with death after surgery. A study of adverse occurrence and failure to rescue. Med Care. 1992;30(7):615–29.

44. Ghaferi AA, Osborne NH, Birkmeyer JD, Dimick JB. Hospital characteristics associated with failure to rescue from complications after pancreatectomy. J Am Coll Surg. 2010;211(3):325–30.

45. Ghaferi AA, Birkmeyer JD, Dimick JB. Complications, failure to rescue, and mortality with major inpatient surgery in medicare patients. Ann Surg. 2009;250(6):1029–34.

46. Ghaferi AA, Birkmeyer JD, Dimick JB. Variation in hospital mortality associated with inpatient surgery. N Engl J Med. 2009;361(14):1368–75.

47. AHRQ Patient Safety Indicators, Technical Specifications, PSI#15 Accidental Puncture or Laceration. Provider-Level Indicator. Version 4.1. 2009: 1–2. Available at: http://www.qualityindicators.ahrq.gov/Downloads/Modules/PSI/V41/TechSpecs/PSI%2015%20Accidental%20Puncture%20or%20Laceration.pdf

48. Kaafarani HM, Borzecki AM, Itani KM, et al. Validity of selected Patient Safety Indicators: opportunities and concerns. J Am Coll Surg. 2011;212(6):924–34.

49. Kin C, Snyder K, Kiran RP, Remzi FH, Vogel JD. Accidental puncture or laceration in colorectal surgery: a quality indicator or a complexity measure? Dis Colon Rectum. 2013;56(2):219–25.

50. Gu J, Stocchi L, Remzi F, Kiran RP. Factors associated with postoperative morbidity, reoperation and readmission rates after laparoscopic total abdominal colectomy for ulcerative colitis. Colorectal Dis. 2013;15(9):1123–9.

51. Sun RC, Button AM, Smith BJ, Leblond RF, Howe JR, Mezhir JJ. A comprehensive assessment of transfusion in elective pancreatectomy: risk factors and complications. J Gastrointest Surg. 2013;17(4):627–35.

52. Greenblatt DY, Rajamanickam V, Mell MW. Predictors of surgical site infection after open lower extremity revascularization. J Vasc Surg. 2011;54(2):433–9.

53. Greenblatt DY, Rajamanickam V, Pugely AJ, Heise CP, Foley EF, Kennedy GD. Short-term outcomes after laparoscopic-assisted proctectomy for rectal cancer: results from the ACS NSQIP. J Am Coll Surg. 2011;212(5):844–54.

54. Halabi WJ, Jafari MD, Nguyen VQ, et al. Blood transfusions in colorectal cancer surgery: incidence, outcomes, and predictive factors: an American College of Surgeons National Surgical Quality Improvement Program analysis. Am J Surg. 2013;206(6):1024–32. discussion 1032–3.

55. Meraney AM, Samee AA, Gill IS. Vascular and bowel complications during retroperitoneal laparoscopic surgery. J Urol. 2002;168(5):1941–4.

56. Bhoyrul S, Vierra MA, Nezhat CR, Krummel TM, Way LW. Trocar injuries in laparoscopic surgery. J Am Coll Surg. 2001;192(6):677–83.

57. Larobina M, Nottle P. Complete evidence regarding major vascular injuries during laparoscopic access. Surg Laparosc Endosc Percutan Tech. 2005;15(3):119–23.

58. Tou S, Malik AI, Wexner SD, Nelson RL. Energy source instruments for laparoscopic colectomy. Cochrane Database Syst Rev. 2011;5, CD007886.

59. Adamina M, Champagne BJ, Hoffman L, Ermlich MB, Delaney CP. Randomized clinical trial comparing the cost and effectiveness of bipolar vessel sealers versus clips and vascular staplers for laparoscopic colorectal resection. Br J Surg. 2011;98(12):1703–12.

60. Marcello PW, Roberts PL, Rusin LC, Holubkov R, Schoetz DJ. Vascular pedicle ligation techniques during laparoscopic colectomy. A prospective randomized trial. Surg Endosc. 2006;20(2):263–9.

61. Halabi WJ, Jafari MD, Nguyen VQ, et al. Ureteral injuries in colorectal surgery: an analysis of trends, outcomes, and risk factors over a 10-year period in the United States. Dis Colon Rectum. 2014;57(2):179–86.

62. Palaniappa NC, Telem DA, Ranasinghe NE, Divino CM. Incidence of iatrogenic ureteral injury after laparoscopic colectomy. Arch Surg. 2012;147(3):267–71.

63. Larach SW, Patankar SK, Ferrara A, Williamson PR, Perozo SE, Lord AS. Complications of laparoscopic colorectal surgery. Analysis and comparison of early vs. latter experience. Dis Colon Rectum. 1997;40(5):592–6.

64. Delacroix SE, Winters JC. Urinary tract injures: recognition and management. Clin Colon Rectal Surg. 2010;23(2):104–12.

65. Speicher PJ, Goldsmith ZG, Nussbaum DP, Turley RS, Peterson AC, Mantyh CR. Ureteral stenting in laparoscopic colorectal surgery. J Surg Res. 2014;190(1):98–103.

66. Delacroix SE, Winters JC. Bladder reconstruction and diversion during colorectal surgery. Clin Colon Rectal Surg. 2010;23(2):113–8.

67. Kashefi C, Messer K, Barden R, Sexton C, Parsons JK. Incidence and prevention of iatrogenic urethral injuries. J Urol. 2008;179(6):2254–7. discussion 2257–8.

68. Rivera R, Barboglio PG, Hellinger M, Gousse AE. Staging rectourinary fistulas to guide surgical treatment. J Urol. 2007;177(2):586–8.

69. Spahn M, Vergho D, Riedmiller H. Iatrogenic recto-urethral fistula: perineal repair and buccal mucosa interposition. BJU Int. 2009;103(2):242–6.

70. Fengler SA, Abcarian H. The York Mason approach to repair of iatrogenic rectourinary fistulae. Am J Surg. 1997;173(3):213–7.

71. Dreznik Z, Alper D, Vishne TH, Ramadan E. Rectal flap advancement—a simple and effective approach for the treatment of rectourethral fistula. Colorectal Dis. 2003;5(1):53–5.

72. Visser BC, McAninch JW, Welton ML. Rectourethral fistulae: the perineal approach. J Am Coll Surg. 2002;195(1):138–43.

73. Culkin DJ, Ramsey CE. Urethrorectal fistula: transanal, transsphincteric approach with locally based pedicle interposition flaps. J Urol. 2003;169(6):2181–3.

74. Bruce RG, El-Galley RE, Galloway NT. Use of rectus abdominis muscle flap for the treatment of complex and refractory urethrovaginal fistulas. J Urol. 2000;163(4):1212–5.

75. Wexner SD, Ruiz DE, Genua J, Nogueras JJ, Weiss EG, Zmora O. Gracilis muscle interposition for the treatment of rectourethral, rectovaginal, and pouch-vaginal fistulas: results in 53 patients. Ann Surg. 2008;248(1):39–43.

76. Remzi FH, El Gazzaz G, Kiran RP, Kirat HT, Fazio VW. Outcomes following Turnbull-Cutait abdominoperineal pull-through compared with coloanal anastomosis. Br J Surg. 2009;96(4):424–9.

77. Lobo DN, Bostock KA, Neal KR, Perkins AC, Rowlands BJ, Allison SP. Effect of salt and water balance on recovery of gastrointestinal function after elective colonic resection: a randomised controlled trial. Lancet. 2002;359(9320):1812–8.

78. Muller S, Zalunardo MP, Hubner M, Clavien PA, Demartines N. A fast-track program reduces complications and length of hospital stay after open colonic surgery. Gastroenterology. 2009;136(3):842–7.

79. Adamina M, Senagore AJ, Delaney CP, Kehlet H. A systematic review of economic evaluations of enhanced recovery pathways for colorectal surgery. Ann Surg. 2015;261(5):e138.

80. Adamina M, Kehlet H, Tomlinson GA, Senagore AJ, Delaney CP. Enhanced recovery pathways optimize health outcomes and resource utilization: a meta-analysis of randomized controlled trials in colorectal surgery. Surgery. 2011;149(6): 830–40.

81. Senagore AJ, Emery T, Luchtefeld M, Kim D, Dujovny N, Hoedema R. Fluid management for laparoscopic colectomy: a prospective, randomized assessment of goal-directed administration of balanced salt solution or hetastarch coupled with an enhanced recovery program. Dis Colon Rectum. 2009;52(12): 1935–40.

82. Allen SJ. Fluid therapy and outcome: balance is best. J Extra Corpor Technol. 2014;46(1):28–32.

83. MacKay G, Fearon K, McConnachie A, Serpell MG, Molloy RG, O'Dwyer PJ. Randomized clinical trial of the effect of postoperative intravenous fluid restriction on recovery after elective colorectal surgery. Br J Surg. 2006;93(12):1469–74.

84. Dumville JC, Gray TA, Walter CJ, Sharp CA, Page T. Dressings for the prevention of surgical site infection. Cochrane Database Syst Rev. 2014;9, CD003091.

85. Horch RE. Incisional negative pressure wound therapy for high-risk wounds. J Wound Care. 2015;24(Suppl 4b):21–8.

86. Anglim B, O'Connor H, Daly S. Prevena, negative pressure wound therapy applied to closed Pfannenstiel incisions at time of caesarean section in patients deemed at high risk for wound infection. J Obstet Gynaecol. 2014;10:1–4.

87. Scalise A, Tartaglione C, Bolletta E, et al. The enhanced healing of a high-risk, clean, sutured surgical incision by prophylactic negative pressure wound therapy as delivered by Prevena Customizable: cosmetic and therapeutic results. Int Wound J. 2015;12(2):218–23.

88. Towfigh S, Clarke T, Yacoub W, et al. Significant reduction of wound infections with daily probing of contaminated wounds: a prospective randomized clinical trial. Arch Surg. 2011; 146(4):448–52.

89. Leaper DJ, Tanner J, Kiernan M, Assadian O, Edmiston Jr CE. Surgical site infection: poor compliance with guidelines and care bundles. Int Wound J. 2015;12(3):357–62.

90. van der Slegt J, van der Laan L, Veen EJ, Hendriks Y, Romme J, Kluytmans J. Implementation of a bundle of care to reduce surgical site infections in patients undergoing vascular surgery. PLoS One. 2013;8(8):e71566.

91. Johnson B, Starks I, Bancroft G, Roberts PJ. The effect of care bundle development on surgical site infection after hemiarthroplasty: an 8-year review. J Trauma Acute Care Surg. 2012;72(5):1375–9.

92. Cima R, Dankbar E, Lovely J, et al. Colorectal surgery surgical site infection reduction program: a national surgical quality improvement program—driven multidisciplinary single-institution experience. J Am Coll Surg. 2013;216(1):23–33.

93. Crolla RM, van der Laan L, Veen EJ, Hendriks Y, van Schendel C, Kluytmans J. Reduction of surgical site infections after implementation of a bundle of care. PLoS One. 2012;7(9): e44599.

94. Regenbogen SE, Read TE, Roberts PL, Marcello PW, Schoetz DJ, Ricciardi R. Urinary tract infection after colon and rectal resections: more common than predicted by risk-adjustment models. J Am Coll Surg. 2011;213(6):784–92.

95. Pronovost PJ, Goeschel CA, Wachter RM. The wisdom and justice of not paying for "preventable complications". JAMA. 2008;299(18):2197–9.

96. Saint S, Meddings JA, Calfee D, Kowalski CP, Krein SL. Catheter-associated urinary tract infection and the Medicare rule changes. Ann Intern Med. 2009;150(12):877–84.

97. Centers for Medicare and Medicaid Services (CMS), HHS. Medicare program; hospital inpatient prospective payment systems for acute care hospitals and the long-term care hospital prospective payment system and fiscal year 2015 rates; quality reporting requirements for specific providers; reasonable compensation equivalents for physician services in excluded hospitals and certain teaching hospitals; provider administrative appeals and judicial review; enforcement provisions for organ transplant centers; and electronic health record (EHR) incentive program. Final rule. Fed Regist. 2014;79(163):49853–50536.

98. Purvis S, Gion T, Kennedy G, et al. Catheter-associated urinary tract infection: a successful prevention effort employing a multipronged initiative at an academic medical center. J Nurs Care Qual. 2014;29(2):141–8.

99. Lo E, Nicolle LE, Coffin SE, et al. Strategies to prevent catheter-associated urinary tract infections in acute care hospitals: 2014 update. Infect Control Hosp Epidemiol. 2014;35(5): 464–79.

100. Nicolle LE, Bradley S, Colgan R, Rice JC, Schaeffer A, Hooton TM. Infectious Diseases Society of America guidelines for the diagnosis and treatment of asymptomatic bacteriuria in adults. Clin Infect Dis. 2005;40(5):643–54.

101. Tambyah PA, Maki DG. Catheter-associated urinary tract infection is rarely symptomatic: a prospective study of 1,497 catheterized patients. Arch Intern Med. 2000;160(5):678–82.

102. Kwaan MR, Lee JT, Rothenberger DA, Melton GB, Madoff RD. Early removal of urinary catheters after rectal surgery is associated with increased urinary retention. Dis Colon Rectum. 2015;58(4):401–5.

103. Wu AK, Auerbach AD, Aaronson DS. National incidence and outcomes of postoperative urinary retention in the Surgical Care Improvement Project. Am J Surg. 2012;204(2):167–71.

104. Coyle D, Joyce KM, Garvin JT, et al. Early post-operative removal of urethral catheter in patients undergoing colorectal surgery with epidural analgesia—a prospective pilot clinical study. Int J Surg. 2015;16(Pt A):94–8.

105. Kennedy GD, Tevis SE, Kent KC. Is there a relationship between patient satisfaction and favorable outcomes? Ann Surg. 2014;260(4):592–8. discussion 598–600.

106. Katz J, Jackson M, Kavanagh BP, Sandler AN. Acute pain after thoracic surgery predicts long-term post-thoracotomy pain. Clin J Pain. 1996;12(1):50–5.

107. Lynch EP, Lazor MA, Gellis JE, Orav J, Goldman L, Marcantonio ER. The impact of postoperative pain on the development of postoperative delirium. Anesth Analg. 1998;86(4):781–5.

108. Benyamin R, Trescot AM, Datta S, et al. Opioid complications and side effects. Pain Physician. 2008;11(2 Suppl):S105–20.

109. Werawatganon T, Charuluxanun S. Patient controlled intravenous opioid analgesia versus continuous epidural analgesia for pain after intra-abdominal surgery. Cochrane Database Syst Rev. 2005;1, CD004088.

110. Rudin A, Flisberg P, Johansson J, Walther B, Lundberg CJ. Thoracic epidural analgesia or intravenous morphine analgesia after thoracoabdominal esophagectomy: a prospective follow-up of 201 patients. J Cardiothorac Vasc Anesth. 2005; 19(3):350–7.

111. Senagore AJ, Delaney CP, Mekhail N, Dugan A, Fazio VW. Randomized clinical trial comparing epidural anaesthesia and patient-controlled analgesia after laparoscopic segmental colectomy. Br J Surg. 2003;90(10):1195–9.

112. Morimoto H, Cullen JJ, Messick Jr JM, Kelly KA. Epidural analgesia shortens postoperative ileus after ileal pouch-anal canal anastomosis. Am J Surg. 1995;169(1):79–82. discussion 82–3.

113. Scott AM, Starling JR, Ruscher AE, DeLessio ST, Harms BA. Thoracic versus lumbar epidural anesthesia's effect on pain control and ileus resolution after restorative proctocolectomy. Surgery. 1996;120(4):688–95. discussion 695–7.

114. Weeks JC, Nelson H, Gelber S, Sargent D, Schroeder G. Short-term quality-of-life outcomes following laparoscopic-assisted colectomy vs open colectomy for colon cancer: a randomized trial. JAMA. 2002;287(3):321–8.

115. Liu H, Hu X, Duan X, Wu J. Thoracic epidural analgesia (TEA) vs. patient controlled analgesia (PCA) in laparoscopic colectomy: a meta-analysis. Hepatogastroenterology. 2014;61(133):1213–9.

116. Levy BF, Tilney HS, Dowson HM, Rockall TA. A systematic review of postoperative analgesia following laparoscopic colorectal surgery. Colorectal Dis. 2010;12(1):5–15.

117. Kuruba R, Fayard N, Snyder D. Epidural analgesia and laparoscopic technique do not reduce incidence of prolonged ileus in elective colon resections. Am J Surg. 2012;204(5):613–8.

118. Day A, Smith R, Jourdan I, Fawcett W, Scott M, Rockall T. Retrospective analysis of the effect of postoperative analgesia on survival in patients after laparoscopic resection of colorectal cancer. Br J Anaesth. 2012;109(2):185–90.

119. Keller DS, Stulberg JJ, Lawrence JK, Delaney CP. Process control to measure process improvement in colorectal surgery: modifications to an established enhanced recovery pathway. Dis Colon Rectum. 2014;57(2):194–200.

120. Favuzza J, Brady K, Delaney CP. Transversus abdominis plane blocks and enhanced recovery pathways: making the 23-h hospital stay a realistic goal after laparoscopic colorectal surgery. Surg Endosc. 2013;27(7):2481–6.

121. Kiran RP, Ahmed Ali U, Coffey JC, Vogel JD, Pokala N, Fazio VW. Impact of resident participation in surgical operations on postoperative outcomes: National Surgical Quality Improvement Program. Ann Surg. 2012;256(3):469–75.

122. Castleberry AW, Clary BM, Migaly J, et al. Resident education in the era of patient safety: a nationwide analysis of outcomes and complications in resident-assisted oncologic surgery. Ann Surg Oncol. 2013;20(12):3715–24.

123. Davis Jr SS, Husain FA, Lin E, Nandipati KC, Perez S, Sweeney JF. Resident participation in index laparoscopic general surgical cases: impact of the learning environment on surgical outcomes. J Am Coll Surg. 2013;216(1):96–104.

124. Gorgun E, Benlice C, Corrao E, et al. Outcomes associated with resident involvement in laparoscopic colorectal surgery suggest a need for earlier and more intensive resident training. Surgery. 2014;156(4):825–32.

125. Englesbe MJ, Pelletier SJ, Magee JC, et al. Seasonal variation in surgical outcomes as measured by the American College of Surgeons-National Surgical Quality Improvement Program (ACS-NSQIP). Ann Surg. 2007;246(3):456–62. discussion 463–5.

126. Gopaldas RR, Overbey DM, Dao TK, Markley JG. The impact of academic calendar cycle on coronary artery bypass outcomes: a comparison of teaching and non-teaching hospitals. J Cardiothorac Surg. 2013;8:191.

127. Birkmeyer JD, Stukel TA, Siewers AE, Goodney PP, Wennberg DE, Lucas FL. Surgeon volume and operative mortality in the United States. N Engl J Med. 2003;349(22):2117–27.

128. Birkmeyer JD, Siewers AE, Finlayson EV, et al. Hospital volume and surgical mortality in the United States. N Engl J Med. 2002;346(15):1128–37.

129. Sutton JM, Wima K, Wilson GC, et al. Factors associated with 30-day readmission after restorative proctocolectomy with IPAA: a national study. Dis Colon Rectum. 2014;57(12):1371–8.

130. Leonard D, Penninckx F, Kartheuser A, Laenen A, Van Eycken E. Effect of hospital volume on quality of care and outcome after rectal cancer surgery. Br J Surg. 2014;101(11):1475–82.

131. Osler M, Iversen LH, Borglykke A, et al. Hospital variation in 30-day mortality after colorectal cancer surgery in Denmark: the contribution of hospital volume and patient characteristics. Ann Surg. 2011;253(4):733–8.

132. Finks JF, Osborne NH, Birkmeyer JD. Trends in hospital volume and operative mortality for high-risk surgery. N Engl J Med. 2011;364(22):2128–37.

133. Drolet S, MacLean AR, Myers RP, Shaheen AA, Dixon E, Buie WD. Elective resection of colon cancer by high-volume surgeons is associated with decreased morbidity and mortality. J Gastrointest Surg. 2011;15(4):541–50.

134. Kirchhoff P, Clavien PA, Hahnloser D. Complications in colorectal surgery: risk factors and preventive strategies. Patient Saf Surg. 2010;4(1):5.

135. Kuwabara K, Matsuda S, Fushimi K, Ishikawa KB, Horiguchi H, Fujimori K. Impact of hospital case volume on the quality of laparoscopic colectomy in Japan. J Gastrointest Surg. 2009;13(9):1619–26.

136. Reames BN, Ghaferi AA, Birkmeyer JD, Dimick JB. Hospital volume and operative mortality in the modern era. Ann Surg. 2014;260(2):244–51.

137. Zhan C, Miller MR. Excess length of stay, charges, and mortality attributable to medical injuries during hospitalization. JAMA. 2003;290(14):1868–74.

138. Dimick JB, Chen SL, Taheri PA, Henderson WG, Khuri SF, Campbell DA. Hospital costs associated with surgical complications: a report from the private-sector National Surgical Quality Improvement Program. J Am Coll Surg. 2004;199(4):531–7.

139. Tang R, Chen HH, Wang YL, et al. Risk factors for surgical site infection after elective resection of the colon and rectum: a single-center prospective study of 2,809 consecutive patients. Ann Surg. 2001;234(2):181–9.

140. Anderson DJ, Kirkland KB, Kaye KS, et al. Underresourced hospital infection control and prevention programs: penny wise, pound foolish? Infect Control Hosp Epidemiol. 2007;28(7):767–73.

141. Gibson A, Tevis S, Kennedy G. Readmission after delayed diagnosis of surgical site infection: a focus on prevention using the American College of Surgeons National Surgical Quality Improvement Program. Am J Surg. 2014;207(6):832–9.

142. Flegal KM, Kit BK, Orpana H, Graubard BI. Association of all-cause mortality with overweight and obesity using standard body mass index categories: a systematic review and meta-analysis. JAMA. 2013;309(1):71–82.

143. Amri R, Bordeianou LG, Sylla P, Berger DL. Obesity, outcomes and quality of care: body mass index increases the risk of wound-related complications in colon cancer surgery. Am J Surg. 2014;207(1):17–23.

144. Dindo D, Muller MK, Weber M, Clavien PA. Obesity in general elective surgery. Lancet. 2003;361(9374):2032–5.

145. Makino T, Shukla PJ, Rubino F, Milsom JW. The impact of obesity on perioperative outcomes after laparoscopic colorectal resection. Ann Surg. 2012;255(2):228–36.

146. Hourigan JS. Impact of obesity on surgical site infection in colon and rectal surgery. Clin Colon Rectal Surg. 2011; 24(4):283–90.

147. Gervaz P, Bandiera-Clerc C, Buchs NC, et al. Scoring system to predict the risk of surgical-site infection after colorectal resection. Br J Surg. 2012;99(4):589–95.

148. Merkow RP, Bilimoria KY, McCarter MD, Bentrem DJ. Effect of body mass index on short-term outcomes after colectomy for cancer. J Am Coll Surg. 2009;208(1):53–61.

149. Kartheuser AH, Leonard DF, Penninckx F, et al. Waist circumference and waist/hip ratio are better predictive risk factors for mortality and morbidity after colorectal surgery than body mass index and body surface area. Ann Surg. 2013;258(5): 722–30.

150. Dionigi G, Rovera F, Boni L, et al. The impact of perioperative blood transfusion on clinical outcomes in colorectal surgery. Surg Oncol. 2007;16 Suppl 1:S177–82.

151. Benoist S. [Perioperative transfusion in colorectal surgery]. Ann Chir. 2005;130(6–7):365–73.

152. Tartter PI. The association of perioperative blood transfusion with colorectal cancer recurrence. Ann Surg. 1992;216(6): 633–8.

153. Guenaga KF, Matos D, Castro AA, Atallah AN, Wille-Jørgensen P. Mechanical bowel preparation for elective colorectal surgery. Cochrane Database Syst Rev. 2005;1, CD001544.

154. Guenaga KK, Matos D, Wille-Jørgensen P. Mechanical bowel preparation for elective colorectal surgery. Cochrane Database Syst Rev. 2009;1, CD001544.

155. Slim K, Vicaut E, Launay-Savary MV, Contant C, Chipponi J. Updated systematic review and meta-analysis of randomized clinical trials on the role of mechanical bowel preparation before colorectal surgery. Ann Surg. 2009;249(2):203–9.

156. Cannon JA, Altom LK, Deierhoi RJ, et al. Preoperative oral antibiotics reduce surgical site infection following elective colorectal resections. Dis Colon Rectum. 2012;55(11):1160–6.

157. Darouiche RO, Wall MJ, Itani KM, et al. Chlorhexidine-alcohol versus povidone-iodine for surgical-site antisepsis. N Engl J Med. 2010;362(1):18–26.

158. Swenson BR, Hedrick TL, Metzger R, Bonatti H, Pruett TL, Sawyer RG. Effects of preoperative skin preparation on postoperative wound infection rates: a prospective study of 3 skin preparation protocols. Infect Control Hosp Epidemiol. 2009;30(10):964–71.

159. Redick EL. Applying FOCUS-PDCA to solve clinical problems. Dimens Crit Care Nurs. 1999;18(6):30–4.

160. Gerard JC, Arnold FL. Performance improvement with a hybrid FOCUS-PDCA methodology. Jt Comm J Qual Improv. 1996;22(10):660–72.

161. Plsek PE. Tutorial: quality improvement project models. Qual Manag Health Care. 1993;1(2):69–81.

162. Reid K, Pockney P, Draganic B, Smith SR. Barrier wound protection decreases surgical site infection in open elective colorectal surgery: a randomized clinical trial. Dis Colon Rectum. 2010;53(10):1374–80.

163. Edwards JP, Ho AL, Tee MC, Dixon E, Ball CG. Wound protectors reduce surgical site infection: a meta-analysis of randomized controlled trials. Ann Surg. 2012;256(1):53–9.

164. Murray BW, Huerta S, Dineen S, Anthony T. Surgical site infection in colorectal surgery: a review of the nonpharmacologic tools of prevention. J Am Coll Surg. 2010;211(6): 812–22.

165. Belda FJ, Aguilera L, García de la Asunción J, et al. Supplemental perioperative oxygen and the risk of surgical wound infection: a randomized controlled trial. JAMA. 2005;294(16):2035–42.

166. Greif R, Akça O, Horn EP, Kurz A, Sessler DI, Group OR. Supplemental perioperative oxygen to reduce the incidence of surgical-wound infection. N Engl J Med. 2000;342(3): 161–7.

167. Pryor KO, Fahey TJ, Lien CA, Goldstein PA. Surgical site infection and the routine use of perioperative hyperoxia in a general surgical population: a randomized controlled trial. JAMA. 2004;291(1):79–87.

168. Meyhoff CS, Wetterslev J, Jorgensen LN, et al. Effect of high perioperative oxygen fraction on surgical site infection and pulmonary complications after abdominal surgery: the PROXI randomized clinical trial. JAMA. 2009;302(14):1543–50.

169. Kurz A, Sessler DI, Lenhardt R. Perioperative normothermia to reduce the incidence of surgical-wound infection and shorten hospitalization. Study of Wound Infection and Temperature Group. N Engl J Med. 1996;334(19):1209–15.

170. Melling AC, Ali B, Scott EM, Leaper DJ. Effects of preoperative warming on the incidence of wound infection after clean surgery: a randomised controlled trial. Lancet. 2001;358(9285): 876–80.

171. Israelsson LA, Jonsson T, Knutsson A. Suture technique and wound healing in midline laparotomy incisions. Eur J Surg. 1996;162(8):605–9.

172. Millbourn D, Cengiz Y, Israelsson LA. Effect of stitch length on wound complications after closure of midline incisions: a randomized controlled trial. Arch Surg. 2009;144(11): 1056–9.

173. Reid K, Pockney P, Pollitt T, Draganic B, Smith SR. Randomized clinical trial of short-term outcomes following purse-string versus conventional closure of ileostomy wounds. Br J Surg. 2010;97(10):1511–7.

174. Sajid MS, Bhatti MI, Miles WF. Systematic review and meta-analysis of published randomized controlled trials comparing purse-string vs conventional linear closure of the wound following ileostomy (stoma) closure. Gastroenterol Rep (Oxf). 2014;3(2):156–61.

175. Waits SA, Fritze D, Banerjee M, et al. Developing an argument for bundled interventions to reduce surgical site infection in colorectal surgery. Surgery. 2014;155(4):602–6.

176. Stevens DL, Bisno AL, Chambers HF, et al. Practice guidelines for the diagnosis and management of skin and soft tissue infections: 2014 update by the Infectious Diseases Society of America. Clin Infect Dis. 2014;59(2):e10–52.

177. Stevens DL, Bisno AL, Chambers HF, et al. Practice guidelines for the diagnosis and management of skin and soft tissue

infections: 2014 update by the infectious diseases society of America. Clin Infect Dis. 2014;59(2):147–59.

178. Nichols RL, Florman S. Clinical presentations of soft-tissue infections and surgical site infections. Clin Infect Dis. 2001;33 Suppl 2:S84–93.

179. Russ AJ, Obma KL, Rajamanickam V, et al. Laparoscopy improves short-term outcomes after surgery for diverticular disease. Gastroenterology. 2010;138(7):2267–274, 2274.e2261.

180. Buchberg B, Masoomi H, Lusby K, et al. Incidence and risk factors of venous thromboembolism in colorectal surgery: does laparoscopy impart an advantage? Arch Surg. 2011; 146(6):739–43.

181. Anderson Jr FA, Wheeler HB, Goldberg RJ, et al. A population-based perspective of the hospital incidence and case-fatality rates of deep vein thrombosis and pulmonary embolism. The Worcester DVT Study. Arch Intern Med. 1991;151(5):933–8.

182. Shapiro R, Vogel JD, Kiran RP. Risk of postoperative venous thromboembolism after laparoscopic and open colorectal surgery: an additional benefit of the minimally invasive approach? Dis Colon Rectum. 2011;54(12):1496–502.

183. Moghadamyeghaneh Z, Hanna MH, Carmichael JC, Nguyen NT, Stamos MJ. A nationwide analysis of postoperative deep vein thrombosis and pulmonary embolism in colon and rectal surgery. J Gastrointest Surg. 2014;18(12):2169–77.

184. Vedovati MC, Becattini C, Rondelli F, et al. A randomized study on 1-week versus 4-week prophylaxis for venous thromboembolism after laparoscopic surgery for colorectal cancer. Ann Surg. 2014;259(4):665–9.

185. Kennedy GD, Rajamanickam V, O'Connor ES, et al. Optimizing surgical care of colon cancer in the older adult population. Ann Surg. 2011;253(3):508–14.

186. McDonald KM, Romano PS, University of California San Francisco-Stanford Evidence-Based Practice Center, United States. Agency for Healthcare Research and Quality. Measures of patient safety based on hospital administrative data—the patient safety indicators. Rockville, MD: U.S. Dept. of Health and Human Services, Public Health Service, Agency for Healthcare Research and Quality; 2002.

187. Sheetz KH, Waits SA, Krell RW, Campbell Jr DA, Englesbe MJ, Ghaferi AA. Improving mortality following emergent surgery in older patients requires focus on complication rescue. Ann Surg. 2013;258(4):614–7. discussion 617–8.

188. Chaudhri S, Maruthachalam K, Kaiser A, Robson W, Pickard RS, Horgan AF. Successful voiding after trial without catheter is not synonymous with recovery of bladder function after colorectal surgery. Dis Colon Rectum. 2006;49(7):1066–70.

189. Delacroix SE, Winters JC. Voiding dysfunction after pelvic colorectal surgery. Clin Colon Rectal Surg. 2010;23(2): 119–27.

190. Waljee A, Waljee J, Morris AM, Higgins PD. Threefold increased risk of infertility: a meta-analysis of infertility after

191. Cornish JA, Tan E, Teare J, et al. The effect of restorative proctocolectomy on sexual function, urinary function, fertility, pregnancy and delivery: a systematic review. Dis Colon Rectum. 2007;50(8):1128–38.

192. Nieuwenhuis MH, Douma KF, Bleiker EM, Bemelman WA, Aaronson NK, Vasen HF. Female fertility after colorectal surgery for familial adenomatous polyposis: a nationwide cross-sectional study. Ann Surg. 2010;252(2):341–4.

193. Juul T, Ahlberg M, Biondo S, et al. Low anterior resection syndrome and quality of life: an international multicenter study. Dis Colon Rectum. 2014;57(5):585–91.

194. How P, Stelzner S, Branagan G, et al. Comparative quality of life in patients following abdominoperineal excision and low anterior resection for low rectal cancer. Dis Colon Rectum. 2012;55(4):400–6.

195. Pachler J, Wille-Jørgensen P. Quality of life after rectal resection for cancer, with or without permanent colostomy. Cochrane Database Syst Rev. 2012;12, CD004323.

196. Bryant CL, Lunniss PJ, Knowles CH, Thaha MA, Chan CL. Anterior resection syndrome. Lancet Oncol. 2012;13(9): e403–8.

197. Emmertsen KJ, Laurberg S. Bowel dysfunction after treatment for rectal cancer. Acta Oncol. 2008;47(6):994–1003.

198. Juul T, Ahlberg M, Biondo S, et al. International validation of the low anterior resection syndrome score. Ann Surg. 2014; 259(4):728–34.

199. Emmertsen KJ, Laurberg S. Low anterior resection syndrome score: development and validation of a symptom-based scoring system for bowel dysfunction after low anterior resection for rectal cancer. Ann Surg. 2012;255(5):922–8.

200. Marijnen CA, van de Velde CJ, Putter H, et al. Impact of short-term preoperative radiotherapy on health-related quality of life and sexual functioning in primary rectal cancer: report of a multicenter randomized trial. J Clin Oncol. 2005;23(9): 1847–58.

201. Stephens RJ, Thompson LC, Quirke P, et al. Impact of short-course preoperative radiotherapy for rectal cancer on patients' quality of life: data from the Medical Research Council CR07/ National Cancer Institute of Canada Clinical Trials Group C016 randomized clinical trial. J Clin Oncol. 2010;28(27): 4233–9.

202. Tevis SE, Kohlnhofer BM, Stringfield S, et al. Postoperative complications in patients with rectal cancer are associated with delays in chemotherapy that lead to worse disease-free and overall survival. Dis Colon Rectum. 2013;56(12):1339–48.

203. Hendren S, Birkmeyer JD, Yin H, Banerjee M, Sonnenday C, Morris AM. Surgical complications are associated with omission of chemotherapy for stage III colorectal cancer. Dis Colon Rectum. 2010;53(12):1587–93.

9

Anastomotic Construction

Steven R. Hunt and Matthew L. Silviera

Key Concepts

- Benign effluent from a peri-anastomotic drain does not rule out anastomotic leak or abscess.
- It is safe practice to leave the mesenteric defect open after constructing an ileocolic anastomosis.
- Fecal diversion reduces septic complications in patients with coloanal anastomoses.
- Diverting loop ileostomy and loop colostomy have similar complication rates.
- Leak testing should be performed on anastomoses to the rectum.

Introduction

The purpose of this chapter is to review the various anastomotic techniques for abdominal and pelvic anastomoses. There are many unique and innovative ways to create anastomoses; however, this chapter will focus on the most common techniques and the problems associated with their construction. It is difficult to overemphasize the importance of judgment and technique in preventing anastomotic complications while still preserving function. Various clinical situations and differing anatomy make it important to be familiar with multiple approaches to the same type of anastomosis. Knowledge of these various techniques is of paramount importance in achieving good outcomes. No matter how well planned the creation of an anastomosis is, problems will arise during execution, and the ability to salvage an anastomosis is a skill every colorectal surgeon must master.

General Principles of Anastomoses

Surgical Staplers

Rudimentary surgical staplers first appeared in the early 1900s, but stapling devices improved dramatically in the 1970s with preloaded disposable cartridges of multiple staggered staple lines. Titanium staples have replaced stainless steel and are found in a variety of staple heights that are bent into a "B" configuration in order to match tissue thickness. Surgical staplers can be divided into two major groups: linear and circular. The simplest linear stapler (TA or thoracoabdominal) applies two rows of staples in a staggered configuration but requires manual transection of the bowel. The linear cutting stapler (GIA or gastrointestinal anastomosis) applies four rows of staggered staples and cuts between the middle two rows of staples, allowing for the division of bowel and the creation of anastomoses. Circular staplers (e.g., EEA or end-to-end anastomosis) have a detachable anvil. Once the anvil and head are coupled together, two circular rows of staggered staples are applied as a circular blade cuts out the interior tissue, allowing communication of the two lumens. EEA staplers come in a variety of diameters, with 25–31 mm staplers being the most common in colorectal surgery [1].

Hand-Sewn Anastomoses

Gastrointestinal anastomoses have been performed by various hand-sewn techniques for many years. Single-layer and double-layer anastomoses have been studied extensively, and a lone randomized controlled trial and three comparative studies have shown no difference in anastomotic leak rates between the two techniques [2–6]. Interrupted and continuous suture techniques have similarly been studied; however, there is not a high level of evidence to support one over the other [6]. With regard to suture material, clinical studies have failed to show benefit of one material over another.

Electronic supplementary material: The online version of this chapter (doi:10.1007/978-3-319-25970-3_9) contains supplementary material, which is available to authorized users.

Anastomoses are frequently constructed with absorbable monofilament suture and absorbable braided suture. Two experimental studies comparing both suture materials showed similar anastomotic burst pressure and histologic characteristics [7, 8]. Given the lack of clear support in the literature for one hand-sewn anastomotic technique, it is the authors' preference to construct hand-sewn anastomoses with a single continuous layer of 3-0 PDS, as the monofilament slides easily through the bowel wall and the anastomosis is quick and easy to construct.

Compression Anastomoses

A compression anastomosis is created when two ends of bowel are held together for a period of time by physical forces during which anastomotic healing takes place. Several days later, the compressed tissue necroses and the device separates and is passed from the body. The anastomosis is held together by the adhesions that form between the tissues adjacent to the area of necrosis. This obviates the need for foreign material (suture/staples) in the anastomosis, which can lead to inflammation, foreign body reaction, and stricture. The idea of compression anastomoses was first reported back in the 1800s but then reemerged in the 1980s with the development of two commercially available products. In the United States, the biofragmentable anastomotic ring (BAR) was developed and studied extensively. Numerous publications, including randomized controlled trials, reported that the BAR was safe and effective [9–14]. Despite the encouraging clinical data that was accumulating, several reports of intraoperative problems with the BAR emerged, and the device never gained widespread acceptance.

A recent advance on this approach utilizes a smart metal (nitinol) that is a temperature-dependent, shape-memory alloy. Two compression rings are mounted on an instrument that is very similar to a conventional EEA stapler (ColonRing). When engaged, the rings are compressed together by nitinol springs, and with the aid of a circular blade, a compression anastomosis is created. Over time, simultaneous healing and necrosis take place, and ultimately the rings detach and pass transanally [15].

Recently a prospective multicenter study of 266 patients who had colorectal compression anastomoses with the nitinol ColonRing was published. The overall anastomotic leak rate was 5.3 % after low anterior resection, with septic complications occurring in 8.3 % [16]. Additionally, a multicenter data registry of 1180 patients was published with an overall leak rate of 3.2 % in all left-sided anastomoses [17]. This data is encouraging, but we are still awaiting a prospective randomized trial comparing the ColonRing to conventional stapled or hand-sewn colorectal anastomoses. At present, it has once again been taken off the market and is not available in the United States.

Tension

One of the tenants of anastomotic creation is that it must be tension-free. With small bowel and ileocolic anastomoses, tension is usually not a problem owing to the mobility of the small bowel. On the other hand, tension can be a significant problem with the pelvic colorectal anastomosis. In order to gain adequate length of the descending colon so that it may reach down into the pelvis, three maneuvers may be employed: (1) high ligation of the IMA, (2) ligation of the IMV at the inferior border of the pancreas, and (3) complete mobilization of the splenic flexure with division of the distal transverse colon mesentery back to the middle colic vessels. Complete mobilization of the splenic flexure is much more than simply dividing the peritoneal attachments at the flexure, and the technical considerations will be discussed in greater detail later in this chapter. It may be tempting to omit complete mobilization of the splenic flexure for an upper colorectal anastomosis, but it is the authors' recommendation to routinely mobilize the splenic flexure after high ligation of both the IMA and IMV in order to consistently create a tension-free colorectal anastomosis.

Blood Supply

Ensuring adequate blood supply to the proximal and distal ends of the bowel that will be anastomosed is of paramount importance. The first step is to confirm that the bowel looks viable and healthy, but this is not entirely sufficient. Sharply cutting an epiploicae at the level of the planned anastomosis and confirming bright red bleeding is reassuring. Additionally, the bowel can be opened sharply (rather than with cautery) to confirm bleeding from the bowel wall. The marginal artery is responsible for proximal colon perfusion for a left-sided anastomosis. We routinely isolate the marginal artery between clamps and "flash" the artery to confirm pulsatile bleeding. Brisk, bright red, pulsatile bleeding nearly guarantees excellent perfusion to the examined colon. Very dark or even black blood from the marginal artery often indicates a problem with the venous outflow and requires a change in the level of the planned anastomosis. Likewise, complete lack of bleeding shows that there is clearly inadequate perfusion to the colon. Both ends of the spectrum are fairly easy to interpret, but it is the gray zone of sluggish bleeding from the marginal artery that is troublesome and should prompt further scrutiny of the blood supply.

A new method of intraoperative perfusion assessment has been developed that uses near-infrared indocyanine green (ICG)-induced fluorescence angiography. The mesentery of the bowel, including the marginal artery, is divided, and the patient is given an intravenous push of ICG. The appropriate platform is used to excite the ICG with near-infrared light to visualize bowel perfusion (Video 9.1). The laparoscopic platform can also be advanced transanally with the aid of a special proctoscope to endoscopically assess mucosal tissue perfusion of the colorectal anastomosis (Video 9.2). Currently, all perfusion assessments performed with this technology are subjective, and no purely objective measure of bowel perfusion exists.

Jafari et al. have published the results of the PILLAR II trial that was a prospective, multicenter, clinical trial that studied the utility of fluorescence angiography on colorectal anastomoses [18]. Nearly 140 patients were analyzed, with the mean level of anastomosis 10 cm from the anal verge. The overall anastomotic leak rate was 1.4 %. Additionally, 8 % of patients had a change in their anastomotic plan due to findings from the perfusion assessment, and none of those patients had an anastomotic leak. The encouraging low leak rate in the PILLAR II trial has paved the way for the current PILLAR III trial, which is a prospective RCT comparing fluorescence angiography to standard of care. This trial will attempt to determine if perfusion assessment with ICG reduces the rate of anastomotic leak.

Prophylactic Drainage

The prophylactic use of drains to avoid anastomotic complications is quite controversial. Drain usage among surgeons is variable. Some surgeons routinely drain anastomoses, others use drains only as dictated by circumstances, and there are others that eschew the practice of drainage. Multiple studies have been conducted with varying results. In general, two types of drains are used to drain anastomoses. The first is an open, or passive, drain. These drains are made of synthetic material and act to provide a route of egress for fluids. The second type is a closed suction drain, consisting of a soft, hollow tube that is placed under negative pressure to actively evacuate fluids. Advocates of drainage maintain that drains will prevent the accumulation of fluid or blood around the anastomosis, permit early detection of a leak, mitigate the consequences of a leak, and provide a "window into the abdomen."

Critics assert that drains provide the surgeon with a false sense of security, that they may cause a leak secondary to negative pressure, or that they may provide an avenue for the introduction of infection. Some detractors feel that drains may cause pain that leads to decreased ambulation, poor inspiratory effort, and associated complications.

The largest meta-analysis of prophylactic drainage includes a heterogenous group of studies with regard to the type of drain used and the location of the anastomoses [19]. In this evaluation of more than 1000 patients in six randomized controlled trials, no difference was seen between the routine drainage group and the group that did not have prophylactic drains. This analysis evaluated clinical anastomotic leak, radiographic anastomotic leak, wound infection, reoperation, and mortality—revealing no difference between the two groups. Many patients included in these studies had open/passive drainage. These studies also included both intraperitoneal and extraperitoneal anastomoses.

A smaller meta-analysis showed no difference in drain-related complications between routine drainage and non-drainage regimens [20]. Interestingly, of the 20 patients with drains that developed anastomotic leaks, only 1 patient (5 %) had any evidence of enteric contents in the drain effluent. This finding certainly disputes the "window into the abdomen" theory and lends credence to the argument that drains may provide surgeons with a false sense of security.

The largest randomized controlled trial of closed suction drainage involved 494 patients that had both intraperitoneal and extraperitoneal colonic anastomoses [21]. There was no difference between the drainage and non-drainage group in anastomotic leak rate, reoperation, mortality, or other abdominal complications.

A more recent systematic review of observational studies looking strictly at extraperitoneal colorectal anastomoses showed that there was a difference in the rate of anastomotic leakage favoring the drained group [22].

While there is scant data to support routine prophylactic drainage, there is no evidence that drains cause adverse events. The decision to drain anastomoses should be left to the discretion of the surgeon. Importantly, if drains are used, benign-appearing effluent in the drain does not rule out an anastomotic leak or abscess. Sound clinical judgment should still prevail when a leak is suspected.

Treatment of Mesenteric Defects

Prior to the popularization of laparoscopic colon resections, routine closure of the mesenteric defect was considered essential to avoid internal herniation leading to obstruction or strangulation. As laparoscopic colectomy propagated, the necessity of closing these defects was questioned. It proved difficult to perform the closure through the small extraction excision, and laparoscopic closure of the defect was cumbersome.

Proponents of leaving the defect open contend that closure of the mesentery creates a risk for bleeding, mesenteric hematoma, and compromise of the anastomosis. While the catastrophic consequences of an open mesenteric defect have been discussed in case reports, studies that have looked at this question specifically have shown that it is safe, and perhaps even prudent, to leave the defect open after creating an ileocolic anastomosis [23, 24].

With ileorectal and ileal pouch anal anastomoses, there is the risk of axial torsion of the small bowel around the free edge of the mesentery. Because this can have devastating consequences if a significant amount of small bowel herniates under this mesenteric edge, some surgeons choose to close this defect by securing the free edge of the small bowel mesentery to the preaortic retroperitoneal fascia. There is no evidence to support this practice.

Diversion

For an in-depth discussion on diversion, see Chap. 55. Briefly, fecal diversion has a role in protecting distal anastomoses that are at high risk for leakage. Commonly, diverting stomas are used to protect low pelvic anastomoses. Any anastomosis within 5 cm of anal verge should be considered for diversion as these anastomoses have a five- to sixfold increase in the rate of clinical anastomotic leakage compared to more proximal anastomoses [25, 26].

Defunctioning stomas can also be used to divert more proximal anastomoses at risk for leakage. These include selected anastomoses in the setting of malnutrition, immunocompromised patients, irradiated tissue, soilage, inflamed tissue, and to protect anastomoses that have been technically difficult to perform. Diversion in these settings should be used judiciously, as proximal diversion itself is not a license to create an anastomosis regardless of the clinical situation. An end ostomy and an interval return to the operating room is the safe option when the integrity of an anastomosis is jeopardized.

While the true value of a diverting stoma is difficult to quantify, it is clear that diversion mitigates the consequences of anastomotic leaks. Given the relatively low rate of anastomotic leaks, the majority of diverting stomas are created unnecessarily. The difficulty lies in predicting which patients are most likely to leak. Diverting stomas and the procedure to reverse them have their own attendant morbidity [27, 28]. In many patients, the diverting stoma is never able to be reversed [29, 30].

A recent analysis of patients included in the National Surgical Quality Improvement Project (NSQIP) examined the use of diverting stomas in patients having a low anterior resection with either a colorectal anastomosis or a coloanal anastomosis [31]. Comparing patients who had a defunctioning stoma to those that did not, they found no difference in sepsis, septic shock, or wound complications after creation of a colorectal anastomosis. In patients with coloanal anastomoses, there was a significant difference favoring diversion for septic complications, reoperation, and length of stay. They also found a significant increase in the incidence of acute renal failure in patients who were diverted.

In theory, proximal diversion decreases the load of contamination in an anastomotic leak and may allow the body to seal off a leak—diminishing clinical consequences. Multiple studies demonstrate that diverted anastomoses have a decreased rate of fecal peritonitis, sepsis, and reoperation [32–36].

The method of diversion is often dependent on the clinical situation. Both loop colostomies (Figure 9-1) and loop ileostomies have advantages and disadvantages. Ileostomies are associated with peristomal dermatitis, pouching difficulties, dehydration, and acute renal failure. Diverting colostomies are more prone to prolapse. Additionally, loop colostomies can be difficult to close through a peristomal incision, and the blood flow through the pre-anastomotic marginal blood vessels can be compromised at the time of loop colostomy closure.

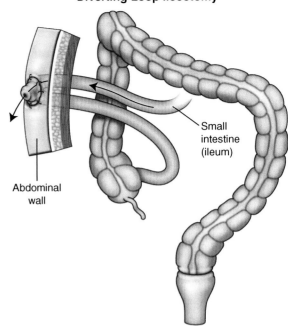

Diverting Loop Ileostomy

Small intestine (ileum)

Abdominal wall

Figure 9-1. Diverting loop ileostomy.

A meta-analysis of randomized controlled trials comparing diverting loop colostomies to loop ileostomies shows no difference between the two groups in complications related to the stoma or in time to ostomy closure [37].

High-Risk Anastomoses

There are certain clinical situations in which clinical judgment precludes the creation of an anastomosis, even with proximal diversion. Such situations include severe malnutrition, significant immunosuppression, gross or long-standing fecal contamination, massively dilated bowel, and the risk of developing hemodynamic instability in the postoperative period. In these situations, even the best technical anastomoses may fail due to factors beyond the surgeon's control. Rather than risk anastomotic failure in these cases, an end ostomy that will allow for future restoration of continuity should be performed.

Abdominal Anastomoses

Small Bowel Anastomoses

Small bowel anastomoses are frequently performed during ileostomy closures, as part of complex adhesiolysis, or during resections for Crohn's disease or small bowel neoplasms. Both stapled and hand-sewn techniques can be used to complete the anastomosis. In creating a stapled side-to-side (functional end-to-end) anastomosis, the bowel should be divided proximally and distally with a linear stapler, taking care to make sure that the staple line is oriented along the axis from the mesentery to the antimesenteric border of the bowel. Additionally, the staple line should be beveled from the mesenteric side away from the specimen. These subtle but simple steps ensure that the mural blood flow to the anastomosis will not be compromised. After the bowel has been divided, the antimesenteric corners of the transverse staple line are removed, and the limbs of the GIA stapler are introduced. As the stapler is closed, the mesentery of each limb of bowel should be pulled laterally to ensure that the stapler is fired on the antimesenteric border of the bowel. The anastomosis is completed by closing the common enterotomy either with a stapler (GIA or TA) or a hand-sewn technique.

Cost can be contained by eliminating two loads of the GIA stapler by creating the anastomosis without dividing the bowel proximal and distal to the resection. Instead, the mesentery to the intended points of transection is divided, and enterotomies are created on the antimesenteric bowel wall proximal and distal to the specimen. The GIA stapler is introduced through these openings and fired along the antimesenteric border. The common enterotomy is closed, and the specimen resected with a single firing of a linear stapler. Alternatively, the bowel can be divided proximal and distal to the specimen with electrocautery, and the GIA stapler can be used to create the anastomosis along the antimesenteric border. The common enterotomy can then be closed with another linear stapler or hand sewn.

During loop ileostomy closure, it can be difficult to adequately mobilize both the proximal and distal limbs of the ileum through the peristomal incision in order to allow for a stapled side-to-side anastomosis. Rather than blindly sweeping down adhesions with your finger and potentially deserosalizing bowel, a hand-sewn anastomosis can be performed. This can be accomplished by resecting the ileostomy and performing a hand-sewn end-to-end anastomosis (one layer, interrupted or continuous) or by unfolding the Brooke ileostomy and simply closing the enterostomy transversely with sutures [38]. A meta-analysis by Leung et al. failed to show any differences between surgical techniques for ileostomy reversal; however, there was a trend toward less postoperative bowel obstruction with stapled small bowel anastomoses [39].

Ileocolic Anastomoses

Ileocolic anastomoses are frequently created after an ileocolic resection for Crohn's disease or a right hemicolectomy for cancer. A recent Cochrane review looked at seven RCTs comprising 1125 patients comparing the techniques of stapled side-to-side anastomoses with hand-sewn anastomoses [40]. The overall leak rate was significantly lower for stapled anastomoses (2.5 %) compared with hand-sewn anastomoses (6 %). In a subgroup of 825 cancer patients, stapled anastomoses remained superior with a significantly lower leak rate (1.3 %) compared to hand-sewn anastomoses (6.7 %).

There were no differences for any other reported outcomes nor were there any differences for the noncancer subgroup that included Crohn's disease.

When contemplating an anastomosis for Crohn's disease, one must take several variables into consideration, including the physiologic and nutritional state of the patient, general condition of the bowel, and presence of additional active disease and peritoneal contamination. Additionally, the chronic use of high-dose immunosuppression may portend an increased risk of anastomotic leak. In some instances, an end ileostomy or even a primary anastomosis protected with a loop ileostomy may be a safe option for the malnourished, immunocompromised Crohn's disease patient. If considering a protective loop stoma, one must be cognizant of how proximal the stoma would be to determine if a persistently high-output stoma is likely. If an ileocolic anastomosis is going to be created, there is no absolute consensus as to the optimal technique for Crohn's disease; however, stapled anastomoses are generally expeditious and easy to construct.

When creating a stapled side-to-side (functional end-to-end) anastomosis, up to four linear stapler firings may be needed to construct the anastomosis. The typical ileocolic anastomosis is created by dividing the small bowel and colon with a GIA at the proximal and distal resection margins, followed by a stapled side-to-side anastomosis along the antimesenteric border of the bowel, and finally the stapled closure of the common enterotomy. Cost can be contained and overlapping staple lines avoided by creating a "Barcelona" anastomosis (Figure 9-2a–d). In this technique, after the mesentery of the bowel has been divided up to the points of proximal and distal resection, two enterotomies are created on the antimesenteric border of the bowel. The limbs of a GIA stapler are advanced into these openings and fired along the antimesenteric border of the bowel. The common enterotomy is then closed and the specimen transected with a second firing of a linear stapler.

Another technique for an ileocolic anastomosis is the stapled end-to-side technique in which an EEA stapler (25–29 mm) is used (Figure 9-3a–d). This has been shown to be a safe and effective anastomotic technique [41]. The terminal ileum is divided, a purse-string suture is placed, and the EEA anvil is secured in the end of the ileum. A colotomy is created within the specimen, and the EEA stapler is advanced through the colotomy in an antegrade fashion to the antimesenteric border of the colon several centimeters distal to the intended margin of transection. The spike is brought out through the antimesenteric wall of the colon, and the anvil within the ileum is connected. The stapler is then closed and fired. The colon is divided with a linear stapler a few centimeters proximal to the EEA anastomosis to ensure that the anastomosis and blind end of the colon are well perfused.

Laparoscopic ileocolic resections and right hemicolectomies are being performed with more frequency. Classically, the colonic mobilization and vascular pedicle ligation are performed laparoscopically. The specimen is resected and

FIGURE 9-2. Barcelona anastomosis. (**a**) Stay sutures are placed and two antimesenteric enterotomies are made. (**b**) A linear stapler is used to construct the common wall. (**c**) An additional firing of the linear stapler is used to complete the anastomosis and resect the specimen. (**d**) Completed anastomosis.

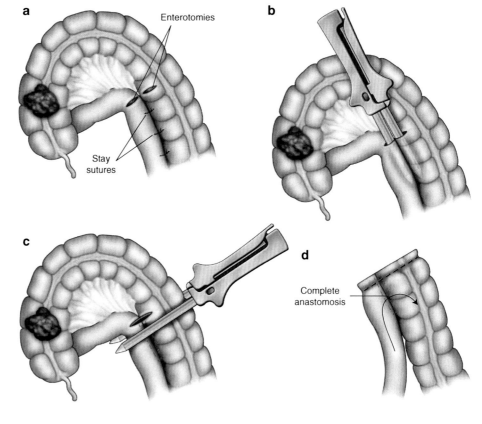

FIGURE 9-3. End-to-side ileocolic anastomosis. (**a**) An EEA anvil is placed into the end of small bowel through a purse string after dividing the bowel. (**b**) A colotomy is made, and the EEA stapler is passed and coupled the spike to the EEA anvil. (**c**) Following the EEA anastomosis, a linear stapler is used to close the colon defect. (**d**) Completed anastomosis.

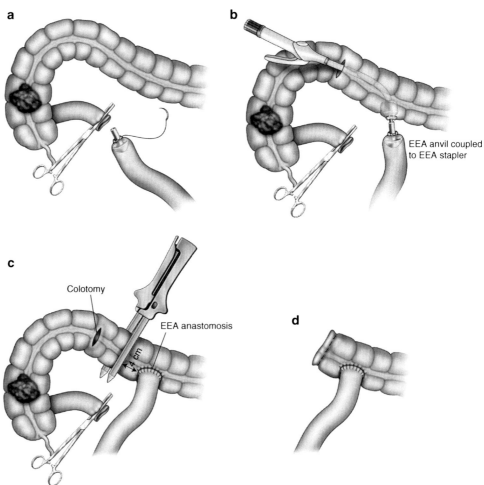

anastomosis created extracorporeally through a small peri-umbilical incision. In recent years, totally laparoscopic right hemicolectomy with intracorporeal anastomosis has gained popularity. Advocates of this technique maintain that there is less bowel manipulation and less traction on the bowel mesentery, which may translate into faster return of bowel function. Additionally, the extraction site can be moved to a location associated with decreased risk of hernia, such as a small Pfannenstiel incision. The most common technique for performing an intracorporeal anastomosis is to create a stapled side-to-side (functional end-to-end) anastomosis using laparoscopic linear staplers. The resultant common enterotomy can then be stapled or sewn closed. Intracorporeal anastomosis may be particularly beneficial in obese patients because they often have thick, foreshortened mesenteries that make extracorporealization particularly difficult and often result in extended extraction site incisions. A meta-analysis of nonrandomized comparative studies looking at intracorporeal anastomosis vs. extracorporeal anastomosis for laparoscopic right hemicolectomies shows no difference in the rate of anastomotic leak, with a trend toward decreased short-term morbidity in the intracorporeal anastomotic group [42]. Given that these are comparative studies and no randomized trials exist, it appears that the intracorporeal anastomosis is safe, but further studies are needed to determine if there is a true benefit [43].

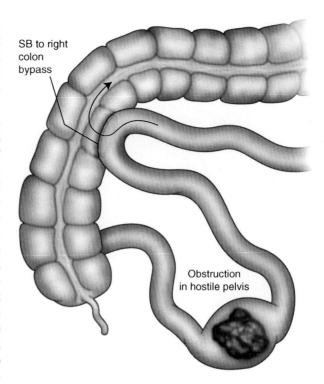

FIGURE 9-4. Intestinal bypass.

Intestinal Bypass

Deep pelvic small bowel obstructions that result from unresectable malignancies or severe radiation damage may be difficult or dangerous to approach surgically. In these situations, options include decompressing gastric tubes, proximal diversion, or intestinal bypass. If the obstructed loop of bowel can be isolated, a simple bypass from the obstructed limb to bowel distal to the obstruction can be performed in either a hand-sewn or side-to-side stapled fashion (Figure 9-4). For distal ileal obstructions, the ascending colon is frequently used as the distal limb of the bypass. If the colon is to be used, mobilization of the ascending colon and hepatic flexure is often necessary to allow the colon to lay alongside the obstructed limb without creating tension on the bypass anastomosis.

When contemplating an intestinal bypass, one must also consider the potential for obstruction of the bowel distal to the bypass. Many of these patients will already have an end colostomy, so bulky pelvic disease or dense pelvic adhesions should not result in an obstruction distal to the bypass. If the patient is in GI continuity, a preoperative contrast enema can assess the distal colon and rectum. One should have a low threshold for creating an ileostomy in a patient who is in GI continuity with bulky pelvic disease. Simply performing an intestinal bypass in this situation may be further complicated by a future distal obstruction in the pelvis.

Pelvic Anastomoses

Basic Principles of Pelvic Anastomoses

Creating an anastomosis in the pelvis can be extremely challenging. Studies have documented that low pelvic anastomoses have a higher rate of leakage than more proximal anastomoses [44, 45]. The increased leak rate highlights the challenges of operating in the pelvis. The space is limited by the unyielding bony structures, making visualization difficult. There are multiple structures within the pelvis that can interfere with or become incorporated into the anastomosis. Tension is a concern with all anastomoses but significantly more so in the pelvis, where anatomic factors can make it a significant challenge to create a tension-free anastomosis. When a low anterior resection is performed, the reservoir function of the rectum is lost proportionally to the length of rectum resected, and anastomotic misadventures can have major consequences on a patient's future quality of life.

Adequate visualization during dissection and creation of the anastomosis is extremely important. It is important to have optimal lighting—accomplished through the use of a headlamp, lighted pelvic retractor, or careful placement of external lights. Because of limited sight lines, it is often not possible for more than one person to visualize pelvic structures simultaneously.

Low Anterior Resection

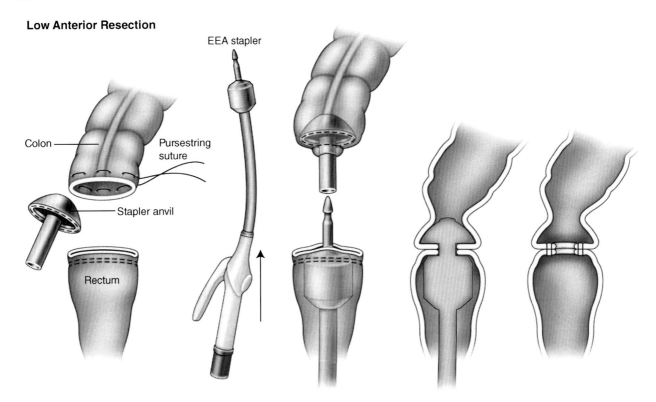

FIGURE 9-5. Stapled colorectal anastomosis. Following a low anterior resection, the EEA stapler is used to construct an end-to-end anastomosis.

When creating a pelvic anastomosis, extraneous structures can be incorporated in the anastomosis. The structure with the greatest consequences of inclusion is the vagina. This should be at the forefront of the surgeon's mind in every female patient. One must be diligent in ensuring that the vagina is out of harm's way during the dissection, rectal division, and anastomotic construction. For anastomoses in the mid- and upper rectum, the surgeon must ensure that the vagina is dissected away from the rectum for several centimeters below the site of the intended anastomosis. Additionally, for stapled anastomoses, the vagina must be visualized and confirmed to be free from the EEA staple line.

In the lower pelvis and especially with coloanal anastomoses, perfect visualization can be difficult to attain. In these situations, it is necessary to use other means to verify that the vagina has not been included in the anastomosis. One of the simplest methods to improve visualization deep in the pelvis is to ask an assistant to break from the sterile field and apply cephalad pressure to the perineum with a fist. If the vagina cannot be visualized after the stapler has been closed, the vaginal wall should be palpated to confirm its independence from the staple line. When performing hand-sewn anastomoses, careful bites should be taken anteriorly to avoid the vaginal wall. As with more proximal anastomoses, the vagina needs to be dissected off of the rectum and anal canal well below the level of intended anastomosis.

Rather than struggle to perform the maneuvers necessary to gain adequate colonic length to reduce anastomotic tension, it can be tempting to use the floppy sigmoid colon as the proximal end of the anastomosis. There are several reasons why the descending colon should be used preferentially to the sigmoid colon when creating the colorectal anastomosis. In a resection for cancer, the inferior mesenteric artery should be divided at its origin for an adequate lymphadenectomy. This high ligation, coupled with the loss of collateral flow from the distal middle rectal vessels, frequently makes the blood supply to the sigmoid colon insufficient. This scant blood flow to the anastomosis puts it at risk for leak or stricture. Additionally, the sigmoid colon's thick muscular wall and diverticulosis make this segment a poor substrate to use in creating what is already a precarious anastomosis. In general, it is better to invest the effort to adequately mobilize the colon to create length for a descending to rectal anastomosis.

Stapled Colorectal Anastomoses

With wide availability of circular EEA staplers, the stapled colorectal anastomosis has gained favor among surgeons (Figure 9-5). Both single-stapled and double-stapled techniques will be described.

In both these techniques, the stapler anvil is secured in the proximal colon with a purse string. The purse-string suture should be placed with small but full-thickness bites of the colon wall, so that there is not a bunching of tissue around the anvil post when the purse string is tied. It is important to ensure that there is not a significant burden of mesenteric or epiploic fat on the stapler anvil. All that is required is to incise the peritoneum overlying any fat that would be incorporated in the staple line. This simple maneuver will allow any extraneous fat to be compressed out of the anastomosis as the stapler is closed, without denuding or devascularizing the colon wall that will be part of the anastomotic staple line.

When the specimen has been removed, preparations should be made prior to creating the anastomosis. Ensure that the pre-anastomotic colon courses to the left of the ligament of Treitz and falls easily into the pelvis. The mesentery of the colon should be straight with no twists. If it appears that the anastomosis will be under *any* tension, further lengthening maneuvers should be performed. These will be described later.

Reevaluate the colon for blood flow—making sure that the colon appears pink and healthy. Confirm that there are no areas of demarcation and that the colon is not hyperemic. The colon must also be scrutinized for signs of venous stasis—mottling or small congested veins containing dark, almost black, blood. If there is any question as to the viability of the pre-anastomotic colon, the anastomosis should not proceed until these concerns have been addressed satisfactorily. A simple method of evaluating blood flow is to sharply incise an epiploic appendage adjacent to the anvil. While rarely pulsatile, bright red bleeding from this incision should be comforting. If there is only dark blood from this incision or any other signs that the blood flow to the anastomosis is compromised, a more proximal site should be chosen to create the anastomosis.

Once matters relating to blood supply and tension have been satisfied, the EEA stapler is gently introduced through the anal canal and remaining rectum by an assistant who is outside of the sterile field. Communication between the surgeon and the assistant is essential. In women, the assistant must confirm that the stapler is not placed in the vagina. As this portion of the procedure is often done with less than optimal visualization of the perineum, the assistant can confirm the rectal location of the stapler by placing a finger in the vagina after the stapler has been introduced. Ideally, the stapler should be advanced all the way to the transverse rectal staple line when creating a double-stapled anastomosis. The abdominal operator must confirm that the stapler is indeed at the end of the rectal stump prior to advancing the stapler spike. If there is any intervening tissue including valves or other gathered rectal tissue, the edges of the stapler will not be well defined at the pouch apex, and the stapler must be repositioned. When navigation of the stapler through the rectum proves difficult, it may be necessary for the abdominal operator to advance the stapler with one hand out of the sterile field and the other hand guiding the device through the rectal pouch.

Once the stapler is in the appropriate position, the spike is advanced slowly under close scrutiny of the abdominal operator. The stapler spike should be delivered near the midpoint of the transverse staple line. After the stapler spike has been fully deployed, the apex of the rectal pouch must be well seated on the stapler. The anvil is secured to the spike and the stapler is closed under direct visualization, taking care to confirm that extraneous tissue is not included. After the stapler has been closed, the abdominal operator must verify that the colonic mesentery is not twisted. This requires following the mesenteric edge all the way back to the middle colic vessels. In laparoscopic procedures where this visualization can be difficult, this might require reestablishment of pneumoperitoneum if necessary. Following this, the abdominal operator directs the assistant to fire the stapler. The stapler is then opened, twisted in order to dislodge from the tissue of the anastomosis, and removed. Any difficulty removing the stapler should generate concern, as this can be a sign of anastomotic failure. The integrity of the anastomosis should then be assessed by one of the various methods discussed later in this chapter.

The single-stapled technique differs from the double-stapled technique in that there is no transverse staple line on the rectal pouch. Instead, the rectum is divided sharply, and a purse string is also placed around the open rectal stump. The stapler is introduced and passed all the way to the proximal end of the rectum. The spike is then introduced through the purse string, and the purse string is tied around the spike. The stapled EEA anastomosis is then created in a similar fashion to the double-stapled anastomosis. While this technique avoids intersecting staple lines, it does leave the rectal stump open briefly, potentially allowing for spillage of stool or even intraluminal tumor cells into the abdominal cavity. For this reason, the single-stapled anastomosis is often used only as a salvage technique.

Rarely, advancing the EEA stapler to the apex of the rectal stump can prove to be extremely difficult, even with bimanual introduction. Excessive force should not be used to advance the stapler. Instead, further circumferential mobilization of the rectum in the mesorectal fascial plane will often eliminate the kinks or folds that inhibit stapler introduction. If this fails, the anastomosis can be created in an end-to-side fashion on the anterior wall of the rectum, several centimeters below the transverse staple line. Should this option be selected, there must be an adequate distance between the upper edge of the circular staple line and the transverse staple line in order to avoid ischemia of the tissue bridge separating the two staple lines. Another option is to attempt to use a smaller caliber stapler, but this requires removal and replacement of the anvil in the pre-anastomotic colon.

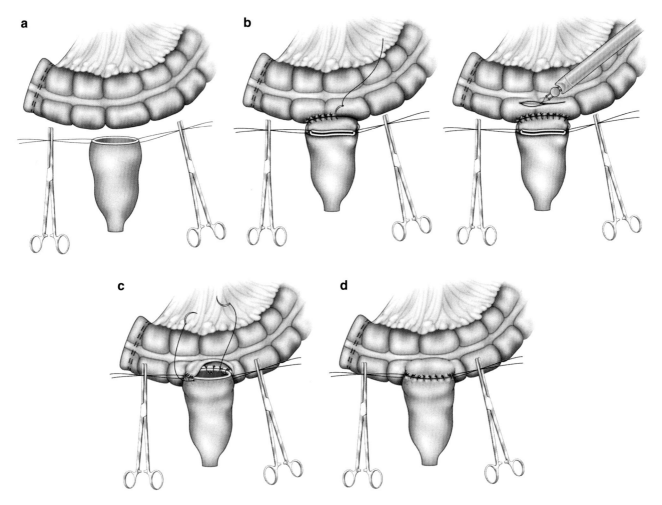

FIGURE 9-6. Hand-sewn colorectal anastomosis. (**a**) The distal end of the colon is closed, and stay sutures are placed on the rectum. (**b**) A posterior layer of sutures are placed (*left*) and a colotomy is made (*right*) to match the size of the opening on the rectal stump. (**c**) The anastomosis is constructed using two continuous running sutures. (**d**) The anterior suture line is oversewn with interrupted sutures.

Hand-Sewn Colorectal Anastomosis

In the upper and mid-rectum, it is possible to create a hand-sewn colorectal anastomosis (Figure 9-6a–d). The evidence suggests that hand-sewn and stapled colorectal anastomoses are equivalent in leak rate. Indeed, the hand-sewn colorectal anastomosis may have a slightly lower rate of stricture [46]. The choice to perform a hand-sewn or stapled anastomosis should be dictated by surgeon preference, patient habitus, clinical circumstances, anatomic accessibility, availability of staplers, and cost. Soilage or spillage of malignant cells is a theoretical problem with this technique, but this has never been borne out scientifically.

If a hand-sewn anastomosis is selected, there is no proven advantage of double-layer over single-layer anastomosis. We will describe a two-layer colorectal anastomosis, but the techniques to create a single-layer anastomosis are similar.

The fatty mesentery of the colon and rectum makes a hand-sewn end-to-end anastomosis difficult to perform. Additionally, there is often a substantial size difference between the proximal bowel and the rectal lumen. For these reasons, a side-to-end colon to rectal anastomosis, as described by Baker, is more practical and allows for better visualization while creating the anastomosis [47]. The distal end of the colon is stapled or sewn closed. The anastomosis will be created several centimeters proximal to this closure on the antimesenteric wall of the colon. In order to set up the anastomosis, two stay sutures should be placed on opposite sides of the anastomosis in order to align the two structures. A posterior layer of interrupted Lembert sutures is placed first. After the posterior row has been placed, a longitudinal antimesenteric colotomy is created to closely approximate the size of the rectal lumen. Two simple running sutures of absorbable monofilament suture are then started at the midpoint of the posterior wall and advanced in opposite directions to create the posterior inner layer. As the sutures proceed onto the anterior aspect of the anastomosis, a Connell suture can be used to create the anterior inner layer closure. The anterior suture line is then oversewn with interrupted Lembert sutures. While other methods exist, this technique is simple and ensures that the mucosa is inverted.

Ileorectal Anastomosis

The ileorectal anastomosis after an abdominal colectomy is performed in the same fashion and following the same precautions as the colorectal anastomosis. Often, the small caliber of the ileum will not accommodate the use of the larger EEA stapler, and a smaller 25 mm stapler diameter is required. Due to the risk of an axial volvulus under the free edge of the small bowel mesentery, some surgeons approximate the free ileal mesenteric edge to the retroperitoneum in the midline.

Ultralow Colorectal and Coloanal Anastomoses

The techniques involved in creating the low anastomoses in the pelvis remain the same as the upper rectal anastomoses. However, in addition to the technical challenges inherent in creating a low anastomosis, the surgeon must be mindful of the functional consequences of resecting the majority of the rectal reservoir. "Anterior resection syndrome" refers to the symptoms of frequency, urgency, stool fragmentation, incontinence, and evacuatory difficulties (see Chap. 56). This syndrome occurs to varying degrees in the majority of patients with low colorectal or coloanal anastomosis [48, 49]. Preoperative radiation and the distance of the anastomosis from the anal verge are risk factors for these symptoms [50]. This syndrome may require patients to take antimotility agents or wear pads or diapers. In the most extreme cases, patients become homebound or request a colostomy.

Neorectal Reservoirs

Many hypothesized that the functional consequences of a low anastomosis could be attributed to the loss of reservoir with straight colorectal or coloanal anastomosis [51]. The colon is less distensible than the native rectum, and it was thought that this low capacitance was responsible for the symptoms. Using techniques developed for restorative proctocolectomy, Lazorthes and Parc both proposed the creation of a colonic reservoir in order to decrease the functional consequences of a low anastomosis [52, 53]. These early studies showed improvement of bowel function in patients with colonic J-pouches.

Over the ensuing years, multiple studies confirmed these findings, demonstrating that the colonic J-pouch was superior to the straight coloanal anastomosis in terms of frequency, incontinence, and quality of life [44, 54–59]. While most studies evaluated function in the first 1–2 years after surgery, the studies evaluating longer-term results show that these functional advantages are durable out to 5 years [60–62]. The superiority of the colonic J-pouch over the straight coloanal anastomosis was also supported by a Cochrane systematic analysis [63].

While almost all defecatory problems improved with a J-pouch reservoir compared to a straight coloanal anastomosis, many patients in the early series reported significant constipation and evacuatory difficulties [53, 64]. The original descriptions of neorectal reservoirs were large, 10–12 cm colonic J-pouches. Some authors theorized that the emptying difficulties were related to large pouch size. Several trials evaluating smaller (5–6 cm) colonic pouches found them to be superior to larger pouches [64, 65].

The creation of the colonic J-pouch first requires confirmation that the colon is adequately mobilized and that the intended apex of the pouch will reach the cuff without tension (Figure 9-7a–c). An antimesenteric colotomy is then created 5–6 cm from the divided end of the colon. A linear cutting stapler is inserted through this colotomy, with one limb of the stapler inserted into the blind end and the other limb delivered up to the proximal limb of the colon. As the stapler is closed, the mesentery of the two limbs is rotated laterally to ensure that the staple line will be centered on the antimesenteric colon. Once the mesentery is oriented and the stapler closed, the pouch is created by firing the stapler. If a stapled anastomosis is to be created, a purse-string suture is then placed around the apical colotomy, and the anvil is secured in the pouch. The anastomosis is then created similarly to other colorectal anastomoses.

Anastomotic leak is a feared complication of low pelvic anastomoses and creates a significant fibrotic reaction in the pelvis that can have disastrous consequences on defecatory function [66]. Some evidence suggests that there may be fewer anastomotic complications with a colonic J-pouch. Doppler flow studies demonstrate that the pouch apex has improved blood flow compared to the colon used for the straight colorectal anastomosis [67]. Indeed, some studies showed a significant decrease in the anastomotic leak rate for the colonic J-pouch when compared to a straight coloanal anastomosis [44, 45].

While colonic reservoirs have benefits for low rectal and coloanal anastomosis, reservoirs anastomosed more than 5–6 cm above the anal verge may actually create problems emptying. It is recommended that a straight colorectal anastomosis be created for mid-rectal and more proximal anastomoses [45, 68, 69].

Occasionally, clinical circumstances make the creation of a colonic J-pouch difficult. Patients with a small pelvis, fatty mesentery, extensive diverticulosis, mucosectomy, or insufficient colonic length are not good candidates for J-pouch creation. Studies have shown that these technical factors preclude J-pouch creation in at least one-quarter of patients [70, 71]. In these situations, a transverse coloplasty offers another option.

Z'graggen was the first to describe the transverse coloplasty as an alternative to the colonic J-pouch, proposing that this technique may provide the functional benefits of the J-pouch reservoir while avoiding the evacuatory difficulties [72]. The coloplasty is created by making an 8 cm longitudinal

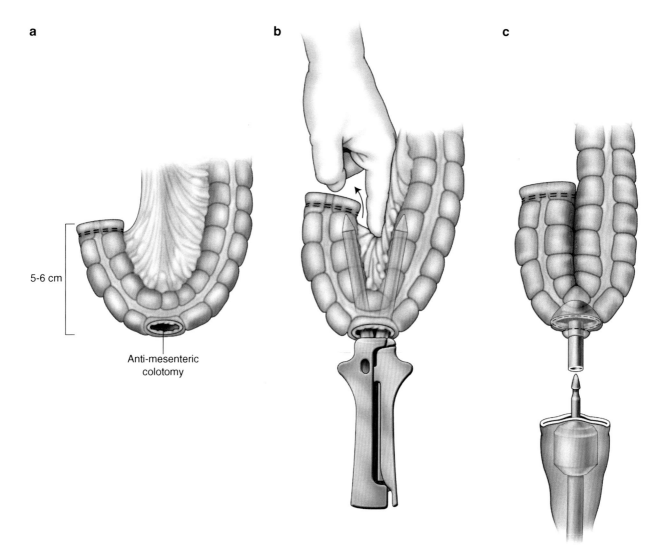

Figure 9-7. Colonic J-pouch. (**a**) A 5–6 cm colonic J-pouch is formed, and a colotomy is made on the antimesenteric portion of the bowel wall. (**b**) The pouch is formed using a linear stapler with 1–2 loads ensuring the colon mesentery is pulled out of the staple line. (**c**) The colorectal anastomosis is constructed using an EEA stapler.

incision in the antimesenteric colon between the tenia coli (Figure 9-8a–d). The incision is created after the purse string and anvil have been placed in the colon, with the distal end of the incision approximately 4 cm proximal to the stapler anvil. Stay sutures are placed on each side of the midpoint of the colotomy to provide lateral traction. The colotomy is then closed transversely, in the fashion of a Heineke-Mikulicz strictureplasty, creating the reservoir. Early studies comparing this technique to the colonic J-pouch found no difference between these two techniques in terms of bowel function, continence, or quality of life, but these studies were small single-center trials [70, 73, 74].

In a large, multicenter randomized controlled trial, Fazio et al. compared the colonic J-pouch to the transverse coloplasty [71]. Taking into account the fact that a significant percentage of patients have technical circumstances that do not allow for J-pouch creation, the authors then compared the transverse coloplasty to the straight coloanal anastomosis

for patients in whom a J-pouch was not possible. After the resection was performed, the surgeon made the determination if a colonic J-pouch was possible. If so, patients were randomized to colonic J-pouch or coloplasty. If a pouch was not feasible, patients were randomized to transverse coloplasty or straight coloanal anastomosis. At 2 years, the colonic J-pouch proved superior to the transverse coloplasty in frequency, clustering, soilage, and continence. Although the sample sizes were smaller, the transverse coloplasty showed no improvement in any functional assessment compared to the straight coloanal anastomosis.

Huber et al. proposed the side-to-end anastomosis as an alternative to the colonic J-pouch for coloanal anastomoses [75] (Figure 9-9a, b). These techniques were compared in a randomized controlled trial of 100 patients [76]. The trial showed that the two techniques had similar frequency, continence, and functional scores at 1 year. At 2 years, the groups remained similar in bowel function, but neorectal volumes

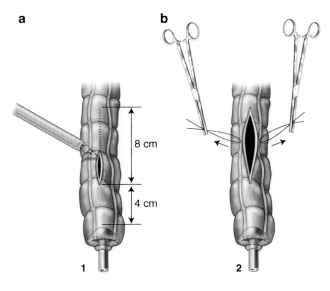

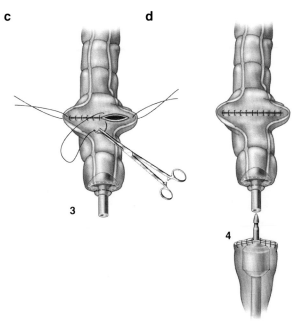

FIGURE 9-8. Transverse coloplasty. (**a**) An 8 cm linear colostomy is made 4 cm from the distal end of the colon. (**b**) The anvil is placed in the end, and stay sutures are placed at the midpoint on each side of the colotomy. (**c**) The longitudinal colotomy is closed in a transverse fashion. (**d**) An end-to-end anastomosis is performed.

were 40 % higher in the colonic J-pouch group compared to the side-to-end anastomosis [77]. A systematic review comparing the side-to-end anastomosis to the colonic J-pouch was also performed [63]. With admittedly small numbers, the analysis did not show any difference in function between these two techniques.

The physiologic basis for the improved function of neorectal reservoirs is not completely understood. Early proponents of the colonic J-pouch touted the increased volume

reservoir, but some have questioned the neorectal "reservoir" theory [78, 79]. Ho et al. were the first to question the reservoir theory based on a small randomized controlled trial. In this study, they compared an 8 cm colonic J-pouch to straight coloanal anastomosis by functional results and anorectal physiology. While the function of the J-pouch was again proven superior, the physiology testing showed that the neorectal capacity was similar for both groups.

In a subsequent study comparing straight coloanal anastomosis to a 5 cm J-pouch, Furst et al. reached the same conclusion—functional improvements with the colonic J-pouch are not the result of an increased reservoir capacitance. These authors suggested that the pouch works by decreasing forward propulsive motility in the J-segment.

Based on these findings, Ho et al. developed a nuclear medicine study using radioactive isotopes designed to mix differentially with either solid or liquid stools [80]. They then conducted a small randomized controlled trial comparing the colonic J-pouch to the straight coloanal anastomosis. As before, while they found better functional results with the J-pouch, the maximal tolerable volumes were similar between the two groups. On scintigraphy, they found that solid stool transport through the colon was the same for both techniques. Interestingly, they found that the J-pouch had significantly better retention of liquid stools in the distal colon above the pouch. While they could not directly prove a link between the retention of liquid stool and decreased motility through the J-pouch segment, their findings support this theory. The better retention of liquid stool certainly explains the superior functional outcomes associated with the colonic J-pouch and may explain why other "reservoir" techniques have not proven as advantageous.

In summary, for low colorectal or coloanal anastomoses, the colonic J-pouch may give the best functional results, but the long-term durability of this benefit is unclear. When the J-pouch is not feasible, the transverse coloplasty or the straight coloanal anastomosis appears to offer similar functional results. The role of the side-to-end coloanal anastomosis is still undefined.

Hand-Sewn Coloanal Anastomosis

The double-stapled coloanal anastomosis is simple and can be created more rapidly than the hand-sewn anastomosis, making stapling the preferred method to create the coloanal anastomosis for most surgeons. There are, however, many circumstances in which a hand-sewn coloanal anastomosis is the only option to avoid an ostomy. Such situations include mucosectomies, failure of the transverse rectal staple line, and tumors that require a combined transabdominal and transanal approach to achieve an adequate margin. Knowledge and expertise in creating a hand-sewn coloanal anastomosis are requisite for any surgeon who performs proctectomies, as it is sometimes difficult to predict when these skills will be called into action.

FIGURE 9-9. Side-to-end coloanal
anastomosis. (**a**) A colotomy is
made proximal to the open end of
the colon. (**b**) The EEA anvil is
passed through this opening.
(**c**) The colonic opening is closed
using a linear stapler, and the
anastomosis is performed using
an EEA stapler.

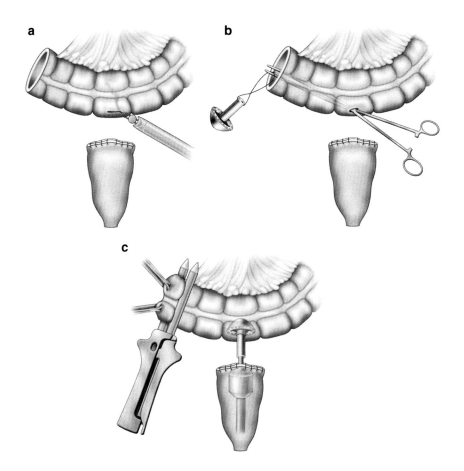

In order to perform a hand-sewn anastomosis, the surgeon must have good visualization of the cut edge of the anal canal. Manufactured self-retaining elastic hook retractors provide effacement of the anus and facilitate exposure of the anastomosis. With larger patients or when visualization is still difficult, better exposure of the anal canal can be achieved by placing multiple circumferential sutures from the anal verge to the skin several centimeters away on the thigh, groin, and buttocks. The transanal dissection, either intersphincteric dissection or mucosectomy, should be performed as appropriate for the pathology. Adequate colon length should be confirmed by assuring that the proximal colon reaches easily below the pubic symphysis. If not, further maneuvers to increase length must be performed before attempting to mature the anastomosis. When ready to perform the anastomosis, the orientation of the colon mesentery should be confirmed, and two noncrushing clamps are passed transanally by the perineal operator. Orientation of the clamps is established, and the open colon specimen is secured into the clamps by the abdominal surgeon while maintaining orientation of the colon. The colon is then coaxed through the pelvis down to the level of the anal anastomosis by rocking it back and forth. The abdominal operator can assist by using both hands to guide the colon into the deep pelvis. A simple full-thickness suture is then placed in each quadrant of the anal canal, making sure that the proximal colon lumen is proportioned equally around the circumference of the anastomosis. The anastomosis is then completed by placing intervening sutures in the remaining gaps.

Baik et al. reported on a case series of patients that had straight hand-sewn coloanal anastomoses after proctectomy for cancer [81]. In their series, 31 % of patients had anal incontinence at 6 months. The percentage of patients with incontinence decreased to 14 % at 1 year. Frequency was also noted, with 20 % of patients reporting more than six bowel movements a day at 1 year.

In the only randomized controlled trial comparing hand-sewn to stapled coloanal J-pouch anastomoses, Laurent et al. randomized 37 patients to the two techniques [82]. While the two groups had tumors at equivalent distances from the anal verge, the hand-sewn anastomoses were constructed nearly a centimeter closer to the anal verge. Functionally, the two groups appeared equivalent, but the very small sample size must be considered in the interpretation of these results.

The hand-sewn coloanal anastomosis can only be performed for very low anastomoses, and when feasible, a stapled anastomosis is preferable to the hand-sewn technique. This technique should be reserved for those anastomoses so low that they cannot be performed using the double-stapled technique.

Assessment of Pelvic Anastomosis

Some form of intraoperative anastomotic assessment should be performed at the time of creation. Multiple tests have been described including endoscopic visual evaluation and mechanical tests such as rectal insufflation with air, betadine, or methylene blue. Mechanical tests of anastomoses demonstrate intraoperative leaks in 5–25 % of anastomoses [83]. The air insufflation test is the simplest to perform. Multiple studies show this test reduces postoperative anastomotic leak rates, leading some to call for insufflation testing to be included as a quality process measure [84–87]. In addition to allowing for an air-leak test, intraoperative flexible endoscopic assessment of the anastomosis allows for visualization of the anastomosis. To date, there is no definitive confirmation that intraoperative endoscopy is more effective than a simple air-leak test [88–90]. Proponents of this technique point out the ability to assess for anastomotic bleeding, mucosal perfusion, and visual defects in the anastomosis.

Whether performing a simple leak test with a proctoscope or as part of an assessment with flexible endoscopy, the principles of the air-leak test remain the same. The bowel several centimeters proximal to the anastomosis should be occluded manually or with a bowel clamp. Saline is added to the pelvis to cover the anastomosis. Air is then insufflated into the rectum. While some feel that insufflation to high pressures may create defects in the anastomosis, it is the authors' opinion that air testing with rigorous rectal insufflation will stress the anastomosis and mimic or exceed the harshest physiologic conditions that may occur in the postoperative period. It is important to visualize the colon proximal to the anastomosis to ensure that it is indeed being distended. During insufflation, the anastomosis should be manipulated in all directions to confirm that a small leak is not being hidden or occluded by extraneous tissue. If there is bubbling, the saline should be slowly removed with suction down to the level of the anastomosis in order to localize the leak.

When an intraoperative leak is discovered, options include suture repair, proximal diversion, or takedown and refashioning of the anastomosis. For small leaks, suture repair is often adequate; however, the anastomosis must be tested again following the repair. Some authors suggest that recreating the anastomosis is the safest way to deal with any positive intraoperative leak test [87, 90]. Recreating the anastomosis usually requires further rectal resection with potential functional consequences. Diversion, rather than reconstruction, remains another option when there is a question about the integrity of the anastomosis. There is no argument that larger leaks, circumferential leaks, and leaks that cannot be visualized or adequately repaired require takedown and refashioning of the anastomosis.

Troubleshooting Problems with Pelvic Anastomoses

Unanticipated Pelvic Anastomosis

Despite thoughtful preoperative planning, situations will arise in which the surgeon must create an unplanned pelvic anastomosis. Frequently, the patient is positioned so that access to the perineum is not possible. If circumstances permit, skin closure and repositioning are an option that allows for the standard double-stapled anastomosis to be created. It is not always necessary or possible to reposition the patient in lithotomy position to create colorectal anastomoses. While a hand-sewn anastomosis remains an option, this becomes more difficult lower in the pelvis. It is also possible to create a stapled side-to-end anastomosis similar to the Baker anastomosis with the patient in supine or even lateral position. This technique requires placement of a purse-string suture in the open end of the rectum in order to secure the anvil for the circular stapler (Figure 9-10a–d). The stapled end of the colon is opened, allowing the circular stapler to be introduced into the colon lumen. The stapler is then guided down the colon over a distance of several centimeters and the stapler spike delivered out through the antimesenteric wall of the colon. The anvil is secured to the stapler, and it is closed and fired. The open end of the colon distal to the anastomosis can then be closed with a transverse stapler.

Inadequate Colonic Length

As emphasized earlier, adequate colonic reach is necessary before anastomotic construction begins. For a left colectomy, adequate reach is usually achieved by performing basic maneuvers including splenic flexure mobilization, division of the inferior mesenteric artery at its origin, and division of the inferior mesenteric vein at the inferior border of the pancreas cephalad to the vein branch that drains the splenic flexure. Splenic flexure mobilization requires more than just freeing the peritoneal attachments of the flexure in the left upper quadrant. Complete mobilization necessitates separation of the omentocolic attachments to the distal transverse colon, deliberate division of the renocolic attachments of the mesentery to Gerota's fascia of the left kidney, and lysis of the gastrocolic attachments between the posterior gastric wall and the transverse colon mesentery. Additionally, the distal transverse colon mesentery can be divided back to the middle colic vessels. These routine maneuvers will almost always allow adequate mobilization to perform any colorectal or coloanal anastomosis.

FIGURE 9-10. Unexpected colorectal anastomosis. (**a**) A purse string is sewn into the open end of the rectum. (**b**) The EEA anvil is placed through the rectal stump and the EEA stapler is passed retrograde through the open end of the colon. (**c**) The anastomosis is completed with firing of the EEA stapler. (**d**) A liner stapler is used to close the open end of the colon.

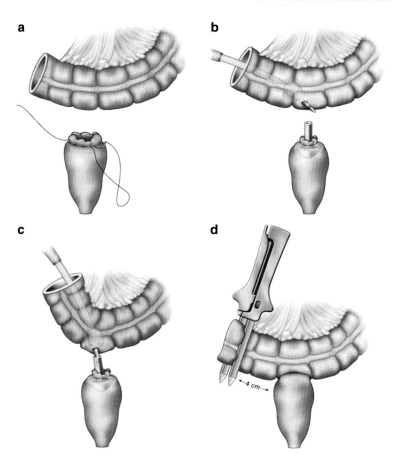

Resection of the splenic flexure as part of an extended left hemicolectomy often presents a challenge in obtaining adequate colonic length to create a tension-free anastomosis. In this case, the transverse colon is tethered by the middle colic vessels, and further mobilization will not increase the reach. In such circumstances, serial ligation of the middle colic vessels proceeding from left to right provides more length. The middle colic pedicles should be divided only as necessary to allow the colon to reach to the level of the anastomosis. After the pedicles have been divided, the blood flow to the distal colon must be reassessed, as the flow through the marginal artery to the anastomosis is frequently dependent on the middle colic vessels. Unfortunately, adequate blood supply and adequate reach sometimes find themselves at odds. If, after division of the middle colic pedicles, there is a compromise of the blood flow to the pre-anastomotic colon, it should be resected back to the point where there is good arterial inflow and satisfactory venous drainage.

Ideally, the colon can be extended around to the left of the ligament of Treitz and delivered into the pelvis to create the anastomosis. If the colon will not reach in this fashion, another route to the pelvis must be pursued. Simply draping the transverse colon over the small bowel is not a good alternative path to the anastomosis. This route rarely provides sufficient length and may lead to avulsion of the anastomosis if the patient develops an ileus and the bowel becomes distended. An option that avoids these pitfalls is to create a window in the terminal ileal mesentery that allows passage of the colon through this retroileal opening (Figure 9-11a, b). The window is created in the space between the ileocolic artery and the distal superior mesenteric artery. This technique, originally described by Rombeau et al., allows an unobstructed path to the anastomosis and also avoids the risk of anastomotic separation should the patient develop a postoperative ileus and small bowel dilation [91]. This technique usually requires mobilization of the proximal transverse colon by dividing the remaining omentocolic and gastrocolic attachments. The window should be large enough to accommodate the colon without causing strangulation. After adequate blood flow to the pre-anastomotic colon is verified, the anastomosis can be created in the usual fashion.

Sometimes, when a significant portion of the transverse colon has been resected, even this retroileal window does not allow adequate reach into the pelvis. In these situations, mobilization of the hepatic flexure and counterclockwise rotation of the colon provide one last opportunity to salvage a colorectal anastomosis (Figure 9-12a–c). This procedure is sometimes referred to as Deloyers' procedure, after the surgeon who published the first description [92]. This technique requires complete mobilization of the hepatic flexure and right colon—including dividing all of the retroperitoneal attachments and mobilization of the small bowel mesentery up to the duodenum. Any remaining middle colic vessels are ligated, leaving the colonic segment's blood supply based off

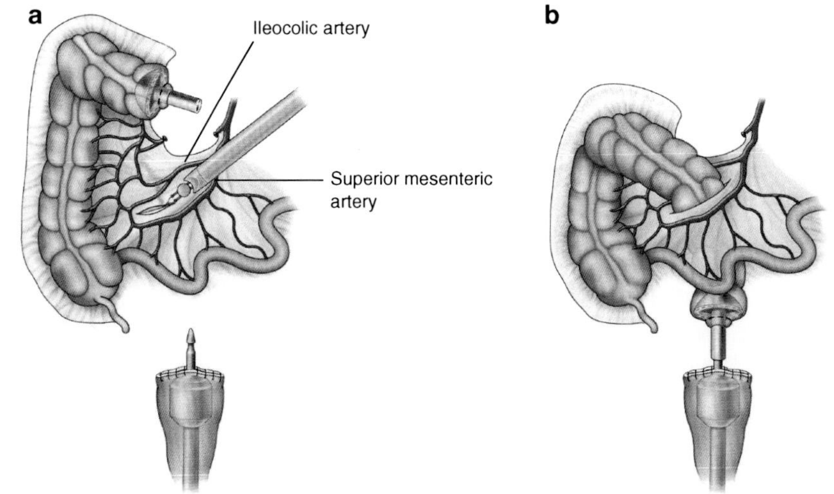

FIGURE 9-11. Retroileal pull-through. (**a**) A window is made on the anterior aspect of the ileocolic pedicle after the terminal ileum is mobilized from the retroperitoneum. (**b**) The colon is passed through this window and into the pelvis to perform the end-to-end anastomosis.

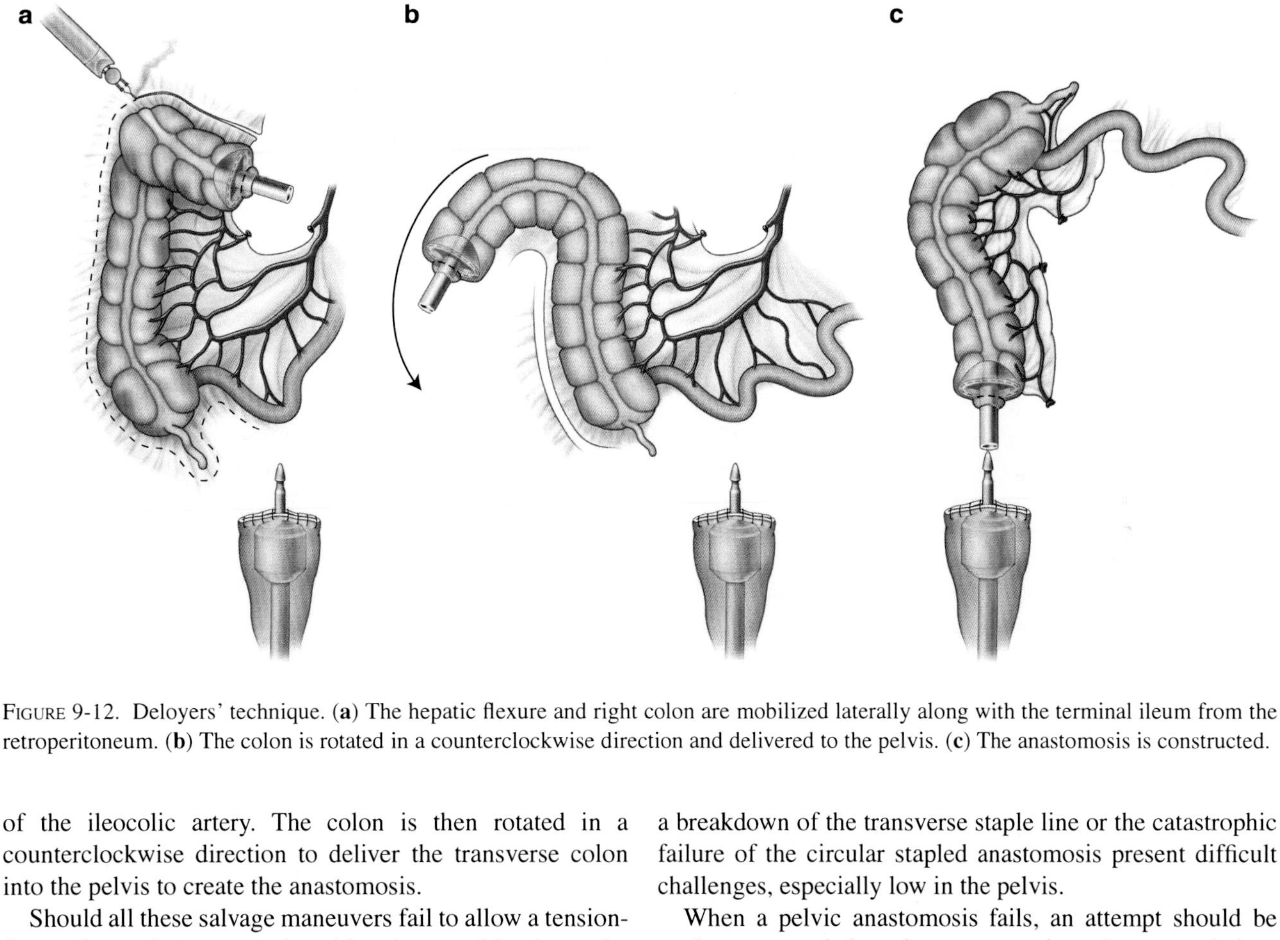

FIGURE 9-12. Deloyers' technique. (**a**) The hepatic flexure and right colon are mobilized laterally along with the terminal ileum from the retroperitoneum. (**b**) The colon is rotated in a counterclockwise direction and delivered to the pelvis. (**c**) The anastomosis is constructed.

of the ileocolic artery. The colon is then rotated in a counterclockwise direction to deliver the transverse colon into the pelvis to create the anastomosis.

Should all these salvage maneuvers fail to allow a tension-free colorectal anastomosis with adequate blood supply, remaining options include a completion colectomy with an ileorectal anastomosis or an end colostomy.

Intraoperative Anastomotic Failure

Unfortunately, failed anastomoses are inevitable in pelvic surgery. The ability to safely and effectively deal with a failure is essential for a colorectal surgeon. Misadventures such as

a breakdown of the transverse staple line or the catastrophic failure of the circular stapled anastomosis present difficult challenges, especially low in the pelvis.

When a pelvic anastomosis fails, an attempt should be made to resect below the anastomosis and recreate it in a standard fashion. In refashioning the anastomosis, care must be taken to further mobilize the rectum from its surrounding structures, specifically the vagina, in order to allow sufficient room to create the new anastomosis.

Sometimes, it is impossible to place the transverse stapler below a failed anastomosis or separated transverse staple line. In this case, the anastomosis or failed staple line should be excised. The open rectal stump should be grasped with long Allis clamps and a purse string placed around the open rectum.

When low in the pelvis, placement of this difficult suture is facilitated by having an assistant apply pressure to the perineum in a cephalad direction. Manipulating a rectal sizer in through the open cuff may also help to better define the tissues and facilitate placement of the purse string. Once the rectal purse string is placed, the stapler anvil should be secured in the colon in the normal manner. The circular stapler is then passed through the anal canal and delivered to the point just below the open end of the rectum and purse string. Slowly, the stapler spike is advanced through the open rectal cuff. Once the spike has been fully deployed, the purse string is tied around the spike and inspected to confirm that the purse string is complete. The anvil is then fixed to the stapler, carefully closed, and fired. The anastomosis is evaluated by the usual means according to the surgeon's preference. As noted earlier, consideration should be given to diversion in these circumstances after an anastomotic mishap.

References

1. Moran BJ. Stapling instruments for intestinal anastomosis in colorectal surgery. Br J Surg. 1996;83(7):902–9.
2. Ceraldi CM, et al. Comparison of continuous single layer polypropylene anastomosis with double layer and stapled anastomoses in elective colon resections. Am Surg. 1993;59(3):168–71.
3. Everett WG. A comparison of one layer and two layer techniques for colorectal anastomosis. Br J Surg. 1975;62(2):135–40.
4. Fielding LP, et al. Anastomotic integrity after operations for large-bowel cancer: a multicentre study. Br Med J. 1980;281(6237):411–4.
5. Reichel K, Rauner P, Guthy E. Clinical and experimental evaluation of single and double layer entero anastomosis. Chirurg Gastroenterol. 1975;9:461–7.
6. Slieker JC, et al. Systematic review of the technique of colorectal anastomosis. JAMA Surg. 2013;148(2):190–201.
7. Andersen E, Sondenaa K, Holter J. A comparative study of polydioxanone (PDS) and polyglactin 910 (Vicryl) in colonic anastomoses in rats. Int J Colorectal Dis. 1989;4(4):251–4.
8. Foresman PA, Edlich RF, Rodeheaver GT. The effect of new monofilament absorbable sutures on the healing of musculoaponeurotic incisions, gastrostomies, and colonic anastomoses. Arch Surg. 1989;124(6):708–10.
9. Bubrick MP, et al. Prospective, randomized trial of the biofragmentable anastomosis ring. The BAR Investigational Group. Am J Surg. 1991;161(1):136–42. discussion 142–3.
10. Corman ML, et al. Comparison of the Valtrac biofragmentable anastomosis ring with conventional suture and stapled anastomosis in colon surgery. Results of a prospective, randomized clinical trial. Dis Colon Rectum. 1989;32(3):183–7.
11. Hardy Jr TG, et al. A biofragmentable ring for sutureless bowel anastomosis. An experimental study. Dis Colon Rectum. 1985;28(7):484–90.
12. Pahlman L, et al. Randomized trial of a biofragmentable bowel anastomosis ring in high-risk colonic resection. Br J Surg. 1997;84(9):1291–4.
13. Seow-Choen F, Eu KW. Circular staplers versus the biofragmentable ring for colorectal anastomosis: a prospective randomized study. Br J Surg. 1994;81(12):1790–1.
14. Thiede A, et al. Overview on compression anastomoses: biofragmentable anastomosis ring multicenter prospective trial of 1666 anastomoses. World J Surg. 1998;22(1):78–86. discussion 87.
15. Kim HR, et al. Early surgical outcomes of NiTi endoluminal compression anastomotic clip (NiTi CAC 30) use in patients with gastrointestinal malignancy. J Laparoendosc Adv Surg Tech A. 2012;22(5):472–8.
16. D'Hoore A, et al. COMPRES: a prospective postmarketing evaluation of the compression anastomosis ring CAR 27()/ColonRing(). Colorectal Dis. 2015;17(6):522–9.
17. Masoomi H, et al. Compression anastomosis ring device in colorectal anastomosis: a review of 1,180 patients. Am J Surg. 2013;205(4):447–51.
18. Jafari MD, et al. Perfusion assessment in laparoscopic left-sided/anterior resection (PILLAR II): a multi-institutional study. J Am Coll Surg. 2015;220(1):82–92.e1.
19. Jesus EC et al. Prophylactic anastomotic drainage for colorectal surgery. Cochrane Database Syst Rev 2004; (4): CD002100.
20. Urbach DR, Kennedy ED, Cohen MM. Colon and rectal anastomoses do not require routine drainage: a systematic review and meta-analysis. Ann Surg. 1999;229(2):174–80.
21. Merad F, et al. Is prophylactic pelvic drainage useful after elective rectal or anal anastomosis? A multicenter controlled randomized trial. French Association for Surgical Research. Surgery. 1999;125(5):529–35.
22. Rondelli F, et al. To drain or not to drain extraperitoneal colorectal anastomosis? A systematic review and meta-analysis. Colorectal Dis. 2014;16(2):O35–42.
23. Cabot JC, et al. Long-term consequences of not closing the mesenteric defect after laparoscopic right colectomy. Dis Colon Rectum. 2010;53(3):289–92.
24. Causey MW, Oguntoye M, Steele SR. Incidence of complications following colectomy with mesenteric closure versus no mesenteric closure: does it really matter? J Surg Res. 2011;171(2):571–5.
25. Rullier E, et al. Risk factors for anastomotic leakage after resection of rectal cancer. Br J Surg. 1998;85(3):355–8.
26. Bertelsen CA, et al. Anastomotic leakage after anterior resection for rectal cancer: risk factors. Colorectal Dis. 2010;12(1):37–43.
27. Platell C, Barwood N, Makin G. Clinical utility of a de-functioning loop ileostomy. ANZ J Surg. 2005;75(3):147–51.
28. Chow A, et al. The morbidity surrounding reversal of defunctioning ileostomies: a systematic review of 48 studies including 6,107 cases. Int J Colorectal Dis. 2009;24(6):711–23.
29. Pokorny H, et al. Predictors for complications after loop stoma closure in patients with rectal cancer. World J Surg. 2006;30(8):1488–93.
30. Chen TA. Loop ileostomy or loop colostomy: which one is better for fecal diversion? Int J Colorectal Dis. 2012;27(1):131–2.
31. Nurkin S, et al. The role of faecal diversion in low rectal cancer: a review of 1791 patients having rectal resection with anastomosis for cancer, with and without a proximal stoma. Colorectal Dis. 2013;15(6):e309–16.
32. Tan WS, et al. Meta-analysis of defunctioning stomas in low anterior resection for rectal cancer. Br J Surg. 2009;96(5):462–72.
33. Shiomi A, et al. Effects of a diverting stoma on symptomatic anastomotic leakage after low anterior resection for rectal

cancer: a propensity score matching analysis of 1,014 consecutive patients. J Am Coll Surg. 2015;220(2):186–94.

34. Chude GG, et al. Defunctioning loop ileostomy with low anterior resection for distal rectal cancer: should we make an ileostomy as a routine procedure? A prospective randomized study. Hepatogastroenterology. 2008;55(86–87):1562–7.

35. Matthiessen P, et al. Defunctioning stoma reduces symptomatic anastomotic leakage after low anterior resection of the rectum for cancer: a randomized multicenter trial. Ann Surg. 2007; 246(2):207–14.

36. Ulrich AB, et al. Diverting stoma after low anterior resection: more arguments in favor. Dis Colon Rectum. 2009;52(3): 412–8.

37. Guenaga KF et al. Ileostomy or colostomy for temporary decompression of colorectal anastomosis. Cochrane Database Syst Rev 2007; (1): CD004647.

38. Goulder F. Bowel anastomoses: the theory, the practice and the evidence base. World J Gastrointest Surg. 2012;4(9):208–13.

39. Leung TT, et al. Comparison of stapled versus handsewn loop ileostomy closure: a meta-analysis. J Gastrointest Surg. 2008; 12(5):939–44.

40. Choy PY et al. Stapled versus handsewn methods for ileocolic anastomoses. Cochrane Database Syst Rev 2011; (9): CD004320.

41. Liu Z, et al. Ileocolonic anastomosis after right hemicolectomy for colon cancer: functional end-to-end or end-to-side? World J Surg Oncol. 2014;12:306.

42. Carnuccio P, Jimeno J, Pares D. Laparoscopic right colectomy: a systematic review and meta-analysis of observational studies comparing two types of anastomosis. Tech Coloproctol. 2014; 18(1):5–12.

43. Tarta C, Bishawi M, Bergamaschi R. Intracorporeal ileocolic anastomosis: a review. Tech Coloproctol. 2013;17(5):479–85.

44. Hallbook O, et al. Randomized comparison of straight and colonic J pouch anastomosis after low anterior resection. Ann Surg. 1996;224(1):58–65.

45. Hida J, et al. Indications for colonic J-pouch reconstruction after anterior resection for rectal cancer: determining the optimum level of anastomosis. Dis Colon Rectum. 1998;41(5):558–63.

46. Neutzling CB et al. Stapled versus handsewn methods for colorectal anastomosis surgery. Cochrane Database Syst Rev 2012; (2): CD003144.

47. Baker JW. Low end to side rectosigmoid anastomosis; description of technique. Arch Surg. 1950;61(1):143–57.

48. Bryant CL, et al. Anterior resection syndrome. Lancet Oncol. 2012;13(9):e403–8.

49. Bloemen JG, et al. Long-term quality of life in patients with rectal cancer: association with severe postoperative complications and presence of a stoma. Dis Colon Rectum. 2009;52(7): 1251–8.

50. Lange MM, van de Velde CJ. Faecal and urinary incontinence after multimodality treatment of rectal cancer. PLoS Med. 2008;5(10):e202.

51. Keighley MR, Matheson D. Functional results of rectal excision and endo-anal anastomosis. Br J Surg. 1980;67(10): 757–61.

52. Lazorthes F, et al. Resection of the rectum with construction of a colonic reservoir and colo-anal anastomosis for carcinoma of the rectum. Br J Surg. 1986;73(2):136–8.

53. Parc R, et al. Resection and colo-anal anastomosis with colonic reservoir for rectal carcinoma. Br J Surg. 1986;73(2):139–41.

54. Dehni N, et al. Long-term functional outcome after low anterior resection: comparison of low colorectal anastomosis and colonic J-pouch-anal anastomosis. Dis Colon Rectum. 1998;41(7): 817–22. discussion 822–3.

55. Joo JS, et al. Long-term functional evaluation of straight colo-anal anastomosis and colonic J-pouch: is the functional superiority of colonic J-pouch sustained? Dis Colon Rectum. 1998;41(6):740–6.

56. Kusunoki M, et al. Function after anoabdominal rectal resection and colonic J pouch--anal anastomosis. Br J Surg. 1991;78(12): 1434–8.

57. Lazorthes F, et al. Late clinical outcome in a randomized prospective comparison of colonic J pouch and straight coloanal anastomosis. Br J Surg. 1997;84(10):1449–51.

58. Ortiz H, et al. Coloanal anastomosis: are functional results better with a pouch? Dis Colon Rectum. 1995;38(4):375–7.

59. Seow-Choen F, Goh HS. Prospective randomized trial comparing J colonic pouch-anal anastomosis and straight coloanal reconstruction. Br J Surg. 1995;82(5):608–10.

60. Portier G, Platonoff I, Lazorthes F. Long-term functional results after straight or colonic J-pouch coloanal anastomosis. Recent Results Cancer Res. 2005;165:191–5.

61. Hida J, et al. Long-term functional changes after low anterior resection for rectal cancer compared between a colonic J-pouch and a straight anastomosis. Hepatogastroenterology. 2007;54 (74):407–13.

62. Harris GJ, Lavery IC, Fazio VW. Function of a colonic J pouch continues to improve with time. Br J Surg. 2001;88(12): 1623–7.

63. Brown CJ, Fenech DS, McLeod RS. Reconstructive techniques after rectal resection for rectal cancer. Cochrane Database Syst Rev 2008; (2): CD006040.

64. Hida J, et al. Functional outcome after low anterior resection with low anastomosis for rectal cancer using the colonic J-pouch. Prospective randomized study for determination of optimum pouch size. Dis Colon Rectum. 1996;39(9):986–91.

65. Lazorthes F, et al. Prospective, randomized study comparing clinical results between small and large colonic J-pouch following coloanal anastomosis. Dis Colon Rectum. 1997;40(12): 1409–13.

66. Hallbook O, Sjodahl R. Anastomotic leakage and functional outcome after anterior resection of the rectum. Br J Surg. 1996;83(1):60–2.

67. Hallbook O, Johansson K, Sjodahl R. Laser Doppler blood flow measurement in rectal resection for carcinoma--comparison between the straight and colonic J pouch reconstruction. Br J Surg. 1996;83(3):389–92.

68. Ramirez JM, et al. Colonic J-pouch rectal reconstruction--is it really a neorectum? Dis Colon Rectum. 1996;39(11):1286–8.

69. Hida J, et al. Comparison of long-term functional results of colonic J-pouch and straight anastomosis after low anterior resection for rectal cancer: a five-year follow-up. Dis Colon Rectum. 2004;47(10):1578–85.

70. Furst A, et al. Colonic J-pouch vs. coloplasty following resection of distal rectal cancer: early results of a prospective, randomized, pilot study. Dis Colon Rectum. 2003;46(9):1161–6.

71. Fazio VW, et al. A randomized multicenter trial to compare long-term functional outcome, quality of life, and complications of surgical procedures for low rectal cancers. Ann Surg. 2007;246(3):481–8. discussion 488–90.

72. Z'Graggen K, et al. A new surgical concept for rectal replacement after low anterior resection: the transverse coloplasty pouch. Ann Surg. 2001;234(6):780–5. discussion 785–7.

73. Ho YH, et al. Comparison of J-pouch and coloplasty pouch for low rectal cancers: a randomized, controlled trial investigating functional results and comparative anastomotic leak rates. Ann Surg. 2002;236(1):49–55.

74. Pimentel JM, et al. Transverse coloplasty pouch and colonic J-pouch for rectal cancer--a comparative study. Colorectal Dis. 2003;5(5):465–70.

75. Huber FT, Herter B, Siewert JR. Colonic pouch vs. side-to-end anastomosis in low anterior resection. Dis Colon Rectum. 1999;42(7):896–902.

76. Machado M, et al. Similar outcome after colonic pouch and side-to-end anastomosis in low anterior resection for rectal cancer: a prospective randomized trial. Ann Surg. 2003;238(2):214–20.

77. Machado M, et al. Functional and physiologic assessment of the colonic reservoir or side-to-end anastomosis after low anterior resection for rectal cancer: a two-year follow-up. Dis Colon Rectum. 2005;48(1):29–36.

78. Ho YH, Tan M, Seow-Choen F. Prospective randomized controlled study of clinical function and anorectal physiology after low anterior resection: comparison of straight and colonic J pouch anastomoses. Br J Surg. 1996;83(7):978–80.

79. Furst A, et al. Neorectal reservoir is not the functional principle of the colonic J-pouch: the volume of a short colonic J-pouch does not differ from a straight coloanal anastomosis. Dis Colon Rectum. 2002;45(5):660–7.

80. Ho YH, et al. Small colonic J-pouch improves colonic retention of liquids – randomized, controlled trial with scintigraphy. Dis Colon Rectum. 2002;45(1):76–82.

81. Baik SH, et al. Hand-sewn coloanal anastomosis for distal rectal cancer: long-term clinical outcomes. J Gastrointest Surg. 2005;9(6):775–80.

82. Laurent A, et al. Colonic J-pouch-anal anastomosis for rectal cancer: a prospective, randomized study comparing handsewn vs. stapled anastomosis. Dis Colon Rectum. 2005;48(4):729–34.

83. Smith S, et al. The efficacy of intraoperative methylene blue enemas to assess the integrity of a colonic anastomosis. BMC Surg. 2007;7:15.

84. Beard JD, et al. Intraoperative air testing of colorectal anastomoses: a prospective, randomized trial. Br J Surg. 1990;77(10):1095–7.

85. Davies AH, et al. Intra-operative air testing: an audit on rectal anastomosis. Ann R Coll Surg Engl. 1988;70(6):345–7.

86. Kwon S, et al. Routine leak testing in colorectal surgery in the Surgical Care and Outcomes Assessment Program. Arch Surg. 2012;147(4):345–51.

87. Ricciardi R, et al. Anastomotic leak testing after colorectal resection: what are the data? Arch Surg. 2009;144(5):407–11. discussion 411–2.

88. Hanna MH, Vinci A, Pigazzi A. Diverting ileostomy in colorectal surgery: when is it necessary? Langenbecks Arch Surg. 2015;400(2):145–52.

89. Kamal T, et al. Should anastomotic assessment with flexible sigmoidoscopy be routine following laparoscopic restorative left colorectal resection? Colorectal Dis. 2015;17:160.

90. Li VK, et al. Use of routine intraoperative endoscopy in elective laparoscopic colorectal surgery: can it further avoid anastomotic failure? Surg Endosc. 2009;23(11):2459–65.

91. Rombeau JL, Collins JP, Turnbull Jr RB. Left-sided colectomy with retroileal colorectal anastomosis. Arch Surg. 1978;113(8):1004–5.

92. Deloyers L. Suspension of the right colon permits without exception preservation of the anal sphincter after extensive colectomy of the transverse and left colon (including rectum). Technic -indications- immediate and late results. Lyon Chir. 1964;60:404–13.

10
Anastomotic Complications

Konstantin Umanskiy and Neil Hyman

Key Concepts

- Patients who develop diffuse peritonitis after intestinal resection with anastomosis should undergo prompt exploratory laparotomy.
- Colorectal anastomoses should be routinely tested prior to abdominal closure.
- Hemodynamically unstable patients who develop a leak after sigmoid resection should undergo a Hartmann procedure.
- Late anastomotic leaks commonly present with subtle and insidious symptoms such as failure to thrive.
- Endoscopic balloon dilation is the procedure of choice for short anastomotic strictures.
- Most cases of anastomotic bleeding resolve with conservative measures.
- Persistent anastomotic bleeding should be treated by colonoscopy with epinephrine injection and/or endoscopic clips.

Anastomotic Leak

Overview

Anastomotic leak is perhaps the most feared and dreaded complication after bowel resection [1]. The consequences of a failed intestinal anastomosis can be devastating to the patient, family, and surgeon alike. Management of an anastomotic leak typically necessitates a lengthy hospitalization with considerable morbidity, suffering, as well as the very real possibility of breathtaking cost and resource utilization [2]. This can include a prolonged stay in the intensive care unit, reoperations in a hostile and hazardous environment to control sepsis, and creation of an intestinal stoma when none was initially expected or planned [3]. Patients often require repeated imaging studies, a wide variety of invasive interventions, and many complex decisions surrounding the necessity, timing, and risk/benefit ratio of the pertinent diagnostic and therapeutic interventions.

Despite the serious and overwhelming burden that can be imposed by an anastomotic leak, we often do not know why the leak occurred in any particular patient or circumstance. There are a wide variety of factors that have been associated with an increased risk of anastomotic dehiscence, some of which may be at least partially remediable [4–10]. In general, sicker patients with more comorbidities are at higher risk. But we seldom know which of the associated factors are actually causative and particularly worthy of focus, since so many of them cluster together in the same patient. For example, patients with Crohn's disease may be considered to be at increased risk for anastomotic complications; but these patients may also be on steroids, other immunomodulatory agents, have preexisting local sepsis, and suffer from hypoproteinemia preoperatively [11].

Despite the critical importance of preventing leaks and understanding the pathophysiology of this potentially devastating problem, relatively little is known about why they actually occur. Avoiding tension on the anastomosis and assuring adequate perfusion to the two ends of the intestine to be joined remain valid and fundamental surgical principles; optimization of comorbid conditions and suspected risk factors is also of value [12]. But leaks often occur when no technical error, defect in surgical judgment, or patient-specific factor can be readily identified. Since we cannot confidently discern the causative element(s) that produced the leak, we are commonly unable to identify opportunities for improvement and devise a strategy to protect the next patient from this complication and its consequences. In short, it seems clear that our present concepts regarding the causes and prevention of anastomotic leak are lacking at best. New paradigms and avoidance strategies are badly needed.

Scope of the Problem

The reported incidence of anastomotic leakage after bowel resection varies from one to more than 20 %, based on the definitions used, location of the anastomosis, and length of

© Springer International Publishing 2016
S.R. Steele et al. (eds.), *The ASCRS Textbook of Colon and Rectal Surgery*, DOI 10.1007/978-3-319-25970-3_10

follow-up [13–21]. A leak rate in the 5–8 % range is perhaps the most commonly reported incidence. Generally speaking, small bowel anastomoses have the lowest leak rate, and low colorectal or coloanal anastomoses carry the highest risk. The importance of definitions and the criteria utilized for diagnosis of a leak when assessing clinical data cannot be overemphasized; standardization of nomenclature across institutions would enable the more robust interpretation of incidence reporting for this key patient outcome. "Anastomotic leak" can signify anything from an apparently trivial, clinically meaningless radiologic finding to a profound septic insult causing a rapid decline, multiorgan failure, and death. In a systematic review, Bruce noted that there were 56 different definitions of "leak" used in the 97 constituent studies of gastrointestinal anastomoses that were reviewed [22].

It seems clear that there is a spectrum of radiologic findings and infectious complications in patients who have undergone an intestinal anastomosis that might reasonably be described as a leak. There is little question about the proper term or diagnosis in a patient who develops peritonitis after bowel resection and is found at laparotomy to have a dehiscence of their anastomotic site. But how should we classify patients who develop an intra-abdominal abscess after surgery? Should the patient who has an abscess around their anastomosis, but no contrast extravasation on an initial imaging study, be considered to have suffered a "leak"? What if a follow-up CT scan now reveals a communication from the abscess to the colorectal anastomosis: did an occult leak cause the abscess or did the abscess erode into the anastomosis? There are countless permutations on this theme, where reasonable surgeons might disagree; in truth, the precise pathophysiology of infectious events after an anastomosis in many patients may be uncertain. This makes comparative analysis of reported outcomes between different studies difficult to interpret.

We have described a spectrum of clinical entities with distinct clinical consequences that can complicate low pelvic anastomoses, for example [23]. These include "free" leaks, anastomotic sinuses, peri-anastomotic abscesses, and fistulas. Interestingly, even patients with "simple" fluid alone in the pelvis on a CT scan without any other evidence of a leak appeared to have impaired long-term function. Anastomotic infectious complications may be divided into leak, surgical site infection (SSI) organ space, and SSI deep. One can reasonably disagree about which category an individual postoperative complication may belong to. But a composite measure such as this may enable meaningful conclusions and avoid the largely arbitrary exercise of trying to distinguish between all of the nuanced findings that the surgeon may encounter in patients who develop an infectious complication associated with an intestinal anastomosis.

Consequences

An anastomotic leak is a potentially life-threatening complication, with a reported mortality in the 10–15 % range [24–29]. Most of these deaths occur in association with sepsis and progressive multiorgan failure, especially for the leaks that present early on in the postoperative course. For this reason, timely diagnosis and treatment prior to the onset of advanced organ dysfunction has been emphasized as a key factor in reducing the mortality rate for anastomotic leaks. However, patients with a more indolent course may also succumb to venous thromboembolic or other indirect complications owing to the prolonged hospital stay, limited mobility, and persistent inflammatory state that commonly occurs in patients who have leaked.

As noted earlier, patients with an anastomotic leak often require difficult and complicated reoperations in a hostile local environment, with considerable additional postoperative morbidity. Lengthy hospitalizations, the need for an intestinal stoma, repeated imaging studies, and trips to interventional radiology for catheter placement/replacement are commonplace [30]. True functional, physical, emotional, and psychological recovery is often measured in months or even years, especially when one considers the need for additional procedures such as stoma reversals even after the acute phase has resolved. Prolonged wound care, ventral hernias, bowel obstructions, and management challenges associated with gastrointestinal adaptation to the altered anatomy may continue to be active considerations for long periods of time, consume an enormous amount of resources, and delay return to the patient's "normal" lifestyle. Further, for many patients, an intestinal stoma is a permanent consequence of the leak [31].

In addition, local sepsis may lead to an impaired functional result, especially after low pelvic anastomosis, where fibrosis can markedly impair the reservoir function of the neorectum and/or be associated with a rigid and unyielding anastomotic stricture [32]. The adverse relationship between anastomotic leak and local recurrence after rectal resection for cancer is intriguing and may have several contributing explanations [33–36]. The leak may impair local and/or systemic immunity or may simply serve as a surrogate for a more aggressive tumor, suboptimal operation, or other host-/tumor-related factors that remain to be fully defined.

Prevention

As in almost any disease process or postoperative complication, prevention is always better than treatment. Unfortunately, we still do not know why most anastomotic leaks occur, and therefore we remain limited in our ability to prevent many of them. Nonetheless, even among high-volume surgeons, significant differences may be found in leak rates, suggesting that technical and/or judgment errors play a causative role in at least some leaks [37]. Time-honored principles such as avoidance of tension on the anastomosis and assuring adequate blood supply to the two ends remain pertinent and important considerations. The role of intraoperative assessment of anastomotic blood supply has received renewed interest in recent years.

TABLE 10-1. Reported risk factors for anastomotic leak

Patient factors
  Overall physiological status
  Steroids
  Need for low rectal/anal anastomosis
  Immunomodulators
  Malnutrition/weight loss
  Emergency surgery
  Obesity
  Male gender
  Advanced age
  Alcohol use
  COPD
  Cigarette smoking
  Previous radiation
  Prior abdominal surgery
  Right vs. left colon (left increased)
  Primary disease (e.g., Crohn's disease, diverticulitis)
Surgeon factors
  Length of surgery
  Blood loss
  Use of pelvic drain
  Bowel preparation
  Use of vasopressors
  Proximal diversion
  Blood supply

Many patient- and surgeon-specific factors have been associated with an increased risk of an anastomotic leak (Table 10-1). However, many are simply markers for a sicker patient or serve as surrogates for various disease processes and/or a compromised host. So, it is unclear how many of the factors on this lengthy list are simply associated with a leak versus actually contributory, and how much effort or emphasis should be placed on trying to remediate them. Further, many factors (e.g., gender, age, disease process) are immutable and just a fact of life. Nonetheless, attention to controlling certain risk factors does seem prudent and worthwhile. These would include smoking cessation, optimization of nutritional status, and weight loss if possible [37–44].

Anastomoses should be tested intraoperatively when feasible, as occult disruptions may be identified and definitively treated [45–47]. A systematic review of the intraoperative assessment of colorectal anastomotic integrity documented an impressive reduction in anastomotic complications when the anastomosis was tested during surgery [11]. When a leak is identified intraoperatively, a sober and disciplined approach is required. Sometimes there is a focal, well-defined defect in an otherwise healthy-appearing anastomosis that can be readily repaired with a suture. However, in other circumstances, such as when there is concern about the blood supply, the defect is poorly visualized or there is a major disruption, it is best to start over, redo the anastomosis entirely, and retest. There is no sense trying to "perfume the pig" by placing a series of sutures into a poorly exposed, amorphous mass of tissue in the hope that the defect will be adequately addressed. With distal anastomoses, this will often include adding a proximal loop ileostomy. Mature surgical

judgment, sometimes including intraoperative consultation with an experienced colleague, can enable optimal and objective decision making.

Intriguing work regarding the relationship of the microbiome and anastomotic leak has been reported by Alverdy and coworkers [48, 49]. It may be that the local microbial environment plays a critical role in anastomotic healing. Specific bacteria that produce locally destructive collagenolytic proteins (e.g., certain *Enterococcus*, *Pseudomonas*, or *Serratia* species) may be an important cause of anastomotic leaks, and perioperative suppression/eradication of these microbes may reduce leak rates. A large multicenter trial is underway to further explore this hypothesis.

Diagnosis

Perhaps one of the biggest fallacies perpetuated over the years about anastomotic leaks is that the diagnosis is typically straightforward and clinically obvious. This misconception is commonly exacerbated by surgical morbidity conferences where these cases are often reviewed. All attendees know or strongly suspect the patient in question suffered a leak (since it is being presented at a complication conference) and are often quick to suggest the diagnosis at the first mention of an abnormal vital sign, laboratory value, or upon review of radiologic studies.

Certainly, there are patients who present in the first few days after surgery with excruciating abdominal pain, hemodynamic instability, diffuse peritonitis, and a rapid and dramatic change in their clinical course; the diagnosis is often plainly evident and requires few if any ancillary studies (even in retrospect). However, in the nuances of actual clinical practice, medical decision making in the setting of a real patient where anastomotic leak is considered is usually far more difficult since, unfortunately, most leaks actually present in a more subtle and insidious manner [50, 51]. We reviewed the clinical course of 452 consecutive patients who had a bowel resection with anastomosis. Even in "uncomplicated" recoveries, tachycardia and tachypnea were almost routine, occurring in more than ½ of the patients frequently throughout the postoperative course. Hypotension, fever, and leukocytosis, factors commonly cited with the benefit of hindsight as reliable evidence of a leak, were also remarkably common in all patients and were poor indicators of a leak. The predictive value for abnormal vital signs or leukocytosis ranged from only 4 to 11 % [52].

Similarly, radiologic findings are often ambiguous and equivocal, commonly requiring careful and considered correlation with the clinical picture. On the one hand, the sensitivity for contrast radiography and CT scan in the setting of a leak has been reported to be in the range of 50 %, so a high index of suspicion must be maintained even when the imaging study appears to be negative [53]. On the other hand, Power has highlighted the broad overlap of radiologic findings in

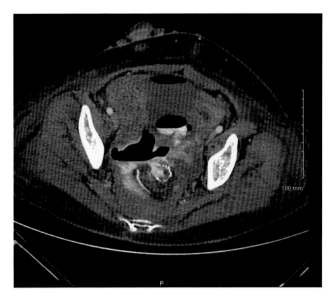

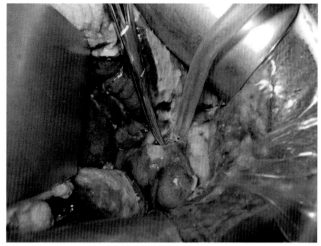

FIGURE 10-2. Diffuse peritonitis after major anastomotic disruption.

FIGURE 10-1. CT scan in a patient with anastomotic leak after low anterior resection.

postoperative patients with or without a leak. For example, free air was seen on CT scan up to 9 days after surgery and localized extraluminal air up to 26 days postoperatively in patients without a leak. Of the many and varied radiologic findings that are often considered to be indicative of a leak, only loculated fluid with air (Figure 10-1) was observed more commonly in patients with an anastomotic leak [54].

With the foregoing as a background, it perhaps should not be surprising that the diagnosis of an anastomotic leak, in its many varied forms and presentations, is often quite delayed. In our review of 1223 patients undergoing an intestinal resection with anastomosis, the leak rate was 2.7 %. Of note, 14/33 leaks were only diagnosed upon readmission to the hospital, and 12 % were identified more than 30 days after surgery. The positive predictive value of CT scan was 89.5 % versus 40 % for contrast enema. However, these studies were used in somewhat different clinical settings, and the CT scans were often thought to be suggestive of a leak, rather than truly definitive [55]. Categorizing CT scans dichotomously into "positive" or "negative" can often seem to be a somewhat contrived exercise, in light of the open-ended and ambiguous terms that are often utilized to describe the radiologic findings.

So, the broad overlap in vital signs, clinical and radiologic findings between patients who have an uncomplicated postoperative course and those who are diagnosed with a leak, and the similarities in presentation between a leak and other common postoperative complications often make the diagnosis challenging in many clinical settings. The fact is that surgeons often worry or even agonize when things turn out to be fine and are commonly led astray by "reassuring" clinical data when patients have actually suffered an anastomotic leak. More reliable clinical, laboratory, and radiologic tools would be of great utility.

Treatment

Many factors need to be considered when deciding on the most appropriate management option for a patient with an anastomotic leak [56]. These include patient-specific factors such as the degree of hemodynamic derangement, physiologic reserve, nutritional status, comorbid complications, initial surgical indications/goals, and the potential need for additional treatments (e.g., chemotherapy for a malignant diagnosis). Similarly, features of the leak such as location (e.g., intraperitoneal vs. extraperitoneal), size of the defect, and the presence of concomitant tissue ischemia also play a major role in the surgeon's decision-making process.

Perhaps the most useful classification in outlining the principles of management is early versus late presentation. Patients with an early leak classically present in the first week after surgery with signs and symptoms of peritonitis, organ dysfunction associated with sepsis, and hemodynamic instability. In this clinical setting with a profoundly sick patient, the diagnosis is generally quite evident, and prompt return to the operating room is required (Figure 10-2). Radiologic studies are often unnecessary and may provide a false sense of reassurance as described above; hoping against hope it will just delay treatment and allow the septic picture to progress. The operating room is often the only place where this pivotal question can be definitively answered and addressed.

However, it bears repeating that even in the early postoperative period, patients with an anastomotic leak will often present with signs and symptoms that lead the surgeon astray and suggest other serious postoperative complications such as a pulmonary embolism, cerebrovascular event, or acute coronary syndrome. This is because patients with a leak will often appear short of breath and develop mental status changes, and the basic acute work-up will commonly reveal an abnormal chest X-ray or EKG. The surgical team must maintain a high index of suspicion for a leak in this setting and remain wary of alternative diagnoses.

Once the diagnosis is established in the first few days after the initial surgery, most patients will require operative exploration. Intravenous antibiotics and close observation may be appropriate in a few highly selected patients with small, contained leaks that otherwise appear reasonably well; most commonly, these are patients who have undergone a low colorectal anastomosis, especially if they have a proximal diversion. Otherwise, at reoperative surgery, the peritoneal cavity is thoroughly irrigated and appropriate cultures obtained. In general, patients with a small bowel to small bowel or ileocolic anastomosis are best treated with resection and repeat anastomosis. Patients who are hemodynamically unstable may be treated with an ileostomy and end-loop stoma, where the distal end is brought out through the same aperture as the ileostomy (Figure 10-3a–c). This markedly simplifies later reconstitution of the gastrointestinal track, which may be done without the need for laparotomy. This "minor" maneuver at the end of a taxing operation may be the difference between later stoma takedown and a permanent ileostomy, as many patients who are candidates for a stoma takedown will not be good candidates for another major laparotomy after a leak. Anastomosis with proximal loop ileostomy is another alternative to address this situation where primary anastomosis alone is deemed unwise.

When a colo-colic anastomosis breaks down, dividing the anastomosis and creating an end colostomy is usually the most appropriate option. Resection with anastomosis and proximal loop ileostomy is another option for hemodynamically stable patients. Performing an anastomosis without diversion in a hemodynamically unstable patient may greatly complicate diagnosing another leak after reoperation, and the second insult may prove too much for the patient to safely tolerate.

A leak after low anterior resection may create some challenging management decisions. If the anastomosis is divided and a colostomy created, then going back months later to attempt another low pelvic anastomosis to a short Hartmann stump may be a formidable endeavor; a pull through with hand-sewn coloanal anastomosis is often required. When there is no ischemia and the leak is relatively small and contained, loop ileostomy and drainage of the anastomosis is usually most appropriate. In stable patients with major disruptions, resection with anastomosis and proximal diversion may also be an option.

Although there is no hard and fast cutoff from "early" to "late" leaks, the management of anastomotic leaks diagnosed beyond the first week to 10 days postoperatively usually differs in many important regards from its earlier counterpart. These patients most commonly have a more insidious, subtle, and nonspecific presentation. Clinical features commonly include a poor appetite, low-grade fever, incomplete resolution of a postoperative ileus, and a generalized failure to thrive. Careful imaging including a CT scan of the abdomen and pelvis with intravenous and enteric (including rectal) contrast is typically the key to diagnosis and treatment planning. Reoperative surgery is usually unnecessary

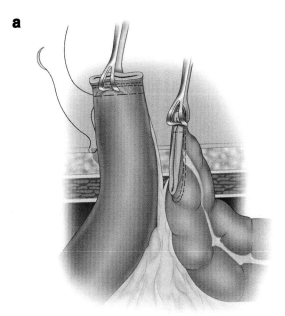

a

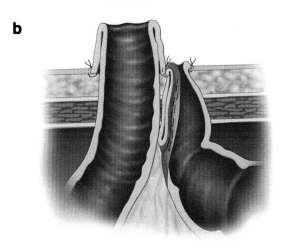

b

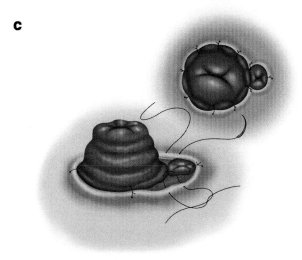

c

FIGURE 10-3. End-loop stoma. (**a**) The bowel is divided and each end is brought up through the opening. (**b**) The proximal portion is completely matured, while the distal end has only a corner matured. (**c**) Side and top view of the matured stoma.

and will quite often make things worse. Beyond a week to 10 days, patients will commonly have an obliterative peritoneal reaction, making dissection difficult and fraught with the danger of extending the damage to adjacent loops of small intestine as well as making the local situation worse. Adhesions are commonly dense and tenacious, leading to prolonged dissection, bleeding, and the need to anastomose, repair, or exteriorize fixed and friable bowel. If surgery is truly needed to control sepsis, the operation must be very carefully planned, focused, disciplined, and goal directed.

Most patients with late presentations are most often best managed by patience, antibiotics, and percutaneous drainage. Even in the presence of a demonstrable leak, percutaneous drainage alone may allow for complete resolution of the local sepsis and ultimate healing of the anastomosis. Unfortunately, this is commonly a slow process, requiring patience, serial imaging, and repeat percutaneous interventions. Both covered stents and vacuum-assisted devices have been used with anecdotal success [57–59].

Nutritional support, using the enteral route whenever possible, should not be neglected. Although patients are commonly restricted to clear liquids or nothing by mouth for prolonged intervals based on surgical custom, it is not at all clear that this enables healing of the anastomosis and may often exacerbate patient discomfort (physical and psychological) and diminish their ability to tolerate a prolonged recovery with repeated imaging studies and invasive interventions.

Anastomotic Stricture

Anastomotic stricture is a relatively common complication of colorectal or pouch-anal anastomosis, occurring in 3–30 % of cases [60], less commonly so following anastomosis elsewhere in the large intestine. The exact pathophysiology underlying anastomotic strictures remains unknown. Ischemia, incomplete "doughnuts" from stapled anastomotic reconstruction, anastomotic leakage, hemorrhage, and radiotherapy are probably contributing factors to this [61–66]. An anastomotic stricture may be defined as a chronic narrowing or obstruction to the flow of intestinal contents resulting in clinical signs or symptoms of complete or partial bowel obstruction [62]. Symptoms most commonly associated with rectal strictures are increasing constipation and partial large bowel obstruction. Other symptoms may include change in stool caliber or overflow diarrhea.

Asymptomatic patients with a stricture and diverting stoma can be identified based on digital rectal examination or upon radiographic or endoscopic evaluation prior to stoma reversal. Diagnosis is typically made by imaging (i.e., contrast enema) or endoscopically—the inability to pass a 12-mm-diameter sigmoidoscope through the anastomotic narrowing [60]. Anastomotic strictures frequently manifest at some delayed interval after surgery, except for cases associated with early postoperative anastomotic edema.

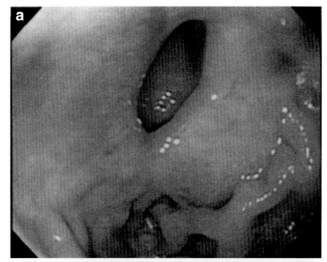
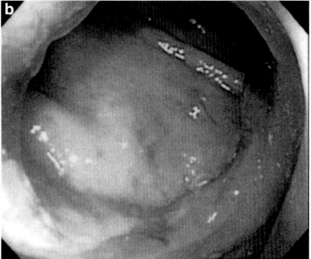

FIGURE 10-4. (**a**) Colorectal anastomotic stricture, before dilation. (**b**) Anastomosis after through the scope balloon dilation.

Luchtefeld [60] found that the stenosis was diagnosed at 1–6 months after surgery in 66 (54 %) of 123 patients, and at more than 6 months after surgery in 17 patients (14 %). Schlegel reported a series of 27 patients with a median time to diagnosis of 7.2 months [62]. Therefore, patients must be followed not only immediately after surgery but the diagnosis must be kept in mind for some time thereafter. Recurrent cancer must be considered as a cause of stricture prior to deciding on the treatment approach.

Short strictures in low colorectal, coloanal, and ileoanal pouch anastomoses can be treated by simple digital dilation, commonly performed in the outpatient setting or under anesthesia. Narrow distal strictures that do not admit the tip of the examining finger can be dilated with Hegar dilators, which are effective in achieving a sufficiently patent anastomosis with a low rate of restenosis.

Endoscopic balloon dilatation is highly effective, and the most commonly used method for treatment of short (<1 cm) colonic and colorectal anastomotic strictures (Figure 10-4a, b).

Several studies of balloon dilation of colonic anastomotic stricture reported success rates that range from 86 to 97 % [5–7]. Two types of balloon can be used for dilation: over the wire (OTW) and through the scope (TTS). The mechanical principles of these techniques are similar resulting in the dilating force being delivered radially and over the entire length of the stricture. Successful dilation is defined as an anastomotic lumen becoming wide enough to allow passage of a standard 12-mm diameter colonoscope and post-procedural relief of obstructive symptoms. Additional dilations may be required if the structure recurs.

The less frequently used method of bougie dilation of anastomotic stricture is accomplished by the radial vector of an axially directed force. Werre [67] treated 15 patients with a benign stricture after low anterior resection by using polyvinyl bougies (Savary-Gilliard). After a mean follow-up of 19 months, normal defecation was restored in ten patients; in five patients, there was only partial improvement, but only three required another form of treatment. No complications were reported. In a case study, Pietropaolo [68] found balloon dilation more effective than bougie dilation with respect to the proportion of patients successfully treated in a single session (76.9 % vs. 51.8 %).

Recurrent cicatricle strictures may be treated with the combination of incision plus balloon dilation [69]. Endoscopic stricturotomy with neodymium-yttrium aluminum garnet laser together with balloon dilation were performed by Luck in ten patients [70]. Treatment was successful, without recurrence or complication, in nine patients (median follow-up 82 months). In the remaining patient, the stricture recurred after 6 years. Brandimarte [71] treated 39 consecutive patients with an anastomotic colorectal stricture endoscopically by making six radial incisions electrosurgically with a precut papillotome. In all cases, satisfactory dilation of the stricture was obtained without complication, and no recurrence was identified at a mean follow-up of 25 months. Complications of electrocautery and laser strictureplasty are very low, with only one group reporting a 2.7 % technical failure rate [72]. Alternatively, transanal endoscopic microsurgical approach (TEM) strictureplasty with electrocautery or laser can be used. Endoscopic, TEM, or strictureplasty approach has been described as effective in 90–100 % of patients with a mean follow-up of 6–92 months [69, 70, 72–74].

Anastomotic strictures that are irregular, markedly angulated, fixed, or longer than 1–2 cm in length, may not be amenable to endoscopic treatment. In the ASCRS survey, surgery was required in 34 patients (28 %), including resection in 18 patients and permanent colostomy in 13 patients [60]. Reoperative rectal dissection in the presence of scarring from previous operations or from ongoing local sepsis is technically demanding and should not be underestimated. Shleigel [62] reported a series of 27 patients who underwent surgical correction of anastomotic stenoses. The authors performed seven colorectal anastomoses for upper rectal anastomotic strictures and 20 coloanal anastomoses for middle and lower rectal strictures (19 Soave's procedures and one colon J-pouch-anal anastomosis). Intestinal continuity was restored in all cases.

In long segment distal rectal strictures or after failure of local therapy, immediate or delayed coloanal anastomosis through a combined abdominal and perineal approach is recommended [75]. A less invasive technique using an end-to-end anastomosis (EEA) stapler may be applied to correct mid- to proximal rectal strictures without the need for laparotomy. Prior to stapling, the rectal anastomotic stricture is dilated and assessed by rigid sigmoidoscopy. Both the anvil and the rod of the circular stapler are introduced transanally, and the instrument positioned until the mural portion of the rectal stricture is caught between the anvil and the rod. The EEA is then fired so that a crescent-shaped rim of the stricture is stapled and resected. The biggest drawback to this method is its inability to treat any tight stricture that would not allow the anvil of the EEA to pass through its opening. An alternative method involves a laparotomy- or laparoscopy-guided approach to introduce the anvil of the stapler from above, via a small colostomy, and inserting the EEA stapler transanally until resistance from the stricture is met. Once positioned correctly, the stapler and anvil are mated and tightened, and the stricture is resected. Long-term results following this technique of stricture resection have been reported as 89–100 % return to normal bowel function with a mean follow-up of 12–49 months [62, 76].

Self-expanding metallic stents (SEMS) have been considered for medium-term symptom relief for recalcitrant benign colorectal strictures in patients who are otherwise unfit for surgery; but their use is associated with a high rate of delayed complications such as perforation, migration, and re-obstruction in up to 38 % of cases [77]. The SEM stents can be considered for short-term relief of acute obstruction and a as a bridge to elective surgery. Newer types of biodegradable stents [78] and fully covered self-expanding stents [79] have been evaluated, but their role in benign colonic and colorectal anastomotic strictures remains undefined.

Finally, diverting ileostomy or colostomy may be the only available treatment option for symptomatic relief of those patients who have failed all treatments or are not candidates for extensive surgical intervention to correct the anastomotic structure.

Anastomotic Bleeding

Anastomotic bleeding following stapled colorectal, colonic, or intestinal anastomosis is a common but usually self-limited complication, with the majority of cases resolving spontaneously with expectant management. Postoperative colorectal anastomotic bleeding can occur in up to 5 % of anastomoses [80–82]. Anastomotic bleeding may occur when the mesentery is incorporated into the staple line and can be further exacerbated by the use of anticoagulant and antiplatelet agents. Continued hemorrhage is rare but, when it occurs, often requires further treatment.

The clinical presentation of anastomotic bleeding is similar to lower gastrointestinal bleeding from other causes, but interventional therapy is more difficult owing to the risk of ischemia or breakdown of the anastomosis. The optimal treatment choices depend on the site of bleeding, patient factors, and skill of the surgeon or endoscopist and may include conservative treatment with packed red blood cells and coagulation factors transfusion, endoscopic therapy, angiographic embolization, locally applied vasoactive substances, or reoperation with anastomotic refashioning.

The risk of postoperative bleeding can be decreased by avoiding the inclusion of mesocolon into the staple line. We also recommend intraoperative assessment of colorectal anastomoses with intraoperative flexible sigmoidoscopy. Ishihara found active and continuous bleeding from the stapled anastomosis intraoperatively in up to 9.6 % of colorectal anastomoses [83]. In the intraoperative setting, an actively bleeding vessel can be visualized and immediate hemostasis achieved by placement sutures under direct inspection, endoscopic injection of 1:200,000 epinephrine, or careful coagulation.

Postoperative anastomotic bleeding can occur from 4 h to 9 days following the operation [84]. Initial management includes correction of any associated coagulopathy and transfusion of blood and blood products if necessary. Attention should be paid to the amount blood and clots that patient is passing as a more accurate measure of the rate of bleeding; the hemoglobin and hematocrit changes may not occur until hours later. Between 2 and 10 units of packed red blood cells may be required in the nonoperative treatment of anastomotic bleeding [16]. It may be important to keep the patient warm by infusing warmed solutions and preventing hypothermia.

If anastomotic bleeding persists, the preferred next step is usually colonoscopic evaluation and management. Colonoscopy allows for direct inspection of the anastomosis with subsequent application of various means of hemostasis. Submucosal peri-anastomotic injection of up to 10 ml of 1:200,000 epinephrine in saline has been shown to result in control of anastomotic bleeding [84]. Cirocco reported the successful use of electrocoagulation, although it was noted that an anastomotic fistula that developed in one of six cases may have been related to this technique [85]. This may be due to the presence of staples at the bleeding site; the dissipation of energy may not be uniform and localized leading to increased tissue damage.

Endoscopic application of clips is an excellent alternative to coagulation and has been shown to be safe and effective in control of anastomotic bleeding [81]. Endoscopic therapy has obvious advantages in terms of less physiological stress on the patient, no requirement for general anesthesia compared with the surgical revision of anastomosis, and is clearly less invasive and more cost-effective. Colonoscopic hemostasis should be performed by a skilled and experienced provider proficient in advanced endoscopic techniques. An alternative course of action should always be entertained in the event endoscopic therapy is unsuccessful, particularly if the bleeding is severe, making a clear endoluminal view of the point of hemorrhage impossible.

Briskly bleeding anastomoses may be amenable to angiographic localization and treatment of the bleeding site. This strategy provides access for vasopressin infusion or embolization to control the hemorrhage. Vasopressin may be associated with significant complications such as myocardial or intestinal ischemia and infarction and therefore has to be carefully considered [86].

Angiographic embolization is an alternative to vasopressin infusion. Although this option avoids myocardial complications, it may precipitate bowel ischemia and infarction by interrupting the distal arterial blood supply [87]. These angiographic methods are best reserved for other intestinal anastomoses, such as in the small bowel, where the endoscopic approach is significantly limited. Although extremely rare, significant anastomotic bleeding after large bowel resection can be severe enough to require reoperation with surgical revision or reconstruction of anastomosis.

References

1. Hyman NH. Managing anastomotic leaks from intestinal anastomoses. Surgeon. 2009;7(1):31–5.
2. Marinatou A, Theodorpoulos GE, Karanika S, et al. Do anastomotic leaks impair postoperative health-related quality of life after rectal cancer surgery? A case-matched study. Dis Colon Rectum. 2014;57(2):181–7.
3. Makela JT, Kiviniemi H, Laitinen S. Risk factors for anastomotic leakage after left-sided colorectal resection with rectal anastomosis. Dis Colon Rectum. 2003;46(5):653–60.
4. Vignali A, Fazio VW, Lavery IC. Factors associated with the occurrence of leaks in stapled rectal anastomoses. A review of 1014 patients. J Am Coll Surg. 1997;185:105–13.
5. Van Geldare D, Fa-Si-Oen P, Noach LA, et al. Complications after colorectal surgery without mechanical bowel preparation. J Am Coll Surg. 2002;194:40–7.
6. Eckman C, Kujath P, Schiedeck THK, et al. Anastomotic leakage following low anterior resection: results of a standardized diagnostic and therapeutic approach. Int J Colorectal Dis. 2004;19:128–33.
7. Griffen FD, Knight CD, Whitaker JM, et al. The double stapling technique for low anterior resection: results, modifications, and observations. Ann Surg. 1990;211:745–52.
8. Yuh Yeh C, Changchien CR, Wang JY, et al. Pelvic drainage and other risk factors for leakage after elective anterior resection in rectal cancer patients. Ann Surg. 2005;241:9–13.
9. Karanjia ND, Corder AP, Bearn P, et al. Leakage from stapled low anastomosis after total mesorectal excision for carcinoma of the rectum. Br J Surg. 1994;81:1224–6.
10. Law WL, Chu KW. Anterior resection for rectal cancer with mesorectal excision. Ann Surg. 2004;240:260–8.
11. Ali UA, Martin ST, Rao AD, Kiran R. Impact of preoperative immunosuppressive agents on postoperative outcomes in Crohn's disease. Dis Colon Rectum. 2014;57(5):663–74.

12. Nachiappan S, Askari A, Currie A, Kennedy R, Faiz O. Intraoperative assessment of colorectal anastomotic integrity: a systematic review. Surg Endosc. 2014;24:2513–30.

13. Golub R, Golub RW, Cantu R, Stein HD. A multi-variate analysis of factors contributing to leakage of intestinal anastomosis. J Am Coll Surg. 1997;184:364–72.

14. Mileski WJ, Joehl RJ, Rege V, Nahrwold DL. Treatment of anastomotic leakage following low anterior colon resection. Arch Surg. 1988;123:968–71.

15. Hansen O, Schwenk W, Hucke HP, Sock W. Colorectal stapled anastomoses. Experiences and results. Dis Colon Rectum. 1996;39:30–5.

16. Jex RK, Van Hcerden JA, Wolff BG, et al. Gastrointestinal anastomoses. Factors affecting early complications. Ann Surg. 1987;206:138–41.

17. Max W, Sweeny WB, Bailey HR, et al. Results of 1000 single layer continuous polypropylene intestinal anastomoses. Am J Surg. 1991;162:461–7.

18. Heald RJ, Leicester RJ. The low stapled anastomosis. Br J Surg. 1981;68:333–7.

19. Marijnen CA, Kapiteijn E, van de Velde CJ, et al. Acute side effects and complications after short term preoperative radiotherapy combined with total mesorectal excision in primary rectal cancer. J Clin Oncol. 2002;20:817–25.

20. Schrock TR, Deveney CW, Dunphy JE. Factors contributing to leak of colonic anastomosis. Ann Surg. 1973;177:513–8.

21. Branagan G, Finnis D. Prognosis after anastomotic leak in colorectal surgery. Dis Colon Rectum. 2005;48:1021–6.

22. Bruce J, Krukowski ZH, Al-Khairy G, et al. Systematic review of the definition and measurement of anastomotic leak after gastrointestinal surgery. Br J Surg. 2001;88:1157–68.

23. Caulfield H, Hyman N. Anastomotic leak after low anterior resection. JAMA Surg. 2013;148(2):177–82.

24. Docherty JG, McGregor JR, Akyol AM, et al. Comparison of manually constructed and stapled anastomoses in colorectal surgery. West of Scotland and Highland Anastomosis Study Group. Ann Surg. 1995;221:176–84.

25. Blumetti J, Chaudhry V, Clintron JR, et al. Management of anastomotic leak: lessons learned from a large colon and rectal surgery training program. World J Surg. 2014;38(4):985–91.

26. Fingerhut A, Hay JM, Elhadad A, et al. Supraperitoneal colorectal anastomosis: hand sewn versus circular staples - a controlled clinical trial. French Associations for Surgical Research. Surgery. 1995;118:479–85.

27. Bokey EL, Chapuis PH, Fung C, et al. Postoperative morbidity and mortality following resection of the colon and rectum for cancer. Dis Colon Rectum. 1995;38:480–7.

28. Alves A, Panis Y, Trancart D, et al. Factors associated with clinically significant anastomotic leakage after large bowel resection: multivariate analysis of 707 patients. World J Surg. 2002;26:499–502.

29. Biondo S, Pares D, Kreisler E, et al. Anastomotic dehiscence after resection and primary anastomosis in left-sided colonic emergencies. Dis Colon Rectum. 2005;48:2272–80.

30. Sarkissian H, Hyman N, Osler T. Postoperative fluid collections after colon resection: the utility of clinical assessment. Am J Surg. 2013;206:551–4.

31. Lim M, Akhtar S, Sasapu K, et al. Clinical and subclinical leaks after low colorectal anastomosis: a clinical and radiologic study. Dis Colon Rectum. 2006;49:1611–9.

32. Nesbakken A, Nygaard K, Lunde OC. Outcome and late functional results after anastomotic leakage following mesorectal excision for rectal cancer. Br J Surg. 2001;88:400–4.

33. Walker KG, Bell SW, Rickard MJ, et al. Anastomotic leakage is predictive of diminished survival after potentially curative resection for colorectal cancer. Ann Surg. 2004;240:255–9.

34. Law WL, Choi HK, Lee YM, et al. Anastomotic leakage is associated with poor long-term outcome in patients after curative colorectal resection for malignancy. J Gastrointest Surg. 2007;11:8–15.

35. Den Dulk M, Marijnen CAM, Collete L, Putter H, Pahlman L, Folkesson J, Bosset J-F, Rödel C, Bujko K, van deVelde CJH. Multicentre analysis of oncological and survival outcomes following anastomotic leakage after rectal cancer surgery. Br J Surg. 2009;96:1066–75.

36. Mirnezami A, Mirnezami R, Chandrakumaran K, et al. Increased local reoccurrence and reduced survival from colorectal cancer following anastomotic leak: systematic review and meta-analysis. Ann Surg. 2011;253(5):890–9.

37. Hyman NH, Osler T, Cataldo P, Burns EH, Shackford SR. Anastomotic leaks after bowel reconstruction: what does peer review teach us about the relationship between postoperative mortality? J Am Coll Surg. 2009;208(1):48–52.

38. Kang CY, Halabi WJ, Chaudhry OO, Nguyen V, Pigazzi A, Carmichael JC, Mills S, Stamos MJ. Risk factors for anastomotic leakage after anterior resection for rectal cancer. JAMA Surg. 2013;148:65–71.

39. Richards CH, Campbell V, Ho C, Hayes J, Elliot T, Thompson-Fawcett M. Smoking is a major risk factor for anastomotic leak in patients undergoing low anterior resection. Colorectal Dis. 2012;14:628–33.

40. Telem DA, Chin EH, Nguyen SQ, Divino CM. Risk factors for anastomotic leak following colorectal surgery: a case-control study. Arch Surg. 2010;145:371–6.

41. Rullier E, Laurent C, Garrelon JL, et al. Risk factors for anastomotic leakage after resection of rectal cancer. Br J Surg. 1997;185:355–8.

42. Lipska M, Bissett IP, Parry BR, et al. Anastomotic leakage after lower gastrointestinal anastomosis: men are at high risk. ANZ J Surg. 2006;76:579–85.

43. Peeters KC, Tollenaar RA, Marijnen CA, et al. Risk factors for anastomotic failure after total mesorectal excision of rectal cancer. Br J Surg. 2005;92:211–6.

44. Park JS, Choi G-S, Kim SH, Kim HR, Kim NK, Lee KY, Kang SB, Kim JY, Lee KY, Kim BC, Bae BN, Son GM, Lee S, Kang H. Multicenter analysis of risk factors for anastomotic leakage after laparoscopic rectal cancer excision: the Korean laparoscopic colorectal surgery study group. Ann Surg. 2013;257(4):665–71.

45. Beard JD, Nicholson ML, Sayers RD, Lloyd D, Everson NW. Intraoperative air testing of colorectal anastomoses: a prospective, randomized trial. Br J Surg. 1990;77:1095–7.

46. Ricciardi R, Roberts PL, Read TE, Marcello PW, Hall JF, Schoetz DJ. How often do patients return to the operating room after colorectal resections? Colorectal Dis. 2012;14:515–21.

47. Jafari MD, Lee KH, Halabi WJ, Mills SD, Carmichael JC, Stamos MJ, Pigazzi A. The use of indocyanine green fluorescence to assess anastomotic perfusion during robotic assisted laparoscopic rectal surgery. Surg Endosc. 2013;27(8):3003–8.

48. Shogan BD, Carlisle EM, Alverdy JC, et al. Do we really know why colorectal anastomoses leak? J Gastrointest Surg. 2013;17(9):1698–707.
49. Shogan BD, An GC, Schardey HM, et al. Proceedings of the first international summit on intestinal anastomotic leak, Chicago, Illinois, October 4-5, 2012. Surg Infect. 2014;15(5):479–89.
50. Pickleman J, Watson W, Cunningham J, et al. The failed gastrointestinal anastomosis: an inevitable catastrophe? J Am Surg. 1999;188:473–82.
51. Platell C, Barwood N, Dorfmann G, et al. The incidence of anastomotic leaks in patient undergoing colorectal surgery. Colorectal Dis. 2006;9:71–9.
52. Larson E, Hyman N, Osler T. Abnormal vital signs are common after bowel resection and do not predict anastomotic leaks. J Am Coll Surg. 2014;218:1195–200.
53. Nesbakken A, Nygaard K, Lunde OC, et al. Anastomotic leak following mesorectal excision for rectal cancer: true incidence and diagnostic challenges. Colorectal Dis. 2005;7:576–81.
54. Power N, Atri M, Ryan S, et al. CT assessment of anastomotic bowel leak. Clin Radiol. 2007;62:37–42.
55. Hyman N, Manchester T, Osler T, et al. Anastomotic leaks after intestinal anastomosis: it's later than you think. Ann Surg. 2007;245:254–8.
56. Landman RG. Surgical management of anastomotic leak following colorectal surgery. Semin Colon Rectal Surg. 2014; 25:58–66.
57. DiMaio CJ, Dorfman MP, Gardner GJ, et al. Covered esophageal self-expandable metal stents in the nonoperative management of postoperative colorectal anastomotic leaks. Gastrointest Endosc. 2012;76(2):431–5.
58. Lamazza A, Fiori E, Schillaci A, Sterpetti AV, Lezoche E. Treatment of anastomotic stenosis and leakage after colorectal resection for cancer with self-expandable metal stents. Am J Surg. 2014;208:465.
59. Weidenhagen R, Gruetzner KU, Wiecken T, Spelsberg F, Jauch KW. Endoscopic of the rectum: a new method. Surg Endosc. 2008;22(8):1818–25.
60. Luchtefeld MA, Milsom JW, Senagore A, Surrell JA, Mazier WP. Colorectal anastomotic stenosis. Results of a survey of the ASCRS membership. Dis Colon Rectum. 1989;32(9):733–6.
61. Orsay CP, Bass EM, Firfer B, Ramakrishnan V, Abcarian H. Blood flow in colon anastomotic stricture formation. Dis Colon Rectum. 1995;38(2):202–6.
62. Schlegel RD, Dehni N, Parc R, Caplin S, Tiret E. Results of reoperations in colorectal anastomotic strictures. Dis Colon Rectum. 2001;44(10):1464–8.
63. Chung RS, Hitch DC, Armstrong DN. The role of tissue ischemia in the pathogenesis of anastomotic stricture. Surgery. 1988;104(5):824–9.
64. Aston NO, Owen WJ, Irving JD. Endoscopic balloon dilatation of colonic anastomotic strictures. Br J Surg. 1989;76(8):780–2.
65. Venkatesh KS, Ramanujam PS, McGee S. Hydrostatic balloon dilatation of benign colonic anastomotic strictures. Dis Colon Rectum. 1992;35(8):789–91.
66. Dinneen MD, Motson RW. Treatment of colonic anastomotic strictures with 'through the scope' balloon dilators. J R Soc Med. 1991;84(5):264–6. Pubmed Central PMCID: 1293221.
67. Werre A, Mulder C, van Heteren C, Bilgen ES. Dilation of benign strictures following low anterior resection using Savary-Gilliard bougies. Endoscopy. 2000;32(5):385–8.
68. Pietropaolo V, Masoni L, Ferrara M, Montori A. Endoscopic dilation of colonic postoperative strictures. Surg Endosc. 1990; 4(1):26–30.
69. Hagiwara A, Sakakura C, Shirasu M, Torii T, Hirata Y, Yamagishi H. Sigmoidofiberscopic incision plus balloon dilatation for anastomotic cicatricial stricture after anterior resection of the rectum. World J Surg. 1999;23(7):717–20.
70. Luck A, Chapuis P, Sinclair G, Hood J. Endoscopic laser stricturotomy and balloon dilatation for benign colorectal strictures. ANZ J Surg. 2001;71(10):594–7.
71. Brandimarte G, Tursi A, Gasbarrini G. Endoscopic treatment of benign anastomotic colorectal stenosis with electrocautery. Endoscopy. 2000;32(6):461–3.
72. Truong S, Willis S, Schumpelick V. Endoscopic therapy of benign anastomotic strictures of the colorectum by electroincision and balloon dilatation. Endoscopy. 1997;29(9):845–9.
73. Kato K, Saito T, Matsuda M, Imai M, Kasai S, Mito M. Successful treatment of a rectal anastomotic stenosis by transanal endoscopic microsurgery (TEM) using the contact Nd:YAG laser. Surg Endosc. 1997;11(5):485–7.
74. Hunt TM, Kelly MJ. Endoscopic transanal resection (ETAR) of colorectal strictures in stapled anastomoses. Ann R Coll Surg Engl. 1994;76(2):121–2. Pubmed Central PMCID: 2502211.
75. Sabbagh C, Maggiori L, Panis Y. Management of failed low colorectal and coloanal anastomosis. J Visc Surg. 2013;150(3): 181–7.
76. Conner WE, Jetmore AB, Heryer JW. Circular stapled rectal strictureplasty with the proximate intraluminal stapler. Dis Colon Rectum. 1995;38(6):660–3.
77. Small AJ, Young-Fadok TM, Baron TH. Expandable metal stent placement for benign colorectal obstruction: outcomes for 23 cases. Surg Endosc. 2008;22(2):454–62.
78. Repici A, Pagano N, Rando G, Carlino A, Vitetta E, Ferrara E, et al. A retrospective analysis of early and late outcome of biodegradable stent placement in the management of refractory anastomotic colorectal strictures. Surg Endosc. 2013;27(7): 2487–91.
79. Caruso A, Conigliaro R, Manta R, Manno M, Bertani H, Barbera C, et al. Fully covered self-expanding metal stents for refractory anastomotic colorectal strictures. Surg Endosc. 2014;29:1175.
80. Lustosa SA, Matos D, Atallah AN, Castro AA. Stapled versus handsewn methods for colorectal anastomosis surgery. Cochrane Database Syst Rev. 2001; (3): CD003144
81. Malik AH, East JE, Buchanan GN, Kennedy RH. Endoscopic haemostasis of staple-line haemorrhage following colorectal resection. Colorectal Dis. 2008;10(6):616–8.
82. Linn TY, Moran BJ, Cecil TD. Staple line haemorrhage following laparoscopic left-sided colorectal resections may be more common when the inferior mesenteric artery is preserved. Tech Coloproctol. 2008;12(4):289–93.
83. Ishihara S, Watanabe T, Nagawa H. Intraoperative colonoscopy for stapled anastomosis in colorectal surgery. Surg Today. 2008;38(11):1063–5.

84. Perez RO, Sousa Jr A, Bresciani C, Proscurshim I, Coser R, Kiss D, et al. Endoscopic management of postoperative stapled colorectal anastomosis hemorrhage. Tech Coloproctol. 2007; 11(1):64–6.

85. Cirocco WC, Golub RW. Endoscopic treatment of postoperative hemorrhage from a stapled colorectal anastomosis. Am Surg. 1995;61(5):460–3.

86. Atabek U, Pello MJ, Spence RK, Alexander JB, Camishion RC. Arterial vasopressin for control of bleeding from a stapled intestinal anastomosis. Report of two cases. Dis Colon Rectum. 1992;35(12):1180–2.

87. Jander HP, Russinovich NA. Transcatheter gelfoam embolization in abdominal, retroperitoneal, and pelvic hemorrhage. Radiology. 1980;136(2):337–44.

Part II
Anorectal Disease

11
Approach to Anal Pain

Amir L. Bastawrous

Key Concepts

- A careful history should direct the diagnosis for patients with anal pain.
- A considerate yet thorough physical exam will usually establish the diagnosis by visualizing pathology or by palpating abnormalities. If not possible in the office, then an exam under anesthesia should be performed.
- Imaging is rarely needed to determine the etiology.
- An anal fissure will typically cause sharp anal pain during and after a hard bowel movement.
- The anal pain associated with a thrombosed external hemorrhoid is usually constant and accompanied by a palpable swelling but without systemic signs of infection.
- Cancer should always be included in the differential diagnosis.

Introduction

One of the more common complaints of patients consulting with colon and rectal surgeons, general surgeons, and primary care physicians is anal pain. In Western culture, the anus is generally taboo to speak about socially. In addition, it is a body region that is difficult for an individual to inspect on himself or herself. Yet anal and rectal pathologies can be inconvenient and are commonly debilitating. It is not unusual to have a patient with an acutely thrombosed external hemorrhoid or a perianal abscess completely incapacitated by their pain. Anal pain as a symptom encompasses a broad spectrum of diagnoses from the benign and self-limited to the neoplastic and life-threatening. A thoughtful and logical methodology is essential to efficiently diagnose and treat patients with anal pain.

Patient History

As with most things in medicine, taking a careful history is foundational when evaluating patients with anal pain. Listening to patients stories in their own words with a focus on their emphasis as much as on their words typically offers clues to the underlying problem. An experienced colorectal surgeon can often surmise the patient's diagnosis prior to any examination just by listening to key descriptions by the patient. An emphasis on pain characteristics is important. One should concentrate on the duration, location (intra-anal, external), character (burning, sharp, dull), causative agents (bowel movement, diarrhea, hard stool, exercise, fecal incontinence, drainage), associated signs and symptoms (fever, chills, weight loss, change in bowel habits), and items that provide any relief (warm water bath, bowel movement, topical creams).

Other elements of the patient history are also important and can provide some guidance. A personal history of diabetes may suggest an anal abscess or Fournier's gangrene. A history of inflammatory bowel disease may hint at anal fissures, fistulae, or abscess. A medication history of infliximab or etanercept may point to psoriasis as a cause for pruritus. A strong family history of colorectal cancer may lead to consideration to rule out rectal cancer as a cause for anal pain. A history of anoreceptive intercourse may raise the concern about sexually communicable infectious diseases, anal dysplasia, or anal cancer.

Finally, one should not be misled by either the patient's or referring physician's working diagnosis; for example, an alternate diagnosis should be considered for the patient who was told they have an anal fissure but whose history doesn't fit. Frequently anal symptoms or signs are called "a hemorrhoid" by default by the non-initiated when in fact the true pathology

© Springer International Publishing 2016
S.R. Steele et al. (eds.), *The ASCRS Textbook of Colon and Rectal Surgery*, DOI 10.1007/978-3-319-25970-3_11

ranges from pruritus to anal cancer, with the occasional correctly diagnosed thrombosed external hemorrhoid.

A few symptom patterns are so common as to be nearly universal.

Anal Fissure (Figure 11-1)

Patients with a diagnosis of anal fissure typically describe sharp, "knife-like," pain during and immediately after a bowel movement [1, 2]. If the pain has not been too chronic, they may recall and describe a precedent hard, constipated bowel movement. They state that the pain may last for minutes or hours after passing stool. Sometimes the pain is so severe; they state they are afraid to have a movement. It isn't uncommon to hear a patient state that he/she will have spotting of blood on the toilet paper after wiping. Some patients will also describe relief with a warm water bath.

Acutely Thrombosed External Hemorrhoid (Figures 11-2 and 11-3)

Patients can usually tell you precisely when they developed an acutely thrombosed external hemorrhoid. They describe

sharp, constant pain after straining, either with a bowel movement (loose or constipated) or lifting something heavy. The pain will coincide with a "bulge" they feel near the anal opening. The pain will last all day, usually increasing gradually, and then decrease over the week [3–6]. Depending on when the patient presents to the office, the pain may be either increasing or decreasing in intensity. They will say it hurts to sit or touch the area. They will not have fever.

Perianal, Perirectal, or Ischiorectal Abscess (Figure 11-4)

Some of the most uncomfortable patients will be those who have an acute abscess [7–11]. Their history is one of gradually worsening pressure and pain. The pain is worse before and during a bowel movement. There may be slight improvement afterward, but the pain lingers. They will typically describe fever and chills. These patients often refuse to sit due to the pain. There can be some similarity of symptoms with patients who have a thrombosed external hemorrhoid, but the primary difference in presenting symptoms is the presence of systemic symptoms of infection. Inability to urinate is a common associated complaint.

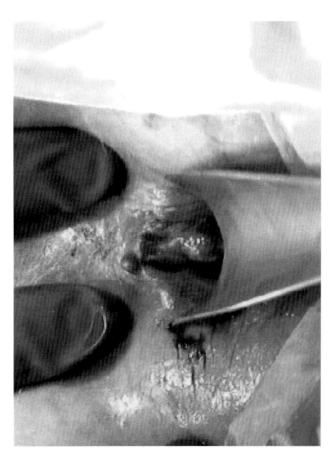

FIGURE 11-1. Anal fissure.

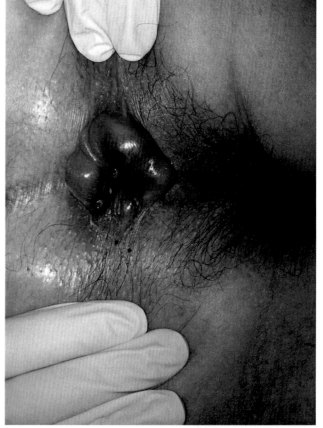

FIGURE 11-2. Acutely thrombosed external hemorrhoid.

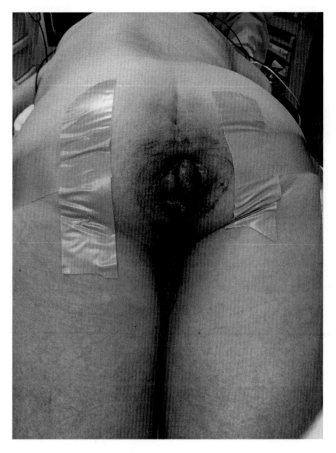

FIGURE 11-3. Hemorrhoidal crisis.

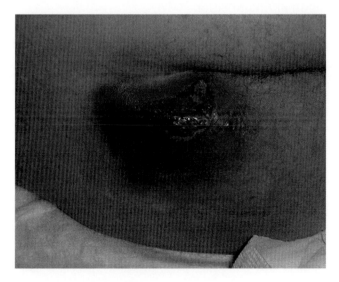

FIGURE 11-4. Perianal abscess.

Pruritus Ani (Figure 11-5)

The symptoms of patients with pruritus ani [12, 13] are occasionally described as painful but not often. Only after further discussion is the pain clarified to be burning or

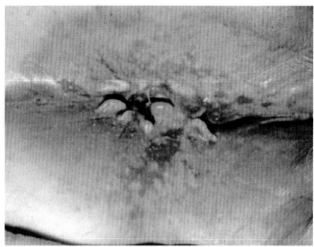

FIGURE 11-5. Pruritus ani.

itching. It is clear that the sensory response of the ano-derm and perianal skin is variable between individuals and may be less discriminatory (or may be just different) than other areas of the body. There does seem to be some overlap in the description of sensations of burning, itching, and pain. The irritation is nearly universally chronic in nature and may be associated with other synchronous diagnoses.

Levator Syndrome

The pain history that patients with pelvic floor dysfunction (levator ani syndrome, proctalgia fugax, outlet obstruction constipation) [14, 15] describe is more variable than for the other diagnoses listed so far. This lack of fitting into a typical pattern itself often points to the diagnosis. The pain may be sharp, dull, burning, or achy. It may be intermittent or constant. The pain may or may not improve with warm water baths. It may be worsened or improved with bowel movement. Often the pain is chronic and worse late in the day. Unless there is associated other pathology, they will not describe fever or bleeding. Some will complain of difficulty with evacuation of stools.

Anal or Rectal Cancer (Figure 11-6)

The fear of malignancy is often part of the reason patients seek medical attention for anal pain. Thankfully, the vast majority of patients who present with anal pain have benign processes; however, the alert physician will always consider cancer within the differential diagnosis. Physicians should not become lulled into complacency after seeing several patients with typical anal fissures, only to misdiagnose a patient with an anal verge squamous

FIGURE 11-6. Anal squamous cell carcinoma.

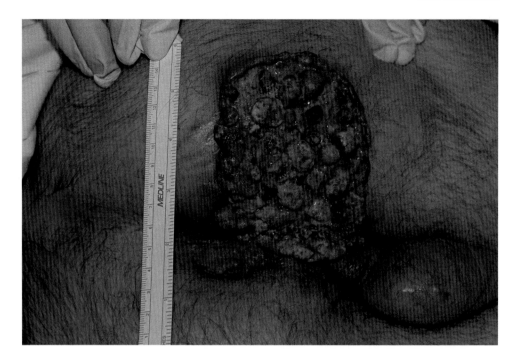

cell carcinoma with a posterior midline ulceration. Anal and rectal cancers can present with pain [16–19]. Rectal cancers can cause pain (especially if low and advanced) with bleeding and change in bowel habits [16]. There is often weight loss associated with the presentation. Anal cancer can present more subtly. Symptoms may overlap with those of anal fissure with pain during and after a bowel movement along with spotting of blood on the toilet paper. There may or may not be an associated mass felt by the patient. Fever, chills, weight loss, and groin adenopathy may also be included in the patient history.

Physical Examination

Although an astute physician can often determine a cause for a patient's anal pain from the history, it takes a careful, systematic examination to confirm the working diagnosis. While a complete physical exam is important, the regional high yield focus of the examination includes the abdomen, inguinal, perianal skin and soft tissue, buttocks and gluteal cleft, anal canal, and rectum.

Abdominal Examination

Anal pathology can on occasion manifest with abdominal findings. An obstructing cancer can cause distention or alteration of bowel sounds. Metastases can present with hepatomegaly. Diverticulitis can manifest with anal abscess or

fistula [20] in addition to abdominal pain or tenderness to palpation. Look for scars of prior operations that may suggest an associated diagnosis. Crohn's disease patients may be very thin and cachectic if they have both anal disease and bowel manifestations.

Inguinal Examination

The inguinal examination may identify adenopathy. Rectal adenocarcinomas can present with inguinal adenopathy if they are located low in the rectal vault or if there is high volume lymphatic metastatic disease in the iliac chains. Anal canal and anal margin squamous cell carcinomas, when metastatic, often present with inguinal adenopathy following anatomic drainage patterns [21–23]. This exam finding has implications for radiotherapy mapping and surveillance of disease regression or recurrence.

Perianal, Gluteal, and Intergluteal Examination

The anal examination requires extreme sensitivity to the patient's physical and psychological condition. They may be embarrassed, in pain, or fearful. Put the patient at ease. Many will appreciate a careful description of the exam as it is performed and an explanation of findings along the way. Take care to warn them before initiating any invasive component of the exam. Putting the patient at ease will foster trust and help the physician obtain more productive data in their analysis.

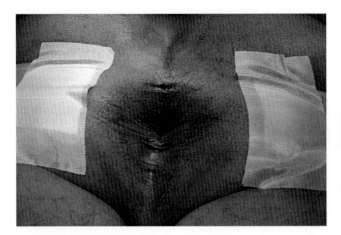

FIGURE 11-7.   Anal fistula.

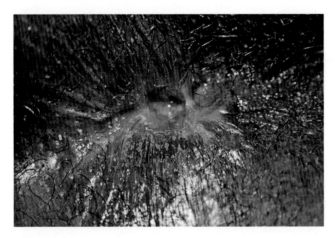

FIGURE 11-8.   Anal stricture.

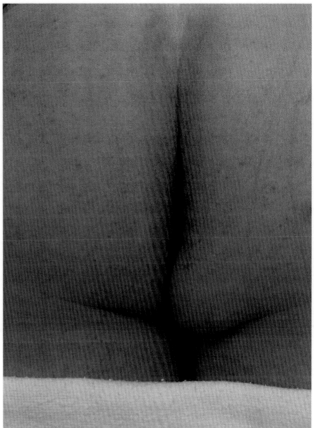

FIGURE 11-9.   Solitary fibrous tumor.

Digital Rectal Examination

Visual examination of the anus is essential. One should look for abnormalities of the skin including color, scaly skin, thickened folds, masses, secondary openings of fistula-*in-ano* (Figure 11-7), evidence of abscess with swelling or redness, skin tags, and external hemorrhoid enlargement. Usually, anal fissure can be diagnosed by visualizing the anoderm before anoscopy with gentle retraction of the buttocks to evert the anoderm and expose the fissure. In the intergluteal cleft, look for sinuses, abscess, and pilonidal pits. Anal stenosis can be seen in some patients after anal surgery (Figure 11-8). The rare subcutaneous mass may be benign or malignant. An assessment of size, fixation, character, firmness, and tenderness is sometimes helpful in establishing the diagnosis (Figure 11-9).

Next, the physician should assess the skin. Is the skin tacky to the touch, consistent with pruritus changes? Specific areas of pain, warmth, or masses should be examined. Prior to the digital rectal examination, the anus should typically be lubricated and a topical anesthetic used, especially if the patient is in pain. If for some reason, *Neisseria gonorrhoeae* is suspected, lubrication should be avoided prior to taking cultures. One should feel for any abnormal anal or distal rectal masses and anal tone. If low resting tone, stool seepage may be a cause for pruritus pain. If tone is high and there is twitching of the anal sphincter, even if there is no visible fissure, a diagnosis of anal fissure disease is likely. The tightness of levator muscles should be assessed bilaterally starting at the coccyx; this will often reproduce the pain or pressure of levator spasm. One should assess for the fluctuant swelling typical of an abscess, and the sacral hollow should be examined for presacral masses or cysts. The coccyx should be distracted to assess for coccydynia; the prostate should be palpated since prostatitis may be the cause of anal pain. If the pain is too intense and the patient cannot tolerate the exam in the office setting, an examination under anesthesia should be scheduled.

Rectal Inspection, Anoscopy, and Sigmoidoscopy

After the digital rectal examination, particularly if the diagnosis is not clear and if the patient tolerated the exam without too much pain, an anoscopic or sigmoidoscopic examination should be performed. These endoscopic tools will help identify intra-anal and rectal lesions. Rarely, an anal melanoma may be seen (Figure 11-10). More common, abnormalities can include lesions from various sexually transmitted infections, mucosal changes of inflammatory bowel disease, internal hemorrhoid disease, or rare conditions, such as melanoma.

Imaging and Diagnostic Testing

The history and examination will occasionally lead to a need to order confirmatory or diagnostic imaging studies. A rare patient whose history is consistent with anorectal abscess, but in whom an abscess cannot be found on exam, may benefit from a CT of the pelvis. A cine-videodefecogram or dynamic MRI of the pelvis may help confirm the diagnosis of a patient with suspected proctalgia fugax or other pelvic floor disorders. High-resolution anorectal manometry [24] and balloon expulsion can be used to differentiate outlet obstruction for patients with constipation. If an anal or rectal cancer is identified on examination, staging with ultrasound, MRI, and CT is appropriate. A pelvic radiograph can identify some foreign bodies (Figure 11-11).

Conclusion

A systematic approach to anal pain will ensure efficient diagnosis and initiation of effective treatments (Figure 11-12). A combination of careful history and detailed examination is nearly universal in obtaining the correct diagnosis. However, in the rare situation where the pain is still of unclear etiology, an examination under anesthesia may be warranted. Even more rarely, would imaging be necessary other than to further delineate an abnormality found on examination.

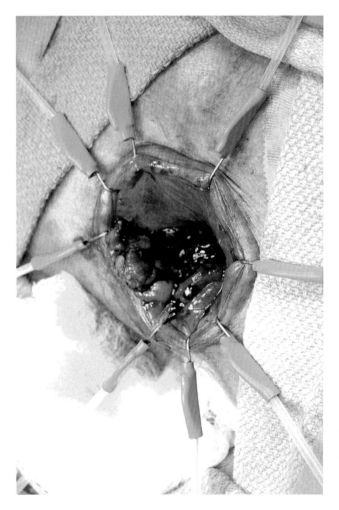

FIGURE 11-10. Anal melanoma.

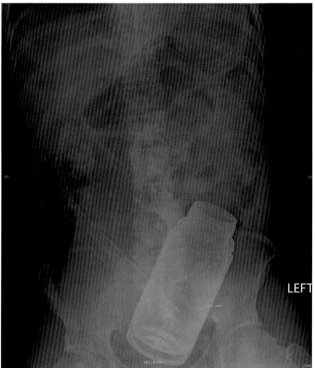

FIGURE 11-11. Foreign body.

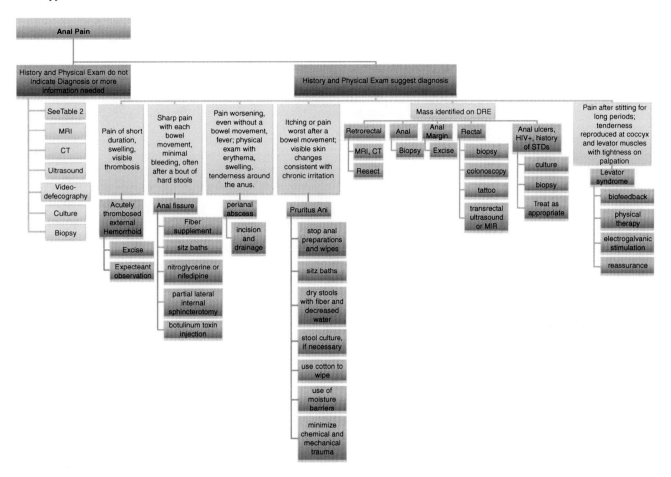

FIGURE 11-12. Systematic approach to anal pain. *With permission from Billingham R. Chronic anal pain. In: Steele, S.R., Maykel, J.A., Champagne, B.J., Orangio, G.R. (Eds). Complexities in Colorectal Surgery. Decision-Making and Management. Springer, New York, 2014. © Springer.*

References

1. Lund JN, Nystrom PO, Coremans G, et al. An evidence-based treatment algorithm for anal fissure. Tech Coloproctol. 2006;10:177–80.
2. Perry WB, Dykes SL, Buie WD, et al. Practice parameters for the management of anal fissures (3rd revision). Dis Colon Rectum. 2010;53:1110–5.
3. Rossi DC, Bastaworus AL. Hemorrhoids. In: Bailey HR, Billingham RP, Stamos MJ, Snyder MJ, editors. Colorectal surgery. Philadelphia, PA: Elsevier; 2012.
4. Rivadeneira DE, Steele SR, Ternent C, et al. Practice parameters for the management of hemorrhoids. Dis Colon Rectum. 2011;54:1059–64.
5. MacRae HM, Temple LK, McLeod RS. A meta-analysis of hemorrhoidal treatments. Semin Colon Rectal Surg. 2002;13:77–83.
6. Loder PB, Kamm MA, Nicholls RJ, et al. Haemorrhoids: pathology, pathophysiology and aetiology. Br J Surg. 1994;81:946–54.
7. Guillaumin E, Jeffrey Jr RB, Shea WJ, et al. Perirectal inflammatory disease: CT findings. Radiology. 1986;161:153–7.
8. Ramanujam PS, Prasad ML, Abcarian H, et al. Perianal abscesses and fistulas. A study of 1023 patients. Dis Colon Rectum. 1984;27:593–7.
9. Gilliland R, Wexner SD. Complicated anorectal sepsis. Surg Clin North Am. 1997;77:115–53.
10. Steele SR, Kumar R, Feingold DL, et al. Practice parameters for the management of perianal abscess and fistula-in-ano. Dis Colon Rectum. 2011;54:1465–74.
11. Bastawrous AL, Cintron JR. Anorectal abscess fistula. In: Cameron J, editor. Current surgical therapy. 8th ed. Philadelphia, PA: Mosby; 2004.
12. Bastawrous AL, Chaudhry V. Specific pruritus ani. Semin Colon Rectal Surg. 2003;14(4):203–12.
13. Chaudhry V, Bastawrous AL. Idiopathic pruritus ani. Semin Colon Rectal Surg. 2003;14(4):196–202.
14. Ternent CA, Bastaworus AL, Morin NA, et al. Practice parameters for the evaluation and management of constipation. Dis Colon Rectum. 2007;50(12):2013.
15. Hull TL, Milsom JW, Church J, Oakley J, Lavery I, Fazio V. Electrogalvanic stimulation for levator syndrome: how effective is it in the long-term? Dis Colon Rectum. 1993;36(8):731–3.
16. Klas JV, Rothenberger DA, Wong WD, Madoff RD. Malignant tumors of the anal canal: the spectrum of disease, treatment, and outcomes. Cancer. 1999;85(8):1686–93.
17. Monson JRT, Weiser MR, Buie WD, et al. Practice parameters for the management of rectal cancer. Dis Colon Rectum. 2013;56:535–50.

18. Blumetti J, Bastawrous AL. Epidermoid cancers of the anal canal: current treatment. Clin Colon Rectal Surg. 2009;22:77–83.

19. Steele SR, Varma MG, Melton GB, Ross HM, Rafferty JF, Buie WD. Standards Practice Task Force of the American Society of Colon and Rectal Surgeons. Practice parameters for anal squamous neoplasms. Dis Colon Rectum. 2012;55(7):735–49.

20. Ben Amor I, Kassir R, Bachir E, et al. Perforated diverticulitis of the sigmoid colon revealed by a perianal fistula. Int J Surg Case Rep. 2015;8:73–5.

21. Lengelé B, Scalliet P. Anatomical bases for the radiological delineation of lymph node areas. Part III: Pelvis and lower limbs. Radiother Oncol. 2009;92(1):22–33.

22. Gretschel S, Warnick P, Bembenek A, et al. Lymphatic mapping and sentinel lymph node biopsy in epidermoid carcinoma of the anal canal. Eur J Surg Oncol. 2008;34(8):890–4.

23. Gerard JP, Chapet O, Samiei F, et al. Management of inguinal lymph node metastases in patients with carcinoma of the anal canal: experience in a series of 270 patients treated in Lyon and review of the literature. Cancer. 2001;92(1): 77–84.

24. Grimaud JC, Bouvier M, Naudy B, Guien C, Salducci J. Manometric and radiologic investigations and biofeedback treatment of chronic idiopathic anal pain. Dis Colon Rectum. 1991;34(8):690–5.

12
Hemorrhoids

Martin Luchtefeld and Rebecca E. Hoedema

Key Concepts

- The classification system of hemorrhoidal disease is based on the degree of clinical prolapse seen on the physical examination.
- Medical therapy for hemorrhoidal symptoms should be the initial treatment recommendation and can include dietary changes, increased water intake, fiber supplementations, and ointment therapy.
- Office-based procedures are offered mainly for internal hemorrhoidal disease with the most common procedure being rubber band ligation.
- Injection sclerotherapy may be performed on an anticoagulated patient due to the fibrotic reaction with almost no increased risk of bleeding.
- Excisional hemorrhoidectomy is the gold standard by which all surgical procedures are compared.
- Postoperative bleeding can occur at one of two different times, right after the procedure itself and delayed hemorrhage occurring 7–10 days post procedure.
- Urgent hemorrhoid surgery is usually reserved for the patient with strangulated, incarcerated, gangrenous hemorrhoids.

Hemorrhoids are one of the most common ailments that will be seen by a colon and rectal surgeon. While hemorrhoids can present in many different ways, there are a number of different conditions that are mistaken by patients and practitioners alike as "hemorrhoids."

Anatomy

Hemorrhoids are a normal part of the anal canal. Our understanding of hemorrhoid anatomy has not changed substantially since 1975 when Thomson published his master's thesis based on anatomic and radiologic studies and first used the term "vascular cushions" [1]. Per Thomson, the submucosa does not form a continuous ring of thickened tissue but instead is a discontinuous series of cushions. Anatomically the three main cushions are located in the left lateral, right anterior, and right posterior positions. Each of these thicker layers has a submucosa filled with blood vessels and muscle fibers. The muscle fibers arise from the internal sphincter and from the conjoined longitudinal muscle. These muscle fibers are thought to be important in maintaining the integrity of the hemorrhoid, and it is the breakdown of this tissue that can contribute to the hemorrhoids becoming symptomatic. The arterial blood supply to hemorrhoids is primarily from the terminal branches of the superior hemorrhoidal artery; branches of the middle hemorrhoidal artery also contribute. Venous outflow is from the superior, middle, and inferior hemorrhoidal veins (Figure 12-1) [2].

Etiology

There are numerous possible reasons why hemorrhoids become symptomatic. Dietary patterns, behavioral factors, anything that can cause excessive straining, and sphincter dysfunction are among the most common reasons. Thompson's vascular cushion theory states that normal hemorrhoidal tissue represents discrete masses of submucosa. During straining, the vascular cushions can become engorged and possibly prevent the escape of fecal material or gas. With the passage of time, however, the anatomic structures supporting the muscular submucosa weaken, allowing the hemorrhoidal tissue to slip or prolapse, leading to typical hemorrhoidal symptoms. Haas et al. noted that supporting tissues can be shown microscopically to deteriorate by the third decade of life [3].

Studies have investigated why this degradation occurs and what are the changes in the local microvasculature. Matrix metalloproteinases (MMPs) are enzymes present in the extracellular space and can degrade collagen, elastin, and

Electronic supplementary material: The online version of this chapter (doi:10.1007/978-3-319-25970-3_12) contains supplementary material, which is available to authorized users.

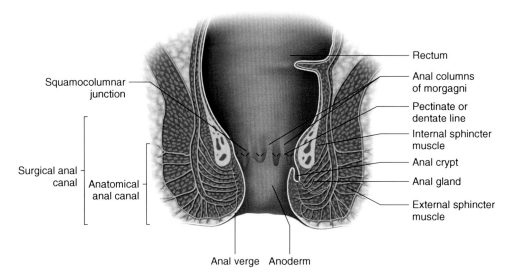

FIGURE 12-1. Hemorrhoid anatomy.

fibronectin. MMP-9 has been found to be overexpressed in hemorrhoid tissue in association with breakdown of elastic fibers [4]. Once the hemorrhoids start to prolapse, the internal sphincter can slow the rate of venous return and increase the hemorrhoid engorgement.

Increased vascular supply and neovascularization may play a role in making hemorrhoids more symptomatic. Aigner found that the terminal branches of the superior hemorrhoidal artery were larger in diameter, had greater flow, and higher peak velocity and acceleration velocity in patients with hemorrhoids compared to normal volunteers [5, 6]. Microvascular density has also been found to be increased in hemorrhoids. Chung et al. found that endoglin (CD105) which is a binding site for TGF-B and is a proliferative marker for neovascularity was found in over half of hemorrhoidal tissue specimens compared to none in normal anorectal mucosa [7]. Other researchers have found higher expression of angiogenesis-related proteins such as vascular endothelial growth factor (VEGF) in hemorrhoidal specimens [4].

Any process that can hinder venous return is thought to increase hemorrhoidal symptoms. Increased sphincter tone by itself can slow venous return [8, 9]; in fact, studies have shown that resting anal canal pressure is higher in patients with symptomatic hemorrhoids compared to normal subjects [10, 11]. Following hemorrhoidectomy, anal canal pressures drop so it is possible that the anal canal pressures are a result of the hemorrhoids rather than a cause [12]. Other possible causes include pregnancy, chronic cough, pelvic floor dysfunction, and simply being erect. Burkitt and Graham–Stewart suggested that Western diets emphasizing low-residue foods lead to increased straining with defecation [13] causing increased venous backflow predisposing to worsening hemorrhoid symptoms.

Despite the many theories that have been proposed, most of these are very speculative, and almost certainly hemorrhoidal symptoms result from a combination of multiple different factors.

Epidemiology

It is difficult to know the true incidence of hemorrhoids. As mentioned earlier, many patients who believe that they have hemorrhoids in fact have some other malady. One study done in 1990 suggested that the prevalence in the United States was 4.4% with the highest rate being in Caucasian patients between 45 and 65 years of age and elevated social economic status [14]. This sort of study has many potential obvious biases. In 2004, the National Institutes of Health noted that the diagnosis of hemorrhoids was associated with 3.2 million ambulatory care visits, 306,000 hospitalizations, and two million prescriptions in the United States [15].

Classification

Hemorrhoids are generally classified as internal, external, or mixed. Internal hemorrhoids are those located above the dentate line, and external hemorrhoids are located below the dentate line. This classification has important implications for treatment as the relative lack of pain fibers in the internal hemorrhoids allows for many more treatment options compared to the external hemorrhoids.

In addition, there is a classification system of the internal hemorrhoids based on the degree of clinical prolapse (Figure 12-2) [16]. This system is useful as it does allow some comparison of treatment methods between studies. Additionally, prolapse is one of the many main driving symptoms for patients to seek treatment. Unfortunately, this system does not address some of the other hemorrhoidal complaints such as pain, bleeding, and thrombosis since most hemorrhoid complaints are a combination of symptoms.

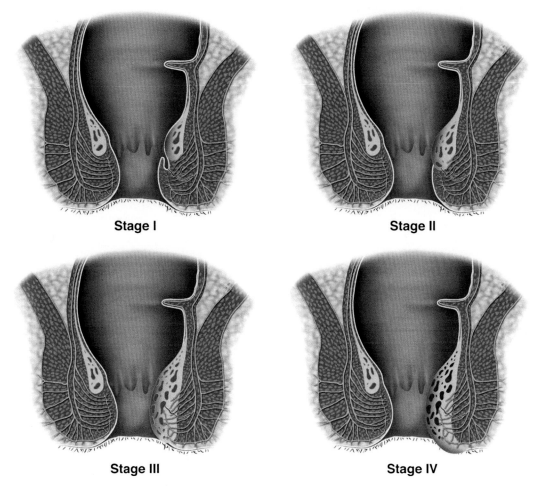

Stage I   Stage II

Stage III   Stage IV

FIGURE 12-2. Hemorrhoid classification table/grading system.

Clinical Presentation

Most patients coming to an outpatient clinic visit with ano-rectal complaints will feel like they have "hemorrhoids." Bleeding, pain, and protrusion are the most common symptoms associated with hemorrhoids. Each of these components can vary in severity based on whether the internal hemorrhoids, external hemorrhoids, or a combination predominates. Itching can also be described, although itching as an isolated symptom is more often the result of pruritus ani.

When internal hemorrhoids are the primary source of the problem, the main symptoms are a combination of rectal bleeding and prolapse. Pain is very rarely associated with internal hemorrhoids, and in fact when this is a significant component of the presenting complaint, the practitioner should be very suspicious of another source of the problem. The bleeding that occurs with hemorrhoids is typically described as bright red in nature with the frequency ranging from rarely to several times per day. The blood can be seen on the toilet paper and in the toilet water, and sometimes patients even describe the sensation of the blood squirting out of the anus. Typically the frequency and severity will increase over time. Although it is very unusual, there can

even be enough bleeding to lead to anemia. Another common symptom of internal hemorrhoids is prolapse. This can range from a simple swelling that quickly reduces after each bowel movement to an internal hemorrhoid that is chronically prolapsed and cannot be reduced. Many of the symptoms of internal and external hemorrhoids overlap. Certainly external hemorrhoids can lead to rectal bleeding in much the same way that internal hemorrhoids can. In addition, the intra-anal portion of the external hemorrhoids can also prolapse out of the anal canal along with the internal hemorrhoid. It can be difficult to distinguish by symptoms alone external hemorrhoids that are engorged and inflamed from prolapsing internal hemorrhoids.

On the other hand, external hemorrhoids are more likely to be associated with pain especially when they are engorged or inflamed. It is the presence of this pain that can help the clinician distinguish whether it is the internal or the external component of the hemorrhoids causing them the most problems.

Thrombosis is one distinct way that hemorrhoids can cause significant symptoms (Figure 12-3). A patient with a thrombosed hemorrhoid will typically describe a sudden onset of pain and swelling in the perianal region. The swell-

FIGURE 12-3. Thrombosed
external hemorrhoid. Courtesy
of Richard Billingham.

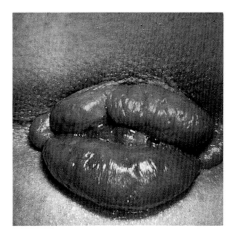

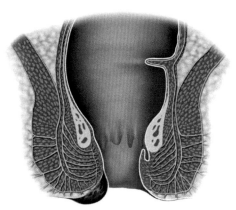

Thrombosed external hemorrhoid

TABLE 12-1. Hemorrhoid symptoms

- Rectal bleeding
- Bright red blood in stool
  - Dripping in toilet
  - On wiping after defecation
- Pain during bowel movements
- Anal itching
- Rectal prolapse (while walking, lifting weights)
- Thrombus
- Extreme pain, bleeding, and occasional signs of systemic illness
  in case of strangulation

ing that occurs will usually last at least days if not weeks, whereas the protrusion that occurs with prolapse or edema usually resolves much quicker. The pain that results from the thrombosed hemorrhoid can vary greatly in severity but is typically constant and unrelenting. Thrombosed hemorrhoids typically occur in the external component but in severe cases can go on to involve the internal hemorrhoids as well. Thrombosed hemorrhoids can occur in patients who have had minimal hemorrhoidal symptoms in the past.

It is important to keep in mind the wide differential diagnosis in patients presenting with anorectal complaints (Table 12-1). Although many of these patients will indeed be found to have hemorrhoids, fissures, or fistulas, they may also harbor a more ominous diagnosis such as anal or rectal carcinoma. The practitioner should keep an open mind and consider other possibilities such as condyloma, Crohn's disease, proctitis, Paget's disease, or other types of dermatoses.

Evaluation and Physical Examination

History

A careful history should be done to guide the clinician to an accurate diagnosis. In addition, it is helpful to know which symptoms bother the patient the most. In some circumstances the patient is satisfied just to know that their symptoms are related to hemorrhoids and not something more

serious. Part of the history should include the patient's bowel habits. If a patient has constipation, treatment of the constipation will be an important part of the treatment plan. Ulcerative colitis and Crohn's disease need to be considered in patients that have had significant diarrhea. If there has been a significant change in bowel habits, one also has to consider the many possibilities that can lead to this change.

For patients with rectal bleeding, the nature, color, and intensity of the bleeding should be noted. If also accompanied by a change in bowel habits, one needs to be suspicious of a malignancy or inflammatory bowel disease.

If pain is a significant component of the presentation, the intensity, frequency, and duration of the pain should be noted. If the pain is severe and described as a tearing sensation primarily at the time of the bowel movement, an anal fissure should be considered. Pain that is constant and has been present for days at a time should elicit consideration of a thrombosed hemorrhoid or perianal abscess as the underlying diagnosis.

Protrusion or swelling in the rectal area can be many different things. If the protrusion has been present constantly for weeks, months, or even years, it can be something as simple as a skin tag. However, one needs to also be mindful of diagnoses such as condyloma and neoplasm in this situation.

Physical Examination

A general physical examination should be conducted with concentration on the abdomen, groin, and perianal area. Typically the patient will be examined in the supine position first before switching to a prone jackknife or left lateral (Sims) position (Figure 12-4). It is important to be as reassuring as possible during this examination as it is inherently embarrassing and uncomfortable. It is always helpful to explain the steps of the examination so as to minimize surprise and discomfort.

The examination begins by gently spreading the buttocks and inspecting the skin, perineum, and the external anal opening. Anal fissures are usually diagnosed just with these

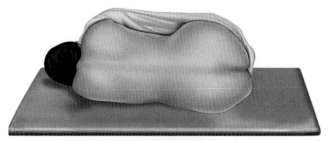

Left lateral position

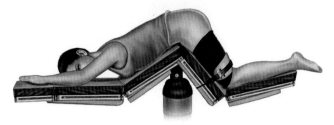

Prone jack knife position

FIGURE 12-4. Patient positioning. (**a**) Left lateral position. (**b**) Prone jackknife position.

simple measures, but if one is not thinking of this possibility, it is easy to miss a fissure. In addition, many other conditions can be identified: dermatitis, fistulas, abscess, anal cancer, skin tags, and condyloma. A digital rectal exam is then performed to assess for masses, pain, and sphincter tone. If there is any component of fecal soiling or incontinence, the sphincter tone should also be investigated by asking the patient to voluntarily squeeze during the digital exam.

Anoscopy is required to fully assess the hemorrhoids (see Figure 4.3). It is important that the anoscope is slotted or allows for side viewing to give the best view of the internal hemorrhoids. Asking the patient to bear down with the anoscope in place can give a better assessment of the severity of the hemorrhoidal problems and specifically the degree of prolapse.

Many patients should also undergo at least a rigid proctoscopy. This allows the surgeon to rule out malignancies or inflammatory conditions that could be mimicking hemorrhoids. This is especially true in older patients with bleeding, weight loss, anemia, or change in bowel habits.

The patient who presents with rectal bleeding should always be considered for full evaluation of the colon. An accurate history is very helpful in determining the need for colonoscopy. The young patient with typical hemorrhoidal bleeding that responds to treatment and with no family history of colon cancer likely does not need further evaluation. In a large series of classic "outlet" bleeding, colonoscopy revealed adenomas in less than 2% and no cancers in patients less than 50 years of age. When considering all age groups, 6.7% of the patients had a significant lesion (e.g., cancer, large polyps, or carcinoma in situ) [17]. Despite this evidence, some clinicians will still recommend colonoscopy in any patient over 40 years of age regardless of the type of bleeding.

Treatment

Treatment aggressiveness is determined by the degree of symptoms. Many patients have large inflamed hemorrhoids but desire nothing other than the reassurance of an accurate diagnosis. Other patients may have symptoms that seem far worse than the physical findings would suggest. The options for the treatment of hemorrhoids can be categorized into medical management, office-based treatments, and operative therapies.

Medical Management

Dietary

The most common problem associated with hemorrhoidal disease is constipation. As a result, the main components of dietary management are geared toward minimizing constipation and consist of a high-fiber diet accompanied by an adequate fluid intake. The recommended dose of dietary fiber is 25 g (for women) to 38 g (for men) per day [18]. This amount of fiber is difficult to attain and far exceeds the mean fiber intake of Americans of 16 g per day. Despite recommendations to increase fiber intake, this figure has not changed over the last 10 years [19]. Many patients find that attempting to reach the maximum amount of fiber leads to bloating and excessive gas, and this can be a limiting factor. Along with the increased fiber, patients should also drink at least 64 oz of fluid per day. The desired outcome of the increased fiber and fluid is a soft but formed bowel movement that can be expelled with minimal effort. Meta-analysis has confirmed that fiber supplementation can alleviate hemorrhoidal bleeding but is not useful for pain, prolapse, and itching [20]. It can take up to 6 weeks for the fiber therapy to show benefit [21].

Other options are available for patients that do not do well with fiber supplementation. Stool softeners are simple and safe and can be very helpful for patients that have exceptionally hard bowel movements. Hyperosmolar laxatives such as polyethylene glycol are a good choice for those patients that do not do well with fiber supplements. The goal of these supplements is ultimately the same as for dietary fiber and water.

For the occasional patient with diarrhea, the dietary focus must change. Evaluation must be carried out to determine the etiology if the diarrhea is significant. Even in the absence of a verified diagnosis, a few basic rules can be applied to the patient with diarrhea. In general, the diet should be high in fiber and low in fat content; caffeine, alcohol, and spicy foods are known to exacerbate diarrhea. Loperamide can be very useful to minimize diarrhea in patients with irritable bowel syndrome.

In many patients, the hemorrhoidal symptoms are tied into their toileting habits. The dietary changes mentioned above are designed to minimize straining and time spent on the toilet. Some patients will continue to have excessive straining time on the toilet despite having soft bowel movements. In this situation, the diagnosis of the obstructed defecation syndrome (ODS) should be considered. ODS will not respond to any type of surgical treatment of hemorrhoids and, in the ideal situation, would be recognized and treated at the outset.

Sitz baths are often used as part of the treatment for hemorrhoids. They are designed to decrease pain, burning, and itching following a bowel movement. They can also aid in hygiene as well as decrease anal canal pressures. Sitz baths tend to be more useful when warm water is used and when performed in the acute setting such as with a thrombosed hemorrhoid or an acute flare-up of hemorrhoidal disease [22]. Some patients with disabilities can have difficulty using them due to an inability to get in and out of a bathtub. In these situations, a portable sitz bath or even a warm shower can be useful. As comfortable as they can be, excessive use can lead to macerated skin and even more discomfort. Soaking time should be limited to 10–15 min two to three times per day.

Topical Therapies

Medical treatments such as topical ointments and suppositories deserve comment. Any trip to a local pharmacy will confirm that there is a vast array of over-the-counter hemorrhoidal treatments. Many of these products will combine a barrier protectant with some other active ingredient. The active ingredients can include vasoconstriction agents, local anesthetics, anti-inflammatory agents, and astringents [23]. There is very little science to support the use of these agents; however, some patients do claim to get relief from these products, and there appears to be little or no harm in their use.

A different approach to treating hemorrhoidal symptoms has been the use of topical nitrates, which have been shown to be beneficial in patients with high sphincter tone and hemorrhoids [24]. Calcium channel blockers are reported to be helpful in the setting of acute thrombosed hemorrhoids [25]. Since both are known to decrease internal sphincter tone, this may be the mechanism of action.

Patients will also sometimes try suppositories or will have them recommended by one of their caregivers. Similar to the ointments described above, suppositories are usually a combination of several different agents. Despite the fact that suppositories are difficult to maintain in the correct anatomic location, some patients do get relief with their use.

Oral Therapy

Flavonoids are a type of plant-based phlebotonics that were first described in the treatment of chronic venous disease and edema. They are reported to increase vascular tone, reduce venous capacity, decrease papillary permeability [26], increase lymphatic drainage [27], and have anti-inflammatory effects [28]. When used as oral therapy for hemorrhoids, a meta-analysis has shown decreased bleeding, pain, and itching with their use [29, 30]. However, many of these agents are not available in pharmaceutical grade in the United States. Calcium dobesilate is one of many synthetic phlebo-

tonics. This agent has also been shown to be effective in decreasing bleeding and inflammation in hemorrhoids [31].

Office-Based Treatments

There are a number of treatments for hemorrhoids that can be carried out in the office. With the exception of a local excision of a thrombosed hemorrhoid, these treatments are all designed to be used for internal hemorrhoids. The relative lack of somatic innervation of the internal hemorrhoids allows such treatments to be considerably less painful than excisional treatments of the external hemorrhoids. Treatments that will be discussed are rubber band ligation, infrared coagulation, and sclerotherapy.

Rubber Band Ligation

Barron first described rubber band ligation of internal hemorrhoids in 1963 [32]. Even before that time, hemorrhoids had been tied off with various types of threads and ligatures [33]. Since Barron's description, it has become one of the most widely used techniques for the treatment of internal hemorrhoid problems. By applying a rubber band at the apex of the internal hemorrhoid, the hemorrhoid is fixed high in the anal canal, correcting the prolapse, and by decreasing the blood flow caudally, the hemorrhoids shrink in size.

The technique of rubber band ligation is straightforward but still must be done with care in order to minimize discomfort (Figure 12-5). No special preparation is required although some surgeons recommend an enema prior to the procedure. The patient is placed in either the prone jackknife or left lateral decubitus position depending on surgeon choice. Anoscopy is then done to determine which hemorrhoids will be banded. An assistant and adequate lighting are critical to get optimal visualization so that the procedure can be done precisely and with little discomfort to the patient. There are a number of different banders available (Figure 12-6). Some banders utilize a grasp, while others use suction to pull the internal hemorrhoid into the banding instrument.

Once the bander is in place, the rubber band is deployed to place it at the base of the internal hemorrhoid. It is important to place the band at least 1–2 cm above the dentate line. The anal transitional zone contains a variable amount of innervation, and bands placed in this area can cause significant pain. Even when proper precautions are taken and the hemorrhoid bands are placed in the appropriate anatomical site, there can be significant pain. Anywhere from 1 to 3 bands can be done at the same setting. Lee et al. found that placing multiple bands increases pain, urinary retention, and vasovagal reactions [34]. Maria et al. also found increased pain with multiple bands [35], and others have noted very similar complication rates [36, 37].

Postoperative care is straightforward. Patients can resume a normal diet and activity shortly after the procedure. They should be warned that there can be a show of blood 5–7 days following the ligation. An office appoint-

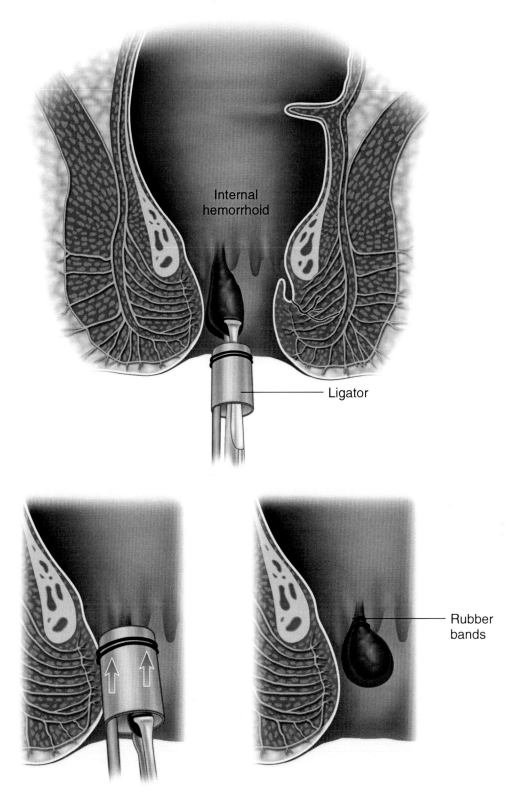

Figure 12-5. Hemorrhoid banding technique.

ment should be made in 2–4 weeks to evaluate the success of the banding.

Complications following banding are unusual, but the patient should be made aware of these possibilities. Delayed rectal bleeding of a significant nature occurs in approximately 1% of the patients [38]. Thrombosis can also occur especially in the remaining external component of the internal hemorrhoidal banding site [38, 39]. Abscess or urinary

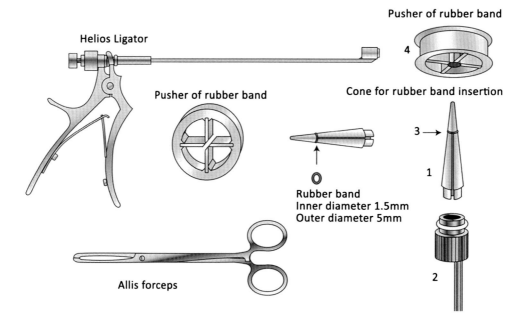

FIGURE 12-6. Hemorrhoid bander. Helio's product is easy to mount a rubber band. It uses a rubber band mounting cone (1), inserts rubber band at the end of cone (2), and pushes the rubber band to the bottom of the cone (3) using rubber band pusher (4). *With permission from Hyung Kyu Yang, Nonsurgical treatment of hemorrhoids. In: Hyung Kyu Yang, ed. Hemorrhoids. Springer, New York, 2014; pp: 47–63.© 2014 Springer.*

dysfunction is very rare [39]. A potentially devastating complication is pelvic sepsis. Although rare, several fatal cases have been reported [40–42].

Sepsis associated with hemorrhoidal banding usually presents with the triad of symptoms: increasing pain, fever, and urinary retention. Any clinician who does hemorrhoidal banding should be aware of this potential complication and be ready to treat it aggressively if it does occur. CT scan of the pelvis may illustrate air outside the rectum and/or inflammation. The diagnosis can also be made in the operating room with an exam under anesthesia. In earlier recognized and milder cases, debridement of the wound with intravenous antibiotics may suffice. In more severe cases, laparotomy with diverting colostomy and pelvic drainage may be necessary.

Rubber band ligation is very effective for the treatment of grade 1–3 hemorrhoids. Meta-analysis of multiple studies reveals that banding is the most effective non-excisional treatment available [43–45]. It should be noted, however, that 18–32% of patients require repeat treatments when followed long term [46, 47]. Still, many patients will find this to be a very acceptable alternative to the excisional treatments.

Infrared Photocoagulation

Energy ablation can be used to treat internal hemorrhoids; these options include infrared photocoagulation, bipolar diathermy, and direct current electrotherapy. Infrared photocoagulation is the most commonly used of these methods (Figure 12-7). Many of the concepts of rubber band ligation apply for infrared photocoagulation as well. Namely, isch-

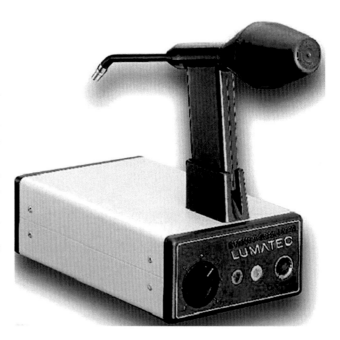

FIGURE 12-7. Infrared photocoagulation machine. *With permission from Hyung Kyu Yang, Nonsurgical treatment of hemorrhoids. In: Hyung Kyu Yang, ed. Hemorrhoids. Springer, New York, 2014; pp: 47–63. © 2014 Springer.*

emia of the internal hemorrhoidal vascular complex leads to scarring and fibrosis in the normal anatomic location [48]. Infrared radiation generates heat that coagulates protein and creates an inflammatory bed. The radiation is applied to the internal hemorrhoid typically at four different locations on

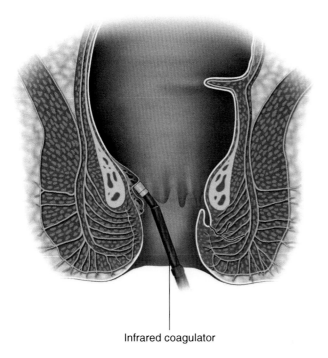

Figure 12-8. Infrared photocoagulation technique.

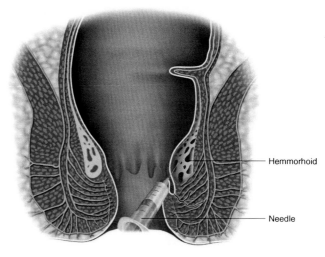

Figure 12-9. Sclerotherapy technique.

each hemorrhoidal complex. The depth of penetration is approximately 3 mm and leads to heat necrosis that causes tissue destruction and eventually fibrosis and scarring.

Positioning in preparation for this procedure is identical to that for hemorrhoidal banding and is based on physician preference (Figure 12-4). Once the patient is positioned, the tip of the infrared coagulator is used 3–4 times at the apex of each internal hemorrhoid. Each application of the photocoagulation is done for 1–1.5 s (although the device allows a range of 0.1–3 s) (Figure 12-8). The precise location of the treatment is just as important as it is for hemorrhoidal banding. If the treatment is done too low or too close to the dentate line, there will be significant post procedure pain. There is usually minimal discomfort once the treatment is complete, and all three hemorrhoid complexes can be treated at the same session [49].

Infrared coagulation is most effective for first- and second-degree hemorrhoids and may be less painful than hemorrhoidal banding [50]. While very effective for the treatment of bleeding, it is less useful for treating significant prolapse of hemorrhoids [41, 51]. Complications are rare following infrared photocoagulation and consist primarily of pain and bleeding due to excessive application of energy.

Bipolar diathermy and direct current electrotherapy have also been reported to be used in the same fashion as infrared coagulation. Bipolar energy does not penetrate as deeply as monopolar energy, and success rates for bipolar diathermy treatment have been reported from 88 to 100% [52]. Despite the good success rates, it has been noted that up to 20% of

patient may require an operative surgical excision for hemorrhoid prolapse [53]. Neither energy ablation technique has been as popular as infrared coagulation.

Sclerotherapy

Injection sclerotherapy was first attempted by John Morgan in 1869 [54]. The concept is analogous to that for infrared photocoagulation and hemorrhoidal banding: this solution is injected at the apex of the internal hemorrhoid complex which leads to scarring and fibrosis and, ultimately, to fixation of the internal hemorrhoidal complex. Many different agents have been tried including phenol, carbolic acid, quinine in urea, sodium morrhuate, and sodium tetradecyl.

The positioning of the patient, exposure, and placement of the sclerosing agent are identical to infrared coagulation. A spinal needle is used to place approximately 1–1.5 mL of the agent in a submucosal fashion at the apex of the internal hemorrhoid (Figure 12-9). The precise injection location into the submucosal space is important as placement too superficial can cause mucosal sloughing, while placing it too deep leads to more risk of infection, abscess, or significant pain. This complication usually occurs due to injection into a surrounding, unintended space [55]. Urinary retention and impotence postinjection sclerotherapy have also been reported [56].

Sclerotherapy is reported to be highly successful but is still not quite as effective as rubber band ligation especially for grade 3 hemorrhoids [57]. The best role for sclerotherapy may be in patients that require anticoagulation since the risk of bleeding is minimal with this technique. This is due to the fibrotic reaction rather than sloughing post procedure and can be safe in patients on anticoagulation. While bleeding is very unusual (approximately 1%) following hemorrhoidal banding, that bleeding risk can be very significant in the anticoagulated patient, and therefore sclerotherapy should be considered an option in this patient population. Multiple repeat attempts should be avoided due to the cumulative risk of stricture.

Operative Management of Hemorrhoids

Operative management of hemorrhoids is usually reserved for those patients who have failed medical management or have recurrent, persistent symptoms despite undergoing some of the internal hemorrhoidal treatments mentioned earlier in this chapter. Typically, only 5–10% of patients with hemorrhoidal complaints require operative hemorrhoidectomy [58]. Occasionally a patient will present with extensive thrombosed hemorrhoids or such advanced disease that it is clear from the initial encounter that a more aggressive approach is necessary. Strangulated, gangrenous hemorrhoids typically need immediate attention and operative intervention (Figure 12-10).

Excisional hemorrhoidectomy has excellent results, minimal recurrence rates, and few complications and remains the gold standard for surgical hemorrhoidal options. Unfortunately, it is also associated with significant postoperative pain. As a result, other newer therapies have been developed to treat hemorrhoids while attempting to minimize postoperative discomfort. The other primary operative management techniques include stapled hemorrhoidopexy and transanal hemorrhoidal dearterialization.

Excisional Hemorrhoidectomy-Closed Technique

Dr. Lynn Ferguson of the Ferguson Clinic first described the closed hemorrhoidectomy technique in the early 1950s [59]. It has remained the most common operation for hemorrhoids in the United States since that time [60]. A mechanical bowel

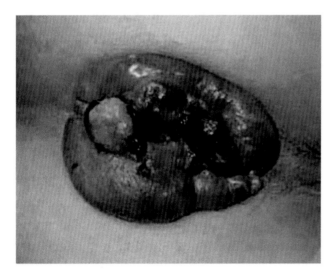

FIGURE 12-10. Strangulated, gangrenous hemorrhoids.

preparation is not necessary, but preoperative enemas are useful to evacuate the rectum. Anesthesia can be tailored to the patient and can range from something as simple as local anesthesia plus intravenous sedation to a full general anesthesia with intubation. Positioning is per surgeon preference and includes the options of lithotomy, prone jackknife, and left lateral decubitus.

The operation starts with a digital exam followed by anoscopy to help clearly define which hemorrhoid complexes should be excised (Figure 12-11). Injecting the perianal skin and hemorrhoids with local anesthetic combined with epinephrine 1: 200,000 can help to decrease bleeding during the procedure. An elliptical incision is made around the hemorrhoid starting at the perianal margin, and a proportional incision should be made so that the length of the incision is approximately 3–4 times longer than its breadth. The hemorrhoid is then elevated off the underlying sphincter muscle fibers. It is useful to place the hemorrhoid under tension to facilitate this dissection. The dissection is carried out past both the external and internal component of the hemorrhoid. Sharp dissection with the scissors or scalpel or even electrocautery can be done to dissect the hemorrhoidal tissue off the underlying sphincter complex.

At the apex of the hemorrhoid, the vascular pedicle is then clamped and then the hemorrhoid excised. The vascular pedicle is then suture ligated with an absorbable suture; the same suture is then used to reapproximate the tissue. As the wound is closed, small bites of the underlying sphincter muscle can be taken in order to close the dead space. If the dissection is relatively bloody, a running locked stitch can be used to maximize hemostasis. Once the first hemorrhoid complex is excised, the remaining hemorrhoidal bundles can be examined to determine if they still need to be excised.

When multiple hemorrhoids are removed, it is important to maintain adequate skin and tissue bridges between the excision sites to minimize the risk of postoperative anal stenosis [61]. If one can still place a medium-sized Hill Ferguson retractor at the end of the procedure, then there is usually very minimal risk of anal stenosis.

A notable variation on the technique is the use of energy devices such as the LigaSure bipolar device or the harmonic device which both can be used to perform the excisional hemorrhoidectomy. The excision and dissection is done in the same fashion. It has been reported that there may be less postoperative discomfort following this approach and will be discussed in more detail later [62].

Excisional Hemorrhoidectomy Open Technique (Milligan–Morgan)

The open technique of excisional hemorrhoidectomy is very popular in the United Kingdom. This technique results in a very similar excision as the Ferguson technique except that the wounds are not closed other than suture ligating the vascular pedicle [63].

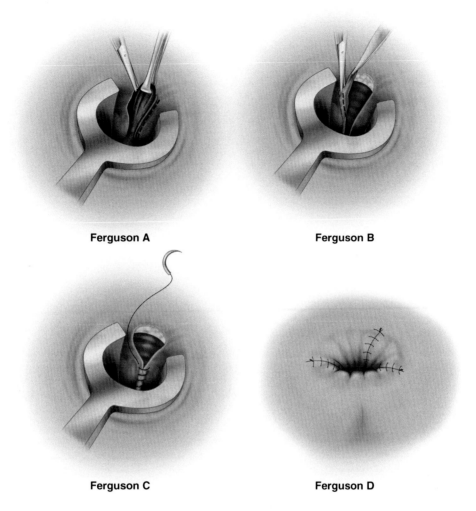

Ferguson A

Ferguson B

Ferguson C

Ferguson D

FIGURE 12-11. Closed hemorrhoidectomy.

The operation commences in a very similar fashion as the Ferguson closed hemorrhoidectomy technique. First, the external hemorrhoidal tissue is grasped, followed by the internal hemorrhoidal tissue and retracting them in a caudal fashion. An excision is then made at the perianal skin and extended into the anal canal. During the dissection it is of utmost importance to leave the sphincter muscles undisturbed. The apex of the vascular pedicle is then suture ligated and the hemorrhoid excised. The excision sites are then left open and allowed to granulate in (Figure 12-12).

Excisional Hemorrhoidectomy (Circumferential or Whitehead)

The Whitehead hemorrhoidectomy was designed to completely remove all the hemorrhoids at the time of surgery

[64]. A circumferential incision is made at the level of the dentate line, and then the submucosal and subdermal hemorrhoidal tissues are dissected out and removed. Any redundant rectal mucosa is excised, and then the remaining proximal rectal mucosa sutured down to the anoderm. This operation is not in common use at this time due to the complication of a Whitehead deformity (Figure 12-13) [65].

Results of Hemorrhoidectomy

Excisional hemorrhoidectomy remains the gold standard for the long-term relief of hemorrhoidal symptoms. Although there are few longitudinal studies, MacRae et al. performed a meta-analysis that confirmed there is very little need for further treatment and that symptoms were well controlled [44].

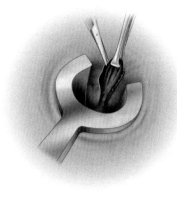

Milligan-Morgan A

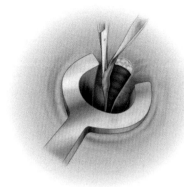

Milligan-Morgan B

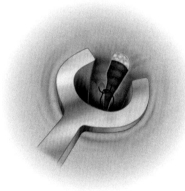

Milligan-Morgan C

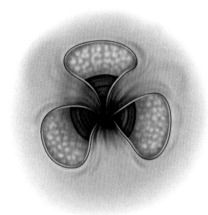

Milligan-Morgan D

FIGURE 12-12. Open hemorrhoidectomy.

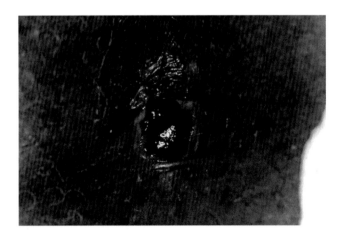

FIGURE 12-13. Whitehead deformity. Courtesy of American Society of Colon and Rectal Surgeons.

Although there has been considerable controversy over the relative merits of opened versus closed techniques, careful analysis in randomized, prospective trials suggests that there is very little difference between the two techniques

[66–69]. One meta-analysis reviewed six trials with almost 700 patients and found no differences in cure rates, length of stay, maximum score, or complication rates [70].

The discomfort with hemorrhoidectomy has led to a search for less painful alternatives [71]. One such approach has been to use energy sources such as the harmonic scalpel or the LigaSure for the tissue dissection. A Cochrane review was done to compare LigaSure hemorrhoidectomy to excisional hemorrhoidectomy [72]. This review confirmed that the early postoperative pain was less when LigaSure™ (Covidien, CT) was used, but this difference disappeared by postoperative day 14. LigaSure hemorrhoidectomy was also found to be slightly faster. The same benefits appear to apply to Harmonic Scalpel™ (Ethicon, Brunswick, NJ) hemorrhoidectomy [73]. It is not clear that the increased cost of the LigaSure device or Harmonic Scalpel device would be offset by the decreased operating room time. Both LigaSure and Harmonic seem to offer patients less postoperative pain, but long-term follow-up data is not yet available. Other approaches in an attempt to decrease pain such as diathermy and the use of lasers have not shown any significant difference [74–76].

There have been other efforts to decrease the pain associated with hemorrhoidectomy. Mathai et al. described doing lateral internal sphincterotomy at the same time as the hemorrhoidectomy [77]. This additional procedure did decrease pain likely by minimizing the sphincter spasm associated with postoperative pain, but division of the sphincter muscle has prevented this approach from being widely accepted. Topical nitroglycerin has also been shown to decrease post hemorrhoidectomy pain [78]. Both oral and topical metronidazole have also been shown to decrease pain although the mechanism is not clear [79].

Complications of Hemorrhoidectomy

Urinary Retention

Urinary retention is one of the most common complications following hemorrhoidectomy and can increase hospital stay [80]. Zaheer found that disease severity, namely, number of quadrants excised, and analgesia requirements were both important risk factors for those patients who underwent hemorrhoidectomy. Although the exact reasons for this complication are not known, it is clear that both fluid restriction and pain control in the perioperative period is important to prevent this complication [81, 82]. There have been a few reports indicating that the stapled hemorrhoidectomy (PPH) is associated with a lower incidence of postoperative urinary retention [83].

Postoperative Hemorrhage

Postoperative hemorrhage is one of the more common complications after hemorrhoidectomy, although the risk is still relatively low. Bleeding typically occurs during one of two time frames post surgery. In approximately 1% of cases, the bleeding will occur in the immediate postoperative period. When this bleeding occurs, it is usually the result of a technical error and most commonly requires a return to the operating room for an exam under anesthesia and control of the bleeding.

Delayed hemorrhage can occur in up to 5.4% of patients and will typically occur 7–10 days after surgery [84, 85].

Post hemorrhoidectomy bleeding has been attributed to sepsis of the ligated pedicle in the past, although Chen et al. found that male patients and the operating surgeon may be risk factors in delayed post hemorrhoidectomy bleeding [86]. If postoperative hemorrhage occurs, immediate packing of the anal canal or tamponade with a Foley balloon catheter will control the bleeding. If the bleeding does not stop, then an exam under anesthesia may be warranted. Patients that require a trip to the operating room can be determined with the aid of rectal irrigation [87]. However, return to the operating room to investigate and control the bleeding is always a safe option.

Anal Stenosis

Anal stenosis can occur if excessive anoderm is removed at the time of the hemorrhoidectomy. The most common setting for this is when an emergency hemorrhoidectomy is done for prolapsed thrombosed hemorrhoids, and inadequate skin bridges remain post surgery. Treatment can be as simple as the use of bulk laxatives but may require dilation and or anoplasty (Figure 12-14) [88, 89].

Postoperative Infection

Postoperative infections are surprisingly uncommon. The risk of postoperative infection occurs less than 1%, but the rate may be underreported due to abscesses spontaneously decompressing. In the rare circumstance when an abscess or cellulitis occurs, it requires operative drainage and/or antibiotics as needed [90]. Prophylactic antibiotic therapy is not indicated for elective hemorrhoid surgery [91].

Fecal Incontinence

Fecal soiling or incontinence can occur following hemorrhoidectomy but is rather unusual. The etiology could be due to a combination of things like sphincter stretch during the procedure due to retraction, direct injury to the sphincter complex, or loss of the hemorrhoidal piles that have been thought to contribute approximately 10–15% of continence.

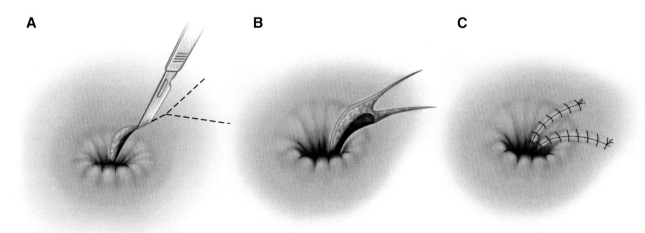

FIGURE 12-14. Y-V Anoplasty.

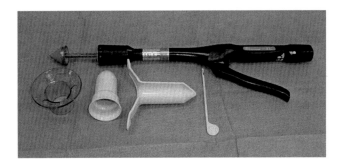

FIGURE 12-15. Stapled hemorrhoidectomy (PPH). *With permission from Schwandner O. Procedure for Prolapse and Hemorrhoids (PPH; Stapled Hemorrhoidopexy). In: Wexner SD, Fleshman JW. Colon and Rectal Surgery: Anorectal Operations. Wolter Kluwers, 2011. © Copyright Wolters Kluwer 2011.*

Stapled Hemorrhoidopexy

Stapled hemorrhoidopexy was developed in Italy as an alternative form of operative therapy for hemorrhoids [92, 93]. It would be mistaken to refer to this procedure as a "hemorrhoidectomy" but is usually referred to as a procedure for prolapse using a hemorrhoidopexy technique (Figure 12-15). In this procedure, an end-to-end circular stapler is used to excise a circumferential ring of internal hemorrhoids, which includes the mucosa and submucosa above the dentate line (Figure 12-16). The result of the operation should be that the remaining hemorrhoids are pulled up into the anal canal and fixed in place. Some of the blood supply to the remaining hemorrhoids is also interrupted so that there is less engorgement of the remaining hemorrhoids.

Because the operation occurs above the dentate line, there has been reported less postoperative pain compared to a hemorrhoidectomy [94–96]. Indications for stapled hemorrhoidopexy include patients with second- or third-degree hemorrhoids who have failed previous nonoperative methods or have severe enough internal disease to go directly to a more aggressive approach. It is generally not used for patients with fourth-degree hemorrhoids or for thrombosed prolapsed hemorrhoids; however, some data do support this procedure in fourth-degree hemorrhoids if they can be reduced in the operating room [97].

Preparation for this operation is the same as for an excisional hemorrhoidectomy. As part of the kit that is provided with the circular stapler, there is a disposable circular translucent anoscope. With the anoscope in place, a purse-string suture is placed in a circumferential fashion into the submucosa approximately 2 cm above the transitional zone. The head of the stapler (similar to an EEA, but the head is not detachable) is then introduced into the rectum past the purse-string suture. The purse string is tied down around the stapler, and then the anvil is very slowly closed while giving gentle traction on the purse-string suture externally. Once closed, the stapler is fired and then removed along with the excised tissue. The staple line should be inspected carefully for bleeding as this is a common occurrence and may require suture ligation.

In female patients the vagina should be inspected and palpated prior to firing the instrument to ensure that there is not a cuff of vaginal tissue included within the stapler.

Soon after the stapled hemorrhoidopexy technique was described, a number of randomized controlled studies were done that confirm there was significantly less postoperative pain compared to excisional hemorrhoidectomy and with equal relief of hemorrhoidal symptoms [94–96].

More long-term follow-up is now being accumulated on patients who have undergone the stapled hemorrhoidopexy. A recent Cochrane review was performed looking at seven trials with 537 patients comparing stapled hemorrhoidopexy to excisional hemorrhoidectomy. Patients undergoing excisional hemorrhoidectomy had fewer recurrences of prolapse and fewer symptoms than those undergoing stapled hemorrhoidopexy [98].

The multiple studies on hemorrhoidopexy confirm that it is a safe alternative to excisional hemorrhoidectomy; however, there are some unique complications that have been reported with this procedure including rectal perforation, persistent rectal pain, retroperitoneal sepsis, rectal obstruction, and rectovaginal fistula. The complication rate is similar between stapled hemorrhoidectomy and conventional hemorrhoidectomy, but stapled hemorrhoidectomy is associated with a higher rate of recurrent disease [99].

Transanal Hemorrhoidal Dearterialization

Transanal hemorrhoidal dearterialization is a relatively new technique first described by Morinaga in 1995 (Figure 12-17) [100]. Doppler is used to guide ligation of the arterial inflow to the hemorrhoids. Although not initially described, suture rectopexy can be done at the same setting to minimize prolapse.

Patient preparation and setup is identical to that for an excisional hemorrhoidectomy. Once proper anesthesia and positioning is accomplished, a specialized anoscope with a Doppler is introduced into the anal canal (Figure 12-18). The Doppler is used as the anoscope is rotated until one of the feeding arteries is identified and suture ligated. The Doppler can also be used to confirm that the artery was adequately ligated. The anoscope is rotated until all of the significant arteries are identified and ligated (generally 4–6 arteries, but this can be quite variable). Depending on the need to correct the prolapse, a suture mucopexy can be performed immediately following the ligation using the same stitch.

The arterial ligation and mucopexy are all done above the dentate line so one would anticipate that the pain would be less following this procedure when compared to excisional hemorrhoidectomy. Early studies seem to confirm that this procedure is less painful than a hemorrhoidectomy and equally as safe [101–104]. There seems to be a relative lack of good data to support this procedure. Giordano performed a systematic review of the available studies in 2009, and although there were 17 trials with 1996 patients, only one of these trials was a randomized controlled study. It was felt

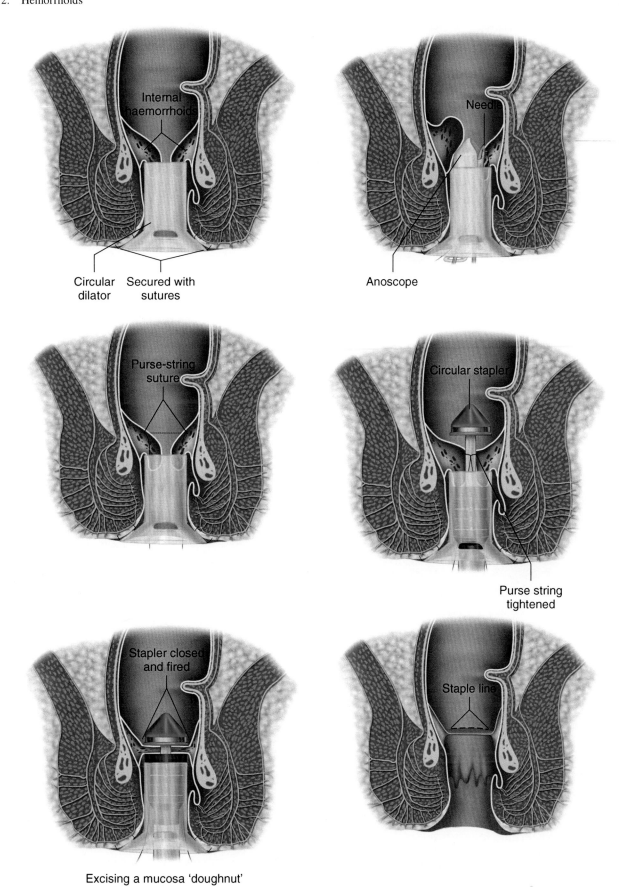

FIGURE 12-16. Stapled hemorrhoidectomy technique.

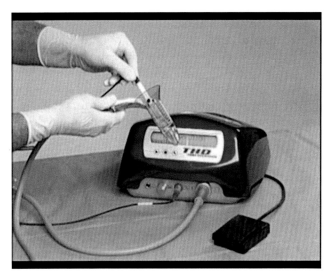

FIGURE 12-17. Transanal hemorrhoidal dearterialization device.

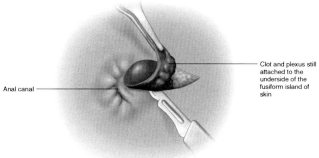

FIGURE 12-19. Enucleation of the thrombosed hemorrhoid.

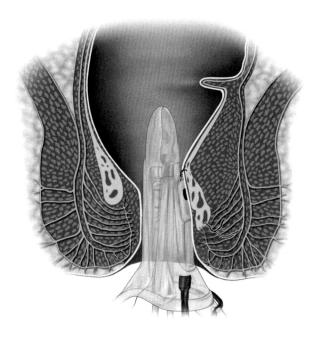

FIGURE 12-18. Transanal hemorrhoidal dearterialization technique.

that the quality of the studies included in this review was low overall. It appears to be a safe alternative with a recurrence rate of 10.8% for prolapse, 9.7% for bleeding, and 8.7% for pain at defecation at follow-up of 1 year or more [105].

Special Clinical Scenarios

Thrombosed External Hemorrhoid

A patient with acute thrombosed external hemorrhoids usually presents with the acute onset of anal pain along with a hard lump in the perianal region (Figure 12-3). Although the

patient may describe a possible precipitating event, such as constipation or excessive straining, most of the time the thrombosis can occur for no apparent reason. The perianal pain and discomfort is constant and can be worse around day 3 or 4. If the patient delays long enough, the thrombosis can sometimes cause pressure ulceration and eventually skin necrosis leading to a spontaneous evacuation of the clot. In these cases, the patient will usually describe an immediate relief of the pain.

The aggressiveness of the treatment is primarily driven by the patient's symptoms. Regardless of the size of the thrombosis, if the patient is relatively comfortable, it is usually best to allow the thrombosis to simply resolve on its own. On the other hand, many patients present to the physician's office due to severe, unrelenting pain, and in this circumstance, enucleation of the thrombus can be very helpful.

This procedure can usually be done under local anesthesia in the office although some patients may require sedation or even general anesthesia (Figure 12-19). In the office setting, local anesthesia can be used at the level of the thrombosed hemorrhoid. Once anesthetized, the skin should be excised overlying the thrombosis to allow as much of the clot to be removed. Bleeding is usually not troublesome and can be controlled with pressure, silver nitrate, and suture ligation if necessary. The wound can be left open or closed with absorbable sutures, depending on the preference of the surgeon (see Video 12-1) [106].

Strangulated (Thrombosed Prolapsed) Hemorrhoids

Strangulated or thrombosed, prolapsed hemorrhoids are internal hemorrhoids that are both incarcerated and irreducible (Figure 12-10). Patients typically have a previous history of prolapsing hemorrhoids and will present with an acute episode of pain and protrusion that is no longer reducible. They may also complain of urinary retention and referred pain. A thorough physical examination will demonstrate both prolapsed incarcerated internal hemorrhoids and thrombosed external hemorrhoids. A significant amount of edema may be present and, if left untreated, may progress to ulceration, necrosis, and eventually gangrene.

Enucleation of the thrombus is inadequate treatment and not appropriate for this clinical scenario. Treatment usually consists of an urgent excisional hemorrhoidectomy in the operating room. The excisional hemorrhoidectomy can be performed in an open or closed technique, although some recommend an open technique in the face of necrosis. A newer option may include the bipolar device hemorrhoidectomy.

An alternative treatment option, if the patient does not wish to go to the OR or does not want surgery or if the OR is unavailable, can be performed in the office or ED setting. This includes using local anesthetic, applying pressure and/ or massage to decrease the edema in the tissues, and then using a combination of rubber band ligations and thrombectomies. This will provide immediate relief for the patient and will not usually require a future surgical hemorrhoidectomy [107].

Portal Hypertension and Hemorrhoids

"Hemorrhoids" or rectal varices in patients with portal hypertension are a distinct entity compared to hemorrhoids in the general population. Rectal varices in patients with portal hypertension provide collateral circulation from the portal system into the systemic venous circulation. As previously mentioned, internal hemorrhoids drain into the middle rectal veins, then the internal iliac veins, and finally the systemic circulation. External hemorrhoids drain into the inferior rectal veins and then the internal iliac veins. The incidence of hemorrhoid symptoms in patients with portal hypertension is similar to the general population [108].

Anorectal varices are very common in patients with portal hypertension. There are reports of anorectal varices present in up to 78% of patients with portal hypertension [109]. Unlike esophageal varices, which are commonly present in this population, anorectal varices rarely bleed. Less than 1% of massive bleeding in these patients is attributed to anorectal varices or "hemorrhoids."

Treatment options for bleeding from the anorectal varices in this patient population are varied. Recommendations include conservative medical management, medical management of the portal pressures, sclerotherapy, suture ligation, stapled anopexy, and, lastly, TIPS and portosystemic shunts [110, 111].

Pregnancy

Hemorrhoid symptoms are not uncommon during pregnancy and can be exacerbated by the physiology of pregnancy, including increased circulating blood volume, impaired venous return, and change in bowel habits, namely, constipation and straining associated with labor. Usually the hemorrhoid symptoms present during pregnancy resolve after delivery and rarely need intervention. Surgical intervention is not warranted during pregnancy unless patients present with strangulated, gangrenous hemorrhoids. Local anesthesia is recommended in the left lateral position in order to rotate the uterus off of the IVC. It has been reported that only approximately 2% of pregnant women require emergent hemorrhoidectomy for strangulated hemorrhoids [112].

Crohn's Disease

Hemorrhoids can occur in patients with Crohn's disease and may require surgical attention; however, patient selection is very important. Hemorrhoid symptoms can be exacerbated in patients with Crohn's disease due to varied bowel habits, namely, diarrhea. Any anorectal surgical intervention must be performed with caution in patients with Crohn's disease due to prolonged wound healing and ulcerations. If the patient has well-controlled Crohn's disease and is not on steroids and there is little active inflammation, then Crohn's disease is not an absolute contraindication to surgical intervention. It has been reported to have a high rate of complications and can precipitate proctectomy for surgical complications not manageable with conservative means [113].

With the advent of newer medical therapies for Crohn's disease, the rate of prolonged healing and associated complications is much less. This was demonstrated in a study by Wolkomir and Luchtefeld where 90% of healing occurred in patients who underwent a hemorrhoidectomy where the ileocolic Crohn's disease was well managed. Hemorrhoidectomy, however, should not be performed in those patients with anorectal Crohn's disease or Crohn's proctitis [114].

Immunocompromised Patients

Immunocompromised patients with hemorrhoidal disease can be a very challenging and difficult clinical dilemma. Similar to the Crohn's disease population, extreme caution should be exercised when considering surgical therapies in this population. Again, poor wound healing and infectious complications are at the forefront of decision making. The HIV/AIDS population does suffer a higher degree of complications post hemorrhoidectomy [115]. Patients who are neutropenic should be offered nonoperative therapies first although the mortality rate in this patient population who undergoes a hemorrhoidectomy is not higher [116].

Symptomatic Hemorrhoids

Figure 12-20 shows a treatment algorithm for symptomatic hemorrhoids.

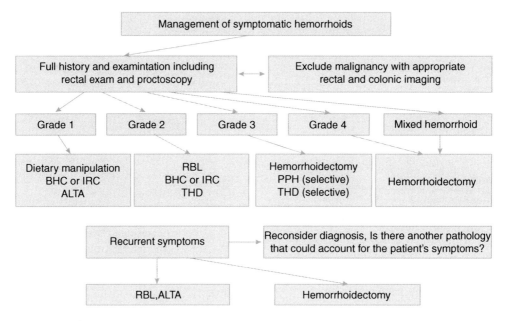

FIGURE 12-20. Treatment algorithm for symptomatic hemorrhoids. *RBL* rubber band ligation; *IRC* infrared coagulation; *THD* transanal hemorrhoidal dearterialization; *PPH* procedure for prolapsing hemorrhoids; *BHC* bipolar hyperthermic coagulation; *ALTA* Aluminum potassium sulfate and tannic acid (sclerotherapy). Adapted from Song G, Kim S. Optimal treatment of Symptomatic Hemorrhoids. J Korean Soc Coloproctol. 2011 Dec; 27(6): 277–81.

References

1. Thomson WH. The nature of haemorrhoids. Br J Surg. 1975;62:542–52.
2. Parnaud E, Guntz M, Bernard A, Chome J. Normal macroscopic and microscopic anatomy of the hemorrhoidal vascular system. Arch Fr Mal App Dig. 1975;65:501–14.
3. Haas PA, Fox TA, Haas GP. The pathogenesis of hemorrhoids. Dis Colon Rectum. 1984;7:442–50.
4. Han W, Wang ZJ, Zhao B, Yang XQ, Wang D, Wand JP, Tang XY, Zhao F, Hung YT. Pathologic change of elastic fibers with difference of microvessel density and expression of angiogenesis-related proteins in internal hemorrhoid tissues. Chin J Gastrointest Surg. 2005;8:56–9.
5. Aigner F, Bodner G, Gruber H, Conrad F, Fritsch H, Margreiter R, Bonatti H. The vascular nature of hemorrhoids. J Gastrointest Surg. 2006;10:1044–50.
6. Aigner F, Gruber H, Conrad F, Eder J, Wedel T, Zelger B, Engelhardt V, Lametschwandtner A, Wienert V, Böhler U, Margreiter R, Fritsch H. Revised morphology and hemodynamics of the anorectal vascular plexus: impact on the curse of hemorrhoidal disease. Int J Colorectal Dis. 2009;1:105–13.
7. Chung YC, Hou YC, Pan AC. Endoglin (CD105) expression in the development of haemorrhoids. Eur J Clin Invest. 2004;34:107–12.
8. Hancock BD. Internal sphincter and the nature of haemorrhoids. Gut. 1977;18:651–5.
9. Loder PB, Kamm MA, Nicholls RJ, Phillips RK. Haemorrhoids: pathology, pathophysiology and aetiology. Br J Surg. 1994;81: 946–54.
10. Sun WM, Read NW, Shorthouse AJ. Hemorrhoids are associated with hypertrophy of internal anal sphincter but with hypertension of the anal cushions. Br J Surg. 1992;79: 592–4.
11. Ho YH, Seow Choen F, Goh HS. Haemorrhoidectomy and disordered rectal and anal physiology in patients with prolapsed haemorrhoids. Br J Surg. 1995;82:596–8.
12. Ho YH, Tan M. Ambulatory anorectal manometric findings in patients before and after haemorrhoidectomy. Int J Colorectal Dis. 1997;12:296–7.
13. Burkitt DP, Graham-Stewart CW. Haemorrhoids--postulated pathogenesis and proposed prevention. Postgrad Med J. 1975;51: 631–6.
14. Johanson JF, Sonnenberg A. The prevalence of hemorrhoids and chronic constipation. An epidemiologic study. Gastroenterology. 1990;98:380–6.
15. Everhart JE. The burden of digestive diseases in the United States. Bethesda, MD: US Department of Health and Human Services. Public Health Service, National Institutes of Health, National Institute of Diabetes and Digestive and Kidney Diseases. NIH Publication; 2008.
16. Banov L, Knoepp LF, Erdman LH, Alia RT. Management of hemorrhoidal disease. J S C Med Assoc. 1985;81:398.
17. Marderstein EL, Church JM. Classic "outlet" rectal bleeding does not require full colonoscopy to exclude significant pathology. Dis Colon Rectum. 2008;51:202–6.
18. Slavin JL. Dietary fiber and body weight. Nutrition. 2005; 21:411–8.
19. McGill CR, Devareddy L. Ten-year trends in fiber and whole grain intakes and food sources for the United States population: National Health and Nutrition Examination Survey 2001-2010. Nutrients. 2015;7:1119–30.
20. Alonso-Coello P, Mills ED, Heels-Ansdell D, Lopez-Yarto M, Zhou Q, Johanson JF, Guyatt G. Fiber for the treatment of hemorrhoids complications: a systematic review and meta-analysis. Am J Gastroenterol. 2006;101:181–8.

21. Moesgaard F, Nielsen L, Hansen JB, Knudsen JT. High-fiber diet reduces bleeding and pain in patients with hemorrhoids. Dis Colon Rectum. 1982;25:454–6.

22. Ryoo S, Song YS, Seo MS, Oh H-K, Choe EK, Park KJ. Effect of electronic toilet system (Bidet) on anorectal pressure in normal healthy volunteers: influence of different types of water stream and temperature. J Korean Med Sci. 2011;26:71–7.

23. Johanson JF. Nonsurgical treatment of hemorrhoids. J Gastrointest Surg. 2002;6:290–4.

24. Tjandra JJ, Tan JJ, Lim JF, Murray-Green C, Kennedy ML, Lubowski DZ. Rectogesic (glyceryl trinitrate 0.2%) ointment relieves symptoms of haemorrhoids associated with high resting anal canal pressures. Colorectal Dis. 2007;9:457–63.

25. Perrotti P, Antropoli C, Molino D, DeStefano G, Antropoli M. Conservative treatment of acute thrombosed external hemorrhoids with topical nifedipine. Dis Colon Rectum. 2001;44:405–9.

26. Labrid C. Pharmacologic properties of Daflon 500 mg. Angiology. 1994;45:524–30.

27. Labrid C. A lymphatic function of Daflon 500 mg. Int Angiol. 1995;14:36–8.

28. Struckmann JR, Nicolaides AN. Flavonoids. A review of the pharmacology and therapeutic efficacy of Daflon 500 mg in patients with chronic venous insufficiency and related disorders. Angiology. 1994;45:419–28.

29. Perera N, Liolitsa D, Iype S, Croxford A, Yassin M, Lang P, Ukaegbu O, Van Issum C. Phlebotonics for haemorrhoids. Cochrane Database Syst Rev. 2012; (8): CD004322.

30. Alonso-Coello P, Zhou Q, Martinex Zapata MJ, Mills E, Heels-Ansdell D, Johanson JF, Guyatt G. Meta analysis of flavonoids for the treatment of haemorrhoids. Br J Surg. 2006;93:909–20.

31. Mentes BB, Gorgul A, Tatlicioglu E, Ayoglu F, Unal S. Efficacy of calcium dobesilate in treating acute attacks of hemorrhoidal disease. Dis Colon Rectum. 2001;44:1489–95.

32. Barron J. Office ligation treatment of hemorrhoids. Dis Colon Rectum. 1963;6:109–13.

33. Ellesmore S, Windsor AC. Surgical history of haemorrhoids. In: Charles MV, editor. Surgical treatment of haemorrhoids. London: Springer; 2002. p. 1–4.

34. Lee HH, Spencer RJ, Beart RW. Multiple hemorrhoidal bandings in a single session. Dis Colon Rectum. 1994;37:37–41.

35. Maria G, Brisinda G, Palermo A, Civello IM. Multiple versus single rubber band ligation for internal hemorrhoids: a review of 450 consecutive cases. Dig Surg. 1992;14:52–5.

36. Chaleoykitti B. Comparative study between multiple and single rubber band ligation in one session for bleeding internal, hemorrhoids: a prospective study. J Med Assoc Thai. 2002;85:345–50.

37. Khubachandani IT. A randomized comparison of single and multiple rubber band ligations. Dis Colon Rectum. 1993;26:705–8.

38. Corman M. Hemorrhoids. In: Colon & rectal surgery. 3rd ed. Philadelphia, PA: JB Lippincott; 1993. p. 68.

39. Bat L, Melzer E, Koler M, Dreznick Z, Shemesh E. Complications of rubber band ligation of symptomatic internal hemorrhoids. Dis Colon Rectum. 1993;36:287–90.

40. O'Hara VS. Fatal clostridial infection following hemorrhoidal banding. Dis Colon Rectum. 1993;23:570–1.

41. Scarpa FJ, Hillis W, Sabetta JR. Pelvic cellulitis: a life-threatening complication of hemorrhoidal banding. Surgery. 1988;103:383–5.

42. Russell TR, Donohue JH. Hemorrhoidal banding. A warning. Dis Colon Rectum. 1985;28:291–3.

43. MacRae HM, McLeod RS. Comparison of hemorrhoidal treatment modalities. Dis Colon Rectum. 1995;38:687–94.

44. MacRae HM, Temple LKF, McLeod RS. A meta-analysis of hemorrhoidal treatments. Semin Colon Rectal Surg. 2002;1:77–83.

45. Johanson JF, Rimm A. Optimal nonsurgical treatment of hemorrhoids: a comparative analysis of infrared coagulation, rubber band ligation, and injection sclerotherapy. Am J Gastroenterol. 1992;87:1600–6.

46. Bayer I, Myslovaty B, Picovsky BM. Rubber band ligation of hemorrhoids: convenient and economic treatment. J Clin Gastroenterol. 1996;23:50–2.

47. Savioz D, Roche B, Glauser T. Rubber band ligation of hemorrhoids: relapse as a function of time. Int J Colorectal Dis. 1998;13:154–6.

48. Dennison A, Whiston RJ, Rooney S, Chadderton RD, Wherry DC, Morris DL. A randomized comparison of infrared photocoagulation with bipolar diathermy for the outpatient treatment of hemorrhoids. Dis Colon Rectum. 1990;33:32–4.

49. Khaliq T, Shah SA, Mehboob A. Outcome of rubber band ligation of haemorrhoids using suction ligator. J Ayub Med Coll Abbottabad. 2004;16:34–7.

50. Poen AC, Felt-Bersma RJ, Cuesta MA, Devillé W, Meuwissen SG. A randomized controlled trial of rubber band ligation versus infra-red coagulation in the treatment of internal hemorrhoids. Eur J Gastroenterol Hepatol. 2000;12:535–9.

51. Quevedo-Bonilla G, Farkas AM, Abcarian H, Hambrick E, Orsay CP. Septic complications of hemorrhoidal banding. Arch Surg. 1988;123:650–1.

52. Hinton CP, Morris DL. A randomized trial comparing direct current therapy and bipolar diathermy in the outpatient treatment of third-degree hemorrhoids. Dis Colon Rectum. 1990;33:931–2.

53. Randall GM, Jensen DM, Machicado GA, Hirabayashi K, Jensen ME, You S, Pelayo E. Prospective randomized comparative study of bipolar versus direct current electrocoagulation for treatment of bleeding internal hemorrhoids. Gastrointest Endosc. 1994;40:403–10.

54. Morgan J. Varicose state of saphenous haemorrhoids treated successfully by the injection of tincture of persulphate of iron. Medical Press and Circular 1869:29–30.

55. Sim AJ, Murie JA, Mackenzie I. Three year follow up study on the treatment of first and second degree hemorrhoids by sclerosant injection or rubber band ligation. Surg Gynecol Obstet. 1983;157:534–6.

56. Bullock N. Impotence after sclerotherapy of haemorrhoids: case reports. BMJ. 1997;314:419.

57. Khoury GA, Lake SP, Lewis MC, Lewis AA. A randomized trial to compare single with multiple phenol injection treatment for haemorrhoids. Br J Surg. 1985;72:741–2.

58. Bleday R, Pena JP, Rothenberger DA, Goldberg SM, Buls JG. Symptomatic hemorrhoids: current incidence and complications of operative therapy. Dis Colon Rectum. 1992;35:477–81.

59. Ferguson JA, Mazier WP, Ganchrow MI, Friend WG. The closed technique of hemorrhoidectomy. Surgery. 1971;70:480–4.

60. Milone M, Maietta P, Leongito M, Pesce G, Salvatore G, Milone F. Ferguson hemorrhoidectomy: is still the gold standard treatment? Updates Surg. 2012;64:191–4.

61. Milsom JW, Mazier WP. Classification and management of post-surgical anal stenosis. Surg Gynecol Obstet. 1986;163:60–4.

62. Xu L, Chen H, Lin G, Ge Q. LigaSure versus Ferguson hemorrhoidectomy in the treatment of hemorrhoids: a meta-analysis of randomized control trials. Surg Laparosc Endosc Percutan Tech. 2015;25:106–10.

63. Milligan ET, Morgan CN, Jones LE, Officer R. Surgical anatomy of the anal canal and operative treatment of haemorrhoids. Lancet. 1937;11:1119–94.

64. Whitehead W. The surgical treatment of hemorrhoids. Br Med J. 1882;1:148–50.

65. Wolff BG, Culp CE. The Whitehead hemorrhoidectomy. An unjustly maligned procedure. Dis Colon Rectum. 1988;31:587–90.

66. Ho YH, Seow-Choen F, Tan M, Leong AF. Randomized controlled trial of open and closed haemorrhoidectomy. Br J Surg. 1997;84:1729–30.

67. Carapeti EA, Kamm MA, McDonald PJ, Chadwick SJ, Phillips RK. Randomized trial of open versus closed day-case haemorrhoidectomy. Br J Surg. 1999;86:612–3.

68. Arbman G, Krook H, Haapaniemi S. Closed vs open hemorrhoidectomy – is there any difference? Dis Colon Rectum. 2000;43:31–4.

69. Gençosmanoğlu R, Sad O, Koç D, Inceoğlu R. Hemorrhoidectomy: open or closed technique? A prospective randomized clinical trial. Dis Colon Rectum. 2002;45:70–5.

70. Ho YH, Buettner PG. Open compared with closed haemorrhoidectomy: meta-analysis of randomized controlled trials. Tech Coloproctol. 2007;11:135–43.

71. Hetzer FH, Demartines N, Handschin AE, Clavien PA. Stapled vs excision hemorrhoidectomy: long term-results of a prospective randomized trial. Arch Surg. 2002;127:337–40.

72. Nienhuijs S, de Hingh I. Conventional versus LigaSure hemorrhoidectomy for patients with symptomatic hemorrhoids. Cochrane Database Syst Rev 2009; (1): CD006761.

73. Sohn VY, Martin MJ, Mullenix PS, Cuadrado DG, Place RJ, Steele SR. A comparison of open versus closed techniques using the Harmonic Scalpel in outpatient hemorrhoid surgery. Mil Med. 2008;73:689–92.

74. Wang JY, Chang-Chien CR, Chen JS, Lai CR, Tang RP. The role of lasers in hemorrhoidectomy. Dis Colon Rectum. 1991;34:78–82.

75. Iwagaki H, Higuchi Y, Fuchimoto S, Orita K. The laser treatment of hemorrhoids: results of a study on 1816 patients. Jpn J Surg. 1989;19:658–61.

76. Senagore A, Mazier WP, Luchtefeld MA, MacKeigan JM, Wengert T. Treatment of advanced hemorrhoidal disease: a prospective, randomized comparison of cold scalpel vs contact ND:YAG laser. Dis Colon Rectum. 1993;36:1042–9.

77. Mathai V, Ong BC, Ho YH. Randomized controlled trial of lateral internal sphincterotomy with haemorrhoidectomy. Br J Surg. 1996;83:380–2.

78. Wasvary HJ, Hain J, Mosed-Vogel M, Bendick P, Barkel DC, Klein SN. Randomized, prospective, double-blind, placebo controlled trial of effect of nitroglycerin ointment on pain after hemorrhoidectomy. Dis Colon Rectum. 2001;44:1069–73.

79. Ala S, Saeedi M, Eshghi F, Mirzabeygi P. Topical metronidazole can reduce pain after surgery and pain on defecation in

80. Zaheer S, Reilly WT, Pemberton JH, Ilstrup D. Urinary retention after operations for benign anorectal diseases. Dis Colon Rectum. 1998;41:696–704.

81. Toyonaga T, Matsushima M, Sogawa N, Jiang SF, Matsumura N, Shimojima Y, Tanaka Y, Suzuki K, Masuda J, Tanaka M. Postoperative urinary retention after surgery for benign anorectal disease: potential risk factors and strategy for prevention. Int J Colorectal Dis. 2006;21:676–82.

82. Hoff SD, Bailey HR, Butts DR, Max E, Smith KW, Zamora LF, Skakun GB. Ambulatory surgical hemorrhoidectomy--a solution to postoperative urinary retention? Dis Colon Rectum. 1994;37:1242–4.

83. Chik B, Law WL, Choi HK. Urinary retention after haemorrhoidectomy: impact of stapled haemorrhoidectomy. Asian J Surg. 2006;29:233–7.

84. Rosen L, Sipe P, Stasik JJ, Riether RD, Trimpi HD. Outcome of delayed hemorrhage following surgical hemorrhoidectomy. Dis Colon Rectum. 1993;36:743–6.

85. Basso L, Pescatori M. Outcome of delayed hemorrhage following surgical hemorrhoidectomy. Dis Colon Rectum. 1994;37:288–9.

86. Chen HH, Wang JY, Changchien CR, Chen JS, Hsu KC, Chiang JM, Yeh CY, Tang R. Risk factors associated with posthemorrhoidectomy secondary hemorrhage: a single-institution prospective study of 4,880 consecutive closed hemorrhoidectomies. Dis Colon Rectum. 2002;45:1096–9.

87. Chen HH, Wang JY, Changchien CR, Yeh CY, Tsai WS, Tang R. Effective management of posthemorrhoidectomy secondary hemorrhage using rectal irrigation. Dis Colon Rectum. 2002;45:234–8.

88. Eu KW, Teoh TA, Seow-Choen F, Goh HS. Anal stricture following haemorrhoidectomy: early diagnosis and treatment. Aust N Z J Surg. 1995;2:101–3.

89. Carditello A, Milone A, Stilo F, Mollo F, Basile M. Surgical treatment of anal stenosis following hemorrhoid surgery. Results of 150 combined mucosal advancement and internal sphincterotomy. Chir Ital. 2002;54:841–4.

90. McCloud JM, Jameson JS, Scott AN. Life-threatening sepsis following treatment for haemorrhoids: a systematic review. Colorectal Dis. 2006;8:748–55.

91. Nelson DW, Champagne BJ, Rivadeneira DE, Davis BR, Maykel JA, Ross HM, Johnson EK, Steele SR. Prophylactic antibiotics for hemorrhoidectomy: are they really needed? Dis Colon Rectum. 2014;57:365–9.

92. Pescatori M, Favetta U, Dedola S, Orsini S. Transanal stapled excision of rectal mucosal prolapsed. Tech Coloproctol. 1997;1:96–8.

93. Longo A. Treatment of hemorrhoidal disease by reduction of mucosa and haemorrhoidal prolapse with a circular stapling device: A new procedure. Proceeding of the 6th World Congress of Endoscopic Surgery, 777–784. 1998.

94. Senagore AJ, Singer M, Abcarian H, Fleshman J, Corman M, Wexner S, Nivatvongs S. A prospective, randomized, controlled multicenter trial comparing stapled hemorrhoidopexy and Ferguson hemorrhoidectomy: perioperative and one-year results. Procedure for Prolapse and Hemorrhoids (PPH) Multicenter Study Group. Dis Colon Rectum. 2004;47:1824–36.

95. Racalbuto A, Aliotta I, Corsaro G, Lanteri R, Di Cataldo A, Licata A. Hemorrhoidal stapler prolapsectomy vs. Milligan-

Morgan hemorrhoidectomy: a long-term randomized trial. Int J Colorectal Dis. 2004;19:239–44.

96. Krska Z, Kvasnièka J, Faltýn J, Schmidt D, Sváb J, Kormanová K, Hubík J. Surgical treatment of haemorrhoids according to Longo and Milligan Morgan: an evaluation of postoperative tissue response. Colorectal Dis. 2003;5:573–6.

97. Boccasanta P, Capretti PG, Venturi M, Cioffi U, De Simone M, Salamina G, Contessini-Avesani E, Peracchia A. Randomised controlled trial between stapled circumferential mucosectomy and conventional circular hemorrhoidectomy in advanced hemorrhoids with external mucosal prolapse. Am J Surg. 2001;182:64–8.

98. Jayaraman S, Colquhoun PH, Malthaner RA. Stapled versus conventional surgery for hemorrhoids. Cochrane Database Syst Rev. 2006; 18: CD005393.

99. Shao WJ, Li GC, Zhang ZH, Yang BL, Sun GD, Chen YQ. Systematic review and meta-analysis of randomized controlled trials comparing stapled haemorrhoidopexy with conventional haemorrhoidectomy. Br J Surg. 2008;95: 147–60.

100. Morinaga K, Hasuda K, Ikeda T. A novel therapy for internal hemorrhoids: ligation of the hemorrhoidal artery with a newly devised instrument (Moricorn) in conjunction with a Doppler flowmeter. Am J Gastroenterol. 1995;90:610–3.

101. Charúa Guindic L, Fonseca Muñoz E, García Pérez NJ, Osorio Hernández RM, Navarrete Cruces T, Avendaño Espinosa O, Guerra Melgar LR. Hemorrhoidal desarterialization guided by Doppler. A surgical alternative in hemorrhoidal disease management. Rev Gastroenterol Mex. 2004;69:83–7.

102. Bursics A, Morvay K, Kupcsulik P, Flautner L. Comparison of early and 1-year follow-up results of conventional hemorrhoidectomy and hemorrhoid artery ligation: a randomized study. Int J Colorectal Dis. 2004;19:176–80.

103. Ramírez JM, Aguilella V, Elía M, Gracia JA, Martínez M. Doppler-guided hemorrhoidal artery ligation in the management of symptomatic hemorrhoids. Rev Esp Enferm Dig. 2005;97:97–103.

104. Felice G, Privitera A, Ellul E, Klaumann M. Doppler-guided hemorrhoidal artery ligation: an alternative to hemorrhoidectomy. Dis Colon Rectum. 2005;48:2090–3.

105. Giordano P, Overton J, Madeddu F, Zaman S, Gravante G. Transanal hemorrhoidal dearterialization: a systematic review. Dis Colon Rectum. 2009;52:1665–71.

106. Grosz CR. A surgical treatment of thrombosed external hemorrhoids. Dis Colon Rectum. 1990;33:249–50.

107. Grosz CR. A surgical treatment of thrombosed external hemorrhoids. Dis Colon Rectum. 1990;33:249–50.

108. Bernstein WC. What are hemorrhoids and what is their relationship to the portal venous system? Dis Colon Rectum. 1983;26:829–34.

109. Chawla Y, Dilawari JB. Anorectal varices--their frequency in cirrhotic and non-cirrhotic portal hypertension. Gut. 1991;32: 309–11.

110. Montemurro S, Polignano FM, Caliandro C, Rucci A, Ruggieri E, Sciscio V. Inferior mesocaval shunt for bleeding anorectal varices and portal vein thrombosis. Hepatogastroenterology. 2001;48:980–3.

111. Rahmani O, Wolpert LM, Drezner AD. Distal inferior mesenteric veins to renal vein shunt for treatment of bleeding anorectal varices: case report and review of literature. J Vasc Surg. 2002;36:1264–6.

112. Saleeby Jr RG, Rosen L, Stasik JJ, Riether RD, Sheets J, Khubchandani IT. Hemorrhoidectomy during pregnancy: risk or relief? Dis Colon Rectum. 1991;34:260–1.

113. Jeffery PJ, Parks AG, Ritchie JK. Treatment of haemorrhoids in patients with inflammatory bowel disease. Lancet. 1977;21: 1084–5.

114. Wolkomir AF, Luchtefeld MA. Surgery for symptomatic hemorrhoids and anal fissures in Crohn's disease. Dis Colon Rectum. 1993;36:545–7.

115. Morandi E, Merlini D, Salvaggio A, Foschi D, Trabucchi E. Prospective study of healing time after hemorrhoidectomy: influence of HIV infection, acquired immunodeficiency syndrome, and anal wound infection. Dis Colon Rectum. 1999;42:1140–4.

116. Grewal H, Guillem JG, Quan SH, Enker WE, Cohen AM. Anorectal disease in neutropenic leukemic patients. Operative vs. nonoperative management. Dis Colon Rectum. 1994;37:1095–9.

13
Anal Fissure

Kim C. Lu and Daniel O. Herzig

Key Concepts

- An acute anal fissure (symptoms <6 weeks) is likely to heal (87%) with dietary modification and supportive care.
- In a chronic anal fissure (symptoms >6 weeks), topical nitroglycerin or calcium channel blockers are slightly better than placebo in inducing healing.
- Injection of botulinum toxin into the internal anal sphincter can heal fissures refractory to topical ointments; though this is not as effective as lateral internal anal sphincterotomy.
- Lateral internal anal sphincterotomy is the most effective therapy in healing fissures; there is an increased risk, however, of fecal incontinence.
- For anal fissures associated with decreased anal sphincter tone, a dermal advancement flap is a reasonable option.

Definition/Clinical Presentation

An anal fissure is a tear in the epithelial lining of the distal anal canal [1]. While this is likely an extremely common condition, it is difficult to know exactly how common. Many people assume this is a hemorrhoidal problem and initially avoid formal evaluation. Further, many fissures will resolve without intervention. Nevertheless, persistent anal pain and bleeding eventually push many patients to seek medical attention. In one single colon and rectal surgery clinic, anal fissures resulted in more than 1200 office visits over a 5-year period [2].

Fissures can be classified as acute vs. chronic and typical vs. atypical. Acute fissures cause bright red bleeding with bowel movements and sharp, burning, tearing anal pain or

spasm that can last for hours after the bowel movement. Physical findings include a linear separation of the anoderm, at times visible with just separation of the buttocks (Figure 13-1). Often, elevated anal resting pressures are appreciated on digital rectal examination. If tolerated by the patient, the suspected diagnosis can be confirmed by visualizing the break in the anoderm with office anoscopy after using an anesthetic lubricant. If only one area can be examined, the posterior midline should be evaluated first, as it is the site of up to 90% of typical anal fissures. The remaining minority of typical fissures are found in the anterior midline [3]. Acute fissures generally resolve within 4–6 weeks of appropriate management; chronic fissures are therefore defined as those producing symptoms beyond 6–8 weeks. Chronic fissures have additional physical findings of an external sentinel tag at the external apex, exposed internal sphincter muscle, and a hypertrophied anal papilla at the internal apex (Figure 13-2).

Typical fissures are usually located in the posterior or anterior midline, have the characteristic findings described above, and are not associated with other diseases. In contrast, atypical fissures can occur anywhere in the anal canal (Figure 13-3), can have a wide variety of findings, and can tend to be associated with other diseases, including malignancy, Crohn's disease, human immunodeficiency virus (HIV) infection, syphilis, and tuberculosis (Figure 13-4).

Pathogenesis

Despite the common nature of this long-standing problem, the exact etiology remains uncertain. Many have described onset of a fissure after the passage of a large, hard stool or anal trauma.

By a mechanical theory, the occurrence in the posterior midline might be because the anorectal angle creates the greatest stress at this location [4]. Sphincter hypertonicity has been frequently described in early reports of the disease

Electronic supplementary material: The online version of this chapter (doi:10.1007/978-3-319-25970-3_13) contains supplementary material, which is available to authorized users.

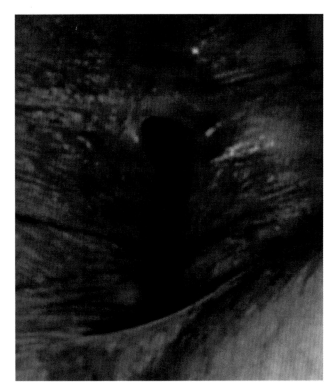

FIGURE 13-1. Acute fissure with clear edges and no signs of chronicity of sphincter hypertrophy. Courtesy of Dr. Richard P. Billingham, MD.

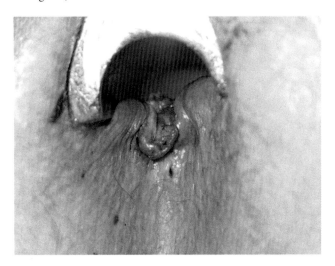

FIGURE 13-2. Chronic fissure with external sentinel tag, internal hypertrophied papilla, and thickened internal anal sphincter muscle.

and has been documented by manometry in multiple studies [5, 6]. It is not clear, however, if the elevated pressures are a cause of the disease or an effect [7].

A second common theory is relative ischemia of the posterior midline. This area of the anal canal has been shown to be relatively ischemic by both arteriographic studies and laser Doppler flowmetry [8, 9]. The theories of hypertonicity and ischemia may be related to some extent, particularly in that hypertonicity may aggravate the relative ischemia.

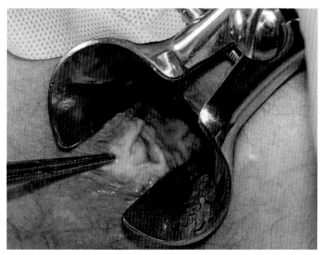

FIGURE 13-3. Atypical fissure with skin changes, broad base, and lateral location. Courtesy of Sam Atallah, MD.

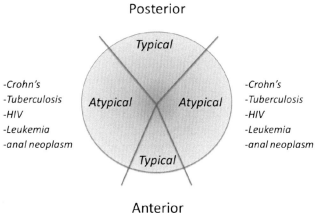

FIGURE 13-4. Type of fissure by location.

Nevertheless, tears in the anoderm undoubtedly occur with a great deal of frequency, whether from a large stool, anorectal intercourse, or instrumentation for surgical procedures, and the evolution to a chronic fissure is likely only seen in a minority of these instances. Furthermore, fissures can occur in the absence of any trauma or constipation.

Nonoperative Treatment

Healing Rates in Acute Anal Fissure

Practice parameters from the American Society of Colon and Rectal Surgeons state that conservative therapy is safe, has few side effects, and should usually be the first step in therapy [10]. Jensen reported a randomized trial done in patients with acute anal fissure. The control group in this trial was instructed to take 10 g of unprocessed bran twice daily and use a warm sitz bath for 15 min twice daily and after bowel movements, if possible. Overall, 91% of patients were able to follow the study protocol. In that control group, the fissure healing rate was 87% [11].

Healing Rates in Chronic Anal Fissure

A more frequent problem for the surgeon is the patient who has had symptoms for several weeks and has failed an initial approach similar to that described by Jensen. In these patients, spontaneous healing rates are likely to be seen in only a minority of patients. A recent Cochrane review of the nonoperative treatment of anal fissure analyzed over 70 randomized trials of chronic anal fissure [12]. Unlike the acute fissure population, the healing rate in the combined placebo group is 35.5%.

Because internal anal sphincter hypertonicity is related to anal fissure, initial nonoperative treatment is targeted to alleviate internal anal sphincter activity through two topical agents, nitroglycerin and diltiazem, and one injectable agent, botulinum toxin A.

Topical

Nitroglycerin

Nitric oxide was reported to be the neurotransmitter mediating relaxation of the internal anal sphincter in the early 1990's [13]. Topical application of 0.2% glyceryl trinitrate ointment (GTN) was subsequently found to result in relaxation of the anal sphincter by manometric studies [14]. A landmark randomized trial was reported in 1997. That showed a healing rate of 68% with GTN treatment, compared with 8% in the placebo group [15]. The recent Cochrane analysis of 18 trials (four including children), however, showed a healing rate of 48.9% with GTN treatment, compared to 35.5% in the placebo or control group. With longer-term follow-up, recurrence varied from 51 to 67% [12].

The most common side effect of topical GTN treatment is headache, at a reported rate of 27% in the pooled analysis and may be as high as 50% [16]. While often minor and temporary, it may lead to discontinuation of therapy in 10–20% of patients [17–19]. In one prospective randomized trial comparing endoanal application vs. perianal application, endoanal application of 0.4% nitroglycerin bid was associated with decreased frequency and severity of headaches [20]. A second potential drawback to topical GTN is tachyphylaxis, which does not respond to escalations in dose or frequency.

There is was not an FDA-approved indication for nitroglycerin in the United States until 2011. The topical form of nitroglycerin was initially supplied as a 2% ointment. To achieve a 0.2% concentration, the prescription often needs to be filled at a compounding pharmacy. Jonas et al. reported that after application of 0.2% GTN, the reduction in mean anal resting pressure lasted only about 2 h, which may

explain some of the treatment failures seen with GTN [16]. In 2011, the FDA approved Rectiv (0.4% nitroglycerin) which is applied endoanally bid for 6–8 weeks. At 24-week follow-up, there was a 77% healing rate [20].

Calcium Channel Blockers

Both diltiazem and nifedipine have been described either orally or topically to cause relaxation of the smooth muscle of the internal anal sphincter. Oral and topical nifedipine have been shown to lower mean resting anal pressure [21]. Similarly, diltiazem has been shown to decrease mean resting anal pressure, although the effect is greater with topical diltiazem [22, 23]. Since studies done with calcium channel blockers have more variability with respect to the medication, dosages, and routes, it is difficult to pool data for analysis. Multiple small trials suggest healing rates equivalent to GTN with fewer side effects [24, 25]. Neither diltiazem nor nifedipine are FDA approved for the treatment of anal fissure. There is no topical formulation available in the United States, so a compounding pharmacy needs to make a topical gel from an oral formulation.

Botulinum Toxin Type A

Botulinum toxins are a family of neuroparalytic proteins synthesized by *Clostridium botulinum*. They inhibit the release of acetylcholine at the neuromuscular junction [26, 27]. These agents can be used to induce a local paralysis that lasts for several months, depending upon the subtype used. The toxins are labeled A through G, according to immunologic specificity, with type A being most commonly used in the United States. Botulinum toxins are Food and Drug Administration approved for treatment of certain spastic disorders, but not anal fissures. They have been used off-label in other disorders, including chronic anal fissures. There is no uniformly recommended dose or site of injection. Botulinum toxin type A is supplied as a powder in 100-unit single-patient-use vials. Once reconstituted, any remaining solution after use must be discarded. Relaxation of the muscle occurs within days and lasts for 2–4 months. This has the theoretical advantage of allowing fissure healing while avoiding permanent fecal incontinence.

After the initial report in 1994, various methods of injection, including injection into the internal or external sphincter, at single or multiple sites, and in various doses, have been described [28]. In one small study of 50 patients with posterior anal fissures, patients were randomized to anterior vs. posterior internal anal sphincter injections. Those injected in the anterior internal anal sphincter were significantly more likely to heal [29].

Botulinum toxin injections of the internal anal sphincter have been compared with placebo, as well as other treatments, with mixed results. In a widely referenced, early, double-blind, placebo-controlled randomized crossover trial of 30 patients, botulinum toxin A injection was found to be superior to saline injection, with a healing rate of 73% with Botox, compared to 13% with placebo ($p=0.003$) [30].

Trials have compared botulinum toxin injection with lateral internal sphincterotomy for fissures refractory to topical medical management. Arroyo et al. reported a randomized controlled trial of 80 patients and showed healing rates of 92.5% for the lateral internal sphincterotomy group, compared with 45% in the botulinum toxin group. They concluded, however, that botulinum toxin was still their preference in patients over 50 or at risk for incontinence due to a higher but not statistically significant incidence of incontinence after sphincterotomy [31]. Other small studies support the finding of higher number of treatment failures, but fewer complications in the botulinum toxin group [32, 33]. In a recent meta-analysis of seven randomized controlled trials, comparing botulinum toxin injection with lateral internal anal sphincterotomy, the healing and recurrence rates were worse with botulinum toxin [34]. In a recent randomized prospective trial comparing lateral internal sphincterotomy with Botox injection/topical diltiazem, 1-year healing rates were far superior with lateral internal anal sphincterotomy (94% vs. 65%) [35].

There is limited data regarding the long-term effectiveness of botulinum toxin. In one retrospective review of 411 patients who failed topical diltiazem, patients were treated with 100 units of botulinum toxin A and underwent fissurectomy under general anesthesia. 74% were healed at 2-year follow-up. Of note, the botulinum toxin was injected into the intersphincteric space.

Operative Treatment

Anal Dilation

One of the earliest forms of treatment was anal dilation, first described in 1829, and studied later in various trials for anal fissure [36, 37]. While extensively studied, there is considerable variability in the technique and a wide range of reported outcomes. Few well-controlled studies exist. The recent Cochrane review included an analysis of seven randomized controlled trials, comparing manual anal stretch to internal sphincterotomy [38]. They demonstrated that dilation was not more effective than sphincterotomy and had a higher rate of incontinence ($OR=4.03$, 95% $CI=2.04$–7.46). A more standardized and objective method of anal stretch, balloon dilation, has been reported. Renzi et al. evaluated the use of balloon dilation compared to lateral internal sphincterotomy in a prospective randomized trial [39]. Healing rates were high in both groups, and there was no difference between the groups. After 24 months of follow-up, however, incontinence was zero in the balloon dilation group, compared to 16% in the lateral internal sphincterotomy

group ($p<0.0001$). While manual dilation is no longer indicated for anal fissure, balloon dilation may be one alternative.

Anal Sphincterotomy (Technique)

While also described in various forms since the early 1800's, isolated division of the internal anal sphincter muscle (sphincterotomy) was first described by Eisenhammer in the 1950's [40]. His technique of posterior internal sphincterotomy at the site of the fissure led to a posterior midline "gutter" or "keyhole" deformity, leading to fecal soiling in 30–40% of patients. Notaras described a simple modification: performing the sphincterotomy laterally, which eliminated this problem [41]. Since then, lateral internal anal sphincterotomy has become the main surgical intervention for failure of medical management. The procedure can be done under local anesthesia, as an outpatient. The variations currently include open vs. closed technique and conservative vs. traditional sphincterotomy. The closed technique is performed by inserting the scalpel blade in the intersphincteric groove and then turning it medially to break the fibers of the internal sphincter (Figure 13-5). The open technique is done through a radial incision overlying the intersphincteric groove. After dissecting the internal anal sphincter away from the anoderm, the distal internal anal sphincter is divided under direct vision (Figure 13-6). Division was originally described to the dentate line, but recent reports describe a more conservative approach, either with division of the muscle to the fissure apex or with division just until the band of hypertrophied muscle is released.

Outcomes Between Closed and Open Anal Sphincterotomy

From the Cochrane Library, a systematic review on the operative procedures for anal fissures was updated in 2011 [38]. The techniques of open and closed sphincterotomy have been compared in multiple reports, including five randomized studies that met inclusion criteria for the Cochrane analysis [42–46]. Combined, these reports show no difference in either persistence of fissure or incontinence with the two techniques. A prospective cohort study evaluated 140 consecutive patients undergoing open or closed sphincterotomy with postoperative endosonography [47]. Postoperative endoanal ultrasounds showed that open sphincterotomy was associated with a significantly higher proportion of complete sphincterotomies. The rate of incontinence and treatment failure was not different between the open and closed groups, but there was a strongly significant increase in incontinence scores ($p<0.001$) and decrease in recurrence rates ($p<0.001$) with increasing length of sphincterotomy.

FIGURE 13-5. Closed lateral sphincterotomy. (**a**) Location of the intersphincteric groove. (**b**) Insertion of the knife blade in the intersphincteric plane. (**c**). Lateral to medial division of the internal anal sphincter (*inset*: medial to lateral division of the muscle).

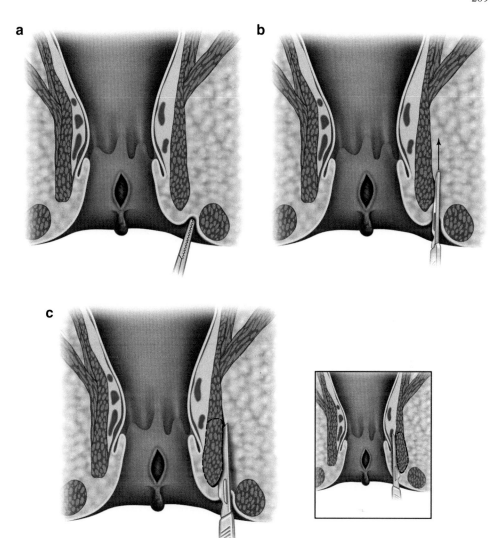

Extent of Sphincterotomy

The decision regarding the extent of sphincterotomy performed in the operating room is a controversial topic. Excessive division increases the risk of incontinence, yet inadequate division increases the risk of persistence or recurrence. While many texts describe division to the dentate line, recent studies have examined a more conservative sphincterotomy. Mentes et al. prospectively randomized 76 patients with chronic anal fissure to lateral internal sphincterotomy to the dentate line or to the apex of the fissure [48]. Treatment failure was zero in the traditional group, and 13% in the conservative group after 1 year of follow-up, with most of the treatment failures occurring after 2 months. There was no statistically significant difference in the postoperative incontinence scores between the two treatment groups. There was, however, an increase in the postoperative incontinence score in the traditional group; this study may have been underpowered to detect a possible difference. In a similar manner, Elsebae et al. prospectively randomized 92 patients to sphincterotomy to the dentate line (traditional) or sphincter-

otomy to the apex of the fissure (conservative) [49]. Treatment failure was zero in the traditional group and 4% in the conservative group (p = NS); persistent incontinence was 4% in the traditional group and 0% in the conservative group (p = NS). The follow-up period, however, was only 18 weeks. In an even more recent study, Magdy et al. randomized 150 patients to traditional sphincterotomy, V-Y advancement flap, or conservative sphincterotomy + V-Y advancement flap. The healing rates were 84% in the traditional group and 94% in the conservative division/advancement flap group. The incontinence rates were 14% vs. 2%, respectively. The low healing rates with traditional sphincterotomy, however, are a bit hard to believe [50].

The techniques of division to the dentate line or to the fissure apex have objective definitions, yet many surgeons approach the sphincterotomy as a more subjective task. The band of hypertrophied internal anal sphincter muscle may or may not relate to either of these two landmarks. While division of the hypertrophied muscle segment is subjective, a subsequent report from Mentes et al. attempted to compare this method by creating a sphincterotomy that achieves an

FIGURE 13-6. Open lateral
internal sphincterotomy. (**a**)
Radial skin incision distal to the
dentate line exposing the
intersphincteric groove. (**b**)
Elevation and division of the
internal sphincter. (**c**) Primary
wound closure.

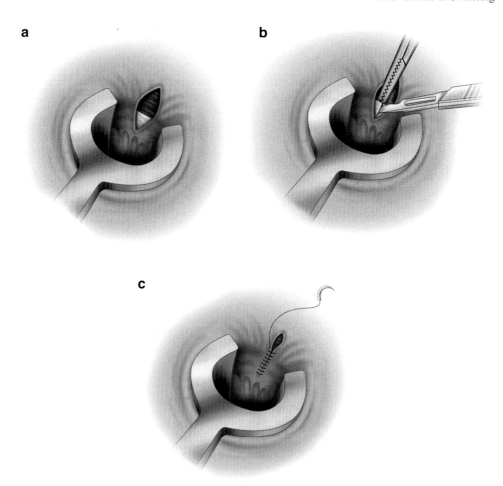

Fissurectomy

The hallmark of chronic fissure is the triad of a hypertrophied internal sphincter, a hypertrophied anal papilla, and an external sentinel tag. Excision of the papilla and tag, or complete fissurectomy, is optional, but particularly useful if the fissure edges appear rolled and epithelialized, as this may promote faster wound healing. Renewed interest in fissurotomy (unroofing of superficial tract extending caudad from fissure) as primary treatment of the fissure has recently been reported [52].

Results of Sphincterotomy

In addition to these randomized controlled trials, a myriad of additional nonrandomized reports are available, describing a

anal caliber of 30 mm. They prospectively compared this technique to division to the apex of the fissure [51]. Their findings showed the average anal caliber was greater in the group that underwent division to the apex, the incontinence rates were higher, and there was no significant difference in treatment failure.

wide range of results from lateral internal sphincterotomy. While most reports cite low rates of treatment failure, the incontinence rate is widely variable and is as high as 30–40 % [53, 54]. With a multimodal approach designed to minimize the risk of permanent incontinence, the trend is clearly moving away from lateral internal sphincterotomy and toward more medical therapy and/or botulinum toxin. It is not clear whether or not this strategy will be the most effective long-term solution with respect to morbidity, costs, and patient satisfaction. The disease, however, is largely measured by the subjective experience of the patient, who is ultimately the best judge of which treatment is worth pursuing and which risks are worth taking. Floyd et al. reported that with multiple options offered to patients, the ultimate time to healing is prolonged, but 72 % of patients can avoid operative treatment, and 97 % of patients can be healed [55].

In a similar report with a median follow-up of 47 months, Lysy et al. reported results from their approach of escalating from topical agents, to botulinum toxin, to sphincterotomy [56]. Like the cohort described by Floyd, 71 % of patients resolved without lateral sphincterotomy. They also noted that the low rate of sphincterotomy came at the price of increased recurrences before complete healing, and a longer time spent in treatment.

Fissures Without Anal Hypertonicity

Treatments directed at relaxation of the anal sphincter, either pharmacologically or surgically, presume that relief of anal hypertonicity will lead to healing. A subset of patients with fissure, however, will not demonstrate hypertonicity, and hypotonicity may actually be found. Giordano et al. recently reported results from their prospective study of simple cutaneous advancement flap in 51 patients over a 6-year period for all patients, regardless of anal tone [57]. They found the procedure to be well tolerated, with a 98% treatment success rate. Nyam and colleagues evaluated 21 patients with fissures and below normal anal pressures. In this group, an island advancement flap resulted in complete healing and no incontinence in all patients [58]. A 2002 report from St. Mark's noted favorable results with advancement flaps for fissures with hypotonicity in a small series, with successful treatment in 7/8 patients with a median follow-up of 7 months [59]. While this technique might not be useful for all patients with refractory fissures, it holds particular promise in addressing the fissure in the setting of a hypotonic anus. Video 13-1 demonstrates the technique of an anal flap. While the video portrays anal stenosis, the technical points of the procedure are well demonstrated.

Crohn's Disease

Fissures are commonly seen in people with Crohn's disease, affecting approximately 30% of patients [60, 61]. When they occur, they tend to be in more atypical locations, deeper, and associated with other pathology, especially fistula. These fissures have atypical appearance as well, often creating deep ulcerations, and potentially creating significant deformity. As with other manifestations of Crohn's, it is reasonable to intervene only as complications dictate. Some authors have reported acceptable outcomes from interventions in these patients [62, 63], but caution should be the rule, and sphincter salvage is prudent. Multidisciplinary care is crucial in addressing anorectal disease in the patient with Crohn's, as appropriate medical management of the disease may lead to resolution of the anorectal disorders in 50% or more of these cases [64, 65].

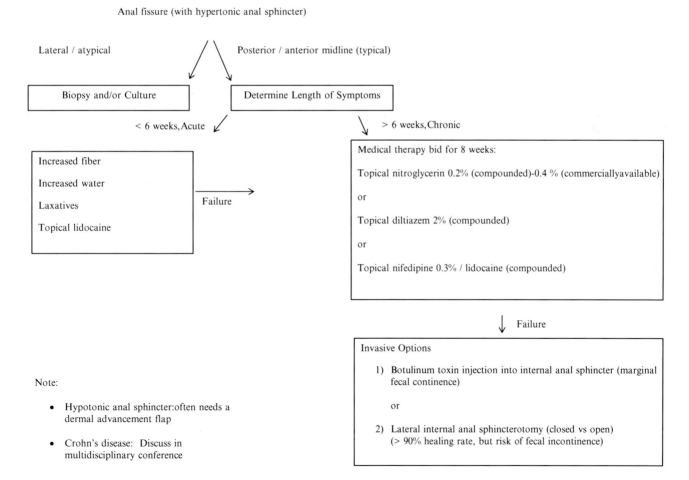

FIGURE 13-7. Treatment algorithm for anal fissure.

Human Immunodeficiency Virus

HIV-related anal disease includes both typical fissures and anorectal ulcers, which can appear as deep, broad-based, or cavitating lesions. Poor sphincter tone and function is a more frequent finding than the hypertonicity that accompanies typical, non-HIV-related fissures. Small studies have reported successful treatment of typical fissures, and the medical treatment of HIV continues to improve [66, 67]. Concerns about delayed wound healing and increased infectious complications, however, remain.

Conclusions

Anal fissure is a common disorder that is effectively treated and prevented with conservative measures in its acute form. Chronic fissures usually require medical therapy that can be effective in a small majority of patients. Initial therapy includes bulking agents, control of constipation, and topical medications to relax the internal anal sphincter. Botulinum toxin and lateral internal sphincterotomy can both be considered for treatment of refractory anal fissures, and the popularity of botulinum toxin is increasing. Sphincterotomy remains an effective operation, with a very high rate of resolution of symptoms, but at the price of some risk of permanent incontinence. A suggested treatment algorithm is provided in Figure 13-7.

References

1. Herzig DO, Lu KC. Anal fissure. Surg Clin North Am. 2010;90:33–44.
2. Ricciardi R, Dykes S, Madoff R. Anal fissure. In: Beck DE, Roberts P, Saclarides TK, Senagore AJ, Stamos MJ, Wexner SD, editors. The ASCRS textbook of colon and rectal surgery. 2nd ed. New York, NY: Springer; 2011. p. 203–18.
3. Hoexter B. Anal fissure. In: Fazio VW, Church J, Delaney CP, editors. Current therapy in colon and rectal surgery. 2nd ed. Philadelphia, PA: Elsevier Mosby; 2005. p. 19–22.
4. Perry GG. Fissure in ano--a complication of anusitis. South Med J. 1962;55:955–7.
5. Farouk R, Duthie GS, MacGregor AB, Bartolo DC. Sustained internal sphincter hypertonia in patients with chronic anal fissure. Dis Colon Rectum. 1994;37:424–9.
6. Nothmann BJ, Schuster MM. Internal anal sphincter derangement with anal fissures. Gastroenterology. 1974;67:216–20.
7. Gibbons CP, Read NW. Anal hypertonia in fissures: cause or effect? Br J Surg. 1986;73:443–5.
8. Klosterhalfen B, Vogel P, Rixen H, Mittermayer C. Topography of the inferior rectal artery: a possible cause of chronic, primary anal fissure. Dis Colon Rectum. 1989;32:43–52.
9. Schouten WR, Briel JW, Auwerda JJ, De Graaf EJ. Ischaemic nature of anal fissure. Br J Surg. 1996;83:63–5.
10. Perry WB, Dykes SL, Buie WD, Rafferty JF. Standards Practice Task Force of the American Society of C, Rectal S. Practice parameters for the management of anal fissures (3rd revision). Dis Colon Rectum. 2010;53:1110–5.
11. Jensen SL. Treatment of first episodes of acute anal fissure: prospective randomised study of lignocaine ointment versus hydrocortisone ointment or warm sitz baths plus bran. Br Med J. 1986;292:1167–9.
12. Nelson RL, Thomas K, Morgan J, Jones A. Non surgical therapy for anal fissure. Cochrane Database Syst Rev. 2012; (2): CD003431.
13. O'Kelly T, Brading A, Mortensen N. Nerve mediated relaxation of the human internal anal sphincter: the role of nitric oxide. Gut. 1993;34:689–93.
14. Loder PB, Kamm MA, Nicholls RJ, Phillips RK. 'Reversible chemical sphincterotomy' by local application of glyceryl trinitrate. Br J Surg. 1994;81:1386–9.
15. Lund JN, Scholefield JH. A randomised, prospective, double-blind, placebo-controlled trial of glyceryl trinitrate ointment in treatment of anal fissure. Lancet. 1997;349:11–4.
16. Jonas M, Barrett DA, Shaw PN, Scholefield JH. Systemic levels of glyceryl trinitrate following topical application to the anoderm do not correlate with the measured reduction in anal pressure. Br J Surg. 2001;88:1613–6.
17. Brisinda G, Maria G, Bentivoglio AR, Cassetta E, Gui D, Albanese A. A comparison of injections of botulinum toxin and topical nitroglycerin ointment for the treatment of chronic anal fissure. N Engl J Med. 1999;341:65–9.
18. Lund JN, Armitage NC, Scholefield JH. Use of glyceryl trinitrate ointment in the treatment of anal fissure. Br J Surg. 1996;83:776–7.
19. Watson SJ, Kamm MA, Nicholls RJ, Phillips RK. Topical glyceryl trinitrate in the treatment of chronic anal fissure. Br J Surg. 1996;83:771–5.
20. Perez-Legaz J, Arroyo A, Moya P, Ruiz-Tovar J, Frangi A, Candela F, et al. Perianal versus endoanal application of glyceryl trinitrate 0.4% ointment in the treatment of chronic anal fissure: results of a randomized controlled trial. Is this the solution to the headaches? Dis Colon Rectum. 2012;55:893–9.
21. Chrysos E, Xynos E, Tzovaras G, Zoras OJ, Tsiaoussis J, Vassilakis SJ. Effect of nifedipine on rectoanal motility. Dis Colon Rectum. 1996;39:212–6.
22. Carapeti EA, Kamm MA, Phillips RK. Topical diltiazem and bethanechol decrease anal sphincter pressure and heal anal fissures without side effects. Dis Colon Rectum. 2000;43:1359–62.
23. Jonas M, Neal KR, Abercrombie JF, Scholefield JH. A randomized trial of oral vs. topical diltiazem for chronic anal fissures. Dis Colon Rectum. 2001;44:1074–8.
24. Bielecki K, Kolodziejczak M. A prospective randomized trial of diltiazem and glyceryltrinitrate ointment in the treatment of chronic anal fissure. Colorectal Dis. 2003;5:256–7.
25. Kocher HM, Steward M, Leather AJ, Cullen PT. Randomized clinical trial assessing the side-effects of glyceryl trinitrate and diltiazem hydrochloride in the treatment of chronic anal fissure. Br J Surg. 2002;89:413–7.
26. Cheng CM, Chen JS, Patel RP. Unlabeled uses of botulinum toxins: a review, part 1. Am J Health Syst Pharm. 2006;63:145–52.
27. Tjandra JJ. Ambulatory haemorrhoidectomy - has the time come? ANZ J Surg. 2005;75:183.
28. Gui D, Cassetta E, Anastasio G, Bentivoglio AR, Maria G, Albanese A. Botulinum toxin for chronic anal fissure. Lancet. 1994;344:1127–8.

29. Maria G, Brisinda G, Bentivoglio AR, Cassetta E, Gui D, Albanese A. Influence of botulinum toxin site of injections on healing rate in patients with chronic anal fissure. Am J Surg. 2000;179:46–50.

30. Maria G, Cassetta E, Gui D, Brisinda G, Bentivoglio AR, Albanese A. A comparison of botulinum toxin and saline for the treatment of chronic anal fissure. N Engl J Med. 1998;338:217–20.

31. Arroyo A, Perez F, Serrano P, Candela F, Lacueva J, Calpena R. Surgical versus chemical (botulinum toxin) sphincterotomy for chronic anal fissure: long-term results of a prospective randomized clinical and manometric study. Am J Surg. 2005; 189:429–34.

32. Iswariah H, Stephens J, Rieger N, Rodda D, Hewett P. Randomized prospective controlled trial of lateral internal sphincterotomy versus injection of botulinum toxin for the treatment of idiopathic fissure in ano. ANZ J Surg. 2005; 75:553–5.

33. Mentes BB, Irkorucu O, Akin M, Leventoglu S, Tatlicioglu E. Comparison of botulinum toxin injection and lateral internal sphincterotomy for the treatment of chronic anal fissure. Dis Colon Rectum. 2003;46:232–7.

34. Chen HL, Woo XB, Wang HS, Lin YJ, Luo HX, Chen YH, et al. Botulinum toxin injection versus lateral internal sphincterotomy for chronic anal fissure: a meta-analysis of randomized control trials. Tech Coloproctol. 2014;18:693–8.

35. Gandomkar H, Zeinoddini A, Heidari R, Amoli HA. Partial lateral internal sphincterotomy versus combined botulinum toxin A injection and topical diltiazem in the treatment of chronic anal fissure: a randomized clinical trial. Dis Colon Rectum. 2015;58:228–34.

36. Saad AM, Omer A. Surgical treatment of chronic fissure-in-ano: a prospective randomised study. East Afr Med J. 1992;69: 613–5.

37. Steele SR, Madoff RD. Systematic review: the treatment of anal fissure. Aliment Pharmacol Ther. 2006;24:247–57.

38. Nelson RL, Chattopadhyay A, Brooks W, Platt I, Paavana T, Earl S. Operative procedures for fissure in ano. Cochrane Database Syst Rev. 2011; (11): CD002199.

39. Renzi A, Izzo D, Di Sarno G, Talento P, Torelli F, Izzo G, et al. Clinical, manometric, and ultrasonographic results of pneumatic balloon dilatation vs. lateral internal sphincterotomy for chronic anal fissure: a prospective, randomized, controlled trial. Dis Colon Rectum. 2008;51:121–7.

40. Eisenhammer S. The evaluation of the internal anal sphincterotomy operation with special reference to anal fissure. Surg Gynecol Obstet. 1959;109:583–90.

41. Notaras MJ. Lateral subcutaneous sphincterotomy for anal fissure--a new technique. Proc R Soc Med. 1969;62:713.

42. Arroyo A, Perez F, Serrano P, Candela F, Calpena R. Open versus closed lateral sphincterotomy performed as an outpatient procedure under local anesthesia for chronic anal fissure: prospective randomized study of clinical and manometric longterm results. J Am Coll Surg. 2004;199:361–7.

43. Filingeri V, Gravante G. A prospective randomized trial between subcutaneous lateral internal sphincterotomy with radiofrequency bistoury and conventional parks' operation in the treatment of anal fissures. Eur Rev Med Pharmacol Sci. 2005;9:175–8.

44. Boulos PB, Araujo JG. Adequate internal sphincterotomy for chronic anal fissure: subcutaneous or open technique? Br J Surg. 1984;71:360–2.

45. Kortbeek JB, Langevin JM, Khoo RE, Heine JA. Chronic fissure-in-ano: a randomized study comparing open and subcutaneous lateral internal sphincterotomy. Dis Colon Rectum. 1992;35:835–7.

46. Wiley M, Day P, Rieger N, Stephens J, Moore J. Open vs. closed lateral internal sphincterotomy for idiopathic fissure-in-ano: a prospective, randomized, controlled trial. Dis Colon Rectum. 2004;47:847–52.

47. Garcia-Granero E, Sanahuja A, Garcia-Botello SA, Faiz O, Esclapez P, Espi A, et al. The ideal lateral internal sphincterotomy: clinical and endosonographic evaluation following open and closed internal anal sphincterotomy. Colorectal Dis. 2009; 11:502–7.

48. Mentes BB, Ege B, Leventoglu S, Oguz M, Karadag A. Extent of lateral internal sphincterotomy: up to the dentate line or up to the fissure apex? Dis Colon Rectum. 2005;48:365–70.

49. Elsebae MM. A study of fecal incontinence in patients with chronic anal fissure: prospective, randomized, controlled trial of the extent of internal anal sphincter division during lateral sphincterotomy. World J Surg. 2007;31:2052–7.

50. Magdy A, El Nakeeb A, el Fouda Y, Youssef M, Farid M. Comparative study of conventional lateral internal sphincterotomy, V-Y anoplasty, and tailored lateral internal sphincterotomy with V-Y anoplasty in the treatment of chronic anal fissure. J Gastrointest Surg. 2012;16:1955–62.

51. Mentes BB, Guner MK, Leventoglu S, Akyurek N. Fine-tuning of the extent of lateral internal sphincterotomy: spasm-controlled vs. up to the fissure apex. Dis Colon Rectum. 2008;51:128–33.

52. Pelta AE, Davis KG, Armstrong DN. Subcutaneous fissurotomy: a novel procedure for chronic fissure-in-ano. a review of 109 cases. Dis Colon Rectum. 2007;50:1662–7.

53. Garcia-Aguilar J, Belmonte C, Wong WD, Lowry AC, Madoff RD. Open vs. closed sphincterotomy for chronic anal fissure: long-term results. Dis Colon Rectum. 1996;39:440–3.

54. Madoff RD, Fleshman JW. AGA technical review on the diagnosis and care of patients with anal fissure. Gastroenterology. 2003;124:235–45.

55. Floyd ND, Kondylis L, Kondylis PD, Reilly JC. Chronic anal fissure: 1994 and a decade later--are we doing better? Am J Surg. 2006;191:344–8.

56. Lysy J, Israeli E, Levy S, Rozentzweig G, Strauss-Liviatan N, Goldin E. Long-term results of "chemical sphincterotomy" for chronic anal fissure: a prospective study. Dis Colon Rectum. 2006;49:858–64.

57. Giordano P, Gravante G, Grondona P, Ruggiero B, Porrett T, Lunniss PJ. Simple cutaneous advancement flap anoplasty for resistant chronic anal fissure: a prospective study. World J Surg. 2009;33:1058–63.

58. Nyam DC, Wilson RG, Stewart KJ, Farouk R, Bartolo DC. Island advancement flaps in the management of anal fissures. Br J Surg. 1995;82:326–8.

59. Kenefick NJ, Gee AS, Durdey P. Treatment of resistant anal fissure with advancement anoplasty. Colorectal Dis. 2002;4: 463–6.

60. Sangwan YP, Schoetz Jr DJ, Murray JJ, Roberts PL, Coller JA. Perianal Crohn's disease. Results of local surgical treatment. Dis Colon Rectum. 1996;39:529–35.

61. Platell C, Mackay J, Collopy B, Fink R, Ryan P, Woods R. Anal pathology in patients with Crohn's disease. ANZ J Surg. 1996;66:5–9.

62. Wolkomir AF, Luchtefeld MA. Surgery for symptomatic hemorrhoids and anal fissures in Crohn's disease. Dis Colon Rectum. 1993;36:545–7.

63. Fleshner PR, Schoetz Jr DJ, Roberts PL, Murray JJ, Coller JA, Veidenheimer MC. Anal fissure in Crohn's disease: a plea for aggressive management. Dis Colon Rectum. 1995;38:1137–43.

64. Ouraghi A, Nieuviarts S, Mougenel JL, Allez M, Barthet M, Carbonnel F, et al. Infliximab therapy for Crohn's disease anoperineal lesions. Gastroenterol Clin Biol. 2001;25: 949–56.

65. Sweeney JL, Ritchie JK, Nicholls RJ. Anal fissure in Crohn's disease. Br J Surg. 1988;75:56–7.

66. Viamonte M, Dailey TH, Gottesman L. Ulcerative disease of the anorectum in the HIV+ patient. Dis Colon Rectum. 1993; 36:801–5.

67. Weiss EG, Wexner SD. Surgery for anal lesions in HIV-infected patients. Ann Med. 1995;27:467–75.

14

Anorectal Abscess and Fistula

Bradley R. Davis and Kevin R. Kasten

Key Concepts

- Successful management of anorectal abscesses requires an in-depth knowledge of pelvic floor anatomy and potential spaces through which sepsis can spread.
- The spaces occupying the anus and their anatomic landmarks will define the nomenclature of abscesses—perianal, perirectal, supralevator, and postanal space.
- Drainage of most abscesses can be performed in the office without drains or setons. If a fistula is encountered it should only be addressed if the anatomy in relationship to the sphincters is clearly identified.
- Necrotizing soft tissue infections are life-threatening emergencies that require aggressive surgical debridement and management of the offending anal gland.
- Fistulas will complicate a significant proportion of perirectal abscesses and are classified based on their relationship with the anal sphincter complex.
- Physical examination is often the only modality needed to determine the fistula track and selection of treatment, and preoperative imaging (MRI, US) is typically unnecessary except for patients with multiple external openings, when the internal opening cannot be identified, or for recurrent cases.
- Goodsall's rule, while being helpful, is accurate in about 60 % of cases and is more accurate for posterior fistulas.
- Fistulotomy is the most successful of the surgical treatments, but is also associated with the highest rates of continence disturbances—several non-cutting techniques have been described—all of which have limitations and varying degrees of success.

Introduction and Epidemiology

It is difficult if not impossible to accurately assess the incidence of anorectal abscesses because they often drain spontaneously or are incised and drained in a physician's office, emergency room, or surgicenter.

Herand Abcarian [1]

While seemingly a benign process, an anorectal abscess can produce significant distress and long-term morbidity. Delay in diagnosis, mismanagement of the disease, or failure to recognize the diagnoses can result in multiple procedures, increased cost, and protracted suffering. Further, confusion regarding the interplay between anorectal abscesses and fistula-in-ano may lead to inappropriate management. As such, it is important that treating clinicians have a good working knowledge of the diagnosis and management or refer the patient to a specialist.

Although the true incidence and prevalence are elusive, data from the operative management of anorectal abscesses provides a floor from which to extrapolate. The incidence of abscess is reportedly between 0.4 and 5 % of patients undergoing operative management [2, 3] translating to 8.6–20 patients per 100,000 population [4, 5], and yielding between 68,000 and 96,000 cases of anorectal abscess each year in the USA [1]. Patients are males at a 3:1 ratio, with both sexes presenting at a mean age of 40 years (range 20–60 years) [6]. Although often asked by patients, there is minimal data to suggest that inadequate hygiene, anal-receptive intercourse, altered bowel habits, diabetes, obesity, or race are associated with increased risk of abscess formation.

Pathophysiology

Anatomy

Management of anorectal abscess requires an in-depth knowledge of pelvic floor anatomy and associated potential spaces whereby purulent material can travel (see Chap. 1). A succinct description of the pelvis (funnel in funnel) illustrates the internal sphincter surrounded by the pelvic floor apparatus (external sphincter, levator ani, and puborectalis), and separated by the intersphincteric plane. The anal canal represents a connection between the anal verge and anorectal junction, with a length of 2–4 cm. At the anal canal's midpoint lies the dentate line, represented by undulating longitudinal folds of columnar endothelium (columns of Morgagni) proximally, and smooth squamous epithelium distally (anoderm). Between the columns of Morgagni, which number between 6 and 14, are unevenly distributed anal crypts whereby anal ducts empty. Importantly, ducts may extend into the internal sphincter, the intersphincteric space, or through the internal sphincter into the external sphincter [7, 8]. As a consequence of these extensions, select anorectal spaces are at risk for transmission of bacteria with subsequent formation of abscess.

The perianal space (Fig. 14-1a) lies immediately around the anal verge, with medial extension to the dentate line and lateral extension to the subcutaneous fat of the buttocks. This space is further connected to the rectal wall above the external sphincter by way of the intersphincteric space. The ischiorectal/ischioanal fossa is a pyramidal shaped potential space between the perineum and levator ani. It is bordered medially by the levator ani and external sphincter, with the obturator internus muscle and fascia along the ischium as its lateral border (Figure 14-1b). Anteriorly it is confined by the transverse perineal muscles. From a posterior standpoint, the ischiorectal fossa is bordered by the gluteus maximus and sacrotuberous ligament. Bilateral ischiorectal fossae are connected via the postanal space, under the anococcygeal ligament (Figure 14-1b). Above the anococcygeal ligament and below the levator ani, these fossae are continuous with the deep posterior anal space. Above the levator ani, between the pelvic wall and rectum, lies the supralevator space. Because this space is superiorly bordered by the peritoneum, abscesses may form from intersphincteric sources that track superiorly, or abdominal sources that track from the peritoneal cavity.

Etiology

Currently identified as vestigial organs with minimal role outside production of odiferous substances, anal crypts are considered the primary source for development of perianal abscesses [9]. The cryptoglandular theory underlying anorectal abscess formation was initially proposed by Eisenhammer [9] and later advocated by Parks [10]. They hypothesized that obstruction of a crypt by foreign body or perianal debris led to abscess formation due to stasis within the ducts. Predisposing factors for the development of cryptoglandular abscesses, which account for 90 % these infections, include liquid stool entering the anal duct, trauma, tobacco abuse, and cystic dilation of the duct resulting in poor emptying. The remaining 10 % are the result of specific disorders such as inflammatory bowel disease (IBD), trauma, and malignancy (Table 14-1).

Classification

Each anorectal abscess is classified based upon the potential space it inhabits (Figure 14-2). In general, perianal and ischiorectal abscesses are the most common, accounting for

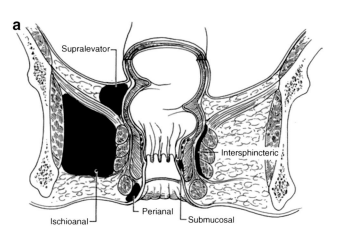
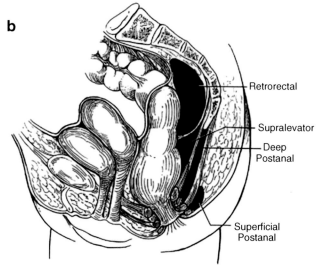

FIGURE 14-1. Anorectal spaces: (a) coronal section; (b) sagittal section. Vasilevsky CA. Anorectal abscess and fistula-in-ano [168] © 1997 David Beck, MD, with permission.

over 80 % of all diagnoses [11]. However, some implicate intersphincteric abscesses as the most common, with the ability to spread in any direction [5]. As expected, supralevator abscesses are the least common. The proverbial "horseshoe abscess" describes a process whereby bilateral disease occurs via connection through the intersphincteric, supralevator, or ischiorectal spaces. Recognition of this process is necessary to prevent undue operative intervention and patient suffering.

Evaluation

History and Symptoms

The patient with an anorectal abscess presents most commonly with acute pain in the perianal or perirectal region. Pain usually prompts an evaluation in the emergency room or physician's office. The pain is usually worsened with

TABLE 14-1. Etiology of anorectal abscess

Nonspecific
   Cryptoglandular
Specific
   Inflammatory bowel disease
      Crohn's disease
      Ulcerative colitis
   Infection
      Tuberculosis
      Actinomycosis
      Lymphogranuloma venereum
   Trauma
      Impalement
      Foreign body
      Surgery
      Episiotomy
      Hemorrhoidectomy
      Prostatectomy
   Malignancy
      Carcinoma
      Leukemia
      Lymphoma
      Radiation

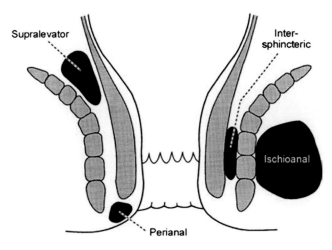

FIGURE 14-2. Classification of anorectal abscesses [169] © 1997 David Beck, MD, with permission.

sitting and defecation. For patient with chronic rectal pain, consideration should be given to an intersphincteric abscess. Further, associated symptoms of urinary dysfunction may distinguish the abscess as supralevator. For supralevator abscesses, pain may be described as a "dull ache" in the pelvic region or lower back. Of note, other symptoms include fever, chills, swelling, erythema, spontaneous drainage, and malaise. Rectal bleeding is unlikely in the majority of patients. Past medical history can alert the clinician to other possible causes of rectal pain including fissure, hemorrhoids, levator spasm, sexually transmitted infections, tuberculosis, human immunodeficiency virus (HIV), IBD,

malignancy, and trauma. Given the possibility of surgical intervention, determining sphincter function and any history of fecal incontinence is important in these patients.

Physical Examination

Physical examination remains the single most important diagnostic study in patients with suspected anorectal abscess. In the prone position, external evaluation will reveal classic signs of infection including erythema, induration, fluctuance, pain, and spontaneous drainage. When completing an examination, ensure evaluation of the contralateral side to determine the existence of horseshoe extensions. For patients with an intersphincteric or supralevator abscess, external review is unlikely to reveal definitive signs. However, upon digital rectal exam, fluctuance or extreme discomfort should alert the clinician to this diagnosis. In this setting, if an internal opening is palpated, purulent drainage may also be noted. Unfortunately, pain oftentimes precludes an adequate rectal exam. When the diagnosis is in doubt, consideration should be given to performance of an exam under anesthesia with anoscopy and possible flexible sigmoidoscopy. In case of suspicion for supralevator abscess, or in patients with complicated medical history, further imaging may be warranted.

Imaging

Classically, imaging was rarely useful in the management of anorectal abscess. Some advocated for barium enema in young patients or those with recurrent fistula disease to rule out inflammatory bowel disease. However, modern techniques including computer tomography (CT), magnetic resonance imaging (MRI), endoanal ultrasound (EAUS), and transperineal sonography (TP-US) are especially helpful in the diagnosis of complicated anorectal abscesses and fistula-in-ano.

Computed Tomography (CT)

The use of CT for anorectal abscess is controversial [12]. However, such imaging is indicated in any patient in whom the diagnosis of anorectal abscess is unclear, those with complex suppurative anorectal conditions, anyone with significant comorbidities in which missing the diagnosis would prove harmful, or as a possible substitution for surgical evaluation. It can also be considered in patients with perianal Crohn's disease to assist delineation of rectal inflammation from anorectal abscess [13]. While high-resolution scanners are important for detailed images, just as important are the techniques utilized to maximize visualization. Triple contrast is often required, to include per os (PO), intravenous (IV), and *per rectum* (PR) modes. Slices of 2.5 mm are used

FIGURE 14-3. Computed
tomography of complex anorectal
abscess extending anteriorly
towards scrotum. Axial images
(**a**), coronal image (**b**), sagittal
image (**c**).

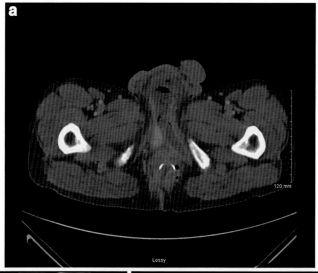

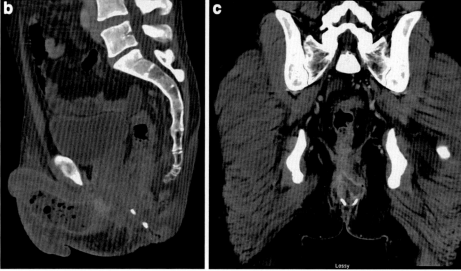

to allow for appropriate reconstruction in sagittal and coronal planes (Figure 14-3a–c). When completed correctly, an abscess appears as an oval-shaped fluid collection with an enhancing wall, with or without demonstration of air. Additionally, fistulous tracts are readily identified by a tubular, air/fluid-filled structure that arises within the anal sphincter [6].

Magnetic Resonance Imaging

MRI for evaluation of anorectal abscess is uncommon, occurring more frequently in complex fistula-in-ano disease. Groups suggest the use of pelvic MRI for any recurrent of incompletely drained abscess to assist identification of horseshoe/postanal, supralevator, and other complex abscesses [14]. However MRI has limited value in the diagnosis of anorectal abscess in the acute setting.

Endoanal Ultrasound

Familiar to most colorectal surgeons, endoanal ultrasound utilizes a probe with 2D or 3D capabilities at a frequency of 5–16 MHz. Similar in discomfort to anoscopy, this technology allows effective characterization of abscesses and fistulae with reported accuracy of 85 % [13]. Normal EAUS demonstrates the interface between the cap and the submucosa (mixed echogenicity), internal sphincter (hypoechoic), intersphincteric space (hyperechoic), and external sphincter (mixed echogenicity) [15]. The probe is covered in a protective sheathing with all air removed, and gently inserted past the puborectalis before slow removal. Fluid is identified by hypoechoic, compressible ovals between or within specific planes. Limitations of this technique include user dependence, limited distance of detection from probe (extrasphincteric, supralevator abscesses), and requirement of intraluminal deployment, which may be precluded by discomfort in acute perianal sepsis.

Transperineal Sonography

A lesser known technique in the colorectal field, TP-US can be quite accurate in diagnosis of fluid collections, internal opening, and even existence and course of a fistulous track. Most importantly, in experienced hands it distinguishes perianal from perirectal abscess and sepsis. Using techniques similar to delineation of vascular structures, patients are evaluated in the left lateral decubitus position. In a comparison of TP-US and MRI, the former was more accurate for superficial fluid collections, while the latter was more accurate for perirectal infection. Overall, concordance between MRI and TP-US was 0.82 for diagnosis of perianal abscess, suggesting a significant advantage for this modality in the acute setting [16]. Clinicians with access to this technology should consider its use in applicable patients to help delineate fluid collection, fistulous tracts, internal openings, and reduce costs compared to MRI and CT studies.

Treatment

Role of Antibiotics

The surgical principles for management of abscesses, in general, hold true for the perianal and perirectal region, with prompt drainage and debridement being the cornerstone. Antibiotics are indicated when associated cellulitis is present, in patients who fail to improve following appropriate drainage, and those with immunosuppressed states. However, medication is rarely adequate in the absence of incision and drainage and at best does nothing to prevent subsequent fistula formation and at worse may increase the risk. In a randomized control trial evaluating treatment of anorectal abscess with and without antibiotics, the risk of fistula formation was unrelated to antibiotic usage. Fistula formation was, however, related to location of the abscess with an eight times higher risk associated with ischiorectal location, and a three times higher risk with intersphincteric compared to the perianal location [17]. (Isolated situations whereby antibiotics may be successful in this setting involve management of perianal Crohn's disease, and will be covered elsewhere.) Coverage is directed towards *Escherichia coli, Enterococcus species*, and *Bacteroides fragilis* in immunocompetent patients, and *Neisseria gonorrhoeae, Chlamydia trachomatis,* cytomegalovirus, and herpes simplex virus in immunocompromised patients [18]. Consider wound culture only in high-risk patient populations, and individuals with recurrent or non-healing disease [13].

Incision and Drainage

The appropriate setting for abscess drainage depends on the location of the abscess and the experience of the clinician. Simple, superficial perianal or ischiorectal abscesses

requiring external drainage at the skin level are amenable to bedside drainage in the office, emergency room, or hospital ward. A simple rule of thumb recommends "outward" drainage whenever an abscess enters, or passes through, skeletal muscle (i.e., levator ani, external sphincter) [19]. All others should be drained internally through the rectum/anus. Standard procedure includes appropriate positioning, use of antiseptic prep, and local anesthesia of choice combined with 1:200,000 epinephrine. Starting with a local field block around the abscess prior to injection of skin overlying the point of maximal tenderness often provides more effective analgesia than injection of the cavity alone. The choice of elliptical incision, or cruciate incision combined with excision of skin flaps, prevents early closure and recurrence (Figure 14-4). When possible, the incision is made as near the anal verge as possible to limit the length of any potential fistula. Additionally, the predominant incision should run parallel to the external sphincter muscle fibers. Packing is not required in this scenario, and its absence yields quicker healing with less pain [20].

Patients requiring internal drainage, those with recurrent or bilateral disease, and those with large abscesses at risk for inadequate bedside drainage, should undergo operative drainage. For abscesses of significant size, consider multiple counter incisions with interposition of setons or Penrose drains to accelerate healing. Drains are removed at 2–3 weeks postoperatively when the base of the cavity has granulated and shrunk. Further candidates for internal drainage include (1) submucosal abscess, (2) intersphincteric abscess, (3) supralevator abscess from intersphincteric fistula, and (4) supralevator abscess from pelvic disease [19]. The diagnosis of intersphincteric fistula should be entertained in patients with pain out of proportion to exam findings. Definitive management involves incision of the internal sphincter along the length of abscess, with or without marsupialization of the wound edges. Individuals with delayed recurrence greater than 2 weeks likely have a fistula, and thus require EUA for delineation and control of fistula track.

Supralevator abscesses require delineation of the track by imaging before surgical correction is undertaken. When the inciting source is intra-abdominal, transrectal drainage is indicated in most scenarios. However, abdominal drainage can be considered depending upon ease of access and directionality of the abscess cavity. When the source is intra-abdominal, percutaneous management may prevent creation of a fistulous track through the levator plate via improper ischiorectal drainage, and is often more successful than transrectal drainage. The scenario of supralevator extension from ischiorectal abscess due to a transsphincteric fistula requires ischiorectal drainage. For instances where a supralevator abscess forms as an upward extension of an intersphincteric fistula, internal drainage via incision of the internal sphincter is best (Figure 14-5).

Bilateral abscess disease, or "horseshoe" abscess, requires operative drainage to delineate and control the source. This difficult-to-treat entity most commonly arises from a deep

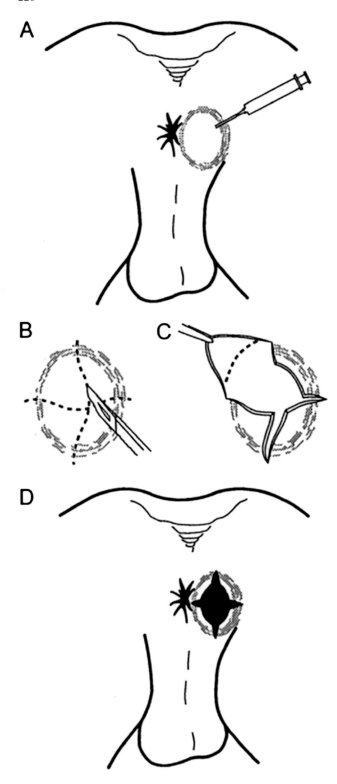

FIGURE 14-4. Drainage of abscess: (**a**) injection of local anesthesia, (**b**) cruciate incision, (**c**) excision of skin, (**d**) drainage cavity.

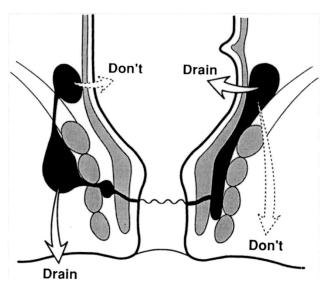

FIGURE 14-5. Drainage of a supralevator abscess.

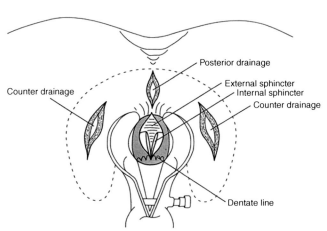

FIGURE 14-6. Drainage of a horseshoe abscess.

postanal space abscess. Many patients present with history of prior drainage procedures, and thus may have complex tracts. Options for management include the Hanley or modified Hanley procedures, consisting of open posterior drainage through the anococcygeal ligament, posterior midline incision of the internal sphincter and inciting anal duct, and open drainage of bilateral ischiorectal fossae to control lateral tracks (Figure 14-6) [21]. Modifications to this procedure include limiting drainage to internal sphincterotomy followed by elliptical incisions over bilateral ischiorectal fossae. If necessary, a seton (cutting or noncutting) is placed in the posterior midline, with subsequent definitive management taking place at a later time (Figure 14-7). More recently, management of deep postanal space abscess was described using an intersphincteric technique. The intersphincteric space is dissected in the posterior midline until identification of the anal duct source, with subsequent continuation into the deep postanal space for drainage and curettage. Benefits included minimization of procedures necessary when using the loose seton technique, reduction in risk of incontinence compared with the cutting seton technique, and ease of learning for the surgeon [22].

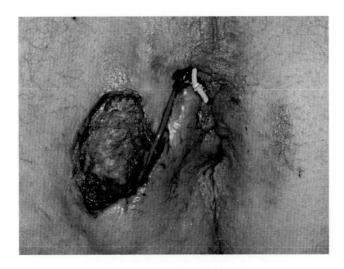

FIGURE 14-7. Horseshoe fistula managed with drainage and seton.

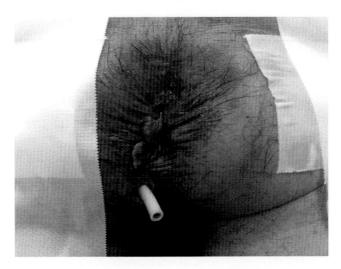

FIGURE 14-8. Pezzer catheter in an ischiorectal fossa abscess.

Catheter Drainage

Minimization of perianal incisions is possible using the placement of a drainage catheter within the abscess cavity. Appropriate size and external fixation of catheter are necessary to ensure adequate drainage, especially in patients with large abscess cavities, patients with severe systemic illness, and those with underlying comorbidities including diabetes mellitus and morbid obesity. To start, a small stab incision is made in anesthetized skin on the medial aspect of the abscess. A mushroom tip catheter (de Pezzer, Malecot, Cook Medical) between 10 and 14 Fr is inserted to full cavity depth. The external portion of the catheter is cut to length, leaving a 2–3 cm area with which you secure it to the perianal skin using a permanent suture (Figure 14-8). Recommendations differ with regard to duration of treatment, ranging from 3 to 21 days. However, removal prior to cessation of drainage usually results in recurrence, and should be avoided.

For non-healing wounds, the catheter is utilized for drain studies to elucidate fistula tracks or other associated pathology.

Drainage with Primary Fistulotomy

Despite a paucity of recent studies on the management of anorectal abscess, controversy abounds regarding the use of primary fistulotomy at the time of abscess drainage. Historically, primary fistulotomy was performed when draining the abscess for source control, thereby increasing the rate of healing without the need for subsequent procedure [11]. In a meta-analysis of six randomized controlled trials, recurrence, persistent abscess/fistula, and repeat surgery were significantly reduced when primary fistulotomy was performed concurrent with abscess drainage (RR=0.13, 95 % CI 0.07–0.24) [23]. However in the acute setting inflammation may inhibit clear determination of muscle involvement and the pooled relative risk of incontinence at 1 year was 3.06 (95 % CI 0.7–13.45), ranging between 2.03 and 4.77 in sensitivity analysis. This did not reach statistical significance when compared to the fistulotomy group and the study authors concluded that a fistulotomy at the time of abscess drainage was warranted. When an accurate estimate of muscle involvement is confounded by acute changes, thereby increasing the risk of excessive muscle incision, placement of seton may be indicated preventing the unintended consequence of incontinence [24, 25].

Despite these recommendations the risk of incontinence with all of the resultant patient morbidity may limit its application [26]. In fact several reports indicate a high rate of spontaneous healing following effective abscess drainage alone [27, 28] with the incidence of recurrent abscess reported to be 30 % and subsequent fistula formation between 26 and 50 % [23, 29, 30]. This may be even lower if the offending duct is identified and opened, confirming a limited role for primary fistulotomy in selected patients [23, 31].

In an effort to identify the crypt of origin when draining an acute abscess a probe can be carefully inserted into the suspected duct by direct visualization. Adjuncts for locating the duct include manual pressure on the abscess cavity while looking for purulent extrusion, identification of inflammation indicating the culprit duct, or simple blind probing. When identified, gentle probe advancement may elucidate the inciting fistula, but care is required to prevent creation of a false track. Unfortunately, a recent study reported successful internal opening (IO) identification of only 36 % using manual abscess cavity compression, consistent with prior published rates of failure exceeding 65 % [32, 33]. Interestingly, one randomized control trial reported 83 % success using simple abscess compression [34]. Because localizing the offending duct is difficult, and misidentification leads to complications, alternative methods are available. In patients who failed identification by abscess compression, injecting

222 B.R. Davis and K.R. Kasten

2 cc of 2 % hydrogen peroxide combined with 1–2 drops of methylene blue into the abscess cavity resulted in localization of the internal opening in 90 % of cases. At median follow-up of 16.5 months, rates of recurrent disease were 2.8 % in those undergoing primary fistulotomy compared with 40 % in patients treated with incision and drainage alone [29].

Unfortunately, there is no clear answer to the question of primary fistulotomy at the time of abscess drainage. In fact, the ASCRS Practice Parameters for management of anorectal abscess advocate, "… weigh[ing] the possible decreased recurrence rate in light of the potential increased risk of continence disturbances" [13]. Surgeons who are inexperienced in the management of anorectal pathology should refrain from searching for a fistula due to higher rates of adverse events and poorer patient outcomes. Healthy patients *without* prior fistulous disease, IBD, or simultaneous anterior fistulas potentially benefit from primary fistulotomy at the time of abscess drainage in the hands of experienced surgeons. Superficial and low transsphincteric (<30–40 % external sphincter involvement) fistulas with minimal sphincter involvement provide the best opportunity for successful fistulotomy at the time of abscess drainage [5].

Postoperative Management

Postoperative care is similar to most anorectal procedures. Local wound care involves sitz baths two to three times daily followed by wound coverage using gauze. Packing is not necessary and should be avoided. Following catheter drainage, a dressing is similarly applied over the catheter end to prevent soiling of clothing. Irrigation of the catheter is not necessary. There is no data to support the use of topical antibiotics. Surgeon follow-up is indicated at 2–3 weeks in patients who undergo incision and drainage, and 7–10 days in those with mushroom-tip catheters. Endpoint for removal is cessation of purulent drainage from the drain, and closure of the wound around catheter. Patients are followed until complete healing of the wound or cavity; especially since recurrence and fistula formation are associated with delay/lack of surgical follow-up. Pain control is obtained with multimodality therapy to include local anesthetic at surgery combined with narcotic and non-narcotic oral medications for home use. Diet is advanced to regular once the patient is aroused from anesthesia, and a bulk-forming fiber supplement is advised for the first month. Activity level may proceed ad lib. Antibiotics are not warranted in the postoperative setting unless cellulitis is present, or in the immunocompromised patient.

Complications

Immediate Postoperative Period

Complications related to abscess drainage and fistulotomy include bleeding and urinary retention. Significant bleeding in the postoperative period following incision and drainage occurs at a rate of 1–2 %. The rate of urinary retention reported in the literature following uncomplicated incision and drainage is 2.3 %, increasing to 6.3 % in patients undergoing fistulectomy/fistulotomy [35]. This compares favorably to the reported incidence of 22 % in patients undergoing hemorrhoidectomy. Universal risk factors for urinary retention in anorectal procedures include age over 50, female sex, and intravenous fluid (IVF) greater than 1 L perioperatively [35].

Abscess Recurrence and Fistula Formation

Rates of abscess recurrence following drainage are estimated at 4–31 %, with a median of 13 % [36]. The only significant prognostic factor for patients presenting with their first abscess without other complicating factors such as IBD was time from disease onset to drainage procedure. Rates of recurrence were higher in those undergoing management more than 7 days after the onset of symptoms [37]. Early recurrence is usually the result of inappropriate technique, early skin apposition, and reformation of the abscess. Insufficient drainage leads to continued inflammation, prolonged healing, and fistula formation [1, 38, 39]. Reasons for semi-acute recurrence include missed loculations, prior intervention with associated scarring, and destruction of natural barriers to infection [26, 40, 41]. Because a large number of recurrent abscesses are due to inadequate treatment in patients who present with spontaneous drainage and receive outpatient care, one group advocated exam under anesthesia for all patients even if the abscess has apparently decompressed [39]. Horseshoe abscesses recur more frequently with a reported incidence between 18 and 50 %, usually requiring multiple operations before healing occurs [42]. The clinician must elucidate site of prior drainage and determine likelihood of horseshoe abscess in order to effectively treat the diagnosis.

Misdiagnosis

When an abscess is not effectively managed despite optimal medical and surgical intervention an alternative diagnosis must be entertained. Pilonidal disease, hidradenitis suppurativa, tuberculosis, herpes simplex virus, HIV, and inflammatory bowel disease (specifically, Crohn's disease) must be part of the differential diagnosis [39]. While the incidence of pilonidal disease is 1:4000, only a few case reports exist detailing its presentation as an anorectal abscess or fistula [43]. In a study of 100 recurrent anorectal abscesses at a large tertiary care colorectal program, 32 % of patients treated for anorectal abscess actually had hidradenitis, underlying the importance of entertaining alternative diagnoses in patients with recurrence [39]. Incidence of HIV and other infectious sources are difficult to estimate, and will be predicated by the surrounding patient population. Between 5 and 19 % of Crohn's patients will demonstrate perianal manifestations prior to any other symptoms, suggesting a significant opportunity to make an early diagnosis.

Special Considerations

Necrotizing Anorectal Infection (Fournier's Gangrene)

Necrotizing anorectal infections are rare, representing less than 0.02 % of hospital admissions with an incidence between 1.6 and 3.3/100,000 [44]. Males outnumber females at a ratio between 9 and 50:1 [45]. Current estimates of mean age are between 45 and 55 years, which steadily increase as the worldwide population ages. The diagnosis is rarely made in children. Some countries report an increasing incidence; however, there is minimal data to support this conclusion in the USA. Medical risk factors commonly associated with necrotizing soft tissue infections include diabetes, hypertension, elderly age, obesity, immunosuppression (especially when due to malnutrition, liver disease, malignancies), drug use, and recent surgery [46]. As expected, rates of necrotizing fasciitis are increased in patients with perianal disease. Commonly, either long-standing or inappropriately managed perianal disease predates an episode of necrotizing fasciitis. In patients diagnosed with Fournier's gangrene, 50–60 % had underlying anorectal abscess as their inciting source [45].

Diagnosis

Presenting symptoms include severe pain out of proportion to exam, fever, chills, erythema, and induration at the site (Figure 14-9). In polymicrobial and clostridial infections, crepitance is often noted. Unfortunately, necrotizing soft tissue infections progress along fascial planes; thus the extent of disease is easily underestimated. Timing of disease progression ranges from 2 to 5 days. Laboratory values are nonspecific, but indicate disease severity. White blood cell count, creatinine kinase, and lactate are most helpful in estimating severity of infection and confirming the diagnosis.

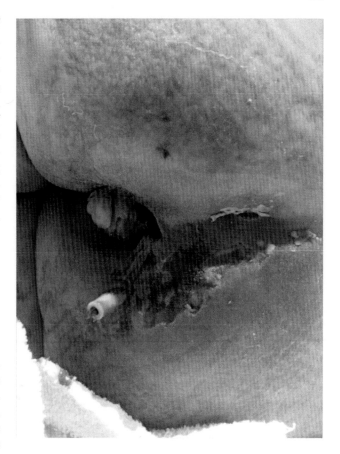

FIGURE 14-9. Necrotizing soft tissue infection in a patient with a supralevator fistula and abscess inadequately drained.

Cultures and gram stain are unhelpful at initial diagnosis, but can guide appropriate postoperative antibiotic therapy. Due to false negatives, bedside biopsy plays a limited role in the diagnosis except in tertiary care centers with experience. When the diagnosis is unclear, imaging is recommended using CT abdomen/pelvis to identify the source and extent of infection.

Treatment

Prompt diagnosis and treatment are necessary to maximize survival. Following diagnosis, treatment involves aggressive fluid resuscitation with crystalloid of choice and initiation of broad-spectrum antibiotics (penicillin g, metronidazole, third-generation cephalosporin, gentamicin). Next, the patient undergoes surgical intervention with wide local excision of affected tissue (Figure 14-10). Due to rapid spread, surgical excision should extend beyond visibly infected tissues. Additionally, the patient should be evaluated on a regular basis in the ICU for any wound changes. It is common to return to the operating room within 24–48 h to re-excise margins, and to ensure appropriate source control.

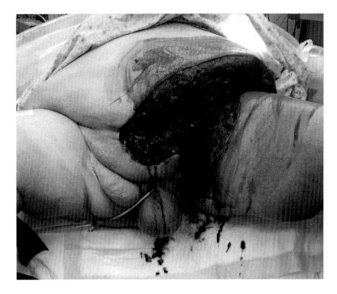

FIGURE 14-10. Extensive soft tissue debridement of necrotizing soft tissue infection starting as an anorectal abscess.

A useful adjunct when anorectal abscess incites necrotizing fasciitis involves the loose-seton technique [47]. Here, multiple radial incisions are made in the external sphincter at its outer margins. The incisions are widened manually, and loose setons placed between every other drainage incision. When combined with standard wide local excision at the outset, trips to the operating room are decreased, as is the overall wound size. Some advocate creation of a colostomy to help with wound care after extensive dissection. While no data currently supports this practice, higher consideration is given to patients with a grossly infected sphincter muscle, and anorectal perforation, or those in an immunocompromised state. Tailoring of antibiotics should occur when culture results return.

Outcomes

Necrotizing fasciitis remains a lethal disease, despite significant advances in diagnosis, surgical care, and supportive management. Mortality rates in the literature span 4–80 %; however, most large studies demonstrate a consistent range of 7–10 %. Death is usually the result of sepsis and sequelae of multi-organ system failure [45]. For survivors, long-term morbidity is dependent upon the extent of wound debridement and recovery of organ systems.

Use of the Fournier's Gangrene Severity Index (FGSI) predicts mortality by combining nine parameters such as temperature, heart rate, and other clinical values. In the sentinel paper, scores >9 predicted probability of mortality at 75 % [48]. Conversely, scores ≤9 predicted probability of survival at 78 %. Since 1995, multiple studies have validated this scoring system [45].

Anorectal Infections in Immunosuppressed Patients

Hematologic Abnormalities in Immunosuppression

In patients with hematologic malignancies, or those treated with myelosuppressive regimens, immunosuppression and low neutrophil count produce an incidence of anorectal sepsis approaching 10 % [49]. Despite the high incidence, diagnosis is often difficult and delayed. This occurs due to low neutrophil counts, whereby non-fluctuant induration with minimal erythema evades untrained eyes, leading to misdiagnosis in half of the patients [50]. If counts increase, normal clinical signs of abscess may occur, allowing for a diagnosis.

Complications of anorectal abscess in hematologically immunosuppressed patients are similar to healthy patients, including recurrence, fistula formation, and incontinence. However, systemic complications of sepsis are more likely in this patient population, including death. When untreated, mortality approaches 60 % [51, 52]. As such, aggressive management is indicated when anorectal sepsis is suspected.

Appropriate treatment of these high-risk patients involves determination of immune status and tailored therapy. Antibiotics are standard of care, aimed at coverage of standard gastrointestinal flora using a local antibiogram. For patients with absolute neutrophil count (ANC) <1000/mm³, antibiotics are first-line therapy with rates of resolution between 30 and 90 % [49, 53]. Patients with higher neutrophil counts will demonstrate an abscess, which requires incision and drainage. Physical exam is limited in these patients, so imaging studies are indicated for delineation of size, extent, and involved structures. CT scans are rapid, easily obtained, and demonstrate supralevator components with high degree of accuracy. If concern exists for more complex anorectal sepsis, and possible necrotizing infection, MRI provides superior imaging for diagnosis. Using T1- and T2-weighted images, physicians can determine abscess vs. inflammation, adjusting treatment accordingly [50].

The decision on timing of surgical intervention is not always clear-cut. Patients with neutropenia suffer higher rates of morbidity following surgery, and mortality was upwards of 45 % in one study vs. 9 % in those treated only with antibiotics [54]. Published rates of failure in neutropenic patients range between 30 and 37 % [50]. If antibiotic therapy fails based on abscess formation, lack of improvement, or development of necrotizing infection, surgical debridement is indicated. While thrombocytopenia is associated with nonoperative management, fluctuance, erythema, and presence of purulent material indicate patients appropriate for surgical drainage [55]. Due to the high risk of morbidity and mortality in patients with incomplete evacuation of purulent material, operative washout is preferred to bedside management. Postoperative care and management proceed similarly to health patients.

Human Immunodeficiency Virus

There is little distinction between the management of HIV patients and otherwise-healthy individuals with anorectal abscess. However, prompt recognition and treatment are required due to concerns of underlying immunosuppression. In this patient population, alternative diagnoses including sexually transmitted infections and CMV are also common. Further, risk of neoplasm requires biopsy of tissue at the time of drainage.

Anal Fistula

The management of anal fistula cannot be undertaken without a thorough understanding of their etiology, and the anatomy of the anal canal and sphincter complex. The disease represents a wide spectrum of complexity and is often misdiagnosed and poorly treated by surgeons and physicians who lack experience. Complexity has certainly increased in large part due to the unwillingness of patients and surgeons to risk continence when managing fistulas, a fact underscored by the significant increase in the use of non-cutting techniques used to treat anal fistulas during the past 30 years [56].

Etiology

A fistula is defined as an abnormal connection between two epithelial lined surfaces such as a set of organs or vessels, which do not normally connect, e.g., the connection between the distal alimentary tract and the integument. The incidence is believed to be 2 per 10,000/year while the prevalence is not truly known [57]. The etiology of anal fistula is cryptoglandular in 90 % of cases, postoperative or traumatic in 3 %, inflammatory bowel disease in 3 %, as a result of anal fissure in 3 %, and tuberculosis related in less than 1 % of cases.

The cryptoglandular cause of anal fistula refers to the presence of the anal crypts, proposed to originate at the bottom of the rectal columns of Morgagni, which are epithelial lined tracts that penetrate to the submucosa and occasionally into and through the internal sphincter. Despite the use of the term "glandular" it is not always the case that these structures are functional and may be vestigial remnants from embryonic growth. Their frequency and location are varied but tend to concentrate posteriorly and are more commonly found in men [7, 58]. Kratzer and Dockerty examined over 100 anatomical specimens histologically, and found anal glands in 55 % of specimens; in 33 % the ducts penetrated the internal sphincter [59]. Parks evaluated 44 specimens and identified 6–10 glands originating from the anal crypts and held the belief that these were mucous producing. The glands terminated variably into the submucosa, internal sphincter, or intersphincteric groove. He postulated that these glands provided a free channel for infection to pass from the anal lumen deep into the sphincter muscles. He believed that chronic infection in the cystic portion of the gland, if deep to the internal sphincter, would result in a sinus forming to the skin. Though technically due to the epithelial lining of the duct it is in fact a fistula [10].

It is believed that the anal crypts become blocked by inspissated debris or stool. As a result, an infection develops at the anal glands, which extends in a path of least resistance, forming an abscess in the intersphincteric space leading to the development of a fistula [9]. Additionally anal fistula can occur as a result of Crohn's disease, malignancy, trauma, tuberculosis, lymphogranuloma venereum, and actinomycosis. Not all cryptoglandular infection results in the development of a fistula. Scoma et al. performed a retrospective analysis of 232 patients who had undergone a drainage procedure and found that 66 % of their patients subsequently developed anal fistula [60]. They did not classify the type of fistula or abscess in their study making generalizations difficult although 77 % of their patients were male. Hamadani et al. performed a similar review of 148 patients with a mean follow-up of 38 months. The cumulative incidence of anal fistula was 36 % with no differences seen in a multivariate analysis among men vs. women, nonsmokers vs. smokers, perioperative antibiotic use, or HIV status. Age less than 40 was the only significant predictor of fistula formation in their study [36]. Wang et al. reviewed the records of 1342 patients with confirmed anal fistula and matched these cases to a separate cohort of patients referred with other anorectal complaints but without fistula disease. Using multivariate analysis BMI exceeding 25 kg/m², prior diabetes, hyperlipidemia, dermatosis, sedentary lifestyle, regular alcohol intake, smoking, non-fistula anorectal surgery, prolonged sitting on the toilet for defecation, and a previous history of enteritis were independently correlated with a risk of anal fistula [61].

It is likely that the true incidence of anal fistula following abscess formation is closer to 30 % and should be suspected in any patient with a recurrent perirectal abscess especially if it occurs at the same site of a previous abscess as fistula-in-ano is thought to be responsible for 40–50 % of recurrent abscesses [39].

Classification

Anal fistula can be characterized as simple or complex. The definition of a complex fistula is not standardized but most authors agree that any fistula that is high transsphincteric or when a fistulotomy would result in incontinence should be considered complex. The definition also includes suprasphincteric, extrasphincteric, all anterior transsphincteric fistulas in women, and those caused by Crohn's disease, malignancy, surgery, and trauma. Roughly 50 % of all fistulas are considered complex giving rise to significant challenges in the treatment of this disease.

Anal fistulas are also classified based on their relationship to the anal sphincter complex. In 1934 Milligan and Morgan suggested a classification of anal fistula based on the position of the internal opening relative to the anorectal ring [62]. This was subsequently modified by Parks et al. (Table 14-2) based on his analysis of 400 cases of treated anal fistula over a 15-year period [63]. He anchored his classification system on the external sphincter due to the importance it played in the surgical management (Figure 14-11a–d).

TABLE 14-2. Classification of fistula-in-ano

Intersphincteric
   Simple low intersphincteric
   High blind tract
   High tract with an opening in the rectum
   High tract with rectal opening, no perineal opening
   Extra-rectal extension
   Secondary to pelvic disease
Transsphincteric
   Uncomplicated
   High blind tract
Suprasphincteric
   Uncomplicated
   Horseshoe extension
Extrasphincteric
   Secondary to anal fistula
   Trauma related
   Pelvic inflammation
   Inflammatory bowel disease or other anal disease

An intersphincteric fistula (Figure 14-11a) occurs in 20–45 % of cases [64] and does not penetrate the external sphincter and "ramifies only in the intersphincteric plane." Parks et al. additionally classified seven subtypes of intersphincteric fistula with the most common having a high blind track, which as its name suggests has an extension in the intersphincteric groove cephalad towards the rectum. The other subtypes are less common.

A transsphincteric fistula (Figure 14-11b) occurs in 30–60 % of cases and penetrates the external sphincter below the level of the puborectalis muscle exiting into varying levels within the ischiorectal fossa. A high blind track may also confound a transsphincteric fistula and can end at the apex of the ischiorectal fossa or alternatively pass through the levator plate into the true pelvic cavity. The latter can be felt if a probe is passed from the opening in the perineal skin, the tip of which will be palpable above the anorectal ring through the wall of the rectum. Care should be taken *not* to iatrogenically perforate the rectum or an extrasphincteric fistula will be the result. The significance of this high blind track is the inability to cannulate the internal opening using a probe passed from the perineal skin as it will preferentially follow the high blind track and not the transsphincteric portion, which comes off at a right angle. It may be possible to cannulate the internal opening through the anus with a right-angle probe in order to secure a seton or if feasible perform a fistulotomy. A flexible tip glide wire can sometimes be used when this sharp angulation is encountered but again care must be taken to avoid creating a false passage (Figure 14-12).

FIGURE 14-11. Classification of anal fistula. (**a**) intersphincteric, (**b**) transsphincteric, (**c**) suprasphincteric, (**d**) extrasphincteric.

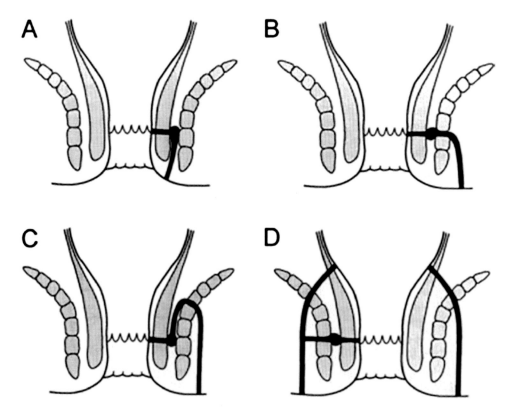

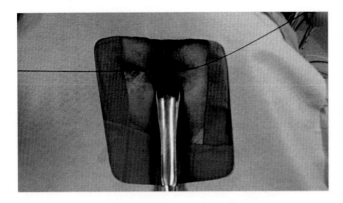

FIGURE 14-12. Flexible glide wire to delineate a transsphincteric fistula with a high blind extension.

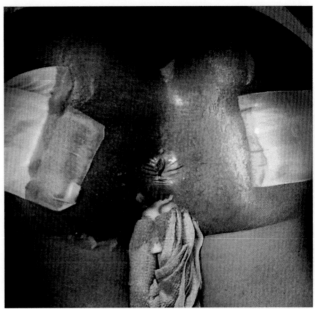

FIGURE 14-13. External opening noted left anterolateral with heaped-up edge.

A suprasphincteric fistula (Figure 14-11c) occurred in 20 % of cases in the series by Parks et al. but has been reported at a much lower frequency by other authors (<2 %) [64, 65] and in this group the track is over the top of the puborectalis, then downward again through the levator plate to the ischiorectal fossa, and finally the skin. As it passes over the puborectalis it is anatomically in the supralevator space and abscess formation here can be palpated by rectal exam. Abscess formation in this space can result in a horse-shoe extension around the rectum.

Lastly extrasphincteric fistula (Figure 14-11d), which only occurs in 2–5 % of cases, passes from the perineal skin through the ischiorectal fat and levator muscles into the rectum. It is outside the external sphincter complex altogether. An extrasphincteric fistula may result from a transsphincteric fistula with a high blind tract that penetrates through the levator plate as described earlier or it may be due to trauma, inflammatory bowel disease, malignancy, or pelvic inflammation that necessitates through the levators to the perineal skin (ruptured appendicitis, terminal ileal Crohn's disease, or diverticulitis are the most common causes).

Submucosal fistulas are likely the result of anal glands that terminate in the submucosa and track just beneath the submucosa not involving the sphincter complex at all. These fistulas may be opened without compromising fecal continence.

Diagnosis

The symptoms of an anorectal fistula will be quite variable based on the location of the external opening, the complexity of the tract, the patient's tolerance, as well as the underlying cause. Fistula that results from cryptoglandular disease will usually be preceded by a history of an anorectal abscess that was drained (either purposefully or spontaneously). Patients will often assume that their symptoms are related to "hemorrhoids" and/or be referred after a biopsy of the external opening by referring physicians. Bleeding is common due to the hyper-granulation tissue that forms on the external

opening and often irritation of the anal margin skin ensues from chronic moisture or from fecal contact. Pain may be a feature for patients with chronic infection or ongoing inflammation and is often cyclical as a result of spontaneous abscess formation and drainage. Severe pain should be a red flag for another etiology of the fistula such as malignancy or Crohn's disease. If a patient has concomitant gastrointestinal symptoms such as abdominal cramping, bloating, early satiety, or weight loss an associated diagnosis such as IBD or malignancy must be excluded.

Physical exam findings are usually pathognomonic for an anal fistula with an opening on the anal margin skin with heaped-up granulation tissue that is tender and often draining (Figure 14-13). The nature of the drainage can vary and may be serous, purulent, or feculent depending on the fistula. Often the location of the fistula can tell the examiner two things: the location of the internal opening and the depth of the fistula through the sphincter muscles. External openings that arise directly in the posterior midline close to the anal verge are usually submucosal while openings off the midline close to the anal verge are frequently intersphincteric. Low transsphincteric fistulas have been shown to occur more often in the anterior location and are less likely to be preceded by an abscess [66]. External openings in the ischiorectal fossa are usually the result of transsphincteric or suprasphincteric fistula and the examiner should suspect that the external sphincter muscle will be involved. In addition Goodsall's rule can be applied to help locate the internal opening. Goodsall described his observations of anal fistula in a book chapter written in 1900 [67]. He subdivided the anal margin skin into quadrants by two lines intersecting at right angles in the center of the anal aperture. The first was

FIGURE 14-14. Goodsall's rule
for anal fistula.

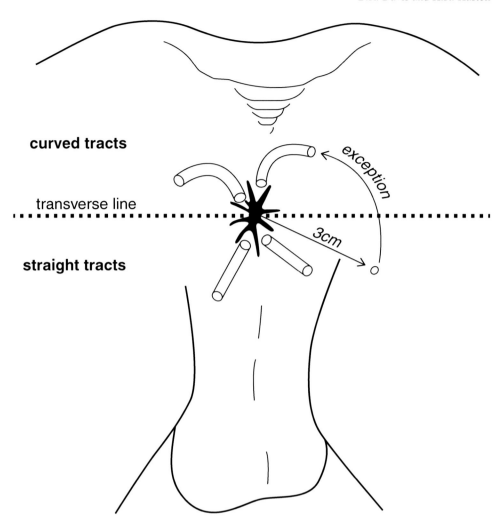

curved tracts

transverse line

straight tracts

drawn connecting the ischial tuberosities and was referred to as the transverse anal line and the second from the coccyx to the pubic symphysis (Figure 14-14). The transverse anal line is of importance as external openings of anal fistulas that are located anteriorly are postulated to drain to an internal opening radially situated while posterior external openings drain to the posterior midline. This observation has proven accurate for external openings situated posteriorly but less so for anterior fistula. Cirocco et al. demonstrated in their retrospective review of 216 patients with transsphincteric fistula that 81 % of all fistulas drained to the midline. They confirmed that posteriorly located fistulas drain to the posterior midline in 90 % of cases (97 % for women, 87 % for men) while 71 % of anteriorly located fistulas drain to the anterior midline [68]. The positive predictive value of Goodsall's rule has been estimated to be 59 % and is more accurate for posteriorly located fistulas [69, 70].

Palpation of the anal canal using the pad of an experienced finger can frequently determine the location of the internal opening by subtle changes in the anoderm [71]. Anoscopy is helpful to exclude inflammatory conditions of the anal canal or other potential causes of the fistula but the internal opening is rarely seen unless pus is draining from it. In patients that have abdominal symptoms or findings in the office concerning for a cause other than cryptoglandular a colonoscopy can be performed. However as a general rule most patients with anal fistula require little if any work-up other than a physical exam.

Preoperative imaging is reserved for patients that present with multiple external openings, those in which an internal opening cannot be identified on physical exam either preoperatively or intraoperative or in cases of recurrence following surgical procedures especially a fistulotomy in which cure would be expected. Increasingly patients presenting with anal pain in the emergency room are undergoing CT scans with rectal contrast that can occasionally demonstrate an anal fistula. However as a rule this is not a helpful test for the evaluation of anal fistula and should not be routinely ordered [72].

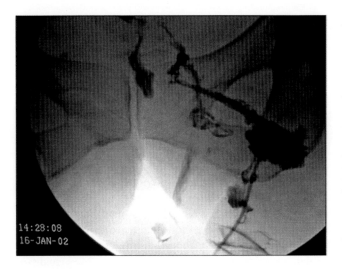

FIGURE 14-15. Fistulography of complex anal fistula (*arrow* on fistula tract).

Fistulography

Water-soluble contrast injected into the external opening under fluoroscopy using a small feeding tube has proved historically to be useful in the evaluation of complex anal fistulas (Figure 14-15). Weisman et al. retrospectively evaluated the utility of fistulography in 27 patients with anal fistula and found that in 13 of the 27 patients (48 %) information obtained from the fistulograms revealed either unexpected pathology (*n*=7) or directly altered surgical management (*n*=6) [73]. However Kuijpers et al. found fistulography to be inaccurate for the detection of internal openings (5/21 patients) and high extensions (9/21 patients) compared to surgical findings [74]. Using a modified technique in which contrast was injected through a Foley catheter inserted into the rectum Pomerri et al. demonstrated an accuracy of 74 % for the detection of internal openings and 92 % for secondary tracks when compared to surgery [75].

Due to the limitation of plane film imaging to delineate anatomic landmarks more recent attempts at fistulography have incorporated CT imaging in combination with contrast injection. Liang et al. prospectively evaluated 18 patients with anal fistula and found that CT fistulography had excellent concordance with intraoperative findings including the identification of the fistula tracks, internal opening, and deep abscesses [72]. They failed to demonstrate that CT fistulography was superior to the intraoperative assessment or compare their findings to other imaging techniques. More data is needed to determine if CT fistulography will be a valid tool to assist in the management of patients with complex anal fistula. However it is likely that fistulography as a diagnostic tool for complex anal fistula will be of limited value given the alternatives available in modern radiology suites or colorectal offices.

Endoanal Ultrasound

Surgeon-performed endoanal ultrasound (EAUS) can be performed in the office as a way to characterize complex fistula and its relationship to the sphincter complex. Fistulas appear as a hypoechoic track, which can be enhanced by the instillation of hydrogen peroxide or a Levovist™ [76]. These agents are injected into the external opening during the ultrasound examination to create air within the tract and increase the hypoechoic signal although the advantage of such agents has not been well established [77, 78]. EUS can also help determine the presence of secondary tracts as well as horseshoe extensions. Muhammed et al. performed a meta-analysis of studies comparing EUS with MRI for the detection and characterization of anal fistula. 240 patients were evaluated in the EUS group. The combined sensitivity and specificity in detecting fistulas were 0.87 (95 % CI: 0.70–0.95) and 0.43 (95 % CI: 0.21–0.69), respectively [79]. EUS performed better in the detection of transsphincteric fistula vs. intersphincteric and suprasphincteric tracts that can be difficult to localize [80, 81]. Buchanan et al. evaluated the utility of EUS compared to *preoperative* clinical assessment in determining the *classification* of anal fistula in 104 patients. EUS was superior to physical exam, which correctly predicted 87 (81 %) vs. 66 (61 %) patients, respectively ($p<0.01$). It was also superior in identifying the internal opening (91 % vs. 78 %), and undrained fluid collections (75 % vs. 33 %) [82]. Nagendranath et al. evaluated the performance of hydrogen peroxide-enhanced EUS in 68 patients undergoing surgery for anal fistula. EUS performed no better than *intraoperative* findings in determining the presence and course of the primary tract. EUS outperformed the surgical findings in detecting the presence of secondary tracts (92.65 vs. 79.41 %; $p<0.001$) and course (91.18 vs. 77.94 %; $p<0.001$) [78]. In 13 patients the findings on the EUS changed the operative approach from fistulotomy to seton placement but the authors do not comment as to the reasoning. Conversely, Toyonaga et al. were able to demonstrate that EUS was superior to *intraoperative* findings in the identification of acute and chronic anal fistula in a prospective series of 400 patients. EUS was superior to physical exam in correctly identifying the fistula track (88.8 % vs. 85.0 %, $p=0.0287$) and horseshoe extension (85.7 % vs. 58.7 %, $p<0.0001$) and in localizing the internal opening (85.5 % vs. 69.1 %, $p<0.0001$) [83]. The concordance with EUS findings intraoperatively has not been demonstrated to improve long-term outcomes of anal fistula surgery [84, 85] but more data is necessary to determine which patients and how often surgeons should perform EUS in the management of anal fistula. The results of these studies are influenced by the expertise and experience of the endosonographer and results may not be reproducible in all surgeons' hands. The images are subject to a high degree of interpretation and standards are not well described. Previous surgery, scars, and trauma as well as the presence of undrained fluid collections can negatively influence the results of EUS. The presence of an abscess can lead to acoustic shadowing and render the results less accurate [86]. As MRI begins to supplant EUS for the evaluation of rectal cancer it is likely that the expertise in evaluating endoanal ultrasounds will diminish.

Magnetic Resonance Imaging

MRI of the sphincter complex has some advantages in diagnosing anal fistulas. No instrumentation of the anus is required and the exam is not operator dependent. The importance of MRI lies in its ability to demonstrate hidden areas of sepsis and secondary extensions, both of which contribute to the high rate of recurrence after surgery. Furthermore, MR imaging can be used to define the anatomic relationships of the fistula to predict the likelihood of postoperative fecal incontinence.

Two types of coils can be used: the endoanal and the external phased array coils. The endoanal coil was utilized to improve the imaging evaluation of perianal fistulas, but anal insertion is not well tolerated by patients [87]. The external phased array coil has a wider field of view and is better for assessing complex tracts, lateral extension, and fistulas crossing the levator ani muscle. Additionally, MR imaging with phased array surface coils requires no patient preparation or insertion of anything inside the anus. The introduction of the 1.5 Tesla (T) and 3.0-T magnets in the acquisition of images has negated the need for the endoanal coil in the evaluation of anal and rectal disease. A prospective trial comparing the use of the endoanal coil to the body coil found that surgical concordance was better using the body coil (96 % vs. 68 %), presumably due to field of view limitations [87]. The 3.0-T imaging improves spatial resolution and diagnostic accuracy over the 1.5-T magnet [88]. The finer detail helps in detecting and characterizing even small fistula tracks. However, comparative studies with 1.5-T or 3.0-T have not been reported.

On axial T2-weighted images, the internal and external anal sphincters appear as circular structures with low signal intensity. After intravenous administration of gadolinium, the internal and external sphincter can be easily distinguished on T1-weighted images by their different contrast enhancement. The internal sphincter muscle enhances to a higher degree than the external sphincter muscle [89]. On T2-weighted MR sequences, active fistulas and abscesses are hyperintense.

The potential of MR imaging in assessment of anal fistulas was demonstrated in a study of 16 patients with cryptoglandular fistulas, when MR imaging findings were compared with the subsequent findings from examination under anesthesia [90]. The authors concluded that MR imaging is the most accurate method for determining the presence and course of anal fistulas and that it may help reduce recurrence due to inaccurate surgical assessment. These conclusions were confirmed in a follow-up study of 35 patients that reported correct MR imaging assessments in 33 of the patients (94 %), including two cases in which examination under anesthesia failed to identify distant sepsis [91]. In a prospective study of 42 patients with suspected anal fistulas [92], the results of digital rectal examination, dynamic contrast-enhanced MR imaging, and surgical exploration were compared. MR imaging had a sensitivity of 97 % and specificity of 100 % for detection of fistulas. In addition, it allowed identification of more secondary tracks and was more accurate in identification of complex fistulas than either digital rectal examination alone or surgical exploration. Beets-Tan et al. reported that preoperative MR imaging provided important additional information in 12 of 56 patients with anal fistulas (21 %). This was further subdivided as 4 of 17 patients with recurrent fistulas (benefit in 24 %) and 6 of 15 patients with Crohn's disease (benefit of 40 %) [93]. In a larger study of 71 patients with recurrent anal fistula in which MR imaging findings were revealed after initial fistula surgery, the postoperative recurrence rate was as low as 16 % when surgeons always acted on the MR imaging findings, suggesting that areas of infection had been missed. By contrast, the rate of recurrence was 30 % when surgeons only sometimes acted on MR imaging results and 57 % when MR imaging results were ignored. Furthermore, in the 16 patients who required further unplanned surgery, MR images had initially correctly indicated the site of disease in all cases [94]. The results of MR imaging, anal endosonography, and clinical examination were compared to determine the optimal technique for classifying perianal fistulas. It was concluded that MR imaging is the optimal technique for distinguishing complex from simple perianal fistulas [95]. Finally in a small series of patients with supralevator abscess MRI was used to correctly characterize the fistula track as transsphincteric or intersphincteric, a distinction that is important in determining the correct drainage procedure (transrectal vs. transperineal) [14].

Taken together, the results of these studies confirm that MR imaging is an accurate modality for evaluation of perianal fistulas and associated complications. The most cost-effective algorithm for managing all patients with anal fistula has yet to be established but preoperative imaging should be considered when recurrent fistulas are encountered following treatment, in cases in which multiple external openings exist and when the anatomy is unclear either in the office or at the time of surgery.

Treatment

Treatment of anal fistulas has always been difficult and apparently the chief reason for the opening of the St Marks Hospital in England in 1836. The goals however of any surgical treatment are summarized as:

1. Elimination of sepsis.
2. Closure of the fistula track.

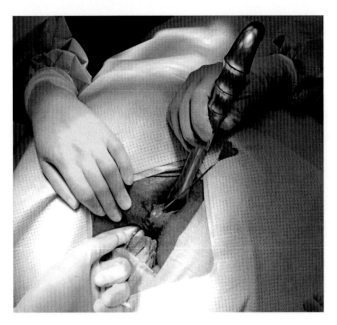

FIGURE 14-16. Probe through the external and internal opening of the anal fistula.

3. Preservation of patient's fecal continence and sphincter function.
4. Minimizing recurrence.

Identification of the external and internal opening is critical and several intraoperative techniques have been described. Physical examination is quite reliable in determining the location of the internal opening in the operating room but if not palpable a catheter can be used to inject either methylene blue or hydrogen peroxide into the external opening with a retractor in the anus. This has been associated with successful identification of the internal opening in 83 % of cases [71].

A gently curved probe inserted into the external opening is an alternative technique for finding the internal opening (Figure 14-16) but care must be taken not to create a false passage and it is better to have an idea of the location of the offending crypt prior to attempts at probing. Chronic tracks will have granulation tissue within them and its absence should raise the suspicion that a false track was created following a fistulotomy.

The ultimate choice of treatment will depend on the amount of sphincter involved in the fistula track with cutting procedures more likely for intersphincteric and low transsphincteric fistula and non-cutting techniques for all others. Patient preference will also influence the procedure choice with most patients opting for sphincter-preserving technique [96]. Surgeons must rely on their experience and comfort for the various non-cutting techniques as the overall quality of evidence to guide decision making is poor [97].

Lay Open Technique (Fistulotomy)

For the confident and successful surgical treatment of fistula-in-ano, one must be practiced and skilled in palpating and recognizing the anorectal ring, for whereas, if this ring be cut, loss of control surely results, yet as long as the narrowest complete ring of muscle remains, control is preserved. All the anal sphincter muscles below this ring may be divided in any manner without harmful loss of control.

Lockhart-Mummery [58]

For simple and most distal or intersphincteric fistula, conventional surgical treatment such as lay open of the fistula tract as a complete transection of the tissue between the fistula tract and anoderm is very effective (Table 14-3). Fistulotomy wounds typically heal after 4–6 weeks, which may be shortened by marsupializing the wound edges [98, 99]. This technique may also reduce the incidence of postoperative bleeding [100].

Recurrence and incontinence are the most significant complication and rates vary widely by author. In a retrospective review of 365 patients, Garcia Aguillar reported recurrence in 4 % of patients with intersphincteric fistula, 7 % with transsphincteric fistula, and 33 % for suprasphincteric and extrasphincteric fistulas [101]. Incontinence after surgical treatment of these fistulas also increased with the complexity of the fistula, lowest being for intersphincteric fistula (37 %) and highest for extrasphincteric fistula (83 %). Factors associated with recurrence included type and extension of the fistula, lack of identification or lateral location of the internal opening, previous fistula surgery, and surgeon experience. Incontinence was associated to female sex, high anal fistula, type of surgery, and previous fistula surgery. Visscher et al. reported on 116 patients who had undergone fistula surgery (both cutting and non-cutting) in whom both a fecal incontinence and quality-of-life questionnaires could be obtained. Median follow-up from the first perianal fistula surgery was 7.8 years (range, 2.1–18.1 years). Thirty-nine patients (34 %) experienced incontinence. Surgical fistulotomy, multiple abscess drainages, and a high transsphincteric or suprasphincteric fistula tract were associated with incontinence. As compared to simple fistula (Wexner score, 1.2 [SD, 2.1]), incontinence was worse after surgery for complex fistula (Wexner score, 4.7 [SD, 6.2], $p = 0.001$), as were quality-of-life elements, including lifestyle ($p = 0.030$), depression ($p = 0.077$), and embarrassment ($p < 0.001$) [102].

Setons

Setons are used to treat anal fistula when a lay open technique is not possible or not advisable. Most complex anal fistulas and fistulas associated with Crohn's disease are specific examples in which a lay open technique would have significant or complete impairment of fecal continence or

TABLE 14-3. Experience with fistulotomy in treating anal fistula

Author	Year	Surgical procedure	# Patients	Outcome	Follow-up
Kronborg	1985	Fistulotomy	26	Recurrence 11 %	12 Months
Hebjorn	1987	Incision and drainage with fistula surgery	20	Recurrence 10 % Minor incontinence 8.3 %	12 Months
Schouten	1991	Incision and drainage with fistula surgery	36	Recurrence 3 % Minor incontinence 39 %	42.5 Months
Tang	1996	Incision and drainage with fistula surgery	24	Recurrence 0 % Minor incontinence 0 %	12 Months
Ho Y	1997	Incision and drainage with fistula surgery	24	Recurrence 0 % Minor incontinence 0 %	15.5 Months
Ho	1998	Fistulotomy	52	Healing time 10 weeks Minor incontinence 11 %	9 Weeks
Belmonte Montes	1999	Fistulotomy	24	Incontinence 5 %	12 Months
Oliver	2003	Incision and drainage with fistula surgery	100	Recurrence 5 % Minor incontinence 6 %	12 Months
Pescatori	2006	Fistulotomy	52	Minor incontinence 8.3 % Recurrence 8.3 %	10 Months
Atkin	2011	Fistulotomy	180		
Tozer	2013	Fistulotomy	50	Recurrence 7 % Minor incontinence 20 %	11 Months
Hall	2014	Fistulotomy	146	Recurrence 6 %	3 Months

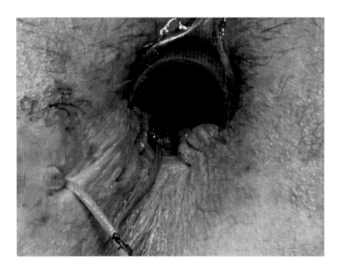

FIGURE 14-17. Seton in an anal fistula.

when healing of the subsequent wound would not be expected to occur (Figure 14-17). A variety of materials have been described for use as setons including wire, non-absorbable suture such as silk, vessel loops, and silastic catheters. Setons can be placed loosely in an effort to promote drainage and fibrosis of the fistula track either as a bridge to a non-cutting repair or as definitive treatment. Alternatively they may be tightened sequentially over time as a cutting seton in an effort to slowly divide the sphincter muscle and preserve continence by allowing a scar to form between the cut ends of the sphincter complex.

With cutting setons, the overlying skin and anoderm are divided at the time of surgery. The seton is then secured tightly around the remaining sphincter complex and is further tightened in the office at varying intervals. A variety of creative ways have been described to facilitate tightening of the seton [103, 104], and intervals vary from days to weeks but in general enough time must lapse for the seton to slowly divide the sphincter muscle. The time to complete healing will depend on the amount of tissue incorporated in the seton and the schedule of visits for tightening and has been reported between 1 month to as long as 1 year [105, 106]. Patients will often experience pain after tightening the seton and must be counseled as to the expected recovery and time frame to healing.

In a meta-analysis of 18 studies including 448 patients who were treated with cutting setons, recurrence rates were reported between 3 and 5 %. Overall fecal incontinence was reported as 5.6 % for patients in whom the internal sphincter was not divided at the initial surgery compared to 25.2 % when it was [107]. In another meta-analysis including 520 patients the average rate of incontinence following cutting seton use was 12 %. The rate of incontinence increased as the location of the internal opening of the fistula moved more proximally in the anal canal. In the studies that described the types of incontinence, liquid stool was the most common followed closely by flatus [108]. In a retrospective review of 112 patients undergoing cutting seton for transsphincteric or suprasphincteric fistulas ($n=84$) and extrasphincteric fistulas ($n=28$) the mean duration the seton was in place was 28.7 days. The mean time to complete wound healing was 9.3 weeks. With a median follow-up of 38.6 months recurrence was noted in one patient (0.9 %). Twenty-seven patients (24.1 %) had continence disorders, including gas incontinence in 21 patients (18.6 %) and liquid stool incontinence in 6 patients (5.4 %). There were no incidents of solid stool incontinence [109].

Non-cutting or draining setons are usually used as a bridge for definitive treatment in an effort to promote fibrosis, decrease the inflammatory response, and aid in identifying the internal opening at the time of the secondary procedure [110]. They can also be left in place to prevent recurrent abscess formation in patients with Crohn's disease or in patients who are not deemed candidates for additional surgery. Setons of any type can fall out due to wear and breaking. Vessel loops tend to be durable and can be left in place for years. If setons are to be left for prolong periods of time they should be loose but not so big that their presence becomes a problem for the patient in terms of hygiene and skin irritation. Setons that are secured in a circular configuration can rotate and the knots can migrate into the fistula track occasionally causing plugging and discomfort. Patient can be advised to twist them occasionally if this happens. The knots themselves can also cause irritation of the contralateral skin if too bulky.

Advancement Flap

Endorectal advancement flap (ERAF) has been advocated as an effective treatment for high transsphincteric or suprasphincteric fistulas. The techniques used are variable but the essential elements include debridement or excision of the fistula tract, mobilization of a vascularized, tension-free mucosal flap, and coverage of the internal opening, which is usually closed with absorbable suture. The procedure can be performed with locoregional anesthesia, but to optimize exposure of the anal canal and lower rectum a spinal anesthetic can be advantageous. A complete bowel preparation with oral purgatives is recommended combined with preoperative antibiotics.

Technique

1. With the patient in prone jackknife position or in lithotomy position, the internal opening of the fistula is exposed—this can be accomplished by everting the anal canal with the Lone Star® retractor system (Figure 14-18a).
2. The internal opening is identified and the crypt-bearing tissue excised.
3. A small rim of the anoderm, below the internal opening, is excised to create a neo-dentate line.
4. The defect in the internal anal sphincter is closed with absorbable sutures (2-0 Vicryl, Ethicon Inc., Somerville, NJ) (Fig. 14-18b).
5. A curvilinear incision is made at the level of the internal opening extending laterally to create a wide tissue flap.
6. Dissection is performed in the submucosal plane consisting of mucosa, submucosa, and few superficial fibers of the internal anal sphincter and then mobilized over a distance of 4–6 cm proximally.
7. The fistulous tract is alternatively curetted or cored out, and the defect in the internal anal sphincter is closed with absorbable sutures.

FIGURE 14-18. (a) Lone star to ever the anal canal. (b) Closing the internal opening. (c) Securing the flap.

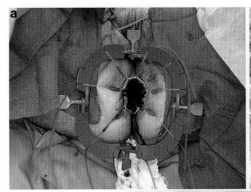
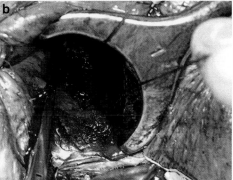
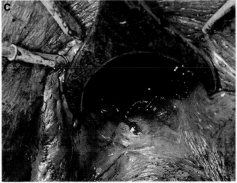

8. The flap is advanced and sutured over the top of the internal opening with absorbable sutures (Figure 14-18c).
9. Vascular supply of the flap is maintained through the submucosal plexus.

The reported healing rates after flap repair vary between 60 and 100 % [111–119]. Ortiz et al. reported on 91 patients who underwent ERAF with a median follow-up of 42 (range 24–65) months. Eighteen patients had recurrence of the fistula during follow-up, with a median time to relapse of 5.0 (range 1.0–11.7) months. There were no recurrences after 1 year [120]. VanOnkelen et al. reported on a series of 252 patients with a high transsphincteric fistula of cryptoglandular origin that underwent ERAF with a median length of follow-up of 21 months (range 6–136 months). Before the procedure, patients underwent endoanal MRI to depict the course of the fistula tract and to determine the presence and location of associated abscesses. Seventeen patient- and fistula-related variables were assessed to determine their influence on recurrence. The failure rate at 3 years was 41 % (95 % CI, 34–48) [121]. Failure was not influenced by age, sex, smoking, or obesity. Nor was it affected by previous attempts at repair, preoperative seton drainage, presence of associated abscesses, location of the internal fistula opening, or postoperative drainage. 46 % of the patients in this series had a horseshoe extension of their fistula. The presence of a horseshoe extension correlated with successful repair 32.0 % [95 % CI, 23–41] vs. 51.0 % [95 % CI, 40.6–61.4]; $p=0.005$.

Despite these findings there are many studies that demonstrate patient, disease, and technical factors associated with either improved or worse outcomes following ERAF repair of complex anal fistula. Which of these are real and which are not can be difficult to discern due to the heterogeneity of patients and methods studied as well as the paucity of high-quality evidence. Knowledge of the literature as well as experience will facilitate discussion with patients regarding the risk of recurrence and complications rates following ERAF repair of complex fistulas.

One study looked at curettage of the fistula track vs. excision by means of "core out" and found no difference in recurrence [116]. In this same study the postoperative maximum squeeze pressure was reduced in patients who had the core out technique but this was not clinically relevant. The location of the internal opening (posterior vs. anterior) has no impact on outcomes of advancement flap repairs in the published literature even though it can be harder to obtain adequate flap length during posterior dissections due to the angulation of the anorectal junction posteriorly [122]. Preoperative seton placement did not impact outcomes of flap repairs in 278 patients with cryptoglandular fistulas reviewed retrospectively. Setons were in place at least 2 months prior to definitive repair [123]. Repeat anorectal advancement flap after recurrence has been shown to be feasible with overall good outcomes [124, 125], but has been shown to be a risk factor for failure [126, 127]. Success of flap advancement was inversely correlated with the number

of prior attempts, and in patients with no or only one previous attempt at repair the healing rate was 87 %. In patients with two or more previous repairs the healing rate dropped to 50 % [126]. The combination of fibrin glue with advancement flap repair has also been associated with worse outcomes when compared to just flap repairs alone [128]. The use of platelet-rich plasma in combination with advancement flap has better outcomes but limited data [129]. Medically induced bowel confinement has not been shown to improve outcomes [130].

Full-thickness flaps have been shown to be superior to partial-thickness flaps in several studies [131, 132]. In one series 34 patients underwent surgery using a partial-thickness flap and 20 a full-thickness flap. Continence was not affected by choice of technique. Recurrence was 35 % and 5 %, respectively.

Patient-related factors that impact outcome include smoking, which both decreases the mucosal blood flow [133] and negatively impacts success of flap repairs [134]. Obesity negatively impacted advancement flap repairs in a study looking at 220 patients with complex anal fistula undergoing advancement flaps. After a median follow-up of 6 months, primary healing rate for the entire cohort was 82 % (180/220). In non-obese patients, recurrence rate was significantly lower than in obese patients (14 % vs. 28 %; $p<0.01$). Moreover, reoperation rate due to recurrent abscess with the need for seton drainage in the failure groups was significantly higher in obese patients when compared to non-obese patients (73 % vs. 52 %; $p<0.01$). Using multivariate analysis, obesity was identified as independent predictive factor of success or failure ($p<0.02$) [135]. Crohn's disease has also been shown to be a risk factor for failure [136].

While anorectal advancement flaps are chosen to preserve the sphincter muscle many reports have demonstrated some degree of fecal incontinence following surgery. Uribe et al. demonstrated significant reductions in maximum resting pressure 3 months after advancement flap repair of complex anal fistula (83.6 ± 33.2 vs. 45.6 ± 18.3, $p<0.001$) and maximum squeeze pressure (208.8 ± 91.5 vs. 169.5 ± 75, $p<0.001$). Before surgery, five patients (8.9 %) reported symptoms of incontinence. After surgery, 78.6 % patients had normal continence, seven patients (12.5 %) complained of minor incontinence, and five (9 %) had major problems with continence [113].

Ligation of Intersphincteric Fistula

The ligation of the intersphincteric fistula track is a sphincter-preserving procedure that can be performed under locoregional, spinal, or general anesthesia. The procedure is appropriate for all patients with high transsphincteric fistulas assuming that a well-formed fistula track has been established. The advantages of the procedure are its simplicity and applicability to most patients with fistula-in-ano (Table 14-4).

TABLE 14-4. Experience with LIFT procedure

Author	Year	# Patients	Procedure	Follow-up (weeks)	Percent healed (%)	Type of study
Rojanasakul et al.	2007	18	LIFT	4	94	Prospective observational
Shanwani et al.	2010	45	LIFT	7	82	Prospective observational
Ellis et al.	2010	31	bioLIFT	6	94	Retrospective
Bleier et al.	2010	39	LIFT	10	57	Retrospective
Ooi et al.	2011	25	LIFT	6	96	Prospective observational
Tan et al.	2011	93	LIFT	4	92	Retrospective review
Steiner et al.		18	LIFT	6	83	Retrospective
Aboulian et al.	2011	25	LIFT	24	68	Retrospective review
Mushaya et al.	2012	25	LIFT	4	68	Prospective randomized
Abcarian et al.	2012	50	LIFT	15	74	Retrospective
Lo et al.	2012	25	LIFT	2	98	Retrospective
van Onkelen et al.	2012	42	LIFT	12	51	Prospective
Chen et al.	2012	10	LIFT	6	100	Retrospective
Lehmann et al.	2013	17	LIFT	4	47	Prospective
Liu et al.	2013	38	LIFT	26	61	Retrospective
Madbouly et al.	2014	35	LIFT	56	74	Prospective randomized
Ye et al.	2015	43	mLIFT	60	87	Retrospective
Bastawrous et al.	2015	66	mLIFT	21	71	Retrospective

bioLIFT: biological LIFT; mLIFT: modified LIFT

Technique

A preoperative rectal enema is given to patients in the morning of surgery. Patients are placed in the prone jackknife position and regional anesthesia is used. The steps involved in the procedure are as follows [137]:

1. Identify the internal opening by injecting peroxide or saline through the external opening.
2. Incise circumanally in the intersphincteric plane at the site of fistula using a 3–4-cm curvilinear incision.
3. Identify the intersphincteric tract using a soft catheter or Lockhart–Mummery and lacrimal probes.
4. Dissect around the intersphincteric portion of the fistula tract being careful not to injure or disrupt the tract. A right-angle probe can be used for this purpose. Using narrow malleable retractors can facilitate exposure of the intersphincteric plane. A Lone Star retractor can also facilitate this exposure.
5. Hook the intersphincteric tract using a small right-angle clamp.
6. Doubly ligate the tract close to the internal and external sphincter with 2-0 Vicryl (Ethicon Inc., Somerville, NJ), and transect it between the sutures. Some surgeons prefer a transfixation suture.
7. Inject the external opening to confirm that the tract was divided completely.
8. Curette the external portion of the fistula tract.
9. Drain the external opening.
10. Re-approximate the intersphincteric incision wound loosely with an interrupted 3-0 Vicryl (Ethicon Inc., Somerville, NJ).

Variations in this technique include orienting the incision in a radial fashion and performing a partial fistulotomy up to the external sphincter [138, 139]. Other modifications include unroofing the fistula from the internal opening to intersphincteric groove, ligating the fistula tract, but preserving the external sphincter [140]. In an effort to increase the success of this procedure the use of biologics has also been examined including inserting a biologic mesh in the intersphincteric groove or as a plug in the external tract [141–143]. Series are small and conclusions cannot be drawn about the efficacy of these approaches.

Postoperatively patients are maintained on a bulk laxative and can be prescribed oral ciprofloxacin and metronidazole although the benefit of antibiotic in the postoperative setting has not been evaluated.

Abcarian et al. reviewed their experience with all-cause transsphincteric fistula treated with the LIFT technique [144]. Median follow-up was 18 weeks and closure was achieved in 74 % of patients. Success of the procedure was inversely correlated with the number of previous attempts at closure, a finding seen by other authors looking at their outcomes with the LIFT procedure [145]. No changes in continence were reported. Hall et al. reported in their multicenter prospective trial of anal fistula procedures a success rate of 79 % at 3 months of follow-up using the LIFT technique. Hospitals that performed more LIFT procedures had higher rates of healing [115].

In a meta-analysis looking at the success of the LIFT procedure 18 studies were reviewed including 592 patients (65 % male). The most common type of fistula was transsphincteric (73.3 % of cases). The mean healing rate reported was 74.6 %. The risk factors for failure were obesity, smoking, multiple previous surgeries, and the length of the fistula tract. The median length of fistula tract was shorter in the healed group compared with the failed group (4 cm vs. 6 cm, $p = 0.004$).

The mean healing time was 5.5 weeks, and the mean follow-up period was 42.3 weeks. The patient satisfaction rates ranged from 72 to 100 %. No de novo incontinence developed secondary to the LIFT procedure. There is not enough evidence that variants in the surgical technique achieve better outcomes (Bio-LIFT, LIFT-Plug, LIFT-Plus) [146].

A more recent meta-analysis of 24 original articles including 1110 patients was performed which included 1 randomized controlled study, 3 case control studies, and 20 case series. Most studies included patients with transsphincteric or complex fistula, not amenable to fistulotomy. During a mean follow-up of 10.3 months, the mean success rate was 76.4 % while incontinence, intraoperative, and postoperative complication rates were negligible (0 %, 0 %, and 5.5 %, respectively). There was no association between pre-LIFT drainage seton and success of the procedure [147].

In another review of 498 patients undergoing the LIFT procedure success rates ranged from 40 to 95 %, with a pooled success of 71 % (352 of 495 patients; 3 of 498 were lost to follow-up). Follow-up ranged from 1 to 55 months, with a reported mean or median of 4–19.5 months. One hundred and eighty-three patients were formally assessed for continence, out of whom 11 (6 %) had a minor disturbance [148].

When the LIFT procedure does fail several authors have noted that the resultant discharge presents at the intersphincteric incision and endoanal ultrasound has confirmed that these were simple fistulas that were subsequently managed with fistulotomy or local wound care [149, 150]. This has been shown in other studies but not as consistently [151].

Fibrin Glue

Fibrin sealants were introduced in the 1990s as an alternative to more invasive surgical procedures in an effort to shorten recovery, prevent incontinence, and simplify surgery in patients with complex anal fistulas. Hjortrup et al. instilled fibrin sealant into the fistula tracks of eight patients who had failed previous surgical attempts at closure and achieved a 50 % success rate after a single injection [152]. The advantages of fibrin glue are that it is simple and repeatable with no significant learning curve and no division of the sphincter muscle.

Generally fibrin sealants consisted of two components: fibrinogen concentrate and thrombin. Factor XIII is added to stabilize the fibrin monomers. Aprotinin is also added to prevent fibrinolysis. The glue is infused into the fistulous tract with the idea that collagen formation within the tract will stimulate healing. It also stimulates the migration and proliferation of fibroblasts and pluripotent endothelial cells to heal the fistula. Between 7 and 14 days postoperatively, plasmin that is present in the surrounding tissue lyses the fibrin clot as the tract is replaced by synthesized collagen [153].

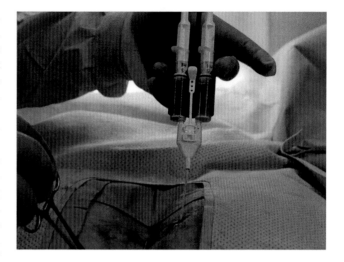

FIGURE 14-19. Fibrin glue injection into an anal fistula.

Technique

1. The patient is placed in the prone jackknife position and anesthesia is introduced (spinal, general, or locoregional).
2. Both openings of the fistula track are identified and mechanically curetted and irrigated with normal saline or hydrogen peroxide.
3. If extensive side branching or undrained abscess is encountered the procedure is aborted and a seton is placed.
4. A double-barreled syringe, containing the two components of the glue, is inserted into the external opening until the tip is seen at the internal opening (Figure 14-19).
5. At this point the internal opening can be variably sutured closed or left opening depending on the surgeon's preference—there is no significant advantage of one technique over the other [154].
6. The syringe is depressed, which mixes the two components as they are injected into the canal while withdrawing the syringe. The tract is filled completely until a bead of glue is seen at the external opening.
7. The glue is allowed to set for 30–60 s to form its stable clot.

Postoperatively, the use of antibiotics and diet restrictions do not seem to confer any benefit to the patient [155], but sitz baths, excessive straining, or vigorous exercise should be avoided to prevent dislodgement of the plug.

The efficacy of fibrin glue injection as a curative procedure remains in question. Success rates vary greatly depending on the etiology and complexity of the fistulas, type of fibrin glue used, and length of patient follow-up (Table 14-5).

Cintron et al. have reported the largest series of patients with perianal fistulas treated with fibrin glue [156]. Seventy-nine consecutive patients in this non-randomized prospective study were treated using one of the three different types of fibrin glue: autologous, Viguard-FS (V. I. Technologies,

TABLE 14-5. Experience with fibrin glue

Author	Year	# Patients	Success rate (%)	Follow-up (months)
Cintron et al.	1999	26	81	3.5
Cintron et al.	2000	79	61	18
Patrlj et al.	2000	69	74	28
Park et al.	2000	29	68	6
Sentovich	2001	20	85	10
Lindsey et al.	2002	42	63	4
Sentovich	2003	48	69	22
Loungnarath et al.	2004	39	31	26
Zmora et al.	2005	60	53	6
Gisbertz et al.	2005	27	33	7
Singer et al.	2005	75	21[a]	27
Maralcan et al.	2006	36	83	12
Ellis and Clark	2006	28	54	22
Dietz	2006	39	31	23
Witte et al.	2007	34	55	7
Adams et al.	2008	36	61	3
de Parades et al.	2010	30	50	12

Inc., New York, NY), and Tisseel VB (Baxter, Deerfield, IL). The majority of fistulas were transsphincteric and 8 % were secondary to Crohn's disease. The overall success rate was 66 %, with a mean follow-up of 1 year. Healing rates correlated with fistula complexity: intersphincteric 82 %, transsphincteric 62 %, and Crohn's related 33 %. The type of glue used did not affect success rates, and the use of commercial glue over autologous was recommended due to ease of preparation, increased strength in laboratory evaluations, and more consistent bonding. The average time to fistula recurrence was 3.3 months while the latest was seen at 11 months. This led the authors to stress the importance of long-term follow-up.

Many authors have suggested reasons for failure of fibrin glue in the treatment of anal fistula but little evidence exists to support these conclusions. Type of glue used, inadequate removal of granulation tissue, incomplete filling of fistula track(s), and track length have all been postulated to play a role in recurrence or persistence of the fistula [153]. In a meta-analysis of 12 published studies of 378 patients with complex anal fistula overall healing rate was 53 % with a wide variation between studies (10–78 %). The only factor that was found to account for this diversity was fistula complexity, with series including a high proportion of complex fistulae reporting worse outcomes [157].

Long-term follow-up of patients who show healing of their fistula tracks at 6 months demonstrated that few recur. Of 60 patients treated with fibrin glue 32 experienced healing. 23 (72 %) of these patients were available for long-term follow-up and 17 (74 %) remained disease free at a mean follow-up of 6.5 years. Six (26 %) patients had variable degrees of recurrence; four needed further surgical interven-

tion and two were treated with antibiotics only. Recurrent disease occurred at an average of 4.1 years (range, 11 months to 6 years) from surgery, and on several occasions was at a different location in the perianal region. None of the patients experienced incontinence following the procedure [158].

Despite the varied success with fibrin glue treatment there is good evidence that patients experience no disturbances in continence as a result of treatment and treatment with fibrin glue does not preclude subsequent treatments of their fistula using alternative approaches. However the heterogeneity of published data regarding the success of this treatment makes it difficult to recommend as a first-line therapy of complex anal fistula.

Anal Fistula Plug

The concept of "filling" the fistula track spurred further innovation in the use of biological materials and in 2006 Johnson et al. performed a prospective trial in which a piece of Surgisis® (Cook Surgical, Inc., Bloomington, IN), a bioabsorbable xenograft, made of lyophilized porcine intestinal submucosa, was fashioned into a plug and secured into the fistula track of 15 patients with complex fistulas achieving an 87 % closure rate. As with the fibrin glue technique no sphincter division is required, so continence is not impaired. Since this initial study the Surgisis Anal Fistula Plug (AFP) (Cook Surgical, Bloomington, IN) has been introduced as a prefabricated cone-shaped device that can be easily secured into the fistula track. It acts as a tissue scaffold for host fibroblasts to promote healing and ingrowth of tissue into the fistula track [159].

TABLE 14-6. Experience with anal fistula plug

Author	Year	Type of study	# Patients	Success rate (%)	Follow-up (months)
Johnson et al.	2006	Prospective	25	87	3
Champagne et al.	2006	Prospective	46	83	12
O'Connor et al.	2006	Prospective	20	80	10
Ellis	2007	Retrospective	13	92	6
Ky et al.	2008	Prospective	45	55	6.5
Christoforidis et al.	2008	Retrospective	47	43	6.5
Safar et al.	2009	Retrospective	36	14	4.2
Ortiz et al.	2009	Prospective randomized	15	20	12
El-Gazzaz et al.	2010	Retrospective	33	25	7.4
van Koperen et al.	2011	Prospective	31	29	11
Chan et al.	2012	Prospective	44	50	10.5
Cintron et al.	2013	Prospective	73	42	15
Tan et al.	2013	Retrospective	26	13	15
Adamina et al.	2014	Prospective	46	43.5	68

Technique

1. The patient is placed in the prone jackknife position and anesthesia is introduced (spinal, general, or locoregional).
2. Both openings of the fistula track are identified and irrigated with normal saline or hydrogen peroxide.
3. The plug is rehydrated, usually in a 0.9 % normal saline solution for 3–5 min, before insertion.
4. The tapered end of the fistula plug is then tied to the anal side of the seton or silk suture and pulled into the fistula tract through the primary opening until it fitted snugly.
5. The plug is then trimmed flush with the primary opening. A 2-0 Vicryl (Ethicon Inc., Somerville, NJ) suture is used to anchor the plug to the mucosa/submucosa and internal sphincter at the primary opening with a figure-of-eight stitch, completely covering it with mucosa at the completion of the stitch.
6. The excess plug protruding from the external opening is trimmed such that the external opening is partially open to allow drainage and prevent infection.

Since introduction of the AFP, success rates have varied widely between 14 and 87 % (Table 14-6). Several technical and perioperative factors have been ascribed to the failures including the absence of preoperative seton placement, overly aggressive curetting of the fistula track resulting in widening of the track, inadequate fixation of the plug into the internal opening, and the presence of multiple tracks. Data is lacking to recommend one surgical technique over another. In one of the largest series by Citron et al. 73 patients underwent anal fistula plug closure of 72 transsphincteric and 1 suprasphincteric fistula [160]. There were eight fistulas secondary to Crohn's disease. Pre-procedure setons were used in patients at the discretion of the operating surgeon. Otherwise all aspects of the procedure were standardized. In their study the plug extrusion rate was 9 % (7/78). There was no difference in closure rates between primary and recurrent fistulas (primary = 20/53 = 38 % and recurrent 8/20 = 40 %).

The overall patient success rate was 38 % (28/73) and the plug success rate was 39.5 % when plug fallouts were eliminated. The fistulas in four out of eight patients with Crohn's disease closed (50 %). There were no intraoperative complications and four postoperative abscesses (4/73; 5 %). Mcgee et al. looked at 41 patients with 42 fistula tracks who underwent AFP closures over a 39-month period. Complete closure was achieved in 18 of 42 (43 %) fistulas at a mean follow-up of 25 months. Closure was not associated with gender, age, tract location, duration of seton, or length of follow-up. Successful closure was significantly associated with increased tract length, because fistulas longer than 4 cm were nearly three times more likely to heal compared with shorter fistulas ((14/23, 61 %) vs. (4/19, 21 %), $p = 0.004$; relative risk = 2.8; 95 % CI 1.14–7.03) [161].

The diversity in study design and outcomes led O'Riordan and his colleagues to summarize the anal fistula plug literature for Crohn's- and non-Crohn's-related fistula-in-ano in a homogenous patient population [162]. Studies were included if results for patients with and without Crohn's disease could be differentiated and reported a mean or median follow-up of more than 3 months. Overall 530 patients were analyzed (488 non-Crohn's and 42 Crohn's patients). The plug extrusion rate was 8.7 % (46 patients). The proportion of non-Crohn's patients achieving fistula closure varied widely between studies, ranging from 0.2 (95 % CI 0.04–0.48) to 0.86 (95 % CI 0.64–0.97). The pooled proportion of patients achieving fistula closure in patients with non-Crohn's fistula-in-ano was 0.54 (95 % CI 0.50–0.59). The proportion achieving closure in patients with Crohn's disease was similar (0.55, 95 % CI 0.39–0.70). The authors noted that the divergent findings make it difficult for surgeons to quote an acceptable success rate during preoperative counseling of patients with anal fistulas considering treatment with the AFP.

A relatively new device for treating anal fistulas is a synthetic anal fistula plug (Figure 14-20) composed of a copolymer (polyglycolic acid:trimethylene carbonate) that is

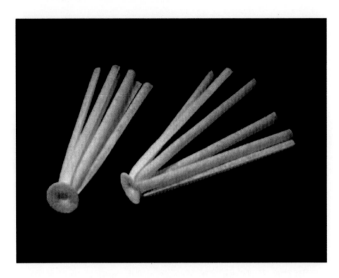

FIGURE 14-20. Bio A absorbable fistula plug (W.L. GORE & Associates, Newark, DE, Courtesy of Michael Stamos, MD, with permission).

gradually absorbed by the body (Gore® Bio-A® Fistula Plug, W.L. Gore & Associates, Elkton, MD). There is limited data to assess the efficacy of this novel technique. Stamos et al. performed a multicenter prospective trial of 93 patients with non-Crohn's-related complex cryptoglandular transsphincteric anal fistulas treated with this device. The primary end point of the study was the healing rate at 6 and 12 months after plug implantation. 13 patients were lost to follow-up and an additional 21 were withdrawn (19 due to recurrence of their fistula prior to 6 months). Of the 66 patients remaining fistula closure at 6 months was 41 % (95 % CI, 30 %–52 %) which improved to 49 % (95 % CI, 38 %–61 %) at 12 months [163].

Novel Techniques

The use of laser in the treatment of anal fistula was initially described in 2011 in a pilot study by Wilhelm [164]. This sphincter-saving technique uses an emitting laser probe [fistula laser closure (FiLaC™), Biolitec, Germany], which destroys the fistula epithelium and simultaneously obliterates the remaining fistula tract. The procedure also includes the closure of the internal opening by means of an anorectal flap. In this pilot study, 11 patients with cryptoglandular fistula underwent FiLaC™ procedure with an overall success of 81 %. A subsequent study of 35 patients demonstrated healing in 71 % [165].

There is limited evidence for the use of adipose-derived stem cells (ADSC) to treat complex anal fistula mostly in patients with Crohn's disease. Autologous ADSC can be easily obtained with liposuction with minimal adverse effects on the patient. In a multicenter randomized controlled trial, Garcia-Olmo et al. [166] used ADSC to treat complex cryptoglandular, rectovaginal, and Crohn's-related fistulas. Initially they achieved a 71 % success rate with ADSC,

compared with 16 % in the control group (fibrin glue only). However, at 1 year this had decreased to 62.5 and to 33 % at 3 years.

An injectable form of Permacol (Tissue Science Laboratories, Covington, GA), a type of porcine acellular collagen matrix, was modified by centrifugation to form a paste and has been used to inject anal fistula in combination with an ERAF. Studies are limited but success rates in non-Crohn's patients have been reported as high as 82 % [167].

References

1. Abcarian H. Anorectal infection: abscess-fistula. Clin Colon Rectal Surg. 2011;24(1):14–21.
2. Shrum RC. Anorectal pathology in 1000 consecutive patients with suspected surgical disorders. Dis Colon Rectum. 1959;2: 469–72.
3. Sl B. Practice proctology. Charles C Thomas: Springfield, IL; 1960.
4. Sainio P. Fistula-in-ano in a defined population. Incidence and epidemiological aspects. Ann Chir Gynaecol. 1984;73(4): 219–24.
5. Ommer A, Herold A, Berg E, Furst A, Sailer M, Schiedeck T. German S3 guideline: anal abscess. Int J Colorectal Dis. 2012;27(6):831–7.
6. Khati NJ, Sondel Lewis N, Frazier AA, Obias V, Zeman RK, Hill MC. CT of acute perianal abscesses and infected fistulae: a pictorial essay. Emerg Radiol. 2015;22(3):329–35. doi:10.1007/s10140-014-1284-3. Epub 2014 Nov 25. PubMed PMID: 25421387.
7. Eglitis J. The glands of the anal canal in man. Ohio J Sci. 1961;61(2):65–79.
8. Seow-Choen F, Ho JM. Histoanatomy of anal glands. Dis Colon Rectum. 1994;37(12):1215–8.
9. Eisenhammer S. The internal anal sphincter and the anorectal abscess. Surg Gynecol Obstet. 1956;103(4):501–6.
10. Parks AG. Pathogenesis and treatment of fistula-in-ano. Br Med J. 1961;1(5224):463–9.
11. McElwain JW, MacLean MD, Alexander RM, Hoexter B, Guthrie JF. Anorectal problems: experience with primary fistulectomy for anorectal abscess, a report of 1,000 cases. Dis Colon Rectum. 1975;18(8):646–9.
12. Sneider EB, Maykel JA. Anal abscess and fistula. Gastroenterol Clin North Am. 2013;42(4):773–84.
13. Steele SR, Kumar R, Feingold DL, Rafferty JL, Buie WD. Practice parameters for the management of perianal abscess and fistula-in-ano. Dis Colon Rectum. 2011;54(12):1465–74.
14. Garcia-Granero A, Granero-Castro P, Frasson M, Flor-Lorente B, Carreno O, Espi A, et al. Management of cryptoglandular supralevator abscesses in the magnetic resonance imaging era: a case series. Int J Colorectal Dis. 2014;29(12):1557–64.
15. Visscher AP, Felt-Bersma RJ. Endoanal ultrasound in perianal fistulae and abscesses. Ultrasound Q 2015;31(2):130–7.
16. Plaikner M, Loizides A, Peer S, Aigner F, Pecival D, Zbar A, et al. Transperineal ultrasonography as a complementary diagnostic tool in identifying acute perianal sepsis. Tech Coloproctol. 2014;18(2):165–71.
17. Sozener U, Gedik E, Kessaf Aslar A, Ergun H, Halil Elhan A, Memikoglu O, et al. Does adjuvant antibiotic treatment after

drainage of anorectal abscess prevent development of anal fistulas? A randomized, placebo-controlled, double-blind, multicenter study. Dis Colon Rectum. 2011;54(8):923–9.

18. Liu CK, Liu CP, Leung CH, Sun FJ. Clinical and microbiological analysis of adult perianal abscess. J Microbiol Immunol Infect. 2011;44(3):204–8.

19. Zinicola R, Cracco N. Draining an anal abscess: the skeletal muscle rule. Colorectal Dis. 2014;16(7):562.

20. Perera AP, Howell AM, Sodergren MH, Farne H, Darzi A, Purkayastha S, et al. A pilot randomised controlled trial evaluating postoperative packing of the perianal abscess. Langenbecks Arch Surg. 2015;400(2):267–71.

21. Hanley PH, Ray JE, Pennington EE, Grablowsky OM. Fistula-in-ano: a ten-year follow-up study of horseshoe-abscess fistula-in-ano. Dis Colon Rectum. 1976;19(6):507–15.

22. Tan KK, Koh DC, Tsang CB. Managing deep postanal space sepsis via an intersphincteric approach: our early experience. Ann Coloproctol. 2013;29(2):55–9.

23. Malik AI, Nelson RL, Tou S. Incision and drainage of perianal abscess with or without treatment of anal fistula. Cochrane Database Syst Rev. 2010;7:Cd006827.

24. Ramanujam PS, Prasad ML, Abcarian H. The role of seton in fistulotomy of the anus. Surg Gynecol Obstet. 1983;157(5):419–22.

25. Cariati A. Fistulotomy or seton in anal fistula: a decisional algorithm. Updates Surg. 2013;65(3):201–5.

26. Schouten WR, van Vroonhoven TJ. Treatment of anorectal abscess with or without primary fistulectomy. Results of a prospective randomized trial. Dis Colon Rectum. 1991;34(1):60–3.

27. Hamalainen KP, Sainio AP. Incidence of fistulas after drainage of acute anorectal abscesses. Dis Colon Rectum. 1998;41(11):1357–61. discussion 61–2.

28. Rizzo JA, Naig AL, Johnson EK. Anorectal abscess and fistula-in-ano: evidence-based management. Surg Clin North Am. 2010;90(1):45–68. Table of Contents.

29. Paydar S, Izadpanah A, Ghahramani L, Hosseini SV, Bananzadeh A, Rahimikazerooni S, et al. How the anal gland orifice could be found in anal abscess operations. J Res Med Sci. 2015;20(1):22–5.

30. Ho YH, Tan M, Chui CH, Leong A, Eu KW, Seow-Choen F. Randomized controlled trial of primary fistulotomy with drainage alone for perianal abscesses. Dis Colon Rectum. 1997;40(12):1435–8.

31. Quah HM, Tang CL, Eu KW, Chan SY, Samuel M. Meta-analysis of randomized clinical trials comparing drainage alone vs primary sphincter-cutting procedures for anorectal abscess-fistula. Int J Colorectal Dis. 2006;21(6):602–9.

32. Read DR, Abcarian H. A prospective survey of 474 patients with anorectal abscess. Dis Colon Rectum. 1979;22(8):566–8.

33. Ramanujam PS, Prasad ML, Abcarian H, Tan AB. Perianal abscesses and fistulas. A study of 1023 patients. Dis Colon Rectum. 1984;27(9):593–7.

34. Oliver I, Lacueva FJ, Perez Vicente F, Arroyo A, Ferrer R, Cansado P, et al. Randomized clinical trial comparing simple drainage of anorectal abscess with and without fistula track treatment. Int J Colorectal Dis. 2003;18(2):107–10.

35. Toyonaga T, Matsushima M, Sogawa N, Jiang SF, Matsumura N, Shimojima Y, et al. Postoperative urinary retention after surgery for benign anorectal disease: potential risk factors and strategy for prevention. Int J Colorectal Dis. 2006;21(7):676–82.

36. Hamadani A, Haigh PI, Liu IL, Abbas MA. Who is at risk for developing chronic anal fistula or recurrent anal sepsis after initial perianal abscess? Dis Colon Rectum. 2009;52(2):217–21.

37. Yano T, Asano M, Matsuda Y, Kawakami K, Nakai K, Nonaka M. Prognostic factors for recurrence following the initial drainage of an anorectal abscess. Int J Colorectal Dis. 2010;25(12):1495–8.

38. Onaca N, Hirshberg A, Adar R. Early reoperation for perirectal abscess: a preventable complication. Dis Colon Rectum. 2001;44(10):1469–73.

39. Chrabot CM, Prasad ML, Abcarian H. Recurrent anorectal abscesses. Dis Colon Rectum. 1983;26(2):105–8.

40. Buchan R, Grace RH. Anorectal suppuration: the results of treatment and the factors influencing the recurrence rate. Br J Surg. 1973;60(7):537–40.

41. Vasilevsky CA, Gordon PH. The incidence of recurrent abscesses or fistula-in-ano following anorectal suppuration. Dis Colon Rectum. 1984;27(2):126–30.

42. Rosen SA, Colquhoun P, Efron J, Vernava 3rd AM, Nogueras JJ, Wexner SD, et al. Horseshoe abscesses and fistulas: how are we doing? Surg Innov. 2006;13(1):17–21.

43. Iqbal CW, Gasior AC, Snyder CL. Pilonidal disease mimicking fistula-in-ano in a 15-year-old female. Case Rep Surg. 2012;2012:310187.

44. Sorensen MD, Krieger JN, Rivara FP, Broghammer JA, Klein MB, Mack CD, et al. Fournier's gangrene: population based epidemiology and outcomes. J Urol. 2009;181(5):2120–6.

45. Wroblewska M, Kuzaka B, Borkowski T, Kuzaka P, Kawecki D, Radziszewski P. Fournier's gangrene – current concepts. Pol J Microbiol. 2014;63(3):267–73.

46. Anaya DA, Dellinger EP. Necrotizing soft-tissue infection: diagnosis and management. Clin Infect Dis. 2007;44(5):705–10.

47. Yang BL, Lin Q, Chen HJ, Gu YF, Zhu P, Sun XL, et al. Perianal necrotizing fasciitis treated with a loose-seton technique. Colorectal Dis. 2012;14(7):e422–4.

48. Laor E, Palmer LS, Tolia BM, Reid RE, Winter HI. Outcome prediction in patients with Fournier's gangrene. J Urol. 1995;154(1):89–92.

49. Buyukasik Y, Ozcebe OI, Sayinalp N, Haznedaroglu IC, Altundag OO, Ozdemir O, et al. Perianal infections in patients with leukemia: importance of the course of neutrophil count. Dis Colon Rectum. 1998;41(1):81–5.

50. Baker B, Al-Salman M, Daoud F. Management of acute perianal sepsis in neutropenic patients with hematological malignancy. Tech Coloproctol. 2014;18(4):327–33.

51. Schimpff SC, Wiernik PH, Block JB. Rectal abscesses in cancer patients. Lancet. 1972;2(7782):844–7.

52. Musa MB, Katakkar SB, Khaliq A. Anorectal and perianal complications of hematologic malignant neoplasms. Can J Surg. 1975;18(6):579–83.

53. Grewal H, Guillem JG, Quan SH, Enker WE, Cohen AM. Anorectal disease in neutropenic leukemic patients.

Operative vs. nonoperative management. Dis Colon Rectum. 1994;37(11):1095–9.

54. Carlson GW, Ferguson CM, Amerson JR. Perianal infections in acute leukemia. Second place winner: Conrad Jobst Award. Am Surg. 1988;54(12):693–5.

55. Badgwell BD, Chang GJ, Rodriguez-Bigas MA, Smith K, Lupo PJ, Frankowski RF, et al. Management and outcomes of anorectal infection in the cancer patient. Ann Surg Oncol. 2009;16(10):2752–8.

56. Blumetti J, Abcarian A, Quinteros F, Chaudhry V, Prasad L, Abcarian H. Evolution of treatment of fistula in ano. World J Surg. 2012;36(5):1162–7.

57. Zanotti C, Martinez-Puente C, Pascual I, Pascual M, Herreros D, Garcia-Olmo D. An assessment of the incidence of fistula-in-ano in four countries of the European Union. Int J Colorectal Dis. 2007;22(12):1459–62.

58. Lockhart-Mummery JP. Discussion of fistula in ano. Proc R Soc Med. 1929;22(9):1331–58.

59. Kratzer GL, Dockerty MB. Histopathology of the anal ducts. Surg Gynecol Obstet. 1947;84(3):333–8.

60. Scoma JA, Salvati EP, Rubin RJ. Incidence of fistulas subsequent to anal abscesses. Dis Colon Rectum. 1974;17(3):357–9.

61. Wang D, Yang G, Qiu J, Song Y, Wang L, Gao J, et al. Risk factors for anal fistula: a case-control study. Tech Coloproctol. 2014;18(7):635–9.

62. Milligan ET, Morgan CN. Surgical anatomy of the anal canal. Lancet. 1934;2:1213.

63. Parks AG, Gordon PH, Hardcastle JD. A classification of fistula-in-ano. Br J Surg. 1976;63(1):1–12.

64. Sileri P, Cadeddu F, D'Ugo S, Franceschilli L, Del Vecchio Blanco G, De Luca E, et al. Surgery for fistula-in-ano in a specialist colorectal unit: a critical appraisal. BMC Gastroenterol. 2011;11:120.

65. Ozkavukcu E, Haliloglu N, Erden A. Frequencies of perianal fistula types using two classification systems. Jpn J Radiol. 2011;29(5):293–300.

66. van Onkelen RS, Gosselink MP, van Rosmalen J, Thijsse S, Schouten WR. Different characteristics of high and low transsphincteric fistulae. Colorectal Dis. 2014;16(6):471–5.

67. Goodsall D. Diseases of the anus and rectum. London: Longman, Green; 1900. 271 p.

68. Cirocco WC, Reilly JC. Challenging the predictive accuracy of Goodsall's rule for anal fistulas. Dis Colon Rectum. 1992;35(6):537–42.

69. Gunawardhana PA, Deen KI. Comparison of hydrogen peroxide instillation with Goodsall's rule for fistula-in-ano. ANZ J Surg. 2001;71(8):472–4.

70. Barwood N, Clarke G, Levitt S, Levitt M. Fistula-in-ano: a prospective study of 107 patients. Aust N Z J Surg. 1997;67(2–3):98–102.

71. Gonzalez-Ruiz C, Kaiser AM, Vukasin P, Beart Jr RW, Ortega AE. Intraoperative physical diagnosis in the management of anal fistula. Am Surg. 2006;72(1):11–5.

72. Liang C, Jiang W, Zhao B, Zhang Y, Du Y, Lu Y. CT imaging with fistulography for perianal fistula: does it really help the surgeon? Clin Imaging. 2013;37(6):1069–76.

73. Weisman RI, Orsay CP, Pearl RK, Abcarian H. The role of fistulography in fistula-in-ano. Report of five cases. Dis Colon Rectum. 1991;34(2):181–4.

74. Kuijpers HC, Schulpen T. Fistulography for fistula-in-ano. Is it useful? Dis Colon Rectum. 1985;28(2):103–4.

75. Pomerri F, Dodi G, Pintacuda G, Amadio L, Muzzio PC. Anal endosonography and fistulography for fistula-in-ano. Radiol Med. 2010;115(5):771–83.

76. Chew SS, Yang JL, Newstead GL, Douglas PR. Anal fistula: Levovist-enhanced endoanal ultrasound: a pilot study. Dis Colon Rectum. 2003;46(3):377–84.

77. Buchanan GN, Bartram CI, Williams AB, Halligan S, Cohen CR. Value of hydrogen peroxide enhancement of three-dimensional endoanal ultrasound in fistula-in-ano. Dis Colon Rectum. 2005;48(1):141–7.

78. Nagendranath C, Saravanan MN, Sridhar C, Varughese M. Peroxide-enhanced endoanal ultrasound in preoperative assessment of complex fistula-in-ano. Tech Coloproctol. 2014;18(5):433–8.

79. Siddiqui MR, Ashrafian H, Tozer P, Daulatzai N, Burling D, Hart A, et al. A diagnostic accuracy meta-analysis of endoanal ultrasound and MRI for perianal fistula assessment. Dis Colon Rectum. 2012;55(5):576–85.

80. Subasinghe D, Samarasekera DN. Comparison of preoperative endoanal ultrasonography with intraoperative findings for fistula in ano. World J Surg. 2010;34(5):1123–7.

81. Choen S, Burnett S, Bartram CI, Nicholls RJ. Comparison between anal endosonography and digital examination in the evaluation of anal fistulae. Br J Surg. 1991;78(4):445–7.

82. Buchanan GN, Halligan S, Bartram CI, Williams AB, Tarroni D, Cohen CR. Clinical examination, endosonography, and MR imaging in preoperative assessment of fistula in ano: comparison with outcome-based reference standard. Radiology. 2004;233(3):674–81.

83. Toyonaga T, Tanaka Y, Song JF, Katori R, Sogawa N, Kanyama H, et al. Comparison of accuracy of physical examination and endoanal ultrasonography for preoperative assessment in patients with acute and chronic anal fistula. Tech Coloproctol. 2008;12(3):217–23.

84. Weisman N, Abbas MA. Prognostic value of endoanal ultrasound for fistula-in-ano: a retrospective analysis. Dis Colon Rectum. 2008;51(7):1089–92.

85. Benjelloun EB, Souiki T, El Abkari M. Endoanal ultrasound in anal fistulas. Is there any influence on postoperative outcome? Tech Coloproctol. 2014;18(4):405–6.

86. Nevler A, Beer-Gabel M, Lebedyev A, Soffer A, Gutman M, Carter D, et al. Transperineal ultrasonography in perianal Crohn's disease and recurrent cryptogenic fistula-in-ano. Colorectal Dis. 2013;15(8):1011–8.

87. Halligan S, Bartram CI. MR imaging of fistula in ano: are endoanal coils the gold standard? Am J Roentgenol. 1998;171(2):407–12.

88. Chang KJ, Kamel IR, Macura KJ, Bluemke DA. 3.0-T MR imaging of the abdomen: comparison with 1.5 T. RadioGraphics. 2008;28(7):1983–98.

89. Schaefer O, Oeksuez MO, Lohrmann C, Langer M. Differentiation of anal sphincters with high-resolution magnetic resonance imaging using contrast-enhanced fast low-angle shot 3-dimensional sequences. J Comput Assist Tomogr. 2004;28(2):174–9.

90. Lunniss PJ, Armstrong P, Barker PG, Reznek RH, Phillips RK. Magnetic resonance imaging of anal fistulae. Lancet. 1992;340(8816):394–6.

91. Lunniss PJ, Barker PG, Sultan AH, Armstrong P, Reznek RH, Bartram CI, et al. Magnetic resonance imaging of fistula-in-ano. Dis Colon Rectum. 1994;37(7):708–18.

92. Beckingham IJ, Spencer JA, Ward J, Dyke GW, Adams C, Ambrose NS. Prospective evaluation of dynamic contrast enhanced magnetic resonance imaging in the evaluation of fistula in ano. Br J Surg. 1996;83(10):1396–8.

93. Beets-Tan RG, Beets GL, van der Hoop AG, Kessels AG, Vliegen RF, Baeten CG, et al. Preoperative MR imaging of anal fistulas: does it really help the surgeon? Radiology. 2001;218(1):75–84.

94. Buchanan G, Halligan S, Williams A, Cohen CR, Tarroni D, Phillips RK, et al. Effect of MRI on clinical outcome of recurrent fistula-in-ano. Lancet. 2002;360(9346):1661–2.

95. Sahni VA, Ahmad R, Burling D. Which method is best for imaging of perianal fistula? Abdom Imaging. 2008;33(1):26–30.

96. Ellis CN. Sphincter-preserving fistula management: what patients want. Dis Colon Rectum. 2010;53(12):1652–5.

97. Gottgens KW, Smeets RR, Stassen LP, Beets G, Breukink SO. Systematic review and meta-analysis of surgical interventions for high cryptoglandular perianal fistula. Int J Colorectal Dis. 2015;30(5):583–93. doi:10.1007/s00384-014-2091-8. Epub 2014 Dec 10. Review. PubMed PMID: 25487858.

98. Jain BK, Vaibhaw K, Garg PK, Gupta S, Mohanty D. Comparison of a fistulectomy and a fistulotomy with marsupialization in the management of a simple anal fistula: a randomized, controlled pilot trial. J Korean Soc Coloproctol. 2012;28(2):78–82.

99. Ho YH, Tan M, Leong AF, Seow-Choen F. Marsupialization of fistulotomy wounds improves healing: a randomized controlled trial. Br J Surg. 1998;85(1):105–7.

100. Pescatori M, Ayabaca SM, Cafaro D, Iannello A, Magrini S. Marsupialization of fistulotomy and fistulectomy wounds improves healing and decreases bleeding: a randomized controlled trial. Colorectal Dis. 2006;8(1):11–4.

101. Garcia-Aguilar J, Belmonte C, Wong WD, Goldberg SM, Madoff RD. Anal fistula surgery. Factors associated with recurrence and incontinence. Dis Colon Rectum. 1996;39(7):723–9.

102. Visscher AP, Schuur D, Roos R, Van der Mijnsbrugge GJ, Meijerink WJ, Felt-Bersma RJ. Long-term follow-up after surgery for simple and complex cryptoglandular fistulas: fecal incontinence and impact on quality of life. Dis Colon Rectum. 2015;58(5):533–9.

103. Durgun V, Perek A, Kapan M, Kapan S, Perek S. Partial fistulotomy and modified cutting seton procedure in the treatment of high extrasphincteric perianal fistulae. Dig Surg. 2002;19(1):56–8.

104. Awad ML, Sell HW, Stahlfeld KR. Split-shot sinker facilitates seton treatment of anal fistulae. Colorectal Dis. 2009;11(5):524–6.

105. Isbister WH, Al Sanea N. The cutting seton: an experience at King Faisal Specialist Hospital. Dis Colon Rectum. 2001;44(5):722–7.

106. Hamalainen KP, Sainio AP. Cutting seton for anal fistulas: high risk of minor control defects. Dis Colon Rectum. 1997;40(12):1443–6. discussion 7.

107. Vial M, Pares D, Pera M, Grande L. Faecal incontinence after seton treatment for anal fistulae with and without surgical division of internal anal sphincter: a systematic review. Colorectal Dis. 2010;12(3):172–8.

108. Ritchie RD, Sackier JM, Hodde JP. Incontinence rates after cutting seton treatment for anal fistula. Colorectal Dis. 2009;11(6):564–71.

109. Chuang-Wei C, Chang-Chieh W, Cheng-Wen H, Tsai-Yu L, Chun-Che F, Shu-Wen J. Cutting seton for complex anal fistulas. Surgeon. 2008;6(3):185–8.

110. Pearl RK, Andrews JR, Orsay CP, Weisman RI, Prasad ML, Nelson RL, et al. Role of the seton in the management of anorectal fistulas. Dis Colon Rectum. 1993;36(6):573–7. discussion 7–9.

111. Kodner IJ, Mazor A, Shemesh EI, Fry RD, Fleshman JW, Birnbaum EH. Endorectal advancement flap repair of rectovaginal and other complicated anorectal fistulas. Surgery. 1993;114(4):682–9. discussion 9-90.

112. Jones IT, Fazio VW, Jagelman DG. The use of transanal rectal advancement flaps in the management of fistulas involving the anorectum. Dis Colon Rectum. 1987;30(12):919–23.

113. Uribe N, Millan M, Minguez M, Ballester C, Asencio F, Sanchiz V, et al. Clinical and manometric results of endorectal advancement flaps for complex anal fistula. Int J Colorectal Dis. 2007;22(3):259–64.

114. Jarrar A, Church J. Advancement flap repair: a good option for complex anorectal fistulas. Dis Colon Rectum. 2011;54(12):1537–41.

115. Hall JF, Bordeianou L, Hyman N, Read T, Bartus C, Schoetz D, et al. Outcomes after operations for anal fistula: results of a prospective, multicenter, regional study. Dis Colon Rectum. 2014;57(11):1304–8.

116. Uribe N, Balciscueta Z, Minguez M, Martin MC, Lopez M, Mora F, et al. "Core out" or "curettage" in rectal advancement flap for cryptoglandular anal fistula. Int J Colorectal Dis. 2015;30(5):613–9.

117. Lee CL, Lu J, Lim TZ, Koh FH, Lieske B, Cheong WK, et al. Long-term outcome following advancement flaps for high anal fistulas in an Asian population: a single institution's experience. Int J Colorectal Dis. 2015;30(3):409–12.

118. Mitalas LE, Gosselink MP, Oom DM, Zimmerman DD, Schouten WR. Required length of follow-up after transanal advancement flap repair of high transsphincteric fistulas. Colorectal Dis. 2009;11(7):726–8.

119. van Koperen PJ, Wind J, Bemelman WA, Bakx R, Reitsma JB, Slors JF. Long-term functional outcome and risk factors for recurrence after surgical treatment for low and high perianal fistulas of cryptoglandular origin. Dis Colon Rectum. 2008;51(10):1475–81.

120. Ortiz H, Marzo M, de Miguel M, Ciga MA, Oteiza F, Armendariz P. Length of follow-up after fistulotomy and fistulectomy associated with endorectal advancement flap repair for fistula in ano. Br J Surg. 2008;95(4):484–7.

121. van Onkelen RS, Gosselink MP, Thijsse S, Schouten WR. Predictors of outcome after transanal advancement flap repair for high transsphincteric fistulas. Dis Colon Rectum. 2014;57(8):1007–11.

122. Mitalas LE, Dwarkasing RS, Verhaaren R, Zimmerman DD, Schouten WR. Is the outcome of transanal advancement flap repair affected by the complexity of high transsphincteric fistulas? Dis Colon Rectum. 2011;54(7):857–62.

123. Mitalas LE, van Wijk JJ, Gosselink MP, Doornebosch P, Zimmerman DD, Schouten WR. Seton drainage prior to transanal

advancement flap repair: useful or not? Int J Colorectal Dis. 2010;25(12):1499–502.

124. Stremitzer S, Riss S, Swoboda P, Dauser B, Dubsky P, Birsan T, et al. Repeat endorectal advancement flap after flap breakdown and recurrence of fistula-in-ano – is it an option? Colorectal Dis. 2012;14(11):1389–93.

125. Mitalas LE, Gosselink MP, Zimmerman DD, Schouten WR. Repeat transanal advancement flap repair: impact on the overall healing rate of high transsphincteric fistulas and on fecal continence. Dis Colon Rectum. 2007;50(10):1508–11.

126. Schouten WR, Zimmerman DD, Briel JW. Transanal advancement flap repair of transsphincteric fistulas. Dis Colon Rectum. 1999;42(11):1419–22. discussion 22–3.

127. Ozuner G, Hull TL, Cartmill J, Fazio VW. Long-term analysis of the use of transanal rectal advancement flaps for complicated anorectal/vaginal fistulas. Dis Colon Rectum. 1996;39(1):10–4.

128. Jacob TJ, Perakath B, Keighley MR. Surgical intervention for anorectal fistula. Cochrane Database of Syst Rev. 2010;5: CD006319.

129. Gottgens KW, Vening W, van der Hagen SJ, van Gemert WG, Smeets RR, Stassen LP, et al. Long-term results of mucosal advancement flap combined with platelet-rich plasma for high cryptoglandular perianal fistulas. Dis Colon Rectum. 2014;57(2):223–7.

130. Nessim A, Wexner SD, Agachan F, Alabaz O, Weiss EG, Nogueras JJ, et al. Is bowel confinement necessary after anorectal reconstructive surgery? A prospective, randomized, surgeon-blinded trial. Dis Colon Rectum. 1999;42(1):16–23.

131. Khafagy W, Omar W, El Nakeeb A, Fouda E, Yousef M, Farid M. Treatment of anal fistulas by partial rectal wall advancement flap or mucosal advancement flap: a prospective randomized study. Int J Surg. 2010;8(4):321–5.

132. Dubsky PC, Stift A, Friedl J, Teleky B, Herbst F. Endorectal advancement flaps in the treatment of high anal fistula of cryptoglandular origin: full-thickness vs. mucosal-rectum flaps. Dis Colon Rectum. 2008;51(6):852–7.

133. Zimmerman DD, Gosselink MP, Mitalas LE, Delemarre JB, Hop WJ, Briel JW, et al. Smoking impairs rectal mucosal blood flow – a pilot study: possible implications for transanal advancement flap repair. Dis Colon Rectum. 2005;48(6):1228–32.

134. Ellis CN, Clark S. Effect of tobacco smoking on advancement flap repair of complex anal fistulas. Dis Colon Rectum. 2007;50(4):459–63.

135. Schwandner O. Obesity is a negative predictor of success after surgery for complex anal fistula. BMC Gastroenterol. 2011; 11:61.

136. Mizrahi N, Wexner SD, Zmora O, Da Silva G, Efron J, Weiss EG, et al. Endorectal advancement flap: are there predictors of failure? Dis Colon Rectum. 2002;45(12):1616–21.

137. Rojanasakul A, Pattanaarun J, Sahakitrungruang C, Tantiphlachiva K. Total anal sphincter saving technique for fistula-in-ano; the ligation of intersphincteric fistula tract. J Med Assoc Thai. 2007;90(3):581–6.

138. Ye F, Tang C, Wang D, Zheng S. Early experience with the modificated approach of ligation of the intersphincteric fistula tract for high transsphincteric fistula. World J Surg. 2015; 39(4):1059–65.

139. Madbouly KM, El Shazly W, Abbas KS, Hussein AM. Ligation of intersphincteric fistula tract versus mucosal advancement flap in patients with high transsphincteric fistula-in-ano: a prospective randomized trial. Dis Colon Rectum. 2014;57(10): 1202–8.

140. Bastawrous A, Hawkins M, Kratz R, Menon R, Pollock D, Charbel J, et al. Results from a novel modification to the ligation intersphincteric fistula tract. Am J Surg. 2015; 209(5):793–8.

141. Tan KK, Lee PJ. Early experience of reinforcing the ligation of the intersphincteric fistula tract procedure with a bioprosthetic graft (BioLIFT) for anal fistula. ANZ J Surg. 2014;84(4): 280–3.

142. Han JG, Yi BQ, Wang ZJ, Zheng Y, Cui JJ, Yu XQ, et al. Ligation of the intersphincteric fistula tract plus a bioprosthetic anal fistula plug (LIFT-Plug): a new technique for fistula-in-ano. Colorectal Dis. 2013;15(5):582–6.

143. Ellis CN. Outcomes with the use of bioprosthetic grafts to reinforce the ligation of the intersphincteric fistula tract (BioLIFT procedure) for the management of complex anal fistulas. Dis Colon Rectum. 2010;53(10):1361–4.

144. Abcarian AM, Estrada JJ, Park J, Corning C, Chaudhry V, Cintron J, et al. Ligation of intersphincteric fistula tract: early results of a pilot study. Dis Colon Rectum. 2012; 55(7):778–82.

145. Campbell ML, Abboud EC, Dolberg ME, Sanchez JE, Marcet JE, Rasheid SH. Treatment of refractory perianal fistulas with ligation of the intersphincteric fistula tract: preliminary results. Am Surg. 2013;79(7):723–7.

146. Vergara-Fernandez O, Espino-Urbina LA. Ligation of intersphincteric fistula tract: what is the evidence in a review? World J Gastroenterol. 2013;19(40):6805–13.

147. Hong KD, Kang S, Kalaskar S, Wexner SD. Ligation of intersphincteric fistula tract (LIFT) to treat anal fistula: systematic review and meta-analysis. Tech Coloproctol. 2014;18(8): 685–91.

148. Yassin NA, Hammond TM, Lunniss PJ, Phillips RK. Ligation of the intersphincteric fistula tract in the management of anal fistula. A systematic review. Colorectal Dis. 2013;15(5):527–35.

149. Tan KK, Tan IJ, Lim FS, Koh DC, Tsang CB. The anatomy of failures following the ligation of intersphincteric tract technique for anal fistula: a review of 93 patients over 4 years. Dis Colon Rectum. 2011;54(11):1368–72.

150. van Onkelen RS, Gosselink MP, Schouten WR. Ligation of the intersphincteric fistula tract in low transsphincteric fistulae: a new technique to avoid fistulotomy. Colorectal Dis. 2013; 15(5):587–91.

151. van Onkelen RS, Gosselink MP, Schouten WR. Is it possible to improve the outcome of transanal advancement flap repair for high transsphincteric fistulas by additional ligation of the intersphincteric fistula tract? Dis Colon Rectum. 2012;55(2): 163–6.

152. Hjortrup A, Moesgaard F, Kjaergard J. Fibrin adhesive in the treatment of perineal fistulas. Dis Colon Rectum. 1991;34(9): 752–4.

153. Hammond TM, Grahn MF, Lunniss PJ. Fibrin glue in the management of anal fistulae. Colorectal Dis. 2004;6(5):308–19.

154. Singer M, Cintron J, Nelson R, Orsay C, Bastawrous A, Pearl R, et al. Treatment of fistulas-in-ano with fibrin sealant in combination with intra-adhesive antibiotics and/or surgical closure of the internal fistula opening. Dis Colon Rectum. 2005;48(4):799–808.

155. de Parades V, Far HS, Etienney I, Zeitoun JD, Atienza P, Bauer P. Seton drainage and fibrin glue injection for complex anal fistulas. Colorectal Dis. 2010;12(5):459–63.

156. Cintron JR, Park JJ, Orsay CP, Pearl RK, Nelson RL, Sone JH, et al. Repair of fistulas-in-ano using fibrin adhesive: long-term follow-up. Dis Colon Rectum. 2000;43(7):944–9. discussion 9–50.

157. Swinscoe MT, Ventakasubramaniam AK, Jayne DG. Fibrin glue for fistula-in-ano: the evidence reviewed. Tech Coloproctol. 2005;9(2):89–94.

158. Haim N, Neufeld D, Ziv Y, Tulchinsky H, Koller M, Khaikin M, et al. Long-term results of fibrin glue treatment for cryptogenic perianal fistulas: a multicenter study. Dis Colon Rectum. 2011;54(10):1279–83.

159. Johnson EK, Gaw JU, Armstrong DN. Efficacy of anal fistula plug vs. fibrin glue in closure of anorectal fistulas. Dis Colon Rectum. 2006;49(3):371–6.

160. Cintron JR, Abcarian H, Chaudhry V, Singer M, Hunt S, Birnbaum E, et al. Treatment of fistula-in-ano using a porcine small intestinal submucosa anal fistula plug. Tech Coloproctol. 2013;17(2):187–91.

161. McGee MF, Champagne BJ, Stulberg JJ, Reynolds H, Marderstein E, Delaney CP. Tract length predicts successful closure with anal fistula plug in cryptoglandular fistulas. Dis Colon Rectum. 2010;53(8):1116–20.

162. O'Riordan JM, Datta I, Johnston C, Baxter NN. A systematic review of the anal fistula plug for patients with Crohn's and non-Crohn's related fistula-in-ano. Dis Colon Rectum. 2012; 55(3):351–8.

163. Stamos MJ, Snyder M, Robb BW, Ky A, Singer M, Stewart DB, et al. Prospective multicenter study of a synthetic bioabsorbable anal fistula plug to treat cryptoglandular transsphincteric anal fistulas. Dis Colon Rectum. 2015;58(3): 344–51.

164. Wilhelm A. A new technique for sphincter-preserving anal fistula repair using a novel radial emitting laser probe. Tech Coloproctol. 2011;15(4):445–9.

165. Giamundo P, Esercizio L, Geraci M, Tibaldi L, Valente M. Fistula-tract laser closure (FiLaC): long-term results and new operative strategies. Tech Coloproctol. 2015;19(8):449–53.

166. Garcia-Olmo D, Herreros D, Pascual I, Pascual JA, Del-Valle E, Zorrilla J, et al. Expanded adipose-derived stem cells for the treatment of complex perianal fistula: a phase II clinical trial. Dis Colon Rectum. 2009;52(1):79–86.

167. Sileri P, Boehm G, Franceschilli L, Giorgi F, Perrone F, Stolfi C, et al. Collagen matrix injection combined with flap repair for complex anal fistula. Colorectal Dis. 2012;14 Suppl 3:24–8.

168. Vasilevsky CA. Anorectal abscess and fistula-in ano. In: Beck DE, editor. Handbook of colorectal surgery. St Louis, Mo: Quality Medical Publishing; 1997.

169. Vasilevsky CA. Fistula-in-Ano and Abscess. In: Beck DE, Wexner SD, editors. Fundamentals of anorectal surgery. London: WB Saunders; 1998.

15

Complex Anorectal Fistulas

Giulio A. Santoro and Maher A. Abbas

Key Concepts

- The history and physical examination are the mandatory first step, providing in most cases the appropriate information to classify a fistula as "simple" or "complex." Anal continence should be evaluated using a validated incontinence score such as the Cleveland Clinic Florida Incontinence Score (CCF-IS) grading system.
- *Imaging procedures include (in order of authors' preference)* two- and three-dimensional endoanal ultrasound (2D/3D EAUS), pelvic magnetic resonance imaging (MRI), computed tomography (CT), and fistulography. Imaging can provide invaluable information on the anatomy of the fistula, including the primary track, internal opening, horseshoe extension, secondary cavities or extensions, and associated sphincter lesions and is a useful guide in surgical management.
- Complex anal fistula is challenging to treat due to the risk of postoperative anal incontinence and the high rate of recurrence. Three factors determine the outcome of surgical treatment: patient-related factors, fistula characteristics, and the surgeon's choice of operation inclusive of its technical conduct.
- Each surgical procedure has advantages and disadvantages, and the choice of operative intervention should be individualized based on patient-related factors and fistula characteristics taking into account success rate as well as impact on patient anal continence.
- Rectourethral fistula is often the result of prostate cancer treatment whether surgical or radiotherapy based. A multidisciplinary approach involving a urologist and a colorectal surgeon is essential. Small distal fistulas and those not radiation induced can be amenable to a local anal repair such as an endorectal advancement flap.

Large fistulas, those induced by radiation, or persistent/recurrent fistulas are best approached by a transperineal approach with a gracilis interposition flap or in select cases by a transabdominal approach with rectal excision. Due to its rarity, rectourethral fistula is best managed in tertiary or quaternary centers with experience managing this condition.

- Ileal-pouch fistula is uncommon and can be extremely challenging to manage due to the morbidity associated with any intervention, failure rate of various surgical options, and long-term consequences to the patient. Simple procedures should be attempted first before more complex procedures are considered. Due to the low incidence of this condition, few centers worldwide have accumulated enough experience with ileal-pouch fistula management. Early referral to such centers is advisable.

Introduction

According to the standards practice task force of the American Society of Colon and Rectal Surgeons (ASCRS), an anal fistula may be termed "complex" when one or more of the following findings are present: the tract crosses more than 30 % of the external anal sphincter (high transsphincteric with or without a high blind tract, suprasphincteric, and extrasphincteric), horseshoe configuration, anterior location in a female, multiple tracts, recurrent, Crohn's disease, prior radiotherapy, or baseline incontinence [1]. In addition, anorectal fistulas with the following anatomical configurations and etiologies are considered complex: rectovaginal fistula, rectourethral fistula, anastomotic fistula following colorectal surgery, posttraumatic fistula, and malignant fistula. In this chapter, the definition, classification, pathophysiology, clinical assessment, diagnostic evaluation, surgical treatment, and outcome of complex anorectal fistula are described. The reader is provided with a comprehensive approach to the management of patients with complex anorectal fistula

Electronic supplementary material: The online version of this chapter (doi:10.1007/978-3-319-25970-3_15) contains supplementary material, which is available to authorized users.

taking into consideration the various factors that influence outcome. Rectovaginal fistula and Crohn's-related fistula are not covered in this chapter but dealt with in other parts of this textbook.

Complex or Recurrent Cryptoglandular Fistulas

Definition, Classification, and Pathophysiology

An anal fistula may be termed "complex" when the tract crosses more than 30 % of the external anal sphincter (high transsphincteric with or without a high blind tract, suprasphincteric, and extrasphincteric), is horseshoe, is anterior based in a female, has multiple tracts, and is recurrent or the patient has preexisting incontinence [1]. The aim of anal fistula treatment is to eradicate the fistulous tract, prevent recurrence, minimize postoperative septic complications, and minimally impact anal continence. The selection of a surgical technique that is both safe and effective can be challenging. Sphincter-preserving operations such as injectable glues or plugs are associated with low risk of incontinence but high rate of persistent or recurrent disease [2]. Non-sphincter-preserving operations such as fistulotomy or fistulectomy have high success rate but can be associated with stool incontinence in some patients. Knowledge of the results of various surgical techniques coupled with good surgical judgment is essential when deciding on a surgical option for a patient.

Clinical Assessment and Diagnostic Evaluation

According to the standards practice task force of the ASCRS, a disease-specific history (demographic characteristics, smoking behavior, previous anorectal surgery, symptoms) and physical examination (inspection, palpation, digital rectal examination, careful probing, anoscopy, and/or rigid proctoscopy) is the mandatory first step, providing in most cases the appropriate information to consider a fistula "simple" or "complex" (strong recommendation based on low-quality evidence: 1C) [1]. The history should include the type of prior anal operations, obstetrical history in females, the presence of gastrointestinal disorders such as inflammatory bowel disease, medical comorbidities such as diabetes, prior radiation therapy to the pelvis, and current smoking status. Inquiry about the patient's bowel habits can provide useful information to guide postoperative care. Anal continence should always be assessed using a validated score such as the Cleveland Clinic Florida Fecal Incontinence Score (CCF-FIS) grading system (Figure 15-1) [3]. The scale reports the various types of incontinence (gas, liquid, solid), pad usage, impact of the incontinence on patient's lifestyle, and frequency of occurrence. A score of 0 corresponds to full

Type of incontinence	Never	Rarely <1/month	Sometimes <1/week >1/month	Usually <1/day >1/week	Always >1/day
Solid	0	1	2	3	4
Liquid	0	1	2	3	4
Gas	0	1	2	3	4
Wears Pad	0	1	2	3	4
Lifestyle Alteration	0	1	2	3	4

FIGURE 15-1. Cleveland Clinic Florida Fecal Incontinence Score (CCF-FIS). 0 = complete continence; 20 = complete incontinence [3].

continence, whereas a score of 20 is indicative of daily incontinence to gas, liquid, and solid. Physical examination can be helpful in delineating the fistula anatomy and reaches a very good accuracy in identifying superficial (100 %) and transsphincteric (100 %) tracts, but it appears inadequate for supralevator (63.6 %) and intersphincteric (33.3 %) tracts [4–6]. Deen and colleagues were able to identify only 50 % of the internal openings and 27.3 % of the horseshoe extensions [4]. Similarly, Poen and colleagues reported a correct diagnosis of primary tracts in only 38 % of patients, with 62 % of patients being unclassified [5]. The limitation of physical examination alone has been highlighted by others with an overall accuracy of 65.4 % for preoperative identification of the primary tract [6]. The additional challenges encountered included inability to identify suprasphincteric or extrasphincteric fistulas, to determine the internal opening, and to delineate ischioanal, pelvirectal, and horseshoe secondary extensions [6].

Considering the limitation of physical examination, the standard practice task force of the ASCRS recommends (strong recommendation based on low-quality evidence: 1C) *performing* imaging procedures (two- and three-dimensional endoanal ultrasound (2D and 3D EAUS), pelvic MRI, and fistulography) for an accurate preoperative classification of the primary tract and its extensions [1]. These assessments can provide information on the anatomy of the fistula, including the primary tract, internal opening, horseshoe extension, secondary cavities or extensions, and associated sphincter lesions [7, 8]. On 2D/3D EAUS, the fistulous tract appears as a hypoechoic structure and can be traced in relationship to the internal and external sphincter muscles (Figure 15-2). Hydrogen peroxide enhancement of the tract can confirm its course as it traverses the anal sphincter complex and can provide accurate classification (Figure 15-3). Similarly, MRI can provide invaluable information to define the exact anatomy of a complex fistula (Figure 15-4). Clear delineation of the fistula anatomy to guide operative intervention can be helpful for surgical planning and may impact surgical outcome [9, 10]. In a large study of patients with recurrent anal

FIGURE 15-2. Recurrent low transsphincteric anal fistula secondary to cryptoglandular disease [3D endoanal ultrasound].

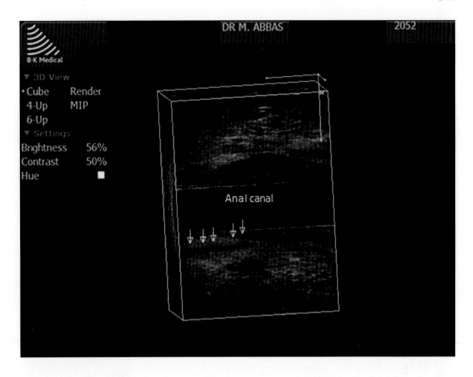

FIGURE 15-3. Persistent high transsphincteric anal fistula secondary to cryptoglandular disease [3D endoanal ultrasound].

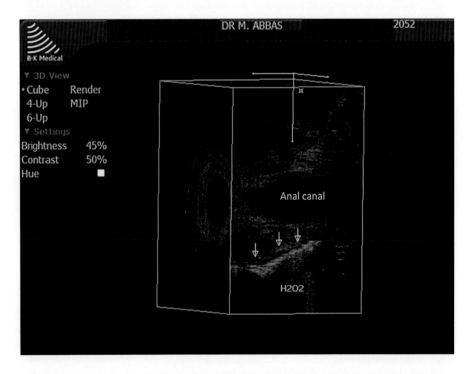

fistulas, the postoperative recurrence rate was low (16 %) when surgeons always guided the patient's treatment based on the MRI findings. However, the recurrence rate rose to 30 % when the surgeons occasionally acted based on the MRI findings and 57 % when the MRI findings were ignored [10]. A variety of investigators have directly compared EAUS (2D/3D both with and without hydrogen peroxide injection through the external opening) with MRI (external phased array/endoanal coil), and these comparisons have found EAUS variously superior [11], equivalent [12–15], or inferior [16]. The difficulty in comparing these modalities is related to the ability to define a true reference standard for fistula-in-ano due to the following potential sources of bias: the operators who perform the assessments can have differing levels of experience with EAUS or with MRI and, similarly, the surgeons who perform the operations have different

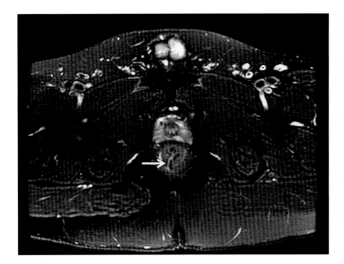

FIGURE 15-4. Suprasphincteric anal fistula secondary to anal trauma [magnetic resonance imaging]. White arrow points to fistula tract.

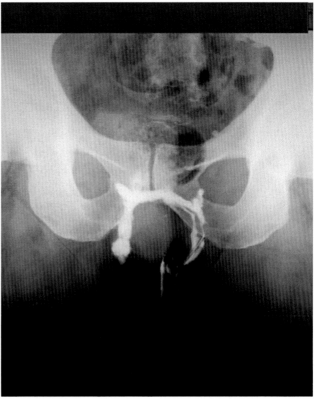

FIGURE 15-5. Fistulogram demonstrating a horseshoe fistula.

levels of experience. For this reason, Buchanan and colleagues proposed the "outcome-derived" reference standard [13]. If there is disagreement between findings at EAUS, MRI, and surgical examination, the findings associated with fistula healing should be assumed to be correct. Sahni and colleagues assessed the optimal technique for fistula classification using an "evidence-based medicine" method [17]. MRI was found to be more sensitive (0.97) than clinical examination (0.75) but comparable to EAUS (0.92) for discriminating between complex and simple fistula. MRI and EAUS can provide complementary information in some cases. However, our preference is to perform EAUS as the initial diagnostic test when available as it is a simpler and less costly modality compared to MRI. In centers where EAUS and MRI expertise is not readily available, fistulography can be performed to delineate tract configurations such as horseshoe fistula, high blind limb extension, or secondary branches (Figure 15-5). However, conventional fistulography is limited in its assessment of muscle involvement by the fistula tract. Computed tomography can be a useful imaging adjunct in select situations to identify recurrent abscesses secondary to complex fistula (Figure 15-6). Under such circumstances, computed tomography can guide drainage procedures to deal with acute sepsis, but in general it is not useful in elective surgical planning geared towards chronic fistula eradication.

In addition to imaging, baseline assessment of sphincter function with anorectal manometry can be helpful in select patients, such as multiparous females or in patients with prior anorectal surgeries [18, 19]. There are two different manometry systems including the low-compliance water perfusion system and the 3D high-resolution anorectal manometry. The low-compliance water perfusion system is equipped with six fluid-filled lumen and radially arranged ports throughout the cross section (Figure 15-7a, b). The pressure is recorded by pressure transducers that are

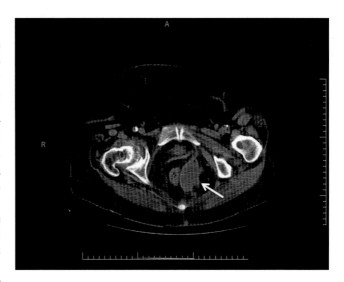

FIGURE 15-6. Computed tomography scan highlights recurrent supralevator abscess with fistula. *White arrow* demonstrates the abscess cavity on the patient's left.

located within each infusion line and are connected to a chart recorder. The 3D high-resolution anorectal manometry can simultaneously provide physiological and topographical data. The registration should include the maximum resting pressure and the maximum squeeze pressure [19].

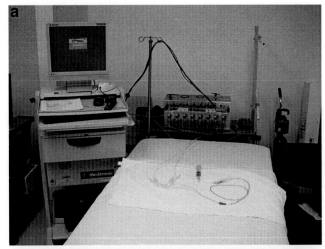

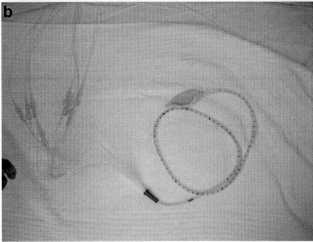

FIGURE 15-7. (**a**) Low-compliance water perfusion anorectal manometry system. (**b**) Anorectal manometry catheter.

Surgical Treatment

Surgical treatment of complex anal fistula involving a significant portion of the muscle can pose significant challenges to the surgeon and have long-term impact on the patient's well-being. The goal to eradicate the fistula should be balanced with the aim to preserve as much of the sphincter integrity to avoid impairment of continence. Similarly, in the case of recurrent fistulas, local structural alterations of the anal canal such as fibrosis or disruption of anal sphincter are often observed. Under such circumstances, surgical options may be limited because of the high risk of incontinence. Sound surgical judgment and familiarity with the outcome data of various operations is of paramount importance in order to pick the appropriate option from a modern armamentarium of surgical interventions [20]. Figure 15-8 provides a comprehensive carepath for a structured approach to guide the care of patients with anorectal fistula. It is based on our extensive experience with treating anorectal fistulas of various etiologies and complexity.

Seton

Seton is an important treatment option that can provide temporary control of fistula symptoms or can serve as a definitive intervention to control or eradicate a chronic fistula. A variety of materials have been used in the placement of setons including suture material (Ethibond, silk, nylon, polypropylene: suture size #2.0 to #2, depending on the tract width), vascular vessel loop, Penrose drain, rubber band, and chemically impregnated material [21]. A draining seton is tied loosely around a fistulous tract to promote drainage, to minimize acute abscess formation, and to allow for scarring of the fistulous tract. While a draining seton can be used as a definitive treatment in some patients [such as patients with multiple complex fistulas, radiation-induced fistula, or active Crohn's disease] (Figures 15-9 and 15-10), it is often a temporary measure as the patient awaits additional definitive fistula surgery. A period of 12 or more weeks is typically advisable during which the patient is assessed periodically to ensure adequate drainage. The seton may be used as a guide for gentle fistula irrigation if needed with solutions such as hydrogen peroxide, saline, antibiotics, or antiseptic. While a draining seton is in place, any new abscess or fistula formation should raise suspicion for inadequate drainage possibly due to having missed the correct fistulous tract at time of seton placement or due to progression of disease. Following an adequate period of drainage, a definitive sphincter-preserving fistula procedure can be performed.

A cutting seton is the second type of seton and typically entails encircling the fistulous tract. The skin and subcutaneous portion of the fistula are divided in the operating room to expose the anal muscle, which is encircled by the seton material (Figure 15-11a). The seton is connected to a Penrose drain which allows the patient over the course of several days to a couple of weeks to gradually pull the seton through the muscular portion of the tract (Figure 15-11b). Progressive cutting by the seton produces a slow fistulotomy, which allows for scarring of the divided tract minimizing wide separation of the divided muscle. An alternative variation of the cutting seton is the multiple seton technique. Two or more setons are passed through the tract, and at various time intervals, each suture is tightened progressively after taking out the previously tightened suture which becomes loose.

Anal Flap

Two types of anal flaps are available to treat anal fistula including transanal endorectal advancement flap and anocutaneous flap. The endorectal advancement flap is a good option for most complex anal fistulas, which typically are higher and involve more of the anal sphincter complex. Usually a noncutting draining seton is placed for 12 or more weeks to allow for fibrosis of the fistulous tract before the definitive flap repair is performed. The endorectal advancement flap is our

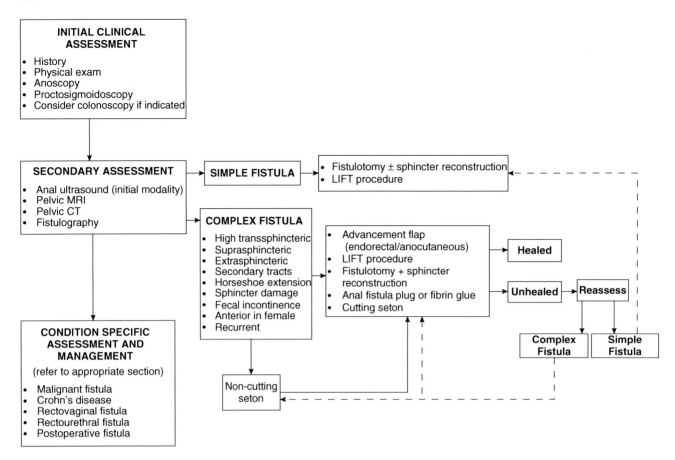

FIGURE 15-8. Carepath for evaluation and treatment of complex anal fistula secondary to cryptoglandular disease.

preferred method to treat most complex anal fistula secondary to cryptoglandular disease, except for posterior-based horseshoe fistula. The operation is typically performed in the prone position under general anesthesia. At time of flap repair, the draining seton is removed. The tract is irrigated with hydrogen peroxide and the tract is traced with a fistula probe. The anorectum is irrigated with Betadine, and the area of the planned flap is outlined and infiltrated with 1 % lidocaine with 1:100,000 epinephrine for hemostasis (Figure 15-12a, b). The subcutaneous portion of the external opening is excised, and the fistula is debrided with a curette (Figure 15-12c). A curvilinear incision is made approximately 1 cm distal to the internal opening and a partial or full thickness broad-based (3–4 cm wide) endorectal flap is raised (Figure 15-12d) [22]. It is important to avoid a mucosa-only based flap as it is associated with a higher failure rate due to ischemia. The flap should be dissected cephalad to ensure enough mobility to reach the lower anal canal. Once the flap is raised, the intramuscular portion of the internal opening is closed with interrupted 3.0 Vicryl suture (Figure 15-12e). The distal portion of the flap containing the mucosal portion of the internal opening is trimmed. The flap is matured over its muscular bed using 3.0 Vicryl single interrupted sutures (Figure 15-12f).

Care is taken to spread any tension across the entire flap to provide adequate coverage of the intramuscular portion of the internal opening. Upon completion of the flap, an antibiotic impregnated gelfoam is placed inside the anal canal.

Ligation of the Intersphincteric Fistula Tract

The ligation of the intersphincteric fistula tract (LIFT) was described in 2007 by Rojanasakul and colleagues from Thailand [23] (Videos 15.1, 15.2, 15.3, 15.4, 15.5, 15.6, 15.7, and 15.8). The LIFT procedure is a sphincter-preserving operation that entails division and ligation of the fistulous tract in the intersphincteric plane. It is a good option for transsphincteric anal fistula. The LIFT procedure is the authors' second preferred surgical option when an endorectal advancement flap is contraindicated (i.e., anal stricture, incontinent patient, prior failed flap). Suprasphincteric and horseshoe fistulas can pose technical challenges and in general are not suitable candidates for the LIFT procedure. A draining seton is not mandatory prior to performing the procedure in fibrotic fistulas. However, wet fistulas with copious drainage and those associated with a cavity can benefit from a draining seton prior to the LIFT procedure. A metallic

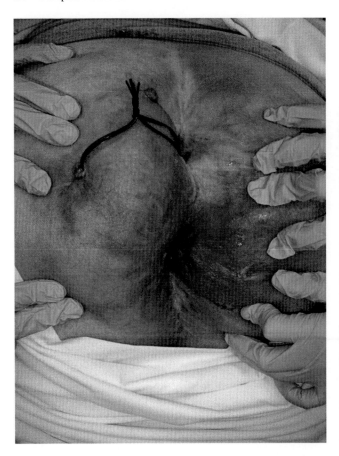

FIGURE 15-9. Draining setons in a patient with multiple complex anorectal fistulas and prior radiation therapy to the pelvis.

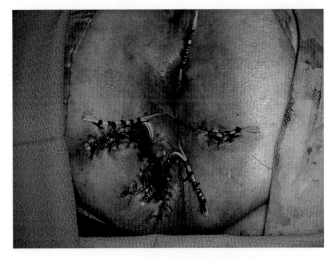

FIGURE 15-10. Draining setons in a patient with long-standing history of multiple fistulas emanating from different internal openings in all 4 anal quadrants.

probe is inserted into the external opening and passed gently through the tract to exit through the internal opening (Figure 15-13a, b). The intersphincteric groove is identified

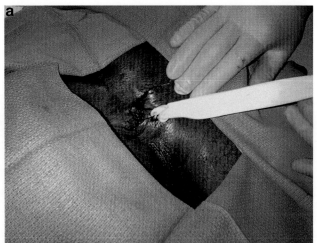

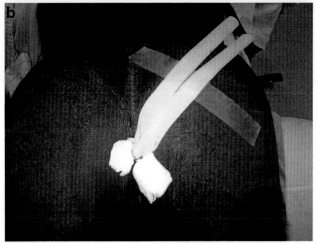

FIGURE 15-11. (a) Cutting seton in a patient with suprasphincteric fistula. The skin and subcutaneous portion of the tract are divided before tightening the seton. (b) The cutting seton is connected to a Penrose drain to allow the patient to gradually pull through the fistula.

externally, and a small circumanal skin incision overlying the fistula is performed to enter the intersphincteric space between the internal and the external sphincter muscles. The dissection in the intersphincteric plane is continued until to fistulous tract is reached and encircled (Figure 15-13c). Care is taken not to divide the tract prior to proper identification and dissection from surrounding sphincter muscle. This is achieved by palpating the fistula probe throughout the dissection. The fistula tract is then encircled by using a right-angle clamp, and two absorbable sutures (2.0 Vicryl) are used to ligate the fistula tract medially and laterally leaving a space in between to sharply divide the fistula (Figure 15-13d). Care is taken not to dislodge the tied sutures (Figure 15-13e). To confirm the integrity of tract division, hydrogen peroxide can be injected from the internal and external orifices while the wound is still open. The intersphincteric plane is closed in two layers (muscle approximation and the skin) by using

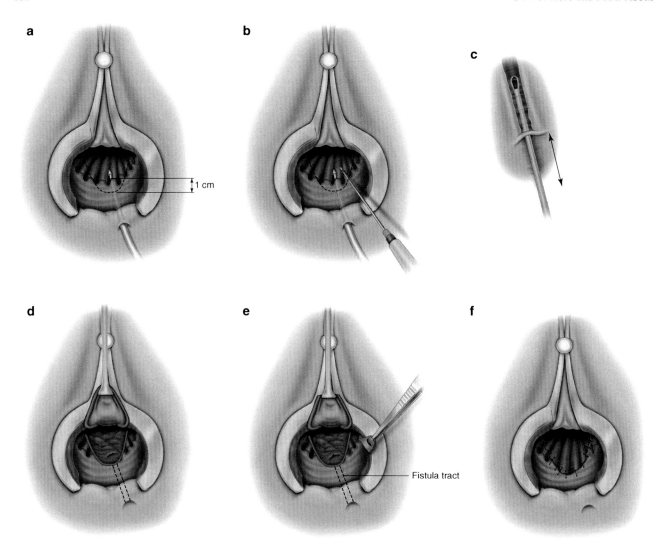

F<small>IGURE</small> 15-12. (**a–d**) Technical steps of endorectal advancement flap.

single interrupted 3.0 Vicryl (Figure 15-13f). Both the internal and external openings are left opened to allow drainage. The external opening nodular induration can be excised and left open. Patients have a normal diet on the day of surgery and are discharged within 24 h. A variation to the conventional LIFT procedure is the BioLIFT procedure which entails the use of a bioprosthetic porcine graft to reinforce the ligation and the closure of the fistula tract [24]. The graft is interposed between the internal and external sphincter muscles to overlap 1–2 cm area of the ligated and divided fistulous tract. Other modifications of the LIFT procedure are the LIFT-PLUS procedure which adds a partial fistulectomy of the subcutaneous portion of the tract from the skin to the external sphincter muscle and the LIFT procedure combined with endorectal advancement flap [25].

Fistulotomy with Sphincter Reconstruction

Fistulotomy with sphincter reconstruction is a suitable technique for complex or recurrent fistulas in incontinent patients or in patients who are at risk for incontinence [26]. Two enemas are given the evening before or the morning of the operation. Prophylactic intravenous antibiotics are given at time of operation and are continued postoperatively for 1 week. The operation is performed under general anesthesia in the prone jack-knife position. If a draining seton has been previously placed, it is removed, and a fistula probe is introduced through the external opening and guided through the tract until it protrudes out of the internal opening (Figure 15-4a). The fistula tract is completely divided using electrocautery (Figure 15-14b). Curettage of the tract and

FIGURE 15-13. (**a–f**)
Intraoperative demonstration of
the LIFT procedure.

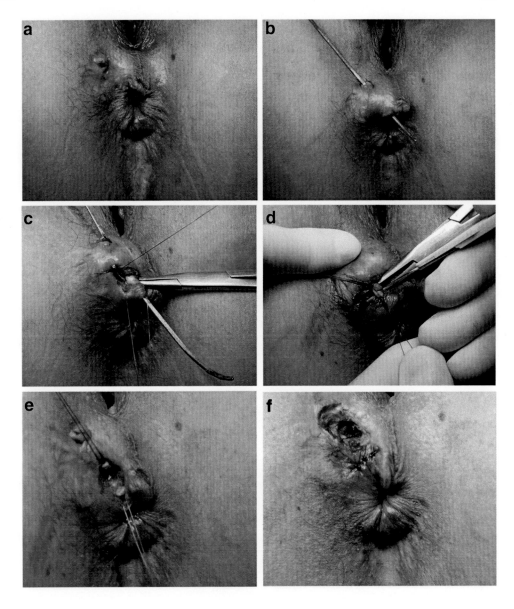

any associated cavities is performed to ensure that all granu-lation tissue is debrided. Excision of the fibrous tract can be performed taking care not to excise any muscle or alterna-tively the fibrous tract is left in situ. The amount of divided sphincter involved in the fistula is carefully assessed, and the edges of the transected muscle are identified for reconstruc-tion. An end-to-end primary sphincteroplasty is performed using a series of horizontal mattress sutures using 2.0 Vicryl or PDS sutures (Figure 15-14c). The fistula bed of the divided fistulous tract is incorporated in the suturing to completely obliterate any potential space behind the muscle reconstruc-tion. The edges of the open wound are finally marsupialized by tacking the divided mucosal and submucosal layer to the muscle repair (Figure 15-14d), keeping the most superficial aspect of the wound open to allow for drainage. 3.0 Vicryl or 3.0 Chromic suture is used for the marsupialization. Stool softeners and analgesic are given as needed.

Anal Fistula Plug

The anal fistula plug is used to close the primary internal opening and serves as a matrix for the obliteration of the fistulous tract. Initially, a bioabsorbable xenograft made of lyophilized porcine intestinal mucosa with conic shape was introduced to the market (Surgisis® AFP, Cook Medical, Bloomington, Indiana, USA) [27]. The tract is traversed with a fistula probe and then curetted. A 2-0 silk suture is tied to the tapered end of the plug and then pulled through the internal opening using the fistula probe until it is snug inside the fistula tract (Figure 15-15a, b). The excess end of the plug is trimmed inside the anal canal side using scissors (Figure 15-15c). The trimmed portion of the plug is fixed to the internal opening and internal anal sphincter muscle using 3.0 Vicryl suture (Figure 15-15d). The mucosal/submucosal

FIGURE 15-14. (**a–d**) Technical steps of fistulotomy with sphincter reconstruction.

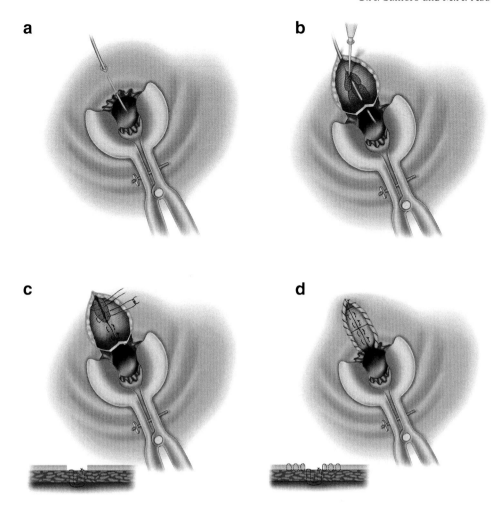

opening at the internal fistula opening is approximated with the same suture. The external opening of the fistula is left open to drain after trimming the tapered end of the plug (Figure 15-15e). Due to the variable results of the Surgisis® AFP with failures related to migration, extrusion, and infection, a new absorbable plug was subsequently introduced (GORE® BIO-A® Fistula Plug, W. L Gore & Associates, Inc., Flagstaff, Arizona, USA) [28]. The plug is designed with a special flat disk head and six plug arms that can allow better anchoring to tissue (Figure 15-16a). The plug is made of 100 % synthetic bioabsorbable material that starts resorption at 6th week and is completed after 6–7 months. The general technical steps of the GORE® BIO-A® Fistula Plug procedure are similar to those of the Surgisis® AFP with some minor variations. After the identification of the fistula, the tract is debrided with a curette. The external opening is cored out to accomplish sufficient drainage. Inside the anal canal, a small submucosal flap is raised in the area of the internal opening. The plug is pulled through the internal opening (Figure 15-16b). In cases where the fistula tract is too narrow for the entire plug, one or more of the six arms can be excised at the junction with the flat disk. The head of

the plug is fixed to the internal sphincter muscle using 2.0 Vicryl suture (Figure 15-16c) and then covered with the small submucosal flap.

Fibrin Glue

Fibrin glue (Tisseel®, Baxter, Deerfield, Illinois, USA) and synthetic glue (cyanoacrylate glue, Glubran® 2, GEM S.R.L., Viareggio, Italy) are injectable products that can be used in the treatment of anorectal fistulas [29]. They act as tissue sealants and are believed to stimulate the growth of fibroblasts and pluripotent endothelial cells into the fistulous tract. This physiologic response triggers collagen deposition and wound healing. Fibrin glue treatment is simple and repeatable and maybe a good initial option in patients with high fistulas. Although associated with an overall low success rate, failure of the glue to eradicate the fistula does not compromise further treatment options, and sphincter function is preserved. The procedure starts by identifying the external fistula opening, followed by the curettage of the fistula tract. Approximately 5 ml of reconstituted fibrin glue is injected through the external opening (Figure 15-17a) until it

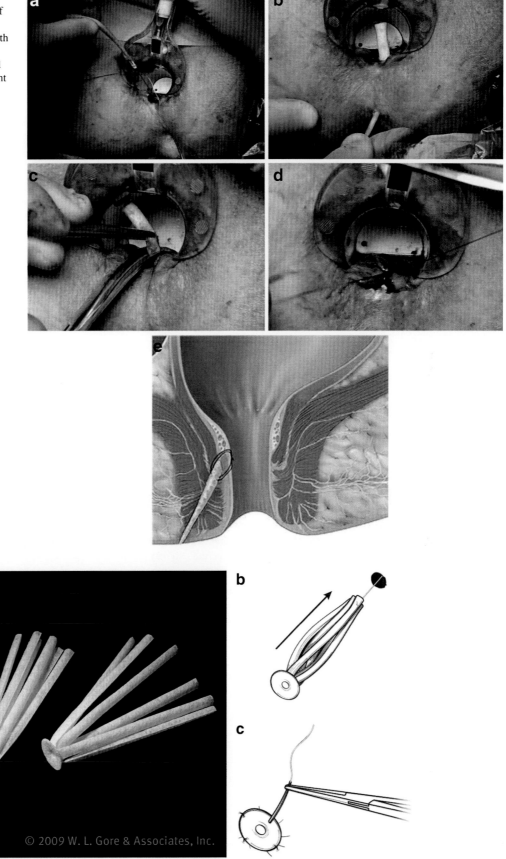

FIGURE 15-15. (a-e) Intraoperative demonstration of the anal fistula plug (Surgisis® AFP) procedure in a patient with high transsphincteric fistula. Anatomical view of obliterated fistula tract following placement of anal fistula plug (Surgisis® AFP).

© 2009 W. L. Gore & Associates, Inc.

FIGURE 15-16. (a) GORE® BIO-A® Fistula Plug. With permission © W. L. Gore and Associates 2009. (b) Pulling of the GORE® BIO-A® Fistula Plug through internal opening. (c) Anchoring the flat top on the GORE® BIO-A® Fistula Plug to covering the internal fistulous opening.

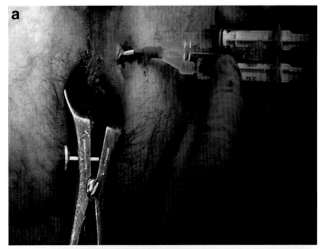

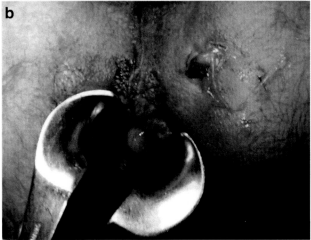

Figure 15-17. (a) Fibrin glue injection of a high transsphincteric fistula through the external fistulous opening. (b) Fistula tract sealed with the fibrin glue. Note the fibrin glue extruding from the internal opening inside the anal canal.

extrudes from the internal opening area (Figure 15-17b). The internal opening is closed with 3-0 Vicryl suture.

Newer and Evolving Technologies: VAAFT, FiLaC, and Stem Cell

The last decade has seen the introduction of three additional new technologies: the video-assisted anal fistula treatment (VAAFT), the fistula laser closure (FiLaC), and stem cell therapy [30–32]. At this stage of development, it is premature to tell what long-term roles these evolving technologies will play in the field of anorectal fistula surgery. The technical expertise with these three procedures has been concentrated in a limited number of centers globally. Thus, they have not formally been incorporated in the management algorithm presented in Figure 15-8, but they are worth describing in this chapter as potential future options pending additional long-term data.

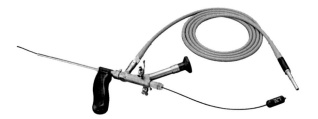

Figure 15-18. Anal fistuloscope (Karl Storz, Tuttlingen, Germany).

The video-assisted anal fistula treatment was initially described by Meinero from Italy [30]. The procedure is performed with a kit, which includes a rigid fistuloscope (Karl Storz, Tuttlingen, Germany) (Figure 15-18), an obturator, a unipolar electrical diathermy probe, an endobrush, an endoscopic grasper, and a synthetic cyanoacrylate glue. The fistuloscope video equipment is an 8°-angled endoscope with an optical working channel to introduce the instruments and an irrigation channel. VAAFT consists of a diagnostic phase followed by an operative phase. In the diagnostic phase, the fistuloscope is inserted through the external opening and advanced by the irrigation of the glycine-mannitol 1 % which expands the fistula tract. Both primary and secondary openings and tracts are explored via the fistuloscope. After the internal opening is located, absorbable sutures are taken at its site in the rectum or anal canal for applying traction. During the next operative phase, the aim is to destroy the fistula tract from the inside by curetting the tract, obliterating it, and closing the internal opening. Through the working channel of the fistuloscope, the fistula tract is cauterized, and necrotic material is removed using an endobrush and irrigation. Finally, the internal opening is closed by either suturing or stapling with a linear or semicircular stapler, or alternatively by advancing an anal flap. In order to reinforce the suture or staple line, 0.5 ml of synthetic cyanoacrylate glue can be applied.

The fistula laser closure is a novel sphincter-saving technique that uses an emitting laser probe [FiLaC™, Biolitec, Germany] to destroy the fistula epithelium and simultaneously obliterate the remaining fistula tract [31]. Since the main reason for operative failure is a persistent fistula tract or remnants of fistula epithelium which were not excised, it is postulated that the benefit of this newly designed radial-emitting laser probe is to eradicate the granulating and fibrous fistula tissue. FiLaC™ eliminates fistula epithelium and granulation tissue in a circular manner causing shrinkage and obliteration of the tract. The first step of the procedure is the identification and localization of the internal opening by hydrogen peroxide or methylene blue injection from the external opening. The fistula tract is debrided with a curette, and a plastic hollow 14 French catheter is inserted using a guide-wire. 400 μm radial-emitting disposable laser fiber is inserted into the catheter with its tip emerging at the internal orifice. The fiber delivers laser energy homogenously at 360°, and by applying continuous energy, the tract is closed while withdrawing it at a speed of 1 mm per second. The procedure includes the closure of the internal opening by means of an anorectal flap. When some scar tissue prevents that, either a mucosal or anodermal flap is used for closure of the internal opening. A modified laser procedure consists of sealing the fistula tract by laser with no need for endorectal flap. The closure of the internal opening is allowed by a laser shrinkage effect.

The potential role of mesenchymal adult stem cells in differentiating into various types of cells may have a role in the treatment of anal fistula, suppressing inflammation and promoting differentiation. Application of autologous expanded adipose-derived stem cells (ASCs) represents a novel approach for enhancing regeneration of damaged tissues [32]. ASCs can be obtained from subcutaneous fat by liposuction, and this process yields 100 times more stem cells than bone marrow aspirates. Following curettage of the fistula tract and suture closure of the internal opening, ASC solution is injected into the tract and into the walls of the fistula. The tract is subsequently sealed with fibrin glue.

Outcome

Complex fistulous disease challenges even the most experienced surgeons. Successful management requires good surgical judgment, knowledge of anorectal anatomy, and technical proficiency in the surgical approaches available to ensure the highest possible postoperative continence and wound healing. Success rate in patients with complex or recurrent anorectal fistulas is lower than in patients with simple anal fistulas. Often more than one procedure is needed to eradicate the fistula. Risk for incontinence is usually higher due to the complexity of the fistula, recurrent or persistent disease, and/or prior failed interventions. A fundamental understanding of the advantages, disadvantages, limitations, and results of the various techniques is essential [33, 34]. The selection of a specific operation for an individual patient based on fistula characteristics, body habitus, gender, baseline continence level, and history of prior interventions if any is of paramount importance.

Seton

According to the standards practice task force of the ASCRS [1], use of a seton and/or staged fistulotomy for the treatment of complex fistula-in-ano has strong recommendation based on moderate-quality evidence [1]. Noncutting seton is usually used as a bridge to additional surgical intervention and typically is not curative. When removed the rate of persistent fistula is very high [35]. A high rate of incontinence (38 %) has been reported with cutting seton. In our practice, we rarely use a cutting seton, which we typically reserve for patients with high complex fistulas who failed multiple prior interventions or in fistulas not amenable to

other techniques such as high posterior-based fistulas in patients with deep buttock cleft. In a study performed by Garcia-Aguilar and colleagues comparing cutting seton with two-stage seton fistulotomy in the management of high anal fistulas, both techniques were equally effective in eradicating the fistula and were associated with similar incontinence rates [36]. When using a tight or cutting seton, the intraoperative preservation of the internal sphincter muscle appears to reduce the postoperative fecal incontinence without a substantial increase in recurrence rates as reported by Vial and colleagues in a systematic review of 19 series and 448 patients [37]. Overall, the fecal incontinence was 5.6 % when the internal anal sphincter was preserved compared to 25.2 % when it was divided. Hasegawa and colleagues reported their results with cutting seton in 32 patients with cryptoglandular fistula (81 % transsphincteric) [38]. Continence disturbance was noted in 54 % of the patients, and the fistula recurrence rate was 29 %. Women with prior vaginal deliveries experienced significant incontinence leading the authors to advice against the use of cutting seton in this subgroup of patients especially in the setting of an anterior fistula. Cutting seton is associated with new onset of gas incontinence. Isbister and Sanea reported their experience with cutting seton in patients with transsphincteric fistula [39]. Frequent gas incontinence developed postoperatively in 9.5 % of the patients, and 21.4 % developed occasional gas incontinence. Mentes and colleagues published their results with cutting seton in transsphincteric fistula involving greater than 50 % of the sphincter complex [40]. Recurrence rate was low (5 %), but the rate of postoperative incontinence was 20 %.

Advancement Flap

According to the standards practice task force of the ASCRS [1], the grade of recommendation for the treatment of complex fistula-in-ano with advancement flap is a strong recommendation based on moderate-quality evidence (1C). The Association of Coloproctology of Great Britain and Ireland (ACPGBI) recommends transanal advancement flap for the treatment of anal fistula when simple fistulotomy is thought likely to result in impaired continence [41]. Endorectal flap has demonstrated a success rate of between 60 and 93 %, and it has been advocated as the treatment of choice for complex fistula-in-ano [41, 42]. It can be technically challenging especially in posterior-based fistula in males and in patients with deep buttock cleft. Postoperative incontinence rate has been reported between 7 and 38 % [43]. Zimmerman and colleagues reported a healing rate of 69 % in patients with transsphincteric fistula at a median follow-up of 14 months [44]. Ortiz and Marzo reported a low recurrence rate of 7 % for high transsphincteric or suprasphincteric fistula [45]. When examining factors affecting success, the level of the fistula did not impact outcome. Continence disturbance was observed in 8 % of cases.

TABLE 15-1. Results of LIFT procedure

	Year	# of patients	Follow-up (months)	Success (%)	Incontinence (%)
Rojanaskul et al. [23]	2007	18	6.5	94	0
Ellis [24]	2010	31	15	94	0
Shanwani et al. [52]	2010	45	9	82	0
Aboulian et al. [53]	2011	25	6	68	0
Tan et al. [54]	2011	93	5.8	85	0
Abcarian et al. [55]	2012	40	4.5	74	0
Mushaya et al. [56]	2012	39	16	92	0
Ooi et al. [57]	2012	25	5.5	68	0
Wallin et al. [58]	2012	93	19	40	31
Han et al. [59]	2013	21	14	95	5
van Onkelen et al. [60]	2013	22	19.5	82	0
Lehmann et al. [61]	2013	17	13.5	65	0
Sirikurnpiboon et al. [25]	2013	41	4.8	83	0
Sileri et al. [62]	2014	26	16	73	0

Abbas and colleagues had an initial success rate of 83 % and a recurrence rate of 14 % during a median follow-up of 30 months [42]. Schouten and colleagues reported a recurrence rate of 25 %, and continence disturbance was observed in 35 % of their patients [46]. Prior drainage with a noncutting seton is believed to increase success rate. Patients who fail an initial flap can be considered for a repeat procedure. Jarrar and colleagues reported their experience in 98 patients treated by an advancement flap [47]. Primary healing occurred in 72 % of patients, and secondary healing (following a second flap after initial failure) occurred in 57 % of cases yielding an overall healing rate 93 %. There was a significant improvement in continence and a decrease in urgency after flap repair. The flap technique can impact success rate. Dubsky and colleagues compared the outcome of full thickness flap with mucosal based flap only [48]. 54 consecutive patients with high anal fistula secondary to cryptoglandular disease were retrospectively reviewed. The overall recurrence rate was 24 % and was much lower in the full thickness subgroup (5 %) compared to the mucosal subgroup (35.3 %). Patients with four or more previous anal surgeries were at highest risk for failure. No difference in postoperative incontinence was noted between subgroups. The addition of autologous platelet-rich plasma can increase success rate as described by van der Hagen and colleagues who reported a 90 % success rate during a follow-up of 26 months [49]. Smoking has been associated with a lower success rate. Zimmerman and colleagues studied the outcome of endorectal advancement flap in 105 patients [50]. During a median time of 14 months, healing rate was 60 % in smokers compared to 79 % in nonsmokers. In another study by the same researchers, blood flow was measured during endorectal advancement flap procedures. Blood flow was significantly lower in smokers compared to nonsmokers [51].

Ligation of the Intersphincteric Fistula Tract

According to the standards practice task force of the ASCRS, data are too preliminary to make a formal recommendation for the LIFT procedure in the treatment of complex fistula-in-ano [1]. The initial reported success rate of the LIFT procedure was 94 % [23]. However, subsequent studies with longer follow-up have shown a wider range of success rate from 40 to 95 % (Table 15.1) [23–25, 52–62]. Wallin and colleagues performed a retrospective review of 93 patients treated by LIFT procedure [58]. Fistula healing rate was initially 40 % and with secondary interventions increased to 57 %. Interestingly, the authors reported that in those patients with recurrence, the LIFT technique had transformed a complex fistula into a simple intersphincteric fistula that could be effectively treated by subsequent intersphincteric fistulotomy. Medialization of the fistula tract or conversion of a transsphincteric fistula into an intersphincteric fistula after LIFT ("downstaging") has been also described by Tan and colleagues in patients with persistent discharge [54]. A recent systematic review including 13 articles and 498 patients reported an overall success rate ranging from 40 to 95 %, with a pooled success of 71 % [63]. Minor continence disturbance was observed in 6 % of cases. The conclusion of this review was that the LIFT procedure appears to be an effective sphincter-conserving approach for the treatment of complex fistula-in-ano. In another review, Vergara-Fernandez and colleagues analyzed 18 studies with 592 patients [64]. The mean healing rate reported was 74.6 %. No de novo incontinence developed secondary to the LIFT procedure. A recent meta-analysis of 24 original articles reported a mean success rate of 76.5 %, an incontinence rate of 0 %, and a postoperative complication rate of 5.5 % (mean follow-up of 10 months) [65]. Lehmann and colleagues assessed the efficacy of the LIFT procedure in 17 recurrent anal fistulas [61].

Table 15-2. Results of the anal fistula plug

	Year	# of patients	Follow-up (months)	Success (%)	Extrusion (%)
Johnson et al. [70]	2006	15	3.5	87	N.R.
Champagne et al. [71]	2006	46	12	83	4
Schwandner et al. [72]	2008	18	9	61	2
Christoforidis et al. [73]	2008	47	5	38	14
Theckkinkattil et al. [74]	2008	36	11	50	10
Starck et al. [75]	2008	32	12	59	N.R.
Lawes et al. [76]	2008	20	7.4	24	N.R.
Safar et al. [77]	2009	35	4.2	13.9	9.7
Ortiz et al. [78]	2009	15	12	20	15
Wang et al. [79]	2009	29	9	34	N.R.
McGee et al. [80]	2010	41	24	44	5
Anyadike et al. [81]	2010	33	14	73	N.R.
Van Koperen et al. [82]	2011	31	11	29	13
Ommer et al. [28]	2012	40	12	57.5	N.R.
O'Riordan et al. [83]	2012	488	3–24.5	54	8.7

The long-term healing rate was 65 %. No de novo incontinence was reported. In a retrospective study, Tan and colleagues compared the LIFT operation with the mucosal advancement flap [66]. The anal flap was more effective than the LIFT operation (93.5 % vs. 62.5 %, respectively). However, a recent prospective randomized trial comparing the LIFT procedure with mucosal advancement flap in patients with high transsphincteric fistula found similar long-term healing rate, recurrence rate, continence, and quality of life [67]. Ellis and colleagues reported a 94 % success rate with the BioLIFT procedure in a prospective study of 31 patients [24]. A lower success rate was noted by Chew and colleagues who reported comparable success of 63 % with both LIFT and BIOLIFT procedures [68]. The LIFT-PLUS procedure was compared to the traditional LIFT procedure in a prospective study on 41 patients [25]. The healing rate in LIFT-PLUS group was 85 % compared to 81 % in the LIFT group. No incontinence was reported.

Anal Fistula Plug

According to the standards practice task force of the ASCRS [1], there is weak recommendation based on moderate-quality evidence (2C) for the treatment of complex fistula-in-ano with AFP. Several studies have reported variable results with this minimally invasive procedure. In an attempt to standardize the indications for use of bioprosthetic Surgisis® AFP and techniques for its placement, a consensus conference was held in 2007 [27]. According to the consensus, the use of the Surgisis® AFP should be recommended in transsphincteric anal fistula without any acute inflammation or infection. It was also suggested that a frequent issue affecting the Surgisis® AFP procedure was a failure in technique of the plug placement [27]. Reported success rate in various studies has ranged from 13.9 to 87 % (Table 15-2) [28, 69–83]. The postoperative abscess/sepsis rate has ranged

from 4 to 29 %. Failures have been related to technical issues, plug extrusion, and infection. O'Riordan and colleagues conducted a systematic review (22 studies included, 488 patients) of the anal fistula plug [83]. Fistula closure was achieved in 54 % of cases. The success rate has been lower in patients with multiple tracts [69]. This can be due to undertreatment of the secondary tracts in which no plug was inserted. In one study, tract length was a predictor of outcome with longer fistula tracts carrying higher success rate [80]. None of studies evaluating the role of the noncutting seton before plug insertion found any significant change in closure rate. However, due to the heterogeneity of patient populations and fistula characteristics described in the various studies, further randomized controlled trial would be needed to settle this issue. Muhlmann and colleagues compared Surgisis® AFP and anal flap for the treatment of complex anal fistulas in 55 patients [84]. The results were disappointing, with 33 % healing rate after flap and 32 % following the plug. van Koperen and colleagues compared the Surgisis® AFP with the mucosal advancement flap for cryptoglandular high transsphincteric fistula in a double-blinded multicenter randomized trial [82]. At a follow-up of 11 months, the recurrence rates were 71 % for the plug and 52 % for the mucosal advancement flap. No significant differences were noted in postoperative pain, pre- and postoperative incontinence scores, soiling, and quality of life. Ortiz and colleagues conducted a randomized clinic trial comparing the Surgisis® AFP with the endorectal advancement flap in patients with high cryptoglandular fistula-in-ano [78]. The trial was closed prematurely due to a high failure rate of the plug (80 %) compared to the flap (12.5 %).

The variable success rates reported with Surgisis® AFP and the inability to reproduce high healing rates in most practice settings provided an opportunity to develop another plug from a different material with the aim to increase success rate. The GORE® BIO-A® Fistula Plug was the second plug introduced in the field of fistula surgery. A German multicenter study investigated the GORE® BIO-A® Fistula Plug in the treatment of high anal fistulas [28]. The overall healing rate in 40 patients was 57.5 % without postoperative impairment of continence. In a retrospective review of 48 patients treated with the same plug, Heydari and colleagues reported an overall healing rate of 69.3 % without change in continence level [85]. No plug dislodgment or postoperative infection was noted. There is a paucity of data comparing the Surgisis® AFP with the GORE® BIO-A® Fistula Plug. Buchberg and colleagues published a retrospective study comparing the two plugs [86]. Twelve patients received the Surgisis® AFP, and ten patients had the GORE® BIO-A® Fistula Plug. The healing rate was 12.5 % in the Surgisis® AFP compared to 54.5 % in GORE® BIO-A® Fistula Plug. Due to the retrospective nature of the study and the small number of patients, it is early to tell whether this trend will be observed when additional data becomes available in the future.

Fibrin Glue

According to the standard practice task force of the ASCRS [1], the grade of recommendation for the treatment of complex fistula-in-ano with debridement and fibrin glue injection is a weak recommendation based on low-quality evidence (2C). The use of fibrin sealant injection initially demonstrated promising results with high success rates between 60 and 80 % [29]. However, subsequent studies with longer follow-up have reported lower success rates of 32–54 % [29]. At 1 year following injection of commercial fibrin sealant, Cintron and colleagues reported a 64 % fistula closure rate [87]. Most recurrences were noted within 3 months of the injection, but some up to 11 months. Sentovich treated 48 fistulas and observed a 60 % healing rate during a median follow-up of 22 months [88]. Retreatment with fibrin glue increased the closure rate to 69 %. Loungnarath and colleagues found that durable healing could not be sustained and was achieved only in 31 % of cases [89]. Most failures were noted within 3 months. The success rate was not different in patients with previous failed treatment. Swinscoe and colleagues reported that following fibrin glue injection, a shorter fistula (<4 cm) tended to recur more frequently than longer fistula (>4 cm) with recurrence rate of 54 % vs. 11 % [29]. A possible explanation is that a short fistula tract does not hold the glue as well as longer tract. van Koperen and colleagues conducted a retrospective study to assess the potential value of fibrin glue in combination with transanal advancement flap compared to advancement flap alone [90]. The overall recurrence rate in their group of cryptoglandular high transsphincteric fistula was 26 %. Recurrence rate for advancement flap alone was 13 % compared to 56 % when fibrin glue was injected in the subgroup of patients without previous fistula surgery and 23 % vs. 41 % in the group with previous fistula surgery. The authors concluded that the

obliteration of the fistula tract with fibrin glue was associated with worse outcome after rectal advancement flap. Singer and colleagues randomized patients to three groups prospectively: group one received injection of antibiotic plus the sealant, group two had surgical closure of the internal opening, and group three had both [91]. At a mean follow-up of 27 months, initial healing was 21, 40, and 31 %, respectively (P=0.38). Therefore, neither of these technical alterations improved the success rate. In a quest to improve the healing rate for the injectable procedure, Jain and colleagues reported good results using cyanoacrylate glue to treat complex fistulas [92]. Seventeen out of 20 patients (85 %) healed following an initial injection, and two patients required one additional injection without further signs of fistula discharge. A second injection can be beneficial as reported by Barillari and colleagues who increased healing rate from 71.4 to 90.2 % after additional injections [93].

The high success rate of fibrin glue injection reported in some series has not been reproducible in the majority of practice settings, and studies that have carefully evaluated patients following fibrin glue injection have reported low success rate. Buchanan and colleagues from St. Mark's hospital conducted a prospective study to evaluate the efficacy of fibrin glue injection in patients with complex anorectal fistula [94]. During a median follow-up time of 14 months, the healing rate was 14 %. Careful long-term assessment of the patients was performed with physical examination and magnetic resonance imaging. The high failure rate associated with fibrin glue injection has been attributed to the difficulty in ensuring the glue remains in the fistula tract, failure of closure of the internal opening, and lack of autologous tissue ingrowth to seal the tract. A Cochrane database systematic review analyzed ten randomized controlled trials [95]. Comparisons were made between various treatment modalities. There was no significant difference in recurrence rate or incontinence rate in any of the studied operation except in the case of advancement flap which carried higher success rate. A higher recurrence rate was noted when fibrin glue injection was added to an endorectal advancement flap, favoring a flap-only technique. Both fibrin glue injection and advancement flap had low incontinence rate, but the higher success rate of the flap favors its use over fibrin glue.

Fistulotomy with Sphincter Reconstruction

Fistulotomy with sphincter reconstruction is an effective surgical treatment for complex anal fistula. Patients with baseline incontinence, those at risk for incontinence (such as patients with previous childbirth, anterior fistula in females, existing sphincter defect from prior anal surgery), and patients with recurrent disease can be suitable candidates for this technique. Overall healing rates range from 83.3 to 97.4 % and the incontinence rates between 3.7 and 21.4 % (Table 15-3) [26, 43, 96–100]. However, studies analyzing

TABLE 15-3. Results of fistulotomy with sphincter reconstruction

	Year	# of patients	Follow-up (months)	Success (%)	Incontinence (%)
Parkash et al. [96]	1985	120	6–60	83.3	3.7
Christiansen and Ronholt [97]	1995	14	12–48	85.7	21.4
Perez et al. [43]	2006	35	32	92.9	12.5
Roig et al. [98]	2010	75	13	89.4	18.3
Kraemer and Picke [99]	2011	38	N.R.	97.4	9.4
Arroyo et al. [100]	2012	70	81	91.4	16.6
Ratto et al. [26]	2013	72	29.4	95.8	11.6

the degree of continence in patients who were treated with this procedure reported a minor degree of incontinence (flatus incontinence and soiling). Ratto and colleagues conducted a prospective study in 72 patients with complex fistulas [26]. The recurrence rate was 4.2 %, and de novo incontinence (soiling) was noted in 11.6 % of patients. In another study of 70 patients with complex anal fistula who underwent fistulotomy with sphincter reconstruction, 70 % of the patients with preoperative anal incontinence improved [100]. The postoperative improvement was assessed subjectively using the CCF-IS scale (*mean score*: 6.75–1.88, $P<0.005$) and objectively measuring anal pressures using anorectal manometry. During a follow-up period of 81 months, recurrence rate was 8.6 % with the majority of recurrences treated successfully with a repeat procedure. Perez and colleagues studied 60 patients in a randomized clinical trial comparing fistulotomy and sphincter reconstruction to fistulectomy and advancement flap [43]. No difference was noted in recurrence rate between the two subgroups (7.1 % vs. 7.4 %) or postoperative incontinence as measured by CCF-IS score. Roig and colleagues retrospectively analyzed 146 patients who underwent endoanal advancement flap (71 patients) or fistulectomy with sphincter repair (75 patients) [98]. Forty-two fistulas (28.7 %) were recurrent, 98 were transsphincteric, and 37 were suprasphincteric. Twenty-six (17.7 %) patients had some degree of preoperative continence disturbances, without significant differences between the two groups ($P=0.47$). After a mean follow-up of 13 months, fistula persisted or recurred in 18.3 % of advancement flap vs. 10.6 % of sphincter reconstruction ($P=0.19$). In 2011, the first German guideline for the treatment of anal fistulas considered "fistula excision with direct reconstruction" to be a therapeutic option [101]. Based on extensive positive experience with this technique (a decade of personal experience of the chapter senior author at Kaiser Permanente Los Angeles Medical Center is pending publication), we concur with the German guideline and do believe that there is a role for fistulotomy with sphincter reconstruction in patients with complex anal fistula. While the majority of available data has been from European centers, we hope that future studies will report results from the United States.

Newer and Evolving Technologies: VAAFT, FiLaC™, and Stem Cell

Using the VAAFT procedure, Meinero and Mori achieved an overall success rate of 73.5 % in 136 patients with non-Crohn's disease-related anal fistula [30]. Recurrence rate was 26.5 % within 2–3 months of follow-up. No worsening in continence was noted in their study. Kochhar and colleagues recently examined the results of the VAAFT procedure in a prospective study in 82 patients [102]. The recurrence rate was 15.8 %. Postoperative pain and discomfort were minimal. Another recent report of the VAAFT procedure revealed a recurrence rate of 17 % without major complications or incontinence [103]. Due to the limited data on VAAFT and its recent introduction, it is premature to draw any firm conclusion about its long-term efficacy, additional benefits, and limitations compared to the existing surgical options. Further studies are needed to determine what future role if any it will play in the management of patients with anal fistula.

Giamundo and colleagues studied the outcome of the FiLaC™ procedure in 35 patients with cryptoglandular and Crohn's disease-related fistulas [31]. The overall success rate was 71 % at 20 months of follow-up. No continence impairment was noted in any of the patients, but significant postoperative pain and anismus were noted in 8 patients (22.9 %) who were treated with the 980 nm diode laser. For this reason, the authors consider that the use of a 1479 nm diode laser for FiLaC™ is preferable to the 980 nm. In addition, they recommend the placement of a draining seton prior to the procedure to help create a more homogenous tract caliber and may contribute to the closure of secondary tracts. More recently, Oztürk and colleagues reported their results in 50 patients treated for intersphincteric and transsphincteric anal fistulas [104]. Healing rate was 82 % during a 12-month follow-up. The FiLaC™ procedure remains investigational at this stage, and additional data is needed prior to making firm recommendations for its use. So far it appears not to impact continence level; however, long-term success rate is unknown. The blind introduction of the laser catheter into the fistulous tract does not provide direct visualization of any secondary tracts which may lead to persistent disease.

Learning curve appears short based on the report of early adapters, but a significant investment in equipment is needed, and this may prove cost ineffective in the long run.

Autologous adipose-derived stem cell is a novel approach for the management of complex anal fistula [32]. A phase III multicenter, randomized, single-blind, add-on clinical trial was performed to investigate the safety and efficacy [105]. In this trial, 200 adult patients from 19 centers were randomly assigned to receive 20 million stem cells (group A), 20 million adipose-derived stem cells plus fibrin glue (group B), or fibrin glue (group C) after closure of the internal opening. Fistula healing was defined as reepithelization of the external opening and absence of collection >2 cm by MR imaging. If the fistula had not healed at 12 weeks, a second dose (40 million stem cells in groups A and B) was administered. Patients were evaluated at 24–26 weeks (primary end point) and at 1 year (long-term follow-up). In treatment of complex anal fistula, a dose of 20 or 60 million adipose-derived stem cells alone or in combination with fibrin glue was considered a safe treatment, achieving healing rates of approximately 40 % at 6 months and of more than 50 % at 1-year follow-up. It was equivalent to fibrin glue alone. No statistically significant differences were found when the three groups were compared [105]. To date, it is difficult to make a judgment of this technique because available data is limited and many questions still remain unanswered.

Rectourethral Fistulas

Definition, Classification, and Pathophysiology

The prostatic urethra is in close proximity to the rectal wall, and it is separated from the rectum by the capsule of the prostate and the Denonvillier's fascia. Rectourethral fistula (RUF) is uncommon and can be congenital or acquired, resulting from surgery, radiation, inflammatory bowel disease, malignant neoplasm, pelvic infections, or trauma. RUF is a very complex condition that negatively impacts the patient's quality of life, can lead to permanent urinary dysfunction, and often requires multiple initial interventions for symptomatic control and additional definitive repair in a significant number of patients (Figure 15-19). In the Western world, the most common mechanism of RUF is multimodality treatment for prostate cancer, including surgery, external radiation therapy (EBRT), or brachytherapy, with an incidence of 0.1–3 % in patients who received these therapies [106]. Less commonly, RUF is the result of rectal or anal cancer treatment. Radiation leads to microvascular injuries and mucosal ischemia. It has been reported that up to 50 % of patients with RUF have a history of irradiation [107]. A review by Hechenbleikner and colleagues reported that

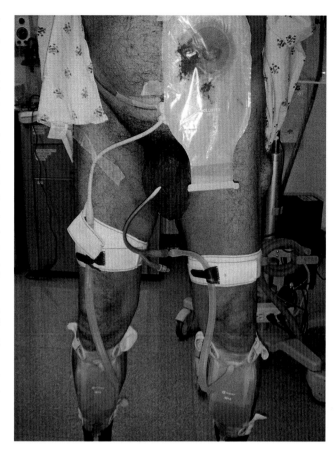

FIGURE 15-19. Patient with radiation-induced rectourethral fistula with diverting colostomy, suprapubic catheter, and urethral catheter.

radiation-induced RUF was due to EBRT in 17.8 % of cases, brachytherapy in 29.6 %, and combination therapy in 42 % [108]. The mean time from the last radiotherapy session and the diagnosis of RUF ranged from 14 months to as long as 14 years, supporting the data that the RUF is a late complication of radiotherapy. It is likely that the increased use of brachytherapy and EBRT for prostate carcinoma will increase the incidence of this condition [109]. Other causes of RUF include surgical intervention (65 %), trauma (22 %), and inflammatory bowel disease (6 %). RUF can occur following open, laparoscopic, or robotic prostatectomy for prostate cancer or abdominoperineal resection for low rectal carcinoma or anal carcinoma. Rectal injury during radical prostatectomy is uncommon with a reported overall incidence ranging from 0.12 to 9 % (0.47–2 % of laparoscopic cases) [110]. RUF can develop if the rectal injury is unrecognized at the time of operation or when primary repair of the rectum fails to heal properly [111]. The main types of trauma-related RUF are penetrating injuries, pelvic trauma/fracture, and motor vehicle accident. The etiology of the fistula greatly affects treatment choice and success, with the greatest difference occurring between irradiated vs. nonirradiated RUF.

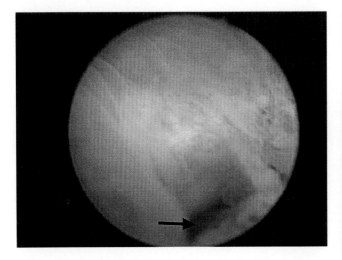

FIGURE 15-20. Cystoscopic view of external beam radiation-induced rectourethral fistula.

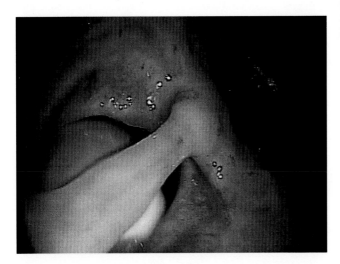

FIG. 15.21 Reflex view during flexible sigmoidoscopy demonstrates post-radical prostatectomy rectourethral fistula. Note the urethral catheter on the bladder side

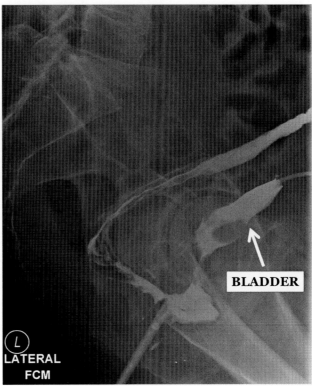

FIGURE 15-22. Gastrografin enema reveals a rectourethral fistula secondary to laparoscopic radical prostatectomy. Note the contrast flow into the bladder (*white arrow*).

Clinical Assessment and Diagnostic Evaluation

A disease-specific history (demographic data, past medical history, previous surgical and trauma history, prior radiation, onset of symptoms) is solicited from the patient. Symptoms of RUF include fecaluria, pneumaturia, hematuria, recturia, rectal bleeding, urinary tract infection, and severe rectal or pelvic pain. Physical examination (inspection, palpation, digital rectal examination) is performed to determine the size and location of the fistula in relationship to anal verge. RUFs related to prostate cancer treatment are anteriorly based and are about 5–6 cm from the anal verge in a normal size adult. The size of the fistula can vary from 5 mm to several centimeters depending on mechanism of injury and prior radiotherapy. Diagnostic modalities include cystoscopy (Figure 15-20), colonoscopy or flexible sigmoidoscopy (Figure 15-21), voiding cystography, retrograde urethrography, gastrografin enema (Figure 15-22), computed tomography scan, and magnetic resonance imaging. These investigations allow a direct visualization of the fistula and provide information of the concomitant colorectal, urethral or bladder pathology [112]. If feasible, urodynamic evaluation can be performed for the preoperative assessment of urinary function. This may impact clinical decision making as those with total urinary incontinence, or severe voiding dysfunction may be treated with a permanent urinary diversion. These diagnostic modalities are useful in the baseline assessment of the patient and are also essential to document healing after conservative management, fecal diversion alone, or definitive RUF repair. It is critical to assess complete healing prior to stoma closure in patients with fecal diversion.

Surgical Treatment

Treatment of RUF poses substantial challenges to the surgeon. Few centers have gathered a large experience in treating this rare condition. A multidisciplinary team approach involving a colorectal surgeon, a urologist, and in some instances a reconstructive surgeon is needed for optimal management. It is important to note that the management of RUF has not been standardized and large variations in treatment approaches exist due the rarity of the condition, surgeon's familiarity with a particular surgical technique, and/or patient population seen at a particular medical institution.

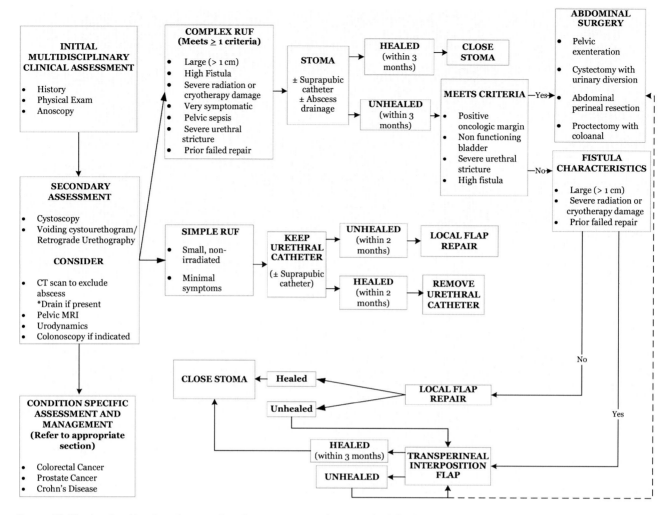

FIGURE 15-23. An algorithm-based approach to the management of rectourethral fistula.

Recently the senior author has proposed an algorithm-based approach to RUF based on his experience managing this rare entity at a tertiary center over a decade period [106].

Figure 15-23 provides the carepath algorithm. RUFs related to malignant neoplasm or Crohn's disease are managed according to these condition-specific treatment algorithms. RUFs related to radiation, cryotherapy, trauma, or prior surgical intervention such as prior prostatectomy are classified according to etiologic factor, degree of symptomatology, presence of pelvic sepsis, degree of urethral stricture, and history of prior repair. Small, minimally symptomatic, nonirradiated RUF can be managed initially with a urethral catheter and if needed suprapubic catheter drainage. Despite extensive recommendations in the literature for routine fecal diversion [113–117], cases meeting the stated criteria do sometime heal spontaneously without fecal diversion. Such cases include post laparoscopic or robotic radical prostatectomy. Chun and Abbas reported that 60 % of RUFs resulting from laparoscopic radical prostatectomy healed spontaneously with urinary +/− fecal diversion [110]. If RUF remains unhealed for 2 or more months, surgical intervention is usually warranted. Local transanal flap repair is a good option for small nonirradiated RUF. If RUF remains unhealed following local flap repair, a diverting stoma followed by additional local flap repair or transperineal repair with gracilis interposition flap or dartos flap would be the next step.

Patients with large RUF (>1 cm), prior radiation or cryotherapy, significant symptoms, severe urethral stricture, or prior failed repair require fecal diversion with suprapubic catheter drainage. Patients with postoperative or trauma-related RUF should undergo computed tomography scan of the pelvis, and if an abscess is present, it should be drained percutaneously under imaging guidance. After 3 months of fecal diversion, the RUF should be reassessed. If healed, the patient can then undergo stoma closure. It is important to reassess the patient with a minimum of two diagnostic studies (endoscopic or imaging) from the bladder and rectal side to confirm complete healing prior to closing the stoma. Patients with unhealed RUF have several options including permanent fecal diversion. Patients who desire definitive repair can be approached via a transabdominal (proctectomy with coloanal with or without omental flap, pelvic exenteration with or without sphincter preservation), transanal flap, transperineal (gracilis flap interposition or dartos flap), transsphincteric, or transsacral technique [106–132]. The first three approaches in our opinion are the most suitable. We consider a transabdominal approach in the form of pelvic exenteration (can be anal sphincter preserving with coloanal) for patients with positive oncologic margins or nonfunctioning bladder. Otherwise, a transanal or transperineal approach is considered. Transanal repair consists of endorectal advancement flap with or without biologic mesh reinforcement [117]. It is most effective for small fistula without extensive tissue damage from radiation or cryotherapy. Patients who fail transanal repair and those with extensive tissue damage, large fistula, or significant urethral stricture are best approached with transperineal repair with gracilis interposition flap. Urethral reconstruction can be achieved with a buccal mucosal flap or biologic mesh. It is important to convey to the patient the expectations and limitations of surgical treatment, including the need for multiple operations, the risk of failure, and the potential poor anorectal and urinary functions.

Transanal Approach

For a nonirradiated small RUF, a transanal approach with rectal advancement flap is a good option in patients without anal stricture [117, 121, 129]. The technical details of the flap operation have been described earlier in this chapter for complex anal fistula. After mobilization of the flap, the urethral opening is identified. Gentle debridement of any granulating tissue is performed. The procedure is typically performed in the Jack-knife prone position under spinal or general anesthesia. A modified technique of biologic mesh reinforcement of the transanal endorectal flap has been previously described [117]. The addition of biologic material can be helpful in patient with larger defect and good vascularized tissue which can facilitate tissue ingrowth. Figure 15-24a–h demonstrates the technical steps of the flap repair with mesh interposition between the prostate and rectal wall. The flap is mobilized, and gentle debridement of the fistula edges on the prostate side is performed. Tissue approximation over the urethral opening is performed if enough pliable tissue is available. Multiple 2.0 Vicryl sutures are introduced into one aspect of the biologic mesh and through the tissue at the apex of the exposed flap bed, ideally one to two centimeters proximal to the fistula opening. The biologic mesh is then parachuted into the exposed flap bed and secured in placed with the sutures. Any excess mesh is trimmed along with distal aspect of the endorectal flap. Finally the flap is secured to the edges of the dissection using 2.0 Vicryl sutures. A urethral catheter is kept for 4–6 weeks postoperatively before assessing fistula healing.

A limitation of the transanal approach is limited exposure in some patients with long anal canal and deep buttock clefts which can make it difficult to adequately mobilize the rectal flap.

Posterior Approach

High RUF can be approached via a posterior approach either through a York-Mason transsphincteric dissection or a Kraske approach [123]. The York-Mason technique involves posterior sagittal division of the anal sphincter and levator muscles as well as the posterior wall of the rectum to gain access to the fistula. Repair of the fistula is performed, followed by closure of the proctotomy and all divided tissue planes. The Kraske approach entails resection of the coccyx, division of the tissues between the coccyx and the sphincters to provide access to the posterior wall of the rectum, which is then opened to provide access to the fistula. The use of a transsphincteric approach has decreased significantly over the past years, because of the risk of fecal incontinence as a complication of anorectal sphincter surgery. Additional concern is poor tissue healing in patients with prior radiotherapy. We rarely consider this approach and favor an abdominal approach if access is needed for a high RUF.

Transperineal Approach

The transperineal approach is the preferred method for most RUFs that require interposition of healthy and well-vascularized tissue. This technique provides a good plane of dissection and exposure for low and mid RUFs. Tissue interposition can be provided with a dartos flap or gracilis muscle for larger irradiated RUF [120, 122, 125, 128, 132, 133]. The dartos flap is harvested from the posterior aspect of the scrotum and rotated inward to interpose between the repaired urethra and rectum. The operation is performed in the prone position. After harvesting the dartos flap, the interposition of the flap is performed through a perineal incision.

The transperineal gracilis muscle interposition flap is an excellent option to repair large irradiated RUFs. The procedure entails two phases: initial harvesting of the gracilis flap in the lithotomy position and then RUF repair through a perineal dissection in the prone position. The gracilis flap is traced externally about 4 cm posterior to the adductor muscle (Figure 15-25a). Three incisions are made over the course of the muscle which is isolated with Penrose drains (Figure 15-25b). The distal insertion of the muscle is then disconnected at the medial aspect of the knee, and the gracilis is dissected off surrounding tissue from distal to proximal, gradually rotating it medially. Small perforators from the superficial femoral vessels are clipped and divided. Care is taken to preserve the major neurovascular bundle which is typically located within 10 cm of the pubic symphysis (Figure 15-25c). The freed portion of the muscle is

FIGURE 15-24. (**a–h**) Transanal endorectal advancement flap with biologic mesh interposition.

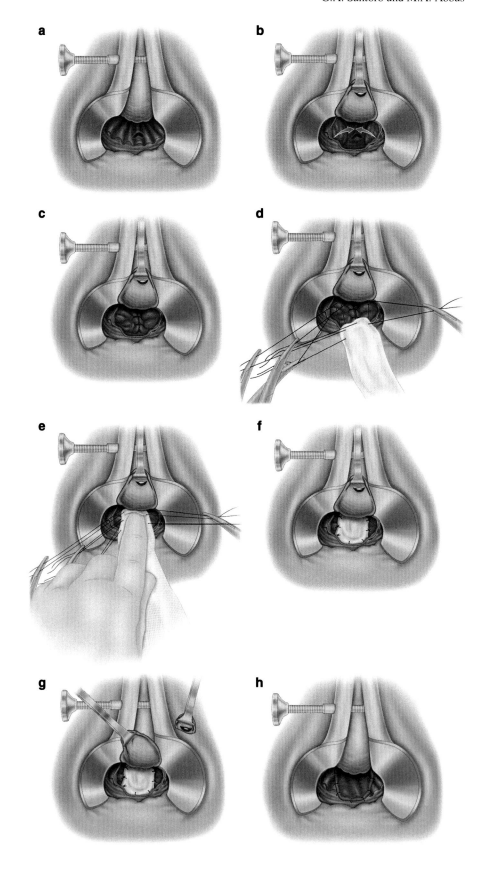

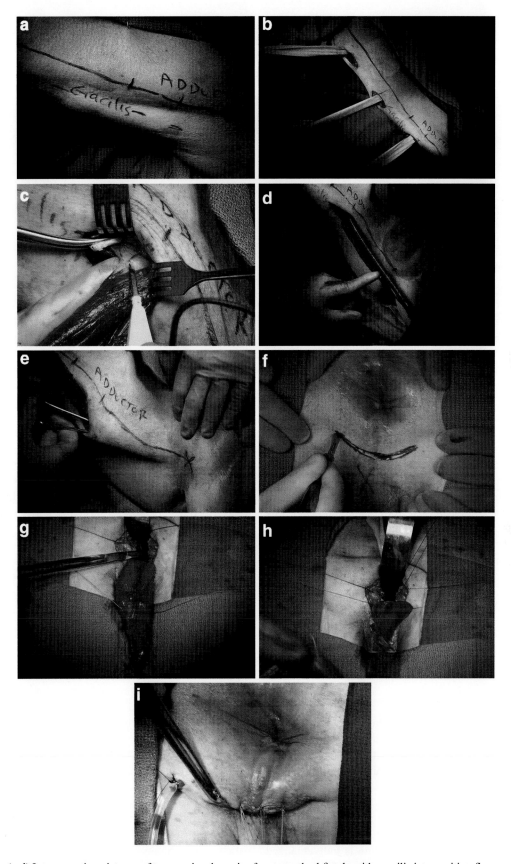

FIGURE 15-25. (a–i) Intraoperative pictures of transperineal repair of rectourethral fistula with gracilis interposition flap.

TABLE 15.4 Outcome of patients with rectourethral fistula in various series

	Year	# of patients	Procedure	Follow-up	Closure (%)
Youssef et al. [120]	1999	12	Dartos flap	9–42 months	69
Garofalo et al. [121]	2003	14	Rectal flap	31 months	68
Lane et al. [107]	2006	22	Transabdominal (68 %)	29 months	88
Wexner et al. [122]	2008	36	Gracilis flap	N.R.	78
Ghoneim et al. [125]	2008	25	Gracilis flap	28 months	100
Gupta et al. [126]	2008	10	Gracilis flap	24 months	100
Ulrich et al. [127]	2009	26	Gracilis flap	22 months	100
Kasraeian et al. [123]	2009	12	Transsphincteric	22 months	75
Vanni et al. [124]	2010	74	Gracilis flap + tissue rectal flap	20 months	92
Samplaski et al. [128]	2011	13	Gracilis flap	2.5 months	92
Hechenbleikner et al. [108]	2013	416	Gracilis flap (72 %)	N.R.	87.5
Keller et al. [106][a]	2015	30	Transperineal (54 %) Transanal (31 %) Transabdominal (15 %)	72 months	90

[a]43 % required definitive fistula repair

exteriorized through the most proximal skin incision and rotated to ensure adequate length for perineal coverage (Figure 15-25d). A subcutaneous passage is created using a large clamp to tunnel the muscle from the medial aspect of the thigh to the perineum (Figure 15-25e). The skin incisions over the medial thigh are closed after placing a subcutaneous drain. The patient is then placed in the prone position. Using curvilinear incision centered over the perineum, dissection is carried anterior to the anal sphincter muscle and through the rectoprostatic plane (Figure 15-25f). Once the plane of the fistula is entered, the dissection is carried another 3–4 cm cephalad. If urethral reconstruction is needed, it is carried out at this phase of the operation using either biologic mesh or buccal mucosa flap harvested from the mouth [124]. The next step is interposing the gracilis flap. Sutures are placed in the muscle edges using 2.0 Vicryl (UR6 needles) and the apex of the dissection cephalad to level of fistula (Figure 15-25g). The muscle is then parachuted into the wound and gently guided to cover the entire bed of the dissection (Figure 15-25h). Additional sutures are placed as needed to secure the muscle in place. The subcutaneous portion of the wound is then closed in layers over a drain and skin is closed (Figure 15-25i).

Transabdominal Approach

In general, we reserve a transabdominal approach for select group of patients with RUF. Patients with postoperative RUF following prostate or rectal surgery and positive oncologic margins can be offered a transabdominal approach. Additional indications include high RUF not accessible to a transanal or transperineal approach, patients with nonfunctioning irradiated bladder or severely stricture urethra which requires excision with urinary diversion, and patients with prior failed repairs. The type of abdominal operation is individualized based on patient- and disease-related factors. Options include cystectomy with urinary diversion, proctectomy with coloanal

anastomosis, abdominoperineal resection, and pelvic exenteration. An omental flap or rectus abdominis flap interposition can be used if needed. The omentum is dissected preserving the left gastroepiploic artery as main blood supply. The flap is placed between the rectum and the urethra after pelvic dissection is carried out to divide and resect the fistula. Primary repair of the rectal wall is performed and covered with the omental flap. If the rectal defect is too large to close and tissue quality is poor, proctectomy with or without sphincter preservation is indicated. Dissection is carried down to the levator muscles to reach below the level of the fistula. For high RUF, the rectum is divided with a stapler at the level of the anorectal junction if technically feasible, and a stapled coloanal anastomosis can be performed. For mid to low RUF, mucosectomy or intersphincteric dissection is performed from below to complete the dissection, and intestinal continuity is restored with a handsewn anastomosis. Abdominoperineal resection can be performed if not sphincter preservation is indicated.

Outcome

The outcome of RUF treatment is difficult to evaluate because published studies with large number of patients are scarce. Significant heterogeneity exists in the various reports due to differences in patient populations and operative techniques. Table 15-4 summarizes the results of several large series [106–108, 120–128]. The reported success rate following definitive operative intervention ranges from 68 to 100 %. However, it is important to emphasize the various management strategies in the published reports. Not all patients require definitive repair. A spontaneous closure rate of 14–46.5 % has been reported after fecal diversion, and some patients can heal small RUF with urethral catheter drainage alone [106]. In a systematic review, Hechenbleikner and colleagues reported similar RUF closure rate in nonirradiated and irradiated patients (89 % vs. 90 %), but the permanent fecal diversion rate was 25 % in irradiated patients compared to 3.8 % in nonirradiated patients [108]. The overall permanent urinary diversion rate was 8.3 % and was significantly higher in irradiated patients (42.5 %) compared to nonirradiated patients (4 %).

The transanal approach with rectal advancement flap is safe and effective in the absence of prior radiation therapy [106, 121]. Garofalo and colleagues reported 85 % closure rate with this technique in 12 patients at the Cleveland clinic [121]. Indication for local flap is small nonirradiated fistula, whereas large fistula requires a more complex procedure. The gracilis muscle interposition is currently the most commonly used method for treating complex, large, recurrent, and/or irradiated RUF. In a systematic review, including 416 patients (40 % with previous pelvic irradiation and/or ablation), most RUFs (90 %) underwent 1 of 4 categories of repair: transanal (5.9 %), transabdominal (12.5 %), transsphincteric (15.7 %), and transperineal (65.9 %) [108]. Tissue interposition flaps, predominantly gracilis muscle, were used in 72 % of repairs. Fistula closure was successful in 87.5 %. Overall permanent fecal and/or urinary diversion rates were 10.6 and 8.3 %. Wexner and colleagues reported their results in 36 males who underwent the gracilis interposition for RUF, mainly due to prostate cancer treatment [122]. Thirteen patients (36 %) had a mean of 1.5 prior failed repairs (range 1–3) [122]. Seventeen patients (47 %) experienced postoperative complications. The initial success rate was 78 %. After a second procedure in 8 patients, the overall clinical healing rate was 97 %.

Proctectomy with coloanal procedure can be considered in select cases in presence of a hostile pelvis, previous radiation therapy, previous attempt at repair, and under a defunctioning stoma. Patsouras and colleagues reported a success rate of 50 % in four patients treated with this technique [118].

Postoperative Fistulas

Definition, Classification, and Pathophysiology

Restorative proctocolectomy (RPC) with ileal-pouch-anal anastomosis (IPAA) has evolved as the mainstay surgical treatment for patients with intractable ulcerative colitis and familial adenomatous polyposis. Ileal-pouch fistula is uncommon but a highly morbid complication. The fistula tract can be classified as pouch anal, pouch vaginal, and pouch perineal. Pouch-anal fistula is defined as a fistulous tract with an internal opening at or above the ileoanal anastomosis and an external opening below the IPAA at the anal canal or perineal skin. Pouch-vaginal fistula may be classified relative to the anastomotic suture line (above, below, or at the level of anastomosis). Fistula is defined as complex if there are multiple tracts and/or the internal opening is at or above the IPAA (high fistula) [134, 135]. Perianal fistula

may occur as a postoperative complication after ultralow anterior resection, coloanal anastomosis, Hartmann reversal procedure, abdominoperineal resection, or transanal endoscopic microsurgery for distal rectal cancer [136, 137]. Major risk factors associated with development of postoperative fistulas include elderly age, diabetes, vasculopathy, smoking, preoperative/postoperative radiotherapy, operative technique, and postoperative pelvic sepsis. Good surgical technique, avoidance of postoperative pelvic sepsis, careful dissection through the rectovaginal septum to avoid incorporating the vagina in the anastomosis when firing the stapler, a tension-free anastomosis with good blood supply, staged procedures, and temporary diversion are of fundamental importance for successful healing of bowel anastomosis and avoidance of such complications.

Clinical Assessment and Diagnostic Evaluation

A disease-specific history includes demographic characteristics, diagnosis at the previous anorectal surgery (inflammatory bowel disease, familial adenomatous polyposis, rectal cancer), and type of surgery (coloanal or colorectal anastomosis; one-stage, two-stage, or three-stage RPC; mean time between the different stages; pouch configuration; stapled or handsewn anastomosis; mean distance of anastomosis from anal verge; postoperative pelvic sepsis), symptoms, and the median time to fistula presentation. Fistulas often present with pelvic and perianal sepsis or drainage and pain. Careful physical examination (inspection, palpation, digital rectal examination, probing) should be performed. Patients with acute pouch-anal sepsis or complicated perianal disease or an inadequate clinical assessment should undergo examination under anesthesia. Preoperative imaging to evaluate the anatomy of the fistula tract includes endoanal ultrasound, pelvic MR imaging, CT scan, pouchography, and fistulography.

Surgical Treatment

Because of the low incidence of these fistulas, the optimal management continues to be controversial. The guiding principles are to control pelvic and perianal sepsis and eliminate the fistulous tract. An acute abscess should be drained, and when necessary, a noncutting seton may be placed to control anorectal infection. Operative techniques include gracilis muscle interposition, lay-open fistulotomy, collagen plug insertion, ileal advancement flap, transvaginal advancement flap, fibrin glue, transperineal repair, Martius (i.e., bulbocavernosus) flap, pouch excision, or redo pouch [134–142]. Pouch-vaginal fistula can persist and recur indefinitely, even after repeated repairs. Simple procedures should be attempted first, if there is a chance of success, before more complex procedures are considered. Temporary diverting ileostomy, permanent end ileostomy with/without pouch excision, and redo-RPC should be considered in patients with ileal-pouch fistulas. Temporary diverting colostomy with/without colo-anal/colorectal anastomoses or permanent end colostomy with/without anastomoses removal or completion proctectomy should be considered in rectal cancer patients [138]. Complex perineal fistula occurring after APR or pelvic exenteration can be treated by the use of an omentoplasty or rectus abdominis musculocutaneous flap to fill the dead space of the pelvis with well-vascularized tissue. If the omentum is not sufficient or the rectus abdominis is not an option due to the presence of a colostomy and urostomy through both muscles, a biological mesh and/or a gluteal flap can be utilized. Medical treatment including anti-TNF agents should be the first-line therapy for patients who present delayed onset of pouch fistula and a suspicion for Crohn's fistula.

Outcome

Gaertner and colleagues conducted a retrospective review on 342 patients who underwent RPC and found 25 patients (7 %) who presented with symptomatic ileal-pouch fistula [140]. Complete fistula healing occurred in 64 % of patients at a median follow-up of 29 months. Operative techniques were heterogeneous, and each patient underwent an average of 2.8 procedures. Mallick and colleagues reviewed the Cleveland Clinic experience with pouch-vaginal fistulas [141]. Fistula occurred in 102 females: 59 at ≤12 months (early fistula) and 43 at > 12 months (late-onset fistula). Local repair was performed in 77.3 % of patients (ileal-pouch advancement flap in 49.5 % of cases and transvaginal repair in 27.8 % of cases). The healing rate after ileal-pouch advancement flap was 42 % when performed as a primary procedure and 66 % when performed secondarily after a different procedure. The healing rate for transvaginal repair was 55 % when done as a primary procedure and 40 % when performed secondarily. Nineteen patients underwent redo ileal-pouch construction, with an overall pouch retention rate of 40 %. At median follow-up of 83 months, 57.7 % of the 102 patients had healed the pouch-vaginal fistula, whereas pouch failure occurred in 34 women (35 %, 12 early onset and 22 late onset). Heriot and colleagues assessed the short-term and long-term outcomes of surgical repair of 68 patients with pouch-vaginal fistula after RPC at St. Mark's Hospital [142]. Surgery was undertaken in 87 % of patients: 24 % pouch excision/diversion or seton drainage and 66 % primary repair. Overall primary healing rate was 40 % at a median follow-up of 19 months. The overall pouch failure rate for patients with pouch-vaginal fistula was 35 %.

References

1. Steele SR, Kumar R, Feingold D, Rafferty JL, Buie WD. The standards practice task force, the American Society of Colon and Rectal Surgeons. Practice parameters for the treatment of perianal abscess and fistula-in-ano. Dis Colon Rectum. 2011; 54:1465–74.

2. Abbas MA, Jackson C, Haigh PI. Predictors of outcome for anal fistula surgery. Arch Surg. 2011;146(9):1011–6.

3. Jorge JM, Wexner SD. Etiology and management of fecal incontinence. Dis Colon Rectum. 1993;36:77–97.

4. Deen KI, Williams JG, Hutchinson R, Keighley MR, Kumar D. Fistulas in ano: endoanal ultrasonographic assessment assists decision making for surgery. Gut. 1994;35:391–4.

5. Poen AC, Felt-Bersma RJF, Eijsbouts QA, Cuesta MA, Meuwissen SG. Hydrogen peroxide-enhanced transanal ultrasound in the assessment of fistula-in-ano. Dis Colon Rectum. 1998;41:1147–52.

6. Ratto C, Gentile E, Merico M, Spinazzola C, Mangini G, Sofo L, Doglietto G. How can the assessment of fistula-in-ano be improved? Dis Colon Rectum. 2000;43:1375–82.

7. Santoro GA, Fortling B. The advantages of volume rendering in three-dimensional endosonography of the anorectum. Dis Colon Rectum. 2007;50:359–68.

8. Vanbeckevoort D, Bielen D, Vanslembrouck R, Van Assche G. Magnetic resonance imaging of perianal fistulas. Magn Reson Imaging Clin N Am. 2014;22:113–23.

9. Weisman N, Abbas MA. Can pre-operative anal ultrasound predict surgical outcome for fistula-in-ano? Dis Colon Rectum. 2008;51:1089–92.

10. Buchanan G, Halligan S, Williams A, Cohen CR, Tarroni D, Phillips RK, Bartram CI. Effect of MRI on clinical outcome of recurrent fistula-in-ano. Lancet. 2002;360:1661–2.

11. Orsoni P, Barthet M, Portier F, Panuel M, Desjeux A, Grimaud JC. Prospective comparison of endosonography, magnetic resonance imaging and surgical findings in anorectal fistula and abscess complicating Crohn's disease. Br J Surg. 1999; 86:360–4.

12. Schwartz DA, Wiersema MJ, Dudiak KM, Fletcher JG, Clain JE, Tremaine WJ, Zinsmeister AR, Norton ID, Boardman LA, Devine RM, Wolff BG, Young-Fadok TM, Diehl NN, Pemberton JH, Sandborn WJ. A comparison of endoscopic ultrasound, magnetic resonance imaging, and exam under anesthesia for evaluation of Crohn's perianal fistulas. Gastroenterology. 2001;121:1064–72.

13. Buchanan GN, Bartram CI, Williams AB, Halligan S, Cohen CR. Value of hydrogen peroxide enhancement of three-dimensional endoanal ultrasound in fistula-in-ano. Dis Colon Rectum. 2005;48:141–7.

14. West RL, Zimmerman DD, Dwarkasing S, Hussain SM, Hop WC, Schouten WR, Kuipers EJ, Felt-Bersma RJ. Prospective comparison of hydrogen peroxide-enhanced three-dimensional endoanal ultrasonography and endoanal magnetic resonance imaging of perianal fistulas. Dis Colon Rectum. 2003;46:1407–15.

15. Ratto C, Grillo E, Parello A, Costamagna G, Doglietto GB. Endoanal ultrasound-guided surgery for anal fistula. Endoscopy. 2005;37:722–8.

16. Buchanan GN, Halligan S, Bartram CI, Williams AB, Tarroni D, Cohen CR. Clinical examination, endosonography and MR imaging in preoperative assessment of fistula in ano: comparison with outcome-based reference standard. Radiology. 2004;233:674–81.

17. Sahni VA, Ahmad R, Burling D. Which method is best for imaging of perianal fistula? Abdom Imaging. 2008;33: 26–30.

18. Soerensen MM, Pedersen BG, Santoro GA, Buntzen S, Bek K, Laurberg S. Long-term function and morphology of the anal

sphincters and the pelvic floor after primary repair of obstetric anal sphincter injury. Colorectal Dis. 2014;16:347–55.

19. Vitton V, Ben Hadj Amor W, Baumstarck K, Behr M, Bouvier M, Grimaud JC. Comparison of three-dimensional high-resolution manometry and endoanal ultrasound in the diagnosis of anal sphincter defects. Colorectal Dis. 2013;15:607–11.

20. Limura E, Giordano P. Modern management of anal fistula. World J Gastroenterol. 2015;21:12–20.

21. Subhas G, Singh Bhullar J, Al-Omari A, Unawane A, Mittal VK, Pearlman R. Setons in the treatment of anal fistula: review of variations in materials and techniques. Dig Surg. 2012;29:292–300.

22. Abbas MA, Sherman M. Endorectal advancement flap. In: Fleshman J, Wexner SD, editors. Master techniques in colon and rectal surgery. 1st ed. Baltimore, USA: Lippincott Williams & Wilkins; 2012.

23. Rojanasakul A, Pattanaarun J, Sahakitrungruang C, Tantiphlachiva K. Total anal sphincter saving technique for fistula-in-ano: the ligation of intersphincteric fistula tract. J Med Assoc Thai. 2007;90:581–6.

24. Ellis CN. Outcomes with the use of bioprosthetic grafts to reinforce the ligation of the intersphincteric fistula tract (BioLIFT procedure) for the management of complex anal fistulas. Dis Colon Rectum. 2010;53:1361–4.

25. Sirikurnpiboon S, Awapittaya B, Jivapaisarnpong P. Ligation of intersphincteric fistula tract and its modification: results from treatment of complex fistula. World J Gastrointest Surg. 2013;5:123–8.

26. Ratto C, Litta F, Parello A, Zaccone G, Donisi L, De Simone V. Fistulotomy with end-to-end primary sphincteroplasty for anal fistula: results from a prospective study. Dis Colon Rectum. 2013;56:226–33.

27. The Surgisis AFP anal fistula plug: report of a consensus conference. Colorectal Dis. 2008;10:17–20.

28. Ommer A, Herold A, Joos A, Schmidt C, Weyand G, Bussen D. Gore BioA Fistula Plug in the treatment of high anal fistulas – initial results from a German multicenter study. Ger Med Sci. 2012;10:1–17.

29. Swinscoe MT, Ventakasubramaniam AK, Jayne DG. Fibrin glue for fistula-in-ano: the evidence reviewed. Tech Coloproctol. 2005;9:89–94.

30. Meinero P, Mori L. Video-assisted anal fistula treatment (VAAFT): a novel sphincter-saving procedure for treating complex anal fistulas. Tech Coloproctol. 2011;15:417–22.

31. Giamundo P, Geraci M, Tibaldi L, Valente M. Closure of fistula-in-ano with laser-FiLaC™: an effective novel sphincter-saving procedure for complex disease. Colorectal Dis. 2014;16:110–5.

32. Georgiev-Hristov T, García-Arranz M, García-Olmo D. Adipose tissue-derived products for complex fistula treatment. Tech Coloproctol. 2013;17:675–6.

33. Beaulieu R, Bonekamp D, Sandone C, Gearhart S. Fistula-in-ano: when to cut, tie, plug, or sew. J Gastrointest Surg. 2013;17:1143–52.

34. Gupta PJ, Gupta SN, Heda PS. Which treatment for anal fistula? Cut or cover, plug or paste, loop or lift. Acta Chir Iugosl. 2012;59:15–20.

35. Zbar AP, Ramesh J, Beer-Gabel M, Salazar R, Pescatori M. Conventional cutting vs. internal anal sphincter-preserving seton for high trans-sphincteric fistula: a prospective randomized manometric and clinical trial. Tech Coloproctol. 2003;7:89–94.

36. García-Aguilar J, Belmonte C, Wong DW, Goldberg SM, Madoff RD. Cutting seton versus two-stage seton fistulotomy in the surgical management of high anal fistula. Br J Surg. 1998;85:243–5.

37. Vial M, Parés D, Pera M, Grande L. Faecal incontinence after seton treatment for anal fistulae with and without surgical division of internal anal sphincter: a systematic review. Colorectal Dis. 2010;12:172–8.

38. Hasegawa H, Radley S, Keighley MR. Long-term results of cutting seton fistulotomy. Acta Chir Iugoslavica. 2000;47:19–21.

39. Isbister WH, Sanea N. The cutting seton: an experience at King Faisal Specialist Hospital. Dis Colon Rectum. 2001;44:722–7.

40. Mentes BB, Oktemer S, Tezcaner T, Azili C, Leventoğlu S, Oğuz M. Elastic one-stage cutting seton for the treatment of high anal fistulas: preliminary results. Tech Coloproctol. 2004;8:159–62.

41. Williams JG, Farrands PA, Williams AB, Taylor BA, Lunniss PJ, Sagar PM, Varma JS, George BD, et al. The treatment of anal fistula: ACPGBI position statement. Colorectal Dis. 2007;9 Suppl 4:18–50.

42. Abbas MA, Lemus-Rangel R, Hamadani A. Long-term outcome of endorectal advancement flap for complex anorectal fistulae. Am Surgeon. 2008;74:921–4.

43. Perez F, Arroyo A, Serrano P, Sánchez A, Candela F, Perez MT, Calpena R. Randomized clinical and manometric study of advancement flap versus fistulotomy with sphincter reconstruction in the management of complex fistula-in-ano. Am J Surg. 2006;192:34–40.

44. Zimmerman DD, Briel JW, Gosselink MP, Schouten WR. Anocutaneous advancement flap repair of transsphincteric fistulas. Dis Colon Rectum. 2001;44:1474–80.

45. Ortiz H, Marzo J. Endorectal flap advancement repair and fistulectomy for high trans-sphincteric and suprasphincteric fistulas. Br J Surg. 2000;87:1680–3.

46. Schouten WR, Zimmerman DD, Briel JW. Transanal advancement flap repair of transsphincteric fistulas. Dis Colon Rectum. 1999;42:1419–23.

47. Jarrar A, Church J. Advancement flap repair: a good option for complex anorectal fistulas. Dis Colon Rectum. 2011;54:1537–41.

48. Dubsky PC, Stift A, Friedl J, Teleky B, Herbst F. Endorectal advancement flaps in the treatment of high anal fistula of cryptoglandular origin: full-thickness vs. mucosal-rectum flaps. Dis Colon Rectum. 2008;51:852–7.

49. van der Hagen SJ, Baeten CG, Soeters PB, van Gemert WG. Autologous platelet derived grow factors (platelet rich plasma) as an adjunct to mucosal advancement flap in high cryptoglandular peri-anal fistulae: a pilot study. Colorectal Dis. 2011;13:784–90.

50. Zimmerman DD, Delemarre JB, Gosselink MP, Hop WC, Briel JW, Schouten WR. Smoking affects the outcome of transanal mucosal advancement flap repair of trans-sphincteric fistulas. Br J Surg. 2003;90:351–4.

51. Zimmerman DD, Gosselink MP, Mitalas LE, Mitalas LE, Delemarre JB, Hop WJ, Briel JW, Schouten WR. Smoking impairs rectal mucosal blood flow- a pilot study: possible implications for transanal advancement flap repair. Dis Colon Rectum. 2005;48:1228–32.

52. Shanwani A, Nor AM, Amri N. Ligation of the intersphincteric fistula tract (LIFT): a sphincter-saving technique for fistula-in-ano. Dis Colon Rectum. 2010;53:39–42.

53. Aboulian A, Kaji AH, Kumar RR. Early result of ligation of the intersphincteric fistula tract for fistula-in-ano. Dis Colon Rectum. 2011;54:289–92.

54. Tan KK, Tan IJ, Lim FS, Koh DC, Tsang CB. The anatomy of failures following the ligation of intersphincteric tract technique for anal fistula: a review of 93 patients over 4 years. Dis Colon Rectum. 2011;54:1368–72.

55. Abcarian AM, Estrada JJ, Park J, Corning C, Chaudhry V, Cintron J, Prasad L, Abcarian H. Ligation of intersphincteric fistula tract: early results of a pilot study. Dis Colon Rectum. 2012;55:778–82.

56. Mushaya C, Bartlett L, Schulze B, Ho YH. Ligation of intersphincteric fistula tract compared with advancement flap for complex anorectal fistulas requiring initial seton drainage. Am J Surg. 2012;204:283–9.

57. Ooi K, Skinner I, Croxford M, Faragher I, McLaughlin S. Managing fistula-in-ano with ligation of the intersphincteric fistula tract procedure: the Western Hospital experience. Colorectal Dis. 2012;14:599–603.

58. Wallin UG, Mellgren AF, Madoff RD, Goldberg SM. Does ligation of the intersphincteric fistula tract raise the bar in fistula surgery? Dis Colon Rectum. 2012;55:1173–8.

59. Han JG, Yi BQ, Wang ZJ, Zheng Y, Cui JJ, Yu XQ, Zhao BC, Yang XQ. Ligation of the intersphincteric fistula tract plus a bioprosthetic anal fistula plug (LIFT-Plug): a new technique for fistula-in-ano. Colorectal Dis. 2013;15:582–6.

60. van Onkelen RS, Gosselink MP, Schouten WR. Ligation of the intersphincteric fistula tract in low transsphincteric fistulae: a new technique to avoid fistulotomy. Colorectal Dis. 2013;15:587–91.

61. Lehmann JP, Graf W. Efficacy of LIFT for recurrent anal fistulas. Colorectal Dis. 2013;15:592–5.

62. Sileri P, Giarratano G, Franceschilli L, Limura E, Perrone F, Stazi A, Toscana C, Gaspari AL. Ligation of the intersphincteric fistula tract (LIFT): a minimally invasive procedure for complex anal fistula: two-year results of a prospective multicentric study. Surg Innov. 2014;21:476–80.

63. Yassin NA, Hammond TM, Lunniss PJ, Phillips RK. Ligation of the intersphincteric fistula tract in the management of anal fistula. A systematic review. Colorectal Dis. 2013;15:527–35.

64. Vergara-Fernandez O, Espino-Urbina LA. Ligation of the intersphincteric fistula tract: what is the evidence in a review? World J Gastroenterol. 2013;19:6805–13.

65. Hong KD, Kang S, Kalaskar S, Wexner SD. Ligation of intersphincteric fistula tract (LIFT) to treat anal fistula: systematic review and meta-analysis. Tech Coloproctol. 2014;18:685–91.

66. Tan KK, Alsuwaigh R, Tan AM, Tan IJ, Liu X, Koh DC. To LIFT or to flap? Which surgery to perform following seton insertion for high anal fistulas? Dis Colon Rectum. 2012;55:1273–7.

67. Madbouly KM, El Shazly W, Abbas KS, Hussein AM. Ligation of intersphincteric fistula tract versus mucosal advancement flap in patients with high transsphincteric fistula-in-ano: a prospective randomized trial. Dis Colon Rectum. 2014;57:1202–8.

68. Chew MH, Lee PJ, Koh CE, Chew HE. Appraisal of the LIFT and BIOLIFT procedure: initial experience and short-term outcomes of 33 consecutive patients. Int J Colorectal Dis. 2013;28:1489–96.

69. Garg P, Song J, Bhatia A, Kalia H, Menon GR. The efficacy of anal fistula plug in fistula-in-ano: a systematic review. Colorectal Dis. 2010;12:965–70.

70. Johnson EK, Gaw JU, Armstrong DN. Efficacy of anal fistula plug vs. fibrin glue in closure of anorectal fistulas. Dis Colon Rectum. 2006;49:371–6.

71. Champagne BJ, O'Connor LM, Ferguson M, Orangio GR, Schertzer ME, Armstrong DN. Efficacy of anal fistula plug in closure of cryptoglandular fistulas: long-term follow-up. Dis Colon Rectum. 2006;49:1817–21.

72. Schwandner O, Stadler F, Dietl O, Wirsching RP, Fuerst A. Initial experience on efficacy in closure of cryptoglandular and Crohn's transsphincteric fistulas by the use of the anal fistula plug. Int J Colorectal Dis. 2008;23:319–24.

73. Christoforidis D, Etzioni DA, Goldberg SM, Madoff RD, Mellgren A. Treatment of complex anal fistulas with the collagen fistula plug. Dis Colon Rectum. 2008;51:1482–7.

74. Thekkinkattil DK, Botterill I, Ambrose NS, Lundby L, Sagar PM, Buntzen S, Finan PJ. Efficacy of the anal fistula plug in complex anorectal fistulae. Colorectal Dis. 2009;11:584–7.

75. Starck M, Bohe M, Zawadzki A. Success rate of closure of high transsphincteric fistula using anal fistula plug. Dis Colon Rectum. 2008;51:692.

76. Lawes DA, Efron JE, Abbas MA, Tejirian T, Hamadani A, Young-Fadok TM, Heppell J. Early experience with the bioabsorbable anal fistula plug. World J Surg. 2008;32:1157–9.

77. Safar B, Jobanputra S, Sands D, Weiss EG, Nogueras JJ, Wexner SD. Anal fistula plug: initial experience and outcomes. Dis Colon Rectum. 2009;52:248–52.

78. Ortiz H, Marzo J, Ciga MA, Oteiza F, Armendáriz P, de Miguel M. Randomized clinical trial of anal fistula plug versus endorectal advancement flap for the treatment of high cryptoglandular fistula in ano. Br J Surg. 2009;96:608–12.

79. Wang JY, Garcia-Aguilar J, Sternberg JA, Abel ME, Varma MG. Treatment of transsphincteric anal fistulas: are fistula plugs an acceptable alternative? Dis Colon Rectum. 2009;52:692–7.

80. McGee MF, Champagne BJ, Stulberg JJ, Reynolds H, Marderstein E, Delaney CP. Tract length predicts successful closure with anal fistula plug in cryptoglandular fistulas. Dis Colon Rectum. 2010;53:1116–20.

81. Anyadike C, Attuwaybi B, Visco J, Butler B, Barrios G. The anal fistula plug in simple and complex fistula-in-ano: a western New York experience. Dis Colon Rectum. 2010;53:575.

82. van Koperen PJ, Bemelman WA, Gerhards MF, Janssen LW, van Tets WF, van Dalsen AD, Slors JF. The anal fistula plug treatment compared with the mucosal advancement flap for cryptoglandular high transsphincteric perianal fistula: a double-blinded multicenter randomized trial. Dis Colon Rectum. 2011;54:387–93.

83. O'Riordan JM, Datta I, Johnston C, Baxter NN. A systematic review of the anal fistula plug for patients with Crohn's and non-Crohn's related fistula-in-ano. Dis Colon Rectum. 2012;55:351–8.

84. Muhlmann MD, Hayes JL, Merrie AE, Parry BR, Bissett IP. Complex anal fistulas: plug or flap? ANZ J Surg. 2011; 81:720–4.

85. Heydari A, Attinà GM, Merolla E, Piccoli M, Fazlalizadeh R, Melotti G. Bioabsorbable synthetic plug in the treatment of anal fistulas. Dis Colon Rectum. 2013;56:774–9.

86. Buchberg B, Masoomi H, Choi J, Bergman H, Mills S, Stamos MJ. A tale of two (anal fistula) plugs: is there a difference in short-term outcomes? Am Surg. 2010;76:1150–3.

87. Cintron JR, Park JJ, Orsay CP, Pearl RK, Nelson RL, Sone JH, Song R, Abcarian H. Repair of fistulas-in-ano using fibrin adhesive: long-term follow-up. Dis Colon Rectum. 2000;43:944–9.

88. Sentovich SM. Fibrin glue for anal fistulas: long-term results. Dis Colon Rectum. 2003;46:498–502.

89. Loungnarath R, Dietz DW, Mutch MG, Birnbaum EH, Kodner IJ, Fleshman JW. Fibrin glue treatment of complex anal fistulas has low success rate. Dis Colon Rectum. 2004;47:432–6.

90. van Koperen PJ, Wind J, Bemelman WA, Slors JF. Fibrin glue and transanal rectal advancement flap for high transsphincteric perianal fistulas; is there any advantage? Int J Colorectal Dis. 2008;23:697–701.

91. Singer M, Cintron J, Nelson R, Orsay C, Bastawrous A, Pearl R, Sone J, Abcarian H. Treatment of fistulas-in-ano with fibrin sealant in combination with intra-adhesive antibiotics and/or surgical closure of the internal fistula opening. Dis Colon Rectum. 2005;48:799–808.

92. Jain SK, Kaza RC, Pahwa M, Bansal S. Role of cyanoacrylate in the management of low fistula in ano: a prospective study. Int J Colorectal Dis. 2008;23:355–8.

93. Barillari P, Basso L, Larcinese A, Gozzo P, Indinnimeo M. Cyanoacrylate glue in the treatment of ano-rectal fistulas. Int J Colorectal Dis. 2006;21:791–4.

94. Buchanan GN, Bartram CI, Phillips RK, Gould SW, Halligan S, Rockall TA, Sibbons P, Cohen RG. Efficacy of fibrin sealant in the management of complex anal fistula. Dis Colon Rectum. 2003;46:1167–74.

95. Jacob TJ, Perakath B, Keighley MR. Surgical intervention for anorectal fistula. Cochrane Database Syst Rev. 2010.

96. Parkash S, Lakshmiratan V, Gajendran V. Fistula-in-ano: treatment by fistulectomy, primary closure and reconstitution. Aust N Z J Surg. 1985;55:23–7.

97. Christiansen J, Rønholt C. Treatment of recurrent high anal fistula by total excision and primary sphincter reconstruction. Int J Colorectal Dis. 1995;10:207–9.

98. Roig JV, García-Armengol J, Jordán JC, Moro D, García-Granero E, Alós R. Fistulectomy and sphincteric reconstruction for complex cryptoglandular fistulas. Colorectal Dis. 2010;12:145–52.

99. Kraemer M, Picke D. Fistulotomy with primary sphincter repair for the treatment of anal fistula. Coloproctology. 2011; 33:104–8.

100. Arroyo A, Perez-Legaz J, Moya P, Armananzes L, Lacueva J, Perez-Vicente F, Candela F, Calpena R. Fistulotomy and sphincter reconstruction in the treatment of complex fistula-in-ano. Long-term clinical and manometric results. Ann Surg. 2012;255:935–9.

101. Ommer A, Herold A, Berg E, Furst A, Sailer M, Schiedeck T. German Society for General and Visceral Surgery. Cryptoglandular anal fistulas. Dtsch Arztebl Int. 2011;108: 707–13.

102. Kochhar G, Saha S, Andley M, Kumar A, Saurabh G, Pusuluri R, Bhise V, Kumar A. Video-assisted anal fistula treatment. JSLS. 2014;18:e2014.00127.

103. Wałęga P, Romaniszyn M, Nowak W. VAAFT: a new minimally invasive method in the diagnostics and treatment of anal fistulas-initial results. Pol Przegl Chir. 2014;86:7–10.

104. Oztürk E, Gülcü B. Laser ablation of fistula tract: a sphincter preserving method for treating fistula-in-ano. Dis Colon Rectum. 2014;57:360–4.

105. Herreros MD, Garcia-Arranz M, Guadalajara H, De-La-Quintana P, Garcia-Olmo D, Collaborative Group FATT. Autologous expanded adipose-derived stem cells for the treatment of complex cryptoglandular perianal fistulas: a phase III randomized clinical trial (FATT 1: fistula Advanced Therapy Trial 1) and long-term evaluation. Dis Colon Rectum. 2012; 55:762–72.

106. Keller DS, Aboseif SR, Lesser T, Abbass MA, Tsay AT, Abbas MA. Algorithm based multidisciplinary team treatment approach to rectourethral fistula. Int J Colorectal Disease. 2015;30:631–8.

107. Lane BR, Stein DE, Remzi FH, Strong SA, Fazio VW, Angermeier KW. Management of radiotherapy induced rectourethral fistula. J Urol. 2006;175:1382–7.

108. Hechenbleikner EM, Buckley JC, Wick EC. Acquired rectourethral fistulas in adults: a systematic review of surgical repair techniques and outcomes. Dis Colon Rectum. 2013; 56:374–83.

109. Hanna JM, Turley R, Castleberry A, Hopkins T, Peterson AC, Mantyh C, Migaly J. Surgical management of complex rectourethral fistulas in irradiated and nonirradiated patients. Dis Colon Rectum. 2014;57:1105–12.

110. Chun L, Abbas MA. Rectourethral fistula following laparoscopic radical prostatectomy. Tech Coloproctol. 2011;15: 297–300.

111. Blumberg JM, Lesser T, Tran VQ, Aboseif SR, Bellman GC, Abbas MA. Management of rectal injuries sustained during laparoscopic radical prostatectomy. Urology. 2009;73(1): 163–6.

112. Thomas C, Jones J, Jager W, Hampel C, Thuroff JW, Gillitzer R. Incidence, clinical symptoms and management of rectourethral fistulas after radical prostatectomy. J Urol. 2010; 183:608–12.

113. Voelzke BB, McAninch JW, Breyer BN, Glass AS, Garcia-Aguilar J. Transperineal management for postoperative and radiation rectourethral fistulas. J Urol. 2013;189:966–71.

114. Bukowski TP, Chakrabarty A, Powell IJ, Frontera R, Perlmutter AD, Montie JE. Acquired rectourethral fistula: methods of repair. J Urol. 1995;153:730–3.

115. Lacarriere E, Suaud L, Caremel R, Rouache L, Tuech JJ, Pfister C. Rectourethral fistulae: diagnosis and management. Review of the literature. Prog Urol. 2011;21:585–94.

116. Choi JH, Jeon BG, Choi SG, Han EC, Ha HK, Oh HK, Choe EK, Moon SH, Ryoo SB, Park KJ. Rectourethral fistula: systemic review of and experiences with various surgical treatment methods. Ann Coloproctol. 2014;30:35–41.

117. Lesser T, Aboseif S, Abbas MA. Combined endorectal advancement flap with alloderm graft repair of radiation and

cryoablation-induced rectourethral fistula. American Surg. 2008;74:341–5.

118. Patsouras D, Yassin NA, Phillips RK. Clinical outcomes of colo-anal pull-through procedure for complex rectal conditions. Colorectal Dis. 2014;16:253–8.

119. Linder BJ, Umbreit EC, Larson D, Dozois EJ, Thapa P, Elliott DS. Effect of prior radiotherapy and ablative therapy on surgical outcomes for the treatment of rectourethral fistulas. J Urol. 2013;190:1287–91.

120. Youssef AH, Fath-Alla M, El-Kassaby AW. Perineal subcutaneous dartos pedicled flap as a new technique for repairing urethrorectal fistula. J Urol. 1999;161:1498–500.

121. Garofalo TE, Delaney CP, Jones SM, Remzi FH, Fazio VW. Rectal advancement flap repair of rectourethral fistula: a 20-year experience. Dis Colon Rectum. 2003;46:762–9.

122. Wexner SD, Ruiz DE, Genua J, Nogueras JJ, Weiss EG, Zmora O. Gracilis muscle interposition for the treatment of rectourethral, rectovaginal, and pouch-vaginal fistulas: results in 53 patients. Ann Surg. 2008;248:39–43.

123. Kasraeian A, Rozet F, Cathelineau X, Barret E, Galiano M, Vallancien G. Modified York-Mason technique for repair of iatrogenic rectourinary fistula: the montsouris experience. J Urol. 2009;181:1178–83.

124. Vanni AJ, Buckley JC, Zinman LN. Management of surgical and radiation induced rectourethral fistulas with an interposition muscle flap and selective buccal mucosal onlay graft. J Urol. 2010;184:2400–4.

125. Ghoniem G, Elmissiry M, Weiss E, Langford C, Abdelwahab H, Wexner S. Transperineal repair of complex rectourethral fistula using gracilis muscle flap interposition--can urinary and bowel functions be preserved? J Urol. 2008;179:1882–6.

126. Gupta G, Kumar S, Kekre NS, Gopalakrishnan G. Surgical management of rectourethral fistula. Urology. 2008;71: 267–71.

127. Ulrich D, Roos J, Jakse G, Pallua N. Gracilis muscle interposition for the treatment of recto-urethral and rectovaginal fistulas: a retrospective analysis of 35 cases. J Plast Reconstr Aesthet Surg. 2009;62:352–6.

128. Samplaski MK, Wood HM, Lane BR, Remzi FH, Lucas A, Angermeier KW. Functional and quality-of-life outcomes in patients undergoing transperineal repair with gracilis muscle interposition for complex rectourethral fistula. Urology. 2011;77:736–41.

129. Lee TG, Park SS, Lee SJ. Treatment of a recurrent rectourethral fistula by using transanal rectal flap advancement and fibrin glue: a case report. J Korean Soc Coloproctol. 2012; 28:165–9.

130. Al-Ali M, Kashmoula D, Saoud IJ. Experience with 30 posttraumatic rectourethral fistulas: presentation of posterior transsphincteric anterior rectal wall advancement. J Urol. 1997;158:421–4.

131. Spotnitz WD. Fibrin sealant: past, present, and future: a brief review. World J Surg. 2010;34:632–4.

132. Takano S, Boutros M, Wexner SD. Gracilis muscle transposition for complex perineal fistulas and sinuses: a systematic literature review of surgical outcomes. J Am Coll Surg. 2014;219:313–23.

133. Varma MG, Wang JY, Garcia-Aguilar J, Shelton AA, McAninch JW, Goldberg SM. Dartos muscle interposition flap for the treatment of rectourethral fistula. Dis Colon Rectum. 2007;50:1849–55.

134. Shah NS, Remzi F, Massmann A, Baixauli J, Fazio VW. Management and treatment outcome of pouch-vaginal fistulas following restorative proctocolectomy. Dis Colon Rectum. 2003;46:911–7.

135. Maslekar S, Sagar PM, Harji D, Bruce C, Griffiths B. The challenge of pouch-vaginal fistulas: a systematic review. Tech Coloproctol. 2012;16:405–14.

136. Kim NK, Lim DJ, Yun SH, Sohn SK, Min JS. Ultralow anterior resection and coloanal anastomosis for distal rectal cancer: functional and oncological results. Int J Colorectal Dis. 2001;16:234–7.

137. Guerrieri M, Gesuita R, Ghiselli R, Lezoche G, Budassi A, Baldarelli M. Treatment of rectal cancer by transanal endoscopic microsurgery: experience with 425 patients. World J Gastroenterol. 2014;20:9556–63.

138. Musters GD, Lapid O, Bemelman WA, Tanis PJ. Surgery for complex perineal fistula following rectal cancer treatment using biological mesh combined with gluteal perforator flap. Tech Coloproctol. 2014;18:955–9.

139. Lolohea S, Lynch AC, Robertson GB, Frizelle FA. Ileal pouch-anal anastomosis-vaginal fistula: a review. Dis Colon Rectum. 2005;48:1802–10.

140. Gaertner WB, Witt J, Madoff RD, Mellgren A, Finne CO, Spencer MP. Ileal pouch fistulas after restorative proctocolectomy: management and outcomes. Tech Coloproctol. 2014;18: 1061–6.

141. Mallick IH, Hull TL, Remzi FH, Kiran RP. Management and outcome of pouch-vaginal fistulas after IPAA surgery. Dis Colon Rectum. 2014;57:490–6.

142. Heriot AG, Tekkis PP, Smith JJ, Bona R, Cohen RG, Nicholls RJ. Management and outcome of pouch-vaginal fistulas following restorative proctocolectomy. Dis Colon Rectum. 2005; 48:451–8.

16
Rectovaginal Fistula

Jamie A. Cannon

Key Concepts

- Repair of rectovaginal fistulas should be tailored to the individual patient based on the anatomy of the fistula and associated conditions.
- Perianal sepsis must be controlled prior to attempting a definitive repair.
- Patients with RVFs from obstetric trauma should be evaluated for concomitant sphincter defects.
- Patients who have a Crohn's-related RVF should have their disease medically optimized prior to repair of the fistula.
- Introduction of healthy, well-vascularized tissue such as a Martius flap or gracilis interposition should be considered in patients who have attenuated tissues or have undergone multiple previous unsuccessful repairs.
- Fecal diversion should be considered in patients undergoing major repairs.

Rectovaginal fistulas (RVFs) are abnormal communications between the anus or rectum and the vagina. RVFs are uncommon in the general population, but are seen frequently by colorectal surgeons. The condition can be extremely disabling and is associated with significant distress in affected women. Patients may present with stool per vagina resulting in frank incontinence, or gas or drainage per vagina. These symptoms can also cause pelvic pain and interfere with intimacy.

Successful treatment of rectovaginal fistulas offers the opportunity to greatly improve a patient's quality of life. Unfortunately, success rates are not on par with other commonly performed operations. Many patients present after having undergone multiple previous attempted repairs, which can be frustrating for the patient and surgeon. Hoexter et al. reported 33% of their patients with previous attempted repairs were in litigation with their surgeons [1].

A number of different factors may contribute to the poor success rates following repair. Anatomically, there is little muscle in the thin rectovaginal septum, which may make it more difficult for this region to heal. Fistulotomy, the most successful

surgery for managing perianal fistulas, is contraindicated as it invariably results in some degree of incontinence, either due to the paucity of sphincteric muscle in women anteriorly or a resulting keyhole defect.

Multiple different approaches have been described to treat rectovaginal fistulas, which reflects the fact that there is not an ideal operation with a uniformly high success rate. Interpreting the literature to determine the best approach can be challenging. Most papers report series with few patients, and the patients are far from uniform. Varied patient presentations make standardizing the multiple different approaches difficult, if not impossible. In addition, surgeons often vary techniques slightly, use different terminologies, or combine approaches, which prohibits a side-to-side comparison. In general, more complicated and extensive repairs are not associated with improved rates of success, which could leave one to believe that a less invasive approach is preferable. However, the complexities of the fistulas selected for a major procedure create a selection bias against these repairs. Preoperative fecal diversion has not been shown consistently to lead to better outcomes, but this again may represent selection bias in those patients chosen for diversion. These compounding factors make the likelihood of a randomized trial comparing different repair types impractical.

Therefore, it is imperative for the surgeon to have a thorough understanding of the patient's anatomy, disease process, and options for repair in order to determine the best approach. In this chapter, we will review the etiologies for rectovaginal fistula, the evaluation of a patient with a rectovaginal fistula, various approaches for repair, and finally discuss the decision making process in choosing the appropriate surgical procedure.

Etiology of Rectovaginal Fistulas

Rectovaginal fistulas can be the result of obstetric injuries, cryptoglandular disease, or Crohn's disease. These etiologies are discussed below. They can also be caused by malignancy,

© Springer International Publishing 2016
S.R. Steele et al. (eds.), *The ASCRS Textbook of Colon and Rectal Surgery*, DOI 10.1007/978-3-319-25970-3_16

radiation therapy, or leaks from a colorectal, coloanal, or ileal pouch-anal anastomosis. These are beyond the scope of this chapter and addressed elsewhere in this book.

Obstetric Injury

Obstetric injury is the most common cause of RVFs. While many published case series have a higher proportion of patients with other etiologies, such as Crohn's disease, this is a reflection of specific referral patterns and the patient populations at different institutions. Rectovaginal fistulas are reported to occur following 0.1–0.5% of all vaginal deliveries [2]. Obstetric fistulas can arise from a fourth-degree tear in which the repair has broken down. This type of fistula will generally become clinically apparent 1–2 weeks after delivery and is most often located at the level of the anal sphincters. Prolonged labor resulting in compression of the rectovaginal septum by the infant's head can lead to necrosis of the RV septum and cause a rectovaginal fistula that presents in a more delayed fashion. These generally occur cephalad to the pelvic floor where the rectovaginal septum is thinnest. Traumatic injury from an instrumented delivery may result in an immediately apparent fistula and also generally occurs in the thin portion of the rectovaginal septum.

Repairs of RVFs caused by obstetric injury tend to be more successful than repairs of fistulas from other causes. Halverson et al. reported on 15 patients with obstetric-related RVFs that had failed previous repairs [3]. All fistulas were eventually able to be repaired for an overall success rate of 100%, but required a total of 23 procedures for a per procedure success rate of 65%. This cohort of patients was compared to patients with recurrent RVF from Crohn's disease that had an overall success rate of only 50% (6 of 12 patients healed with a total of 21 procedures).

Cryptoglandular Disease

Cryptoglandular disease, which is the most common cause of simple anorectal fistulas, can also cause rectovaginal fistulas. This occurs when an anteriorly located anal gland or its associated duct becomes occluded; the resulting abscess may form in the rectovaginal septum and decompress into the vagina. If the communication fails to heal, a rectovaginal fistula results. These are generally located at the level of the dentate line on the rectal side and course through the anal sphincters to the low vagina or introitus.

Crohn's Disease

Rectovaginal fistulas caused by Crohn's disease are variable in their presentation and location. As they are the result of transmural inflammation from the anorectum, they are frequently associated with perianal sepsis, branching fistula tracts, additional rectocutaneous fistulas, and scarring and stricturing of the anorectum. Approximately 10% of women with Crohn's disease will develop a rectovaginal fistula, and they are more common in those who suffer from colonic Crohn's disease [4, 5].

Surgical repair of rectovaginal fistulas caused by Crohn's disease is not as successful as repair of fistulas of obstetric or cryptoglandular origin. Prior to attempting any repair, control of perianal sepsis is required. This may require abscess drainage and seton placement. A discrete, epithelialized tract should be present before attempting repair, which is best achieved with initial seton placement. Multiple fistula tracts, a watering can perineum, or active inflammation of the rectal mucosa are contraindications to repair. Figure 16-1 shows a rectovaginal fistula from Crohn's disease. Multiple external openings with stool present are visible in the perineum. This patient would benefit from placement of a seton to allow the fistula to mature prior to definitive repair.

Repair should not be undertaken in the presence of active inflammation of the rectum as the repair is unlikely to heal. Those with significant Crohn's-related pathology of the anorectum are unlikely to be good candidates for repair and should be managed either medically, with a seton, or with a proctectomy. Athanasiadis et al. found

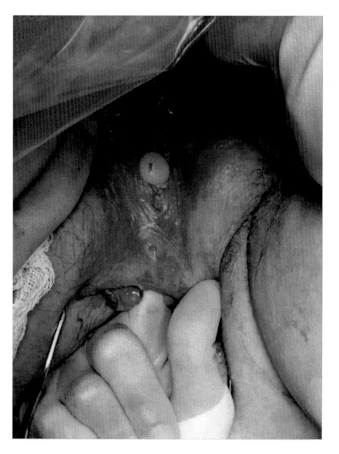

FIGURE 16-1. Large Crohn's-related rectovaginal fistula with multiple external openings in the perineum.

that of patients presenting with Crohn's disease and a rectovaginal fistula, only 51% were deemed appropriate for attempted repair [6]. Overall, 19% of patients eventually underwent a proctectomy for management of their disease.

The use of infliximab has been shown to lead to spontaneous healing of fistulas in Crohn's disease. Kraemer et al. reported healing of symptomatic fistulas in 8 of 19 patients with Crohn's-associated anorectal fistulas treated with infliximab prior to surgery [7]. Its role in the management of rectovaginal fistulas specifically is not well delineated, but multiple reports have shown spontaneous healing of RVFs. These results may not be durable once immunomodulators have been discontinued [8], but are promising enough to warrant a trial of medical therapy prior to surgical intervention. If the fistula does not close spontaneously, reducing the amount of associated inflammation will likely improve the chance of success with surgical repair. Sands et al. reviewed the ACCENT II trial which studied infliximab in patients with fistulizing Crohn's disease [8]. Twenty-nine patients in this trial had rectovaginal fistulas. Patients were evaluated at week 14 of treatment with infliximab, and 13 of those patients (44.8%) were found to have healed fistulas. While this success rate has not been duplicated in other studies, healing with infliximab therapy alone has been demonstrated elsewhere as well. Table 16-1 summarizes these findings.

Successful surgical treatment of Crohn's-related RVF varies in the literature, with success rates ranging from 30 to 70%. Selection bias may be responsible for some of this variation; the more highly selected the candidates the greater the chance of success. Patients most likely to have a successful repair are those with an isolated RVF without other perianal diseases and in whom their Crohn's disease is quiescent. The success rates reported below for repair of Crohn's-related RVFs can be compared to a success rate of 74% in simple fistulas that are not related to Crohn's [9].

Luffler et al. reported on 45 patients with Crohn's-related RVFs [10]. The patients underwent a total of 95 interventions, averaging 2.1 interventions per patient. Their long-term success rate was 53%, but 10 patients (22.2%) required proctectomy. They found levatorplasty and endorectal advancement flaps to have similar rates of success at approximately 50%.

Drs. Hull and Fazio reported on 48 Crohn's patients with RVF. [11] Nine required proctectomy and five were treated with a seton only. Of the 35 who underwent

attempted definitive repair, 19 were successful (54%). Five of the failures underwent subsequent successful procedures for an overall success rate of 24/35 (69%). They also found that success was more likely among the patients who had fecal stream diversion, with 8/9 diverted patients having successful repairs.

El-Gazzaz et al. reported on 65 women with Crohn's disease who underwent RVF repair [12]. They had 30 successes (46.2%). They noted that many of the failures were late failures and thus recommended long-term follow-up in order to accurately determine success. It is difficult, however, to discern between actual treatment failures and recurrent disease with the development of new Crohn's-related fistulas.

Evaluation of a Patient with a Rectovaginal Fistula

The etiology of the fistula can often be determined from the patient's history. History taking should be directed toward the patients obstetric history, previous abdominal and anorectal operations, history of radiation treatment, and signs and symptoms of Crohn's disease or diverticulitis. Physical examination begins with a visual external examination. Care should be taken to search for signs of continuing perianal sepsis, such as undrained abscesses or purulent perineal drainage. Evidence of perianal Crohn's disease should be sought. Cloacal-type defects can be seen following severe obstetric injury.

On digital rectal examination, the condition of the perineal body and rectovaginal septum should be noted. Care should be taken to assess the quality and strength of the anal sphincters. Large rectovaginal fistulas may be readily apparent on rectal examination. Bimanual examination may be required to detect smaller fistulas. Careful palpation of the entire rectovaginal septum between the fingers of each hand may reveal the presence of a small fistula. Note should also be made of any strictures or scarring of the anal canal from previous or active Crohn's disease. The location of the fistula relative to the sphincter muscles and pelvic floor should be determined as this can affect the type of repair chosen.

If the fistula is not palpable, further investigations are needed. Baig et al. found that physical examination was successful in identifying the fistula in 74% of patients [9]. If it cannot be identified on examination, alternate etiologies to explain the patient's symptoms should be considered, such as a colovaginal fistula rather than a rectovaginal fistula. Colovaginal fistulas from diverticulitis are a more common condition, and a contrasted CT scan of the abdomen and pelvis will demonstrate inflammation of the sigmoid colon directly overlying the vagina if this is the case. However, very small or high RVFs may not be palpable on exam.

While other imaging studies are often employed, RVFs can be difficult to detect on routine imaging. Options include

TABLE 16-1. Medical therapy for Crohn's-related RVFs

Author	Year of publication	Drug utilized	No. of patients	No. of successful closures (%)
Present [45]	1980	6-MP	6	2 (33.3)
Ricart [46]	2001	Infliximab	15	5 (33.3)
Bodegraven [47]	2002	Infliximab	4	0 (0)
Sands [8]	2004	Infliximab	29	13 (44.8)
Parsi [48]	2004	Infliximab	14	2 (14.2)

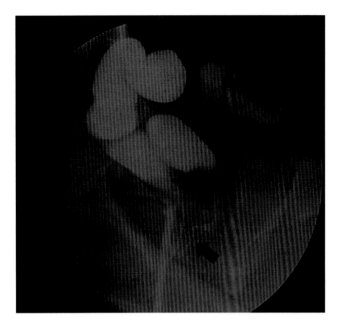

FIGURE 16-2. Gastrografin enema showing contrast passing through a rectovaginal fistula. © 2015 Kobayashi and Sugihara; licensee Springer. This is an Open Access article distributed under the terms of the Creative Commons Attribution License (http://creativecommons.org/licenses/by/4.0), which permits unrestricted use, distribution, and reproduction in any medium, provided the original work is properly credited [53].

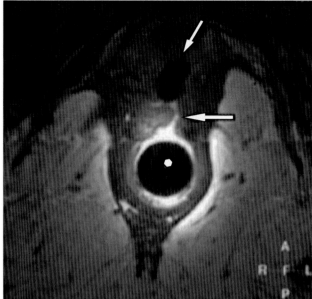

FIGURE 16-3. Rectovaginal fistula as seen on MRI.

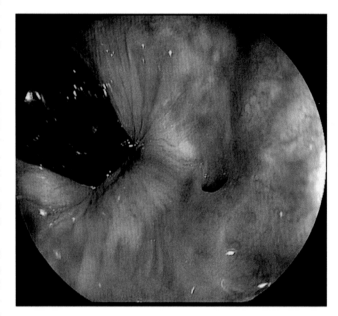

FIGURE 16-4. Rectovaginal fistula on retroflexed view on colonoscopy. © 2015 Kobayashi and Sugihara; licensee Springer. This is an Open Access article distributed under the terms of the Creative Commons Attribution License (http://creativecommons.org/licenses/by/4.0), which permits unrestricted use, distribution, and reproduction in any medium, provided the original work is properly credited [53].

gastrografin enema and vaginography. These have a low yield, however, and are rarely successful in imaging distal fistulas. They rely on occlusion of the anal canal or vaginal introitus in order to generate enough pressure to show passage of contrast through the fistula, and balloon placement may occlude the fistulous opening itself. Figure 16-2 shows an RVF on gastrografin enema. Baig et al. found vaginography did not identify the fistula in any of the five patients in whom it was performed [9]. Defecography may rarely be useful, but may identify other pelvic floor pathologies.

Endoanal ultrasound and MRI are the most useful imaging studies to identify a fistula [13]. MRI also has the advantage of identifying other disease within the pelvis. Figure 16-3 shows the appearance of an RVF on MRI. Endoanal ultrasound has been reported to identify the tract in 73% of patients [9]. Injection of hydrogen peroxide through the tract may aid in identification [14]. Ultrasound is also useful in that it enables assessment of the anal sphincters. It should be performed routinely in patients with an RVF secondary to obstetric trauma as they may have associated sphincter damage. Anal manometry may be considered as well. Patients with Crohn's disease should undergo a complete evaluation of their Crohn's disease, to include colonoscopy and CT or MR enterography. While the fistula itself is rarely seen on colonoscopy, colonoscopy allows for identification of active disease and other Crohn's-related complications. Figure 16-4 demonstrates the appearance of an internal opening on colonoscopy.

The best option for identifying an occult RVF is an examination under anesthesia. This allows for probing of the rectovaginal septum with a fistula probe to elucidate the location (Figure 16-5). It also allows for inspection of the anal canal and rectal and vaginal mucosa to identify areas of inflamma-

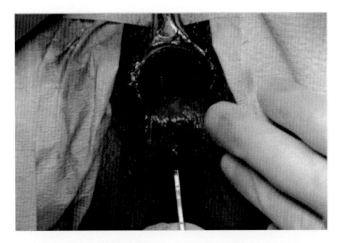

FIGURE 16-5. Fistula probe passing through a rectovaginal fistula.

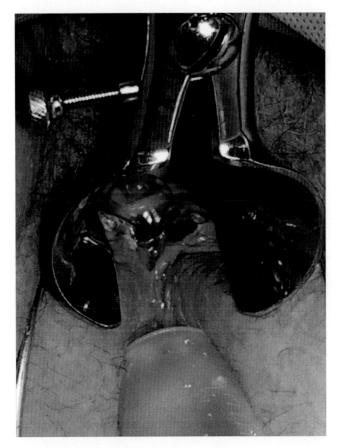

FIGURE 16-6. With the patient in Trendelenburg position, saline is placed in the vagina. An asepto syringe is used to inject air in the rectum. Bubbling in the vagina reveals the location of the recto-vaginal fistula.

tion or dimpling for more targeted inspection. If this is not successful, other techniques may be employed. With the patient in Trendelenburg and lithotomy position, the vagina can be filled with saline while the rectum is insufflated with air (Figure 16-6). Air bubbling through the RV septum can

elucidate the fistula's location. Alternatively, a tampon or operative sponge may be placed in the vagina. Saline with methylene blue dye can be introduced into the rectum via a flexible sigmoidoscope. Blue staining on the gauze within the vagina confirms that a fistula is present, but may not show the actual location.

Surgical Approaches to Repair of Rectovaginal Fistulas

A number of different techniques have been employed to repair a rectovaginal fistula, and for many patients more than one attempt at repair is necessary. For simple rectovaginal fistulas, defined as located in the mid or lower vagina and without Crohn's disease, Baig et al. reported successful repair in 14/19 patients (74%) using a variety of techniques. [9] For recurrent fistulas of various etiologies, Halverson and colleagues reported 23/48 procedures successful (48%) in 29 patients, for an overall healing rate of 79% [3]. Pinto and associates looked at 118 patients with RVF and found an overall success rate of 58.8% per procedure, with 103 patients eventually healing completely (87.3%) [15]. Among those with Crohn's, success was only 44.2% per procedure, but 78% of patients were eventually healed. They found recurrence rates were similar after various types of repairs. Tobacco use was identified as a risk factor for recurrence.

A list of the many surgical approaches to rectovaginal fistulas would be quite extensive. While the various approaches can be grouped into categories based on their similarities, each individual series will often describe a slight modification to previous reports. Patients are also frequently managed with more than one type of repair as treatments are customized to the fistula. For example, a rectal advancement flap may be combined with a transperineal repair or sphincteroplasty. This makes direct comparison of the various techniques difficult. The types of repairs are grouped together here for review as endorectal (rectal advancement flaps or sleeve advancements), transperineal (episioproctotomy or sphincteroplasty), tissue transposition (Martius flap or gracilis), transvaginal, and transabdominal.

Endorectal Repairs

Endorectal advancement flaps are the most commonly performed procedure for the management of a rectovaginal fistula. The procedure as described by Rothenberger et al. in 1982 [16] remains similar to what is described in most reports today with only minor variations in technique. The patient is placed in the jackknife prone position. A Pratt bivalve anoscope is used to expose the anterior rectal wall. Distal to the location of the fistula, an incision is made through the mucosa, submucosa, and down to the internal sphincter. A flap is raised in the rectum proximally. While some describe only raising mucosa and submucosa, fibers of the circular muscle (internal sphincter) are generally included, and this is how Rothenberger described the procedure. The flap is raised for a distance of 4 cm proximal to the location of the fistula in order to allow for a tension-free anastomosis. Once the flap has been raised, the fistula itself is closed by approximating the fibers of the internal sphincter. This may require some lateral mobilization in order to bring the edges of the internal sphincter into approximation. The distal-most portion of the flap that contains the fistula is excised. The healthy flap is brought down to cover the fistula opening and secured in place. Figure 16-7 depicts these steps.

The most common cause for failure is thought to be flap retraction or necrosis. Therefore, it is essential that enough flap be mobilized so there is no tension on the anastomosis. The base of the flap should be at least twice the width of the apex of the flap in order to ensure adequate blood supply. Rothenberger reported overall good success with this technique. Out of 35 patients, 30 were successfully repaired with this approach (86%). This success rate is similar to that reported by Lowry et al. from the same institution with 43/49 (88%) successful [17].

Others, however, have not reported the same high degree of success with this technique. Ellis reported a

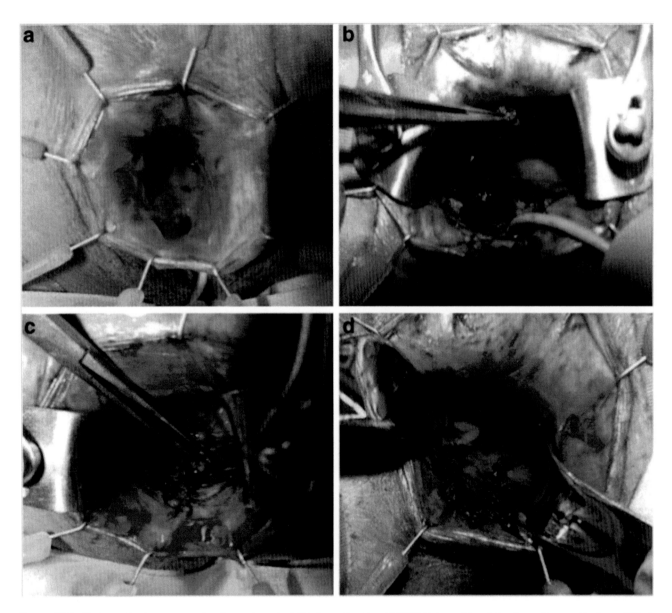

FIGURE 16-7. Endorectal advancement flap for rectovaginal fistula. Rectovaginal fistula is seen from the anus (a). The flap of mucosa, submucosa, and circular muscle is raised (b). Circular muscle is sutured by horizontal mattress manner (c). The flap is advanced over the repaired area (d). The flap is sutured in place at its apex and along its sides. © 2015 Kobayashi and Sugihara; licensee Springer. This is an Open Access article distributed under the terms of the Creative Commons Attribution License (http://creativecommons.org/licenses/by/4.0), which permits unrestricted use, distribution, and reproduction in any medium, provided the original work is properly credited [53].

TABLE 16-2. Endorectal advancement flaps

Author	Year of publication	No. of patients	No. of successful closures (%)
Rothenberger [16]	1982	35	30 (86)
Jones [49]	1987	23	16 (70)
Lowry [17]	1988	44	56 (78)
Watson [50]	1995	12	7 (58)
Sonoda [19]	2002	37	16 (43)
Ellis [18]	2008	44	29 (66)
Hull [20]	2011	37	23 (62)

66% success rate in 44 patients [18]. Sonoda et al. reported success in 16/37 (43.2%) [19], while Hull and colleagues in 23/37 (62%) in a population that excluded Crohn's disease [20].

Athanasiadis and associates compared endorectal advancement flaps to multiple other closure techniques in a Crohn's population [6]. While the numbers are few, they reported disappointing success with this technique. Only 2/7 rectal advancement flaps were successful (29%), while the success rate for all other repair types combined was 37/49 (76%). Available data on endorectal advancement flaps is summarized in Table 16-2. There have been other modifications of the described procedure. Schwandner et al. described using a biologic graft as part of this procedure [21, 22]. Once the endorectal flap was raised, a 2 × 2 cm graft from porcine small intestine mucosa was placed in the rectovaginal space, and the flap sutured over the graft. They report successful healing in 15/21 patients (71%).

Of note, the likelihood of a successful repair with an endorectal advancement flap decreases if patients have undergone previous repairs [18, 23–26]. Halverson et al. reported only 9 successes in 30 patients who had undergone previous repairs with this technique (30%) [3]. Similarly, while Lowry had 88% success with a first repair, they found the success rate fell to 55% in those who had had two previous repairs [17].

Transperineal Repairs

A number of variations in technique exist in performing a transperineal repair, and terminology in the literature is diverse. For the purpose of this discussion, we have grouped together a variety of techniques that all share some common key points. Such techniques include episioproctotomy with layered closure, transperineal repair with levatorplasty, the LIFT procedure, and sphincteroplasty. These procedures all begin with an incision in the perineum that may be circumlinear around the anus, transverse, or vertical. Dissection continues cephalad along the rectovaginal septum. The rectum and vagina are separated from one another and the fistula tract divided, as seen in Figure 16-8. The incision is closed in layers. Ideally, some

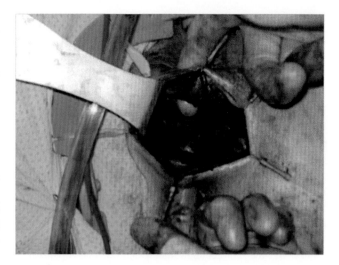

FIGURE 16-8. Transperineal repair where the rectum and vagina have been separated and the defects in each are visible.

TABLE 16-3. Transperineal repairs

Author	Year of publication	No. of patients	No. of successful closures (%)
Athanasiadis [6]	2007	20	14 (70)
Hull [20]	2011	50	39 (78)
Wiskind [51]	1992	21	21 (100)

tissue, preferentially muscle, is interposed between the rectum and vagina. This may be done via levatorplasty or sphincteroplasty. The repaired areas of the rectum and vagina can also be imbricated. A rectal advancement flap can be added to the procedure.

Athanasiadis and colleagues reported good success with this technique in a Crohn's population with 14/20 (70%) undergoing successful repairs [6]. Lowry had success in 22 of 25 patients who underwent a combined sphincteroplasty and endorectal advancement flap (88%), which was an improvement over the 78% success with advancement flap alone [17]. Hull and associates reported success in 39/50 patients who underwent a transperineal repair (78%) [20]. Of note, patients with Crohn's disease were excluded. Important in this study is they found that the rate of post-repair incontinence was only 8%, as compared to 38% in those undergoing endorectal advancement flaps. A transperineal repair with sphincteroplasty is the most appropriate type of repair in women who have a sphincter defect (most often from obstetric injury), as this is addressed simultaneously.

Following repair, some authors advocate placement of a biologic graft to separate the vagina and rectum. Ellis described a transperineal repair with a graft made from porcine intestinal submucosa placed in the rectovaginal septum [18]. He reported an 81% success (22/27). The available data for transperineal repairs is summarized in Table 16-3.

Tissue Transposition Repairs

Tissue transposition repairs offer the advantage of interposing healthy, well-perfused tissue between the rectum and vagina. They add bulk to the rectovaginal septum and physically increase the distance between the rectum and vagina, and by bringing their own blood supply may aid in healing. These types of repairs have the highest success rate of all transperineal repairs; however, these repairs may be accompanied by pain, delayed healing, and unsatisfactory cosmesis at the donor site.

Patients that are appropriate candidates for transposition repairs are those who have failed less invasive techniques or who have inadequate native tissue. Due to the complexity of the operation, fecal diversion is generally performed prior to or at the time of surgery. The operation is most often conducted jointly by the colorectal surgeon and a plastic surgeon. Colorectal surgeons trained in these techniques may perform the entire operation. The labial fat pad with bulbocavernosus muscle (Martius flap) or gracilis muscle transposition are the most commonly used tissues for transposition and are reviewed here. Use of other muscles including the sartorius and gluteal muscle has also been described. The choice of a Martius flap versus gracilis muscle for the donor tissue is based on the desired bulk of tissue and individual surgeon experience.

Martius Flap

The Martius flap was initially described by Dr. Heinrich Martius in 1928 and uses the bulbocavernosus muscle and labial fat pad for transposition [27]. The technical details of the operation are well described by Kniery et al. in 2015 [28]. The initial incision is made in the vaginal introitus distal to the fistula opening in order to expose the rectovaginal septum. Dissection continues in the rectovaginal septum cephalad to the fistula (Figure 16-9). The fistula tract is curetted and closed primarily on the rectal side. The vaginal portion of the fistula is excised from the vaginal flap. In order to harvest the donor tissue, a vertical incision is made in the labia majora (Figure 16-10). The labial fat pad and underlying bulbocavernosus muscle are dissected out from the surrounding tissues. The amount of muscular tissue varies from patient to patient and may not be visible in some. The blood supply to the flap comes in inferiorly and posteriorly from the posterior labial vessels. Dissection ensues in a lateral to medial direction taking care not to injure the blood supply. The flap is transected superiorly and tunneled to the rectovaginal septum. It should be rotated carefully so as not to kink the blood supply (Figures 16-11 and 16-12). The flap is laid within the RV septum and the vaginal flap sutured over the Martius flap (Figure 16-13). Figure 16-14 shows

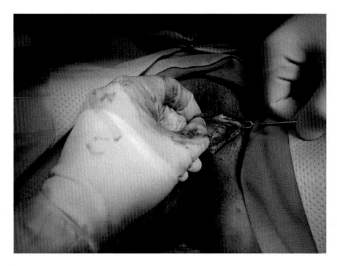

FIGURE 16-10. Martius flap repair. Incision over the left labia majora to expose the fat pad and bulbocavernosus. Courtesy of Drs. Eric Johnson and Scott Steele.

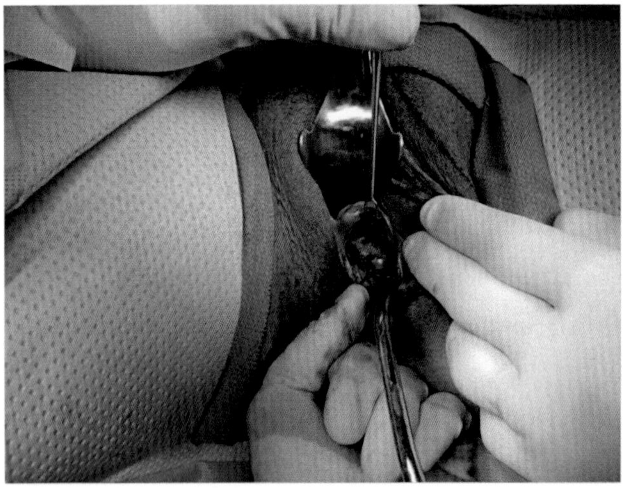

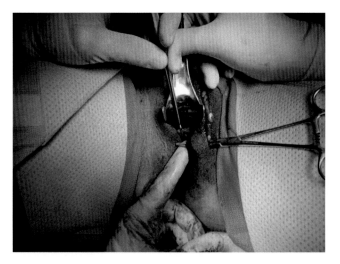

FIGURE 16-9. Martius flap repair. The vaginal flap has been raised revealing the rectovaginal fistula. Courtesy of Drs. Eric Johnson and Scott Steele.

FIGURE 16-11. Martius flap. A tunnel is created from the origin of the bulbocavernosus to the vaginal incision. Courtesy of Drs. Eric Johnson and Scott Steele.

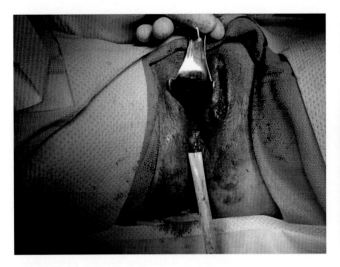

FIGURE 16-12. Martius flap. The donor tissue has been brought into the rectovaginal septum. Courtesy of Drs. Eric Johnson and Scott Steele.

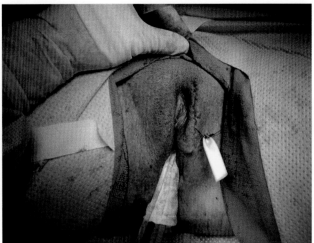

FIGURE 16-14. Appearance after the Martius flap. Courtesy of Drs. Eric Johnson and Scott Steele.

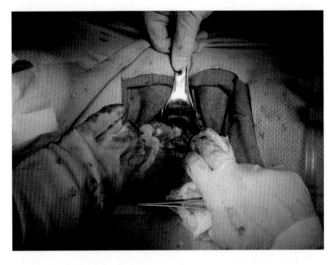

FIGURE 16-13. Martius flap. The vaginal incision has been closed over the Martius flap. Courtesy of Drs. Eric Johnson and Scott Steele.

TABLE 16-4. Martius flap

Author	Year of publication	No. of patients	No. of successful closures (%)
White [27]	1982	14	13 (93)
Aartsen [30]	1988	14	13 (93)
McNevin [31]	2007	16	15 (94)
Songne [32]	2007	14	13 (93)
Pitel [29]	2011	23	15 (65)
Kniery [28]	2015	5	3 (60)

the postoperative appearance. The authors report successful healing in 3/5 patients, all of whom had failed previous repairs. The largest case series using the Martius flap was published by Pitel et al. in 2011 [29]. They reported a 65% success rate in 23 patients. Other small case studies report success rates ranging from 92 to 100% [27, 30–34]. Complications are rare but include local wound dehiscence and dyspareunia. The available data is summarized in Table 16-4.

Gracilis Muscle Transposition

Repair using a gracilis muscle transposition offers the advantage of providing a large bulk of well-vascularized muscle to separate the vagina and rectum. Its origin is near the perineum, which makes it a convenient donor. It is, however,

associated with higher morbidity due to the mobilization and transposition of this large muscle. Success rates are quite promising, and this repair should be considered in patients who have had multiple recurrences or poor native tissue. Fecal diversion is generally performed prior to or at the time of the procedure.

The operation involves a transperineal incision, in which the rectum and vagina are separated. The fistula is divided and both the rectum and vagina are closed primarily. Dissection should continue cephalad to the fistula until healthy tissue is reached. An endorectal advancement flap can be added to the procedure as well. The perineal incision created is seen in Figure 16-15 and does not differ from that in other transperineal approaches. The gracilis muscle is then harvested. This can be performed with a long incision the length of the gracilis, or with separate smaller incisions near the muscle's origin and insertion. The muscle is mobilized with division of the perforating vessels. It is divided just above its insertion. It is tunneled from the proximal-most portion of the incision to the perineal incision, as seen in Figure 16-16. Care must be taken that the flap is not rotated excessively and its blood supply not kinked. The muscle is secured to the apex of the rectovaginal dissection and the transperineal incision closed, as seen in Figure 16-17. Reported success rates range from 47% [35] to 92% [35, 36]. The largest

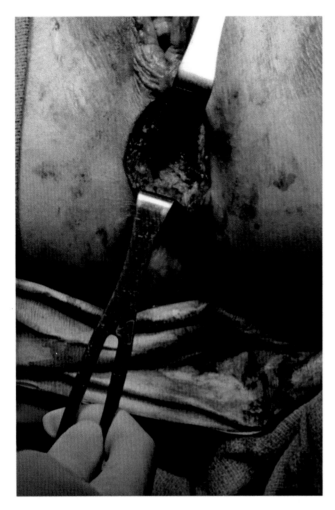

FIGURE 16-15. Gracilis transposition. A transperineal incision is made to separate the rectum and the vagina. Courtesy of Drs. Jamie Cannon, Andre Levesque, and James Long.

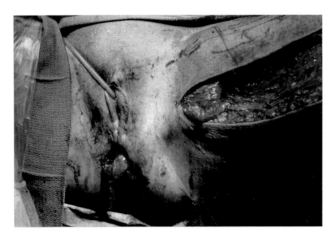

FIGURE 16-16. Gracilis transposition. The gracilis muscle has been tunneled from the left thigh to the transperineal incision. Courtesy of Drs. Jamie Cannon, Andre Levesque, and James Long.

series was published by Pinto et al. [15]. They reported a 79% success in 24 patients. Table 16-5 summarizes the available data.

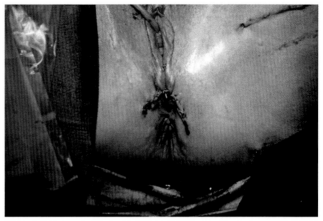

FIGURE 16-17. Gracilis transposition. Postoperative appearance. Courtesy of Drs. Jamie Cannon, Andre Levesque, and James Long.

Transvaginal Repairs

Transvaginal repairs are infrequently reported in the literature and usually found more often in the gynecologic literature than the colorectal literature; however, there is good evidence that repair through the vagina has acceptable success rates. Proponents of a transvaginal repair emphasize the relative ease and better exposure gained through the vagina as compared to the anus. The initial incision is usually made in healthy tissue, as the origin of disease is on the rectal side. However, as the rectum is the higher-pressure side of the fistula, any repair is unlikely to be successful if the rectal side is not addressed. Therefore transvaginal repairs should involve closure of the rectum and not just of the vagina.

Sher et al. report on the use of a transvaginal flap for Crohn's-related RVF [37]. They describe their technique, which is quite similar to an endorectal advancement flap. An incision is made in the vagina distal to the fistula. A flap is raised exposing the rectovaginal septum. Both the rectal and vaginal side are closed. The levators are approximated in the midline in between the repair. The fistula is then excised from the vaginal flap and the flap is sutured in place over the repair. In their study, all patients had fecal diversion and they reported that 13/14 patients healed (93%).

Transabdominal Repair

Transabdominal repairs are generally reserved for fistulas that are located in the mid-rectum with an internal opening at the fornix of the vagina, as these are difficult to access from a perineal or endoluminal approach. Transabdominal repair generally involves a low anterior resection, where the segment of rectum containing the fistula is resected and a colorectal or coloanal anastomosis performed. Depending on the height of the fistula, this may be done transabdominally only, or with a transabdominal transanal (TATA) approach and colonic pull-through. The vaginal side of the defect can be closed primarily.

TABLE 16-5. Gracilis muscle transposition

Author	Year of publication	No. of patients	No. of successful closures (%)
Furst [36]	2008	12	11 (92)
Wexner [35]	2008	17	9 (53)
Lefevre [52]	2009	8	6 (75)
Pinto [15]	2010	24	19 (79)

Van der Hagen and colleagues reported their experience with a transabdominal approach where a formal resection was not undertaken [38]. They laparoscopically separated the rectum and vagina and repaired each primarily. The omentum was mobilized and laid in between the rectum and the vagina. They reported successful repair in 38/40 patients. The same approach was described by Chu and associates who reported success in 6/6 patients [39]. Mukwege reported similar successful results using a laparoscopic transabdominal approach in ten patients [40]. While techniques differed from patient to patient and included traditional LAR, TATA, and fistula excision with omentum interposition, overall 9/10 repairs were successful.

Alternate Repairs

A variety of alternate techniques exist as well. The use of a fistula plug has been described but should be limited to those with a long-tract RVF. Ellis reported their protocol, which is to use a plug as first-line treatment if the length of the RVF is 1 cm or greater [18]. The plug is brought from the rectal to vaginal side, excess length on the plug is trimmed, and it is sutured in place with absorbable suture. He noted success in 6/7 patients with this technique (86%). Gajsek et al. also reported on plug use with 4/9 repairs being successful (44%) [41]. Failures were treated with repeat plug placement, but none of the repeat procedures were successful. Weerd et al. described the successful injection of fat into the tissue surrounding the fistula in a very small case series [42]. D'Ambrosio performed the repair via a transanal endoscopic microsurgical (TEMS) approach and reported success in 12/13 patients undergoing this procedure [43].

Choice of Technique for Repair

The number of types of repairs discussed above demonstrates that a one-size-fits-all approach is not practical. It is also reflective of the fact that this is a difficult condition to treat.

In deciding on a surgical approach, the surgeon should evaluate the patient for continuing inflammation or ongoing pelvic sepsis. These must be controlled prior to surgical repair or the chance of success is dismal. Ongoing pelvic sepsis should be managed with abscess drainage, antibiotics, and seton placement until resolved. The patient is reassessed 6 weeks after seton placement to confirm the sepsis has resolved. If there is evidence of residual abscess or branching fistula tracts, these must be addressed. Once a mature isolated fistula tract is present, definitive repair can be considered.

Treatment with anti-TNF agents should be considered preoperatively in all patients with Crohn's disease. If active Crohn's disease persists, the patient should undergo medical management and possible temporizing measures rather than attempting to cure the fistula. Seton placement is ideally suited. Not all patients with Crohn's disease and RVF will be candidates for repair. Repair should be considered for those who develop a mature isolated tract without branching, without other draining areas, and with healthy rectal mucosa. If this is not possible, non-cutting seton placement can be a long-term method of controlling symptoms. Proctectomy is considered for those with severe disease refractory to seton placement and maximized medical therapy. The presence of an anal stricture with quiescent disease is not a contraindication for repair, as the stricture can be addressed simultaneously with the fistula with endorectal techniques such as flap construction or sleeve advancement [44–65]. A portion of the circumference of the stricture can be removed along with the fistula when an endorectal advancement flap is performed. If this does not result in correction of the stricture, a sleeve advancement with circumferential resection of the stricture is an alternative option.

The surgeon must also decide whether preoperative diversion is indicated. As discussed above, diversion has not been shown to decrease the rate of fistula recurrence, although this may well be because the patients that undergo fecal diversion have more complicated disease. The surgeon should estimate the likelihood of success with the repair chosen, as well as the magnitude of the operation. When low rates of success are anticipated (e.g., multiple prior repairs, poor tissue compliance), preoperative fecal diversion should be considered. This is not generally necessary in the repair of simple rectovaginal fistulas. Patients undergoing major transabdominal resections, or muscle transposition procedures, should have fecal diversion.

The anatomic location of the fistula will dictate a local repair versus a transabdominal approach. Fistulas located in the mid-rectum and upper vagina will not be accessible via a local approach and should therefore be managed with a transabdominal approach.

For local repairs, the quality of the patient's tissue should be assessed. If the patient's tissues are healthy, have normal compliance, and lack scarring, an endorectal advancement flap is an appropriate first approach. If the RVF is secondary to obstetric injury, endorectal ultrasound is used to determine if a sphincter defect is also present. If a sphincter defect is identified, a transperineal repair with sphincteroplasty is performed simultaneously. The chance of success with an advancement flap decreases with each attempt at repair;

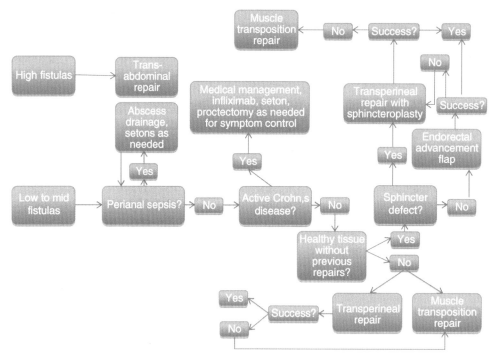

FIGURE 16-18. Algorithm for management of rectovaginal fistulas.

therefore a transperineal approach should be considered in those who have failed previous endoanal advancement flaps. For either endoanal advancement flaps or transperineal repairs, the surgeon may also consider the use of biologic grafts to reinforce the repair. If the local tissues are not adequate for repair, then transposition of healthy tissue should be considered. The most common tissues used for transposition are the Martius flap or gracilis muscle. Figure 16-18 provides an algorithm that summarizes the above recommendations.

Conclusions

Rectovaginal fistulas are distressing conditions to patients and present a therapeutic challenge to surgeons. Whether the etiology of the fistula is obstetric, Crohn's related, or cryptoglandular, a thorough evaluation of the patient's anatomy is required in order to select the right repair. While not all patients will be candidates for surgical repair, the majority of patients will eventually undergo successful treatment of their RVF. Familiarity with the various surgical techniques described and the ability to apply the appropriate surgery to the right patient will increase the chance of a successful intervention.

References

1. Hoexter B, Laboow SB, Moseson MD. Transanal rectovaginal fistula repair. Dis Colon Rectum. 1985;28:572–5.
2. Venkatesh KS, Ramanujam PS, Larson DM, Haywood MA. Anorectal complications of vaginal delivery. Dis Colon Rectum. 1989;32:1039–41.
3. Halverson AL, Hull TL, Fazio VW, Church J, Hammel J, Floruta C. Repair of recurrent rectovaginal fistulas. Surgery. 2001;130(4):753–7.
4. Radcliffe AG, Ritchie JK, Hawley PR, et al. Anovaginal and rectovaginal fistulas in Crohn's disease. Dis Colon Rectum. 1988;31:94–9.
5. Schwartz DA, Loftus Jr EV, Tremaine WJ, et al. The natural history of fistulizing Crohn's disease in Olmsted County, Minnesota. Gastroenterology. 2002;122:875–80.
6. Athanasiadis S, Yazigi R, Kohler A, Helmes C. Recovery rates and functional results after repair for rectovaginal fistula in Crohn's disease: a comparison of different techniques. Int J Colorectal Dis. 2007;22:1051–60.
7. Kraemer M, Kirschmeier A, Marth T. Perioperative adjuvant therapy with infliximab in complicated anal crohn's disease. Int J Colorectal Dis. 2008;23:965–9.
8. Sands BE, Blank MA, Patel K, van Deventer SJ. Long-term treatment of rectovaginal fistulas in Crohn's disease: response to infliximab in the ACCENT II Study. Clin Gastroenterol Hepatol. 2004;2:912–20.
9. Baig MK, Zhao RH, Yuen CH, Nogueras JJ, Singh JJ, Weiss EG, Wexner SD. Simple rectovaginal fistulas. Int J Colorectal Dis. 2000;15:323–7.
10. Luffler T, Welsch T, Muhl S, Hinz U, Schmidt J, Kienle P. Long-term success rate after surgical treatment of anorectal and rectovaginal fistulas in Crohns' disease. Int J Colorectal Dis. 2009; 24:521–6.
11. Hull TL, Fazio VW. Surgical approaches to low anovaginal fistula in Crohn's disease. Am J Surg. 1997;173(2):95–8.
12. El-Gazzaz G, Hull T, Mignanelli E, Hammel J, Gurland B, Zutshi M. Analysis of function and predictors of failure in women undergoing repair of crohn's related rectovaginal fistula. J Gastrointest Surg. 2010;14:824–9.

13. Stoker J, Rociu E, Schouten WR, et al. Anovaginal and recto-vaginal fistulas: endoluminal sonography versus endoluminal MR imaging. Am J Roentgenol. 2002;178:737–41.

14. Maconi G, Parente F, Bianchi PG. Hydrogen peroxide enhanced ultrasound fistulography in the assessment of enterocutaneous fistulas complicating Crohn's disease. Gut. 1999;45:874–8.

15. Pinto RA, Peterson TV, Shawki S, Davila GW, Wexner SD. Are there predictors of outcome following rectovaginal fistula repair? Dis Colon Rectum. 2010;53:1240–7.

16. Rothenberger DA, Christenson CE, Balcos EG, Schottler JL, Nemer FD, Nivatvongs S, Goldberg S. Endorectal advancement flap for treatment of simple rectovaginal fistula. Dis Colon Rectum. 1982;25:297–300.

17. Lowry AC, Thorson AG, Rothenberger DA, Goldberg SM. Repair of simple rectovaginal fistulas. Influence of previous repair. Dis Colon Rectum. 1988;31:676–8.

18. Ellis CN. Outcomes after repair of rectovaginal fistulas using bioprosthetics. Dis Colon Rectum. 2008;51:1084–8.

19. Sonoda T, Hull T, Piedmonte MR, Fazio VW. Outcomes of primary repair of anorectal and rectovaginal fistulas using the endorectal advancement flap. Dis Colon Rectum. 2002;45:1622–8.

20. Hull TL, El-Gazzaz G, Gurland B, Church J, Zutshi M. Surgeons should not hesitate to perform episioproctotomy for rectovaginal fistula secondary to cryptoglandular or obstetrical origin. Dis Colon Rectum. 2011;54:54–9.

21. Schwandner O, Fuerst A, Kunstreich K, Scherer R. Innovative technique for the closure of rectovaginal fistula using Surgisis mesh. Tech Coloproctol. 2009;13:135–40.

22. Schwandner O, Fuerst A. Preliminary results on efficacy in closure of transsphincteric and rectovaginal fistulas associated with crohn's disease using new biomaterials. Surg Innov. 2009;16(2):162–8.

23. Roberts PL. Rectovaginal fistula. Semin Colon Rectal Surg. 2007;18:69–78.

24. Mazier WP, Senegore AJ, Schiesel EC. Operative repair of anovaginal and rectovaginal fistulas. Dis Colon Rectum. 1995;38:4–6.

25. Ozuner G, Hull TL, Cartmill J, Fazio VW. Long-term analysis of the use of transanal rectal advancement flaps for complicated anorectal/vaginal fistulas. Dis Colon Rectum. 1996;39:10–4.

26. Penninckx F, Moneghi D, D'Hoore A, Wyndaele J, Coremans G, Rutgeerts P. Success and failure after repair of rectovaginal fistula in Crohn's disease; analysis of prognostic factors. Colorectal Dis. 2007;3:406–11.

27. White AJ, Buchsbaum HJ, Blythe JG, Lifshitz S. Use of the bulbocavernosus muscle (Martius procedure) for repair of radiation-induced rectovaginal fistulas. Obstet Gynecol. 1982;60:114–8.

28. Kniery K, Johnson EK, Steele SR. How I do It: Martius flap for rectovaginal fistulas. J Gastrointest Surg. 2015;19:570–4.

29. Pitel S, Lefevre JH, Parc Y, Chafai N, Shields C, Tiret E. Martius advancement flap for low rectovaginal fistula: short- and long-term results. Colorectal Dis. 2011;13:e112–5.

30. Aartsen EJ, Sindram IS. Repair of the radiation induced recto-vaginal fistulas without or with interposition of the bulbocaver-nosus muscle (Martius procedure). Eur J Surg Oncol. 1988;14:171–7.

31. McNevin MS, Lee PY, Bax TW. Martius flap: an adjunct for repair of complex, low rectovaginal fistula. Am J Surg. 2007;193:597–9.

32. Songne K, Scotté M, Lubrano J, et al. Treatment of anovaginal or rectovaginal fistulas with modified Martius graft. Colorectal Dis. 2007;9:653–6.

33. Cui L, Chen D, Chen W, Jiang H. Interposition of vital bulbo-cavernosus graft in the treatment of both simple and recurrent rectovaginal fistulas. Int J Colorectal Dis. 2009;24:1255–9.

34. Kin C, Gurland B, Zutshi M, Hull T, Krummel T, Remzi F. Martius flap repair for complex rectovaginal fistula. Pol Przegl Chir. 2012;84:601–4.

35. Wexner SD, Ruiz DE, Genua J, Nogueras JJ, Weiss EG, Zmora O. Gracilis muscle interposition for the treatment of rectoure-thral, rectovaginal, and pouch-vaginal fistulas. Results in 53 patients. Ann Surg. 2008;248:39–43.

36. Furst A, Schmidbauer C, Swol-Ben J, Iesalnicks I, Schwandner O, Agha A. Gracilis transposition for repair of recurrent anovaginal and rectovaginal fistulas in Crohn's disease. Int J Colorectal Dis. 2008;23:349–53.

37. Sher ME, Bauer JJ, Gelernt I. Surgical repair of rectovaginal fistulas in patients with Crohn's disease: trans-vaginal approach. Dis Colon Rectum. 1991;34:641–8.

38. Van der Hagen SJ, Soeters PB, Baeten CG, van Gemert WG. Laparoscopic fistula excision and omentoplasty for high rectovaginal fistulas: a prospective study of 40 patients. Int J Colorectal Dis. 2011;26:1463–7.

39. Chu L, Wang J, Li L, Tong XW, Fan BZ, Guo Y, Li HF. Laparoscopic repair of iatrogenic vesicovaginal and rectovagi-nal fistula. Int J Clin Exp Med. 2015;8(2):2364–70.

40. Mukwege D, Mukanire N, Himpens J, Cadiere GB. Minimally invasive treatment of traumatic high rectovaginal fistulas. Surg Endosc. 2015 Apr 7. [Epub ahead of print]

41. Gajsek U, McArthur DR, Sagar PM. Long-term efficacy of the button fistula plug in the treatment of ileal pouch-vaginal and crohn's related rectovaginal fistulas. Dis Colon Rectum. 2011;54:999–1002.

42. Weerd D, Weum S, Norderval S. Novel treatment for recalci-trant rectovaginal fistulas: fat injection. Int Urogynecol J. 2015;26(1):139–44.

43. D'Ambrosio G, Paganini AM, Guerrieri M, et al. Minimally invasive treatment of rectovaginal fistula. Surg Endosc. 2012;26:546–50.

44. Simmang CL, Lacey SW, Huber PJ. Rectal sleeve advancement. Repair of rectovaginal fistula associated with anorectal stricture in Crohn's disease. Dis Colon Rectum. 1998;41:787–9.

45. Present DH, Korelitz BI, Wisch N, Glass JL, Sachar DB, Pastermack BS. Treatment of Crohn's disease with 6-mercapto-purine. A long-term randomized, double-blind study. N Engl J Med. 1980;302:981–7.

46. Ricart E, Panaccione R, Loftus EV, Tremaine WJ, Sandborn WJ. Infliximab for Crohn's disease in clinical practice at the Mayo Clinic: the first 100 patients. Am J Gastroenterol. 2001;96:722–9.

47. Van Bodegraven AA, Sloots CE, Felt-Bersma RJ, Meuwissen SG. Endosonographic evidence of persistence of Crohn's disease associated fistulas after infliximab treatment, irrespective of clinical response. Dis Colon Rectum. 2002;45:39–45.

48. Parsi M, Lashner B, Achkar JP, Connor JT, Brzezinski A. Type of fistula determines response to infliximab in patients with fistulous Crohn's Disease. Am J Gastroenterol. 2004;99:445–9.

49. Jones IT, Fazio VW, Jagelman DG. The use of transanal rectal advancement flaps in the management of fistulas involving the anorectum. Dis Colon Rectum. 1987;30:919–23.

50. Watson SJ, Philips RKS. Non-inflammatory rectovaginal fistula. Br J Surg. 1995;82:1641–3.

51. Wiskind AK, Thompson JD. Transverse transperineal repair of rectovaginal fistulas in the lower vagina. Am J Obstet Gynecol. 1992;167:694–9.

52. Lefèvre JH, Bretagnol F, Maggiori L, Alves A, Ferron M, Panis Y. Operative results and quality of life after gracilis muscle transposition for recurrent rectovaginal fistula. Dis Colon Rectum. 2009;52:1290–5.

53. Kobayashi H, Sugihara K. Successful management of rectovaginal fistula treated by endorectal advancement flap: report of two cases and literature review. Springerplus. 2015;4:21.

54. Takano S, Boutros M, Wexner S. Gracilis transposition for complex perineal fistulas: rectovaginal fistula and rectourethral fistula. Dis Colon Rectum. 2014;57:538.

55. Rius J, Nessim A, Nogueras JJ, Wexner SD. Gracilis transposition in complicated perianal fistula and unhealed perineal wounds in Crohn's disease. Eur J Surg. 2000;166:218–22.

56. Cohen JL, Stricker JW, Schoetz DJ, Coller JA, Veidenheimer MC. Rectovaginal fistula in Crohn's disease. Dis Colon Rectum. 1989;32:825–8.

57. Andreani SM, Dang HH, Grondona P, Zhan AZ, Edwards DP. Rectovaginal fistula in Crohn's disease. Dis Colon Rectum. 2007;50:2215–22.

58. O'Leary DP, Milroy CE, Durdey P. Definitive repair of anovaginal fistula in Crohn's disease. Ann R Coll Surg Engl. 1998;80:250–2.

59. Hull TL, Bartus C, Bast RN, Floruta C, Lopez R. Success of episioproctotomy for cloaca and rectovaginal fistula. Dis Colon Rectum. 2006;50:97–101.

60. Chew SS, Reiger NA. Transperineal repair of obstetric- related anovaginal fistula. Aust N Z J Obstet Gynaecol. 2004;44:68–71.

61. MacRae HM, McLeod RS, Cohen Z, Stern H, Reznick R. Treatment of rectovaginal fistulas that has failed previous repair attempts. Dis Colon Rectum. 1995;38:921–5.

62. Gottgens KW, Smeets RR, Stassen LP, Beets G, Breukin SO. The disappointing quality of published studies on operative techniques for rectovaginal fistulas: a blueprint for a prospective multi-institutional study. Dis Colon Rectum. 2014;57:888–98.

63. Ulrich D, Roos J, Jakse G, Pallua N. Gracilis muscle interposition for the treatment of recto-urethral and rectovaginal fistulas: a retrospective analysis of 35 cases. J Plast Reconstr Aesthet Surg. 2009;2:352–6.

64. Zmora O, Tulchinsky H, Gur E, Goldman G, Klausner JM, Rabau M. Gracilis muscle transposition for fistulas between the rectum and urethra or vagina. Dis Colon Rectum. 2006;49:1316–21.

65. Reichert M, Schwandner T, Hecker A, Behnk A, Baumgart-Vogt E, Wagenlehner F, Padberg W. Surgical approach for repair of rectovaginal fistula by modified martius flap. Geburtshilfe Frauenheilkd. 2014;74(10):923–7.

17

Pilonidal Disease and Hidradenitis Suppurativa

Eric K. Johnson

Key Concepts

- Pilonidal disease presents with a wide range of symptoms and multiple treatment options exist. Treatment should be tailored to the severity of disease, anatomy of disease, and patient expectations.
- Because of the wide array of available surgical options, the surgeon treating pilonidal disease should master 3–4 approaches that are applicable to a wide range of disease presentations.
- Treatments applied to both pilonidal disease and hidradenitis suppurativa should not be more disabling for the patient than the disease itself.
- There are numerous medical options available to treat hidradenitis suppurativa. They should be investigated and attempted prior to aggressive radical surgical management.
- Radical excision of hidradenitis suppurativa with surgical reconstruction offers the best hope to avoid disease recurrence.

Background

The term "pilonidal" is derived from the root words "pilus" (a hair) and "nidus" (nest). Since 1880 when Dr. R.M. Hodges coined the term pilonidal sinus [1], the diagnoses of pilonidal cyst, sinus, and abscess have been used interchangeably and somewhat indiscriminately to mean the same thing, though they most certainly do not—in the case of abscess. It is largely for this reason that the more modern nomenclature of "pilonidal disease" (PD) is used to describe the spectrum of disorders that may be encountered. The first published description of this disease occurred in 1847 when Dr. A.W. Anderson described a case of "hair extracted from an ulcer" [2]. The first pilonidal abscess was described in 1854 [3], though there is no question that this condition was encountered earlier. It wasn't until World War II that surgeons became much more familiar with this disease entity, likely because of the large number of cases seen in members of the military. In fact, the disorder was known as "jeep disease" and was thought to be related to modern mechanized warfare, which required soldiers to ride in vehicles for extended periods of time [4].

It is clear from early publications that little has changed in terms of the issues that confront both the patient and surgeon. A 1955 publication from the Veteran's Administration health system reveals that the debate over open and closed wound management is not new [5]. In this study, patients managed with primary wound closure developed recurrence 40% of the time and required hospital stays of approximately 17 days, while those managed with open technique stayed for 30 days and had a recurrence rate of 35%! While we have seen significant reductions in both length of hospital stay and recurrence, it is clear that we still do not have the ideal answer for this condition.

Etiology

There has been considerable debate over whether PD is congenital or acquired, but most would currently agree that it is an acquired disease. It is generally believed that the initiating event is traumatization of the skin and surrounding hair follicles in the natal cleft. This occurs secondary to trapping of hairs, not necessarily those arising locally in the natal cleft. The local anatomy creates an unfavorable environment where friction, warmth, moisture, and perhaps local hypoxia lead to local trauma secondary to the barbed texture of the hair. A granulomatous foreign body-type reaction results. There is even some histological and immunohistochemical evidence that PD may represent a unilocalized type of hidradenitis suppurativa [6]. Disease typically begins as

Electronic supplementary material: The online version of this chapter (doi:10.1007/978-3-319-25970-3_17) contains supplementary material, which is available to authorized users.

© Springer International Publishing 2016

S.R. Steele et al. (eds.), *The ASCRS Textbook of Colon and Rectal Surgery*, DOI 10.1007/978-3-319-25970-3_17

289

a small sinus that may drain fluid but then can progress to numerous sinuses with associated cystic dilation and potential abscess formation. In some cases, unless the process is interrupted, it can become more widespread leading to worsening symptoms. Disease can range from the asymptomatic single sinus found incidentally up to a severe locally destructive process associated with significant disability.

PD is not limited to the natal cleft area, and there are several reports of disease occurring in the interdigital areas in hair dressers [7], as well as in other areas such as the umbilicus [8]. The presence of disease in these atypical areas further supports the above theory. PD has been reported to affect males more commonly than females; however recent data from the armed forces suggests that the incidence rates are similar at 1.9 and 1.7 per 1000 person-years, respectively [9]. There are several risk factors that have been implicated in the development of PD including positive family history of disease, elevated body mass index (BMI>25), poor hygiene, hirsutism, deep natal cleft anatomy, occupation that requires prolonged sitting, and excessive sweating [10–12]. It is not uncommon to see disease affect an individual who lacks many or most of these factors however. A prospective study comparing 587 patients with PD to 2780 healthy controls showed that hirsute individuals that sit down for more than 6 h per day and who bathe two or fewer times per week have a 219-fold increased risk for sacrococcygeal PD [12]. A positive family history may not only predispose to disease occurrence, but may also be associated with increased recurrence rates after surgery as well as earlier onset of disease [11].

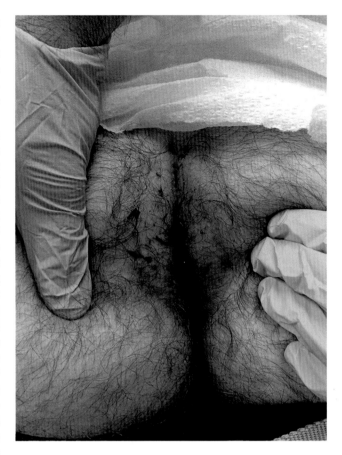

FIGURE 17-1. This image shows a hirsute individual with midline "pits" that could go unnoticed. Note the poor hygiene.

Clinical Presentation/Diagnosis

Patient presentation can range from a referral for completely asymptomatic and incidentally discovered disease to a person who is significantly disabled by locally destructive disease. Commonly encountered scenarios are the patient who has an acute pilonidal abscess that requires drainage, and the surgical office visit to discuss definitive surgical therapy after either acute abscess drainage or persistent disease of moderate severity impacting the patient's quality of life. Often, in the military setting, disease that would otherwise be ignored requires operative management secondary to its impact upon an individual's ability to perform at a high physical level or live in an austere environment.

Establishing a diagnosis is rather simple and does not require extensive testing or imaging. Simple history taking and a physical exam will in most cases solidify the diagnosis. Patients will often complain of pain over the sacrococcygeal area with drainage of clear fluid or bleeding. In the case of acute abscess, fever may also occur. Physical exam will reveal "pits" in the midline. There may be several pits, or only one small pit that could be easily overlooked if the examiner does not consider this diagnosis (Figure 17-1). Examination may also often reveal induration just lateral to

midline that can be unilateral or bilateral. This may also be associated with additional draining sinuses. In more significant cases, there may be open wounds that can have a large range in size (Figure 17-2a–c). Acute abscess is typically associated with overlying erythema, fluctuance, and severe local tenderness (Figure 17-3). In a less common scenario, the examiner may mistake PD as an anorectal fistula if a sinus is present close to the anus. It is important to examine the midline overlying the sacrum for pits. If they are present, then pilonidal sinus should be included in the differential diagnosis in these individuals (Figure 17-4a, b).

Recurrent disease in the patient who has already undergone surgical excision is another commonly encountered scenario (Figure 17-5). Recurrence may occur either early (within 1 year) or late. Early recurrence is often actually persistence of an open wound that never healed after surgery. This may be thought of as PD, but in many cases is actually nothing more than a non-healing midline sacrococcygeal wound. Wounds placed in the midline often demonstrate delayed healing or non-healing. The pathophysiology related to a non-healing wound may actually be different than that related to PD; however the methods we use to treat these maladies are similar. Recurrence presents similarly to primary PD, and may be related to poor surgical technique,

FIGURE 17-2. (**a–c**) These images show a range of open wounds that may be seen with pilonidal disease.

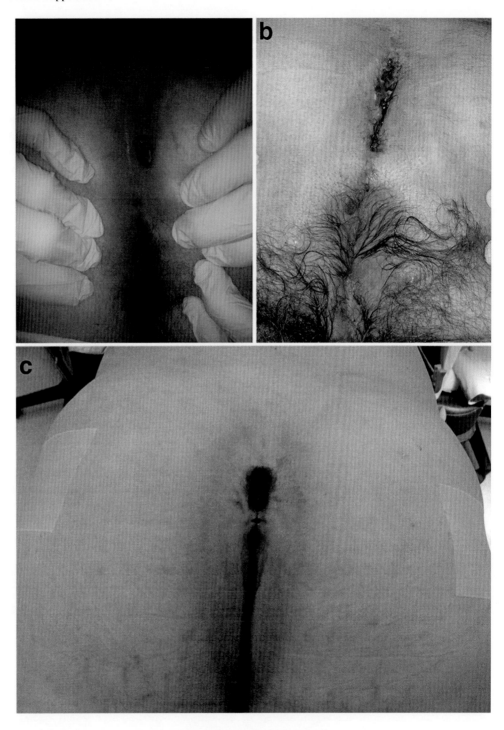

patient noncompliance, or failure to modify the pre-existing risk factors that led to disease in the first place. Recurrence may also simply be the natural history of disease.

Treatment

There are numerous treatment options available to address PD. An important overriding concept that should be completely clear is that the treatment should be tailored to the patient's expectations, disease anatomy, and disease severity. Options range from nonoperative therapies up to wide local excision with local flap reconstruction. The debate of open wound management versus closed management remains, and even when primary closure is performed, wound care and physical limitations may be required for an extended period of time. Given the large number of operative choices available, it is likely not practical to be well versed in all. A good recommendation would be to be familiar with three or four operative options that range from simple to complex and provide a solution for several different anatomic configurations of disease.

Nonoperative Management

It is first important to recognize when PD requires no invasive management at all. As stated earlier, some patients are referred based simply upon the incidental finding of midline pits in the natal cleft. If the patient is asymptomatic, and physical examination reveals no concerning findings, they require no operative management. You never want the treatment to be worse than the disease, and that is exactly what one will discover in this setting. The patient may still benefit from counseling regarding ways to reduce their risk of developing symptomatic disease. Risk factor modification such as weight loss, avoidance of prolonged sitting at work, improved hygiene, and weekly clipping of hair in and adjacent to the natal cleft may reduce the chance that a patient will develop symptoms related to PD. These are also appropriate in the setting of active and symptomatic disease. These measures may lead to either improvement in symptoms or quiescence in mild cases. A study published in 1994 showed that these measures combined with limited lateral incision and drainage in the setting of acute abscess led to fewer occupied hospital bed days when compared to excisional procedures [13]. Over a 17-year follow-up, only 23 of 101 cases went on to require excisional therapy.

Given that weekly shaving has been associated with success, many have advocated laser hair removal as a long-lasting alternative for the conservative management of PD. Despite the interest in this mode of therapy, we lack any robust data to support its use. Small studies of 6–14 patients have shown some benefit to laser epilation in the setting of recurrent PD [14, 15]. This procedure is uncomfortable for the patient and often requires local anesthetic. Treatments are performed over 3–11 sessions at 6–8-week intervals and can be quite costly. A study of laser epilation in teenagers with PD, 25/28 of which were managed initially with surgery, showed only one recurrence over a mean follow-up of 2 years [16]. The authors concluded that use of the laser was a safe method for addressing intergluteal hair that may reduce recurrence rates.

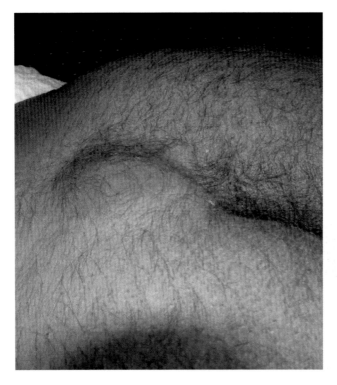

FIGURE 17-3. This image depicts an acute pilonidal abscess.

FIGURE 17-4. (**a, b**) These images show two different patients that presented with draining perianal sinuses. Note the midline pits over the sacrum that make one more suspicious of pilonidal disease as the cause.

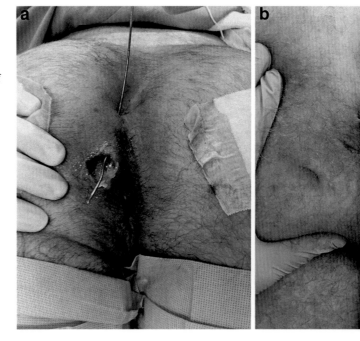

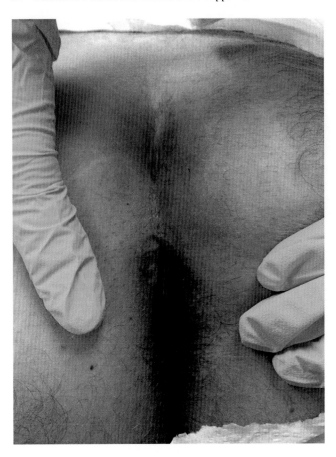

FIGURE 17-5. This image shows a patient who developed recurrence after an attempt at a cleft lift procedure. Incorrect performance of the distal portion of the procedure may have led to this recurrence.

A randomized trial comparing laser hair removal to traditional methods as an adjunctive therapy after surgery for PD demonstrated a lower recurrence rate in the laser-treated group [17]. This appeared to be related to noncompliance with traditional hair removal methods after 1 year. There is however some debate over the benefit of hair removal in the setting of PD that has been managed operatively. A retrospective analysis of patients that had undergone surgery to treat PD was performed with focus on those who performed razor hair removal vs. those that did not [18]. Recurrence was observed in 30% of those who shaved vs. 19% of those who did not shave ($p=0.01$). This would suggest a potential negative effect of postoperative razor epilation. Future studies should likely focus on a comparison between laser hair removal and no hair removal in the adjunctive setting.

While some form of hair removal may lead to reduced recurrence rates as well as reduced requirement for excisional therapy, this method alone is unlikely to lead to disease cure—especially in the setting of more significant or severe disease. Often the hair that is found inside of sinus tracts is clearly noted to be long hair from other parts of the body. It is theorized that longer hairs can fall into the natal cleft,

become trapped, and result in disease. Clearly, local epilation alone will not eliminate this threat.

Although not necessarily considered nonoperative (maybe non-excisional) therapy, methods employing the use of phenol or fibrin glue injection to ablate sinus tracts have been investigated in small series by many [19–26]. These techniques often employ tract curettage, debridement, and hair removal, which contribute significantly to success. Use of phenol as an ablative agent has been associated with success rates of 60–95% [19–21]. Fibrin glue injection combined with a variety of techniques has shown success in the range of 90–100% [22–25]. A recent evaluation of individuals treated with fibrin glue revealed that 79% of patients were satisfied, 71% were back to normal activities within 2 weeks, and 74% required no further treatment [26]. A video-assisted ablative technique has also been described using a 4 mm rigid hysteroscope with a five french working channel [27]. Continuous irrigation is used, hair is removed, and the cavity and tracts are ablated using a bipolar electrode. Only one recurrence was detected over 12 months in 27 patients. This may represent a potential option for minimally invasive/non-excisional therapy. The potential advantages of these therapies over excisional methods are more rapid recovery and less post-procedural pain.

Operative/Excisional Management

There are numerous methods available for the operative management of PD. The literature is filled with a large number of publications reporting results from various procedures. The typical manuscript is a retrospective review examining the results from a small series of patients that have undergone one specific type of operative procedure. There are several randomized trials comparing one surgical method vs. another with variable results. Essentially, it is possible to find evidence to support whatever procedure one prefers to perform. Results are likely related to variations in how patients are cared for postoperatively as well as differences in surgical technique. It is best to review some of the more common methods of operative management beginning with those that are considered simple and progressing to the complex. A well-prepared surgeon will be familiar with most of these methods, and will tailor their management to disease severity, disease anatomy, and patient expectations.

Basic Procedures

Outside of incision and drainage of a pilonidal abscess, the simplest procedure to perform is laying open of the cyst and all sinus tracts. This may also be termed "unroofing" of disease. This and wide local excision of all disease down to the post-sacral fascia were the procedures performed most commonly in the early days of PD management. Often, unroofing was combined with marsupialization of the wound. Recurrence rates of 15–35% [5] led many to seek out more effective methods of surgical management. It is important to ensure that as much of the surgical wound as possible be kept

FIGURE 17-6. (a–c) These
images show yet another patient
who presented with what was
thought to be an anal fistula.
Midline pits were noted and the
disease was treated with a
lay-open technique, which
resulted in rapid healing. Of note,
this could potentially represent
hidradenitis suppurativa.

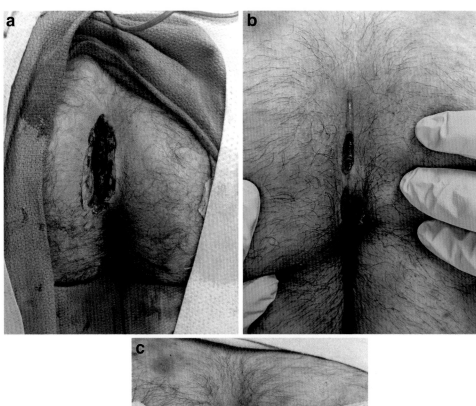

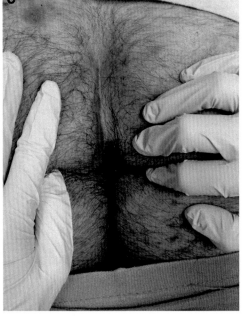

off the midline, as midline wounds tend to have some difficulty with healing. Simple tract unroofing and curettage are
particularly helpful in the setting of minor disease affecting
the perianal area (often mistaken as an anal fistula). The bulk
of this wound will lie off the midline and will heal quickly
(Figure 17-6a–c). There continues to be debate over which
approach is superior, though recent data would suggest that a
higher volume of excised specimen is associated with a
higher surgical site infection rate and likely a higher risk of
recurrent disease [28]. The next logical step was to perform
excision combined with primary wound closure which can
often require the mobilization of minor skin flaps.

Primary closure has been combined with drainage in some
settings with a wide variation in results. The use of a drain in
this setting has been studied, but has not been shown to result
in improved results as far as patient satisfaction, healing, or
infection is concerned [29]. A meta-analysis of this subject
showed that there were no statistically significant differences
in outcomes with or without the use of a drain in the setting
of primary wound closure [30]. A recent randomized
controlled trial comparing the laying open method to wide
excision with primary closure showed that healing occurred
faster in the primary closure group with no differences in the
groups noted at 1 year of follow-up [31]. Interestingly, this

group of investigators made no effort to keep the majority of the wound off the midline. Rao and colleagues in 2010 published a prospective randomized study comparing the lay-open technique to primary closure augmented by the placement of gentamicin-impregnated collagen [32]. The antibiotic-impregnated material was placed in the base of the wound with overlying tissue closure. The results showed improved healing at 4 weeks, improved postoperative pain, and lower cost in the primary closure group. Recurrence rates were no different at 5 years.

Another group performed a 4-arm randomized trial comparing primary closure, primary closure with hydrogen peroxide irrigation, wide local excision, and wide local excision with hydrogen peroxide irrigation [33]. The wide local excision combined with peroxide irrigation group showed the lowest recurrence rate and the fastest time to healing. The investigators attributed this to the ability to clearly delineate all tracts and disease with peroxide irriga-tion, allowing them to perform a more precise and low-volume excision. Similarly, another group performed a retrospective analysis of PD patients that had undergone surgery and concluded that use of methylene blue injection to delineate disease was associated with a lower recurrence rate [34].

There have been several descriptions of "pit picking" procedures over the years. These procedures are relatively minor in terms of the amount of tissue excised; they result in small wounds, and may be ideal for those suffering with mild to moderate levels of disease. These procedures are not suit-able for the patient with a large open wound or in those with severe recurrent disease. The basic premise of this method is that the central pits are excised with minimal surrounding tissue, hair and debris are removed, the old adjacent abscess cavity or "cyst" is excised through a lateral incision using an undermining technique, the pit excision sites are closed pri-marily, and the lateral incision is closed partially to allow for drainage. This results in a good cosmetic result with minimal pain, early return to work, and rapid healing (Figure 17-7) [35]. A punch biopsy knife of appropriate size may be used to perform the pit excision and is ideal for this application. This procedure has been modified slightly by many, but the basic tenets remain in the various methods. The use of phenol as a sclerosing agent has been combined with pit excision and has resulted in good outcomes [36].

Complex Procedures

The common thread among all "complex" procedures is the mobilization of adjacent tissue to achieve primary wound closure—in effect, the creation of a local flap. Some of these procedures combine wide local excision of diseased tissue with flap reconstruction, while others preserve as much local tissue as possible. These procedures also range from simple to complex. While there are numerous options, attention will be devoted to the discussion of the Karydakis flap, the Bascom cleft-lift procedure, and the rhomboid or Limberg flap procedure and its modifications. There are additional

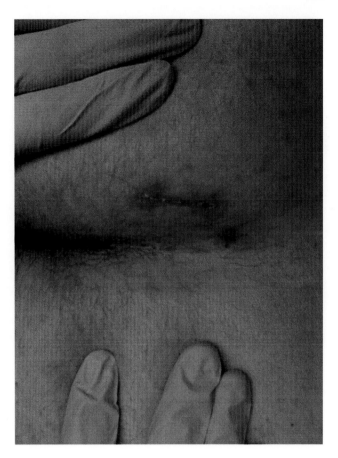

FIGURE 17-7. This image shows a patient 2 weeks after a simple Bascom, or "pit picking" operation.

flap procedures such as the z-plasty, V-Y advancement flap, and other rotational flap techniques that will not be discussed. Many support the use of flap procedures in primary PD, while others believe that they should only be used in the setting of disease recurrence after primary surgery. It is possible that these procedures are more effective in curing disease, because they result in a modification of the natal cleft anatomy. The majority of these techniques result in a flattening of the natal cleft, which may prevent disease recurrence.

Karydakis Flap

This procedure is performed first by excising the affected tissue in the midline, typically leaving an elliptical defect. A beveled skin flap is then created and mobilized across the midline to facilitate a primary closure that is lateral of midline (Figure 17-8). A closed suction drain may be used or omitted. The purported advantages of this procedure are the tension-free closure that is out of the midline coupled with some flattening of the natal cleft. This is probably the easiest flap procedure to perform. This procedure has been shown to be superior to simple primary midline closure in terms of patient satisfaction, recurrence rate, and rate of postoperative complications [37]. It has also been reported to be comparable to other more complex flap procedures such as the modified Limberg flap [38, 39].

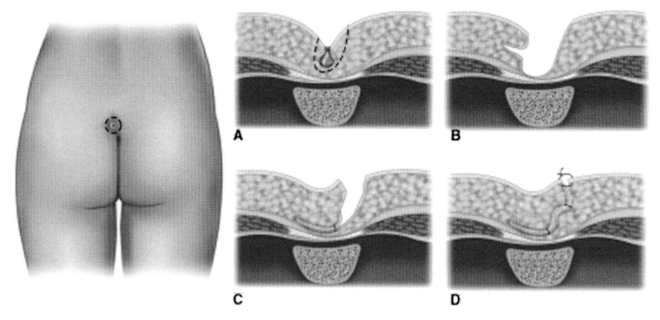

FIGURE 17-8. This drawing depicts one method of performing a Karydakis flap.

Cleft Lift Procedure (See Video 17-1)

The cleft lift procedure was originally described and popularized by Dr. John Bascom, and is often referred to as the Bascom cleft lift. This is a simple but intricate procedure that is designed to "lift" the natal cleft and result in an incision that is closed off the midline. Interestingly, wide excision is not required—in fact, the only tissue that is excised is the overlying skin on one side of the natal cleft. This procedure requires that the patient be marked prior to incision to establish a "safe zone," beyond which no dissection is performed. The patient is placed in the prone position and the buttocks are squeezed together (Figure 17-9). The area where the skin on both sides of the natal cleft touches is marked with a magic marker. This establishes the safe zone. The buttocks are then taped apart exposing the disease (Figure 17-10). After skin preparation, the area to be excised is marked with another marking pen (Figure 17-11). This proposed incision will be partially elliptical and should extend from the midline pits out to one side of the safe zone. The distal portion of this incision is scimitar shaped in order to facilitate closure near the anus without causing local deformity.

Local anesthetic is injected and the incision is made down to the level of the subcutaneous fat. The overlying skin is excised taking care to leave the subcutaneous fat in place. A flap is then raised across the midline out to the opposite safe zone border (Figure 17-12). The thickness of this flap should approximate that of a breast flap that would be created during a mastectomy. When creating the flap down toward the distal portion of the incision (near the anus), the flap should be thicker to prevent dimple formation near the anus. Any disease-related debris or granulation tissue should be gently debrided with a surgical sponge and irrigation with saline

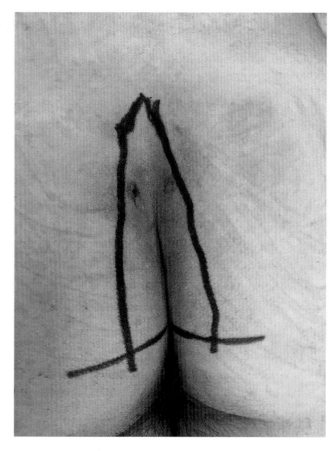

FIGURE 17-9. After squeezing the buttocks together and marking the safe zone.

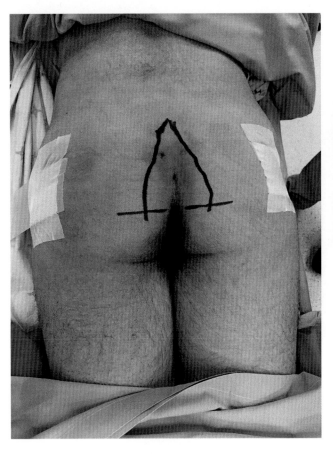

FIGURE 17-10. Image showing the buttocks taped apart under tension providing excellent operative exposure.

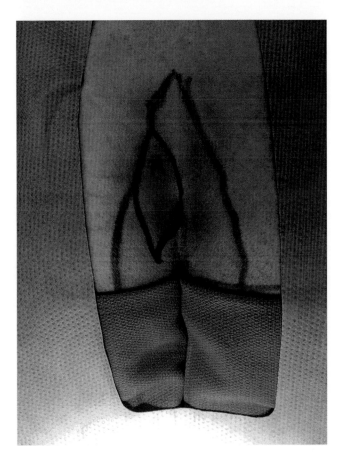

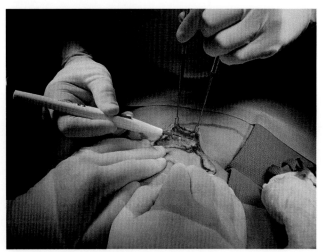

FIGURE 17-12. This image shows the operative creating the flap to be used for the cleft lift.

should be undertaken. Any remaining "cyst wall" or tissue contracture can be divided into squares with a scalpel or electrocautery device. The subcutaneous tissue is then closed in layers with an absorbable suture. The superficial layers are reapproximated in layers, lastly with a subcuticular suture (Figure 17-13a,b). Use of a drain is optional, but certainly not necessary.

A case-control study published in 2011 compared the results of the cleft lift procedure to wide excision and packing in 70 patients [40]. A total of 97% of patients undergoing cleft lift healed completely while only 73% of wide excision patients healed. Three of nine patients with chronic wounds underwent subsequent cleft lift with a 100% success rate. Recurrence was noted in 2.5% of cleft lifts and in 20% of wide excisions. Others have shown similar success in rates of healing with the cleft lift procedure as compared to wide excision and packing and excision and primary midline closure [41]. This technique has also been compared to the Limberg flap in a randomized prospective fashion [42]. Short-term outcomes of 122 patients were analyzed and revealed that those undergoing the cleft lift had shorter operative durations, less excised tissue weight, improved pain scores, and fewer physical limitations on postoperative day 10. There were no differences in healing, complications, or early recurrences.

There is little question that this technique is easier to perform, takes less time, and removes less tissue than the more complex flap procedures such as the rhomboid flap. It results in flattening of the natal cleft, which is likely desirable. Unfortunately, not every patient with PD is a candidate for this procedure. Those with complex recurrent disease and large open wounds may not be ideal candidates, and may require more extensive flap procedures. Disease that is very close to the anus may cause difficulty with this technique, though if open wounds are able to be moved off the midline, they may still heal.

FIGURE 17-11. The area to be excised is marked. Typically this excision is performed on the side where induration or a "cyst" is located.

FIGURE 17-13. (**a, b**) These images show the procedure at the completion of the case and at 3-week follow-up with complete healing.

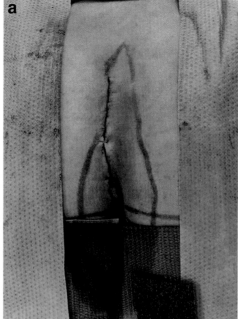 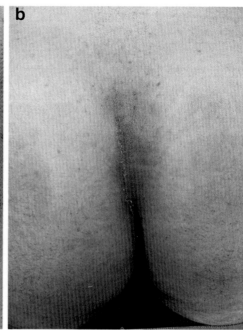

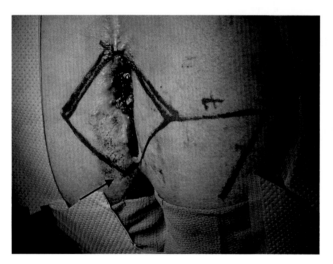

FIGURE 17-14. This image shows the planned lines of incision for the rhomboid flap. Note that the caudal tip is NOT located directly over the anus. This modification results in a wound that does not come to a point at the location of highest risk.

Rhomboid/Limberg Flap (See Video 17-2)

The rhomboid flap is a useful but more complex procedure that can be used in any setting of PD, but is typically reserved for more severe cases. The procedure involves a "diamond-" or rhombus-shaped area of wide excision encompassing all disease in the midline (Figure 17-14). While most will excise tissue down to the level of the post-sacral fascia, this is not entirely necessary. One must ensure however that the thickness of the mobilized lipocutaneous flap approximates the thickness of the tissue that is excised. This technique works particularly well in the setting of complex recurrent disease. The planned incision is marked, and the flap is raised with

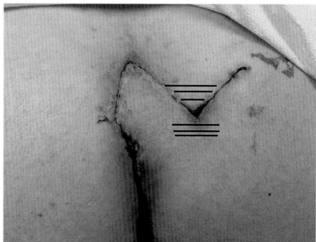

FIGURE 17-15. This image shows areas at the point of maximal tension that must be undermined to facilitate closure.

electrocautery. It is recommended to handle the flap gently during mobilization. It is important to take care to undermine the areas adjacent to the flap so that the most tension-free closure can be obtained (Figure 17-15). Once the flap is mobilized completely (Figure 17-16), it is anchored to the post-sacral tissues with an absorbable suture. A closed-suction drain is placed and a layered closure takes place using absorbable suture. The skin can be closed using a variety of techniques, none of which has proven to be superior. Some will cover the final closure with glue to create a watertight seal (Figure 17-17). A modification of this procedure was created in order to keep the caudal point of the incision away from the anus (Figure 17-14).

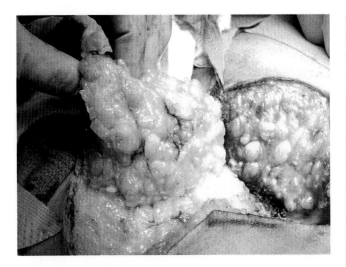

FIGURE 17-16. The Limberg flap after full mobilization, just prior to closure.

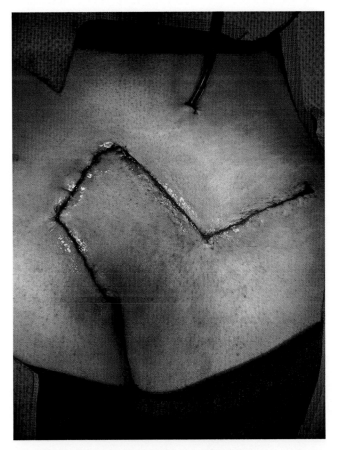

FIGURE 17-17. The appearance at the completion of the Limberg flap procedure. The wound has been covered with glue.

The drain can be left in place for 48 h or until it has produced 30 ml or less daily for 2 consecutive days. The patient should avoid any strenuous activity for 2–4 weeks. It is not uncommon for these wounds to separate slightly in one or two areas over the ensuing 2 weeks (Figure 17-18). This will require some minor wound care and is typically well

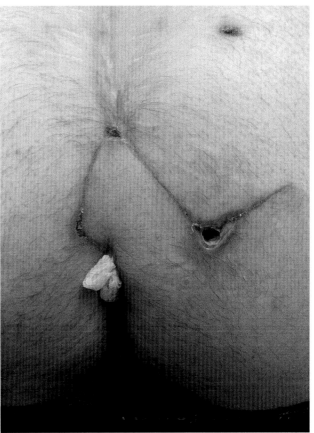

FIGURE 17-18. Follow-up will often reveal areas of minor wound separation that will require some ongoing basic wound care.

tolerated. Occasionally it will take 4–8 weeks for the wound to completely heal. In some cases, the disease spans a very large area over the sacrum extending from the perianal area for a long-distance cephalad. Many are uncomfortable creating such a large area of excision and flap in this setting. When this is the case, the technique can still be used but may be modified. The most difficult area in which to achieve healing is the caudal midline. An excision can be performed, and flap created such that the caudal midline is covered leaving an open wound cephalad (Figure 17-19). The remaining wound can be managed in a variety of ways, but the use of a negative pressure wound therapy device makes this management easy (Figure 17-20a, b). This device can be used in the standard fashion until the remaining wound is small enough to manage using standard dressings. The area will typically heal quickly, and does not impair the flap in any way.

Potential surgical site-related postoperative complications include wound dehiscence, flap necrosis, hematoma, wound infection, and seroma. These occur at rates of 4%, 0–2%, 1%, 3–5%, and 3%, respectively [43, 44]. Recurrence can be seen in approximately 4% [44]. Several series have compared outcomes associated with the Limberg flap (LF), modified Limberg flap (MLF), and excision with primary midline closure [45–48]. The evidence indicates that the LF or MLF is associated with faster return to work, lower rates of surgical

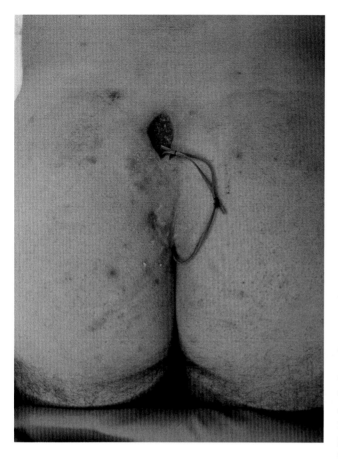

FIGURE 17-19. This image shows a patient with recurrent disease that resulted in a large abscess that was drained superiorly and required some tissue debridement. This resulted in a large area of disease to be addressed.

site infection, lower recurrence, and lower rates of wound dehiscence. Comparisons of the MLF, LF, and Karydakis flap show similar superiority for the LF and MLF [49, 50], while others have shown equivalence [51].

Disease Recurrence

Given that there are several known risk factors that predispose to the occurrence of PD, many have attempted to investigate factors that may predict disease recurrence. Familial history of disease, increased sinus number, larger cavity diameter, and primary wound closure have been shown to be associated with higher rates of recurrence [52]. Interestingly, tobacco smoking and body mass index > 25 have NOT been shown to increase recurrence [53]. Recurrence has been shown to be lower in those that undergo surgical incision and drainage prior to definitive surgery as compared to those who have spontaneous abscess rupture [54]. Along these lines, surgery performed in the "after-hours" and potentially emergent setting has been associated with higher recurrence rates [55]. Many publications that report on recurrence are criticized secondary to a lack of long-term follow-up. Doll and colleagues analyzed data from German military members and performed a telephone survey specifically investigating for recurrence [56]. They were able to demonstrate recurrence rates that were 22% higher than previously reported through collection of data over a longer period of follow-up. Recurrences up to 20 years after surgery were seen, and they recommended that studies investigating long-term outcomes should have at least 5 years of follow-up.

FIGURE 17-20. (a, b) This image shows a patient similar to that in Figure 17-19. The flap was created and closed leaving an open wound superiorly that was treated with negative pressure wound therapy and healed easily.

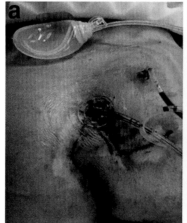
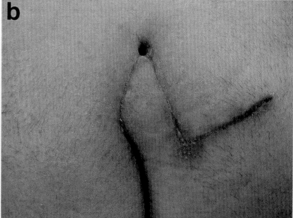

Hidradenitis Suppurativa

Background

The term hidradenitis suppurativa (HS), also known as acne inversa, was coined in 1864 by Verneuil [57] and literally refers to "sweat gland inflammation producing pus." The disease is a chronic inflammatory disorder involving the skin of apocrine gland-bearing areas, typically the perineum, inguinal, inframammary, and axillary regions. Colorectal surgeons are often consulted for assistance in managing those with perianal and perineal disease. Individuals afflicted with HS suffer a tremendous impact upon their quality of life with effects on both their physical and mental health [58, 59]. Practitioners in Europe have suggested that HS has the highest impact upon quality of life among all assessed dermatologic diseases [60].

The prevalence of HS is estimated to be 127.8 per 100,000 or 0.13%, with a higher prevalence among women, based on data from the Rochester epidemiology project [61]. This translates to fewer than 200,000 affected patients in the USA, 93% of which are between the ages of 18 and 64 years [62]. The reported mean age of onset is between 20 and 24 years of age, with less than 8% of affected individuals developing disease earlier than 13 years of age [63]. Early-onset disease seems to be correlated with family history of disease. When compared to psoriasis, another chronic skin disease, HS patients consume more health care and generate higher health care costs [64].

Etiology/Presentation/Diagnosis

Much like with pilonidal disease, the etiology of HS has been debated for quite some time. It was once thought purely to be secondary to infection of the apocrine sweat glands, but there is now general agreement that this is not true. The disease is characterized by chronic follicular occlusion resulting in secondary inflammation of the apocrine glands [65]. The initial inciting event is believed to be hyperkeratosis that leads to follicular occlusion [66, 67]. Others have proposed that the follicular occlusion occurs as a result of a defect in the follicular support system [68]. In any case, there is ultimate dysfunction in the entire folliculopilosebaceous unit (FPSU) that leads to follicular rupture and secondary bacterial infection involving the apocrine glands. Disease manifests initially as open comedones, typically with a few "heads," and tender subcutaneous papules [69]. In many this leads to a chronic and progressive worsening of symptoms in which additional nodules form, rupture, and drain a thick mucopurulent foul-smelling liquid. Over time this leads to sinus tract formation, fibrotic subcutaneous scarring, and potentially disabling contractures of the affected limb [69].

There are a number of variables that have been identified as risk factors for disease. Tobacco smoking and obesity have been associated with both the presence of disease and lower remission rates [70]. Weight loss has been shown to be temporally associated with remission [71, 72], with one report demonstrating disease quiescence with rapid weight loss after gastric bypass surgery. Sweating, shaving, deodorant use, and friction have also been implicated as potential exacerbating factors [73]. It is also believed that there may be dietary triggers that worsen disease (high carbohydrate diet, milk consumption) [74].

Diagnosis is typically made based on common physical exam findings including skin thickening, induration, abscess formation, the presence of draining sinuses, and contractures in the regions of the body considered at risk. There are several other diagnoses in the differential that should be considered (Table 17-1). The diagnosis can be confirmed histologically with a biopsy specimen. Given that disease can present with a wide range of severity, there have been two classification or staging systems proposed to grade disease, the Hurley system and the Sartorius system (Tables 17-2 and 17-3). The Hurley system is used more commonly as it seems to be better suited to clinical as opposed to research use. Because of some criticism related to the simplicity of the Hurley staging system, a French group have introduced a latent classification system, which better groups HS patients into three distinct phenotypes (Table 17-4) [75]. Despite its weaknesses however, the Hurley system seems to be most useful to physicians making treatment recommendations for affected individuals.

Several comorbid conditions have well-known association with HS. There is a well-established link between acne and HS, as well as with pilonidal disease [66]. Some other commonly

TABLE 17-1. A list of diagnoses that should be considered in the differential diagnosis of hidradenitis suppurative [67]

Diseases to be considered in the differential diagnosis
Acne
Actinomycosis
Anal fistula
Carbuncles
Cat scratch disease
Cellulitis
Crohn's disease
Cutaneous blastomycosis
Dermoid cyst
Granuloma inguinale
Erysipelas
Furuncles
Inflamed epidermoid cyst
Lymphadenopathy
Lymphogranuloma venereum
Nocardia infection
Noduloulcerative syphilis
Perirectal abscess
Pilonidal disease
Tuberculous abscess
Tularemia

TABLE 17-2. Description of the Hurley classification of hidradenitis suppurativa, likely the most useful in the clinical setting

Hurley staging system of hidradenitis suppurativa	
Stage I	Abscess formation, single or multiple, without scarring or sinus tracts
Stage II	Recurrent abscesses with tract formation and scarring, single or multiple, with widely separated lesions
Stage III	Multiple interconnected tracts and abscesses throughout an entire region

TABLE 17-3. The Sartorius scoring or staging system

Sartorius staging system/Sartorius score	
Involvement in specific body areas	3 points for each area involved
Nodules	2 points for each
Fistulas	4 points
Scars	1 point
Other findings	1 point
Longest distance between two lesions	2–4 points
If lesions are separated by normal skin	Yes—0 points, No—6 points

Some have modified the system by adding value to the presence of pain, drainage, or odor. This may be a more useful system in the research setting to quantify severity of disease

TABLE 17-4. Latent or phenotypic classification proposed by Canoui-Poitrine et al. [75]

Latent classification	Phenotype	Affected region
LC1	Axillary-mammary	Axilla, breast, perineum, inguinal
LC2	Follicular	Ears, chest, back, legs, axillary, breast
LC3	Gluteal	Gluteal fold

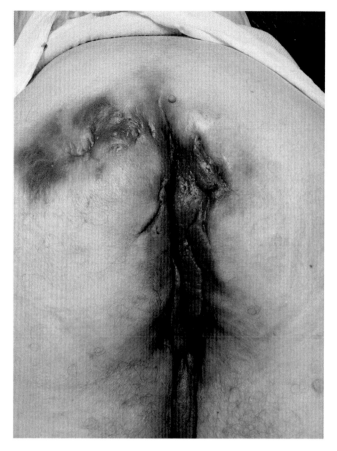

FIGURE 17-21. This image shows a patient with Hurley stage III hidradenitis suppurativa.

associated diseases include inflammatory bowel disease (particularly Crohn's disease), spondyloarthropathy, genetic keratin disorders, and squamous cell carcinoma [76]. In some cases it can be difficult to differentiate between the diseases, particularly in pilonidal disease and Crohn's disease with anal involvement. It is not entirely surprising that there can be considerable overlap in how all of these associated diseases are treated.

Treatment

As with treatment of any disease, it is important to identify the goals of therapy and patient expectations of the outcome, as well as what they will have to go through to achieve the desired end point. Medical therapy with the ultimate goal of suppression, coupled with the occasional procedure to drain an abscess, may suit a patient with Hurley stage I or II disease quite well. Conversely, the patient with Hurley stage III (Figure 17-21) disease may be so affected by their disease that they may be willing to undertake a radical surgical procedure to achieve "cure." The best way to achieve the lowest recurrence rate is to aggressively remove all apocrine gland-bearing tissue in the affected area, which will often require a complex reconstructive approach [67].

Medical Therapy

There are several different forms of medical therapy that can be considered, many of which work via different mechanisms. It appears that treatment is most successful when used in combined fashion as opposed to monotherapy [66]. Forms of medical therapy include antibacterial washes, topical antibiotics, systemic antibiotics, topical and systemic retinoids, antiandrogens, intralesional and systemic corticosteroids, and immunosuppressives [77]. Oral metformin has also been shown to be useful in treating individuals that have been unresponsive to traditional treatments [78]. Systemic antibiotics cannot be used for extended periods of time secondary to the selection of resistant strains of bacteria. While bacterial infection may be a secondary event in HS, it is clear from published research that persistence of bacterial colonization, likely in the form of biofilms, plays some role in the progression of disease [79]. Retinoids are likely beneficial secondary to their effect on normalization of epithelial cell proliferation and differentiation, which in turn may reduce the occurrence of follicular occlusion [80]. While these drugs are very effective in women of child-bearing age, their use must be cautioned due to their risk of teratogenicity. There are several reports of treatment success associated with their use [81, 82]. While antiandrogen therapy is often used (estrogen/progestin combinations, finasteride, spironolactone), the evidence to support its use is fairly weak [83].

Given the association of HS with inflammatory bowel disease, some have suggested that HS is a systemic process and could be treated similarly [84–86]. There are several reports of the use of tumor necrosis alpha (TNF alpha) inhibitors in the treatment of HS, with infliximab supported by the majority of available data [87–94]. There is also support for the use of other TNF alpha inhibitors [95]. It may be useful to employ these newer drugs if the effect of infliximab seems to fade or if the patient develops a sensitivity to the medication. Newer reports show some success with the use of photodynamic therapy [96, 97], as well as the use of intense pulsed light therapy [98]. Lasers have been used to treat HS both superficially [99] and when used as an instrument for excision in lieu of a scalpel or other energy devices [100].

Surgical/Excisional Therapy

For patients intolerant of or unwilling to undergo medical therapy, or for those with disease of significant severity, surgical excisional therapy may present the only viable option. Excisional therapy is based on the premise that wide excision of all apocrine gland-bearing tissue in the affected region is the best method to sustain low recurrence rates. This is typically achieved through a radical approach whereby all affected skin and subcutaneous fat is excised down to the fascial level. This will often result in a very large defect that cannot be addressed through simple primary closure. Local flap closure or split-thickness skin grafting (Figure 17-22a–d) is commonly necessary to achieve adequate tissue coverage of the wound. This may require the involvement of a plastic surgeon. Attempts at simple unroofing of sinus tracts seem to be associated with higher rates of recurrence. A technique referred to as STEEP (skin tissue-sparing excision with electrosurgical peeling) has been proposed as an alternative to the above techniques [101, 102]. In this technique the sinus roof is incised with a wire-loop electrosurgical instrument, which is similar to the "unroofing" technique. Affected tissue is then tangentially excised which results in sparing of the sinus floors and surrounding subcutaneous tissue. Wounds are left to heal by secondary intention. The premise behind this technique is that it is "tissue sparing" and leads to faster healing with improved outcomes.

There are several case series reporting the outcomes associated with the use of a wide variety of radical excisional procedures employing the use of different reconstructive techniques [103–105]. Whatever technique is chosen should be based on the anatomy of disease, patient expectations, risk of recurrence, and possibility of functional limitations. Vacuum-assisted closure devices can also be helpful in wounds that are too large to close primarily, but may not require more complex reconstructive options [106]. In cases where skin grafting may be used, a two-stage approach has been described [107]. The radical excision is performed initially which is immediately followed by coverage with artificial dermis. This allows for formation of granulation tissue as well as some surrounding wound contraction which may lead to a requirement for less grafting as well as improved graft take. In almost every case, the skin graft must be placed in an area subject to high levels of motion and

FIGURE 17-22. (a–d) This series of images shows a patient with Hurley stage III disease who underwent radical excision and closure with split-thickness skin grafting.

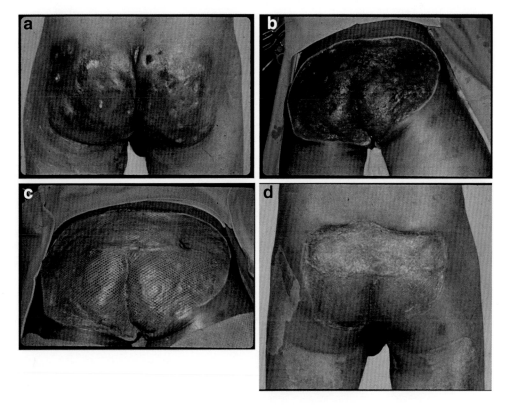

potential friction—none of which are good for a fresh skin graft. Perhaps staging the grafting approach decreases motion under the graft, which can potentially lead to improved outcomes.

Conclusion

Both pilonidal disease and hidradenitis suppurativa represent chronic inflammatory processes that can present with a wide spectrum of severity, but invariably disable those affected and result in a substantial decrease in their quality of life. While treatment of these disease processes may not seem to be surrounded in glamour, it most certainly results in a grateful patient. Pilonidal disease is quite common, while HS is much less so, but any colorectal surgeon can be expected to care for a number of individuals afflicted with these diseases. In order to ensure optimal treatment and outcomes, it is critical to tailor recommendations to the severity of disease, anatomy of disease, and our patient's expectations of risks and expected outcomes.

References

1. Hodges RM. Pilonidal sinus. Boston Med Surg J. 1880;103:485–6.
2. Anderson AW. Hair extracted from an ulcer. Boston Med Surg J. 1847;36:74.
3. Warren JM. Abscess, containing hair, on the nates. Am J Med Sci. 1854;28:113.
4. Buie LA. Jeep disease (pilonidal disease of mechanized warfare). South Med J. 1944;37:103–9.
5. Close AS. Pilonidal cysts: an analysis of surgical failures. Ann Surg. 1955;141:523–6.
6. Von Laffert M, Stadie V, Ulrich J, Marsch WC, Wohlrab J. Morphology of pilonidal sinus disease: some evidence of its being a unilocalized type of hidradenitis suppurativa. Dermatology. 2011;223:349–55.
7. Uysal AC, Alagoz MS, Unlu RE, Sensoz O. Hair dresser's syndrome: a case report of an interdigital pilonidal sinus and review of the literature. Dermatol Surg. 2003;29:288–90.
8. Coskun A, Bulus H, Akinci OF, Ozgonul A. Etiological factors in umbilical pilonidal sinus. Indian J Surg. 2011;73:54–7.
9. Armed Forces Health Surveillance Center (AFHSC). Pilonidal cysts, active component, U.S. Armed Forces, 2000–2012. MSMR. 2013;20:8–11.
10. Bolandparvaz S, Moghadam DP, Salahi R, Paydar S, Bananzadeh M, Abbasi HR, Eshraghian A. Evaluation of the risk factors of pilonidal sinus: a single center experience. Turk J Gastroenterol. 2012;23:535–7.
11. Doll D, Matevossian E, Wietelmann K, Evers T, Kriner M, Petersen S. Family history of pilonidal sinus predisposes to earlier onset of disease and a 50% long-term recurrence rate. Dis Colon Rectum. 2009;52:1610–5.
12. Harlak A, Mentes O, Kilic S, Coskun K, Duman K, Yilmaz F. Sacrococcygeal pilonidal disease: analysis of previously proposed risk factors. Clinics. 2010;65:125–31.
13. Armstrong JH, Barcia PJ. Pilonidal sinus disease. The conservative approach. Arch Surg. 1994;129:914–7.
14. Odili J, Gault D. Laser depilation of the natal cleft—an aid to healing the pilonidal sinus. Ann R Coll Surg Engl. 2002;84:29–32.
15. Landa N, Aller O, Landa-Gundin N, Torrontegui J, Azpiazu JL. Successful treatment of recurrent pilonidal sinus with laser epilation. Dermatol Surg. 2005;31:726–8.
16. Lukish JR, Kindelan T, Marmon LM, Pennington M, Norwood C. Laser epilation is safe and effective therapy for teenagers with pilonidal disease. J Pediatr Surg. 2009;44:282–5.
17. Ghnnam WM, Hafez DM. Laser hair removal as adjunct to surgery for pilonidal sinus: our initial experience. J Cutan Aesthet Surg. 2011;4:192–5.
18. Petersen S, Wietelmann K, Evers T, Huser N, Matevossian E, Doll D. Long-term effects of postoperative razor epilation in pilonidal sinus disease. Dis Colon Rectum. 2009;52:131–4.
19. Schneider IH, Thaler K, Kockerling F. Treatment of pilonidal sinus by phenol injections. Int J Colorectal Dis. 1994;9:200–2.
20. Dogru O, Camci C, Aygen E, Girgin M, Topuz O. Pilonidal sinus treated with crystallized phenol: an eight-year experience. Dis Colon Rectum. 2004;47:1934–8.
21. Hegge HG, Vos GA, Patka P, Hoitsma HF. Treatment of complicated or infected pilonidal sinus disease by local application of phenol. Surgery. 1987;102:52–4.
22. Stansby G, Greatorex R. Phenol treatment of pilonidal sinuses of the natal cleft. Br J Surg. 1989;729–30.
23. Lund JN, Leveson SH. Fibrin glue treatment of pilonidal sinus: results of a pilot study. Dis Colon Rectum. 2005;48:1094–6.
24. Seleem MI, Al-Hashemy AM. Management of pilonidal sinus using fibrin glue: a new concept and preliminary experience. Colorectal Dis. 2005;7:319–22.
25. Greenberg R, Kashtan H, Skornik Y, Werbin N. Treatment of pilonidal sinus disease using fibrin glue as a sealant. Tech Coloproctol. 2004;8:95–8.
26. Elsey E, Lund JN. Fibrin glue in the treatment for pilonidal sinus: high patient satisfaction and rapid return to normal activities. Tech Coloproctol. 2013;17:101–4.
27. Milone M, Musella M, Di Sardo Spiezio A, Bifulco G, Salvatore G, Sosa Fernandez LM, Bianco P, Zizolfi B, Nappi C, Milone F. Video-assisted ablation of pilonidal sinus: a new minimally invasive treatment—a pilot study. Surgery. 2014;155:562–6.
28. Alptekin H, Yilmaz H, Kayis SA, Sahin M. Volume of excised specimen and prediction of surgical site infection in pilonidal sinus procedures (surgical site infection after pilonidal sinus surgery). Surg Today. 2013;43:1365–70.
29. Milone M, Musella M, Salvatore G, Leongito M, Milone F. Effectiveness of a drain in surgical treatment of sacrococcygeal pilonidal disease. Results of a randomized and controlled clinical trial on 803 consecutive patients. Int J Colorectal Dis. 2011;26:1601–7.
30. Milone M, Di Minno MN, Musella M, Maietta P, Ambrosino P, Pisapia A, Salvatore G, Milone F. The role of drainage after excision and primary closure of pilonidal sinus: a meta-analysis. Tech Coloproctol. 2013;17:625–30.
31. Lorant T, Ribbe I, Mahteme H, Gustafsson UM, Graf W. Sinus excision and primary closure versus laying open in pilonidal disease: a prospective randomized trial. Dis Colon Rectum. 2011;54:300–5.

32. Rao MM, Zawislak W, Kennedy R, Gilliland R. A prospective randomized study comparing two treatment modalities for chronic pilonidal sinus with a 5-year follow-up. Int J Colorectal Dis. 2010;25:395–400.

33. Aldagal SM, Kensarah AA, Alhabboubi M, Ashy AA. A new technique in management of pilonidal sinus, a university teaching hospital experience. Int Surg. 2013;98:304–6.

34. Doll D, Novotny A, Rothe R, Kristiansen JE, Wietelmann K, Boulesteix AL, Dusel W, Petersen S. Methylene Blue halves the long-term recurrence rate in acute pilonidal sinus disease. Int J Colorectal Dis. 2008;23:181–7.

35. Colv EP, Bertelsen CA. Short convalescence and minimal pain after out-patient Bascom's pit pick operation. Dan Med Bull. 2011;58:A4348.

36. Olmez A, Kayaalp C, Aydin C. Treatment of pilonidal disease by combination of pit excision and phenol application. Tech Coloproctol. 2013;17:201–6.

37. Can MF, Sevinc MM, Yilmaz M. Comparison of Karydakis flap reconstruction versus primary midline closure in sacrococcygeal pilonidal disease: results of 200 military service members. Surg Today. 2009;39:580–6.

38. Can MF, Sevinc MM, Hancerliogullari O, Yilmaz M, Yagci G. Multicenter prospective randomized trial comparing modified Limberg flap transposition and Karydakis flap reconstruction in patients with sacrococcygeal pilonidal disease. Am J Surg. 2010;200:318–27.

39. Bessa SS. Comparison of short-term results between the modified Karydakis flap and the modified Limberg flap in the management of pilonidal sinus disease: a randomized controlled study. Dis Colon Rectum. 2013;56:491–8.

40. Gendy AS, Glick RD, Hong AR, Dolgin SE, Soffer SZ, Landers H, Herrforth M, Rosen NG. A comparison of the cleft lift procedure vs wide excision and packing for the treatment of pilonidal disease in adolescents. J Pediatr Surg. 2011;46:1256–9.

41. Dudink R, Veldkamp J, Nienhuijs S, Heemskerk J. Secondary healing versus midline closure and modified Bascom natal cleft lift for pilonidal sinus disease. Scand J Surg. 2011;100:110–3.

42. Guner A, Boz A, Ozkan OF, Ileli O, Kece C, Reis E. Limberg flap versus Bascom cleft lift techniques for sacrococcygeal pilonidal sinus: prospective, randomized trial. World J Surg. 2013;37:2074–80.

43. Altintoprak F, Gundogdu K, Ergonenc T, Dikicier E, Cakmak G, Celebi F. Retrospective review of pilonidal sinus patients with early discharge after limberg flap procedure. Int Surg. 2014;99:28–34.

44. Kaya B, Eris C, Atalay S, Bat O, Bulut NE, Mantoglu B, Karabulut K. Modified Limberg transposition flap in the treatment of pilonidal sinus disease. Tech Coloproctol. 2012;16:55–9.

45. Osmanoglu G, Yetisir F. Limberg flap is better for the surgical treatment of pilonidal sinus. Results of a 767 patients series with an at least five years follow-up period. Chirurgia (Bucur). 2011;106:491–4.

46. Horwood J, Hanratty D, Chandran P, Billings P. Primary closure or rhomboid excision and Limberg flap for the management of primary sacrococcygeal pilonidal disease? A meta-analysis of randomized controlled trials. Colorectal Dis. 2012;14:143–51.

47. Khan PS, Hayat H, Hayat G. Limberg flap versus primary closure in the treatment of primary sacrococcygeal pilonidal disease; a randomized clinical trial. Indian J Surg. 2013;75:192–4.

48. Dass TA, Zaz M, Rather A, Bari S. Elliptical excision with midline primary closure versus rhomboid excision with limberg flap reconstruction in sacrococcygeal pilonidal disease: a prospective, randomized study. Indian J Surg. 2012;74:305–8.

49. Sit M, Aktas G, Yilmaz EE. Comparison of the three surgical flap techniques in pilonidal sinus surgery. Am Surg. 2013;79:1263–8.

50. Arslan K, Said Kokcam S, Koksal H, Turan E, Atay A, Dogru O. Which flap should be preferred for the treatment of pilonidal sinus? A prospective randomized study. Tech Coloproctol. 2014;18:29–37.

51. Saylam B, Balli DN, Duzgun AP, Ozer MV, Coskun F. Which surgical procedure offers the best treatment for pilonidal disease? Langenbecks Arch Surg. 2011;396:651–8.

52. Onder A, Girgin S, Kapan M, Toker M, Arikanoglu Z, Palanci Y, Bac B. Pilonidal sinus disease: risk factors for postoperative complications and recurrence. Int Surg. 2012;97:224–9.

53. Sievert H, Evers T, Matevossian E, Hoenemann C, Hoffman S, Doll D. The influence of lifestyle (smoking and body mass index) on wound healing and long-term recurrence rate in 534 primary pilonidal sinus patients. Int J Colorectal Dis. 2013;28:1555–62.

54. Doll D, Matevossian E, Hoenemann C, Hoffman S. Incision and drainage preceding definitive surgery achieves lower 20-year long-term recurrence rate in 583 primary pilonidal sinus surgery patients. J Dtsch Dermatol Ges. 2013;11:60–4.

55. Doll D, Evers T, Krapohl B, Matevossian E. Is there a difference in outcome (long-term recurrence rate) between emergency and elective pilonidal sinus surgery? Minerva Chir. 2013;68:199–205.

56. Doll D, Krueger CM, Schrank S, Dettmann H, Petersen S, Duesel W. Timeline of recurrence after primary and secondary pilonidal sinus surgery. Dis Colon Rectum. 2007;50:1928–34.

57. Verneuil A. De l'hidrosadenite phlegmoneuse et des asbces sudoripares. Arch Gen Med. 1864;2:537–57.

58. Alavi A, Anooshirvani N, Kim WB, Coutts P, Sibbald RG. Quality-of-life impairment in patients with hidradenitis suppurativa. A Canadian study. Am J Clin Dermatol. 2015;16:61–5.

59. Shavit E, Dreiher J, Freud T, Halevy S, Vinker S, Cohen AD. Psychiatric comorbidities in 3207 patients with hidradenitis suppurativa. J Eur Acad Dermatol Venereol. 2015;29:371–6.

60. Zouboulis CC, Desai N, Emtestam L, Hunger RE, Ioannides D, Juhasz I, Lapins J, Matusiak L, Prens EP, Revuz J, Schneider-Burrus S, Szepietowski JC, van der Zee HH, Jemec GB. European S1 guideline for the treatment of hidradenitis suppurativa/acne inversa. J Eur Acad Dermatol Venereol. 2015. doi:10.1111/jdv.12966. [Epub ahead of print].

61. Shahi V, Alikhan A, Vazquez BG, Weaver AL, Davis MD. Prevalence of hidradenitis suppurativa: a population-based study in Olmstead County, Minnesota. Dermatology. 2014;229:154–8.

62. McMillan K. Hidradenitis suppurativa: number of diagnosed patients, demographic characteristics, and treatment patterns in the United States. Am J Epidemiol. 2014;179:1477–83.

63. Deckers IE, van der Zee HH, Boer J, Prens EP. Correlation of early-onset hidradenitis suppurativa with stronger genetic susceptibility and more widespread involvement. J Am Acad Dermatol. 2015;Pii:S0190-9622(14)02202-6. doi:10.1016/j.jaad.2014.11.017.

64. Kirby JS, Miller JJ, Adams DR, Leslie D. Health care utilization patterns and costs for patients with hidradenitis suppurativa. JAMA Dermatol. 2014;150:937–44.

65. Micheletti RG. Hidadenitis suppurativa: current views on epidemiology, pathogenesis, and pathophysiology. Semin Cutan Med Surg. 2014;33(3 suppl):S48–50.

66. Gill L, Williams M, Hamzavi I. Update on hidradenitis suppurativa: connecting the tracts. F1000Prime Rep. 2014;6:112.

67. Asgeirsson T, Nunoo R, Luchtefeld MA. Hidradenitis suppurativa and pruritus ani. Clin Colon Rectal Surg. 2011;24:71–80.

68. Danby FW, Jemec GB, Marsch WC, von Laffert M. Preliminary findings suggest hidradenitis suppurativa may be due to defective follicular support. Br J Dermatol. 2013;168:1034–9.

69. Micheletti RG. Natural history, presentation, and diagnosis of hidradenitis suppurativa. Semin Cutan Med Surg. 2014;33(3 suppl):S51–3.

70. Kromann CB, Deckers IE, Esmann S, Boer J, Prens EP, Jemec GB. Risk factors, clinical course and long-term prognosis in hidradenitis suppurativa: a cross-sectional study. Br J Dermatol. 2014;171:819–24.

71. Thomas CL, Gordon KD, Mortimer PS. Rapid resolution of hidradenitis suppurativa after bariatric surgical intervention. Clin Exp Dermatol. 2014;39:315–7.

72. Kromann CB, Ibler KS, Kristiansen VB, Jemec GB. The influence of body weight on the prevalence and severity of hidradenitis suppurativa. Acta Derm Venereol. 2014;94:553–7.

73. Von der Werth JM, Williams HC. The natural history of hidradenitis suppurativa. J Eur Acad Dermatol Venereol. 2000;14:389–92.

74. Melnik BC. Acneigenic stimuli converge in phosphoinositol-3 kinase/Akt/Foxo 1 signal transduction. J Clin Exp Dermatol Res. 2010;1:101.

75. Canoui-Poitrine F, Le Thaut A, Revuz JE, Vialette C, Gabison G, Poli F, Pouget F, Wolkenstein P, Bastuji-Garin S. Identification of three hidradenitis suppurativa phenotypes: latent class analysis of a cross-sectional study. J Invest Dermatol. 2013;133:1506–11.

76. Fimmel S, Zouboulis CC. Comorbidities of hidradenitis suppurativa (acne inversa). Dermatoendocrinology. 2010;2:9–16.

77. Rambhatla PV, Lim HW, Hamzavi I. A systematic review of treatments for hidradenitis suppurativa. Arch Dermatol. 2012;148:439–46.

78. Verdolini R, Clayton N, Smith A, Alwash N, Mannello B. Metformin for the treatment of hidradenitis suppurativa: a little help along the way. J Eur Acad Dermatol Venereol. 2013;27:1101–8.

79. Jahns AC, Killasli H, Nosek D, Lundskog B, Lenngren A, Muratova Z, Emtestam L, Alexeyev OA. Microbiology of hidradenitis suppurativa (acne inversa): a histological study of 27 patients. APMIS. 2014;122:804–9.

80. Blok JL, van Hattem S, Jonkmann MF, Horvath B. Systemic therapy with immunosuppressive agents and retinoids in hidradenitis suppurativa: a systematic review. Br J Dermatol. 2013;168:243–52.

81. Matusiak L, Bieniek A, Szepietowski JC. Acitretin treatment for hidradenitis suppurativa: a prospective series of 17 patients. Br J Dermatol. 2014;171:170–4.

82. Verdolini R, Simonacci F, Menon S, Pavlou P, Mannello B. Alitretinoin: a useful agent in the treatment of hidradenitis suppurativa, especially in women of child bearing age. G Ital Dermatol Venereol. 2014. [Epub ahead of print].

83. Alikhan A, Lynch PJ, Eisen DB. Hidradenitis suppurativa: a comprehensive review. J Am Acad Dermatol. 2009;60:539–61.

84. Marzano AV, Borghi A, Stadnicki A, Crosti C, Cugno M. Cutaneous manifestations in patients with inflammatory bowel diseases: pathophysiology, clinical features, and therapy. Inflamm Bowel Dis. 2014;20:213–27.

85. Kelly G, Sweeney CM, Tobin AM, Kirby B. Hidradenitis suppurativa: the role of immune dysregulation. Int J Dermatol. 2014;53:1186–96.

86. Dessinioti C, Katsambas A, Antoniou C. Hidradenitis suppurativa (acne inversa) as a systemic disease. Clin Dermatol. 2014;32:397–408.

87. Grant A, Gonzalez T, Montgomery MO, Cardenas V, Kerdel FA. Infliximab therapy for patients with moderate to severe hidradenitis suppurativa: a randomized, double-blind, placebo-controlled crossover trial. J Am Acad Dermatol. 2010;62:205–17.

88. Sullivan TP, Welsh E, Kerdel FA, Burdick AE, Kirsner RS. Infliximab for hidradenitis suppurativa. Br J Dermatol. 2003;149:1046–9.

89. Fernandez-Vozmediano JM, Armario-Hita JC. Infliximab for the treatment of hidradenitis suppurativa. Dermatology. 2007;215:41–4.

90. Usmani N, Clayton TH, Everett S, Goodfield MDJ. Variable response of hidradenitis suppurativa to infliximab in four patients. Clin Exp Dermatol. 2007;32:204–5.

91. Bahillo Monne C, Honorato Guerra S, Schoendorff Ortega C, Gargallo Quintero AB. Management of hidradenitis suppurativa with biological therapy: report of four cases and review of the literature. Dermatology. 2014;229:279–87.

92. Kerdel FA. Current and emerging nonsurgical treatment options for hidradenitis suppurativa. Semi Cutan Med Surg. 2014;33(3 suppl):S57–9.

93. Zhang J, Reeder VJ, Hamzavi IH. Use of biologics in the treatment of hidradenitis suppurativa: a review of the Henry Ford hospital experience. Br J Dermatol. 2014;171:1600–2.

94. Moriarty B, Jiyad Z, Creamer D. Four-weekly infliximab in the treatment of severe hidradenitis suppurativa. Br J Dermatol. 2014;170:986–7.

95. Diamantova D, Lomickova I, Cetkovska P. Adalimumab treatment for hidradenitis suppurativa associated with Crohn's disease. Acta Dermatovenerol Croat. 2014;22:291–3.

96. Fadel MA, Tawfik AA. New topical photodynamic therapy for treatment of hidradenitis suppurativa using methylene blue niosomal gel: a single-blind, randomized, comparative study. Clin Exp Dermatol. 2014. doi:10.1111/ced.12459. [Epub ahead of print].

97. Scheinfeld N. The use of photodynamic therapy to treat hidradenitis suppurativa a review and critical analysis. Dermatol Online J. 2015;21(1):Pii:13030/qt62j7j3c1.

98. Piccolo D, DiMarcantonio D, Crisman G, Cannarozzo G, Sannino M, Chiricozzi A, Chimenti S. Unconventional use of intense pulsed light. Biomed Res Int. 2014;2014:618206. doi:10.1155/2014/618206. Epub 2014 Sep 3.

99. Tierney E, Mahmoud BH, Hexsel C, Ozog D, Hamzavi I. Randomized controlled trial for the treatment of hidradenitis suppurativa with a neodymium-doped yttrium aluminum garnet laser. Dermatol Surg. 2009;35:1188–98.

100. Hazen PG, Hazen BP. Hidradenitis suppurativa: successful treatment using carbon dioxide laser excision and marsupialization. Dermatol Surg. 2010;36:208–13.

101. Blok JL, Spoo JR, Leeman FWJ, Jonkman MF, Horvath B. Skin-tissue-sparing excision with electrosurgical peeling (STEEP):

a surgical treatment option for severe hidradenitis suppurativa Hurley stage II/III. J Eur Acad Dermatol Venereol. 2014.

102. Blok JL, Boersma M, Terra JB, Spoo JR,Leeman FW, van den Heuvel ER, Huizinga J, Jonkman MF, Horvath B. Surgery under general anesthesia in severe hidradenitis suppurativa: a study of 363 primary operations in 113 patients. J Eur Acad Dermatol Venereol. 2015. doi:10.1111/jdv.12952. [Epub ahead of print].

103. Alharbi Z, Kauczok J, Pallua N. A review of wide surgical excision of hidradenitis suppurativa. BMC Dermatol. 2012;12:9.

104. Mizukami T, Fujiwara M, Ishikawa K, Aoyama S, Fukamizu H. Reconstruction for extensive groin hidradenitis suppurativa using combination of inferior abdominal flap and medial thigh-lift: a case report. Aesthetic Plast Surg. 2014;38:745–8.

105. Chen ML, Odom B, Santucci RA. Surgical management of genitoperineal hidradenitis suppurativa in men. Urology. 2014;83:1412–7.

106. Chen YE, Gerstle T, Verma K, treiser MD, Kimball AB, Orgill DP. Management of hidradenitis suppurativa wounds with an internal vacuum-assisted closure device. Plast Reconstr Surg. 2014;133:370e–7.

107. Yamashita Y, Hashimoto I, Matsuo S, Abe Y, Ishida S, Nakanishi H. Two-stage surgery for hidradenitis suppurativa: staged artificial dermis and skin grafting. Dermatol Surg. 2014;40:110–5.

18
Dermatology and Pruritus Ani

Wolfgang B. Gaertner and Genevieve B. Melton

Key Concepts

- Pruritus ani is a dermatologic condition characterized by itching or burning at the perianal area.
- Pruritus ani can be either primary (idiopathic) or secondary.
- Primary pruritus ani is the most common form of pruritus ani. The most common causes of secondary pruritus ani are local irritants and common anorectal conditions.
- All chronic perianal dermatoses require a detailed history and physical exam, including all past diagnostic tests and forms of treatment.
- The single most valuable diagnostic test in patients with recurrent or ongoing pruritus ani is skin biopsy.
- Treatment options for pruritus ani are numerous. Management should focus on the underlying or suspected etiology, following an evidenced-based stepwise diagnostic and treatment algorithm.

Introduction

Dermatologic diseases of the anus are a group of inflammatory, infectious, and neoplastic conditions that are difficult to diagnose and challenging to manage. While patients often do not openly discuss the associated symptoms with medical professionals, these conditions can often have a significant impact on their quality of life. Patients presenting with anal dermatologic disease are often seen by a diverse group of providers, including general practitioners, gastroenterologists, dermatologists, and colorectal surgeons. Some providers such as primary care physicians may encounter these conditions less commonly, thus making efficient and evidence-based treatment strategies highly important.

In 1660, Samuel Hafenreffer defined "itch" as "an unpleasant sensation that elicits the desire or reflex to scratch" [1]. More specifically, pruritus ani is defined as a dermatologic condition characterized by persistent and unpleasant itching or burning sensation in the perianal region [2]. The incidence of pruritus ani is estimated to range from 1 to 5 % in the general population, with men being affected more than women in a 4:1 ratio and most commonly diagnosed in the fourth–sixth decades of life [3–5].

Pruritus ani can be classified into primary or idiopathic (accounting for 50–90 % of cases) and secondary [6]. It may be caused by a wide spectrum of conditions, among which perianal eczema is probably the most common. Because pruritus ani often has a multifactorial etiology and high chronicity, most patients have symptoms for many years, as well as a long list of prescribed or over-the-counter treatments. Appropriate management can be difficult and requires a detailed evaluation in search for its etiology.

Pathophysiology of Perianal Signs and Symptoms

The sensation of itch is elicited as a surface phenomenon mediated by nonmyelinated C-fibers in the epidermis and subdermis and can be also classified as pruritoceptive (C-fiber mediated), neuropathic (i.e., after herpes zoster infection), and central or neurogenic. Itch has long been considered as a sub-modality of pain. The intensity hypothesis postulates that neurons are activated by both painful and pruritogenic stimuli, but weaker activation of nociceptive receptors can also result in itch [7]. Recent evidence suggests that the overall neurophysiology of itch is much more complex than initially thought. For example, when algogens are applied topically in lower concentrations, they typically result in low-intensity pain and not pruritus [8].

Microneurography experiments conducted by Schmelz et al. [9] identified afferent C-nerve fibers that were histamine sensitive but insensitive to mechanical stimuli. These findings support the labeled line theory of pruritus, which hypothesizes that discrete and mutually exclusive afferent

© Springer International Publishing 2016
S.R. Steele et al. (eds.), *The ASCRS Textbook of Colon and Rectal Surgery*, DOI 10.1007/978-3-319-25970-3_18

fibers are able to detect either itch or pain [10]. The stimulation of these histamine-sensitive C-nerve fibers demonstrates a central response in a subset of spinothalamic tract neurons [11]. In contrast, subdermally injected histamine-induced pruritus has been shown to activate multiple sites in the brain, overall indicating that itch is a multidimensional sensation, and there is not a single neurologic itch center [12].

Biochemically, histamine, kallikrein, bradykinin, papain, and trypsin can experimentally and individually produce itching. This may explain the lack of effectiveness of antihistamine medications against itching. While multiple itch mediators have been identified, the antagonism of these mediators produces varied clinical results (Table 18-1). This strongly suggests that specific neuronal pathways are involved at both peripheral and central levels in mediating itch.

Scratching is thought to produce inadequate feedback to inhibit further itching. Persistent scratching causes skin trauma, which is an additional stimulus for itching and additional scratching; therefore, this can lead to a chronic vicious cycle. Substituting scratching for other stimuli such as heat, cold, pain, or stinging by applying alcohol or pepper extract (capsaicin) may cause inhibitory feedback and then can decrease the urge to scratch.

TABLE 18-1. Itch mediators and corresponding antipruritic agents

Itch mediator	Antipruritic agent
Histamine	Antihistamines
Acetylcholine	Doxepin (mainly antihistaminic mechanism)
Serotonin	Paroxetine, fluoxetine (SSRIs)
	Mirtazapine (serotonin inverse agonist)
	Ondansetron (5HT3 antagonist)
Opioids	Naloxone, naltrexone (μ-receptor antagonists)
	Nalfurafine, butorphanol (kappa-receptor agonists)
Leukotrienes	Zafirlukast, zileuton
Prostaglandins	NSAIDs
Substance P	Aprepitant
TRPV1	Capsaicin
TRPM8	Menthol
TNF-alpha	Thalidomide
GABA	Gabapentin, pregabalin

SSRI selective serotonin reuptake inhibitor, *TRPV1* transient receptor potential vanilloid 1, *TRPM8* transient receptor potential melastatin 8, *TNF* tumor necrosis factor, *GABA* gamma-aminobutyric acid, *NSAIDs* nonsteroidal anti-inflammatory drugs, *5HT* 5-hydroxytryptamine

Itching associated with healing is also common after the inflammatory response caused by common anorectal conditions (i.e., fissure and hemorrhoids), as well as after anorectal operations and trauma. The release of histamine and various kinins and prostaglandins is a contributing factor in this situation; therefore, antihistamines, topical anti-inflammatory agents (steroids), and topical anesthetics have shown beneficial effects in these patients [13].

The complexity of the neurophysiological mechanisms causing pruritus as well as the extensive range of peripheral as well as central mediators of pruritus suggests that an effective antipruritic strategy would require a diverse approach.

Etiology and Contributing Factors

Although the overall differential diagnosis of anal dermatoses includes a long list of inflammatory, infectious, sexually transmitted, and neoplastic diseases, in this section, we will focus on the most common primary and secondary etiologies. Proposed etiologies of primary or idiopathic pruritus ani include a variety of associated factors, including anatomic, dietary, hygienic, psychogenic, local irritants and medications (Table 18-2). In many cases, both primary and secondary etiologies coincide, but a careful history and full physical examination will help elucidate the most significant contributing factor. For example, a patient with pruritus ani may present with irritable bowel syndrome, diarrhea, and fecal incontinence. Both primary and secondary etiologies in this patient may include fecal contamination, anal leakage, anxiety, dietary, and hygiene; and some of these may be directly related to one another. One must therefore individualize each case and focus on the most significant contributing factor for that patient taking into consideration the overlap of different etiologies. The causes of secondary pruritus ani can be divided into several broad categories: infectious, dermatologic, systemic disease and anorectal causes (Table 18-3) [3, 4].

In the absence of a primary cutaneous disorder, pruritus ani is thought to have two probable causes: (1) irritation from mucus, fecal material, or other perineal moisture (such as urine in an elderly patient with urinary incontinence) and (2) nerve impingement in the sacral region that causes a neuropathic itch or notalgia paresthetica. While there is good

TABLE 18-2. Proposed etiologies of primary or idiopathic pruritus ani

Anatomic factors	Obesity, deep clefts, hirsutism, tight clothing
Diet	Coffee (including decaffeinated), chocolate, spicy and heavily condimented foods, citrus fruits, tomatoes, beer, dairy products, vitamin A and D deficiencies, fat substitutes, consumption of large volumes of liquids
Personal hygiene	Poor cleansing habits, excessive perianal hygiene causing trauma
Local irritants	Fecal contamination, moisture, soaps, perfumes, topical medications, toilet paper, wet wipes, alcohol, witch hazel
Drugs	Quinidine, colchicine, IV steroids
Psychogenic	Anxiety, neurosis, psychosis, neurodermatitis, neuropathy, "itch syndromes"

Modified from Stamos MJ, Hicks TC, Pruritus ani: diagnosis and treatment. In: Perspectives in Colon and Rectal Surgery, 1998;11(1):1–20. Thieme Medical Publishers [17]

TABLE 18-3. Causes of secondary pruritus ani

Infectious
  Bacterial
  Fungal/yeast
  Viral
  Parasitic
Dermatologic
  Psoriasis
  Lichen planus, lichen simplex chronicus
  Lichen sclerosus
  Contact dermatitis
  Atopic dermatitis
  Local malignancy (squamous cell carcinoma, Paget's and Bowen's disease)
Systemic disease
  Diabetes mellitus
  Leukemia, lymphoma, polycythemia vera
  Liver disease (jaundice)
  Chronic renal failure
  Thyroid disorders
Colorectal and anal causes
  Hemorrhoids (internal and external)
  Rectal prolapse (mucosal and full thickness)
  Fissure
  Fistula-in-ano
  Diarrhea (infectious, inflammatory bowel disease, irritable bowel syndrome)
  Secreting villous tumors
Other
  Radiation dermatitis
  Fecal incontinence and anal leakage
  Gynecologic conditions (pruritus vulvae, vaginosis, vaginal discharge)

evidence supporting fecal contamination as a cause of anal pruritus, this seems to produce more of an irritant effect rather than an allergic effect [14]. The perianal skin also seems to be more susceptible to fecal contamination as a cause of perianal skin irritation compared to other sites of the body [14]. Anal leakage alone is frequently associated with anal pruritus, and this has been correlated with a pronounced anal inhibitory reflex in patients with pruritus ani [15]. Anxiety, stress, and fatigue, as well as personality, coping skills, and obsessive-compulsive disorders, probably play a role in the exacerbation of pruritus ani [16].

Irritants

Pruritus ani can result from several products including lanolin, neomycin, parabens, topical anesthetics from the "caine" family, and certain toilet papers [18]. Bowyer and McColl [19] studied 200 consecutive patients with pruritus ani and found that topical local anesthetics were the most commonly found causative factor. The enzymes responsible for perianal skin irritation from fecal contamination include lipase, elastase, and chymotrypsin [20]. Further skin irritation is often exacerbated by multiple and diverse treatment attempts and excessive hygiene measures. This allows for sensitization of

the perianal area, which may then be followed by allergic contact dermatitis or perianal eczema.

There are six common foods that often are associated with and thought to cause perianal irritation and pruritus: coffee, tea, cola, beer, chocolate, and tomato (ketchup). In some cases, total elimination will result in remission of itching in 2 weeks [21]. After a 2-week elimination period, foods may be reintroduced to determine the association and potentially the threshold exposure with the appearance of symptoms.

Steroid-Inducing Itching

Although anogenital itching has been reported with both topical and systemic steroids, it commonly occurs as a rebound phenomenon after withdrawal of steroids [22, 23]. Application of topical steroids for as little as 2 weeks can produce acute dermatitis resembling that seen with a blister that has been unroofed and exposed to air [24]. Steroids should only be used to achieve specific effects to the anogenital area. The potency and dosing of steroids should be tapered in a planned fashion with the goal of eliminating steroids altogether from a maintenance regimen. Allergic contact dermatitis to topically applied steroids has been well documented and is class specific. Switching to desoximetasone (a less commonly used agent in steroid class) may be a solution, but the ideal solution would be elimination of all steroids. Calcineurin inhibitors (tacrolimus and pimecrolimus) offer excellent anti-inflammatory effect without many of these steroidal side effects.

Infectious

Perianal infections associated with pruritus can be bacterial, viral, fungal, or parasitic in origin. Overall, infections have been commonly described as rare causes of pruritus ani [25]. However, emerging data demonstrates that fungal infections may be more prevalent in patients with pruritus ani than once thought [26].

Common bacterial causes include beta-hemolytic *streptococci*, *Staphylococcus aureus*, and *Corynebacterium minutissimum* [27], with beta-hemolytic *streptococcus* being the leading cause of perianal dermatitis in children [28]. *Staphylococcus aureus* perianal infections are more commonly reported in the adult population and typically present as a refractory and prolong dermatitis [29]. Erythrasma, a superficial infection of the intertriginous skin caused by *Corynebacterium minutissimum*, has been reported to cause up to 18 % of cases of pruritus ani in warm climates [27].

Fungal infections may account for 10–43 % of secondary infectious pruritus ani cases [4, 26, 27]. *Candida albicans* is the most common fungi identified in patients with pruritus ani [26, 30]. *Candida*, however, often colonizes the skin and

Dermatologic

Several dermatologic conditions may present as pruritus ani. These conditions include psoriasis, seborrheic dermatitis, atopic dermatitis, contact dermatitis, lichen planus, lichen sclerosus, lichen simplex chronicus, and local malignancies. Accurate diagnosis largely depends on a thorough history and physical examination of the perianal skin as well as the skin of the entire body [18].

Anal eczema, probably the most common dermatologic cause of pruritus ani, is generally considered to primarily represent contact dermatitis to chemicals and medications that are applied to the anal area. These substances are used by up to 57 % of patients with anogenital complaints and include popular hemorrhoid ointments that contain potent sensitizers (local anesthetics, *Myroxylon pereirae*, bufexamac), dyes, and perfumes used in scented toilet paper and soaps, feminine hygiene sprays and deodorants, and medicated talcum powders and skin cleansers [31–33]. Patients with anal eczema are also more likely to have asthma and hay fever. Most studies evaluating the role of specific allergens causing anal eczema have identified local anesthetics, aminoglycoside antibiotics, and thimerosal as the most common causative agents [26, 31, 34]. It is also important to test the patients' own products, as some studies have found these to be common and clinically relevant allergens. Although the role of dry, moist, or recycled toilet paper has been looked at, well-designed studies have not shown toxic effects of its components [33, 35, 36].

For example, Kranke et al. [26] prospectively studied 126 patients with a presumptive diagnosis of anal eczema over a 4-year period. All patients followed a diagnostic algorithm that involved medical history, physical examination, biochemical and microbiology testing, patch tests, proctoscopy, and biopsy if appropriate. The majority of patients had symptoms for over 1 year. Fifty-eight patients (46 %) were confirmed to have contact eczema, and the leading noneczematous etiology was intertrigo dermatitis with *Candida* spp. in 54 patients (43 %). The most common positive contact allergen identified was thimerosal.

Atopic dermatitis may be the most common hereditary cause of pruritus ani, with a frequency of 15–20 % of the population. Atopic dermatitis is caused by disruption of the epidermal barrier function. Filaggrin, the cement of the epidermis, is defective or absent in patients with atopic dermatitis because of mutations of the filaggrin gene [37]. Complete loss of the filaggrin gene is seen in ichthyosis vulgaris, a common keratinizing disorder frequently associated with atopic dermatitis and seen at the buttocks and perianal skin [38]. Psoriasis affects 1–3 % of the general population and is an important etiology of secondary pruritus ani, with reports varying from 5.5 to 55 % [19, 39–41].

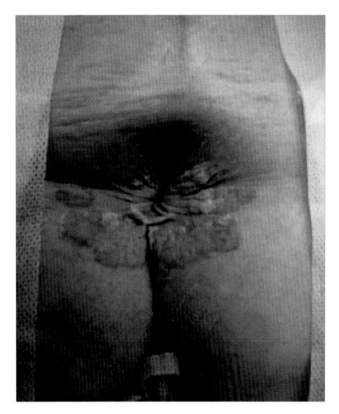

FIGURE 18-1. Patient with external anal condyloma acuminata and perianal fungal infection that presented with anal pruritus. Condyloma fulguration and antifungal treatment were effective at resolving pruritus.

can also be cultured from the perianal skin in normal subjects. *Dermatophytes* can cause pruritus ani less frequently but should be considered pathogenic and treated appropriately when found in patients with pruritus ani [27].

Several viral and sexually transmitted diseases (STD) can present as pruritus ani. These include herpes syndromes, syphilis, gonorrhea, molluscum contagiosum, and condyloma accuminata. Condyloma accuminata, which is associated with human papillomavirus infection (see section of "Neoplasm"), is a common cause of itching (Figure. 18-1). The diagnosis of condyloma acuminata is easy to recognize and should not be confused with primary or idiopathic causes. Herpes syndromes are typically characterized by pain and burning with red macules that progress to vesicles that rupture, ulcerate, and may become secondarily infected. Although parasite infections are a rare infectious cause of pruritus ani, they should be considered when clinically appropriate. Common perianal parasites include *Enterobius vermicularis* (pinworms), *Sarcoptes scabiei*, and pediculosis pubis [3]. Pinworms, in particular, are a common cause of nocturnal and post-defecation pruritus ani, especially in children.

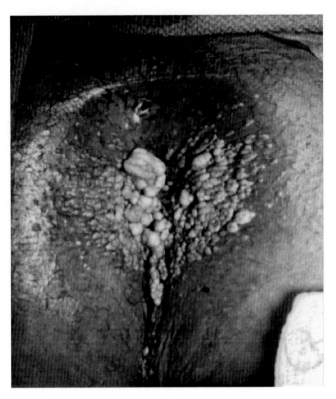

FIGURE 18-2. External anal condylomata acuminata presenting with perianal pruritus. Condyloma fulguration was effective at resolving pruritus.

Other less common dermatologic causes of pruritus ani include seborrheic dermatitis, lichen planus, lichen sclerosus, and lichen simplex chronicus. Seborrheic dermatitis is an uncommon cause of pruritus ani, characterized by extensive, moist erythema in the perineum [4]. Lichen planus is a relatively common inflammatory disease that affects the skin and mucous membranes and is thought to be caused by an altered, cell-mediated immune response. It is commonly seen in patients with other disease processes, such as ulcerative colitis, primary biliary cirrhosis, hepatitis C infection, and myasthenia gravis [42]. It is typically self-limited, resolving after 8–12 months.

Lichen sclerosus is a disease of unknown cause, seen more frequently in women, and involves the vulva extending posteriorly to the perianal region [4, 18, 43]. When it occurs on the penis, it is termed balanitis xerotica obliterans. Lichen simplex chronicus, also known as neurodermatitis, is a secondary skin manifestation that develops in an area of repetitive trauma from scratching or rubbing. A primary etiology may not be found in many cases, and the pruritus is typically intermittent and worsens at night or when a patient is quiet or still [44].

Neoplasms

Although uncommon, pruritus ani can be a presenting symptom of dermatologic neoplasms, such as condylomata, Paget's disease, and Bowen's disease. Condyloma acuminata

with anal intraepithelial neoplasia is the sequel to human papillomavirus infection and refers to premalignant changes in the area of the dentate line and anal transitional zone. Although pruritus has not been well studied in large studies evaluating patients with AIN [45, 46], it is commonly identified in patients with a history of anal warts (Figure 18-2). Extra-mammary Paget's disease (cutaneous adenocarcinoma in situ) is rare and occurs more often during the sixth decade of life, in white patients, and in women compared to men (3–4:1 ratio) [47]. The perianal region is the most commonly involved extra-mammary site, and pruritus is a common presenting symptom [48]. When diagnosed, it may be indicative of and associated with an underlying apocrine or eccrine carcinoma. In particular, the rate of anorectal malignancy associated with perianal Paget's disease ranges from 33 to 86 % [48, 49]. Therefore, investigations of the gastrointestinal, urinary, and gynecologic systems should be performed for a potential associated malignancy. Intraepithelial squamous cell carcinoma in situ, also known as Bowen's disease, of the anus is also rare but frequently presents with pruritus as the main symptom [50].

Anorectal Conditions

Hemorrhoidal disease, skin tags, and chronic anal fissure in ano are commonly seen pathologies in patients with pruritus ani [51, 52]. These conditions alone can cause pruritus but also are often associated with varying degrees of leakage, prolapse, and soiling. Correcting these disorders in patients with pruritus ani is typically warranted. However, the response to treatment and the impact of correcting these conditions on pruritus ani symptoms are unclear and have only been reported in small retrospective studies [39, 40, 52]. Treatment modalities have included both office-based and operative strategies with varying degrees of success.

For example, Murie et al. [52] found that pruritus was more common in 82 patients with hemorrhoids than in age- and sex-matched controls without hemorrhoids and that correction (with banding or hemorrhoidectomy) usually eliminated itching. Bowyer and McColl [19] reported that hemorrhoids were the sole cause of itching in 16 of 200 patients and contributory in 27 others. Correction of fissure was required in five patients before symptoms were relieved. Five others had skin tags which when removed, eliminated symptoms. In general it is difficult to know whether anorectal conditions are the cause or a contributing factor of pruritus ani. Operative management that avoids further scaring or corrects fecal incontinence or leakage should be offered to pruritus patients in most cases.

Systemic Diseases

Several systemic diseases have been associated with pruritus ani; however, the precise causative factors remain unknown. Diabetes mellitus is the most commonly reported systemic disease. Other frequently reported associated conditions include liver disease, lymphoma, leukemia, pellagra, vitamin A and D deficiencies, renal failure, iron-deficiency anemia, and hyperthyroidism [3, 4, 27].

Diagnoses of Perianal Disease

Establishing an exact diagnosis may be difficult mainly because the clinical presentation is frequently nonspecific. This often results in dissatisfied patients, who may be seen multiple times and by several doctors in different specialties. Consequently patients can have symptoms for many years, as well as a long list of prescribed and over-the-counter medications [53].

To pinpoint the cause of dermatologic diseases of the anus, it is recommended that patients be asked about their current diet, current and previous medications, personal history of atopy, information about bowel habits, and perianal hygiene regimen, including how they routinely clean the anal area after a bowel movement. A review of the patient's medical history, including any history of anorectal conditions or operations, is essential. Other pertinent history includes previous skin infections, especially mycotic infections of the genitalia, STDs, anal seepage, and symptoms of fecal and urinary incontinence.

A diagnostic algorithm, including a full history and physical examination, biochemical and microbiology testing, proctoscopy, and patch tests (including the patient's own products), is strongly recommended (Figure 18-3).

Physical Examination

The morphology of a lesion is a starting point for diagnosis, but may not be specific, and some diseases may present with a number of different appearances. Physical examination should also include evaluation of other related sites of skin manifestations including the groins, axillae, buttock cleft, and other intertriginous areas or skin folds. Response to treatment at these areas should also be documented at follow-up examinations. Washington Hospital classifies pruritus ani based on physical exam findings: stage 0 is normal skin, stage 1 is red and inflamed skin, stage 2 has lichenified skin, and stage 3 has lichenified skin, coarse ridges, and ulcerations [18]. This classification system is practical and useful for communicating with other providers.

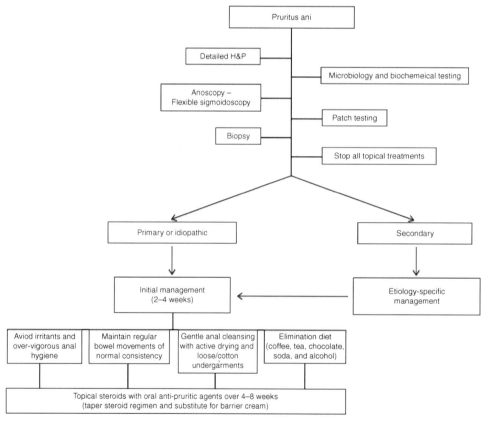

FIGURE 18-3. Diagnostic and treatment algorithm for patients presenting with pruritus ani.

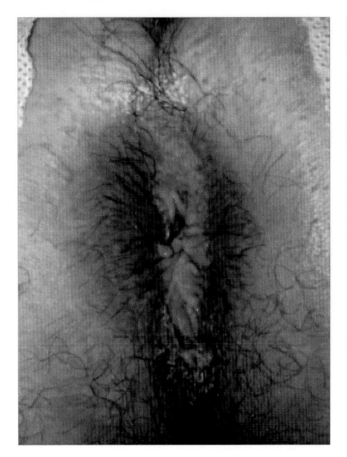

FIGURE 18-4. Hyperpigmentation and perianal skin lichenification seen in a patient with erythrasma.

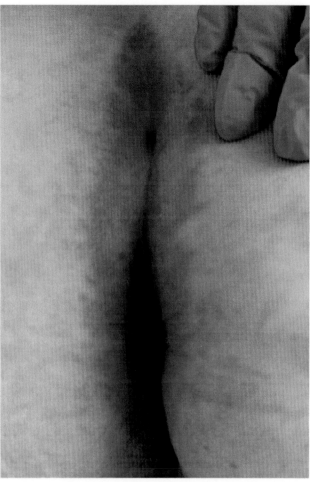

FIGURE 18.5. Perianal fungal infection in a patient with anal seepage and fecal incontinence. This infection is characterized by a bright red rash at the perianal area and intergluteal fold in a "butterfly" distribution.

Infectious

In the setting of bacterial perianal dermatitis, the perianal skin typically shows a moist, bright, and erythematous eruption with distinct borders and no satellite lesions. Patients usually do not have upper respiratory symptoms [28]. Chronic infected discharge from the anus may lead to hyperpigmentation of the anorectal cleft. This finding is commonly seen in patients with long-standing anorectal conditions, including pilonidal disease, anorectal fistulas, and hidradenitis suppurativa. Erythrasma is often associated with scaly, well-defined patches of initially reddish and then brownish-colored lesions at other intertriginous areas (Figure 18-4) [54, 55]. When caused by *Corynebacterium minutissimum*, these lesions show a characteristic coral-red fluorescence when examined with a Wood's lamp. *C. minutissimum* is commonly present and pathogenic at other body folds (axillae, groin, inframammary) and toe webs [54].

Molluscum contagiosum has a distinct presentation with clusters of small, palpable, flesh-colored papules with central umbilication. In general, human immunodeficiency virus (HIV)-associated lesions rarely present with itching except for secondary fungal infections. Perianal fungal infections are characterized by a bright red rash without the cheesy exudate

sometimes seen in other parts of the body (Figure. 18-5). These infections may present following treatment with systemic antibiotics and topical or systemic steroids [56]. *Candida* is commonly found in patients with pruritus secondary to common anorectal conditions (i.e., hemorrhoids, fissure) and is typically eliminated with adequate treatment of the underlying condition [57]. Infections where *dermatophytes* are cultured almost always present with pruritus and are considered pathogenic, as compared to infections caused by *C. albicans* [30]. Topical steroids may render direct scrapings negative for hyphae but frequently facilitate *dermatophyte* growth.

Dermatologic

Anal eczema or contact dermatitis is characterized by erythema, scaling, and vesicles. Similar findings may be located on the face, neck, dorsum of the hands, as well as popliteal and antecubital fossas. Atopic dermatitis presents as nonspecific and diffuse erythema, often seen with signs of

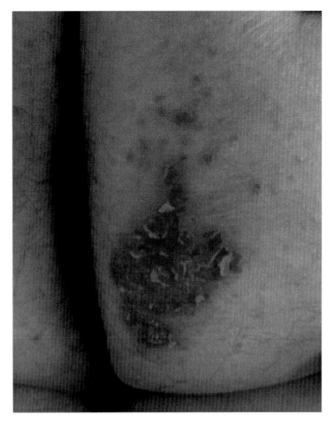

FIGURE 18-6. Perianal psoriasis or psoriasis inversa showing a well-demarcated, scaly, bright red, plaque-like lesion.

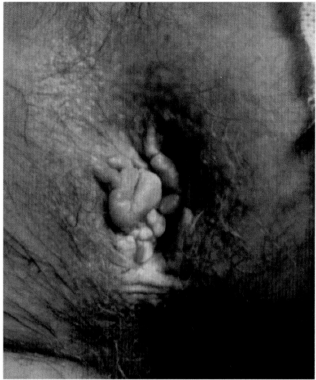

FIGURE 18-7. Lichen sclerosus of the anus with chronic healing showing replacement by chronic inflammation, sclerosis, and atrophy of the affected area.

skin excoriation. Associated findings include: keratosis pilaris (rough sandpaper-like texture over the posterior biceps and thighs), Morgan's folds or Morgan–Dennie lines (redundant creases beneath the eyes), "sniffers" lines (a subtle transverse crease across mid-nose), urticaria, and white dermatographism. With the loss of an adequate epidermal barrier, secondary infections and irritation by contact agents are common in patients with atopic dermatitis.

Psoriasis typically appears as well-demarcated, scaly, plaque-like lesions that are bright red in color (Figure 18-6). Typical lesions are commonly found on the scalp, elbows, knees, knuckles, and penis [18], but perianal psoriasis may also present as an isolated lesion. In the perianal region, lesions tend to be poorly demarcated, pale, and non-scaling because of persistent maceration, hence the term inverse psoriasis [4, 18]. With seborrheic dermatitis, excessive perianal moisture is the common denominator, and special attention should be directed to the scalp, chest, ears, beard, and suprapubic areas since these regions are commonly affected as well.

Lichen planus presents as shiny, flat-topped papules that are darker than the surrounding skin and begin on the volar aspects of the wrists and forearms. Genital and mucous

membrane involvement are common [18]. Wickham striae are intersecting gray lines that can be seen if mineral oil is applied to the plaques and help to establish the diagnosis. Lichen sclerosus mainly involves the vulva but typically extends posteriorly toward the perianal region. The first phase of this condition begins as ivory-colored, atrophic papules that break down and expose underlying erythematous raw tissue. This process is severely pruritic and painful. As this heals, the area is replaced by chronic inflammation, sclerosis, and atrophy of the affected area (Figure 18-7). The classical finding is white patches around the vulva and anus [4, 18]. Histologically, these lesions are consistent with a chronic scar, lacking a lymphocytic interface (Figure 18-8) [41, 58–61]. Because of a reported 4–6 % risk of developing squamous cell carcinoma, all nonresponders or those with recurrent sclerosis should have a skin biopsy to rule out malignancy [27, 62]. Treatment of the disease does not appear to modify this risk [63].

Lichenification is the characteristic finding seen in patients with lichen simplex chronicus or neurodermatitis. The perianal skin appears thickened and is commonly described as cracking and scaling. Patients frequently have a history of an anorectal operation that involved a chronic wound or delayed healing.

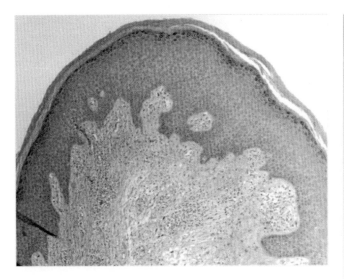

FIGURE 18-8. Photomicrograph of lichen sclerosus showing signs of chronic scaring and lack of lymphocytic interface dermatitis.

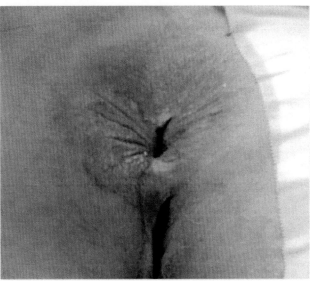

FIGURE 18-9. Perianal Paget's disease presenting with anal pruritus.

Neoplasms

The presentation of dermatologic malignancies, such as Paget's and Bowen's disease, may vary from a mild rash to a florid type of eczema at times associated with indurated skin. The classic presentation is an erythematous and eczematoid perianal plaque (Figure 18-9). Infiltrative processes may be less well defined in Paget's disease with the same caveat about margins. Pruritus and bleeding are the most common complaints [48]. Other symptoms include pain, mucous seepage, lump, and difficulty with defecation [64].

Biochemical Testing

After failed topical management and if systemic disease is suspected, biochemical testing is warranted. Common laboratory tests to rule out systemic and infectious causes include liver and kidney function tests, blood glucose level, white blood cell count with differential, C-reactive protein, and erythrocyte sedimentation rate. These tests are most useful in patients with decompensated chronic systemic disease like hepatic and renal failure and severe perianal infections.

Microbiology Testing

Cultures of perianal skin exudates and infectious material are simple and straightforward but can be misleading if not performed adequately. Infected material should be aspirated with a syringe and expelled into a sterile container. Alternatively, a swab may be used to collect a specimen but this is less than ideal. Culture specimens should be placed in appropriate media (anaerobic, bacterial, fungal, and viral) and refrigerated without delay. Viral cultures should be kept

on ice. Fluid from vesicular lesions should be aspirated or taken with a swab from the base of an unroofed lesion and placed on a cell culture media or a microscopic slide for Tzanck smears if herpes zoster is suspected [65]. Swabs should be lubricated with saline if lubricated at all because conventional water-soluble lubricant is bactericidal for some organisms including *Neisseria gonorrhoeae*. Skin scrapings may be submitted for fungus culture. Scrapings can also be examined for hyphae with KOH prep, but this test is rarely available because of the lack of trained and experienced personnel. It is essential to have discussed the proper arrangements with the laboratory and nursing personnel (clinic and operating room) to assure adequate specimen handling and testing well before obtaining a specimen.

In patients with diarrhea, bacterial stool cultures as well as ova and parasites on three different stool samples can be useful. In patients with suspected or confirmed streptococcal or staphylococcal perianal infections, nasal or throat swabs rarely detect the offending bacteria and therefore are unnecessary [42]. If pinworms are suspected, a cellophane or scotch tape test in the early morning identifies adult worms and their eggs and confirms the diagnosis [4].

Patch Testing

Patients with an extensive list of allergies, both dietary and drug related, are good candidates for patch testing. This usually involves a dermatologic consultation, which can be very helpful when the staff has a particular interest in perianal dermatology. As part of a diagnostic algorithm in a prospective study of patients with clinical suspicion of anal eczema, Kranke and colleagues [26] found that patch testing was confirmatory in 33 of 58 patients (57 %), with at least one positive

Table 18-4. Patch test findings in 58 consecutive patients suspected of having allergic contact anal eczema [26]

Contact allergen	N (%)
Thimerosal	11 (19)
Patients own products	6 (10)
Balsam of Peru (*Myroxylon pereirae*)	5 (9)
Amerchol	3 (5)
Lanolin alcohol	3 (5)
Nickel sulfate	3 (5)
Fragrances/perfumes	3 (5)
Lidocaine, benzocaine	2 (3)
Propolis	1 (2)
Neomycin	1 (2)

allergic reaction (Table 18-4). It is important to also test the patient's own products as these have been shown to be a significant etiology in pruritus ani [1, 26].

Endoscopic Evaluation

All patients with pruritus ani should undergo anoscopy and flexible sigmoidoscopy. These exams are especially useful in patients with anorectal pathology and inflammatory bowel disease. Full colonoscopy is indicated for patients who are age-appropriate for colorectal cancer screening and those with hematochezia, iron-deficiency anemia, and positive family history of colorectal cancer.

Biopsy

Skin lesions not responding to treatment or suspicious for malignancy require biopsy. This is the single most valuable test in patients with primary pruritus ani and should include an area of the lesion with adjacent normal skin. Specific query should be made to a pathologist with expertise in dermatologic pathology with clinically suspected diagnoses. Biopsy may conveniently be done with either an 11 blade or skin punch blades (Keyes dermal punches) that come in numerous sizes in separate sterile packages. Bleeding is readily controlled with silver nitrate or topical thrombin-based hemostatic agents.

Evidence-Based Management

The management of dermatologic diseases of the anus in practice is particularly challenging for several reasons. These conditions are hidden on a part of the body often associated with embarrassment, and therefore patients may have advanced disease before they present to a doctor for help. Additionally, there is limited class A data regarding the management of pruritus ani.

Aims of Treatment

The aims of treatment for any form of anal dermatitis are rapid relief of symptoms, healing of dermatitis, and prevention of recurrence. Long-term recurrence can be prevented in many patients by avoiding contact with allergens and irritants, as well as curing the underlying anorectal disease or condition. The choice of treatment must take into account the different causative factors: irritation from contact, allergic contact, infection, primary inflammatory disease, and neoplasia. Treatment of underlying anorectal conditions (hemorrhoids, fistula, incontinence, etc.) should be initiated from the first patient visit.

Primary Pruritus Ani

Because primary or idiopathic pruritus ani is more common, a therapeutic trial of generic management is recommended. This will be effective in more than 90 % of patients [6]. This management strategy focuses on reestablishing ideal anal hygiene and providing reassurance that there is no underlying condition causing the symptoms. Treatment begins with avoiding known irritants such as soaps, lotions, creams, perfumed powders, medicated baby wipes, and any product with witch hazel. The patient must also know to avoid further trauma to the perianal skin, which may be caused by scratching, dry toilet paper, and vigorous scrubbing with bathing. Gently blotting the skin clean with moist toilet paper, a cotton ball, or a soft, unscented, and non-medicated baby wipe is recommended. Generally, baby wipes of all types should be avoided, especially when contact and atopic dermatitis is suspected. An important part of the initial management of primary pruritus ani is to avoid moisture and keep the perianal area dry. Patients should avoid tight-fitting, synthetic undergarments and may also use a small piece of cotton or makeup removal pad to help soak up any excess moisture. The brief use of a hair dryer with cool air is an excellent way to keep the perianal skin dry after cleansing. Unscented Dove® (Unilever, London, UK) is free of conventional soap and is the preferred bathing agent. It is also important for patients to maintain regular bowel movements of normal consistency. This is especially useful to avoid seepage and fecal contamination of the perianal skin. A high-fiber diet without excessive fluid intake and the judicious use of loperamide or cholestyramine is recommended, as needed. As mentioned earlier in this chapter, an elimination diet excluding "high-risk" dietary components such as coffee, tea, chocolate, soda, and alcohol for 2 weeks can be strongly considered in most patients with primary pruritus ani. Smith et al. [39] showed that an elimination diet gave partial or complete relief in 27 of 56 (48 %) of their patients.

In those patients in whom the initial management strategy is not effective after 4–6 weeks, attention is directed toward excluding the multiple potential causes of secondary pruritus

TABLE 18-5. Marketed topical products most commonly prescribed for the treatment of perianal dermatitis [66]

Active ingredients	Brand name(s)
Single active agents	
Hydrocortisone	Procto-Kit, DermoPosterisan
Tribenoside	Borraza-G
Cinchocaine	Dolapostern
Glyceryl trinitrate	Rectogesic
Corticosteroids + local anesthetics	
Hydrocortisone + pramocaine or cinchocaine or lidocaine or benzocaine + amylocaine + esculin	Pramosone, Proctofoam, Proctocream-HC, Proctosedyl, Xyloproct
Prednisolone + cinchocaine or + desonide + lidocaine + heparin + vitamins A and E	Scheriproct, Cirkan
Diflucortolone + lidocaine	Neriproct
Fluocinonide + lidocaine	Jelliproct
Fluocortolone + lidocaine or cinchocaine	Doloproct, Ultraproct
Fluocinolone + lidocaine (+ menthol + bismuth)	Synalar Rectal
Corticosteroids + antimicrobials/antiseptics	
Hydrocortisone + benzyl benzoate + Peru balsam + bismuth + zinc with or without resorcinol	Anusol-HC
Corticosteroids + local anesthetics + antimicrobials/antiseptics	
Hydrocortisone + cinchocaine with neomycin + esculin or framycetin	Proctosedyl
Local anesthetics + antimicrobials/antiseptics	
Cinchocaine + policresulen	Faktu
Other combinations	
Trimebutine + ruscogenin	Proctolog
Peru balsam + bismuth + zinc	Anusol
Hydrocortisone + *Escherichia coli* suspension	Posterisan
Hydrocortisone + phenylephrine + paraffin oil + fish oil	Preparation H
Lidocaine + carraginates + zinc	Titanoreine

Products with >10,000 prescriptions in 2011 according to IMS data for Brazil, France, Germany, Japan, the UK, and the USA [66]

ani. If no secondary cause can be found, topical therapy is recommended (Table 18-5). After generic management and proper anal hygiene are assured, topical steroids are an effective and safe treatment option. First-line topical treatment includes preparations with a low-potency topical steroid such as 1 % hydrocortisone, which should not be given for more than 8 weeks. In a double-blinded, randomized trial, 11 patients with primary pruritus ani received 1 % hydrocortisone or placebo for 2 weeks followed by the opposite treatment for another 2 weeks [67]. There was a washout period of 2 weeks between treatments. Treatment with 1 % hydrocortisone resulted in a 68 % reduction of itch using a visual analogue score, and 75 % showed significant improvements in quality of life. Potent or extended use of topical steroids should be avoided as they can lead to skin atrophy, infections, and worsened pruritus ani (Figure 18-10) [18, 27]. Capsaicin has also been studied in a randomized fashion in 44 patients with primary pruritus ani [68]. This topical agent decreases levels of substance P, a neuropeptide that triggers itching and burning pain. Topical capsaicin (0.006 %) showed relief of symptoms in 70 % of patients as compared to 2 % patients who received placebo (1 % menthol).

The majority of patients with moderate symptoms and minimal skin changes will respond well to low-dose topical steroids or topical capsaicin. These preparations are applied at night and in the morning after bathing. If topical steroids are used, a tapering regimen should be set in place ending with substitution of a barrier cream such as Calmoseptine® (Calmoseptine, Inc., Huntington Beach, CA). Patients with chronic perianal skin changes should be managed with a medium- or high-potency steroid (Table 18-6). It is important to emphasize to patients that a high-potency steroid should be used for a limited period of time, generally 4–8 weeks. Once normalization of the skin has occurred, patients are switched to a mild steroid that can be further tapered down to bi-weekly applications until total elimination.

Non-irritating cleansers are highly recommended during the initial therapeutic trial, especially when patients do not have a bath or shower directly available. Dilute white vinegar (one tablespoon in an 8-oz glass of water) on a cotton ball is a cheap and effective non-soapy cleanser. It is our personal preference to use tea tree oil, a volatile oil with antibacterial and antifungal properties, in patients with moist perianal skin and pruritus. Patients who come to the office with acute moderate to severe changes of the perianal skin may be treated with Berwick's dye (crystal violet 1 % + brilliant green 1 % + 95 % ethanol 50 % + distilled H2O q.s.ad. 100 %), which is dried with a hair dryer, and subsequently covered with benzoin tincture as a barrier and dried similarly. This topical treatment will stay in place for several days if only water is used to cleanse, relieves symptoms rapidly, and allows for re-epithelialization of broken-down skin. Application of Berwick's dye to the perianal skin is especially useful for pruritus ani occurring after anorectal operations.

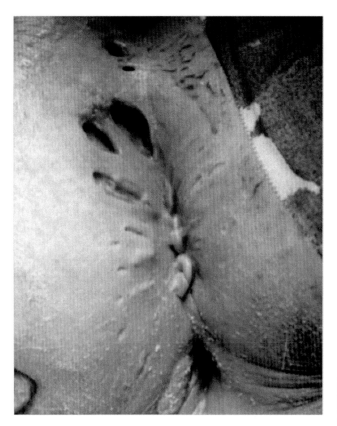

FIGURE 18-10. Chronic skin changes of atrophy and ulcerations secondary to pruritus ani with associated left buttock infection in a patient who had been taking steroids for 8 years.

Skin breakdown or maceration caused by scratching or over vigorous cleansing efforts must be avoided. A combination of topical and systemic medications has shown the best results compared to either alone. Doxepin (both topical and oral) and hydroxyzine are effective adjuncts to reduce or eliminate itching. Doxepin, a tricyclic antidepressant, possesses both anti-H1 and anti-H2 activity. Hydroxyzine, a potent H1 receptor inverse agonist, has shown to have equal antipruritic efficacy compared to oral doxepin but with higher sedation effects [70]. Although centrally acting agents such as gabapentin and paroxetine have shown to be effective antipruritic agents in uremic and cholestatic patients [71], their efficacy in patients with pruritus ani has not been studied. Our experience with gabapentin in severe refractory pruritus ani has been quite rewarding. Patients may not be aware of nocturnal scratching and this can be a serious contributing factor in many cases of primary pruritus ani. Patients who are awakened by the urge to scratch should gently cleanse the perianal skin and reapply their barrier ointment.

For intractable cases or primary pruritus ani, intradermal injection of methylene blue has been described with some efficacy (Figure 18-11) [27, 72]. The presumed mechanism of symptomatic improvement is through the destruction of nerve endings. This treatment modality was initially

TABLE 18-6. Relative potency of topical steroids

Group 1 (most potent)
  Betamethasone dipropionate 0.05 % (Diprolene®)
  Clobetasol propionate 0.05 % (Temovate®)
Group 2
  Desoximetasone 0.25 % (Topicort®)
  Fluocinonide 0.05 % (Lidex®)
Group 3
  Betamethasone valerate ointment 0.1 % (Valisone®)
  Triamcinolone acetonide 0.5 % (Aristocort®)
Group 4
  Desoximetasone 0.05 % (Topicort LP®)
  Flurandrenolide 0.05 % (Cordran®)
Group 5
  Betamethasone valerate cream 0.1 % (Valisone®)
  Hydrocortisone butyrate 0.1 % (Locoid®)
  Triamcinolone acetonide 0.1 % (Kenalog®)
Group 6 (least potent)
  Alclometasone dipropionate 0.05 % (Aclovate®)
  Hydrocortisone 1 %

Finne CO, Fenyk JR, Dermatology and pruritus ani. In: Fleshman JW, Wolff BG, editors. The ASCRS textbook of colon and rectal surgery. New York: Springer; 2007. p. 277–294) [69]. © Springer

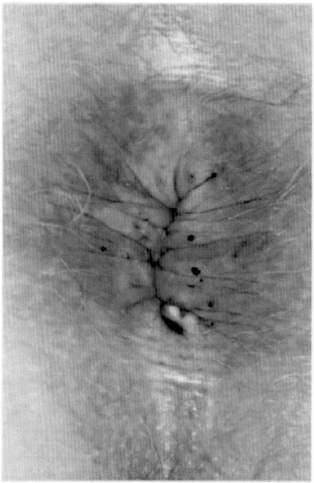

FIGURE 18-11. Tattooing with methylene blue for severe refractory idiopathic pruritus ani. Courtesy of C.O. Finne, St. Paul, MN.

described by Eusebio and colleagues [72] and involved the intracutaneous and subcutaneous injection of 30 mL of 0.25 % bupivacaine with 1:200,000 epinephrine mixed with equal volumes of 0.5 % lidocaine at the anoderm and perianal areas, with the patient under deep sedation in the operating room. After this, 20–30 mL of 0.5 % methylene blue was injected at the same sites using a 25-G spinal needle. Twenty-one of 23 patients reported good short- and long-term results. However, the authors also reported full-thickness skin necrosis in three patients. Mentes et al. [73] used a slightly different technique in 30 patients with intractable primary pruritus ani. Patients underwent intradermal and subcutaneous injection of a mixture of 7–8 mL of 2 % methylene blue with equal volumes of 0.5 % lidocaine without previous local anesthesia or sedation. For patients who had a partial response at 1-month follow-up, a "rescue treatment" was offered. At 1 month, 80 % of patients were free of symptoms. Five patients underwent an additional "rescue" injection and four of five had complete relief of symptoms. No major complications or cases of skin necrosis were reported. The authors attributed this to a smaller injected volume.

Secondary Pruritus Ani

Infectious

Bacterial infections of the perianal region should be treated with systemic antibiotics. If a specific agent has not been identified, antibiotic coverage should include Gram-positive and Gram-negative cocci. Parenteral antibiotics have been reported to be especially useful with *Staphylococcus aureus* infections [74]. When refractory pruritus ani is associated with cultures that show growth of *Candida albicans*, antifungals should be given, especially in patients who are immunosuppressed, who are diabetic, or who were recently treated with systemic steroids or antibiotics [27]. We have seen good results with a combination of oral fluconazole and topical luliconazole 1 %, given for 2–3 weeks. Again, when *dermatophytes* are found in the setting of pruritus ani, this associated fungal infection should also be treated appropriately [27]. The treatment of erythrasma involves systemic antibiotics, typically erythromycin 250 mg *qid* for 10 days. Tetracycline may be used as a second alternative [54, 55]. Silver sulfadiazine is an effective topical adjunct in patients with bacterial perianal dermatitis, especially in patients with ulcerations and fissuring skin as it sooths and promotes re-epithelialization. It should be noted that when topical therapy is given with systemic antibiotics and antifungals, it should be for symptom relief but not as the primary antibacterial or antifungal agent.

Dermatologic

With regard to anal eczema, both the European and American Academy of Allergy, Asthma, and Immunology guidelines recommend starting treatment with basic skin care. Keys to success include avoiding allergens, irritants, and tight constricting undergarments, liberal use of warm sitz baths for comfort, and keeping the affected area dry at all other times. As mentioned above, gentle but thorough cleansing of the perianal area with soap substitutes (i.e., Dove) is recommended during bathing [75]. When these methods fail, mild-to-moderately potent topical corticosteroids for 2–3 weeks periods are recommended. The efficacy of topical steroids compared to placebo has been studied in a small, double-blinded, randomized controlled trial, favoring topical steroid treatment [66]. Topical calcineurin inhibitors such as tacrolimus and pimecrolimus are also effective for reducing inflammation and itch in patients with anal eczema and also avoid skin atrophy. Two randomized controlled trials comparing topical tacrolimus 0.1 % to placebo in a total of 53 patients with chronic idiopathic pruritus ani showed significant symptomatic improvement up to 6 weeks follow-up [76, 77]. One of these studies failed to show significant differences in quality of life as assessed by the Dermatology Life Quality Index questionnaire [77]. Although systemic gamma interferon and narrowband UVB therapy have shown promising results in patients with atopic dermatitis as well as cholestatic and uremic pruritus [78, 79], no evidence in patients with pruritus ani exists. Of importance, bacterial and fungal infections should be suspected after multiple or prolonged unsuccessful treatments.

Treatment of atopic dermatitis begins with providing a barrier such as Vaseline® (white petrolatum USP) or Calmoseptine® (Calmoseptine, Inc., Huntington Beach, CA), the use of anti-inflammatory agents (systemic and topical) and antipruritic agents. Psoriasis is not a curable condition, but symptoms can be well controlled with mild topical steroid preparations (i.e., 1 % hydrocortisone cream). Seborrheic dermatitis responds well to 2 % sulfur with 1 % hydrocortisone or miconazole lotion [80]. Keeping the perianal area clean and dry is essential for treatment success.

Lichen sclerosus is initially managed with topical steroids. Potent topical steroid creams, such as clobetasol 0.05 %, for a short course (4–6 weeks) followed by less potent hydrocortisone cream are the mainstay of treatment. Systemic steroids are given only for very severe cases [18, 42]. Topical calcineurin inhibitors are effective alternatives in the treatment of lichen sclerosus in patients who have failed therapy with potent corticosteroids or who have a contraindication for the use of corticosteroids [81]. Treatment with retinoid and testosterone creams may be useful in selective cases [28, 43]. Patients should be followed periodically for raised lesions or ulcers that fail to heal, and it is important to explain to patients that the appearance of the vulvar and perianal lesions may never change even if the symptoms are relieved [43]. The treatment of lichen simplex chronicus or neurodermatitis begins with topical steroids to decrease the inflammation and break the itch-scratch-itch cycle. Antihistamines, doxepin, or capsaicin creams are effective adjuncts to topical steroids. For patients who have a poor response to topical steroids, topical acetylsalicylic acid/dichloromethane or immunomodulators, such as tacrolimus, have shown positive results [44].

Treatment of perianal Paget's disease requires wide local excision. Adequate microscopically clear margins and ruling out invasive disease are important to avoid clinical recurrence [82]. Positive skin margins are a common occurrence after excision; therefore, preoperative and intraoperative planning should involve a detailed discussion with an experienced pathologist regarding specimen location and orientation. Invasive disease is treated with abdominoperineal resection and delayed margin positivity requires re-excision. Soft-tissue and skin reconstruction frequently requires V–Y gluteal flaps or skin grafting, with the assistance of plastic surgery. It is important for the patient to be aware of the possibility of radical resection, delayed re-excision of margins, and stoma. Recurrence of disease is common and may occur up to a decade after initial excision [18]; therefore, regular and long-term follow-up is imperative.

Systemic Diseases

Effective treatment of pruritus ani in patients with poorly controlled or exacerbated systemic disease involves appropriate management of the underlying disease. Occasionally, pruritus will be the presenting symptom in patients with liver failure and diabetes mellitus. Appropriate skin cleansing, application of a topical barrier, and antipruritic agents are the mainstay of treatment. Cimetidine has been reported to eliminate itching induced by lymphoma and polycythemia vera. In our experience, doxepin and gabapentin are also effective antipruritic agents in patients with systemically induced pruritus ani. Chronic itching in these patients may also lead to lichenification and secondary infections. Appropriate systemic antibiotic or antifungal therapy is warranted.

In summary, perianal dermatologic conditions include a wide variety of diagnoses that require comprehensive and stepwise diagnostic and management algorithms. These conditions are likely to be much more common than estimated in the current literature, mainly because of the embarrassment associated with seeking medical attention as well as the relapsing and chronic nature of idiopathic etiologies. Patients with primary pruritus ani refractory to treatment should be aware of this chronicity and focus on symptom control instead of symptom eradication and also understand the potential need for treatment strategies for relapsing disease or flares.

References

1. Hafenreffer S. Nosodochium, in quo cutis, eique adaerentium partium, affectusomnes, singulari methodo, et cognoscendi e curandi fidelisime traduntur. Ulmae(Westphalia) Kühnen; 1660. p. 98–102.
2. Billingham RP, Isler JT, Kimmins MH, et al. The diagnosis and management of common anorectal disorders. Curr Probl Surg. 2004;33(7):586–645.
3. Hanno R, Murphy P. Pruritus ani: classification and management. Dermatol Clin. 1987;5(4):811–6.
4. Zuccati G, Lotti T, Mastrolorenzo A, et al. Pruritus ani. Dermatol Ther. 2005;18(4):355–62.
5. Mazier WP. Hemorrhoids, fissures, and pruritus ani. Surg Clin North Am. 1994;74(6):1277–92.
6. Metcalf A. Anorectal disorders. Five common causes of pain, itching and bleeding. Postgrad Med. 1995;98(5):81. –4, 87–9, 92–4.
7. Ikoma A, Steinhoff M, Ständer S, Yosipovitch G, Schmelz M. The neurobiology of itch. Nat Rev Neurosci. 2006;7: 535–47.
8. Steinhoff M, Bienenstock J, Schmelz M, Maurer M, Wei E, Biro T. Neurophysiological, neuroimmunological, and neuroendocrine basis of pruritus. J Invest Dermatol. 2006;126: 1705–18.
9. Schmelz M, Schmidt R, Bickel A, Handwerker HO, Torebjork HE. Specific C-receptors for itch in human skin. J Neurosci. 1997;17:8003–8.
10. Patel KN, Dong X. Itch: cells, molecules, and circuits. ACS Chem Neurosci. 2011;2:17–25.
11. Andrew D, Craig AD. Spinothalamic lamina I neurons selectively sensitive to histamine: a central neural pathway for itch. Nat Neurosci. 2001;4:72.
12. Yosipovitch G, Greaves M, Schmelz M. Itch. Lancet. 2003; 36:690–4.
13. Verbov J. Pruritus ani and its management – a study and reappraisal. Clin Exp Dermatol. 1984;9:46–52.
14. Caplan RM. The irritant role of feces in the genesis of perianal itch. Gastroenterology. 1966;50:19–23.
15. Eyers AA, Thomson JP. Pruritus ani: is anal sphincter dysfunction important in aetiology? Br Med J. 1979;2:1549–51.
16. Koblenzer CS. Psychologic and psychiatric aspects of itching. In: Bernhard JD, editor. Itch: mechanisms and management of pruritus. New York, NY: McGraw-Hill; 1994. p. 347–65.
17. Stamos MJ, Hicks TC. Pruritus ani: diagnosis and treatment. Perspect Colon Rectal Surg. 1998;11(1):1–20. Thieme Medical Publishers.
18. Gordon PH, Nivatvongs S. Perianal dermatologic disease. In: Gordon PH, editor. Principles and practice of surgery for the colon, rectum and anus. 3rd ed. New York, NY: Informa Healthcare; 2007. p. 247–73.
19. Bowyer A, McColl I. A study of 200 patients with pruritus ani. Proc R Soc Med. 1970;63(Suppl):96–8.
20. Andersen PH, Bucher AP, Saeed I, Lee PC, Davis JA, Maibach HI. Faecal enzymes: in vivo human skin irritation. Contact Dermatitis. 1994;30(3):152–8.
21. Friend WG. The cause and treatment of idiopathic pruritus ani. Dis Colon Rectum. 1977;20:40–2.
22. Andrews D, Grunau VJ. An uncommon adverse effect following bolus administration of intravenous dexamethasone. J Can Dent Assoc. 1986;52:309–11.
23. Kligman AM, Frosch PJ. Steroid addiction. Int J Dermatol. 1979;18:23–31.
24. Goldman L, Kitzmiller KW. Perianal atrophoderma from topical corticosteroids. Arch Dermatol. 1973;107:611–2.
25. Markell KW, Billingham RP. Pruritus ani: etiology and management. Surg Clin North Am. 2010;90(1):125–35.
26. Kranke B, Trummer M, Brabek E, Komericki P, Turek TD, Aberer W. Etiologic and causative factors in perianal dermatitis:

results of a prospective study in 126 patients. Wien Klin Wochenschr. 2006;118(3-4):90–4.

27. Siddiqi S, Vijay V, Ward M, et al. Pruritus ani. Ann R Coll Surg Engl. 2008;90(6):457–63.

28. Sheth S, Schechtman AD. Itchy perianal erythema. J Fam Pract. 2007;56(12):1025–7.

29. Weismann K, Sand Petersen C, Roder B. Pruritus ani caused by beta-haemolytic streptococci. Acta Derm Venereol. 1996;76(5): 415.

30. Dodi G, Pirone E, Bettin A, et al. The mycotic flora in procto-logical patients with and without pruritus ani. Br J Surg. 1985;72(12):967–9.

31. Bauer A, Geier J, Elsner P. Allergic contact dermatitis in patients with anogenital complaints. J Reprod Med. 2000;45(8): 649–54.

32. Goldsmith PC, Rycroft RJ, White IR, Ridley CM, Neill SM, McFadden JP. Contact sensitivity in women with anogenital dermatoses. Contact Dermatitis. 1997;36(3):174–5.

33. Blecher P, Korting HC. Tolerance to different toilet paper prep-arations: toxicological and allergological aspects. Dermatology. 1995;191(4):299–304.

34. Wilkinson JD, Hambly EM, Wilkinson DS. Comparison of patch test results in two adjacent areas of England. II. Medicaments. Acta Derm Venereol. 1980;60(3):245–9.

35. Minet A, Eggers S, Willocx D, Bourlond A, Lachapelle JM. Allergic contact dermatitis from Kathon CG in moist toilet paper. Contact Dermatitis. 1989;21(2):107–8.

36. de Groot AC, Baar TJ, Terpstra H, Weyland JW. Contact allergy to moist toilet paper. Contact Dermatitis. 1991;24(2):135–6.

37. Smith FJ, Irvine AD, Terron-Kwiatkowski A, Sandilands A, Campbell LE, Zhao Y, et al. Loss-of-function mutations in the gene encoding filaggrin cause ichthyosis vulgaris. Nat Genet. 2006;38:337–42.

38. Segre JA. Epidermal differentiation complex yields a secret: mutations in the cornification protein filaggrin underlie ichthyo-sis vulgaris. J Invest Dermatol. 2006;126:1202–4.

39. Smith LE, Henrichs D, McCullah RD. Prospective studies on the etiology and treatment of pruritus ani. Dis Colon Rectum. 1982;25:358–63.

40. Dasan S, Neill SM, Donaldson DR, Scott HJ. Treatment of per-sistent pruritus ani in a combined colorectal and dermatological clinic. Br J Surg. 1999;86:1337–40.

41. Habif TP. Clinical dermatology: a color guide to diagnosis and therapy. 4th ed. Philadelphia, PA: Mosby; 2004.

42. Chuang TY, Stitle L. Lichen planus. Emedicine website. http://emedcine.medscape.com/article/1123213-overview. Accessed 18 Apr 2008.

43. Meffert J. Lichen sclerosus et atrophicus. Emedicine website. http://emedicine.medscape.com/article/1123316-overview. Accessed 29 Jan 2009.

44. Hogan DJ, Mason SH, Bower SM. Lichen simplex chronicus. Emedicine website. http://emedicine.medscape.com/article/1123423-overview. Accessed 10 Oct 2008.

45. Chang GJ, Berry JM, Jay N, Palefsky JM, Welton ML. Surgical treatment of high-grade anal squamous intraepithelial lesions: a prospective study. Dis Colon Rectum. 2002;45:453–8.

46. Goldstone SE, Winkler B, Ufford LJ, Alt E, Palefsky JM. High prevalence of anal squamous intraepithelial lesions and squamous-cell carcinoma in men who have sex with men as seen in a surgical practice. Dis Colon Rectum. 2001;44:690–8.

47. Berardi RS, Lee S, Chen HP. Perianal extramammary Paget's disease. Surg Gynecol Obstet. 1988;167:359–65.

48. Perez DR, Trakarnsanga A, Shia J, Nash GM, Temple LK, Paty PB, Guillem JG, Garcia-Aguilar J, Weiser MR. Manage-ment and outcome of perianal Paget's disease: a 6-decade institutional experience. Dis Colon Rectum. 2014;57(6): 747–51.

49. Sarmiento JM, Wolff BG, Burgart LJ, Frizelle FA, Ilstrup DM. Paget's disease of the perianal region—an aggressive dis-ease? Dis Colon Rectum. 1997;40:1187–94.

50. Marchesa P, Fazio VW, Oliart S, Goldblum JR, Lavery IC. Perianal Bowen's disease: a clinicopathologic study of 47 patients. Dis Colon Rectum. 1997;40:1286–93.

51. Daniel GL, Longo WE, Vernava III AM. Pruritus ani causes and concerns. Dis Colon Rectum. 1994;37:670–4.

52. Murie JA, Sim AJ, Mackenzie I. The importance of pain, pruritus and soiling as symptoms of haemorrhoids and their response to haemorrhoidectomy or rubber band ligation. Br J Surg. 1981; 68:247–9.

53. Weichert GE. An approach to the treatment of anogenital pruri-tus. Dermatol Ther. 2004;17(1):129–33.

54. Sindhuphak W, MacDonald E, Smith EB. Erythrasma: over-looked or misdiagnosed? Int J Dermatol. 1985;24(2):95–6.

55. Bowyer A, McColl I. Erythrasma and pruritus ani. Acta Derm Venereol. 1971;51(6):444–7.

56. Alexander S. Dermatological aspects of anorectal disease. Clin Gastroenterol. 1975;4:651–7.

57. Pirone E, Infantino A, Masin A, Melega F, Pianon P, Dodi G, et al. Can proctological procedures resolve perianal pruritus and mycosis? A prospective study of 23 cases. Int J Colorectal Dis. 1992;7:18–20.

58. Meffert JJ, Davis BM, Grimwood RE. Lichen sclerosus. J Am Acad Dermatol. 1995;32:393–416. quiz 417–398.

59. Neill SM, Tatnall FM, Cox NH. Guidelines for the management of lichen sclerosus. Br J Dermatol. 2002;147:640–9.

60. Powell JJ, Wojnarowska F. Lichen sclerosus. Lancet. 1999;353:1777–83.

61. Wong YW, Powell J, Oxon MA. Lichen sclerosus: a review. Minerva Med. 2002;93:95–9.

62. Val I, Almeida G. An overview of lichen sclerosus. Clin Obstet Gynecol. 2005;48:808–17.

63. Carli P, Cattaneo A, De Magnis A, Biggeri A, Taddei G, Giannotti B. Squamous cell carcinoma arising in vulval lichen sclerosus: a longitudinal cohort study. Eur J Cancer Prev. 1995;4:491–5.

64. Lock MR, Katz DR, Parks A, Thomson JP. Perianal Paget's dis-ease. Postgrad Med J. 1977;53:768–72.

65. McClatchey KD. Clinical laboratory medicine. 2nd ed. Philadelphia, PA: Lippincott Williams & Wilkins; 2002.

66. Health Inc IMS. Prescribing insights. Danbury, CT: IMS; 2011.

67. Al-Ghnaniem R, Short K, Pullen A, et al. 1% Hydrocortisone ointment is an effective treatment of pruritus ani: a pilot randomized controlled crossover trial. Int J Colorectal Dis. 2007;22(12):1463–7.

68. Lysy J, Sistiery-Ittah M, Israelit Y, et al. Topical capsaicin—a novel and effective treatment for idiopathic intractable pruritus ani: a randomized, placebo controlled, crossover study. Gut. 2003;52(9):1323–6.

69. Finne CO, Fenyk JR. Dermatology and pruritus ani. In: Fleshman JW, Wolff BG, editors. The ASCRS textbook of

colon and rectal surgery. New York, NY: Springer; 2007. p. 277–94.

70. Shohrati M, Davoudi SM, Keshavarz S, Sadr B, Tajik A. Cetirizine, doxepine, and hydroxyzine in the treatment of pruritus due to sulfur mustard: a randomized clinical trial. Cutan Ocul Toxicol. 2007;26(3):249–55.

71. Siemens W, Xander C, Meerpohl JJ, Antes G, Becker G. Drug treatments for pruritus in adult palliative care. Dtsch Arztebl Int. 2014;111(50):863–70.

72. Eusebio EB, Graham J, Mody N. Treatment of intractable pruritus ani. Dis Colon Rectum. 1990;33(9):770–2.

73. Mentes BB, Akin M, Leventoglu S, et al. Intradermal methylene blue injection for the treatment of intractable idiopathic pruritus ani: results of 30 cases. Tech Coloproctol. 2004;8(1): 11–4.

74. Baral J. Pruritus ani and Staphylococcus aureus [letter]. J Am Acad Dermatol. 1983;9(6):962.

75. Schneider L, Tilles S, Lio P, et al. Atopic dermatitis: a practice parameter update 2012. J Allergy Clin Immunol. 2013; 131:295–9.

76. Ucak H, Demir B, Cicek D, Dertlioglu SB, Akkurt ZM, Ucmak D, Halisdemir N. Efficacy of topical tacrolimus for the treatment of persistent pruritus ani in patients with atopic dermatitis. J Dermatolog Treat. 2013;24(6):454–7.

77. Suys E. Randomized study of topical tacrolimus ointment as possible treatment for resistant idiopathic pruritus ani. J Am Acad Dermatol. 2012;66(2):327–8.

78. Decock S, Roelandts R, Steenbergen WV, Laleman W, Cassiman D, Verslype C, Fevery J, Pelt JV, Nevens F. Cholestasis-induced pruritus treated with ultraviolet B phototherapy: an observational case series study. J Hepatol. 2012;57(3):637–41.

79. Panahi Y, Davoudi SM, Madanchi N, Abolhasani E. Recombinant human interferon gamma (Gamma Immunex) in treatment of atopic dermatitis. Clin Exp Med. 2012;12(4):241–5.

80. Alexander-Williams J. Causes and management of anal irritation. Br Med J (Clin Res Ed). 1983;287(6404):1528.

81. Fistarol SK, Itin PH. Diagnosis and treatment of lichen sclerosus: an update. Am J Clin Dermatol. 2013;14(1):27–47.

82. Beck DE, Fazio VW. Perianal Paget's disease. Dis Colon Rectum. 1987;30:263–6.

19
Sexually Transmitted Infections

Cindy Kin and Mark Lane Welton

Key Concepts

- Nucleic acid amplification tests are superior to culture to screen for *Chlamydia trachomatis* and *Neisseria gonorrhoeae* infections. The best specimens are vaginal or endocervical swabs from women and first catch urine samples from men.
- Nucleic acid amplification tests for *Chlamydia trachomatis* and *Neisseria gonorrhoeae* can be used for rectal and oropharyngeal specimens in addition to genital sites to increase the sensitivity of testing.
- If one suspects failure of standard antibiotic treatment for gonococcal infection then a culture needs to be performed to evaluate antibiotic susceptibility.
- Male and female patients with infections causing rectal or genital ulcerations are at increased risk for HIV infection, compared to patients with non-ulcerative STIs.
- Patients diagnosed with syphilis should be tested for HIV. Patients with HIV should be regularly screened for syphilis.
- Empiric treatment for proctitis in populations at high risk for STIs should be given at the time of evaluation rather than waiting for test results, and should consist of treatment for gonorrhea, chlamydia/lymphogranuloma venereum, and genital herpes.
- Herpes simplex virus is a common cause of proctitis in men who have sex with men and often present without visible external ulcerations.

Introduction

This chapter discusses sexually transmitted infections (STIs) that are likely to be encountered by colorectal surgeons. Clinicians must maintain a high level of suspicion for STIs to avoid delays or errors in diagnosis. A frank discussion of the patient's sexual history should direct STI testing and empiric therapy.

A substantial proportion of patients with STIs are completely asymptomatic. Overall, 7 % of men who have sex with men (MSM) undergoing screening for STI test will be positive for at least one infection. Asymptomatic MSM who report an STI exposure have a 17 % chance of testing positive for at least one STI. An HIV-positive MSM with an STI is twice as likely to be asymptomatic from the STI than an HIV-negative MSM with an STI [1].

"Sexually transmitted diseases" and "sexually transmitted infections" are interchangeably used terms, but the latter has been increasingly adopted to emphasize that infections may not cause symptoms of disease, nor may they result in development of disease. For example, infection with the human papillomavirus may not develop into the diseases of cervical cancer or anal cancer. This term is also regarded as less stigmatizing and thus may result in improved testing rates.

This chapter will discuss the diagnosis and management of STIs, as well as the risk factors for infection and public health concerns related to the infections.

Screening Guidelines for Asymptomatic High-Risk Patients

The predominant risk factor for contracting STIs is high-risk sexual behavior. Other risk factors include current infection with ulcerative STIs and HIV seropositivity. MSM, especially those who engage in unprotected receptive anal intercourse, represent the demographic group at greatest risk for STIs and should undergo regular universal testing for STIs. People in high-risk sexual networks such as swingers are also at very high risk for STIs and should also undergo universal testing for STIs. A policy of universal testing can help to stop the cycle of ongoing transmission of STIs within these networks [2].

Furthermore, MSM and other high-risk populations including prostitutes and swingers should undergo testing for STIs (mainly, chlamydia and gonorrhea) at anorectal,

© Springer International Publishing 2016
S.R. Steele et al. (eds.), *The ASCRS Textbook of Colon and Rectal Surgery*, DOI 10.1007/978-3-319-25970-3_19

TABLE 19-1. Initial sexually transmitted infections (STI) testing and empiric therapy by symptom

Symptom	Suspected etiology	Testing	Empiric therapy
Genital, anal, perianal ulcers	Herpes Syphilis Chancroid Donovanosis	Syphilis serology HSV culture or PCR HIV *H. ducreyi* testing in settings where chancroid is prevalent	Treatment for HSV or syphilis depending on clinical suspicion
Proctitis	Gonorrhea Chlamydia Syphilis Herpes	Intra-anal swabs for chlamydia and gonorrhea and HSV culture or PCR	Treatment for gonorrhea, chlamydia/LGV, and herpes depending on clinical suspicion and risk factors
Proctocolitis	*Campylobacter, Shigella*, and *Entamoeba histolytica* LGV	Stool studies NAAT for chlamydia	
Enteritis	*Giardia*	Stool studies	

HSV herpes simplex virus, *LGV* lymphogranuloma venereum, *PCR* polymerase chain reaction, *NAAT* nucleic acid amplification tests

oropharyngeal, and urogenital sites, as isolated non-urogenital infections represent the majority of infections in both MSM and high-risk women. With testing at multiple anatomic sites, over 10 % of MSM had chlamydia and 6 % had gonorrhea, while 7 % of female prostitutes and swingers had chlamydia and 3 % had gonorrhea. Given that most of these infections were isolated non-urogenital infections, the practice of coincidental treatment is an inadequate strategy for controlling transmission of these infections [3].

Screening Guidelines for Symptomatic Patients

Symptoms of STIs may include painful or painless perianal or genital lesions; rectal, vaginal, or urethral discharge; or proctitis. Table 19-1 details the suspected etiologies, recommended testing, and empiric therapy by symptom class.

Perianal or Genital Lesions

Lesions or other symptoms involving the anus and perianal skin may be easily mistaken for other diagnoses, such as fissure or hemorrhoid disease, delaying appropriate treatment. Lesions in the perianal skin may also be misdiagnosed as a perianal fistula or abscess, folliculitis, hidradenitis, or pruritus ani. Patients (and sometimes their physicians) are likely to assume that any discomfort in the anal region can be attributed to hemorrhoids and will start empiric treatment for hemorrhoids without confirming the diagnosis. Thus, it is imperative to perform at least a visual inspection of the perianal skin and anal canal when evaluating any anorectal complaint. Digital exam with anoscopy should also be performed if the patient can tolerate it.

Genital lesions in young sexually active patients are most likely to be genital herpes or syphilis. Less commonly, chancroid and donovanosis may also be the cause of genital ulcers.

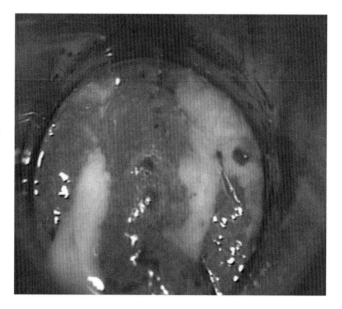

FIGURE 19-1. Patients with STIs may present with proctitis, characterized by anorectal pain, tenesmus, and mucopurulent discharge. Proctoscopy may not be possible due to pain.

Patients should undergo serologic testing for syphilis and HSV culture or PCR, as well as HIV testing. Empiric treatment of the most likely pathogen should be started. Painless lesions may be condyloma or other HPV-related dysplasia. The genital lesions of molluscum contagiosum may cause pruritus.

Proctitis

Proctitis is inflammation of the rectum, causing symptoms of anorectal pain, tenesmus, and discharge (Figure 19-1). The suspected etiologic agents are *N. gonorrhea, C. trachomatis, T. pallidum*, and HSV. Patient discomfort may preclude a proctoscopic examination, but intra-anal swabs for chlamydia and gonorrhea and HSV can and should be performed. Swabs should be taken before doing a rectal exam with lubricant given its bacteriostatic properties. Infectious proctitis is often misdiagnosed as inflammatory bowel disease so it is important to elicit a clear sexual history to help distinguish between the two. Anorectal pain and bleeding may also signal the presence of a malignancy such as anal or rectal cancer.

Patients who present with both symptoms of proctitis as well as anal ulceration are very likely to have HSV (83 %) or gonorrhea [4]. However, as over two-thirds of MSM with HSV proctitis do not have a concomitant external ulceration, it is important to test for HSV in these patients without the classic herpetic ulcer [4].

HIV-positive MSM presenting with proctitis are more likely than their HIV-negative counterparts with proctitis to be infected with HSV-1 (14 % vs. 7 %) or HSV-2 (22 % vs. 12 %), lymphogranuloma venereum (8 % vs. 0.7 %), or multiple STIs (18 % vs. 9 %). They are equally likely to have chlamydia or gonorrhea [4]. Empiric treatment for proctitis should be given at the time of evaluation rather than waiting for test results and should consist of treatment for gonorrhea (ceftriaxone 250 mg intramuscular × 1 day), chlamydia/LGV (doxycycline 100 mg bid × 21 days), and HSV (valacyclovir 1 g bid × 10 days). Symptom management with topical anesthetics and stool softeners will also be helpful. When test results come back, the medication regimen can be adjusted.

Proctocolitis

Proctocolitis causes symptoms of proctitis (anorectal pain, tenesmus, and discharge) along with diarrhea and abdominal cramps. Lower endoscopy reveals inflammation of the rectal and distal colonic mucosa. Stool studies may reveal fecal leukocytes. The suspected etiologic agents include *Campylobacter*, *Shigella*, and *Entamoeba histolytica*. LGV serovars of *C. trachomatis* may also cause proctocolitis. The route of transmission may be oral or oral-anal.

Enteritis

Symptoms of enteritis include diarrhea and abdominal cramping; since the rectum is not involved, patients will not present with proctitis symptoms. Enteritis acquired as an STI can be attributed to oral-anal contact. The most common etiologic agent is *Giardia lamblia*.

Diagnosis and Management of Sexually Transmitted Bacterial Infections

Testing for Chlamydia and Gonorrhea

Nucleic acid amplification tests (NAATs) are 86 % sensitive and 97 % specific for detecting gonorrhea and chlamydia, regardless of the specimen type used [5]. NAATs are also superior to other forms of testing due to the increased ease of specimen transport. The Centers for Disease Control (CDC) recommends that NAATs be used in all circumstances to detect chlamydia and gonorrhea, except for special circumstances involving prepubescent patients, and potential treatment failures in which cultures are indicated [6].

Gonorrhea

Epidemiology

Neisseria gonorrhoeae is the causative agent in gonococcal infections and represent the second most common notifiable communicable disease in the US with over 300,000 cases reported to the CDC in 2011. This is likely a gross underestimation of the actual disease burden due to underdiagnosis and underreporting. While US public health efforts have made great strides in controlling gonococcal infection, there are still groups within the population suffering from particularly high rates of gonorrhea, including MSM, HIV-positive patients, African Americans, adolescents, and young adults [7].

Clinical Presentation

Most men infected with gonorrhea experience urethritis manifesting as painful urination. They may also experience epididymitis or disseminated infection. Proctitis can also occur in those who engage in anal receptive intercourse. Gonococcal infections in women tend to be asymptomatic although they can cause cervicitis, urethritis, proctitis, and, later, pelvic inflammatory disease.

Screening and Testing for *N. gonorrhoeae*

MSM with high-risk sexual practices such as multiple anonymous partners and unprotected oral and anal intercourse are at higher risk for gonococcal infections affecting the oropharynx and rectum. For this reason, the CDC recommends routine screening of oropharyngeal, anorectal, and urogenital sites for all MSM who are sexually active and at risk for STI.

NAATs are the recommended testing method given their high sensitivity and specificity [5]. First catch urine or urethral swab is the recommended sample type for men. In women, the recommended sample types are vaginal swabs that can be either self- or clinician-collected or endocervical swab if a pelvic examination is also indicated. First catch urine in women may miss 10 % of infections compared to the other sample types [6]. Rectal and oropharyngeal specimens can also be tested with NAATs. The CDC recommends testing extragenital sites to increase the sensitivity of screening. Patients who test positive by NAAT do not need to undergo routine repeat testing as this does not improve the positive predictive value of the test [6].

Treatment and Management of Gonorrhea

For uncomplicated gonococcal infections, the CDC recommends combination therapy with ceftriaxone 250 mg intramuscular injection plus a single dose of oral azithromycin 1 g, or a 7-day course of oral doxycycline 100 mg twice daily [8]. Azithromycin is preferred due to the high prevalence of tetracycline resistance. Patients with allergies to cephalosporins can be treated with a single oral dose of azithromycin 2 g, but *N. gonorrhoeae* isolates have demonstrated resistance to azithromycin (Figure 19-2).

N. gonorrhoeae culture testing to evaluate for antibiotic susceptibility with rectal or oropharyngeal swab, endocervical swab for women, or urethral swab for men should be performed if treatment failure is clinically suspected, or NAAT positivity persists [6].

Patients who have undergone treatment for gonorrhea should be referred to programs to reduce STI risk and also undergo retesting for gonorrhea at 3 months. Sexual partners of infected patients in the preceding 2 months should also undergo treatment with ceftriaxone and azithromycin [9].

FIGURE 19-2. Treatment algorithm for patients with *N. gonorrhoeae* infection.

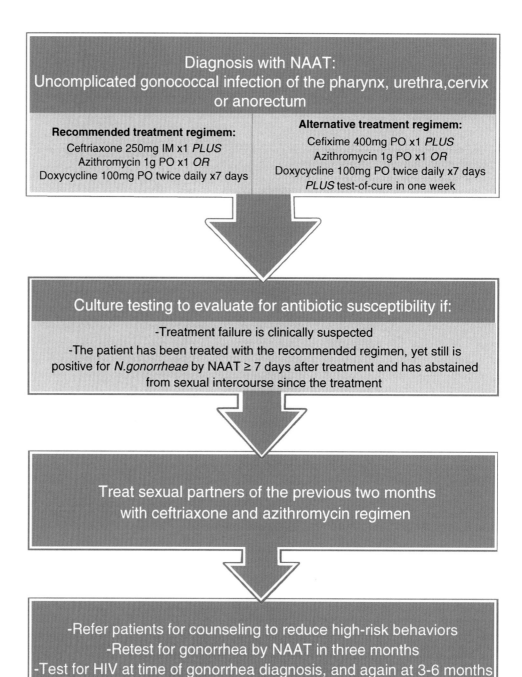

As patients with gonococcal infection have a higher risk of HIV infection, they should also undergo testing for HIV at the time of gonorrhea detection and 3–6 months later.

Emerging Antibiotic Resistance

N. gonorrhoeae has a record of developing antibiotic resistance—to penicillins and tetracyclines in the 1980s and then to fluoroquinolones in the 2000s [7]. Resistance to cephalosporins is developing as well, limiting treatment options to third-generation cephalosporins [9, 10]. MSM are more likely than heterosexual men to be infected with resistant strains of *N. gonorrhoeae* [11]. As antimicrobial susceptibility testing is not routinely performed, clinicians need to maintain a high suspicion for treatment failure and must report treatment failures [12].

Chlamydia

Epidemiology

Infection with *Chlamydia trachomatis* is the most common notifiable disease in the USA with over 1.3 million cases reported to the CDC in 2010. The prevalence of urogenital chlamydia is over 11 % and anorectal chlamydia is over 8 % among women undergoing STI evaluation [13].

Clinical Presentation

Most patients with chlamydia are asymptomatic or have such mild nonspecific symptoms that a visit to a physician never occurs, and they never become aware that they are infected. Therefore, screening is crucial to controlling this disease and preventing the severe potential sequelae of pelvic inflammatory disease that increases the risk of infertility (20 %), chronic pelvic pain (18 %), and ectopic pregnancy (9 %). Men with chlamydia infection most commonly have symptoms of urethritis; a smaller proportion has epididymitis and an even smaller proportion experiences infertility as a result of the infection. Infections affecting the rectum are usually asymptomatic and can be attributed to unprotected anal receptive intercourse (Figure 19-3). However, some patients may develop proctocolitis. Ocular infection and reactive arthritis can also occur.

Screening and Testing for *C. trachomatis*

As for gonorrhea, the recommended testing method for *C. trachomatis* is the NAAT. The recommended sample type for men is a first catch urine or urethral swab. For women, vaginal swab is recommended and if a pelvic examination is indicated then endocervical swab is also an acceptable sample type. Urine samples from women are less sensitive. Rectal and oropharyngeal specimens should also be used for screening

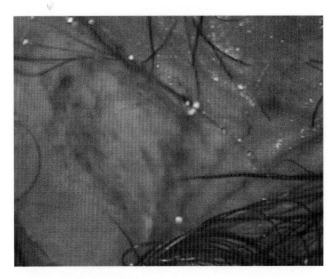

FIGURE 19-3. Chlamydia infection may present with no symptoms, mild symptoms, urethritis, ulcerations, or proctitis. Pictured is an ulcer due to chlamydia infection. Photograph courtesy of Stephen Goldstone, MD.

to increase the sensitivity of the test. Positive NAATs do not need to be routinely repeated [5, 6].

There is a high incidence of co-occurrence of anorectal and urogenital chlamydia in women—over 94 % of women with anorectal infection also have urogenital chlamydia, and over 71 % of women with urogenital infection also have anorectal infection [13].

Due to its high prevalence and serious sequelae and the potential to reduce the incidence of pelvic inflammatory disease, the CDC and the US Preventive Services Task Force recommend screening sexually active women aged 24 and younger for chlamydia, as well as older women at increased risk for infection [5, 14]. Selective testing based on symptoms and sexual history is an inadequate strategy for identifying most cases of chlamydia infection [13].

Routine universal screening for men is not recommended, as complications from chlamydia infection in men is rare. Chlamydia screening is recommended for certain high-risk male populations based on prevalence data. These populations include men in STI clinics, National Job Training Programs, and juvenile detention facilities, as well as men under 30 years old who are in the military or in jail, and men whose partners have been diagnosed with chlamydia [15]. For all MSM reporting receptive anorectal intercourse, rectal chlamydia screening is recommended [16].

Treatment and Repeat Testing

A single oral dose of 1 g of azithromycin is the recommended treatment for *C. trachomatis* infection and should be given empirically for acute nongonococcal urethritis or for suspected or proven infection in women. A 7-day course of twice daily doxycycline 100 mg is equally effective [17].

TABLE 19-2. Centers for Disease Control recommended antibiotic regimens for bacterial sexually transmitted infections (STIs) [18]

Infection	Recommended regimens	Alternative regimens
Chlamydia trachomatis	Azithromycin 1 g PO × 1 dose or doxycycline 100 mg PO twice daily × 7 days	Erythromycin base 500 mg PO four times daily × 7 days or erythromycin ethylsuccinate 800 mg PO four times daily × 7 days or levofloxacin 500 mg PO once daily × 7 days or ofloxacin 300 mg PO twice daily × 7 days
Neisseria gonorrhoeae	Ceftriaxone 250 mg IM injection × 1 dose *plus* azithromycin 1 g PO × 1 dose *or* doxycycline 100 mg PO twice daily × 7 days	Cefixime 400 mg PO × 1 *plus* azithromycin 1 g PO × 1 *or* doxycycline 100 mg PO twice daily × 7 days plus test-of-cure in 1 week
Acute proctitis in patient with recent receptive anal intercourse, with anorectal exudate or WBCs on gram-stained smear	Treat empirically with: ceftriaxone 250 mg IM × 1 dose plus doxycycline 100 mg PO twice daily × 7 days	
LGV proctitis/proctocolitis (MSM with anorectal chlamydia and proctitis or HIV)	Doxycycline 100 mg PO twice daily × 3 weeks	Erythromycin base 500 mg orally four times daily for 3 weeks
Primary, secondary, or early latent syphilis	Penicillin G benzathine 2.4 million units IM × 1 dose	Doxycycline 100 mg orally twice daily for 2 weeks or tetracycline 500 mg four times daily for 2 weeks (Penicillin-allergic pregnant women with syphilis should undergo desensitization and be treated with penicillin regimen)
Tertiary or late latent syphilis or syphilis of unknown duration	Penicillin G benzathine 2.4 million units IM once per week × 3 weeks	
Neurosyphilis	Aqueous crystalline penicillin G 18–24 million units per day, administered as 3–4 million units IV every 4 h or as a continuous infusion, × 10–14 days	
Chancroid	Ceftriaxone 250 mg IM × 1 dose or azithromycin 1 g PO × 1 dose or ciprofloxacin 500 mg PO twice daily × 3 days or erythromycin base 500 mg PO three times daily × 7 days	
Granuloma inguinale (Donovanosis)	Doxycycline 100 mg PO twice daily[a]	Azithromycin 1 g PO once per week[a] or ciprofloxacin 750 mg PO twice daily[a] or erythromycin base 500 mg PO four times daily[a] or trimethoprim/sulfamethoxazole 800 mg/160 mg PO twice daily[a]

WBC white blood count, *HIV* human immunodeficiency virus, *MSM* men who have sex with men, *LGV* lymphogranuloma venereum

[a]All regimens are for at least 3 weeks duration and should be continued until all lesions have healed

Alternative regimens include 7-day courses of erythromycin, levofloxacin, or ofloxacin (Table 19-2) [18]. Azithromycin is also effective treatment for the other infectious causes of nongonococcal urethritis aside from *C. trachomatis*, including *Mycoplasma genitalium* and *Ureaplasma urealyticum* [19]. The single dose of azithromycin is preferred as it can be given directly to the patient at the time of testing to maximize compliance. Patients should be instructed not to engage in sexual intercourse for 7 days after the single dose of azithromycin (or until they complete the full 7-day course of the other antibiotic regimens), and they should also avoid having sexual intercourse until their partners are treated as well to avoid reinfection [18]. Patients should be counseled to refer anyone with whom they have had sexual contact in the 60 days prior to chlamydia diagnosis or symptom onset for testing and treatment.

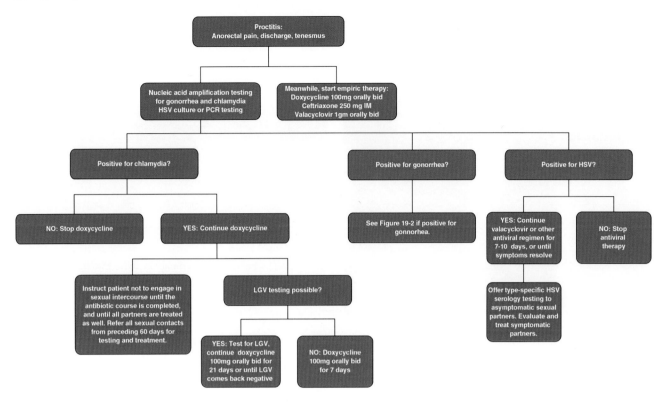

FIGURE 19-4. Management algorithm for MSM with proctitis reporting receptive anal intercourse.

Routine test-of-cure several weeks after treatment for chlamydia is not recommended by the CDC if the patient has undergone appropriate treatment and is asymptomatic with no suspicion of reinfection. However, as recurrent chlamydial infections are common in both men and women after treatment due to reinfection, repeat testing should be performed three months after treatment [15, 18].

Lymphogranuloma Venereum

Epidemiology

C. trachomatis serovars L1, L2, and L3 cause lymphogranuloma venereum. L2b has been identified as the main causative agent of the recent epidemic [20]. While anorectal infection with non-LGV C. trachomatis serovars A-K is mild and often asymptomatic, the LGV serovars cause severe inflammation and invasive infection. LGV has reemerged recently in its anorectal form due to outbreaks within MSM sexual networks. Infection has been associated with attendance at sex parties as well as HIV seropositivity. Hemorrhagic proctitis due to LGV has only been reported in MSM [21–24]. Risk factors for LGV proctitis include HIV seropositivity and chlamydia with concurrent ulcerative disease, previously diagnosed STI, unprotected receptive anal intercourse with casual partners, MSM,

having sex at sex parties, and having sex with HIV-positive partners [16, 25]. MSM with anorectal chlamydia should undergo LGV testing; if it is not available, then MSM with anorectal chlamydia and either proctitis, >10 white blood cells per high-power field on anorectal smear, or HIV seropositivity should be treated empirically for LGV [16]. A recommended algorithm for testing and treatment of chlamydia and LGV for MSM reporting anal intercourse is detailed in Figure 19-4.

Clinical Presentation

Depending on the site of primary inoculation (genital vs. anorectal), patients will manifest different syndromes. Patients with the inguinal syndrome (genital inoculation) experience unilateral painful inguinal or femoral lymphadenopathy (buboes), possibly with a genital ulcer. Patients with the anorectal syndrome experience ulcerative proctocolitis or proctitis characterized by mucopurulent discharge and tenesmus, along with systemic constitutional symptoms (Figures 19-5 and 19-6) [20]. Untreated LGV infection can result in severe complications including colorectal fistulas and strictures, elephantiasis, infertility, and pelvic fibrosis [21].

The proper diagnosis of LGV is frequently delayed because symptoms can be misleading, physicians may be unfamiliar with the disease, and there is no routine diagnostic

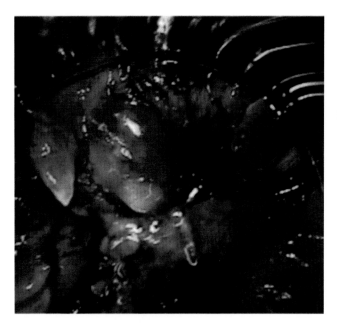

FIGURE 19-5. Proctitis due to lymphogranuloma venereum, demonstrating marked inflammation one week after treatment started. Photograph courtesy of Stephen Goldstone, MD.

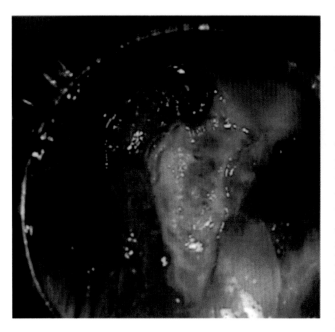

FIGURE 19-6. After two months of treatment for lymphogranuloma venereum, proctitis has resolved and ulcerations are healing. Photograph courtesy of Stephen Goldstone, MD.

test for LGV serovars [20]. Since LGV proctocolitis presents with bleeding, pain, and tenesmus, it can be mistaken as inflammatory bowel disease [21, 22]. Even pathologic specimens from endoscopic examination can be confusing, as mucosal ulcers, cryptitis, crypt abscesses, and granulomas are common histological findings that can also be attributed to inflammatory bowel disease [22, 23].

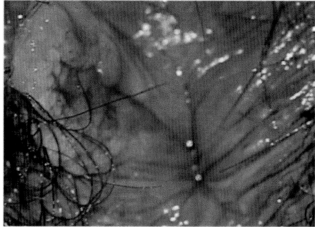

FIGURE 19-7. Chancre due to primary syphilis. Photograph courtesy of Stephen Goldstone, MD.

Treatment

The recommended treatment for LGV proctitis is twice daily doxycycline 100 mg orally for 3 weeks or for as long as anorectal symptoms persist. Buboes may require aspiration or incision and drainage to prevent ulcerations. Clinical follow-up should be continued until signs and symptoms have resolved. Sex partners from the preceding 60 days should undergo testing for chlamydia and be treated for chlamydia (one oral dose of azithromycin 1 g or one week of doxycycline) (Table 19-2) [20].

Syphilis

Epidemiology

Rates of primary and secondary syphilis, after declining for many years to a nadir of 2.1 cases per 100,000 in the year 2000, have experienced a concerning resurgence to over double that rate to 5.3 per 100,000 in 2013. Over 90 % of cases of primary and secondary syphilis occur in men, and the rise in syphilis rates is attributable to increases in men [26, 27]. Men in their 20s, MSM, black men, and Hispanic men have had the greatest increases. Rates of syphilis among women increased in the mid 2000s but have since decreased again. Similar to their male counterparts, the rate among black and Hispanic women is higher than in white women [27]. Half to a third of MSM infected with syphilis are coinfected with HIV, and the rates of HIV seroconversion following syphilis infection are high [27].

Clinical Presentation

Syphilis, caused by the spirochete *Treponema pallidum*, presents classically in its primary form as a solitary nontender genital chancre, but it can also present with multiple chancres or proctitis with bleeding, pain, and tenesmus (Figures 19-7, 19-8, and 19-9). Only a third of patients are

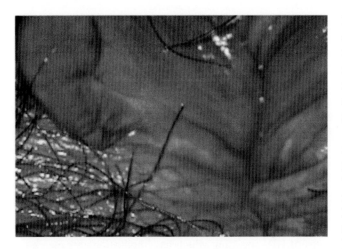

FIGURE 19-8. Healed chancre after resolution of primary syphilis. Photograph courtesy of Stephen Goldstone, MD.

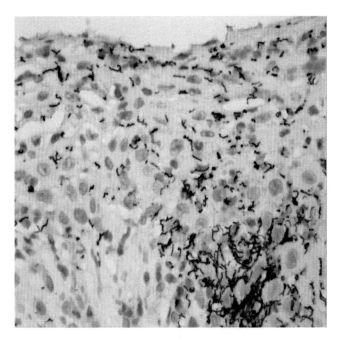

FIGURE 19-9. Immunohistochemistry staining for spirochetes, indicative of syphilis infection. Photograph courtesy of Stephen Goldstone, MD.

diagnosed during the primary infection as the primary chancre can be quite small and unnoticeable. HIV-positive patients have a higher rate of asymptomatic primary syphilis, may experience more aggressive secondary infection, and are at increased risk of developing neurosyphilis [28].

Testing Recommendations

Two types of serologic tests are used to make a presumptive diagnosis of syphilis. The nontreponemal tests include the Venereal Disease Research Laboratory (VDRL) and RPR tests and are used for screening as they become positive within

3 weeks of the primary chancre. Dark field examination to detect *T. pallidum* in lesion exudate or tissue may be successful in diagnosing early syphilis, as the nontreponemal tests may be negative in these early stages. Some patients may manifest a serofast reaction, causing the nontreponemal test to be elevated for a long period of time [26]. Treponemal tests include the fluorescent treponemal antibody absorbed tests, *T. pallidum* passive particle agglutination assay, and other immunoassays. These tests usually remain reactive for life in patients who have had a reactive test at one point. Patients with a positive nontreponemal test should undergo a confirmatory treponemal test. Patients with a negative VDRL or RPR but with strong clinical indicators of primary syphilis should undergo repeat nontreponemal testing two weeks later [18, 26]. Confirmed cases of syphilis must be reported to local and state health departments.

Due to the rebound in syphilis rates disproportionately affecting MSM, all sexually active MSM should be screened at least annually for syphilis, more frequently if they engage in high-risk sexual practices such as having multiple or anonymous sex partners [18, 27]. Due to the high rate of coinfection with HIV, patients with syphilis should undergo HIV testing, and all patients with HIV should undergo regular syphilis screening [18, 28].

Treatment

The CDC recommends a single intramuscular dose of 2.4 million units of penicillin G benzathine for primary, secondary, and early latent syphilis [18, 26]. Patients coinfected with HIV should be treated with the regimen recommended for the treatment of neurosyphilis and should be closely monitored due to increased rates of relapse [28]. The Jarisch-Herxheimer reaction, an acute febrile reaction characterized by headache, myalgia, and fever, may develop within 24 h of treatment and occurs most commonly in patients with early syphilis. Patients with penicillin allergy should be treated with doxycycline, tetracycline, ceftriaxone, or azithromycin. Pregnant women with syphilis and a penicillin allergy should undergo desensitization and treated with penicillin. Sexual contacts of patients with primary, secondary, or early latent syphilis should undergo presumptive treatment.

Treatment of primary and secondary syphilis should result in a decline of the nontreponemal test titers over the ensuing months. Repeat testing with nontreponemal tests should be performed at 6 and 12 months after treatment [18]. Retreatment for relapse should consist of 2.4 million units of intramuscular penicillin G benzathine weekly for three weeks (Table 19.2) [18].

Chancroid

Chancroid, caused by *Haemophilus ducreyi*, has declined worldwide but is a common cause of genital ulcer disease, a risk factor for HIV transmission. It usually presents with multiple painful purulent genital ulcers that progress through pustular and ulcerative stages, as well as painful regional lymphadenopathy with bubo formation. Perianal chancroid is less common than genital chancroid but can occur in MSM. Diagnosis can be difficult due to its rarity. There are no FDA-approved tests for it in the USA. Thus, diagnosis of chancroid is made based on symptoms of painful genital ulceration and regional lymphadenopathy in the absence of syphilis and HSV [18].

First-line treatment of chancroid includes azithromycin, erythromycin, ceftriaxone, and ciprofloxacin, detailed in Table 19.2 [29]. HIV-positive patients may have a higher risk of treatment failure with single-dose regimens. Inguinal bubo formation requires at least a two-week course of antibiotic therapy and may also require aspiration or incision and drainage to prevent spontaneous rupture [30, 31].

Granuloma Inguinale (aka Donovanosis)

Granuloma inguinale is a rare tropical genitoulcerative disease caused by *Klebsiella granulomatis* (formerly *Calymmatobacterium granulomatis*), endemic in Papua New Guinea, South Africa, India, Brazil, and Australia. The mode of transmission is via sexual contact, fecal contamination, and autoinoculation [32]. Clinical presentation includes papules or nodules that progress into a painless ulcer, usually in the genital area. Disseminated disease may cause cervical ulceration, pelvic lymphadenopathy, and septic arthritis and can be mistaken for cervical and ovarian cancer [32, 33]. Coinfection with HIV may worsen the course of the disease with more ulceration and tissue damage and thus the need for prolonged antibiotic therapy. Malignant transformation can also occur in HIV-positive patients [34, 35]. Testing is performed using tissue smears from the lesions and microscopic identification of characteristic intracytoplasmic inclusion bodies (Donovan bodies). PCR has recently become available as well. Treatment regimens include three-week courses of doxycycline, ciprofloxacin, erythromycin base, or trimethoprim/sulfamethoxazole [32].

Diagnosis and Management of Sexually Transmitted Viral Infections

Herpes

Epidemiology

Herpes simplex virus types 1 and 2 (HSV-1 and HSV-2) are common in the population with a seroprevalence of 54 % and 15.7 %, respectively [36]. Both may cause anogenital herpes infection. While most cases are caused by HSV-2, HSV-1 is an increasing etiologic agent in anogenital herpes, especially among heterosexual women and young MSM [37, 38]. The overall seroprevalence of HSV-2 has decreased among the

14–49-year-old population in the USA over the last two decades—from 21.2 % in the late 1980s and early 1990s to 15.5 % in the late 2000s. However, this decrease is due mainly to decreases among whites while the rates in black men and women have not changed, thus representing increased racial disparity. Over 90 % of patients with genital herpes are unaware that they have it [39]. Primary prevention of genital herpes is difficult due to the high rates of unrecognized infection [40]. HSV has been found to be frequently reactivated for short periods of time (less than 12 h) and then rapidly cleared without causing clinical symptoms, likely by the peripheral mucosal immune system. These subclinical reactivations may also contribute to increased transmission [41, 42]. Men with HSV infection, even when asymptomatic, also have higher rates of HIV shedding which has implications for increased HIV transmission.

Clinical Presentation

HSV infections classically present with multiple painful vesicular ulcers, although not all infected patients have these symptoms (Figure 19-10). HSV is the most common cause of proctitis among HIV-positive men, occurring in more than a third of HIV-positive MSM with proctitis. HSV is the cause of proctitis in 20 % of HIV-negative men with proctitis [4]. Only a third of patients with HSV proctitis have external ulcers as well, thus underscoring the need to test and treat for herpes in MSM with proctitis, regardless of the presence of ulcers [4]. HSV-2 infection is more likely to cause recurrences than HSV-1 infection. Patients who also have HIV are more likely to have more severe and painful lesions, and increased HSV shedding, even when they are asymptomatic.

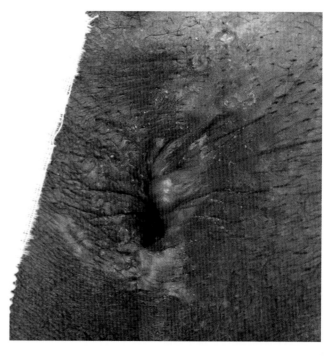

FIGURE 19-10. Perianal herpes lesions that have started to resolve.

Testing and Screening

HSV testing can be performed with cell culture or PCR, although a negative result may be attributed to intermittent viral shedding. Type-specific HSV serologic assays are also available and can be used to evaluate patients with symptoms of genital herpes but with negative HSV cultures, patients who have a partner with genital herpes, patients seeking an STI evaluation, HIV-positive patients, and MSM at high risk for being infected with HIV. Routine screening of the general population is not recommended.

Treatment

The first clinical episode of genital herpes can cause severe ulcerations as well as systemic symptoms. Therefore, treatment with antiviral therapy—acyclovir, famciclovir, or valacyclovir—is recommended to shorten the course of the episode. Suppressive antiviral therapy can decrease the number of recurrences in patients with frequent recurrences (at least four per year) [43]. Suppressive therapy may also be indicated to decrease the risk for transmission to sexual partners, especially when the patient's sexual partner is not positive for HSV, or if the patient has multiple partners [44]. Condom use and avoidance of sexual activity during recurrences offer additional protection against transmission to HSV-negative partners [45]. Another option for recurrent genital herpes is the use of episodic treatment. Recommended regimens for treatment of the first clinical episode, suppressive therapy, and episodic therapy are detailed in Table 19-3. Rarely, HSV can cause severe complicated disease requiring hospitalization and intravenous acyclovir therapy. For patients coinfected with HIV, suppressive herpes treatment with valacyclovir has also been shown to decrease rectal, seminal, and plasma HIV levels [46–51]. HSV resistance to acyclovir, valacyclovir, and famciclovir may result in persistent infections, which will need to be treated with alternative regimens such as foscarnet or cidofovir. Asymptomatic sex partners should be offered type-specific serologic testing for HSV infection, and symptomatic sex partners should be evaluated and treated accordingly.

Human Papillomavirus

Epidemiology

Over 40 different HPV types can cause genital infection, and most infections are asymptomatic and self-limited. Sexually active people have at least a 50 % risk of becoming infected at least once in their lifetime, if they are not vaccinated. Low-risk HPV types include HPV types 6 and 11, and these are the most common etiologic agents for genital warts, while the high-risk HPV types 16 and 18 are associated with cancers of the anus, cervix, penis, vulva, and vagina. Genital

warts may also harbor more high-risk HPV types 16, 18, 31, 33, and 35 and may contain areas of high-grade dysplasia. These precursor lesions are common among high-risk populations such as MSM- and HIV-positive patients, occurring in over half of HIV-positive MSM and over a third of HIV-negative MSM [52].

Clinical Presentation

While the majority of infections with HPV are asymptomatic and self-limited, some patients may develop genital warts, dysplastic lesions, or cancer depending on the virus type. Genital warts, or condyloma, present as growths on the genital mucosa, anal mucosa, and perianal skin (Figure 19-11). Patients with warts within the anal canal may have a history of receptive anal intercourse but not necessarily. Symptoms may include pain, pruritus, discomfort, or bleeding, depending on the location and size of the warts. Patients with HIV infection or another source of immunosuppression are more likely to develop genital warts, and these warts are less likely to respond to treatment and more likely to recur.

The high-risk HPV types can cause invasive squamous cell cancers of the anus. Squamous cell carcinoma occurs more frequently in patients who are immunosuppressed, especially in patients who are coinfected with HIV. Disturbances in the peripheral immune function in the anal mucosa may explain this increased risk to progress to invasive anal cancer [53–56].

Testing

HPV testing can be used to screen women for cervical cancer, but screening for HPV is not indicated for men, sex partners of women with known HPV, adolescent women, or for other HPV-related malignancies such as anal cancer [18].

As certain high-risk populations such as HIV-positive MSM have seen a rise in incidence of invasive anal squamous cell carcinoma, screening programs to detect precursor lesions have been developed to prevent progression to invasive cancer [52]. Liquid-based anorectal cytology specimens are the preferred specimen type to screen for high-grade anal dysplasia [57]. Self-collected samples are less sensitive than clinician-collected samples [52]. Patient with positive findings should be referred to a specialist for high-resolution anoscopy or routine anoscopy and monitoring.

Treatment

The indication to treat anogenital warts is to relieve symptoms. Untreated genital warts may self-resolve or worsen. Treatment does not affect the risk of transmission of HPV. External genital warts can be treated in a variety of ways (Table 19-3). Patients may apply their own treatment at home

TABLE 19-3. Centers for Disease Control recommended treatment regimens for viral STIs [18]

Infection	Recommended regimens
Genital herpes (HSV-1 or HSV-2): first clinical episode	Acyclovir 400 mg PO three times daily for 7–10 days or acyclovir 200 mg PO five times daily for 7–10 days or famciclovir 250 mg PO three times daily for 7–10 days or valacyclovir 1 g PO twice daily for 7–10 days
Suppressive therapy for recurrent genital herpes (frequent recurrences)	Acyclovir 400 mg PO twice daily or famciclovir 250 mg PO twice daily or valacyclovir 500 mg PO once daily[a] or valacyclovir 1 g PO once daily
Suppressive therapy for patients coinfected with HSV and HIV	Acyclovir 400–800 mg PO twice to three times per day or famciclovir 500 mg PO twice day or valacyclovir 500 mg PO twice daily
Episodic therapy for recurrent genital herpes	Acyclovir 400 mg PO three times daily for 5 days or acyclovir 800 mg PO twice daily for 5 days or acyclovir 800 mg PO three times daily for 2 days or famciclovir 125 mg PO twice daily for 5 days or famciclovir 1000 mg PO twice daily for 1 day or famciclovir 500 mg once, then 250 mg PO twice daily for 2 more days or valacyclovir 500 mg PO twice daily for 3 days or valacyclovir 1 g PO once daily for 5 days
Episodic therapy for patients coinfected with HSV and HIV	Acyclovir 400 mg PO three times daily for 5–10 days or famciclovir 500 mg PO twice daily for 5–10 days or valacyclovir 1 g PO twice daily for 5–10 days
External genital warts (HPV) Patient applied	Podofilox 0.5 % solution or gel: application with cotton swab twice daily for 3 days, then 4 days without therapy; can repeat cycle up to four times (max 0.5 mL per day) or imiquimod 5 % cream: apply three times per week up to 16 weeks, washing treated area with soap and water 6–10 h afterward or sinecatechins 15 % ointment: apply three times daily for up to 16 weeks
External genital warts (HPV) Provider administered	Cryotherapy with liquid nitrogen or cryoprobe or podophyllin resin 10–25 % in a compound tincture of benzoin or trichloroacetic acid (TCA) or Bichloroacetic acid (BCA) 80–90 % or surgical removal
Anal warts (HPV) Provider administered	Cryotherapy with liquid nitrogen or trichloroacetic acid (TCA) or bichloroacetic acid (BCA) 80–90 %: can be applied weekly as needed or surgical removal

HIV human immunodeficiency virus, *HSV* herpes simplex virus, *HPV* human papillomavirus

[a]This regimen may be less effective than the others for patients with over ten recurrences per year

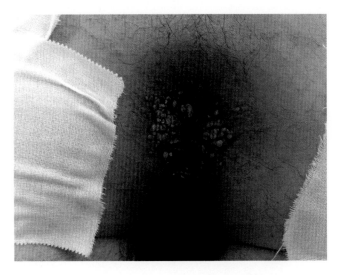

FIGURE 19-11. Perianal condyloma due to HPV infection.

using podofilox solution or gel, imiquimod cream, or sine-catechins ointment. Provider-administered options include cryotherapy, podophyllin resin, or trichloroacetic or bichloroacetic acid. The latter compounds should be applied sparingly to avoid adjacent tissue damage, and if the treatment causes pain or if too much acid is accidentally applied, soap, talc, or sodium bicarbonate (baking soda) can be used to neutralize the acid. Patients with extensive genital warts may warrant surgical management.

Anal condyloma—including warts in the anal canal and the distal rectum—can be treated with cryotherapy, TCA or BCA, or surgical therapy. High-resolution anoscopy may be indicated to inspect for high-grade dysplasia as well.

The management of high-grade anal dysplasia, the precursor to invasive squamous cell carcinoma, remains a controversial topic. While some clinicians view ablation or destruction of high-grade dysplasia as an important strategy to prevent progression to invasive cancer, others disagree with this approach. Patients with high-grade intra-anal dysplasia who undergo ablation have recurrence rates of about 50 % overall (higher in HIV-positive patients) but a low risk of developing anal cancer [58–62]. This controversy is discussed more thoroughly in the chapter on Anal Malignancies.

Vaccine

The two HPV vaccines available are the bivalent vaccine, which protects against high-risk oncogenic HPV types 16 and 18, and the quadrivalent vaccine which protects against HPV types 6, 11, 16, and 18 and should be given before one become sexually active. Both are approved for girls and boys aged 9–26 years old [18]. The quadrivalent vaccine has been shown to reduce the rates of high-grade anal dysplasia among MSM and may help to reduce the risk of anal cancer [63].

HIV and AIDS

Epidemiology

Over one million people in the USA have HIV, and over half of those infected are MSM. A quarter of those patients reported high-risk sexual practices such as unprotected sexual intercourse with a casual partner, or sex in exchange for money or drugs, and almost half of those patients reported using noninjection drugs over the past year [64].

Testing

HIV screening is recommended for all patients who present for STI testing. Positive screening tests for HIV antibody require confirmatory testing before a diagnosis can be made. If patient is suspected of having acute HIV infection, then a nucleic acid test should be performed in addition to the antibody test, and the patient should be referred immediately to an infectious disease specialist [18]. The FDA has recently approved combination tests detecting both HIV antigen and antibody, as well as tests that differentiate HIV-1 from HIV-2 [65].

Anorectal Issues

Anorectal complaints such as pain due to fissures may be the presenting symptom of patients with HIV infection. Fissures in HIV-positive patients may be a manifestation of HIV but could also represent coinfection with other STIs such as HSV or syphilis. Treatment of fissures in patients with HIV should consist of the same treatment undertaken for fissures in the general population. Special attention should be given to controlling diarrhea symptoms as well as avoidance of anal receptive intercourse.

Anal ulcers are another source of anal pain in patients with HIV and are located in a more proximal location within the anal canal—often above the dentate line—and are broader and more ulcerative than fissures. There may be evidence of destruction of the underlying sphincter muscle.

Perianal abscesses and fistulas are common in patients with HIV or AIDS. Patients with well-controlled HIV and normal CD4 counts who develop abscesses and fistulas can be treated with the same surgical techniques as one would do for patients without HIV. However, abscesses in patients with AIDS should be treated with smaller incisions, favoring drain placement over larger incisions. Fistulas in patients with advanced or poorly controlled AIDS should be treated with placement of draining setons rather than fistulotomy to avoid the creation of a nonhealing wound.

External thrombosed hemorrhoids in patients with HIV or AIDS should be treated in the same manner as those occurring in patients without HIV. Symptomatic internal hemorrhoids should be treated with first-line therapy with fiber and improvement of bowel habits. A more proximal source of

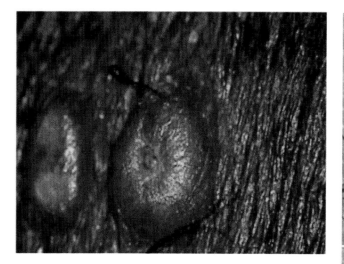

FIGURE 19-12. Molluscum contagiosum lesions present as waxy dome-shaped umbilicated papules.

bleeding should be ruled out with lower endoscopy. Patients who fail nonoperative management may safely undergo rubber band ligation of internal hemorrhoids. Hemorrhoidectomy is safe in HIV-positive patients without AIDS; patients with advanced or poorly controlled AIDS and severe hemorrhoids not amenable to banding may have wound healing problems.

Molluscum Contagiosum

Molluscum contagiosum is a common cutaneous viral infection caused by the *Molluscipoxvirus*, causing small, waxy, dome-shaped umbilicated papules (Figure 19-12). It is second only to genital warts as the most common nonulcerative STI, affecting up to 5 % of the population, 18 % of patients with immunosuppression, and 30 % of patients with advanced AIDS [66]. Secondary bacterial infection may occur especially if patients tend to scratch the lesions. Mollusca contagiosa occur frequently in young children, but their occurrence in adults is usually considered an STI and involves the pubic area. Risk factors include shaving. Transmission occurs through skin-to-skin contact, and autoinoculation can also occur to spread to other sites, especially in the 30 % of patients who develop an eczematous reaction around the lesions, which cause pruritus. Sexual contact can lead to transmission from the genitalia to the oral mucosa, conjunctiva, and cornea [67]. Diagnosis can be made by visual inspection although if there is difficulty then dermatoscopy revealing orifices, vessels, and specific vascular patterns can help confirm the diagnosis [68]. A recent PCR test has been developed as well for the molluscum contagiosum virus [69].

Immunocompetent patients will self-resolve these lesions over a period of months to years, so most patients prefer treatment. Treatment consists of removal of the lesions, similar to the treatment of genital warts. Curettage excision and

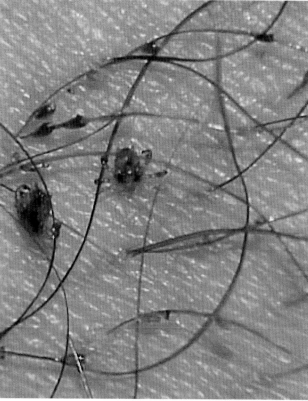

FIGURE 19-13. Pubic lice infestation causes severe pruritus and can be treated with permethrin 1 % cream. Photograph courtesy of Stephen Goldstone, MD.

cryotherapy are the most common methods of treatment [70, 71]. These treatments should not be performed in patients with immunosuppression due to the risk of nonhealing wounds and superinfection with other bacterial, viral, or fungal organisms. For these patients topical treatments such as imiquimod 5 % cream may be helpful without incurring the risk of open surgical wounds [72].

Pubic Lice: *Phthirus pubis*

Pubic lice are obligate blood-sucking parasites and infestation is diagnosed by finding lice on pubic hair (Figure 19-13). As lice can neither jump nor fly, transmission is due to close contact. Therefore, the diagnosis of pubic lice should prompt testing for other STIs. Pubic lice infestation affects 2–10 % of the population worldwide [73]. The increased incidence of pubic hair removal has been associated with a lower incidence of pubic lice infections due to destruction of their natural habitat [74].

The CDC recommends permethrin 1 % cream or pyrethrins 0.3 %/piperonyl butoxide 4 % cream as the first-line therapy for pubic lice. Alternative regimens include malathion 0.5 % lotion or oral ivermectin. Permethrin should be used on the day of diagnosis and again 7–10 days later to completely

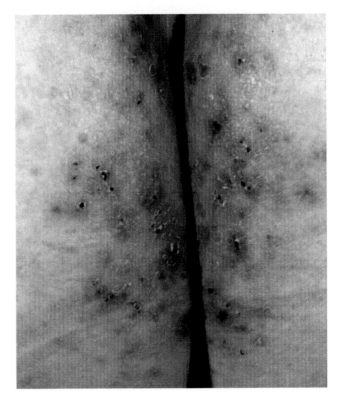

FIGURE 19-14. Scabies infestation causing an intensely pruritic rash can be treated with permethrin 5 % cream. Photograph courtesy of Stephen Goldstone, MD.

eradicate the infestation as the treatment does not kill the eggs. Laundering clothes and bedding in hot water should be done as well to prevent reinfection and transmission [18, 75].

Scabies

Scabies is caused by the mite *Sarcoptes scabiei* var. *hominis*. Scabies transmission is via skin-to-skin contact, as the mites neither jump nor fly. Scabies most commonly occurs in young children but can also occur in patients subject to overcrowded conditions, poor hygiene, homelessness, and via sexual contact. The mites burrow into the skin, creating wavy scaly lines on the skin surface, usually located on the hands and feet, typically in finger webs. The infestation causes an intense pruritic rash localized in a characteristic distribution in the armpits, elbow creases, wrists, and groin areas (Figure 19-14). Infants, children, and immunosuppressed patients may develop a more severe vesicular and pustular rash. Diagnosis can be made by visual inspection and history. Skin scrapings of the burrows, papules, and vesicles can be performed by applying mineral oil to the skin and scraping laterally across the lesion with a scalpel and examining the scraping microscopically for mites, eggs, and fecal pellets.

First-line treatment of scabies is with topical permethrin 5 % cream, which is rather effective as there is not much resistance [76]. The cream should be applied to all areas of the body from the neck down, and then washed off 8–14 h later. Reapplication of the cream should be performed 1 week later to ensure eradication. The pruritus may persist for up to 2 weeks after treatment. Oral ivermectin can also be used as first-line therapy or second-line therapy if the permethrin cream does not work [18]. Clothing and bedding should be washed in hot water and dried in a hot dryer to prevent re-infestation and transmission. Crusted scabies results when uncomplicated scabies goes untreated. Treatment involves both ivermectin orally on days 1, 2, 8, 9, and 15, as well as permethrin 5 % cream daily for 1 week, then twice a week until the disease is cured [77].

References

1. Mimiaga MJ, Helms DJ, Reisner SL, Grasso C, Bertrand T, Mosure DJ, et al. Gonococcal, chlamydia, and syphilis infection positivity among MSM attending a large primary care clinic, Boston, 2003 to 2004. Sex Transm Dis. 2009;36(8):507–11.
2. van Liere GA, Hoebe CJ, Niekamp AM, Koedijk FD, Dukers-Muijrers NH. Standard symptom- and sexual history-based testing misses anorectal Chlamydia trachomatis and neisseria gonorrhoeae infections in swingers and men who have sex with men. Sex Transm Dis. 2013;40(4):285–9.
3. van Liere GA, Hoebe CJ, Dukers-Muijrers NH. Evaluation of the anatomical site distribution of chlamydia and gonorrhea in men who have sex with men and in high-risk women by routine testing: cross-sectional study revealing missed opportunities for treatment strategies. Sex Transm Infect. 2014;90(1):58–60.
4. Bissessor M, Fairley CK, Read T, Denham I, Bradshaw C, Chen M. The etiology of infectious proctitis in men who have sex with men differs according to HIV status. Sex Transm Dis. 2013;40(10):768–70.
5. Zakher B, Cantor AG, Pappas M, Daeges M, Nelson HD. Screening for gonorrhea and Chlamydia: a systematic review for the U.S. Preventive Services Task Force. Ann Intern Med. 2014;161(12):884–93.
6. Prevention CfDCa. Recommendations for the laboratory-based detection of Chlamydia trachomatis and Neisseria gonorrhoeae – 2014. MMWR Recomm Rep. 2014;63(RR-02):1–19.
7. Workowski KA, Berman SM, Douglas JM. Emerging antimicrobial resistance in Neisseria gonorrhoeae: urgent need to strengthen prevention strategies. Ann Intern Med. 2008;148(8):606–13.
8. (CDC) CfDCaP. Update to CDC's sexually transmitted diseases treatment guidelines, 2010: oral cephalosporins no longer a recommended treatment for gonococcal infections. MMWR Morb Mortal Wkly Rep. 2012;61(31):590–4.
9. Bolan GA, Sparling PF, Wasserheit JN. The emerging threat of untreatable gonococcal infection. N Engl J Med. 2012;366(6):485–7.
10. (CDC) CfDCaP. Cephalosporin susceptibility among Neisseria gonorrhoeae isolates – United States, 2000–2010. MMWR Morb Mortal Wkly Rep. 2011;60(26):873–7.
11. Kirkcaldy RD, Zaidi A, Hook EW, Holmes KK, Holmes KH, Soge O, et al. Neisseria gonorrhoeae antimicrobial resistance among men who have sex with men and men who have sex exclusively with women: the Gonococcal Isolate Surveillance Project, 2005–2010. Ann Intern Med. 2013;158(5 Pt 1):321–8.

12. Kovari H, de Melo Oliveira MD, Hauser P, Läuchli S, Meyer J, Weber R, et al. Decreased susceptibility of Neisseria gonorrhoeae isolates from Switzerland to Cefixime and Ceftriaxone: antimicrobial susceptibility data from 1990 and 2000 to 2012. BMC Infect Dis. 2013;13:603.

13. van Liere GA, Hoebe CJ, Wolffs PF, Dukers-Muijrers NH. High co-occurrence of anorectal chlamydia with urogenital chlamydia in women visiting an STI clinic revealed by routine universal testing in an observational study; a recommendation towards a better anorectal chlamydia control in women. BMC Infect Dis. 2014;14:274.

14. LeFevre ML. Force USPST. Screening for Chlamydia and gonorrhea: U.S. Preventive Services Task Force recommendation statement. Ann Intern Med. 2014;161(12):902–10.

15. Geisler WM. Diagnosis and management of uncomplicated Chlamydia trachomatis infections in adolescents and adults: summary of evidence reviewed for the 2010 Centers for Disease Control and Prevention sexually transmitted diseases treatment guidelines. Clin Infect Dis. 2011;53 Suppl 3:S92–8.

16. Van der Bij AK, Spaargaren J, Morré SA, Fennema HS, Mindel A, Coutinho RA, et al. Diagnostic and clinical implications of anorectal lymphogranuloma venereum in men who have sex with men: a retrospective case-control study. Clin Infect Dis. 2006;42(2):186–94.

17. Stamm WE, Hicks CB, Martin DH, Leone P, Hook EW, Cooper RH, et al. Azithromycin for empirical treatment of the nongonococcal urethritis syndrome in men. A randomized double-blind study. JAMA. 1995;274(7):545–9.

18. Workowski KA, Berman S, (CDC) CfDCaP. Sexually transmitted diseases treatment guidelines, 2010. MMWR Recomm Rep. 2010;59(RR-12):1–110.

19. Stamm WE, Batteiger BE, McCormack WM, Totten PA, Sternlicht A, Kivel NM, et al. A randomized, double-blind study comparing single-dose rifalazil with single-dose azithromycin for the empirical treatment of nongonococcal urethritis in men. Sex Transm Dis. 2007;34(8):545–52.

20. Martin-Iguacel R, Llibre JM, Nielsen H, Heras E, Matas L, Lugo R, et al. Lymphogranuloma venereum proctocolitis: a silent endemic disease in men who have sex with men in industrialised countries. Eur J Clin Microbiol Infect Dis. 2010; 29(8):917–25.

21. Gallegos M, Bradly D, Jakate S, Keshavarzian A. Lymphogranuloma venereum proctosigmoiditis is a mimicker of inflammatory bowel disease. World J Gastroenterol. 2012; 18(25):3317–21.

22. Arnold CA, Limketkai BN, Illei PB, Montgomery E, Voltaggio L. Syphilitic and lymphogranuloma venereum (LGV) proctocolitis: clues to a frequently missed diagnosis. Am J Surg Pathol. 2013;37(1):38–46.

23. Soni S, Srirajaskanthan R, Lucas SB, Alexander S, Wong T, White JA. Lymphogranuloma venereum proctitis masquerading as inflammatory bowel disease in 12 homosexual men. Aliment Pharmacol Ther. 2010;32(1):59–65.

24. Pathela P, Blank S, Schillinger JA. Lymphogranuloma venereum: old pathogen, new story. Curr Infect Dis Rep. 2007; 9(2):143–50.

25. de Vries HJ, van der Bij AK, Fennema JS, Smit C, de Wolf F, Prins M, et al. Lymphogranuloma venereum proctitis in men who have sex with men is associated with anal enema use and high-risk behavior. Sex Transm Dis. 2008;35(2):203–8.

26. Mattei PL, Beachkofsky TM, Gilson RT, Wisco OJ. Syphilis: a reemerging infection. Am Fam Physician. 2012;86(5):433–40.

27. Patton ME, Su JR, Nelson R, Weinstock H, (CDC) CfDCaP. Primary and secondary syphilis – United States, 2005–2013. MMWR Morb Mortal Wkly Rep. 2014;63(18):402–6.

28. Lynn WA, Lightman S. Syphilis and HIV: a dangerous combination. Lancet Infect Dis. 2004;4(7):456–66.

29. Kemp M, Christensen JJ, Lautenschlager S, Vall-Mayans M, Moi H. European guideline for the management of chancroid, 2011. Int J STD AIDS. 2011;22(5):241–4.

30. Lewis DA. Epidemiology, clinical features, diagnosis and treatment of Haemophilus ducreyi – a disappearing pathogen? Expert Rev Anti Infect Ther. 2014;12(6):687–96.

31. Ernst AA, Marvez-Valls E, Martin DH. Incision and drainage versus aspiration of fluctuant buboes in the emergency department during an epidemic of chancroid. Sex Transm Dis. 1995;22(4):217–20.

32. Basta-Juzbašić A, Čeović R. Chancroid, lymphogranuloma venereum, granuloma inguinale, genital herpes simplex infection, and molluscum contagiosum. Clin Dermatol. 2014; 32(2):290–8.

33. Barroso LF, Wispelwey B. Donovanosis presenting as a pelvic mass mimicking ovarian cancer. South Med J. 2009; 102(1):104–5.

34. Sethi S, Sarkar R, Garg V, Agarwal S. Squamous cell carcinoma complicating donovanosis not a thing of the past! Int J STD AIDS. 2014;25(12):894–7.

35. Sardana K, Garg VK, Arora P, Khurana N. Malignant transformation of donovanosis (granuloma inguinale) in a HIV-positive patient. Dermatol Online J. 2008;14(9):8.

36. Bradley H, Markowitz LE, Gibson T, McQuillan GM. Seroprevalence of herpes simplex virus types 1 and 2 – United States, 1999–2010. J Infect Dis. 2014;209(3):325–33.

37. Xu F, Sternberg MR, Kottiri BJ, McQuillan GM, Lee FK, Nahmias AJ, et al. Trends in herpes simplex virus type 1 and type 2 seroprevalence in the United States. JAMA. 2006;296(8): 964–73.

38. Ryder N, Jin F, McNulty AM, Grulich AE, Donovan B. Increasing role of herpes simplex virus type 1 in first-episode anogenital herpes in heterosexual women and younger men who have sex with men, 1992–2006. Sex Transm Infect. 2009;85(6):416–9.

39. Fanfair RN, Zaidi A, Taylor LD, Xu F, Gottlieb S, Markowitz L. Trends in seroprevalence of herpes simplex virus type 2 among non-Hispanic blacks and non-Hispanic whites aged 14 to 49 years – United States, 1988 to 2010. Sex Transm Dis. 2013; 40(11):860–4.

40. Mertz GJ. Asymptomatic shedding of herpes simplex virus 1 and 2: implications for prevention of transmission. J Infect Dis. 2008;198(8):1098–100.

41. Mark KE, Wald A, Magaret AS, Selke S, Olin L, Huang ML, et al. Rapidly cleared episodes of herpes simplex virus reactivation in immunocompetent adults. J Infect Dis. 2008;198(8): 1141–9.

42. Mark KE, Wald A, Magaret AS, Selke S, Kuntz S, Huang ML, et al. Rapidly cleared episodes of oral and anogenital herpes simplex virus shedding in HIV-infected adults. J Acquir Immune Defic Syndr. 2010;54(5):482–8.

43. Le Cleach L, Trinquart L, Do G, Maruani A, Lebrun-Vignes B, Ravaud P, et al. Oral antiviral therapy for prevention of genital

herpes outbreaks in immunocompetent and nonpregnant patients. Cochrane Database Syst Rev. 2014;8, CD009036.

44. Corey L, Wald A, Patel R, Sacks SL, Tyring SK, Warren T, et al. Once-daily valacyclovir to reduce the risk of transmission of genital herpes. N Engl J Med. 2004;350(1):11–20.

45. Martin ET, Krantz E, Gottlieb SL, Magaret AS, Langenberg A, Stanberry L, et al. A pooled analysis of the effect of condoms in preventing HSV-2 acquisition. Arch Intern Med. 2009; 169(13):1233–40.

46. Zuckerman RA, Lucchetti A, Whittington WL, Sanchez J, Coombs RW, Zuñiga R, et al. Herpes simplex virus (HSV) suppression with valacyclovir reduces rectal and blood plasma HIV-1 levels in HIV-1/HSV-2-seropositive men: a randomized, double-blind, placebo-controlled crossover trial. J Infect Dis. 2007;196(10):1500–8.

47. Zuckerman RA, Lucchetti A, Whittington WL, Sánchez J, Coombs RW, Magaret A, et al. HSV suppression reduces seminal HIV-1 levels in HIV-1/HSV-2 co-infected men who have sex with men. AIDS. 2009;23(4):479–83.

48. Mugwanya K, Baeten JM, Mugo NR, Irungu E, Ngure K, Celum C. High-dose valacyclovir HSV-2 suppression results in greater reduction in plasma HIV-1 levels compared with standard dose acyclovir among HIV-1/HSV-2 coinfected persons: a randomized, crossover trial. J Infect Dis. 2011;204(12): 1912–7.

49. Perti T, Saracino M, Baeten JM, Johnston C, Diem K, Ocbamichael N, et al. High-dose valacyclovir decreases plasma HIV-1 RNA more than standard-dose acyclovir in persons coinfected with HIV-1 and HSV-2: a randomized crossover trial. J Acquir Immune Defic Syndr. 2013;63(2):201–8.

50. Nagot N, Ouédraogo A, Foulongne V, Konaté I, Weiss HA, Vergne L, et al. Reduction of HIV-1 RNA levels with therapy to suppress herpes simplex virus. N Engl J Med. 2007; 356(8):790–9.

51. Baggaley RF, Griffin JT, Chapman R, Hollingsworth TD, Nagot N, Delany S, et al. Estimating the public health impact of the effect of herpes simplex virus suppressive therapy on plasma HIV-1 viral load. AIDS. 2009;23(8):1005–13.

52. Chin-Hong PV, Berry JM, Cheng SC, Catania JA, Da Costa M, Darragh TM, et al. Comparison of patient- and clinician-collected anal cytology samples to screen for human papillomavirus-associated anal intraepithelial neoplasia in men who have sex with men. Ann Intern Med. 2008;149(5):300–6.

53. Guimarães AG, da Costa AG, Martins-Filho OA, Pimentel JP, Zauli DA, Peruhype-Magalhães V, et al. CD11c + CD123Low dendritic cell subset and the triad TNF-α/IL-17A/IFN-γ integrate mucosal and peripheral cellular responses in HIV patients with high-grade anal intraepithelial neoplasia: a systems biology approach. J Acquir Immune Defic Syndr. 2015;68(2):112–22.

54. Yaghoobi M, Le Gouvello S, Aloulou N, Duprez-Dutreuil C, Walker F, Sobhani I. FoxP3 overexpression and CD1a + and CD3+ depletion in anal tissue as possible mechanisms for increased risk of human papillomavirus-related anal carcinoma in HIV infection. Colorectal Dis. 2011;13(7):768–73.

55. Guimarães AG, Silva Junior RM, Costa OT, Silva IT, Gimenez FS, Araujo JR, et al. Morphometric analysis of dendritic cells from anal mucosa of HIV-positive patients and the relation to intraepithelial lesions and cancer seen at a tertiary health institution in Brazil. Acta Cir Bras. 2011;26(6):521–9.

56. Sobhani I, Walker F, Aparicio T, Abramowitz L, Henin D, Cremieux AC, et al. Effect of anal epidermoid cancer-related viruses on the dendritic (Langerhans') cells of the human anal mucosa. Clin Cancer Res. 2002;8(9):2862–9.

57. Bean SM, Chhieng DC. Anal-rectal cytology: a review. Diagn Cytopathol. 2010;38(7):538–46.

58. Goldstone SE, Johnstone AA, Moshier EL. Long-term outcome of ablation of anal high-grade squamous intraepithelial lesions: recurrence and incidence of cancer. Dis Colon Rectum. 2014;57(3):316–23.

59. Burgos J, Curran A, Tallada N, Guelar A, Navarro J, Landolfi S, et al. Risk of progression to high-grade anal intraepithelial neoplasia in HIV-infected MSM. AIDS. 2015;29(6):695–702.

60. Tong WW, Jin F, McHugh LC, Maher T, Sinclair B, Grulich AE, et al. Progression to and spontaneous regression of high-grade anal squamous intraepithelial lesions in HIV-infected and uninfected men. AIDS. 2013;27(14):2233–43.

61. Sendagorta E, Herranz P, Guadalajara H, Bernardino JI, Viguer JM, Beato MJ, et al. Prevalence of abnormal anal cytology and high-grade squamous intraepithelial lesions among a cohort of HIV-infected men who have sex with men. Dis Colon Rectum. 2014;57(4):475–81.

62. Darwich L, Videla S, Cañadas MP, Piñol M, García-Cuyàs F, Vela S, et al. Distribution of human papillomavirus genotypes in anal cytological and histological specimens from HIV-infected men who have sex with men and men who have sex with women. Dis Colon Rectum. 2013;56(9):1043–52.

63. Palefsky JM, Giuliano AR, Goldstone S, Moreira ED, Aranda C, Jessen H, et al. HPV vaccine against anal HPV infection and anal intraepithelial neoplasia. N Engl J Med. 2011;365(17):1576–85.

64. Finlayson TJ, Le B, Smith A, Bowles K, Cribbin M, Miles I, et al. HIV risk, prevention, and testing behaviors among men who have sex with men – National HIV Behavioral Surveillance System, 21 U.S. cities, United States, 2008. MMWR Surveill Summ. 2011;60(14):1–34.

65. (CDC) CfDCaP. National HIV testing day and new testing recommendations. MMWR Morb Mortal Wkly Rep. 2014; 63(25):537.

66. Villa L, Varela JA, Otero L, Sánchez C, Junquera ML, Río JS, et al. Molluscum contagiosum: a 20-year study in a sexually transmitted infections unit. Sex Transm Dis. 2010;37(7):423–4.

67. Nguyen HP, Franz E, Stiegel KR, Hsu S, Tyring SK. Treatment of molluscum contagiosum in adult, pediatric, and immunodeficient populations. J Cutan Med Surg. 2014;18(5):299–306.

68. Ianhez M, Cestari SC, Enokihara MY, Seize MB. Dermoscopic patterns of molluscum contagiosum: a study of 211 lesions confirmed by histopathology. An Bras Dermatol. 2011; 86(1):74–9.

69. Hošnjak L, Kocjan BJ, Kušar B, Seme K, Poljak M. Rapid detection and typing of Molluscum contagiosum virus by FRET-based real-time PCR. J Virol Methods. 2013;187(2):431–4.

70. Simonart T, De Maertelaer V. Curettage treatment for molluscum contagiosum: a follow-up survey study. Br J Dermatol. 2008;159(5):1144–7.

71. Tyring SK. Molluscum contagiosum: the importance of early diagnosis and treatment. Am J Obstet Gynecol. 2003;189(3 Suppl):S12–6.

72. Liota E, Smith KJ, Buckley R, Menon P, Skelton H. Imiquimod therapy for molluscum contagiosum. J Cutan Med Surg. 2000;4(2):76–82.

73. Anderson AL, Chaney E. Pubic lice (Pthirus pubis): history, biology and treatment vs. knowledge and beliefs of US college students. Int J Environ Res Public Health. 2009; 6(2):592–600.

74. Dholakia S, Buckler J, Jeans JP, Pillai A, Eagles N. Pubic lice: an endangered species? Sex Transm Dis. 2014;41(6): 388–91.

75. Gunning K, Pippitt K, Kiraly B, Sayler M. Pediculosis and scabies: treatment update. Am Fam Physician. 2012;86(6): 535–41.

76. Strong M, Johnstone P. Interventions for treating scabies. Cochrane Database Syst Rev. 2007;3, CD000320.

77. Wolf R, Davidovici B. Treatment of scabies and pediculosis: facts and controversies. Clin Dermatol. 2010;28(5):511–8.

20
Anal Intraepithelial Neoplasia

Rocco Ricciardi

Key Concepts

- Anal intraepithelial neoplasia is a dysplastic condition of squamous tissue and is considered to be a premalignant stage of anal cancer.
- The histological findings and cellular abnormalities mirror cervical dysplasia.
- Anal cytology is a useful method to identify anal neoplasia in high-risk groups.
- When cytology is concerning, the evaluation of anal neoplasia can proceed with anal cytology and high-resolution microscopy, a technique similar to colposcopy.
- A targeted approach to dysplasia ablation through microscopy is more sparing than historically practiced wide local excisions and flap advancements.
- Treatment should be tailored to the patient's degree of dysplasia, risk factors, immune status, continence, symptoms, and likelihood of progression.

Introduction

Anal intraepithelial neoplasia is a dysplastic condition of the squamous tissue and is considered to be a premalignant stage of anal cancer. Anal intraepithelial neoplasia (AIN) is further stratified into three grades: AIN I, AIN II, and AIN III, defined as low-, moderate-, and high-grade dysplasia, respectively (Figure 20-1). The histological findings, including the cytologic changes, mitotic activity, nuclear membrane changes, and cellular abnormalities [1, 2], mirror cervical dysplasia grading. Terminology can be confusing as anal intraepithelial neoplasia is referred to by many names including anal dysplasia, intraepithelial carcinoma, intramucosal carcinoma, squamous cell carcinoma in situ, and Bowen's disease. In addition, recently the terms high-grade anal intraepithelial neoplasia (HGAIN) and low-grade anal intraepithelial neoplasia (LGAIN) have been proposed that correspond to AIN III/II and AIN I, respectively [1].

In this chapter we will use the terms anal intraepithelial neoplasia which parallel the pathophysiology of cervical intraepithelial neoplasia, vulvar intraepithelial neoplasia, and perineal intraepithelial neoplasia.

Symptoms

The vast majority of individuals will experience no outward manifestation of human papillomavirus (HPV) infection, and similarly most patients with AIN have no clear symptoms. A small subset of patients will describe occasional rectal bleeding, and an even smaller group will experience pain with bowel movements. As AIN progresses to anal cancer, symptoms become more frequently reported. In fact, 50 % of patients with invasive cancer describe pain and bleeding [3, 4]. A minority of patients with anal intraepithelial neoplasia describe a palpable lesion on the non-hair-bearing portion of the anal skin, but the majority have no outward sign of disease. However, those patients with signs of external genital warts and immunosuppression have a very high risk of AIN.

Epidemiology

Anal intraepithelial neoplasia develops from HPV contact generally through direct exposure [1, 5, 6]. It is estimated that there are more than 100 subtypes of HPV but not all have been implicated as disease causing. In fact, as stated in the prior section, most patients who come into contact with HPV have no actual symptoms and experience no untoward effects. For those who come into contact with the virus, about 90 % of all patients remain asymptomatic and those that have infection resolve without any treatment within 2 years [7]. A small number develop persistent asymptomatic infections, while a smaller number of patients will develop condyloma. It is unclear why a fraction of patients develop neoplasia in the form of AIN that then may progress to squamous cell cancer.

© Springer International Publishing 2016
S.R. Steele et al. (eds.), *The ASCRS Textbook of Colon and Rectal Surgery*, DOI 10.1007/978-3-319-25970-3_20

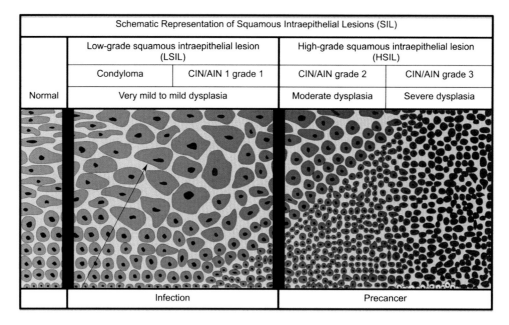

Schematic Representation of Squamous Intraepithelial Lesions (SIL)				
	Low-grade squamous intraepithelial lesion (LSIL)		High-grade squamous intraepithelial lesion (HSIL)	
	Condyloma	CIN/AIN 1 grade 1	CIN/AIN grade 2	CIN/AIN grade 3
Normal	Very mild to mild dysplasia		Moderate dysplasia	Severe dysplasia
	Infection		Precancer	

FIGURE 20-1. Schematic representation of squamous intraepithelial lesions (SIL). As shown in this illustration, with increasing severity of SIL of the anus, the proportion of the epithelium replaced by immature cells with large nuclear-cytoplasmic ratios increases. Invasive cancer probably arises from the one or more foci of high-grade SIL (HSIL) as depicted in the drawing by epithelial cells crossing the basement membrane below the region of HSIL. With permission from Brickman C, Palefsky JM Human papillomavirus in the HIV-infected host: epidemiology and pathogenesis in the antiretroviral era Curr HIV/AIDS Rep 2015;12:6–15. Copyright Springer [73].

Explanations for why the virus causes condyloma or neoplasia in some patients but not in others are speculative. It is likely related to patient immune function, subtype of HPV, repetitive inoculation, and/or potentially concomitant infections such as other sexually transmitted infections. For example, among HPV subtypes, types 6 and 11 cause 90 % of genital warts [8] as compared to those subtypes that are associated with cancer (i.e., types 16, 18). We do know that almost all patients with anal squamous cell cancer, and presumably AIN, have been exposed to HPV at some time in their life. The HPV exposure was likely years prior to the development of actual squamous tissue changes.

HPV, the causative exposure to AIN, is quite prevalent in both the developed and developing world. Estimates indicate that at any point in time, one in ten women worldwide harbors the HPV virus [9]. Prior to the introduction of the HPV vaccine, there had been a steady rise in the rate of HPV infections across the nation and the globe. However, with the introduction of the HPV vaccine, the prevalence of HPV types 6, 11, 16, and 18 identified by cytology specimens decreased by over 50 % among teens and young women. In addition and as expected, HPV prevalence has not been declining in older women who would not have received the vaccine [10]. Data from the National Disease and Therapeutic Index suggest that although cases of genital warts as measured by initial visits to physicians' offices increased during the late 1990s through 2011, genital wart cases appear to have decreased since 2011 [11], presumably because of increased vaccination (Figure 20-2).

Incidence data characterizing trends of HPV infection and condyloma are easily obtainable, yet it is unclear whether the rate of AIN has changed in the last several years. There are no public records and cancer surveillance data do not record incidence or treatment of dysplastic lesions. National cancer incidence data do reveal that the rate of anal cancer has been increasing for several years. Using statistical models for analysis, rates for new anal cancer cases have been rising on average 2.2 % each year over the last 10 years [12]. The number of new cases of anal cancer was 1.8 per 100,000 people per year based on 2007–2011 cases, and the cancer is still slightly more common in women than in men [12].

Much of what is known regarding the transformation of AIN to squamous cell cancer has been extracted from the cervical cancer literature. A recent review of medical records of men who developed anal cancer revealed a common history of precursor high-grade squamous intraepithelial lesions, i.e., anal intraepithelial neoplasia [13]. Because the virus has been detected in many asymptomatic patients, it is likely that viral persistence after integration of the viral genome into the host [14] occurs in order to produce genetic change. Viral oncogenes are then ultimately responsible for directly coupling to oncogenic enhancers and promoters permitting continued expression through integration and immortalization [14]. A number of genetic changes are proposed to

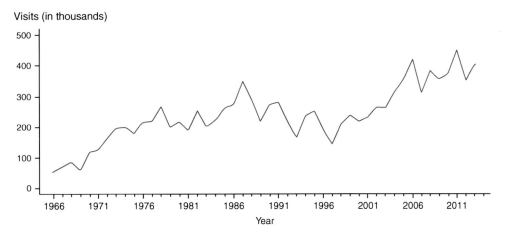

FIGURE 20-2. Genital warts. Initial visits to Physicians' Offices, United States, 1966–2013 http://www.cdc.gov/std/stats13/figures/49.htm. *Source*: IMS Health, Integrated Promotional Services™. IMS Health Report, 1966–2013.

occur after viral integration leading to phenotypic changes of the squamous epithelium. Abnormalities to chromosomes 1, 3, 7, 8, 11, 15, and 20 have all been reported with varying frequency [15, 16]. One of the most frequently reported changes in chromosomal structure is a gain in the long arm of chromosome 3q [17], which is also reported to occur in the transition from low-grade to severe cervical dysplasia and/or cervical cancer [15]. Although it is unclear which gene mediates this transformation, the mechanism may be through phosphatidylinositol 3-kinase, an oncogene on chromosome 3 that phosphorylates other proteins involved in cellular growth. This oncogene has been similarly implicated in the tumorigenesis of ovarian [18] and cervical [19] cancer but not in anal cancer at this time.

Following incorporation of the viral genome into host DNA, cellular changes and atypia of squamous tissues occur [1, 13, 20]. Ultimately these changes correspond to AIN I which then can progress to AIN II and AIN III and ultimately dedifferentiate into squamous cell cancer. It is unclear whether the development of anal neoplasia must traverse all these steps or if squamous cell cancer can skip one or more phases, i.e., from AIN I directly to AIN III. The degree of cellular abnormality and the level of cellular changes correspond to each phase; AIN I has minor changes to the epithelial cells and AIN III corresponds to full-thickness changes to the epithelium with aberrant structure and cellular atypia (Figure 20-1). Ultimately, the oncogenetic pathway is similar to the pathway described in cervical cancer, which degenerates from cervical intraepithelial neoplasia.

Screening/Surveillance

Most patients at risk for anal neoplasia undergo screening with digital rectal examination, anal cytology, and anoscopy. Anal cytology is akin to cervical cytology, providing cellular material for review of intraepithelial lesions. The technique is performed as part of a full physical examination and generally includes a digital rectal examination and anoscopic examination. The cytology must be performed before any instrumentation of the anus and before lubrication is used. The procedure is performed with a moist swab in the anal canal and without any preparation. Following completion, a digital rectal examination and anoscopy can be performed. Obvious condylomatous lesions are concerning if found, particularly in immunosuppressed patients, and should be removed or treated topically with close follow-up.

The anal cytology smear is graded by a cytologist with the same classification used in gynecologic samples. Anal cytology may return as insufficient, normal, atypical squamous cells of undetermined significance, low-grade squamous intraepithelial lesion, high-grade squamous intraepithelial lesion, or anal cancer. Based on these results and prior medical history, the recommendation is either continued surveillance or more detailed evaluation with high-resolution anoscopy. Lesions classified as atypical squamous cells of undetermined significance or higher are generally referred for high-resolution anoscopy. However, a large number of patients have abnormal cytology results leading to a considerably large population of patients to evaluate in microscopy. In addition, given that the sensitivity of anal cytology ranges from 69 to 93 % and specificity ranges from 32 to 59 % [21–23], results can be difficult to interpret. It is important to remember that anal cytology in high-risk cohorts such as men who have sex with men has false-negative rates of up to 23 % in HIV-negative patient and 45 % if HIV positive [24]. Therefore, close follow-up of all high-risk patients is likely to be the best strategy (see Figure 20-3).

Defining the population that is high risk and requiring evaluation is challenging because of societal and other behavioral concerns. Overall, the risk of anal neoplasia is highest in immunosuppressed individuals as they appear to have great difficulty in clearing the virus from their body. Rates of anal dysplasia in HIV-infected patients of all sexual

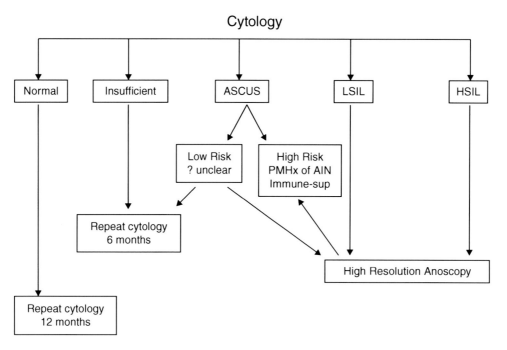

FIGURE 20-3. Management algorithm for anal cytology results. General guidelines provided. Individual case management is based on many factors, which may increase or decrease the interval of evaluation.

risk groups are substantial indicating some value for anal cancer screening in all HIV-infected patients regardless of sexual practices [25, 26]. The immunosuppressed group should also include those with organ transplants [27, 28], as well as other medically induced suppressive conditions. Men who have sex with men and a concomitant diagnosis of HIV pose the greatest risk of HPV-related illnesses and thus anal neoplasia [29]. Patients with prior history of HPV infection are also likely to be at high risk for anal dysplasia and cancer as well as those patients who practice anal receptive intercourse or persons with a high lifetime number of sexual partners [30].

One of the highest-risk groups is women with a past history of cervical, vulvar, or perineal neoplasia. A number of population-based studies report an increase in anal neoplasia risk among women with a history of invasive cervical cancer [31, 32]. In addition to invasive cervical cancer, a recent review of Surveillance, Epidemiology, and End Results data identified a significant association between gynecologic neoplasm and anal cancer for both in situ and invasive cancers of the cervix and vulva and in situ neoplasm of the vagina. In that study, the highest risk for anal cancer was identified in those women with evidence of either in situ or invasive squamous cell cancer of the vulva [33]. The proximity of the anus to the vulva may explain why patients with vulvar neoplasia were at highest risk for anal cancer, yet the increased risk with in situ neoplasia was also remarkable. Thus, patients with gynecologic neoplasia, and especially vulvar neoplasia,

should be followed closely for potential anal cancer development.

Individuals with a past history of sexually transmitted infections may also represent an important screening population. A past history of condyloma is generally a sign of prior contact with human papillomavirus. At this time, it is unclear whether those individuals who tend to develop condyloma (without any sign of dysplasia) have a tendency to develop benign warts rather than cancer. Further studies are needed to investigate the link between prior history of condyloma and anal neoplasia. In addition, it is difficult to prove any synergy between human papillomavirus and other sexually transmitted infections that might act in an additive way to speed up transformation to AIN. However, the presence of HIV with anal coinfection with syphilis, gonococci, Epstein-Barr virus, cytomegalovirus, or herpes simplex was identified as an independent risk factor for dysplasia and cancer [34]. These data point to association between the herpes virus and HPV, yet the effect of these infections on anal neoplasia pathogenesis is certainly unclear.

The value of anal cancer screening is difficult to quantify. There are several studies using computer models to determine the benefit of these tests. Screening HIV-positive homosexual and bisexual men for anal dysplasia with anal cytology offers quality-adjusted life expectancy benefits at a cost comparable with other accepted clinical preventive interventions [35]. Others have not come to the same conclusion indicating that many of the criteria for assessing the need for a screening program were not met for anal neoplasia screening and that cost-effectiveness remained unacceptable [36]. The lack of concordance for these models may be related to the lack of agreement with uncertainties in modeling clinical scenarios in the face of poor evidence. For those patients with a past history of high-grade dysplasia and immunosuppression, a role for surveillance is likely to be of some benefit given the high rate of recurrent disease in this population [17]. It is thought that a combination of surveillance high-resolution anoscopy and anal cytology at 6 and 12 months is cost-effective after treatment of anal neoplasia in HIV-infected men who have sex with men [37].

At this time, a review of 30 regional and national guidelines for screening in HIV patients revealed that only two societies recommended digital and anorectal examination [38]. The "European AIDS Clinical Society Guidelines" recommends digital examination every 1–3 years for HIV-positive men who have sex with men. In New York State, the Department of Health has recommended annual anal cancer screening for HIV-positive men who have sex with men, HIV-positive patients with history of condyloma, and HIV-positive women with a history of gynecologic neoplasia. However, the US Guidelines for the prevention and treatment of opportunistic infections in HIV-infected adults and adolescents recommended only an annual digital examination for the HIV-positive population in general [38].

Diagnosis

Most patients are diagnosed with anal neoplasia through investigation with digital rectal examination, anal cytology, anoscopy, and/or endoscopy. The sensitivity of digital rectal examination in identifying anal neoplasia is fairly low as many AIN lesions are not palpable. Anoscopy is routinely performed by colon and rectal surgeons and can be used to identify macroscopic areas of AIN, which often appear to be benign condylomata, but may return with AIN on biopsy (Figure 20-4). In addition, endoscopic identification of AIN occurs quite commonly particularly during the retroflexed view of the anus. A biopsy of the lesion should lead to a consult with a surgeon who has experience with these lesions. Last, a large number of patients are identified with anal dysplasia on cytologic evaluation during routine screening. These patients are best evaluated with microscopic examination and referred to a facility with appropriate knowledge and capacity.

During diagnostic evaluation, it is imperative to remember that patients with AIN should have a complete and thorough history and physical examination. It is important to remember the link between anal dysplasia and other HPV-related diseases such as oral cancer, gynecologic neoplasia [33], and other genital lesions. In our practice, we refer all female patients for gynecologic evaluation and inquire about dental examinations. The physical exam should include a head to

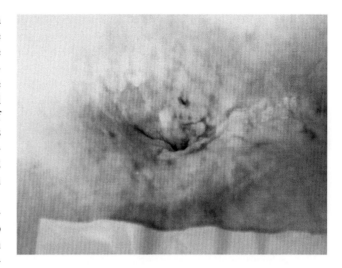

FIGURE 20.4. AIN 3. Courtesy of Richard Billingham, MD.

toe evaluation for squamous cell lesions, considering the mouth and all lymph node basins. Referral to gynecology or a urologic service should also be considered when applicable based on findings and history.

Following examination of the entire body, the evaluation of AIN can proceed with anal cytology and high-resolution microscopy, a technique similar to colposcopy of gynecologic neoplasia. In fact, the colposcopic appearance of variable grades of anal squamous intraepithelial lesions is similar to those described for the cervix [39]. In high-resolution anoscopy, a colposcope or another microscope is used to examine the anal verge and anal canal in close detail. The procedure can be performed in any position, but left or right lateral positioning provides greater visualization of difficult areas, such as under the prostate in men. No bowel or anorectal preparation is necessary and the procedure is most commonly performed without analgesia. After positioning, the tissues to be examined are swabbed with a 3–5 % acetic acid solution for 2–5 min. Some colposcopists choose to add an iodine-based Lugol's solution to further assist with detection of dysplastic tissue. The mechanism for Lugol's utility is that only healthy epithelial tissue absorbs the compound which causes normal tissue to appear wood-like. However, dysplastic tissues do not absorb the solution leaving these tissues with a yellowish hue. Although used by many colposcopists, our protocol is to avoid Lugol's solution as it interferes with proper dysplasia differentiation (i.e., AIN I versus AIN II or III).

For those who do not use Lugol's solution, the acetowhitening from acetic acid with microscopic assistance is sufficient to identify dysplastic tissues. The entire anal canal and anal verge should be examined, but we find that dysplastic tissues are most commonly found within the transition zone, as this area has the greatest area of susceptible and immature squamous tissues. The acetowhitening is particularly helpful in characterizing the degree of dysplasia. Dysplastic epithelium will absorb acetic acid and appear scaly white as

compared to columnar tissues. The characterization of
dysplastic tissue and differentiation of AIN I, II, or III can
then be performed without biopsies and in real time under
high magnification. Dysplastic tissues are characterized by
scaly white plaques and with greater disarray of vascular
patterns, the higher the grade of dysplasia. We also find that
high-grade dysplasia tends to be quite friable when in contact with the anoscope or a swab (Figure 20-5).

The equipment used for the evaluation of AIN is expensive
and the high-resolution microscopy procedure is time intensive and difficult to learn. Others have taken to diagnose AIN
with simple anoscopy or endoscopic methods. At this time,
data have not demonstrated that high-resolution anoscopy is
superior to other methods. However, a multicenter randomized trial is underway to demonstrate the value of close surveillance. Interestingly, a recent study from Ohio revealed no
difference in anal cancer progression with simple observation
versus high-resolution anoscopy [40]. However, the length of
follow-up, diagnostic accuracy, and follow-up protocols were
unclear as the study was underpowered to detect smaller outcome differences. Others have demonstrated a very low rate
of anal cancer progression with an intense surveillance strategy involving anal cytology, digital anorectal examination,
and oncogenic HPV testing in men who have sex with men.
Abnormalities on screening lead to high-resolution anoscopy
and ablation as indicated [41].

Treatment

It should be clear that there is no proven treatment for HPV
infection. As stated earlier, the infection is self limited such
that treatment is directed only to the macroscopic (i.e., genital warts) or pathologic (i.e., precancerous) lesions caused by
infection [42, 43]. It is thought that all subclinical HPV
infections resolve without treatment, and thus, any attempt at
antiviral therapies is not indicated [43, 44]. When dysplasia
is present, whether in the anus, vulva, or cervix, there are a
number of methods to manage or treat these neoplastic tissues ranging from no intervention to very aggressive care. At
this time there is no clear best treatment option for all types
of patients and all degrees of anal dysplasia. Ultimately the
best method of treatment must be efficacious in preventing
the progression of anal intraepithelial neoplasia to cancer
while reducing the morbidity of treatment and preserving
function. In addition, one other consideration in treatment
should be reducing the rate of virus transmission to others
(Table 20-1).

Observation may be the best option for patients with low-
grade dysplasia. In particular, this may be the least difficult
technique for patients with no symptoms and with low likelihood of conversion to anal cancer. Management would consist of surveillance every 4–12 months [45]. Supporters
of this "watch and wait" strategy cite overall low rates of
disease progression and malignant potential (especially for

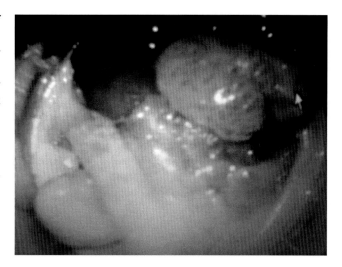

FIGURE 20.5. AIN on high-resolution anoscopy. The *pointer* denotes
area of high-grade dysplasia. Courtesy of Rocco Ricciardi, MD.

low-grade disease) and the increased morbidity associated
with excision and repeated focal destruction [1]. Certainly,
the risk of progression is fairly low in patients with low-
grade dysplasia with evidence indicating that some proportion of patients will exhibit regression of disease without
treatment [45, 46]. It is our practice to recommend observation in select cases depending on risk factors, comorbidities,
and available resources. In a recent review of cases observed
for anal neoplasia, patients followed with expectant
management or high-resolution anoscopy rarely develop
squamous cell cancer if they were compliant with treatment
protocols [40].

Topical treatments have demonstrated effectiveness for
both high- and low-grade dysplasia. These agents include
imiquimod and 5-FU. Imiquimod is one of the most tested
agents [47–49] and is considered to be efficacious by those
who use it regularly. Despite its effectiveness in both immunosuppressed [47] and immunocompetent patients, there is a
high rate of recurrence when treatment is discontinued [47,
48]. Many of the recurrent lesions are unrelated to the primary dysplastic lesion but rather due to undetected HPV
types [48]. Interestingly a recent meta-analysis failed to
demonstrate any statistically significant effect of imiquimod
in the management of anal intraepithelial neoplasia, but there
was a trend for imiquimod to downgrade high-grade AIN to
a lower-risk stage [50]. As compared to imiquimod, 5-FU
has fewer trials but is similarly effective in reducing dysplasia
with complete response in 39 % [50]. Unfortunately, patients
treated with 5-FU similarly had high rates of recurrence
(50 %) and even higher rates of side effects [50, 51]. There
are a smattering of reports demonstrating efficacy for other
topical agents such as trichloroacetic acid [52], cidofovir
[53], as well as photodynamic therapy [54].

Surgery is an effective option to treat anal neoplasia. Data
reveal that electrocautery is highly effective in inducing
complete response of AIN especially in immunocompetent

TABLE 20-1. Common options used in treatment of anal dysplasia

Treatment	Advantages	Disadvantages	Cure	Recurrence
Observation	Cost cheap No side effects	Low cure rate Time intense	Poor	High
Imiquimod	Minimal pain Easy to use	Burning Moderate cost	Poor	High with DC
5-FU	Easy to use	Burning Moderate cost	Poor	High with DC
Infrared coagulation	Clinic use	Need equipment	Good	Moderate in immunosuppressed
Ablation	One application	Painful Costly	Good	Moderate in immunosuppressed
Wide local excision	Removes all tissue	Disfiguring Painful	Good	Low

individuals (72 %) as compared to immunosuppressed individuals (51 %) [55]. Ablation is generally performed in the operating room with electrocautery in conjunction with high-resolution anoscopy; yet, others perform the procedure in the clinic with local anesthesia. The technique is highly selective with targeting of only those areas with evidence of dysplasia. The operating surgeon should remember that the disease is limited to the epidermis and does not require destruction of deeper dermal tissues. In addition, margins are unnecessary with ablation, so the electrocautery can be highly targeted without damage of healthy neighboring tissues. In fact, healthy skin bridges should be preserved as much as possible. During ablation, the surgeon should be mindful of potential scarring, stricture formation, and the need to preserve as much healthy tissue as possible. The preservation of the patients' gastrointestinal function and continence is critical. In addition, the patient will likely require further observation, and limiting electrocautery burns will lead to reduced scarring and ease of further examination in microscopy clinic.

In addition to ablation or excision, infrared coagulation can also be used to destroy lesions. Infrared devices use a beam of infrared light delivered through a light guide covered with a disposable plastic sheath to ablate tissue and coagulate blood in the immediate surface area in contact with the tip [56]. The infrared beam can be pulsed at varying intervals to prevent trauma to deeper tissues. A 1 s pulse penetrates the tissue to a depth of approximately 1 mm targeting the epithelium and destroying dysplastic tissue [56]. The other advantage of infrared coagulation is the ability to perform the technique within the clinic setting and without general anesthesia [57]. The technique is reportedly as effective as electrocautery and considered to be associated with less pain [1].

In the past, mapping biopsies with wide local excision was recommended for patients with anal intraepithelial neoplasia. Unfortunately, much healthy and uninvolved tissue was removed with the dysplastic tissues, and this treatment option was associated with high rates of recurrence between 13 and 63 % [58–60]. In addition, because of the extensive tissue destruction, wide local excision was associated with

high rates of local wound complications such as stenosis and incontinence [59]. Although anal mapping with wide local excision was once routinely performed [61], it is generally not required to treat even the most challenging and diffuse disease.

When selecting which of the above options is best for an individual patient, the physician should consider patient treatment goals, symptoms, history of immunosuppression, past history of dysplasia, and bowel function. At this time, it is unclear what role HPV subtype, concurrent sexually transmitted infections, and other concerns should play in selecting treatment options. There is one trial comparing imiquimod, topical fluorouracil, and electrocautery in HIV-positive men that revealed higher rates of complete response and fewer side effects in the electrocautery group [62]. However, an attempt at Cochrane review failed to provide guidelines for treatment in anal intraepithelial neoplasia because of lack of high-quality randomized controlled trials [50].

Management Strategies

For AIN I, a minimalist approach may be the most effective strategy. Again, in the cervical literature, a large number of patients will regress to normal epithelium but similar data are unavailable in the anus. Given the lack of data regarding progression of low-grade dysplasia in healthy immunocompetent patients, most clinicians would advocate observation. However, the high likelihood of cure after ablation or other interventions makes a surgical approach attractive, particularly if the patient does not wish to return to a microscopy clinic on a regular basis. Low-grade dysplasia in an immunosuppressed patient presumably has a higher likelihood of progression but a high likelihood of recurrence as well. Thus, repeated ablative attempts to the anus with the potential development of scarring, stenosis, bleeding, and chronic pain render an aggressive approach difficult for patients. For immunocompetent patients with high-grade dysplasia, the simplest method of treatment is ablation. There are some who would attempt topical therapy, but surgical ablation is efficient, is effective, and can be targeted with high-resolution

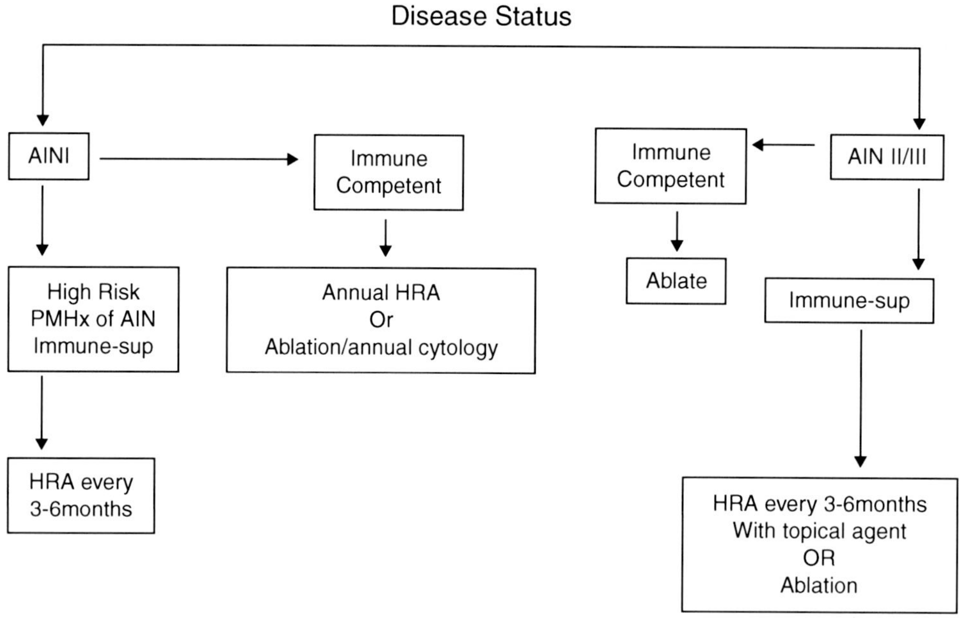

Disease Status

FIGURE 20.6. Algorithm for the treatment of AIN based on immune status and biopsy results.

anoscopy in the right hands. For immunosuppressed individuals with high-grade dysplasia, the best treatment is unclear (Figure 20-6). These patients have high likelihood of recurrence, multifocal disease, other comorbidities and health concerns, and other difficulties. Our approach is to combine therapies with topical therapy, close observation with high-resolution anoscopy, and ablation when the disease appears to be worsening or when patient follow-up is questionable. Our office chooses to limit the ablative interventions for these high-risk patients but follow closely and ablate only those areas that appear most ominous. In addition, the role of wide local excision in the surgical armamentarium is unclear.

Progression

Progression of anal intraepithelial neoplasia to squamous cell cancer of the anus parallels the pathway of cervical dysplasia to cervical cancer [63]. Once established in the anal epithelium, dysplasia of the anus rarely regresses [64] causing substantial concern for patients and their caregivers. The persistence of disease is particularly troubling for those with symptoms, but data proving persistence is incomplete as not all cases with anal dysplasia present for workup. In addition, it is unclear why anal dysplasia is thought to be more persistent than equivalent degrees of cervical dysplasia given the common pathogenic cause of these two conditions. In fact, it is estimated that approximately 60 % of low-grade cervical lesions will spontaneously regress in the cervix [45, 46]. Despite the favorable results in the cervix, similar anal disease is seen as prognostically worse. There are no natural

history studies of untreated anal dysplasia, although case reports do detail a high rate of progression of the precursor lesions to anal cancer with lack of follow-up [65, 66]. The high rate of progression is particularly true for immunosuppressed patients as compared to immunocompetent patients [65].

Prevention

As with all infectious diseases that are transmissible by sexual contact, the best method of prevention is safe sexual practices or limiting sexual contact [67]. In addition to monogamy, proper and consistent use of prophylactic condoms has been shown to reduce the transmission of HPV [68]. Although latex condoms can prevent infection most of the time, the virus can still cause infection by infecting areas that are not covered by a condom. In addition to condoms, educational interventions targeting socially and economically disadvantaged women in which information provision is complemented by sexual negotiation skill development can encourage at least short-term sexual risk reduction behavior [69]. Thus, educational interventions do have the potential to reduce the transmission of HPV and possibly reduce the incidence of squamous carcinoma [69].

In addition to primary prevention techniques, vaccines have also been efficacious in reducing the incidence of HPV infection. In the general screening population, HPV vaccine efficacy was almost 100 % for cervical intraepithelial neoplasia, vulvar and vaginal intraepithelial neoplasia, and anogenital condyloma [70]. In men who have sex with men, the use of quadrivalent HPV vaccine significantly reduced the rates of moderate and high-grade anal intraepithelial neoplasia [42]. Although the vaccinated populations were HPV naïve, there are some data indicating effectiveness of HPV vaccines in preventing reinfection or reactivation of disease [71]. Along the same reasoning, a nonconcurrent cohort study of HPV-vaccinated men who had been previously treated with high-grade anal intraepithelial neoplasia was noted to have a reduction in anal intraepithelial neoplasia recurrence [72].

Conclusions

Anal cancer incidence is rising in the United States indicating increased prevalence of AIN; therefore, screening programs are under development to identify disease earlier. There is a growing body of data indicating that high-resolution anoscopy with ablation leads to a low rate of anal cancer development [41]. However, optimal therapy of anal intraepithelial neoplasia is unclear. Multiple modalities exist and the clinician should balance factors such as symptoms, disease severity, dysplasia multifocality, immunosuppression, and past history of disease into account. Ultimately, the condition should be treated with the intent to preserve continence and reduce postoperative scarring and strictures while reducing the potential for disease progression to invasive cancer.

References

1. Steele SR, Madhulika GV, Melton GB, Ross HM, Rafferty JF, Buie WD, on behalf of the Standards Practice Task Force of the American Society of Colon and Rectal Surgeons. Practice parameters for anal squamous neoplasms. Dis Colon Rectum. 2012;55:735–49.
2. Bean SM, Chhieng DC. Anal-rectal cytology: a review. Diagn Cytopathol. 2010;38:538–46.
3. Robb BW, Mutch MG. Epidermoid carcinoma of the anal canal. Clin Colon Rect Surg. 2006;19:54–60.
4. Ryan DP, Compton CC, Mayer RJ. Carcinoma of the anal canal. N Engl J Med. 2000;342:792–800.
5. Holly EA, Ralston ML, Darragh TM, Greenblatt RM, Jay N, Palefsky JM. Prevalence and risk factors for anal squamous intraepithelial lesions in women. J Natl Cancer Inst. 2001;93:843–9.
6. Chin-Hong PV, Berry JM, Cheng SC, et al. Comparison of patient and clinician collected anal cytology samples to screen for human papillomavirus-associated anal intraepithelial neoplasia in men who have sex with men. Ann Intern Med. 2008;149:300–6.
7. Ho GYF, Bierman R, Beardsley L, Chang CJ, Burk RD. Natural history of cervicovaginal papillomavirus infection in young women. N Engl J Med. 1998;338:423–8.
8. Garland SM, Steben M, Sings HL, James M, Lu S, Railkar R, et al. Natural history of genital warts: analysis of the placebo arm of 2 randomized phase III trials of a quadrivalent human papillomavirus (types 6, 11, 16, and 18) vaccine. J Infect Dis. 2009;199:805–14.
9. Forman D, de Martel C, Lacey CJ, Soerjomataram I, Lortet-Tieulent J, Bruni L, Vignat J, Ferlay J, Bray F, Plummer M, Franceschi S. Global burden of human papillomavirus and related diseases. Vaccine. 2012;30 Suppl 5:F12–23.
10. Markowitz LE, Hariri S, Lin C, Dunne EF, Steinau M, McQuillan G, et al. Reduction in human papillomavirus (HPV) prevalence among young women following HPV vaccine introduction in the United States, National Health and Nutrition Examination Surveys, 2003–2010. J Infect Dis. 2013;208:385–93.
11. 2013 STD Surveillance – Figure 49. IMS Health, Integrated Promotional Services™. IMS Health Report, 1966–2013. http://www.cdc.gov/std/stats13/figures/49.htm. Accessed 3 Aug 2015.
12. SEER Stat Fact Sheet-Anal Cancer. http://seer.cancer.gov/statfacts/html/anus.html. Accessed on 7 Aug 2015.
13. Berry JM, Jay N, Cranston RD, Darragh TM, Holly EA, Welton ML, Palefsky JM. Progression of anal high-grade squamous intraepithelial lesions to invasive anal cancer among HIV-infected men who have sex with men. Int J Cancer. 2014;134:1147–55.
14. Arends MJ, Buckley CH, Wells M. Aetiology, pathogenesis, and pathology of cervical neoplasia. J Clin Pathol. 1998;51:96.
15. World Health Organization, International Agency for Research on Cancer. IARC monographs on the evaluation of carcinogenic risks to humans. Monographs.iarc.fr/ENG/Monographs/vol90/mono90.pdf. 3. Accessed 10 Sept 2013.
16. Gagne SE, Jensen R, Polvi A, et al. High-resolution analysis of genomic alterations and human papillomavirus integration in anal intraepithelial neoplasia. J Acquir Immune Defic Syndr. 2005;40:182–9.
17. Ricciardi R, Burks E, Schoetz DJ, Verma Y, Kershnar E, Kilpatrick MW, Tsipouras P, Walat RJ. Is there a gain in chromosome 3q in the pathway to anal cancer? Dis Colon Rectum. 2014;57:1183–7.
18. Shayesteh L, Lu Y, Kuo WL, Baldocchi R, et al. PIK3CA is implicated as an oncogene in ovarian cancer. Nat Genet. 1999;21:99–102.
19. Ma YY, Wei SJ, Lin YC, et al. PIK3CA as an oncogene in cervical cancer. Oncogene. 2000;19:2739–44.
20. Welton ML, Varma MG. Anal cancer. In: Wolff BG, Fleshman JW, Beck DE, et al., editors. The ASCRS textbook of colon and rectal surgery. New York, NY: Springer; 2007. p. 482–500.
21. Arain S, Walts AE, Thomas P, Bose S. The anal Pap smear: cytomorphology of squamous intraepithelial lesions. CytoJournal. 2005;2:4.
22. Palefsky JM, Holly EA, Hogeboom CJ, Berry JM, Jay N, Darragh TM. Anal cytology as a screening tool for anal squamous intraepithelial lesions. J Acquir Immune Defic Syndr Hum Retrovirol. 1997;14:415–22.
23. Fox PA, Seet JE, Stebbing J, et al. The value of anal cytology and human papillomavirus typing in the detection of anal intraepithelial neoplasia: a review of cases from an anoscopy clinic. Sex Transm Infect. 2005;81:142–6.
24. Chin-Hong PV, Vittinghoff E, Cranston RD, et al. Age related prevalence of anal cancer precursors in homosexual men: the EXPLORE study. J Natl Cancer Inst. 2005;97:896–905.

25. Gaisa M, Sigel K, Hand J, Goldstone S. High rates of anal dysplasia in HIV-infected men who have sex with men, women, and heterosexual men. AIDS. 2014;28:215–22.

26. Gandra S, Azar A, Wessolossky M. Anal high-risk human papillomavirus infection and high-grade anal intraepithelial neoplasia detected in women and heterosexual men infected with human immunodeficiency virus. HIV/AIDS (Auckl NZ). 2015;7:29–34.

27. Palefsky JM, Rubin M. The epidemiology of anal human papillomavirus and related neoplasia. Obstet Gynecol Clin North Am. 2009;36:187–200.

28. Sillman FH, Sentovich S, Shaffer D. Anogenital neoplasia in renal transplant patients. Ann Transplant. 1997;2:59–66.

29. Del Amo J, Gonzalez C, Geskus RB, et al. What drives the number of high-risk human papillomavirus types in the anal canal in HIV-positive men who have sex with men? J Infect Dis. 2013;207(8):1235–41.

30. National Cancer Institute. Anal cancer treatment. cancer.gov/cancertopics/pdq/treatment/anal/HealthProfessional. Accessed on 7 Aug 2015.

31. Edgren G, Sparen P. Risk of anogenital cancer after diagnosis of cervical intraepithelial neoplasia: a prospective population based study. Lancet Oncol. 2007;8:311–6.

32. Hemminki K, Dong C, Vaittinen P. Second primary cancer after in situ and invasive cervical cancer. Epidemiology. 2000;11:457–61.

33. Saleem AM, Paulus JK, Shapter AP, Baxter NN, Roberts PL, Ricciardi R. Risk of anal cancer in a cohort with human papillomavirus-related gynecologic neoplasm. Obstet Gynecol. 2011;117:643–9.

34. Sobhani I, Walker F, Roudot-Thoraval F, Abramowitz L, Johanet H, Hénin D, Delchier JC, Soulé JC. Anal carcinoma: incidence and effect of cumulative infections. AIDS. 2004;18:1561–9.

35. Goldie SJ, Kuntz KM, Weinstein MC, et al. The clinical effectiveness and cost-effectiveness of screening for anal squamous intraepithelial lesions in homosexual and bisexual HIV-positive men. JAMA. 1999;281:1822–9.

36. Czoski-Murray C, Karnon J, Jones R, Smith K, Kinghorn G. Cost-effectiveness of screening high-risk HIV-positive men who have sex with men (MSM) and HIV-positive women for anal cancer. Health Technol Assess. 2010;14(53):3–4, 9–10.

37. Assoumou SA, Mayer KH, Panther L, Linas BP, Kim JJ. Cost-effectiveness of surveillance strategies after treatment for high-grade anal dysplasia in high risk patients. Sex Transm Dis. 2013;40:298–303.

38. Ong JJ, Chen M, Grulich AE, Fairley CK. Regional and national guideline recommendations for digital ano-rectal examination as a means for anal cancer screening in HIV positive men who have sex with men: a systematic review. BMC Cancer. 2014;14:557.

39. Jay N, Berry JM, Hogeboom CJ, Holly EA, Darragh TM, Palefsky JM. Colposcopic appearance of anal squamous intraepithelial lesions: relationship to histopathology. Dis Colon Rectum. 1997;40:919–28.

40. Crawshaw BP, Russ AJ, Stein SL, Reynolds HL, Marderstein EL, Delaney CP, Champagne BJ. High-resolution anoscopy or expectant management for anal intraepithelial neoplasia for the prevention of anal cancer: is there really a difference? Dis Colon Rectum. 2015;58:53–9.

41. Goldstone SE, Johnstone AA, Moshier EL. Long-term outcome of ablation of anal high-grade squamous intraepithelial lesions: recurrence and incidence of cancer. Dis Colon Rectum. 2014;57:316–23.

42. Palefsky JM, Giuliano AR, Goldstone S, Moreira Jr ED, Aranda C, Jessen H, Hillman R, Ferris D, Coutlee F, Stoler MH, Marshall JB, Radley D, Vuocolo S, Haupt RM, Guris D, Garner EI. HPV vaccine against anal HPV infection and anal intraepithelial neoplasia. N Engl J Med. 2011;365:1576–85.

43. Division of STD Prevention, National Center for HIV/AIDS, Viral Hepatitis, STD, and TB Prevention, Centers for Disease Control and Prevention. www.cdc.gov/std/stats13/other.htm. Accessed 1 Mar 2015.

44. Devaraj B, Cosman BC. Expectant management of anal squamous dysplasia in patients with HIV. Dis Colon Rectum. 2006;49:36–40.

45. Ostor AG. Natural history of cervical intraepithelial neoplasia: a critical review. Int J Gynecol Pathol. 1993;12:186–92.

46. Melnikow J, Nuovo J, Willan AR, Chan BK, Howell LP. Natural history of cervical squamous intraepithelial lesions: a meta-analysis. Obstet Gynecol. 1998;92(4 Pt 2):727–35.

47. Wieland U, Brockmeyer NH, Weissenborn SJ, Hochdorfer B, Stücker M, Swoboda J, Altmeyer P, Pfister H, Kreuter A. Imiquimod treatment of anal intraepithelial neoplasia in HIV-positive men. Arch Dermatol. 2006;142:1438–44.

48. Kreuter A, Potthoff A, Brockmeyer NH, Gambichler T, Stücker M, Altmeyer P, Swoboda J, Pfister H, Wieland U. Imiquimod leads to a decrease of human papillomavirus DNA and to a sustained clearance of anal intraepithelial neoplasia in HIV-infected men. J Invest Dermatol. 2008;128:2078–83.

49. Fox PA, Nathan M, Francis N, Singh N, Weir J, Dixon G, Barton SE, Bower M. A double-blind, randomized controlled trial of the use of imiquimod cream for the treatment of anal canal high-grade anal intraepithelial neoplasia in HIV-positive. AIDS. 2010;24:2331–5.

50. Macaya A, Munoz-Santos C, Balaguer A, Barbera MJ. Interventions for anal canal intraepithelial neoplasia. Cochrane Database Syst Rev. 2012;12, CD009244.

51. Richel O, Wieland U, de Vries HJ, Brockmeyer NH, van Noesel C, Potthoff A, Prins JM, Kreuter A. Topical 5-fluorouracil treatment of anal intraepithelial neoplasia in human immunodeficiency virus-positive men. Br J Dermatol. 2010;163:1301–7.

52. Singh JC, Kuohung V, Palefsky JM. Efficacy of trichloroacetic acid in the treatment of anal intraepithelial neoplasia in HIV positive and HIV negative men who have sex with men. J Acquir Immune Defic Syndr. 2009;52:474–9.

53. Tristram A, Hurt CN, Madden T, Powell N, Man S, Hibbitts S, Dutton P, Jones S, Nordin AJ, Naik R, Fiander A, Griffiths G. Activity, safety, and feasibility of cidofovir and imiquimod for treatment of vulval intraepithelial neoplasia (RT³VIN): a multicentre, open-label, randomised, phase 2 trial. Lancet Oncol. 2014;15:1361–8.

54. van der Snoek EM, Amelink A, van der Ende ME, et al. Photodynamic therapy with topical metatetrahydroxychlorin (Fosgel) is ineffective for the treatment of anal intraepithelial neoplasia, grade iii. J Acquir Immune Defic Syndr. 2009;52:141–3.

55. Goldstone RN, Goldstone AB, Russ J, Goldstone SE. Long-term follow-up of infrared coagulator ablation of anal high-grade dysplasia in men who have sex with men. Dis Colon Rectum. 2011;54:1284–92.

56. Goldstone SE, Kawalek AZ, Huyett JW. Infrared coagulator: a useful tool for treating anal squamous intraepithelial lesions. Dis Colon Rectum. 2005;48:1042–54.

57. Sirera G, Videla S, Piñol M, Coll J, García-Cuyás F, Vela S, Cañadas M, Darwich L, Pérez N, Gel S, Cobarsi P, Clotet B, HIV-HPV Study Group. Long-term effectiveness of infrared coagulation for the treatment of anal intraepithelial neoplasia grades 2 and 3 in HIV-infected men and women. AIDS. 2013;27(6):951–9.

58. Margenthaler JA, Dietz DW, Mutch MG, et al. Outcomes, risk of other malignancies, and need for formal mapping procedures in patients with perianal Bowen's disease. Dis Colon Rectum. 2004;47:1655–61.

59. Brown SR, Skinner P, Tidy J, Smith JH, Sharp F, Hosie KB. Outcome after surgical resection for high-grade anal intraepithelial neoplasia (Bowen's disease). Br J Surg. 1999;8:1063–6.

60. Marchesa P, Fazio VW, Oliart S, Goldblum JR, Lavery IC. Perianal Bowen's disease: a clinicopathologic study of 47 patients. Dis Colon Rectum. 1997;40:1286–93.

61. Cleary RK, Schaldenbrand JD, Fowler JJ, Schuler JM, Lampman RM. Perianal Bowen's disease and anal intraepithelial neoplasia: review of the literature. Dis Colon Rectum. 1999;42:945–51.

62. Richel O, de Vries HJ, van Noesel CJ, Dijkgraaf MG, Prins JM. Comparison of imiquimod, topical fluorouracil, and electrocautery for the treatment of anal intraepithelial neoplasia in HIV-positive men who have sex with men: an open-label, randomised controlled trial. Lancet Oncol. 2013;14:346–53.

63. Schiffman MH, Castle P. Epidemiologic studies of a necessary causal risk factor: human papillomavirus infection and cervical neoplasia. J Natl Cancer Inst. 2003;95, E2.

64. Palefsky JM, Holly EA, Ralston ML, et al. Anal squamous intraepithelial lesions in HIV-positive and HIV-negative homosexual and bisexual men. J Acquir Immune Defic Syndr Hum Retrovirol. 1998;17:320–6.

65. Scholefield JH, Castle MT, Watson NF. Malignant transformation of high-grade anal intraepithelial neoplasia. Br J Surg. 2005;92(9):1133–6.

66. Watson AJ, Smith BB, Whitehead MR, Sykes PH, Frizelle FA. Malignant progression of anal intra-epithelial neoplasia. ANZ J Surg. 2006;76(8):715–7.

67. Centers for Disease Control and Prevention. Sexually transmitted diseases. 1600 Clifton Rd Atlanta, GA 30329-402. cdc.gov/std/treatment/default.htm. Accessed 7 Aug 2015.

68. Winer RL, Hughes JP, Feng Q, et al. Condom use and the risk of genital human papillomavirus infection in young women. N Engl J Med. 2006;354(25):2645–54.

69. Shepherd J, Weston R, Peersman G, Napuli IZ. Interventions for encouraging sexual lifestyles and behaviours intended to prevent cervical cancer. Cochrane Database Syst Rev. 2000;2, CD001035.

70. The FUTURE I/II Study Group. Four year efficacy of prophylactic human papillomavirus quadrivalent vaccine against low grade cervical, vulvar, and vaginal intraepithelial neoplasia and anogenital warts: randomised controlled trial. BMJ. 2013;341:3493.

71. Muñoz N, Kjaer SK, Sigurdsson K, Iversen OE, Hernandez-Avila M, Wheeler CM, Perez G, Brown DR, Koutsky LA, Tay EH, Garcia PJ, Ault KA, Garland SM, Leodolter S, Olsson SE, Tang GW, Ferris DG, Paavonen J, Steben M, Bosch FX, Dillner J, Huh WK, Joura EA, Kurman RJ, Majewski S, Myers ER, Villa LL, Taddeo FJ, Roberts C, Tadesse A, Bryan JT, Lupinacci LC, Giacoletti KE, Sings HL, James MK, Hesley TM, Barr E, Haupt RM. Impact of human papillomavirus (HPV)-6/11/16/18 vaccine on all HPV-associated genital diseases in young women. J Natl Cancer Inst. 2010;102:325–39.

72. Swedish KA, Factor SH, Goldstone SE. Prevention of recurrent high-grade anal neoplasia with quadrivalent human papillomavirus vaccination of men who have sex with men: a nonconcurrent cohort study. Clin Infect Dis. 2012;54:891–8.

73. Brickman C, Palefsky JM. Human papillomavirus in the HIV-infected host: epidemiology and pathogenesis in the antiretroviral era. Curr HIV/AIDS Rep. 2015;12:6–15.

Part III
Malignant Disease

21

Anal Cancer

Tushar Samdani and Garrett M. Nash

Key Concepts

- Chemoradiotherapy (CRT) is the primary treatment for patient with anal squamous cell carcinoma (mitomycin + 5-FU + radiotherapy). The dosage of radiotherapy varies based on the size of the tumor and presence of lymph node involvement.
- Surgery (local excision) can be used to remove some small squamous cell carcinomas (usually measuring <1 cm or ½ in.) that do not involve the anal sphincter musculature.
- Following primary treatment with chemoradiotherapy, patients are evaluated with repeat physical examination of the anal area at approximately 8–12 weeks after completion of treatment, and then at 6- to 8-week intervals until resolution of any suspicious findings. Patients with persistent but nonprogressive disease may be followed up to 6 months after chemoradiotherapy for assessment of complete remission.
- Patients with progressive disease or recurrence after chemoradiotherapy are considered for salvage abdominoperineal resection (APR).
- Dosage of radiotherapy and chemotherapy may be modified based on CD4 count and blood count in immunocompromised patients.
- Anal melanoma is very aggressive, and is generally treated with local excision (LE).
- Anal adenocarcinoma is treated with APR and usually with neoadjuvant chemoradiotherapy, as in treatment for distal rectal adenocarcinoma.

Introduction

Anal cancer accounts for only a small percentage (4 %) of all cancers of the lower alimentary tract [1]. Approximately 0.2 % of men and women will be diagnosed with anal cancer at some point during their lifetime, based on 2009–2011 data. As per the American Cancer Society: Cancer Facts and Figures 2015, estimated new cases of anal cancer in the USA will be approximately 7270 in 2015; the estimated deaths from anal cancer in 2015 will be approximately 1010 (Tables 21-1 and 21-2) [2].

Risk Factors

The incidence of anal cancer appears to have risen over the last few years. This may be due to a higher incidence in persons engaging in receptive anal intercourse, or having multiple sexual partners. These practices increase the likelihood of infection with human papillomavirus (HPV), which is strongly associated with premalignant anal squamous intraepithelial lesions and the development of anal squamous cell cancer [3].

Risk factors associated with anal cancer:

- Sexually transmitted disease.
- Anal receptive intercourse.
- More than ten sexual partners.
- The presence of precancerous anal lesions such as condylomas or high-grade anal intraepithelial neoplasia, and cervical, vulvar, or vaginal cancers.
- Immunosuppression secondary to solid organ transplantation or chronic glucocorticoid therapy.
- HIV seropositivity, low CD4 count.
- Smoking.

Anatomy of the Anal Canal

Complete knowledge of anatomical landmarks and histological features of the anal canal is crucial in order to understand the origins of different types of anal neoplasms and determine their management (see Chap. 1). The surgical anal canal extends from the puborectal sling to the intersphincteric groove (the white line of Hilton). It is histologically divided into two unequal

© Springer International Publishing 2016

S.R. Steele et al. (eds.), *The ASCRS Textbook of Colon and Rectal Surgery*, DOI 10.1007/978-3-319-25970-3_21

sections (the upper two-thirds and lower one-third) by the dentate line (pectinate line), which is the site of fusion of the proctodeum below and the post-allantoic gut above (Fig. 21-1).

TABLE 21-1. WHO histological classification of malignant tumors of the anal canal

• Carcinoma	• Carcinoid tumor
– Squamous cell carcinoma	• Malignant melanoma
– Adenocarcinoma	• Nonepithelial tumors
Rectal type	• Secondary tumors
Of anal glands	
Within anorectal fistula	
– Mucinous adenocarcinoma	
– Small-cell carcinoma	
– Undifferentiated carcinoma	
– Others	

WHO World Health Organization
Source: AJCC Cancer Staging Manual plus EZTNM, 6th edition

- The anal canal just above the dentate line (for about 1–2 cm) is known as the anal transition zone (ATZ). Beyond this transition zone, the [surgical] anal canal is lined with columnar epithelium. Its lower ends are joined together by folds of mucus membranes known as anal valves. The upper two-thirds of the anal canal are supplied by the superior rectal artery, which is a branch of the inferior mesenteric artery.
- The lower one-third of the anal canal is lined by stratified squamous epithelium that blends with the skin. The lower one-third is supplied by the inferior rectal artery, which is a branch of the internal pudendal artery.

The anal margin extends laterally from the intersphincteric groove to a radius of approximately 5 cm, and is characterized by keratinized stratified squamous epithelium. The intersphincteric groove indicates the junction between keratinized

TABLE 21-2. TNM classification for anal cancer

	Primary tumor (T)
TX	Primary tumor cannot be assessed
T0	No evidence of primary tumor
Tis	Carcinoma in situ (Bowen's disease, high-grade squamous intraepithelial lesion HISL), AIN II–III
T1	Tumor 2 cm or less in greatest dimension
T2	Tumor more than 2 cm but not more than 5 cm in greatest dimension
T3	Tumor more than 5 cm in greatest dimension
T4	Tumor of any size invades adjacent organ(s), e.g., vagina, urethra, bladder (direct invasion of rectal wall, perirectal skin, subcutaneous tissue, or sphincter muscle is not classified as T4)
	Regional lymph node (N)
NX	Regional lymph nodes cannot be assessed
N0	No regional lymph node metastasis
N1	Metastasis in perirectal lymph nodes(s)
N2	Metastasis in unilateral internal iliac and/or unilateral inguinal lymph node(s)
N3	Metastasis in perirectal and inguinal lymph nodes and/or bilateral internal iliac and/or inguinal lymph nodes
	Distant metastases (M)
M0	No distant metastasis
M1	Distant metastasis

Source: AJCC Cancer Staging Manual plus EZTNM, 6th edition

FIGURE 21-1. Anal canal anatomy.

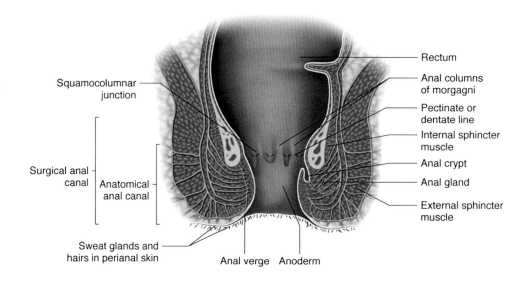

stratified squamous epithelium and the non-keratinized strati-fied squamous epithelium [4, 5]. Anal squamous cell carci-noma commonly arises from either squamous epithelium of the lower part of the anal canal. Rarely does it arise from the ATZ. On the other hand, histological variants of SCC, such as transitional, basaloid, and cloacogenic variants, arise from ATZ. Adenocarcinoma of the anal canal originates from the colorectal zone in the upper portion of the anal canal or from the glandular cells of the ATZ mucosa whereas anal margin squamous cell carcinoma arises lateral to intersphincteric groove. Of note, histological features of anal melanoma are similar to cutaneous melanoma arising from basal cell layer of stratified squamous epithelium.

Some authors have simplified classification of the anal region, dividing it into three easily identifiable regions based on visual examination [6].

Intra-anal lesions are lesions that cannot be visualized on perianal examination until gentle traction is applied on the buttocks.

Perianal lesions are completely visible, without traction on the buttocks, extending within 5 cm of the anal margin.

Skin lesions fall outside the 5 cm radius from the anal opening. Hence, some have classified this into three distinct regions: intra-anal (visualized with gentle traction on the buttocks), perianal, and skin tumors (beyond a 5 cm radius from the anal opening).

Squamous Cell Carcinoma of the Anal Canal

In the USA, the median age at diagnosis of squamous cell carcinoma of the anal canal (SCAC) is 60–65 years, and there is slightly higher incidence in women [3, 7].

Symptoms

Approximately one-third of patients with SCAC are asymp-tomatic, or have nonspecific symptoms on presentation. Clinical manifestations of anal canal tumors are mainly related to tumor size and extent of infiltration. The most common symptom is rectal bleeding, which is seen in approximately 45 % of cases, followed by anal pain or sensa-tion of anal mass, seen in 30 % [8, 9]. Other symptoms include anal pruritus, discomfort in sitting, a change in bowel habits, incontinence (due to tumor infiltration into the sphincter), discharge, bleeding, fissure, or fistula. Diagnosis may be delayed because initial symptoms are nonspecific, and the anal canal is often a difficult location for examina-tion. Moreover, because anal cancer is rare, many primary care practitioners have little experience in diagnosing it.

The clinical diagnosis of an anal tumor should be con-firmed by histologic examination. A forceps or needle biopsy may be done to establish the diagnosis. It is very important to document an exact description of location and appearance of the biopsy site, as this will help in planning radiation fields and posttreatment surveillance. If the lesion is large or involves the sphincter, an excisional biopsy is inadvisable because the subsequent wound healing may delay optimal chemoradiation treatment (CRT). Enlarged lymph nodes may be excised or biopsied with needle aspiration, under radiological guidance [3, 10].

Examination

Detailed physical examination is very important, as a lesion in the anal canal may be easily missed on cursory exam. Physical examination includes inspection to assess for tumor location, size, and extent, and direct visualization of the mass via anos-copy, rigid proctoscopy, or flexible sigmoidoscopy, which may be retroflexed in the rectum. Digital rectal exam should be done to assess sphincter function, and relation of tumor to the sphincter (Figs. 21-2 and 21-3a, b). The tumor may pres-ent as a small ulcer or fissure with slightly exophytic and indu-rated margins, and irregular thickening of the anal canal. If a thorough anal canal examination is not possible due to signifi-cant perianal pain or spasm, examination under anesthesia may be done to assess the tumor. Along with local examina-tion of the anal canal, groin lymph nodes (LNs) should be examined to rule out involvement. It has been traditionally recommended that patients with an anal cancer should undergo colonoscopy to evaluate for synchronous colorectal lesions [3, 10]; however, it should be noted that there are no definitive data demonstrating an association between SCAC and adenomatous neoplasia of the colon or rectum. In women

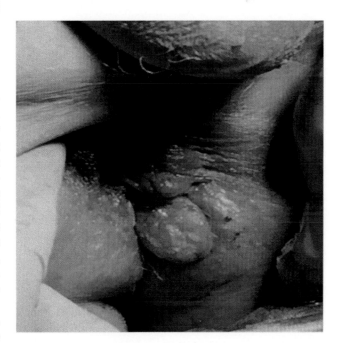

FIGURE 21-2. Anal cancer.

FIGURE 21-3. Anal squamous cell carcinoma invading rectal mucosa. (**a**) Low power view; (**b**) higher power view.

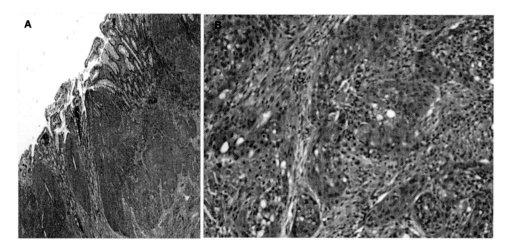

with anal cancer, a pelvic examination may be performed to determine the extent of invasion of an anterior lesion into the posterior vagina. Female patients should have routine gynecologic evaluations, given the risk of other HPV-associated diseases such as cervical dysplasia (Fig. 21-4) [11].

Investigation

Treatment of anal cancer is based on the stage of the tumor. Therefore, a comprehensive physical exam should be complemented with imaging, to determine the possibility of locoregional or systemic spread.

Investigation of Choice

- Locoregional staging: MRI of the rectum/pelvis, with or without endoscopic ultrasound.
- Distant metastasis: CT scan of the chest, abdomen, or pelvis; or FDG PET/CT.

MRI of the Rectum/Pelvis

MRI provides high-resolution, multiplanar information regarding the location, size, circumferential and craniocaudal extent of the primary tumor, and involvement of adjacent structures, including the sphincter (Fig. 21-5). The sensitivity of MRI in identifying SCAC has been reported to approach 90–100 % [12]. Along with evaluation of the primary tumor, MRI can be used to assess involvement of the pelvis and inguinal LNs. MRI determines LN involvement based on various criteria such as LN size, loss of the normal bean-shaped morphology and fatty hilum, internal T1 and T2 signal heterogeneity with central necrosis, and inhomogeneous enhancement. Short-axis threshold values of 8 mm, 5 mm, and 10 mm have been suggested for pelvic, perirectal, and inguinal LNs, respectively [13, 14].

Transanal Endoscopic Ultrasound

Transanal endoscopic ultrasound may be used to assess local staging of anal cancer (Fig. 21-6). This modality may be

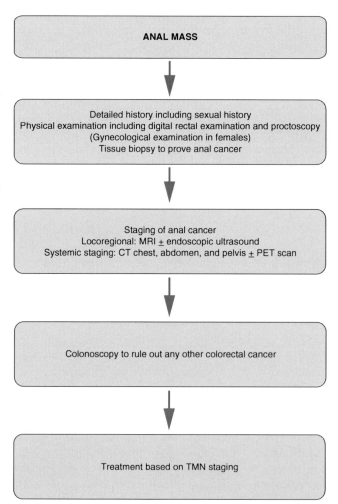

FIGURE 21-4. Algorithm for anal mass evaluation and work-up.

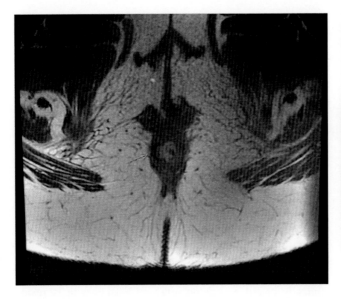

FIGURE 21-5. Anal cancer: pretreatment MRI T2 oblique, suspicion for focal tumor invasion into the right lateral internal anal sphincter (green arrow).

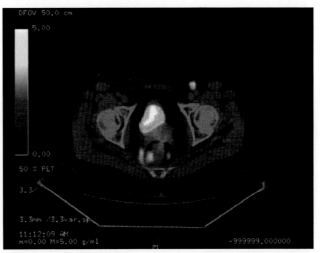

FIGURE 21-7. Anal cancer: left inguinal adenopathy and mesorectal adenopathy seen on PET/CT.

CT Scan of Chest, Abdomen, and Pelvis with IV Contrast

CT scanning of the chest, abdomen, and pelvis is used to identify possible metastatic disease [16].

FDG PET/CT

Approximately 98 % of anal tumors are FDG avid. Hence, FDG PET/CT has assumed an increasing role in the staging and assessment of treatment response [17]. PET/CT may be used to evaluate primary tumor size, LN status, and distant metastasis, and may help in planning radiation therapy by clearly defining the site of metabolically active tumor. It may also be useful in posttreatment surveillance (Fig. 21-7). PET/CT is indicated for node-positive and T2–T4 anal canal and anal margin cancer to verify staging before treatment. PET/CT has become part of the standard work-up, particularly for evaluating LNs that appear ambiguous on CT, to aid in management, and to serve as a pretreatment baseline. PET/CT has demonstrated a sensitivity of >90 % and a specificity of 80 %. PET/CT has been shown to alter the staging of anal carcinoma in approximately 20 % of cases, and treatment intent in approximately 3–5 %. The main impact of PET/CT on therapy stems from its superiority in detecting involved pelvic or inguinal nodes, prompting the radiation oncologist to include these in the RT field [18, 19, 20]. PET/CT has also impacted posttreatment management in 18 % of anal cancer patients (Fig. 21-8). It may confirm persistence of disease or local recurrence, and influence decision making regarding the use of chemotherapy in patients with metastatic disease [3, 21]. The high negative predictive value of PET-CT may dictate avoidance of unnecessary biopsy after chemoradiotherapy.

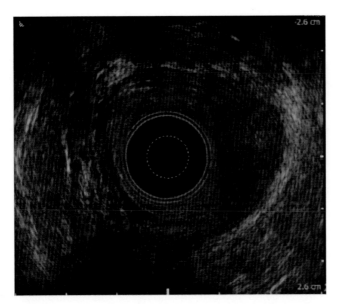

FIGURE 21-6. Transanal endoscopic ultrasound can be used to assess local staging of anal cancer.

superior to MRI in evaluating small superficial tumors [15]. However, the limitations of transanal endoscopic ultrasound include an inability to ascertain involvement of the proximal pelvis or groin LNs, and it may be difficult to use in assessing a stenotic or painful anal lesion. Lastly, its accuracy is highly operator dependent.

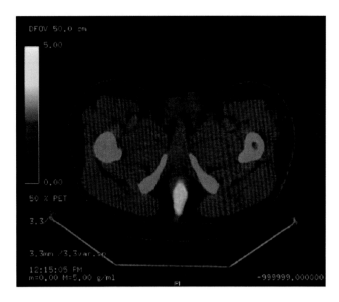

FIGURE 21-8. Anal cancer: pretreatment SUV = 18.1.

Summary of the Initial Work-Up of Anal Cancer

1. In the setting of a T1 tumor, after a thorough physical exam, MRI of the rectum/pelvis or transanal endoscopic ultrasound may be used for additional local staging. In the absence of nodal disease, a CT scan of the chest and abdomen may be used for distant staging.
2. In the setting of a T2–T4 tumor or node-positive anal cancer, PET/CT may be used in addition to MRI or transanal endoscopic ultrasound to screen for distant metastases, to assess response to CRT, and as a tool in subsequent cancer surveillance.

Treatment of Anal Cancer

Until three decades ago, abdominoperineal resection (APR) of the rectosigmoid and anus was the preferred surgical procedure for most cancers of the anal canal. This radical operation was performed in order to achieve adequate margins of resection [8]. Local resection was done for smaller lesions. Surgical treatment alone was associated with local failure in 27–47 % of cases [22]. Early tumors could be cured by APR, with 5-year survival rates of 50–70 %. However, APR entails a permanent intestinal stoma and is associated with substantial morbidity. Over the last three decades, there has been significant change in the management of epidermoid anal carcinomas, with more patients undergoing nonsurgical treatment.

Evolution in the Management of Anal Cancer (Fig. 21-9)

Radiotherapy

Dosage

Dosage of RT varies based on the size of the tumor and presence of suspected LN involvement. In general, larger cancers require higher doses of radiation. The database of the RTOG 9811 trial suggests that size >5 cm is a poor prognostic factor [29]. Doses in the range of 30 Gy, with concurrent mitomycin C and 5-FU, have been shown to control small tumors (CCR rate of 86 %) and subclinical disease effectively. The preliminary results of the ACCORD-03 trial compared 45 Gy in 25 patients plus a 15 Gy boost with a higher dose, but found no benefit in CFS, and higher toxicity, at >59 Gy [30]. Similar results were reported in the RTOG 92-08 trial [31].

Patients with SCAC receive a minimum RT dose of 45 Gy to the primary cancer. The recommended initial dose is 30.6 Gy to the pelvis, anus, perineum, and inguinal nodes. Following initial dose of 30.6 Gy, field of radiation should be reduced from L5–S1 junction to bottom of sacroiliac joints. In patients without nodal metastasis, inguinal nodes are not included in radiation field after 36 Gy. Patients with disease clinically staged as node positive or T3–T4 or with T2 residual disease after 45 Gy should receive an additional boost of 9–14 Gy [28].

Field of Radiotherapy

Multi-field techniques with supervoltage radiation (photon energy >6 mV) are used to deliver a minimum dose of 45 Gy in 1.8 Gy fractions (25 fractions over 5 weeks) to the primary cancer. The RTOG panel established three elective clinical target volume (CTV) areas: CTVa targets the perirectal, presacral, and internal iliac regions; CTVb targets the iliac LNs; and CTVc targets the inguinal LNs; inclusion of all is recommended in RT for anal cancer. The superior field border includes the rectosigmoid junction (L5–S1 junction); the inferior border includes the anus, with a minimum 2.5 cm margin around the anus and tumor; the lateral border includes the lateral inguinal nodes, based on imaging or body landmarks. An attempt should be made to reduce the dose to the femoral heads [32, 33] (Fig. 21-10).

Side Effects [34–36]

The short-term side effects of RT include:

- Dermatitis.
- Temporary anal swelling and pain.
- Frequency and urgency in defecation.
- Nausea, weakness.
- Vaginal discomfort and discharge.

These side effects often improve after radiation stops. Long-term side effects include:

- Anal stenosis.
- Pelvic fracture.
- Chronic radiation proctitis.
- Vaginal stenosis (female patients should be encouraged to use a vaginal dilator).

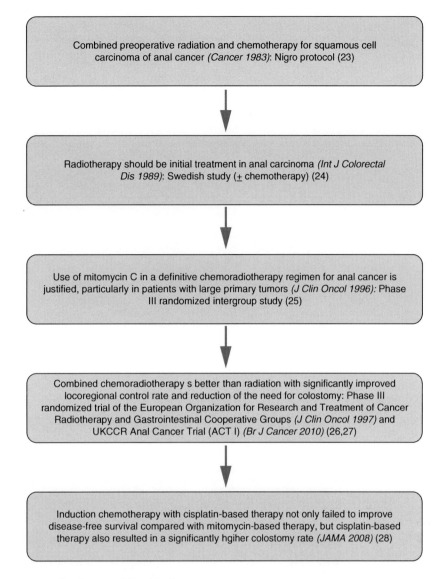

FIGURE 21-9. Evolution of management of anal cancer (algorithm).

- Radiation may affect fertility in both women and men (patients should be informed about sperm and ovarian tissue banking).
- Dyspareunia.
- Lymphedema.

Special Considerations

Intensity-Modulated Radiation Therapy

Intensity-modulated radiation therapy (IMRT) utilizes detailed beam shaping, enabling precision in targeting tumor and sparing normal tissue. Compared with conventional three-dimensional (3D) CRT (Figs. 21-11 and 21-12), IMRT may spare the perineal skin, external genitalia, and bladder, reducing toxicity to surrounding anatomic structures, and preventing toxicity-related delay in completion of treatment—thereby improving treatment outcomes [3, 72, 73]. In a retrospective study from Memorial Sloan Kettering Cancer Center of 221 patients with anal SCC treated with CRT between 1991 and 2007, 44 patients received IMRT and 177 received 3DCRT. The 2-year local recurrence-free survival, distant metastasis-free survival, colostomy-free survival, and overall survival were 88 %, 83 %, 96 %, and 92 %, respectively, in the IMRT group, and 81 %, 88 %, 91 %, and 89 %, respectively, in the 3DCRT group, demonstrating no significant difference between the groups [74].

FIGURE 21-10. External beam radiotherapy.

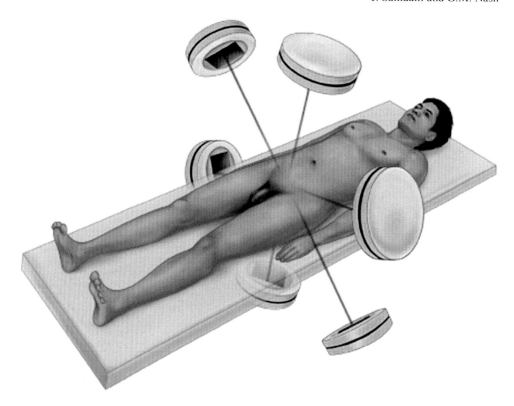

FIGURE 21-11. T1N0 anal SCC—IMRT: 4500cGy in 180cGy fractions to pelvic nodes (*orange*); 5000cGy in 200cGy fractions to primary tumor (*red*).

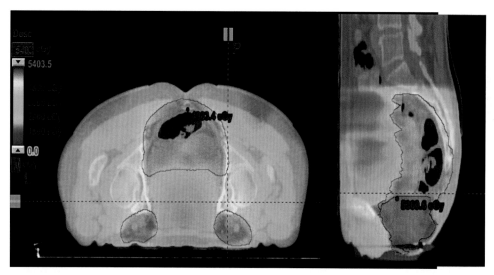

FIGURE 21-12. T3N1 anal SCC—IMRT: 4500cGy in 180cGy fractions to pelvic nodes (*brown*); 5000cGy in 200cGy fractions to primary tumor (*red*); additional boost of 600cGy in 200cGy fractions to the primary tumor (*red*).

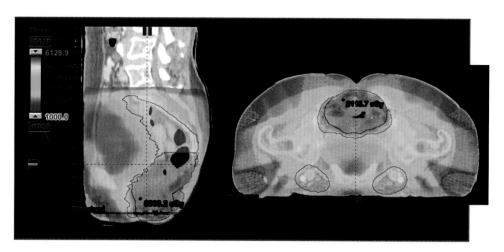

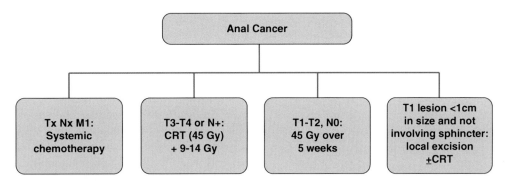

Figure 21-13. Anal cancer treatment.

Current Management Protocol (Fig. 21-13)

Limited Localized Disease: Stages I–III (Any T, Any N, M0)

LE can be used to remove some small tumors (usually measuring <1 cm or ½ in.) that do not involve the sphincter. In some cases, this may be followed with chemotherapy and RT, which is especially recommended in the setting of a positive margin. The standard treatment for anal cancers that cannot be removed without harming the anal sphincter is RT combined with chemotherapy (CRT).

Current primary recommendations for the treatment of non-metastatic anal cancer include CRT; commonly used therapeutic drugs include 5-FU and mitomycin.

Mitomycin + 5-FU + RT

This regimen consists of 5-FU 1000 mg/m²/day delivered via IV continuous infusion on days 1–4 and 29–32 (maximum daily dose of 5-FU = 2000 mg/day), plus mitomycin 10 mg/m² via IV bolus on days 1 and 29 (maximum = 20 mg per dose) [28]. RT may be included in all stages of disease, with a minimum 45 Gy delivered over 5 weeks. Additional RT of 9–14 Gy may be considered for patients with T3, T4, or node-positive disease, or those with residual disease after an initial dose of 45 Gy [37, 38].

Metastatic Disease (Stage IV): Any T, Any N, M1

Metastatic disease is commonly treated with cisplatin-based (5-FU + cisplatin) chemotherapy.

Cisplatin + 5-FU

The regimen consists of 5-FU 1000 mg/m²/day via IV continuous infusion on days 1–5, plus cisplatin 100 mg/m² via IV on day 2, repeated every 28 days [39]. Patients with meta-static disease receiving systemic chemotherapy have approximate survival rates of 60 % at 1 year and 32 % at 5 years, respectively [8, 39].

In some patients with metastatic disease, surgical intervention may be required for relief of symptoms such as pain, bleeding, or fecal incontinence.

Prognostic Factors

The size of the primary tumor and the presence of nodal or distant metastases are the principal determinates of outcome. Patients with de novo tumors >5 cm are at significantly increased risk of requiring an APR with permanent colostomy, and such tumors are associated with inferior disease-free and overall survival. Male gender and HIV-positive status may portend an unfavorable long-term outcome [8, 40, 41].

Evaluation of Treatment Response

The mainstay in assessment of tumor response is clinical follow-up. Patients are evaluated by repeat physical examination of the anal area at approximately 8–12 weeks after completion of chemoradiotherapy, and at 6- to 8-week intervals until resolution of any suspicious findings. Based on evaluation, patients are classified with respect to remission, as follows:

- *Persistent disease*: Patients with persistent disease but no progression are followed closely to see if further regression occurs. Based on the ACT II study, patients with persistent but nonprogressive disease may be followed up to 6 months after chemoradiotherapy, until determination of complete remission.
- *Complete remission*: Patients with complete remission should undergo evaluation every 3–6 months for 5 years. This should include digital rectal examination, endoscopic examination, and examination of the groin. CT

scan of the chest, abdomen, and pelvis, or PET/CT, is performed annually for 3 years in patients with slow disease regression, and those who initially had locally advanced disease (T3/T4) or node-positive cancer.

- *Progressive or persistent disease at 6 months*: If the patient has persistent disease at 6 months, or progressive disease develops in the meantime, biopsy may be done to confirm cancer. Biopsy is recommended earlier in the setting of tumor mass progression or unsatisfactory response to treatment [3, 8, 10, 36]. However, unnecessary biopsy should be avoided to minimize the risk of soft tissue infections, tissue necrosis, or impairment of anal function.

Salvage Treatment

Approximately 10–30 % of patients have persistent or recurrent disease after initial CRT. Risk factors associated with failure of initial treatment include:

- HIV-positive status.
- High T and N stage at original presentation.
- Interruption of treatment during CRT.

Progressive disease is biopsied and restaged before salvage treatment [42–44]. Some studies recommend an additional RT of 9 Gy, rather than resorting to APR immediately. However, salvage surgery is generally recommended for persistent anal cancer. Surgical treatment is based on the extent of the persisting tumor. Patients with very limited residual tumor may be able to undergo LE. Others with larger residual disease should undergo salvage APR. Salvage APR is associated with 5-year locoregional control in 30–77 % of patients [43, 45, 46]; overall survival at 5 years ranges from 30 to 60 %. Wound complications are common, and may be seen in as many as 80 % of patients who undergo salvage APR after CRT. In order to reduce wound complications, muscle flap reconstruction of the perineum may be considered [47].

Treatment of Recurrent Anal Cancer

If anal cancer recurs locally after initial treatment, restaging is performed to rule out systemic metastasis; this includes CT chest, abdomen, and pelvis or PET/CT based on institutional preference. Local recurrence after CRT is commonly managed with salvage APR. Isolated recurrence in an inguinal node may be treated with RT to the groin, with or without chemotherapy, if there is no history of previous RT to the groin. If isolated recurrence develops in an inguinal node despite previous RT, inguinal node dissection may be performed without an APR [25, 48] (Table 21-3).

Treatment of HIV-Positive Patients

HIV is associated with a markedly increased incidence of anal cancer, most likely due to immunosuppression, and HPV infection secondary to anal-receptive intercourse [49, 50]. Initial treatment of anal cancer is CRT; however, certain factors such as a patient's CD4 count play a role in modifying the dose of RT; doses range from 32 to 63 Gy; chemotherapy may be delivered in conventional dose regimens, including 5-FU combined with mitomycin or cisplatin. Studies have shown that patients with CD4 >200 have acceptable treatment-related toxicity and may achieve very good disease control. On the other hand, patients with CD4 <200 have a markedly higher incidence of treatment-related morbidities. However, this is not associated with decreased overall survival. The chemotherapy dose may need to be altered, based on the patient's blood counts.

Mitomycin + 5-FU: If nadir WBC count is <2400 but >1000, or if nadir platelet count is >50,000 but <85,000, the second dose of mitomycin is reduced to 7.5 mg/m^2, from 10 mg/m^2.

If nadir WBC count is <1000 or if platelet count is <50,000, the second dose of mitomycin is reduced to 5 mg/m^2, from 10 mg/m^2.

On day 28, if the WBC count is <2400 or the platelet count is <85,000, chemotherapy is delayed for 1 week [25].

There is a higher incidence of in situ anal cancer among homosexual and bisexual men, irrespective of their HIV status. Data suggest that anal cytology screening in these men every 2–3 years may be cost effective and yield benefits in life expectancy [51].

Anal Melanoma

Anal melanoma represents 1–4 % of all anorectal malignancies. It is the third most common site of melanoma, after the skin and retina, accounting for less than 1 % of all melanomas [52, 53]. It is most commonly seen in females, and the mean age of presentation is 60 years [54]. These tumors arise from the transitional epithelium of the anal canal, the anoderm, or the mucocutaneous junction.

Symptoms

The most common symptom of anal melanoma is bleeding per rectum. However, as in the setting of any other anal lesion the patient may present with pain, change in bowel habits, or tenesmus. Early lesions may be mistaken as thrombosed hemorrhoids [53].

Physical Examination

A thorough physical exam, including assessment of the groin, should be done. Anal melanoma may be pigmented, and either polypoid or ulcerated, with raised edges. Satellite lesions may also be present.

Histopathological Diagnosis

The features of anal melanoma resemble those of cutaneous melanomas. The majority shows a junctional component adjacent to the invasive tumor, which proves that the lesion is primary in nature. The tumor cell expresses S-100, HMB-45, and Melan A. Perineural invasion is an important prognostic factor (Figs. 21-14 and 21-15) [5, 55].

Treatment

The overall prognosis of anal melanoma is dismal, with a 10- to 19-month survival after diagnosis [56, 57]. Melanoma does not respond well to chemotherapy or RT; thus, surgery is the principal treatment when disease is localized. The extent of surgical resection is a matter of debate. Anal melanoma is very aggressive, and up to 35 % of patients initially pres-

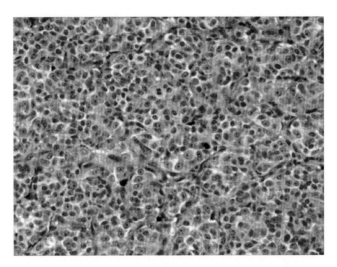

FIGURE 21-14. Anal melanoma with epithelioid morphology.

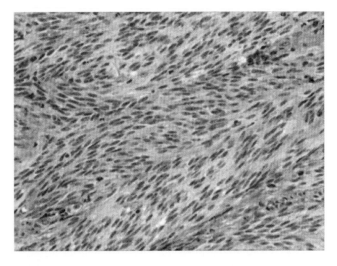

FIGURE 21-15. Anal melanoma with spindle cell morphology.

ent with metastatic disease. Patients with tumor >1 cm are unlikely to be cured by any type of treatment. Some authors claim that APR is the first choice of treatment, particularly for patients with small tumors and no evidence of nodal metastasis. However, as most patients with anal melanoma die of distant metastasis, major operative intervention like abdominoperineal resection may not offer a survival advantage; hence some author prefer local excision as initial treatment for melanoma. Melanoma of anal canal is sometimes detected as an incidental tumor when local excision is done for hemorrhoids. If R0 resection is achieved during local excision for hemorrhoids, patients do not need further intervention and have shown acceptable cure rates. Palliative local excision should be considered for patients with local symptoms due to anal melanoma (Table 21-3) [53, 54, 58–62].

Anal Margin Squamous Cell Carcinoma (Fig. 21-16)

The anal margin begins at the margin of hair-bearing perianal skin, extending onto the perianal skin for a 5 cm radius. SCC at the anal margin behaves like any other SCC of the skin, and drains into regional LNs such as the inguinal nodes. Anal margin SCC accounts for one-fourth to one-third of all anal SCC [63–65].

Epidemiology

SCC of the anal margin generally presents in patients between 65 and 75 years of age. There is no gender predilection [63, 64].

Symptoms

Like other anal canal tumors, diagnosis of SCC of the anal margin is delayed because of nonspecific symptoms, and difficult location. The most common presentation is a symptomatic mass in the perianal region, or persistent pruritus. Any person with persistent pruritus in the perianal region should be thoroughly examined for a perianal mass; suspicious lesions should be biopsied.

Examination

A thorough exam including assessment of the groins should be performed in patients with anal canal tumors. The relationship of tumor to the anal sphincter must be ascertained [68].

Staging

A CT of the chest, abdomen, and pelvis should be performed to rule out distant metastasis.

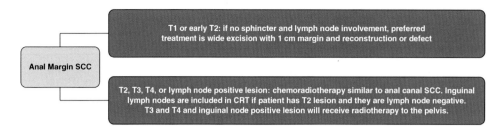

T1 or early T2: if no sphincter and lymph node involvement, preferred treatment is wide excision with 1 cm margin and reconstruction or defect

Anal Margin SCC

T2, T3, T4, or lymph node positive lesion: chemoradiotherapy similar to anal canal SCC. Inguinal lymph nodes are included in CRT if patient has T2 lesion and they are lymph node negative. T3 and T4 and inguinal node positive lesion will receive radiotherapy to the pelvis.

FIGURE 21-16. Algorithm for management of anal margin cancer.

Lymph node involvement: Studies have shown that the chance of LN involvement in a T1 lesion is extremely low. However, the chance of LN involvement in a T2 lesion is 24 %, and as high as 67 % in a T3 lesion [63].

Management (Fig. 21-6)

Management depends upon:

- Size of tumor.
- LN involvement.
- Sphincter involvement.

T1 N0 lesions: If there is no sphincter or LN involvement, the preferred treatment is wide excision with a 1 cm margin, when possible. The defect may be closed primarily; however, a large defect may require a V-Y advancement flap or skin graft. If the defect cannot be closed with an advancement flap, a pedicle flap may be necessary.

T2 N0 lesions: Early T2 lesions may be treated with surgery if no LN involvement is present; however, advanced lesions may be treated with CRT, as the chance of occult LN involvement is higher. Surgery to achieve a clear margin may result in an unacceptably large defect.

T3, T4, or LN-positive lesions: CRT protocols similar to those given for anal canal SCC are used. Inguinal LNs are included in CRT. T3 and T4 and inguinal node-positive lesions should receive radiotherapy (RT) to the pelvis [63–69].

Anal Adenocarcinoma

Primary mucinous adenocarcinoma of the anus is a rare malignancy, accounting for approximately 3 % of anal cancers. Most anal adenocarcinomas originate from the colorectal zone in the upper portion of the anal canal, or from the glandular cells of the ATZ mucosa.

Adenocarcinoma of the anal canal can be categorized based on origin (Fig. 21-17).

- Colorectal-type adenocarcinoma: Macroscopically and histologically, these lesions are indistinguishable from ordinary colorectal adenocarcinoma. However, they carry

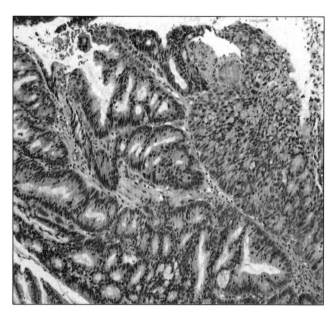

FIGURE 21-17 Superficial portion of an anal adenocarcinoma showing a low-grade gland forming component and a high-grade component with more solid growth.

a higher risk of nodal disease along the inguinal and femoral nodal chains. Immunohistology shows positivity for cytokeratin (CK) 20 and CDX2, and negativity for CK7, which is compatible with colorectal subtype anal adenocarcinoma.

- Adenocarcinoma within an anorectal fistula: Anorectal fistulae can be developmental or acquired due to inflammatory conditions such as Crohn's disease.
- Adenocarcinoma of the anal glands: This diagnosis is given if the tumor is primary to the anal canal and centered within the wall of the anorectal area, without a preexisting fistula and without surface mucosa dysplasia, irrespective of the extent of mucin production. Anal gland adenocarcinoma is CK7 positive [5].

Clinical Features and Diagnosis

Anal adenocarcinoma presents with symptoms similar to those of any other anal mass. Thorough physical examination and biopsy are required to confirm the diagnosis.

TABLE 21-3. Types of anal cancer and preferred treatment

Type of anal cancer	Preferred treatment
Recurrent SCC	Local recurrences after treatment with radiation therapy and chemotherapy are treated with salvage APR
Anal melanoma	Local excision
Anal adenocarcinoma	Combined modality treatment including APR with adjuvant CRT to be optimal treatment

Staging

Staging is similar to that done for anal canal SCC.

Prognostic Factors

Prognostic factors in anal adenocarcinoma are [70]:

- T stage.
- N stage.
- Histologic grade.
- Treatment modality.

Management (Table 21-3)

Due to the rarity of this disease, very few studies have been published reporting on management of anal adenocarcinoma. Management options include LE, radical surgery (APR) with or without chemotherapy, or CRT. Historically, APR was the preferred treatment; however, with recent advances in CRT, a combined modality treatment including APR plus adjuvant CRT is considered optimal [70–77].

Biologicals

SCC of the anus commonly overexpresses EGFR. EGFR and KRAS mutations appear rare (76, 77). In a study by Lukan et al. the potential role of EGFR inhibition was supported by partial remission, minor remission, or no progression in five patients with wild-type KRAS anal cancer treated with either cetuximab as a single agent or cetuximab with irinotecan. Two patients with KRAS mutation did not respond to cetuximab, and had progression of disease. The authors concluded that cetuximab-based treatment can be used in patients with metastatic KRAS wild-type anal cancer after failure of, or as an alternative to, cisplatin/5-fluorouracil (FU)-based therapy [77].

Conclusions

Anal cancer is an uncommon gastrointestinal cancer. A thorough clinical examination and high index of suspicion are needed for diagnosis. Chemoradiotherapy, using 5-FU/mitomycin C with RT, is the mainstay of treatment for patients with anal SCC; early T1 tumors may be treated surgically, if excision does not compromise sphincter function. Patients with metastatic anal SCC are most commonly treated with cisplatin-based chemotherapy. Improvements in current treatment modalities including IMRT, and biologics such as cetuximab, may provide more refined and successful treatments for patients with anal cancer.

References

1. Simpson JAD, Scholefield JH. Diagnosis and management of anal intraepithelial neoplasia and anal cancer. BMJ. 2011; 343:d6818.
2. American Cancer Society. Cancer facts and figures 2015. Atlanta, GA: American Cancer Society; 2015. Last accessed April 1, 2015.
3. Chin JY, Hong TS, Wo JY. Anal cancer: current and future treatment strategies. Gastrointest Canc Targets Therapy. 2013;3: 19–27.
4. Drake RL, Wayne Vogl A, Mitchell AWM. Gray's anatomy for students. 3rd ed., vol 5; 2014. pp. 463–4.
5. Shia J. An update on tumors of the anal canal. Arch Pathol Lab Med. 2010;134(11):1601–11.
6. Pineda CE, Welton ML. Management of anal squamous intraepithelial lesions. Clin Colon Rectal Surg. 2009;22(2):94–101.
7. Ryan DP, Compton CC, Mayer RJ. Carcinoma of the anal canal. N Engl J Med. 2000;342:792–800.
8. Osborne MC, Maykel J, Johnson EK, Steele SR. Anal squamous cell carcinoma: an evolution in disease and management. World J Gastroenterol. 2014;20(36):13052–9.
9. Tanum G, Tveit K, Karlsen KO. Diagnosis of anal carcinoma – doctor's finger still the best? Oncology. 1991;48:383–6.
10. Glynne-Jones R, Northover JMA, Cervantes A. Anal cancer: ESMO clinical practice guidelines for diagnosis, treatment and follow-up. Ann Oncol. 2010;21 Suppl 5:v87–92.
11. Frisch M, Glimelius B, van den Brule AJ, et al. Sexually transmitted infection as a cause of anal cancer. N Engl J Med. 1997;337(19):1350–8.
12. Tonolini M, Bianco R. MRI and CT of anal carcinoma: a pictorial review. Insights Imaging. 2013;4(1):53–62.
13. Parikh J, Shaw A, Grant LA, et al. Anal carcinomas: the role of endoanal ultrasound and magnetic resonance imaging in staging, response evaluation and follow-up. Eur Radiol. 2011;21: 776–85.
14. Roach SC, Hulse PA, Moulding FJ, et al. Magnetic resonance imaging of anal cancer. Clin Radiol. 2005;60:1111–9.
15. Otto SD, Lee L, Buhr HJ, et al. Staging anal cancer: prospective comparison of transanal endoscopic ultrasound and magnetic resonance imaging. J Gastrointest Surg. 2009;13(7):1292–8.
16. Cummings BJ, Ajani JA, Swallow CJ. Cancer of the anal region. In: DeVita Jr VT, Lawrence TS, Rosenberg SA et al. Cancer:

principles & practice of oncology. 8th ed. Philadelphia, PA: Lippincott, Williams & Wilkins; 2008.

17. Nguyen BT, Joon DL, Khoo V, et al. Assessing the impact of FDG-PET in the management of anal cancer. Radiother Oncol. 2008;87(3):376–82.

18. Bhuva NJ, Glynne-Jones R, Sonoda L, Wong WL, Harrison MK, To PET or not to PET? That is the question. Staging in anal cancer. Ann Oncol. 2012;23(8):2078–82.

19. Caldarella C, Annunziata S, Treglia G, Sadeghi R, Ayati N, Giovanella L. Diagnostic performance of positron emission tomography/computed tomography using fluorine-18 fluorodeoxyglucose in detecting locoregional nodal involvement in patients with anal canal cancer: a systematic review and meta-analysis. Sci World J. 2014;2014:196068.

20. Mistrangelo M, Pelosi E, Bellò M, Ricardi U, et al. Role of positron emission tomography-computed tomography in the management of anal cancer. Int J Radiat Oncol Biol Phys. 2012;84(1):66–72.

21. Vercellino L, Montravers F, de Parades V, et al. Impact of FDG PET/CT in the staging and the follow-up of anal carcinoma. Int J Colorectal Dis. 2011;26(2):201–10.

22. Wayne F, Bhayani N, Ford D, Yang G, Thomas C. Anal carcinoma. Curr Cancer Ther Rev. 2009;5:142–50.

23. Nigro N, Seydel H, Considine B, Vaitkevicius V, Leichman L, Kinzie J. Combined preoperative radiation and chemotherapy for squamous cell carcinoma of the anal canal. Cancer. 1983;51:1826–9.

24. Goldman S, Glimelius B, Glas U, Lundell G, Påhlman L, Ståhle E. Management of anal epidermoid carcinoma – an evaluation of treatment results in two population-based series. Int J Colorectal Dis. 1989;4(4):234–43.

25. Flam M, John M, Pajak TF, et al. Role of mitomycin in combination with fluorouracil and radiotherapy, and of salvage chemoradiation in the definitive nonsurgical treatment of epidermoid carcinoma of the anal canal: results of a phase III randomized intergroup study. J Clin Oncol. 1996;14(9):2527–39.

26. Bartelink H, Roelofsen F, Eschwege F, et al. Concomitant radiotherapy and chemotherapy is superior to radiotherapy alone in the treatment of locally advanced anal cancer: results of a phase III randomized trial of the European Organization for Research and Treatment of Cancer Radiotherapy and Gastrointestinal Cooperative Groups. J Clin Oncol. 1997;15(5):2040–9.

27. Northover J, Glynne-Jones R, Sebag-Montefiore D, et al. Chemoradiation for the treatment of epidermoid anal cancer, 13-year follow-up of the first randomised UKCCCR Anal Cancer Trial (ACT I). Br J Cancer. 2010;102(7):1123–8.

28. Ajani JA, Winter KA, Gunderson LL, et al. Fluorouracil, mitomycin, and radiotherapy vs fluorouracil, cisplatin, and radiotherapy for carcinoma of the anal canal: a randomized controlled trial. JAMA. 2008;299(16):1914–21.

29. Ajani JA, Winter KA, Gunderson L, et al. Prognostic factors derived from a prospective database dictate clinical biology of anal cancer: the intergroup trial (RTOG 98-11). Cancer. 2010;116(17):10.

30. Peiffert D, Tournier-Rangeard L, Gerard JP, et al. Induction chemotherapy and dose intensification of the radiation boost in locally advanced anal canal carcinoma: final analysis of the randomized UNICANCER ACCORD 03 trial. J Clin Oncol. 2012;30:1941–8.

31. John M, Pajak T, Flam M, Hoffman J, Markoe A, Wolkov H, et al. Dose escalation in chemoradiation for anal cancer: preliminary results of RTOG 92-08. Cancer J Sci Am. 1996;2(4):205–11.

32. Scher ED, Ahmed I, Yue NJ, Jabbour SK. Technical aspects of radiation therapy for anal cancer. J Gastroint Oncol. 2014;5(3):198–211.

33. Myerson RJ, Garofalo MC, El Naqa I, et al. Elective clinical target volumes for conformal therapy in anorectal cancer: a radiation therapy oncology group consensus panel contouring atlas. Int J Radiat Oncol Biol Phys. 2009;74:824–30.

34. Allal AS, Sprangers MAG, Laurencet F, Reymond MA, Kurtz JM. Assessment of long-term quality of life in patients with anal carcinomas treated by radiotherapy with or without chemotherapy. Br J Cancer. 1999;80(10):1588–94.

35. De Bree E, van Ruth S, Dewit LG, Zoetmulder FA. High risk of colostomy with primary radiotherapy for anal cancer. Ann Surg Oncol. 2007;14(1):100–8.

36. Shridhar R, Shibata D, Chan E, Thomas CR. Anal cancer: current standards in care and recent changes in practice. CA Cancer J Clin. 2015;65:139–62.

37. Ferrigno R, Nakamura RA, Dos Santos Novaes PE, et al. Radiochemotherapy in the conservative treatment of anal canal carcinoma: retrospective analysis of results and radiation dose effectiveness. Int J Radiat Oncol Biol Phys. 2005;61(4):1136–42.

38. Huang K, Haas-Kogan D, Weinberg V, Krieg R. Higher radiation dose with a shorter treatment duration improves outcome for locally advanced carcinoma of anal canal. World J Gastroenterol. 2007;13(6):895–900.

39. Faivre C, Rougier P, Ducreux M, et al. 5-Fluorouracil and cis-platinum combination chemotherapy for metastatic squamous-cell anal cancer. Bull Cancer. 1999;86(10):861–5.

40. Cummings BJ, Keane TJ, O'sullivan B, Wong CS, Catton CN. Epidermoid anal cancer: treatment by radiation alone or by radiation and 5-fluorouracil with and without mitomycin C. Int J Radiat Oncol Biol Phys. 1991;21(5):1115–25.

41. Czito BG, Willett CG. Current management of anal canal cancer. Curr Oncol Rep. 2009;11(3):186–92.

42. Ben-Josef E, Moughan J, Ajani JA, Flam M, Gunderson L, Pollock J, et al. Impact of overall treatment time on survival and local control in patients with anal cancer: a pooled data analysis of Radiation Therapy Oncology Group trials 87-04 and 98-11. J Clin Oncol. 2010;28:5061–6.

43. Papaconstantinou HT, Bullard KM, Rothenberger DA, Madoff RD. Salvage abdominoperineal resection after failed Nigro protocol: modest success, major morbidity. Colorectal Dis. 2006;8:124–9.

44. Glynne-Jones R. James R, Meadows H, Begum R, Cunningham D, Northover J, Ledermann JA, Beare S, Kadalayil L, Sebag-Montefiore D. May 20 Supplement, 2012. ASCO Annual Meeting Abstracts. J Clin Oncol. 30(Suppl 15). Optimum time to assess complete clinical response (CR) following chemoradiation (CRT) using mitomycin (MMC) or cisplatin (CisP), with or without maintenance CisP/5FU in squamous cell carcinoma of the anus: Results of ACT II; 2012. p. 4004.

45. Van der Wal BC, Cleffken BI, Gulec B, Kaufman HS, Choti MA. Results of salvage abdominoperineal resection for recurrent anal carcinoma following combined chemoradiation therapy. J Gastrointest Surg. 2001;5:383–7.

46. Ghouti L, Houvenaeghel G, Moutardier V, Giovannini M, Magnin V, Lelong B, et al. Salvage abdominoperineal resection after failure of conservative treatment in anal epidermoid cancer. Dis Colon Rectum. 2005;48:16–22.

47. Chessin DB, Hartley J, Cohen AM, Mazumdar M, Cordeiro P, Disa J, et al. Rectus flap reconstruction decreases perineal wound complications after pelvic chemoradiation and surgery: a cohort study. Ann Surg Oncol. 2005;12:104–10.

48. Longo WE, Vernava 3rd AM, Wade TP, et al. Recurrent squamous cell carcinoma of the anal canal. Predictors of initial treatment failure and results of salvage therapy. Ann Surg. 1994;220(1):40–9.

49. Frisch M, Biggar R, Goedert J, et al. Human papillomavirus-associated cancers in patients with human immunodeficiency virus infection and acquired immunodeficiency syndrome. J Natl Cancer Inst. 2000;92(18):1500–10.

50. Machalek DA, Poynten M, Jin F et al. Anal human papillomavirus infection and associated neoplastic lesions in men who have sex with men: a systematic review and meta-analysis. Lancet Oncol. 2012;3(5):487–500.

51. Goldie SJ, Kuntz KM, Weinstein MC, Freedberg KA, Welton ML, Palefsky JM. The clinical effectiveness and cost-effectiveness of screening for anal squamous intraepithelial lesions in homosexual and bisexual HIV-positive men. JAMA. 1999;281(19):1822–9.

52. Chang AE, Karnell LH, Menck HR. The National Cancer Data Base report on cutaneous and noncutaneous melanoma: a summary of 84,836 cases from the past decade: the American College of Surgeons Commission on Cancer and the American Cancer Society. Cancer. 1998;83(8):1664–78.

53. Parra RS, de Almeida ALNR, Badiale GB, da Silva Moraes MMF, Rocha JJR, Féres O. Melanoma of the anal canal. Clinics. 2010;65(10):1063–5.

54. Zhong J, Zhou JN, Xu FP, Shang JQ. Diagnosis and treatment of anorectal malignant melanoma: a report of 22 cases with literature review. Ai Zheng. 2006;25:619–24.

55. Pirenne Y, Bouckaert W, Vangertruyden G. Rectal melanoma: a rare tumor. Acta Chir Belg. 2008;108:756–8.

56. Brady MS, Kavolius JP, Quan SH. Anorectal melanoma. A 64 year experience at Memorial Sloan Kettering Cancer Center. Dis Colon Rectum. 1995;38:146–51.

57. Stroh C, Manger T. Primary amelanotic anorectal melanoma – a case report. Zentralbl Chir. 2007;132:560–3.

58. David AW, Perakath B. Management of anorectal melanomas: a 10-year review. Trop Gastroenterol. 2007;28:76–8.

59. Roviello F, Cioppa T, Marrelli D, Nastri G, De Stefano A, Hako L, et al. Primary ano-rectal melanoma: considerations on a clinical case and review of the literature. Chir Ital. 2003;55:575–80.

60. Roumen RM. Anorectal melanoma in the Netherlands: a report of 63 patients. Eur J Surg Oncol. 1996;22:598–601.

61. Droesch JT, Flum DR, Mann GN. Wide local excision or abdominoperineal resection as the initial treatment for anorectal melanoma? Am J Surg. 2005;189:446–9.

62. Homsi J, Garrett C. Melanoma of the anal canal: a case series. Dis Colon Rectum. 2007;50:1004–10.

63. Newlin HE, Zlotecki RA, Morris CG, Hochwald SN, Riggs CE, Mendenhall WM. Squamous cell carcinoma of the anal margin. J Surg Oncol. 2004;86(2):55–62.

64. Mendenhall WM, Zlotecki RA, Vauthey JN, Copeland EM. III Squamous cell carcinoma of the anal margin. Oncology (Williston Park). 1996;10(12):1843–8. Discussion 1848, 1853–1854.

65. Quan S. Anal cancers squamous and melanoma. Cancer. 1992;70 Suppl 5:1384–9.

66. Welton M, Varma M. In: Wolff B, Fleshman J, Beck D, Pemberton J, Wexner S, et al., editors. The ASCRS textbook of colon and rectal surgery. New York: Springer Science + Business Media; 2007. Anal Cancer. pp. 482–500.

67. Chawla AK, Willett CG. Squamous cell carcinoma of the anal canal and anal margin. Hematol Oncol Clin North Am. 2001;15(2):321–44.

68. Wietfeldt ED, Thiele J. Malignancies of the anal margin and perianal skin. Clin Colon Rectal Surg. 2009;22(2):127–35.

69. Chapet O, Gerard JP, Mornex F, et al. Prognostic factors of squamous cell carcinoma of the anal margin treated by radiotherapy: the lyon experience. Int J Colorectal Dis. 2007;22(2):191–9.

70. Belkacémi Y, Berger C, Poortmans P, et al. Management of primary anal canal adenocarcinoma: a large retrospective study from the rare cancer network. Int J Radiat Oncol Biol Phys. 2003;56(5):1274–83.

71. Chang GJ, Gonzalez RJ, Skibber JM, et al. A twenty-year experience with adenocarcinoma of the anal canal. Dis Colon Rectum. 2009;52(8):1375–80.

72. Kachnic LA, Winter K, Myerson RJ, et al. RTOG 0529: a phase II evaluation of dose-painted intensity modulated radiation therapy in combination with 5-fluorouracil and mitomycin-C for the reduction of acute morbidity in carcinoma of the anal canal. Int J Radiat Oncol Biol Phys. 2013;86(1):27–33.

73. DeFoe SG, Beriwal S, Jones H, et al. Concurrent chemotherapy and intensity-modulated radiation therapy for anal carcinoma – clinical outcomes in a large National Cancer Institute-designated integrated cancer centre network. Clin Oncol (R Coll Radiol). 2012;24(6):424–31.

74. Rothenstein DA, Dasgupta T, Chou JF, et al. Comparison of outcomes of intensity-modulated radiotherapy and 3-D conformal radiotherapy for anal squamous cell carcinoma using a propensity score analysis. (2011 ASCO Annual Meeting abstract number 3555). J Clin Oncol. 2011;29:2011.

75. Alvarez G, Perry A, Tan BR, Wang HL. Expression of epidermal growth factor receptor in squamous cell carcinomas of the anal canal is independent of gene amplification. Mod Pathol. 2006;19(7):942–9.

76. Le LH, Chetty R, Moore MJ. Epidermal growth factor receptor expression in anal canal carcinoma. Am J Clin Pathol. 2005;124:20–3.

77. Lukan N, Ströbel P, Willer A, et al. Cetuximab-based treatment of metastatic anal cancer: correlation of response with KRAS mutational status. Oncology. 2009;77(5):293–9.

22
Presacral Tumors

John Migaly and Christopher R. Mantyh

Key Concepts

- Unless contraindicated, presacral tumors should be surgically excised because of the risk of malignancy.
- MRI should be performed to characterize the lesions and to plan surgery.
- Lesions that are below sacral level S4 can be excised through a posterior/perineal approach.
- Complete, non-piecemeal excision is critical to avoiding recurrence or infection.

Introduction

Retrorectal masses are a group of lesions that encompass a wide spectrum of disease processes, ranging from congenital lesions (with varied malignant potential) to inflammatory disease processes and overt malignancy [1, 2]. In general, retrorectal tumors are extremely rare, with the incidence of the tumors varying in the reported literature [1–3]. The Mayo Clinic has reported that retrorectal tumors represent 1 in 40,000 hospital admissions [4]. Diagnosis of these lesions is usually incidental on physical exam or on imaging studies, as symptomatology is usually vague [4]. Imaging remains the key to preoperative characterization of these lesions in addition to preoperative planning. Although the majority of patients will have undergone computed tomography (CT scan), magnetic resonance imaging (MRI) is an essential element in the preoperative evaluation. Although the role of preoperative biopsy has been a source of debate, because of the fear of recurrence at or seeding of biopsy tracts, there is a good single institutional data to support its selective use [5].

Anatomic Considerations

The presacral or retrorectal space is not a true space but rather a potential space (see Chap. 1). It is a unique area in that it represents a developmentally critical location where several types of embryological distinct cell lines converge for the final steps prior to the completion of ontogeny. It is these changes that produce the variety of benign and malignant and solid and cystic growths that can occur in this space [1]. The retrorectal space is the area posterior to the rectum, but, more specifically, its superior extent is the pelvic peritoneal reflection, its lateral limits are the ureters and iliac vessels, posteriorly it is defined by the sacrum, and anteriorly it is defined as the posterior wall of the rectum. The inferior border is the levator complex and the coccygeal muscles (Figure 22-1) [3].

The retrorectal space presents a multitude of challenges to the surgeon, and this subset of procedures is not recommended for those uninitiated in pelvic surgery. The sacral nerve rootlets are located in this retrorectal space, and thus injury to and sacrifice of these structures can have substantial implications on rectoanal and sexual function. In cases requiring the unilateral sacrifice of all of the sacral nerve rootlets, the patient will likely retain normal anorectal and sexual function. Bilateral sacrifice of the third sacral nerve rootlet will usually result in fecal incontinence [6, 7].

Classification

Histology/Pathology

The classification of presacral masses encompasses a wide variety of etiologies and tissue types (Table 22-1). The classification of these retrorectal lesions, first elaborated by Uhlig and Johnson in 1975, divides these lesions broadly into congenital, acquired, neurogenic, osseous, and "others" [3]. Understanding the various subtypes, disease behavior, and malignant potential is essential to tailor treatment regimens.

Congenital Lesions

Congenital lesions represent two-thirds of all retrorectal lesions, which are thought to arise from various combinations of the three embryonic cell layers. These congenital

© Springer International Publishing 2016
S.R. Steele et al. (eds.), *The ASCRS Textbook of Colon and Rectal Surgery*, DOI 10.1007/978-3-319-25970-3_22

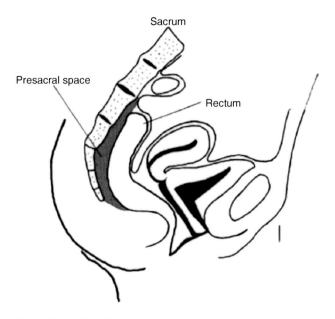

FIGURE 22-1. Location of the presacral space (Reprinted with permission from Ghosh J, Eglinton T, Frizelle FA, Watson AJ. Presacral tumours in adults. Surgeon. 2007 Feb;5(1):31–8 © 2007, Elsevier Ltd. [30]).

TABLE 22-1. Classification of retrorectal tumors

Congenital
  Developmental cyst
    Epidermoid cyst
    Dermoid cyst
  Teratoma
  Teratocarcinoma
  Chordoma
  Anterior meningocele
  Rectal duplication
  Adrenal rest tumors
Neurogenic tumors
  Neurofibroma
  Neurilemmoma
  Ependymoma
  Ganglioneuroma
  Neurofibrosarcoma
  Malignant peripheral nerve sheath tumors
Osseous
  Osteoma
  Osteogenic sarcoma
  Sacral bone cyst
  Ewing's tumor
  Giant-cell tumor
  Chondrosarcoma
  Chondromyxosarcoma
Miscellaneous
  Metastatic or recurrent disease
  Lipoma
  Fibroma
  Leiomyoma
  Hemangioma
  Desmoid
  Liposarcoma
  Leiomyosarcoma
  Fibrosarcoma
  Endothelioma
  Granuloma
  Perineal abscess
  Fistula

lesions can be cystic or solid [8]. In general, these lesions are more common in females than males [4, 8].

Dermoid and Epidermoid Cysts

Dermoid and epidermoid cysts are lined with squamous epithelial cells and may contain various skin appendages such as hair or nails (Figure 22-2). These lesions are thought to arise from the ectodermal layer in embryonic development. Patients can have a postanal dimple or sinus that can be mistaken for an abscess and errantly drained [9, 10]. This also accounts for the high rate of infection of these cysts.

Enterogenous

Unlike dermoid and epidermoid cysts, enterogenous cysts are multilocular. Enterogenous cysts arise from the endoderm of the primitive hindgut. These lesions can also undergo malignant degeneration.

Tailgut Cysts

Tailgut cysts are also referred to as retrorectal cystic hamartomas which arise from the persistence of the hindgut. Rectal duplication cysts contain all of the layers of the intestinal tract (Figure 22-3). Rectal duplication cysts can also undergo malignant change [11].

Teratomas

Teratomas also contain cells from all three germ layers, but, more importantly, these lesions are true neoplasms. They can contain both solid and cystic components. Up to 10 % of these lesions contain cancer, and thus aggressive extirpation should be pursued. Because of the diverse germ cell layers, these lesions can become squamous cell carcinomas, rhabdomyosarcomas, or anaplastic tumors [1]. These tumors can contain tissues from almost any organ system including digestive and respiratory or bony tissue. Similar to other congenital lesions, teratomas are more common in females. They are also more common in children than adults. Factors that are associated with malignant degeneration and/or recurrence are incomplete resection and resections where the coccyx is not removed [1, 12].

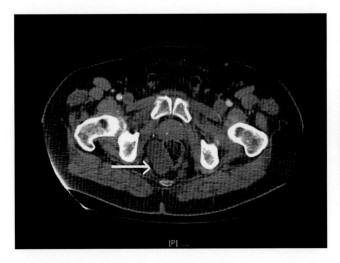

FIGURE 22-2. CT image of an epidermoid cyst.

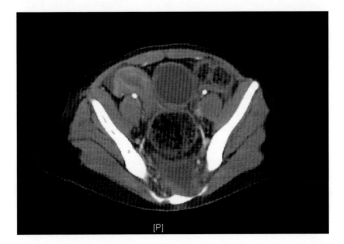

FIGURE 22-3. CT image of rectal duplication cyst.

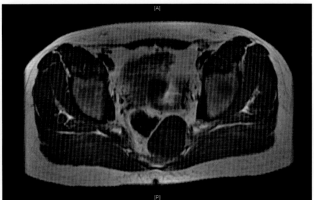

FIGURE 22-4. MRI image of a ganglioneuroblastoma.

Chordomas

The most common malignant tumor of the presacral space is the sacrococcygeal chordoma. These tumors arise from what is believed to be vestigial notochord tissue. These lesions are more common in male patients under 40 with an incidence of about 0.08 per 100,000. These lesions can occur almost anywhere on the spinal cord but are most commonly found in the presacral area. The patients present with vague symptomatology including low back pain. The 5- and 10-year survival rates are 67 and 40 %, respectively, and though surgery remains a mainstay of treatment, it is associated with a high recurrence rate [13].

Anterior Sacral Meningocele

These lesions arise from protrusions of the dural sac through a defect in the sacrum. The classic radiologic finding of the "scimitar sign" can often be seen on plain films. Patients often have vague symptomatology including

headaches related to postural changes and Valsalva [4, 14]. Magnetic resonance imaging usually easily characterizes these lesions, and percutaneous biopsy should be avoided for fear of bacterial contamination of the cerebrospinal fluid and iatrogenic meningitis.

Neurogenic Tumors

Neurogenic tumors represent about 10 % of all retrorectal tumors (Figure 22-4). They arise from peripheral nerves and include neurofibromas, schwannoma, ganglioneuroma, neuroblastomas, ganglioneuroblastoma, and ependymoma. Ependymomas are the most common of these tumors [4, 15]. Differentiation between benign and malignant variants can be difficult, and these tumors can produce significant neuropathy as a presenting symptom.

Osseous Lesions

Osseous lesions include giant-cell tumors, osteoblastoma, aneurysmal bone cysts, osteogenic sarcoma, Ewing's sarcoma, myeloma, and chondrosarcomas. These lesions represent 10 % of all retrorectal tumors. These may be the most aggressive of all the retrorectal tumors and can be very locally destructive and have pronounced metastatic potential [1, 16].

Diagnosis

History and Physical

Because of the location of these tumors in the presacral space, the symptomatology tends to be vague and nonspecific. Many of these tumors are diagnosed incidentally on rectal examination, and in fact 97 % of presacral lesions are palpable on digital rectal examination [4]. Many patients will have lower back pain or pelvic pain; however, in general, there is not a plethora of common findings. Patients with congenital cysts/tumors may have a postanal sinus; however, the most likely etiology of a postanal sinus is perianal fistulous disease. Therefore the lesions may be diagnosed after several unsuccessful attempts at treatment of a perianal fistula that usually culminates in cross-sectional imaging as the true manner of identification. Patients with advanced tumors can have constipation, sexual dysfunction, urinary incontinence, and other leg and gluteal symptoms related to local extension and mass effect. Neurologic exams with attention to these symptoms in addition to gluteal and lower extremity dysfunction allow for preoperative documentation of these defects and aid in assessing the locally invasive nature of the lesion.

Imaging Studies

The preoperative assessment of a retrorectal tumor should include intraluminal evaluation of the rectum via flexible sigmoidoscopy. Understanding the extent of the mass of the tumor on the rectum and the ability to assess the mucosal integrity of the rectum are both important elements of the preoperative preparation. Flexible sigmoidoscopy allows for a better assessment of the upper and lower extents of these tumors, in addition to the relationship of the lesion to the sphincter complex. Endorectal ultrasound (ERUS) can be utilized to assess the relationship of tumors to the muscular layers of the rectum and the anal sphincters; despite the fact that majority of the lesions are well circumscribed, the subset of tumors that are not can be quite locally advanced and destructive. ERUS can also allow a very preliminary assessment of sacral bony destruction by tumors.

Plain films have limited utility but can sometimes demonstrate osseous destruction of the sacrum or calcifications within the tumor itself. In patients with anterior sacral meningocele, the classic "scimitar sign" can often be seen on plain films, but usually cross-sectional imaging is a requirement for confirmation. Magnetic resonance imaging (MRI) with gadolinium is the imaging modality of choice for retrorectal tumors. MRI is critical in the management of these tumors by facilitating accurate diagnosis, determining the anatomic extent of the lesion, and selecting the optimal surgical approach. Information that can be extracted from an MRI is much more granular in comparison to other modalities, including key elements such as location, size, morphology, margins, and interface [17]. MRI determination of the location of lesions in relation to the sacral vertebral bodies allows for planning of abdominal versus posterior versus combined surgical approaches. Characterization of the lesion as solid or cystic is easily achievable via MRI, but subtle nodularity or septation of these lesions allows for further characterization of these lesions into their various subtypes (Figure 22-5). Threatened margins can be more easily identified via MRI

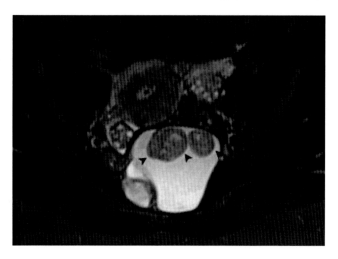

FIGURE 22-5. MRI of presacral cyst. T2-weighted imaging of an epidermoid cyst shows a bilobulated cystic lesion with pools of keratin debris (*arrows*) inside the larger cyst (Reprinted Loock MT, Fornès P, Soyer P, Rousset P, Azizi L, Hoeffel C. MR imaging features of nongynaecologic cystic lesions of the pelvis. Clin Imaging 2013;37(2):211–8 © 2013 Elsevier Ltd, with Permission from Elsevier. [31]).

such as bony erosion, or invasion of tumors and pelvic side wall invasion are more clearly definable. Arterial and venous anatomy is seen in much greater detail. What MRI excels at in comparison to CT scan is defining invasion of the muscular walls of the rectum, particularly in cases of sacrococcygeal chordoma [18]. These details, in total, make multimodality and multispecialty planning for operative interventions requiring en bloc resection of the rectum, partial sacrectomy, and arterial reconstruction or endovascular techniques much easier.

Preoperative Biopsy

Biopsy of presacral tumors presents a twofold question. First, is biopsy associated with a higher rate of local recurrence? Second, does biopsy have proven utility in the management of presacral tumors, i.e., does it changes the management? In general, biopsy of cystic lesions should only be undertaken in situations where there is some question of the characterization of the lesion *after* a high-quality MRI interpreted by an experienced radiologist. To be clear, it is universally acknowledged that biopsy of presacral lesions via the transrectal or transvaginal route is strongly discouraged, as it is possible to infect a sterile cystic lesion. In addition, biopsy via these routes necessitates either partial or complete proctectomy or vaginectomy to remove the biopsy tract in continuity with the presacral tumor in order to prevent recurrence. Biopsy of a meningocele via any route should be avoided for fear of an infection of the cerebrospinal fluid and resultant meningitis.

Early work from several authors discouraged biopsy of these tumors for fear of local recurrence [19–21]. More recent data suggests that percutaneous biopsy of retrorectal tumors can be performed without an increased risk of recurrence. In a single institutional series of 87 patients, Messick et al. performed biopsy of 24 patients (28 %) prior to surgical extirpation with no postoperative tumor recurrences. In this same series, only 4 of the 24 patients underwent excision of their biopsy site, also without any reported recurrences [5]. In our current practice, we do not biopsy all solid presacral lesion and even fewer mixed solid or cystic lesions. There is a role for biopsy in unresectable, sizeable, or aggressive tumors such as Ewing's sarcoma or osteogenic sarcoma where preoperative radiation or chemotherapy could be of value for systemic or local control or to improve the likelihood of resectability. It is our current practice to excise the biopsy tract and site at the time of definitive surgery.

Management

Role of Preoperative Neoadjuvant Therapy

Retrorectal tumors can exhibit a diverse set of behaviors and can be quite large and locally advanced by the time they are diagnosed. In addition, the subset of pelvic sarcomas has fairly significant systemic metastatic potential. With this in mind, there is a definite role for neoadjuvant chemotherapy for some of these tumors. In cases of large locally advanced presacral tumors, where resectability is at issue, neoadjuvant radiotherapy may render some benefit in decreasing tumor size and increasing resectability.

Surgical Treatment

Unless the lesion is unresectable or there is evidence of systemic metastasis, presacral tumors should be resected, as 30–40 % of the lesions will be malignant and benign lesions can undergo malignant change. Furthermore, approximately up to 10 % of cystic lesions will become chronically infected and can complicate any planned operative intervention [2–5].

Preoperative Planning

The key to preoperative planning is understanding the extent of the resection field. In patients that have direct invasion of the muscular wall of the rectum, proctectomy must be anticipated. In cases of bony invasion, partial sacrectomy is planned. Pelvic sidewall involvement may necessitate intraoperative radiotherapy and vascular or ureteric reconstruction. The assembly of a multispecialty team of colorectal, urologic, neurosurgical, orthopedic, vascular, and plastic surgeon is a prerequisite for many of these undertakings.

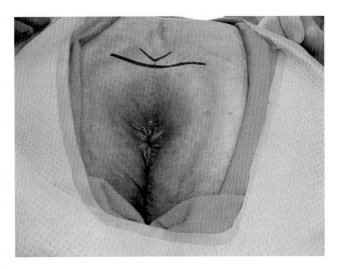

FIGURE 22-6. Transverse incision marked, as well as the sacrum and coccyx, for a posterior approach.

Surgical Approach

The location, the morphology, and the impingement or involvement of other pelvic structures dictate the operative approach. In general, a well-circumscribed presacral lesion whose uppermost extent can be palpated on digital rectal examination can usually be approached via a posterior approach. Several single institutional series also seem to share consensus where the S4 level is the line of division between abdominal and posterior approaches [3, 5, 22–25]. In lesions above the S4 level of the spine, a purely abdominal approach can be considered, while lesions below S4 can be approached posteriorly. Lesions spanning both above and below are best approached via a combined abdominal and posterior approach.

Posterior Approach

Patients are given a mechanical, cathartic bowel preparation the night before in preparation for this procedure. After intubation, the patient is placed in the prone jackknife position atop a large bolster. The rectum is irrigated with a dilute solution of betadine and saline; after this the buttocks are taped apart. While the incision for this procedure is usually described as a midline incision from the lower portion of the sacrum down to the anus, while yet others describe a transverse incision (Figure 22-6), our practice is different. The technique used by our group involves making a curvilinear incision; the incision is placed just to the left of the lower portion of the sacrum and carried in a curvilinear caudad direction around the lateral aspect of the coccyx toward the midline and the intergluteal fold just below the tip of the coccyx. Once the intergluteal fold is reached (below the tip of the coccyx), the incision is extended downward in the midline to a point approximately 2–3 cm short of the anal orifice (Figure 22-7). The reason for this type of incision is that the

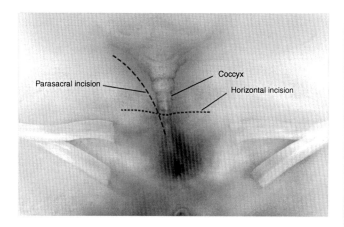

FIGURE 22-7. Posterior approach for the removal of a presacral tumor and placement of incision. The patient is in prone jackknife position, and the incision can either be horizontal on the anococcygeal ligament or curvilinear to the left of the lower sacrum/coccyx and into the intergluteal fold (With permission from Ludwig KA, Kalady MF. Transsacral approaches for presacral cyst: rectal tumor. Operative Techniques in General Surgery 2005;7:3-126-136 © 2005 Elsevier Ltd. [32]).

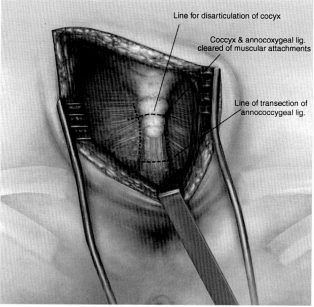

FIGURE 22-8. The anococcygeal ligament is divided, and the coccyx is subsequently cleared of its lateral attachments and removed; this facilitates dissection along the sacrum (With permission from Ludwig KA, Kalady MF. Transsacral approaches for presacral cyst: rectal tumor. Operative Techniques in General Surgery 2005;7:3-126-136 © 2005 Elsevier Ltd. [32]).

curvilinear incision allows for easier access to the lateral aspect of the coccyx, which is routinely removed.

Once the skin incision is completed, the dissection is deepened until the coccyx and the anococcygeal ligament are visualized. The anococcygeal ligament is divided, and extreme care is taken to identify the posterior aspect of the sphincter complex in order to preserve it. After this, the coccyx is freed along both sides of its lateral aspects and then the coccyx is removed (Figures 22-8 and 22-9). It is our practice to routinely remove the coccyx for two reasons. The first is that many of the congenital cysts are tethered to and originate at the coccyx, and it is thought that preserving the coccyx results in a higher recurrence rate [3, 26]. The second reason we routinely remove the coccyx is that removal allows for better visualization of the retrorectum and the mass, which creates a somewhat wider operative field, which facilitates removal of these tumors. This technique allows for intact removal of the lesion and reduces the likelihood of inadvertent perforation of the lesion, which is linked to a higher rate of recurrence and infection.

The lesion can be usually "shelled out" by dissecting it off of the sacrum and then slowly rolling the most proximal aspect of the tumor toward the incision from a cephalad to a caudad direction and then slowly dissecting it off the rectum (Figures 22-10, 22-11, and 22-12). There is quite often a feeding vessel that is encountered on the proximal aspect of many of these lesions that needs to be controlled; this can be safely and easily accomplished with a long handled bipolar energy source. After the removal of the tumor (Figure 22-13), the operative field is submerged beneath irrigant, and a

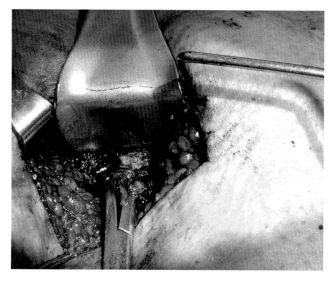

FIGURE 22-9. The tip of the coccyx is removed en bloc with the specimen.

proctoscope is used to insufflate the rectum to check for an air leak and assure that the rectum has not been violated. The soft tissue and the incision are closed in multiple layers over a closed suction drain (Figure 22-14).

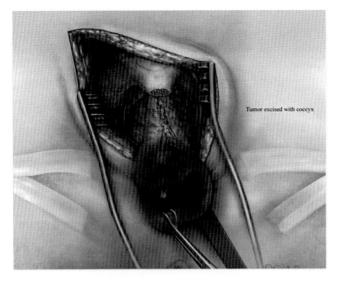

FIGURE 22-10. Now with access to the presacral space, the surgeon can carefully dissect the cyst off of the sacrum and "roll" it toward himself from cephalad to caudad (With permission from Ludwig KA, Kalady MF. Transsacral approaches for presacral cyst: rectal tumor. Operative Techniques in General Surgery 2005;7:3-126-136 © 2005 Elsevier Ltd. [32]).

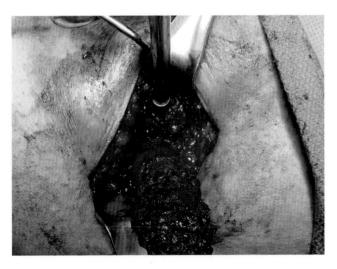

FIGURE 22-11. The presacral mass is mobilized off the rectal wall.

Combined Abdominal and Perineal Approach

Although there are subsets of tumors that are appropriate for a purely abdominal approach, it is advisable to prepare the patient as if a combined abdominal approach is planned to allow for all contingencies. The patients should be placed in lithotomy so that if a perineal or posterior approach is needed, access to the area has been anticipated and facilitated. Ureteric stents can be placed in bulky, high tumors.

A standard midline incision is utilized, and a thorough examination of all quadrants of the abdomen should be performed to assure that there are no metastases. The sigmoid

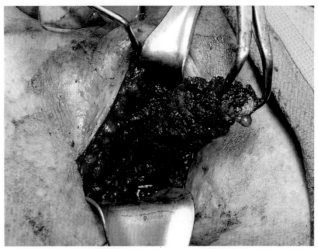

FIGURE 22-12. Side view of the coccyx tip and mass en bloc dissection from the rectal wall.

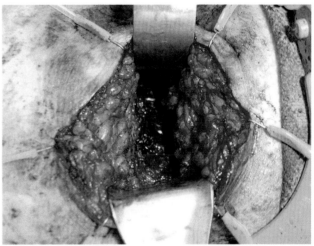

FIGURE 22-13. With the specimen out, a large cavity is present, and the posterior rectal wall can be visualized.

colon is mobilized along the white line of Toldt, and the presacral space is entered at the level of the sacral promontory in the same fashion as a total mesorectal excision. The left and right hypogastric nerves are identified and preserved. The rectum is pulled forward. The lesion can then be dissected away from the mesorectum with preservation of the rectum.

When the lesion is large (Figure 22-15) and the space is small or visualization posteriorly is less than ideal, there are several maneuvers that can aid with visualization and facilitate posterior dissection. The lateral stalks can be taken down to the level of the levators, and the rectum can be mobilized anteriorly to the pelvic floor; in addition the superior rectal artery can be divided at the level of the sacral promontory to take tension of the mesentery, and the root of sigmoid and left colon mesentery can be detached from the retroperitoneum and aorta all the way to the root of the inferior mesenteric

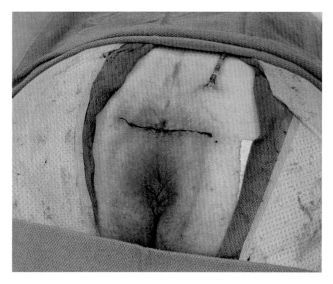

FIGURE 22-14. The incision is closed in multiple layers over a suction drain.

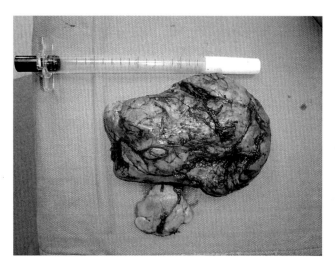

FIGURE 22-15. A large presacral mass.

artery. These maneuvers, in combination, allow the rectum to be pulled up and out of the pelvis to allow easier visualization of the dissection planes and better retraction. There is often a feeding vessel to the tumor in the midline, and ligating the middle sacral vessels can often help stem potential blood loss. The tumor is then dissected anteriorly off of the rectum and posteriorly off of the sacrum and laterally off of the sidewalls. In situations where tumor is densely adherent to the posterior rectum, a proctectomy should be performed for en bloc removal with the tumor. Most of the time, a stapled low colorectal anastomosis can be performed, but on occasion a hand-sewn coloanal anastomosis may be necessary.

If the internal iliac artery or vein needs to be sacrificed, communication with the anesthesiologist in advance of ligation is ideal, as the sacrifice of these vessels can sometimes be associated with large-volume bleeding misadventures and

blood products should be on hand. If the involvement of these vessels is identified preoperatively, catheter-based venous or arterial embolization can be considered in advance of surgery.

In situations where the lowermost portion of the tumor cannot be reached from the abdominal approach, there are two options: the first is to place the patient in high lithotomy and proceed via a posterior approach, and the second is to close the abdomen and place the patient in prone jackknife position. The visualization and performance of the posterior approach with the patient placed in high lithotomy are challenging, and it is our preference to close the abdomen and subsequently flip the patient to the prone jackknife position. The visualization is superior, and the incidence of cyst perforation is much lower. In addition, partial sacrectomy of the lower sacrum including nerve rootlets can be accomplished via this approach when necessary.

In patients where the tumor is quite large and the anticipated pelvic or perineal defect is quite large, there are several options for tissue interposition or reconstruction. A transabdominal rectus abdominis myocutaneous (TRAM) flap can be transposed into the pelvis to fill fairly impressive defects. For more modest defects, less morbid options may be V-Y fasciocutaneous flap closure and unilateral or bilateral gracilis transposition.

Closed suction drainage of the pelvis and the perineum should be performed in these patients.

Outcomes

Malignant Lesions

In a single institutional report, Messick et al. reported on 87 patients who had excision of retrorectal tumors; the overall recurrence rate was 16 %, with the recurrence rate of malignant tumors being 30 %. In this particular series, all of the recurrences in the malignant cohort were distant, and the median survival was 47.5 months [5]. In series where the tumors are extracted piecemeal or the tumors are violated, the recurrence rate can be as high as 65 % or higher [21, 27].

Although retrorectal sarcomas tend to be locally advanced, half of all patients have reasonable long-term survival. Dozois et al. reported a median survival of 4.7 years with survival at 2 and 5 years reported at 75 and 55 %, respectively [24]. In other data acquired from the Surveillance, Epidemiology, and End Results (SEER) program, McMaster and colleagues reported on sacral chordomas, which represent 29 % of all chordomas. In this study, the 5- and 10-year survival rates for sacral chordomas were 74 and 32 %, respectively [13]. Another series of 39 patients with malignant retrorectal tumors by Cody and associates reported a 5- and 10-year survival of 50 and 37 %, respectively. In this series, 38 % of these tumors were chordomas and 15 % were neurogenic tumors [2].

Finally, Wang and colleagues reported a series of 45 patients with presacral tumors, in which 48 % of the patient had malignant tumors. Incomplete resections were associated with inferior outcomes. The 5-year survival rate for malignant tumors was 41 % [28].

Benign/Cystic Lesions

The Cleveland Clinic series of tumors located strictly below S4 reported that 95 % were approached via a posterior approach only, and the local recurrence rate for the benign cohort was 11 %. Coccygectomy was performed in 51 % of patients; however, there was no difference in the recurrence rates between patients that underwent coccygectomy and those that did not [5]. Glasgow et al. published a series of 34 patients with retrorectal tumors where 26 patients had benign tumors. At a mean follow-up of 22 months, none of the patients in the benign group had recurred [29]. Another series by Jao and associates reported on a series of presacral lesions, of which 66 were benign retrorectal tumors. Of note, there was a 15:1 ratio of females to males. The overwhelming majority of the lesions were resected through a posterior approach, with 10 of 66 patients experiencing a recurrence [4].

Conclusion

Presacral tumors represent a diverse set of tumors with a strong predominance of the congenital cysts. The symptomatology of these tumors is often vague, and early diagnosis is an unusual event. Many of these tumors are found on digital rectal examination, and many are found incidentally on imaging or in the workup of nonspecific symptomatology. The tumors can have solid, cystic, or mixed features. Surgical extirpation is recommended for almost all tumors, as they a third can contain a malignancy and they can undergo malignant degeneration. MRI is essential in preoperative planning, as in a multidisciplinary team. Biopsy of lesions should only be reserved for lesions that are thought to be unresectable or metastatic. The majority of lesions that are below the S4 level can be approached via a posterior approach. Larger or more locally advanced lesions may require both an abdominal and perineal approach with en bloc resections of a portion of the sacrum or rectum. Lesions that are resected completely without disruption have a better prognosis than those that are not.

References

1. Hobson KG, Ghaemmaghami V, Roe JP, Goodnight JE, Khatri VP. Tumors of the retrorectal space. Dis Colon Rectum. 2005;48(10):1964–74.
2. Cody 3rd HS, Marcove RC, Quan SH. Malignant retrorectal tumors: 28 years' experience at Memorial Sloan-Kettering Cancer Center. Dis Colon Rectum. 1981;24(7):501–6.
3. Uhlig BE, Johnson RL. Presacral tumors and cysts in adults. Dis Colon Rectum. 1975;18(7):581–9.
4. Jao SW, Beart Jr RW, Spencer RJ, Reiman HM, Ilstrup DM. Retrorectal tumors. Mayo Clinic experience, 1960-1979. Dis Colon Rectum. 1985;28(9):644–52.
5. Messick CA, Hull T, Rosselli G, Kiran RP. Lesions originating within the retrorectal space: a diverse group requiring individualized evaluation and surgery. J Gastrointest Surg. 2013;17(12):2143–52.
6. Gunterberg B, Kewenter J, Petersen I, Stener B. Anorectal function after major resections of the sacrum with bilateral or unilateral sacrifice of sacral nerves. Br J Surg. 1976;63(7):546–54.
7. Gunterberg B, Petersen I. Sexual function after major resections of the sacrum with bilateral or unilateral sacrifice of sacral nerves. Fertil Steril. 1976;27(10):1146–53.
8. Bullard Dunn K. Retrorectal tumors. Surg Clin North Am. 2010;90(1):163–71. Table of Contents.
9. Singer MA, Cintron JR, Martz JE, Schoetz DJ, Abcarian H. Retrorectal cyst: a rare tumor frequently misdiagnosed. J Am Coll Surg. 2003;196(6):880–6.
10. Abel ME, Nelson R, Prasad ML, Pearl RK, Orsay CP, Abcarian H. Parasacrococcygeal approach for the resection of retrorectal developmental cysts. Dis Colon Rectum. 1985;28(11):855–8.
11. Springall RG, Griffiths JD. Malignant change in rectal duplication. J R Soc Med. 1990;83(3):185–7.
12. Hickey RC, Martin RG. Sacrococcygeal teratomas. Ann N Y Acad Sci. 1964;114:951–7.
13. McMaster ML, Goldstein AM, Bromley CM, Ishibe N, Parry DM. Chordoma: incidence and survival patterns in the United States, 1973-1995. Cancer Causes Control. 2001;12(1):1–11.
14. Williams B. Cerebrospinal fluid pressure changes in response to coughing. Brain. 1976;99(2):331–46.
15. Stewart RJ, Humphreys WG, Parks TG. The presentation and management of presacral tumours. Br J Surg. 1986;73(2):153–5.
16. Freier DT, Stanley JC, Thompson NW. Retrorectal tumors in adults. Surg Gynecol Obstet. 1971;132(4):681–6.
17. Hosseini-Nik H, Hosseinzadeh K, Bhayana R, Jhaveri KS. MR imaging of the retrorectal-presacral tumors: an algorithmic approach. Abdom Imaging. 2015;40(7):2630–44.
18. Sung MS, Lee GK, Kang HS, Kwon ST, Park JG, Suh JS, et al. Sacrococcygeal chordoma: MR imaging in 30 patients. Skeletal Radiol. 2005;34(2):87–94.
19. Luken 3rd MG, Michelsen WJ, Whelan MA, Andrews DL. The diagnosis of sacral lesions. Surg Neurol. 1981;15(5):377–83.
20. Bohm B, Milsom JW, Fazio VW, Lavery IC, Church JM, Oakley JR. Our approach to the management of congenital presacral tumors in adults. Int J Colorectal Dis. 1993;8(3):134–8.
21. Lev-Chelouche D, Gutman M, Goldman G, Even-Sapir E, Meller I, Issakov J, et al. Presacral tumors: a practical classification and treatment of a unique and heterogeneous group of diseases. Surgery. 2003;133(5):473–8.
22. Macafee DA, Sagar PM, El-Khoury T, Hyland R. Retrorectal tumours: optimization of surgical approach and outcome. Colorectal Dis. 2012;14(11):1411–7.
23. Sagar AJ, Tan WS, Codd R, Fong SS, Sagar PM. Surgical strategies in the management of recurrent retrorectal tumours. Tech Coloproctol. 2014;18(11):1023–7.
24. Dozois EJ, Jacofsky DJ, Billings BJ, Privitera A, Cima RR, Rose PS, et al. Surgical approach and oncologic outcomes

following multidisciplinary management of retrorectal sarcomas. Ann Surg Oncol. 2011;18(4):983–8.

25. Merchea A, Dozois EJ. Lesions originating within the retrorectal space. J Gastrointest Surg. 2014;18(12):2232–3.

26. Aktug T, Hakguder G, Sarioglu S, Akgur FM, Olguner M, Pabuccuoglu U. Sacrococcygeal extraspinal ependymomas: the role of coccygectomy. J Pediatr Surg. 2000;35(3):515–8.

27. Kaiser TE, Pritchard DJ, Unni KK. Clinicopathologic study of sacrococcygeal chordoma. Cancer. 1984;53(11):2574–8.

28. Wang JY, Hsu CH, Changchien CR, Chen JS, Hsu KC, You YT, et al. Presacral tumor: a review of forty-five cases. Am Surg. 1995;61(4):310–5.

29. Glasgow SC, Birnbaum EH, Lowney JK, Fleshman JW, Kodner IJ, Mutch DG, et al. Retrorectal tumors: a diagnostic and therapeutic challenge. Dis Colon Rectum. 2005;48(8): 1581–7.

30. Ghosh J, Eglinton T, Frizelle FA, Watson AJ. Presacral tumours in adults. Surgeon. 2007;5(1):31–8.

31. Loock MT, Fornès P, Soyer P, Rousset P, Azizi L, Hoeffel C. MR imaging features of nongynaecologic cystic lesions of the pelvis. Clin Imaging. 2013;37(2):211–8.

32. Ludwig KA, Kalady MF. Transacral approaches for prescral cyst: rectal tumor. Oper Tech Gen Surg. 2005;7: 3-126-136.

23

Molecular Basis of Colorectal Cancer and Overview of Inherited Colorectal Cancer Syndromes

Matthew F. Kalady and Y. Nancy You

Key Concepts

- Colorectal cancer is a genetically heterogeneous disease that arises via at least three main oncogenic pathways: chromosomal instability, microsatellite instability, and the methylator phenotype. Each pathway produces distinct but overlapping clinical phenotypes. These pathways are represented in sporadic colorectal cancer as well as in hereditary colorectal cancer syndromes.
- Identification and diagnosis of a hereditary colorectal cancer syndrome require a high level of suspicion and appropriate knowledge to evaluate the patient and at-risk family members. These syndromes have distinct genetic and clinical traits and are broadly classified into polyposis (adenomatous, hamartomatous, serrated polyps) and non-polyposis (HNPCC and Lynch syndrome).
- Familial adenomatous polyposis is a multisystem disease that confers a near 100 % colorectal cancer malignancy risk. Close endoscopic surveillance and timely prophylactic surgery are required to limit colorectal cancer formation. Desmoid disease and duodenal adenocarcinoma are other leading causes of morbidity and mortality.
- *MutYH*-associated polyposis (MAP) is a recessively inherited syndrome that carries an approximately 75 % lifetime risk of colorectal cancer. Annual colonoscopic surveillance is necessary, and surgery is indicated for uncontrolled polyp burden or the development of adenocarcinoma. Extended colectomy should be offered in healthy patients.
- The hamartomatous syndromes (Peutz-Jeghers syndrome, juvenile polyposis syndrome, and PTEN hamartoma syndrome) are rare but are associated with significant colorectal cancer and extracolonic multisystem malignancy. Early recognition and extensive screening and surveillance protocols are required.
- Serrated polyposis syndrome is characterized by numerous and/or large serrated polyps. Although no genetic etiology has been identified, it carries an approximately 25 % risk of developing colorectal cancer. Annual colonoscopic surveillance is necessary and surgery is indicated for uncontrolled polyp burden or the development of adenocarcinoma. Extended colectomy should be offered in healthy patients.
- Lynch syndrome is the most common of the hereditary syndromes and is responsible for about 3 % of all colorectal cancers. Universal screening and systematic molecular analysis of newly diagnosed colorectal cancer for DNA mismatch repair deficiency provide an effective approach to identifying patients at risk for Lynch syndrome.
- Patients with Lynch syndrome face significantly elevated risks for colorectal and extracolonic cancers in multiple organs. Lynch syndrome patients benefit from colonoscopic screening and participation in a hereditary registry.
- After the development of an initial colorectal cancer, patients with Lynch syndrome have high risk for metachronous colorectal neoplasia. Extended resection (total abdominal colectomy for colon cancer and total proctocolectomy for rectal cancer) should be considered weighing risks of future malignancy and quality of life.

Introduction

Our understanding of the genetic and molecular changes leading to colorectal cancer (CRC) development continues to evolve. A complex system of checks and balances maintains normal colorectal mucosa homeostasis and integrity during cell division and replication. Alterations in these mechanisms can lead to malignant change. In general, CRC is a multistep process that entails the accumulation of genetic and epigenetic changes over time. Mutations in oncogenes may result in overexpression of a gene or pathway, leading to constitutive cellular signaling or proliferation. Conversely, mutations or loss of tumor suppressor genes may remove an inhibitory signal that produces uncontrolled cell growth.

© Springer International Publishing 2016
S.R. Steele et al. (eds.), *The ASCRS Textbook of Colon and Rectal Surgery*, DOI 10.1007/978-3-319-25970-3_23

Furthermore, mutations in caretaker genes may result in oncogenesis by losing the ability to induce apoptosis or repair damaged DNA. The underlying genetic and epigenetic changes leading to CRC influence the disease course including clinical phenotype, prognosis, and response to therapy.

Clinical management and research must be executed with the knowledge that CRC is not a single entity but rather a heterogeneous disease, different in each person. Understanding CRC in this context and classifying tumors based on their molecular underpinnings are needed to truly study the disease and meaningfully stratify clinical management. This applies to both sporadic CRC as well as CRC arising within a hereditary syndrome. There are at least three major molecular pathways that have been described for the development of CRC: chromosomal instability, microsatellite instability, and the methylator phenotype. Each pathway has unique characteristics, but there is some overlap between the pathways and two or more pathways may exist in the same patient. This chapter is not a comprehensive review of cancer genetics or even CRC genetics but provides an overview of the current understanding of both sporadic and hereditary CRC for the practicing surgeon.

Chromosomal Instability

Chromosomal instability is the most common form of genomic instability in CRC, accounting for about 75 % of all CRC [1]. Chromosomal instability refers to an alteration in the chromosome copy number or structure. Physical loss of a chromosome segment may delete entire genes and produce loss of heterozygosity for those genes. That is, as one allele is lost, only one functional copy of the gene exists and there is no longer redundancy for that gene. Loss of the second allele results in complete loss of that gene function. *APC* and *p53* are examples of tumor suppressor genes, whose loss via this mechanism results in chromosomal unstable CRC.

The traditional adenoma-to-carcinoma sequence as described by Vogelstein and Fearon is characterized by the accumulation of genetic changes over time and the prototype

chromosomal instability CRC [2]. An overview of this pathway is given in Figure 23-1. Clinically, CRCs arising via chromosomal instability tend to be located in the left colon, have male predominance, and develop later in life. Genetically, key genes mutated in this pathway include *APC*, *KRAS*, and *p53*.

APC

The adenomatous polyposis coli (*APC*) gene, a tumor suppressor, has been called the gatekeeper gene because it is the key initiating step to malignant transformation for many colorectal adenocarcinomas. The APC protein regulates the WNT signaling pathway via intracellular binding of β-catenin. Mutations in *APC* lead to transcription of no protein or a protein without normal function. Decreased quantity or function of APC protein allows for intracellular accumulation of β-catenin and thus increased translocation into the nucleus where it serves as a transcription factor responsible for proteins involved in cell signaling, proliferation, and cell-to-cell adhesion. Inherited *APC* mutations are the cause of familial adenomatous polyposis (FAP), which is discussed elsewhere in this chapter.

KRAS

KRAS is an oncogene involved in the mitogen-activated protein kinase (MAPK) pathway whose upstream signaling receptor is the epidermal growth factor receptor (EGFR). This pathway drives nuclear transcription of cellular proliferation. Oncogenic mutations turn on the KRAS signal and drive uncontrolled cell growth, regardless of upstream signaling. Thus, KRAS mutation status is an important factor when deciding to use monoclonal antibodies that target the EGFR signaling pathway to treat CRC. Mutant KRAS provides constitutive MAPK signaling and upstream blockage of EGFR is not effective in blocking MAPK [3]. RAS mutations are present in nearly 40 % of CRC [4]. In practical terms, the tumor should be tested for the KRAS mutation if the patient is being considered for anti-EGFR therapy

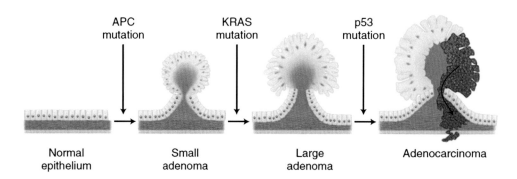

FIGURE 23-1. Schematic representation of the traditional adenoma-to-carcinoma sequence resulting in chromosomal instability.

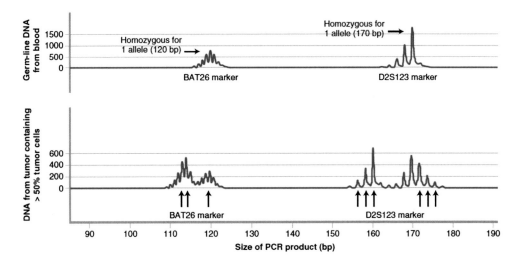

FIGURE 23-2. Example of DNA fragment lengths from polymerase chain reaction (PCR) products used to determine microsatellite instability. Two markers, BAT26 and D2S123, are shown here. The upper track readout is from germline DNA derived from patient blood. The lower track readout is from a portion of the patient's tumor that was histologically confirmed to contain at least 50 % cancer cells. In the germline track, BAT26 displays a single peak (*arrow*), indicating that the patient is homozygous for this marker. In the tumor DNA, there are two peaks for the BAT26 marker. The second peak represents a new allele (*double arrows*) in the tumor that is approximately five nucleotides smaller than the normal allele. This constitutes microsatellite instability for that marker. Marker D2S123 is homozygous in the germline (*arrow*), but two different new alleles exist in the tumor DNA (*triple arrows*). The allele on the left has lost approximately ten nucleotides and the allele on the right has gained two nucleotides. Thus, this marker also demonstrates microsatellite instability.

(e.g., cetuximab), and such therapy should not be instituted if the patient is found to have mutated KRAS CRC, as anti-EGFR therapy has been shown to be no more effective than supportive care in this situation.

p53

p53 is encoded by the gene *TP53* and preserves the cell cycle and genomic stability. As a tumor suppressor, p53 stops the cell cycle in G1/S phase to allow mutations or replications errors to be repaired. If the damage cannot be repaired, p53 may induce apoptosis. p53 is thought to be necessary to drive invasiveness of the lesion. It is rarely found in adenomas (5 %) and increased in malignant polyps (50 %) and is present in 75 % of invasive CRC [5].

Microsatellite Instability

Microsatellite instability results from faulty DNA mismatch repair (MMR) function. Routine DNA replication is associated with high infidelity, with specific sites along the DNA strand that are prone to errors. These sites are areas of repetitive DNA sequences, called microsatellites. Microsatellites are noncoding segments of DNA that contain repetitive sequences of one to four nucleotides. There are hundreds of thousands of microsatellites in the genome, and microsatellite patterns provide a unique DNA fingerprint. When these errors are not repaired due to MMR deficiency, the length of the microsatellite regions are altered and the fingerprint changes; i.e., there are different lengths of the DNA fragments. Thus, the pattern of fragments detected by PCR techniques produces a different pattern of microsatellites and thus the term microsatellite unstable or microsatellite instability high (MSI-H). An example of a DNA fragment length fingerprint is shown in Figure 23-2.

Functionally, loss of MMR function leads to an accumulation of unrepaired errors. Several key tumor suppressor genes have multiple short repetitive sequences that make them prone to DNA mismatch. Loss of MMR function allows the accumulation of mutations in these genes that subsequently lead to adenoma and cancer formation. Examples include TGF-β receptor II, BAX, and IGF2R. Cancers arising through this molecular pathway are termed the mutator phenotype as these tumors tend to be hypermutated and account for approximately 15 % of CRC [4]. Inherited mutations in one of the DNA mismatch repair genes result in Lynch syndrome, which is discussed elsewhere in this chapter.

CpG Island Methylator Phenotype (CIMP)

Epigenetic mechanisms such as hypermethylation of DNA promoter regions can affect gene expression and protein translation without changing the inherent DNA sequence.

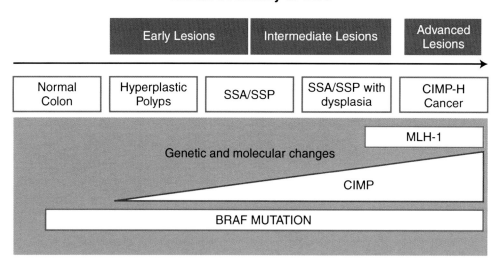

FIGURE 23-3. Schematic representation of proposed serrated pathway to colorectal cancer.

Methylation of cytosine is a common biological phenomenon that occurs throughout the genome and controls multiple processes. Several key tumor suppressor genes contain cytosine-guanine (CpG) repetitive sequences, which are prone to hypermethylation in the promoter region. Hypermethylation in the promoter region silences transcription of that gene, and thus no functional protein is made. As the areas prone to hypermethylation contain regions rich in cytosine and guanine dinucleotide repeats or CpG islands, they have been termed CpG island methylator phenotype (CIMP or CIMP high). The exact definition of CIMP is still debated, but it is characterized by the hypermethylation of a panel of markers [6]. This pattern is reproducible in approximately 20 % of CRCs and is associated with aberrant methylation of the mismatch repair gene, *MLH1*. Approximately 85 % of MSI-H CRCs develop via loss of the expression of the MMR gene, *hMLH1* caused by DNA hypermethylation. Methylation of other key genes and their contribution to CRC initiation are an area of intense study and research.

In contrast to CRC arising via chromosomal instability in which the precursor lesions are adenomatous polyps, the precursor lesions in CIMP cancers are serrated polyps. The sequence of mutations and contributions of specific mutations as initiators and drivers of oncogenic change continue to be defined. The most common initial mutation occurs in the *BRAF* oncogene [7]. *BRAF* mutations support the transformation of normal mucosa to aberrant crypt foci or a hyperplastic polyp or sessile serrated polyp (SSP). These altered cells become senescent as a protective mechanism so as not to propagate mutated cells. Senescence is controlled by p16. As methylation becomes more prevalent, loss of p16 via promoter methylation which keeps the cells senescent allows progression to more advanced polyps [8]. Increasing methylation gives rise to CIMP and eventual methylation of

MLH1, which in turn silences transcription. Loss of MLH1 results in MMR deficiency and thus the development of an MSI-H CRC. As CIMP CRCs develop through serrated polyp intermediates, this pathway is called the serrated pathway. An overview of this process is shown in Figure 23-3. Clinically, CIMP CRC tends to develop in the right colon, at advanced age, and is more common in females [9].

General Approach and Classification of Suspected Hereditary Syndromes

Awareness and suspicion are the keys to identifying hereditary CRC syndromes. Although only about 5–10 % of all CRCs arise with a known hereditary syndrome, recognizing these cases and making the correct diagnosis impact care of that particular patient and their family including future generations. Clinical evaluation should include a personal and family history, physical examination, documentation of gastrointestinal polyps or cancers, and identification of extracolonic manifestations. If the patient or family members have colorectal polyps, note should be made of the histology, size, location, and age at diagnosis. Family history can provide clues to the inheritance patterns and thus also the syndrome. This information can be used to broadly characterize the syndrome into polyposis or nonpolyposis. The histologic types of polyps (adenomas, hamartomas, or serrated polyps) further refine the possible syndromes. The main adenomatous polyposis syndromes are familial adenomatous polyposis (FAP) and *MUTYH*-associated polyposis (MAP). The more common of the extremely rare hamartomatous polyp syndromes include Peutz-Jeghers syndrome (PJS), juvenile polyposis syndrome (JPS), and PTEN hamartoma syndrome. A predominance of serrated polyps or large serrated polyps

TABLE 23-1. Classification and overview of hereditary colorectal cancer syndromes

Polyposis syndromes

Syndrome	Gene(s)	Main polyp type	Inheritance	Predominant clinical findings	Approximate CRC risk
FAP					
Classical	*APC*	Adenoma	AD	100–1000 adenomas; duodenal adenomas and carcinomas; gastric fundic gland polyps, desmoid tumors, epidermoid cysts, extra teeth, osteomas	100 %
Profuse	*APC*	Adenoma	AD	>1000 adenomas; duodenal adenomas and carcinomas; gastric fundic gland polyps, desmoid tumors, epidermoid cysts, extra teeth, osteomas	100 %
Attenuated	*APC*	Adenoma	AD	<100 adenomas; gastric fundic gland polyps, desmoid tumors, epidermoid cysts, extra teeth, osteomas	80 %
MAP	*MYH*	Adenoma	AR	0–1000 adenomas, CRC <50 years; gastric fundic gland polyps, duodenal adenomas, and carcinomas	80 %
JPS	*BMPR1A* *SMAD4*	Hamartoma	AD	≥5 juvenile polyps; any juvenile polyp and JPS family history; HHT	40 %
PJS	*STK11*	Hamartoma	AD	Peutz-Jeghers polyps Orocutaneous pigmentation Family history of PJP; cancer of small bowel, colon, stomach, pancreas, breast, ovary, testis	40 %
PHTS	*PTEN*	Hamartoma	AD	Colorectal adenomas, lipomas, fibromas, ganglioneuromas, juvenile hamartomas; colorectal cancer; macrocephaly, trichilemmomas	10 % (Cowden)
SPS	Unknown	Serrated polyps	Unknown	>20 serrated polyps Any serrated polyp and family history of SPS >5 serrated polyps proximal to the sigmoid, 2 are >1 cm diameter	25–40 %
Nonpolyposis syndromes					
Lynch syndrome	*MLH1, MSH2, MSH6, PMS2, EPCAM*	Adenoma	AD	Microsatellite-unstable CRC, advanced adenomas; gastric, duodenal, small bowel, transitional cell, gall bladder, pancreas, endometrial, ovarian	60–80 %
Familial CRC type X	Unknown	Adenoma	AD	Amsterdam criteria positive, microsatellite stable tumors	12 %

FAP familial adenomatous polyposis, *MAP* MUTYH-associated polyposis, *JPS* juvenile polyposis syndrome, *PJP* Peutz-Jeghers polyposis, *PHTS* PTEN hamartoma tumor syndromes, *SPS* serrated polyposis syndrome, *CRC* colorectal cancer, *HHT* hereditary hemorrhagic telangiectasia, *AD* autosomal dominant, *AR* autosomal recessive
With permission from Kalady MF, Heald B. Diagnostic approach to hereditary colorectal cancer syndromes. Clin Colon Rectal Surg. In press. © Thieme [223]

should raise suspicion for serrated polyposis syndrome (SPS), which is defined by clinical criteria. Nonpolyposis syndromes are generically referred to as hereditary nonpolyposis colorectal cancer (HNPCC) and are defined by patterns of cancer within the family. HNPCC is defined clinically by Amsterdam criteria, while Lynch syndrome is characterized by a genetic proclivity to colorectal and extracolonic cancers [10, 11].

A specific diagnosis is warranted to assign risk for cancer development and guide surveillance and prophylactic interventions. Information gained from the initial evaluation can guide the specific diagnostic tests required to make a diagnosis. Genetic counseling is a critical component to this evaluation and is recommended before genetic testing to discuss potential implications of the results. An overview of the classification of hereditary CRC syndromes is given in Table 23-1. Key distinguishing points about each of these syndromes are discussed in the remainder of this chapter.

Adenomatous Polyposis Syndromes

Familial Adenomatous Polyposis

Clinical Presentation

FAP is an autosomal dominant inherited disease that occurs in approximately 1:10,000 live births and affects both genders equally and all races. Patients with FAP may be asymptomatic or may present with bleeding, diarrhea, abdominal pain, or mucous discharge. Other symptoms such as anemia, obstruction, or weight loss usually occur as polyps grow larger in size or number and may foreshadow the presence of cancer. The hallmark feature of FAP is colorectal adenomatous polyposis, but the phenotype varies per patient, even within the same family. Severe FAP is characterized by thousands of colorectal adenomas. Oftentimes there is little normal mucosa between the adenomatous polyps. Mild

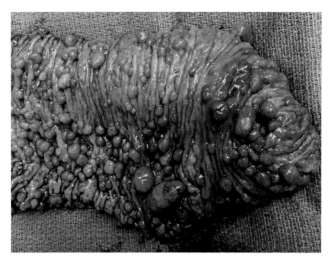

FIGURE 23-4. Moderate to severe polyposis in the resected specimen of a 22-year-old woman with familial adenomatous polyposis. Photo is courtesy of Matthew F. Kalady, MD.

polyposis is described as having between 100 and 1000 colorectal adenomas. Patients with fewer than 100 adenomas are considered to have attenuated FAP. Nearly 100 % of patients with FAP will develop CRC if left untreated. Figure 23-4 provides an example of moderate to severe polyposis.

FAP is a multisystem disease and may present with various extracolonic lesions. These include gastroduodenal adenomas and carcinoma, desmoid disease, osteomas, epidermoid cysts, papillary thyroid carcinoma, small bowel polyps and carcinoma, congenital hyperplasia of the retinal pigment epithelium (CHRPE), and dental anomalies. These extracolonic manifestations and their management recommendations are discussed later.

Two specific subtypes of FAP are based on a specific constellation of extracolonic manifestations. Gardner's syndrome is FAP with desmoid tumors, osteomas, epidermoid cysts, or extranumerary teeth [12]. Turcot syndrome is FAP associated with malignant tumors of the central nervous system [13]. Both syndromes are also caused by mutations in *APC*.

Underlying Genetics

FAP is caused by an inherited mutation in the *APC* gene on chromosome 5q21. As patients are born with only one functional copy of the "gatekeeper" gene, loss of the second allele via sporadic mechanisms leads to rapid development of hundreds to thousands of colorectal adenomas. More than 850 different mutations have been described, most of which produce a stop codon that ceases protein translation which yields a truncated APC protein. Depending on the location of the "stop," the truncated protein has variable functional abilities, likely accounting for some of phenotypic variation seen with different mutations. About 25 % of patients with FAP have a de novo mutation and thus have no family history.

Diagnosis

FAP may be diagnosed genetically or clinically. Genetic testing reveals an *APC* germline mutation in approximately 80 % of cases. Indications for genetic counseling referral and testing include a family history of FAP, personal history of more than ten adenomas, personal history of adenomas, and an extracolonic manifestation of FAP. For at-risk individuals in families with a known mutation, genetic testing is directed for that mutation. Approximately 20 % of patients will not have an identified germline mutation but still have the clinical phenotype. Additionally, some patients or families refuse genetic testing for various reasons. In this situation, a clinical diagnosis of adenomatous polyposis is made.

CRC Risk

FAP carries a near 100 % CRC risk. Cancers develop at a median age of 39. The goal of surveillance and intervention is to reduce the risk of death from colorectal cancer via colectomy or proctocolectomy before cancers develop. The risk of CRC in attenuated FAP is approximately 70 %, and cancers develop at a relatively later age (average 58 years) compared to classical FAP [14].

FAP Extracolonic Manifestations

Upper Gastrointestinal Tract

Approximately 90 % of patients with FAP develop duodenal adenomas. Despite the high incidence of adenomas, only about 5–10 % of patients will develop periampullary cancer [15]. Nonneoplastic gastric fundic gland polyps are a common finding, occurring in about 50 % of patients. These have a minimal risk of malignancy [16]. Rare gastric cancers in FAP are felt to develop from gastric adenomas that form in the gastric antrum in about 10 % of FAP patients.

Desmoids

Desmoid disease affects approximately 5 % patients with FAP. About half of FAP-associated desmoid tumors arise intra-abdominally in bowel mesentery and 40 % develop in the abdominal wall. The remainder present in the back, neck, or limbs. Desmoids can manifest as flat, fibrous, sheetlike lesions or as defined discrete masses (see Figure 23-5). Desmoids have been associated with female gender, a family history of desmoids, and *APC* mutations at the 3′ end of codon 1440. The majority of desmoids develop within 5 years after abdominal surgery, presumably as part of an inflammatory response [17, 18]. Church has proposed a desmoid risk factor score to delineate desmoid risk which incorporates gender, extracolonic FAP manifestations, and family history of desmoids, both with and without using genotype [19]. A recent study from the Cleveland Clinic reported that desmoid disease can occur with nearly any *APC* mutation,

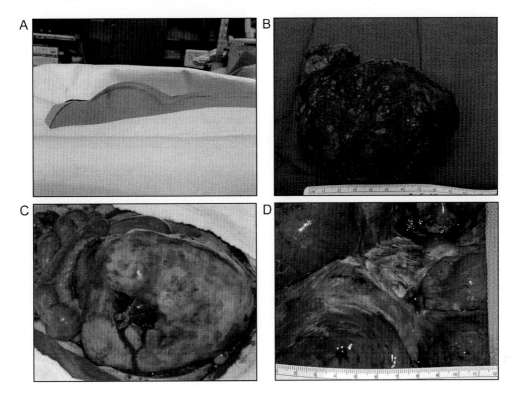

FIGURE 23-5. Different manifestations of desmoid disease. (a) Abdominal wall desmoid occurring 1 year after total proctocolectomy for familial adenomatous polyposis. (b) Resected abdominal wall desmoid. (c) Large intra-abdominal desmoid arising from the root of the small bowel mesentery. (d) Sheetlike desmoid tumor arising in the mesentery with associated desmoid reaction. Photos in (a) and (b) are courtesy of Matthew F. Kalady, MD. Photos in (c) and (d) are courtesy of Dr. James Church.

regardless of the location of the mutation in the gene. However, there is an increased propensity to develop desmoids, and clinically more severe desmoids, when the mutation is at the 3' end of the gene [20].

Thyroid Cancer

Although the risk of thyroid cancer in FAP is only 2 %, it is double the risk of that for the general population. The incidence is 17 times higher in women than in men and it develops at a young mean age of 27 years. The primary histology is papillary carcinoma [21–24].

Other Malignant Tumors

There are several rare extracolonic malignant tumors associated with FAP that have a higher incidence than the general population. These include pancreatic adenocarcinomas (relative risk 4.5; lifetime risk 1.7 %) [25], hepatoblastoma in children (RR 750–7500; absolute risk 2 %) [26, 27], and medulloblastoma (RR 7; lifetime risk (0.025 %) [28].

Other Benign Lesions

Several benign lesions are associated with FAP that do not necessarily require intervention but can be used to help make a diagnosis. Congenital hypertrophy of the retinal pigment epithelium (CHRPE) is characterized as well-delineated grayish-black or brown oval spots seen in 60–85 % of FAP patients [29]. Boney lesions including dental abnormalities and mandibular and skull osteomas are found in approximately 20 % of patients. Multiple cutaneous and subcutaneous lesions are associated with FAP including epidermoid cysts, lipomas, and fibromas. These are benign and intervention is not necessary unless they cause symptoms. The presence of these on the face, scalp, and extremities rather than on the back in young patients should raise suspicion for possible FAP.

Management

Screening

Colorectal: The goal of colorectal screening and surveillance in FAP is to limit CRC risk by timely intervention and surgical referral. Screening should be done on all individuals with a genetic diagnosis or in first-degree relatives of persons with a clinical diagnosis of FAP. If no genetic mutation is found in a family but they have a clinical diagnosis, all first-degree relatives should be screened. Screening begins at age 12 and can be initiated with flexible proctosigmoidoscopy. If polyps are seen, a full colonoscopy is warranted. If no polyps are identified on the initial proctosigmoidoscopy, the exam should be repeated every

TABLE 23-2. Scores of duodenal adenoma characteristics and management recommendations according to Spigelman criteria

Duodenal disease grading scale (points assigned)			
Assigned points	1	2	3
Number of polyps	1–4	5–20	>20
Size of polyps (mm)	1–4	5–10	>10
Histology	Tubular	Tubulovillous	Villous
Dysplasia	Mild	Moderate	Severe
Recommendations based on Spigelman score			
Total points	Spigelman stage	Recommendation	
0	0	Repeat endoscopy in 5 years	
1–4	I	Repeat endoscopy in 5 years	
5–6	II	Repeat endoscopy in 2–3 years	
7–8	III	Repeat endoscopy in 6–12 months	
9–12	IV	Surgical evaluation	

1–2 years or earlier if symptoms develop. For those without a genetic diagnosis, first-degree relatives who are not found to have any polyps by age 40 can safely be transitioned to screening guidelines for the general population.

Duodenal and gastric: Upper gastrointestinal endoscopic screening is a key part of FAP disease management. Screening is done with a side-viewing endoscope and should begin at age 20–25 years. Screening intervals are based on the Spigelman staging system (Table 23-2).

Desmoids: There are not recommendations for routine screening for desmoid disease.

Thyroid: Annual thyroid screening by ultrasound should be recommended to FAP patients. In a prospective study utilizing annual thyroid ultrasound on 192 asymptomatic patients with FAP, five patients (2.6 %) were found to have a thyroid cancer. Four of the five cancers were papillary carcinoma. Importantly, an additional 72 patients (30 %) had other thyroid nodules discovered during the screening examination [24].

Other neoplasia: Due to the overall low incidence of other rare tumors in FAP, routine screening is not recommended. Specific examinations may be considered if there is high penetrance of a particular extraintestinal cancer type within a family.

Treatment

Colorectal

The goals of FAP treatment are to remove or limit the CRC risk while maximizing quality of life. As CRC is near certain, surgical removal is the mainstay of treatment. The timing of surgery and choice of operation require consideration of multiple aspects of the disease and the patient. These choices are discussed below.

Timing of Surgery

Decisions for colorectal surgery in FAP depend on the presence of symptoms, the age at diagnosis, and personal patient circumstances. Patients with symptoms should be offered surgery both to treat the symptoms and to prophylactically treat potential occult cancer. For asymptomatic teenagers with FAP, surgery can be reasonably delayed until the late teen years or early twenties when they have reached physical and emotional maturity. CRC before the age of 20 is extremely rare and is usually accompanied by symptoms. Since cancer risk increases with age, patients diagnosed in their third decade or beyond should be offered surgery at the time of diagnosis.

Delaying surgery in an asymptomatic patient may be considered in specific circumstances. Examples include women with a low polyp burden who wish to have children. Since pelvic surgery decreases fecundity [30], it is reasonable to delay proctectomy as long as the patient remains in a strict surveillance program. Morbidly obese patients who wish to undergo ileal pouch-anal anastomosis (IPAA) may delay surgery, if they are able to lose weight, so that a restorative proctectomy may be more feasible. Also, patients who have desmoids in their family or have risk factors may delay surgery, as most desmoids develop after surgery. Deferral of surgery should only be done in patients who are asymptomatic, motivated, and adherent to surveillance protocols.

Extent of Resection

For patients without evidence of rectal cancer, surgical options include colectomy with ileorectal anastomosis (IRA) or total proctocolectomy (TPC) with or without restoration of the gastrointestinal tract. There are oncologic and functional implications of both procedures. Decisions are made based on balancing future cancer risk with quality of life associated with bowel function, as valued by both the patient and surgeon. TPC removes all or nearly all at-risk mucosa and almost completely eliminates future CRC risk. Restoration of the gastrointestinal tract via an ileal pouch-anal anastomosis (IPAA) results in more frequent bowel movements, higher incidence of incontinence, and decreased quality of life compared to colectomy and IRA [31–33]. The improved function of an IRA is countered by cancer risk in the residual rectum.

Patient selection is key to minimizing risk. An IRA is the preferred approach for patients who have a relatively low colorectal polyp burden. Church et al. have used polyp burden as one guide in determining the extent of resection. At a median follow-up of 12 years, of 95 patients treated with colectomy and IRA who had fewer than 1000 adenomas in the colon and fewer than 20 adenomas in the rectum, none required proctectomy. Conversely, of 33 patients who underwent an IRA and had more than 1000 colon adenomas and more than 20 rectal adenomas, 56 % underwent subsequent proctectomy for symptoms, uncontrolled polyp burden, or advanced neoplasia [34]. The genotype-phenotype correlation potentially influences decisions regarding the extent of resection. *APC* mutations at codons 1309 and 1328 are associated with severe polyposis and are independent risk factors for proctectomy after TAC in FAP [35].

In the presence of colon cancer and metastatic disease, decisions regarding whether to proceed with proctocolectomy instead of just colectomy should be based on the likelihood of cure and risk of metachronous cancer in the rectum if left in situ. Patients with locally advanced primary tumors (or those with possible metastatic disease) with minimal rectal polyp burden may be better served by abdominal colectomy and IRA (or proctocolectomy and ileostomy) vs. restorative proctocolectomy—where complications of surgery are more common and may delay administration of adjuvant chemotherapy. For patients who develop rectal cancer, total proctocolectomy should be performed with restoration of the gastrointestinal tract via an IPAA when possible. In the presence of stage IV disease with limited life expectancy, a proctectomy may be considered if there is no cancer in the colon and the polyp burden is minimal or controlled. If the rectal cancer is locally advanced and radiotherapy is required, it should be utilized in the preoperative period or not at all if a restorative proctocolectomy is planned, as postoperative radiotherapy is associated with toxicity and risk of ileal pouch loss. If an IPAA is not planned and radiotherapy is not given preoperatively, an omental pedicle flap or pelvic inlet mesh should be considered to occlude the small bowel from the pelvis in case postoperative radiotherapy is unexpectedly required. Adjuvant chemotherapy is given for stage III cancer.

Morbidity and quality of life should be considered when deciding the extent of surgery. Compared to colectomy and IRA, proctectomy is associated with increased urinary and sexual and urinary dysfunction complications [32], decreased fecundity in females [30], and reduced quality of life scores [33]. Given the fact that many of these operations are performed in young patients, the potential complications can be even more devastating. Therefore, an abdominal colectomy alone is favored, if appropriate from an oncologic standpoint and the patient is felt to be reliable with regard to surveillance.

Despite the argument that TPC removes the risk of CRC, a small percentage of patients may develop cancer in the anal transition zone or in the ileal pouch [36]. Debate exists over the use of mucosectomy and hand-sewn anastomosis vs. double-stapled anastomosis during TPC and IPAA as a means of reducing the risk of subsequent cancer. Mucosectomy to the dentate line theoretically removes all colorectal mucosa at risk for neoplasia. However, this technique potentially fails if an incomplete mucosectomy results in residual cells of rectal mucosa. Residual nests of rectal mucosa have been found either outside the ileal pouch or adjacent to the pouch-anal anastomosis in up to 21 % of patients undergoing prior mucosectomy [37].

This risk must be balanced against the cancer risk from a small anal transition zone that remains following a stapled IPAA. It may be preferable to have any at-risk mucosa in the lumen of the gut, where it can be observed over time, rather than implanted outside the ileal pouch at the time of mucosectomy, where it cannot be observed. In cases of rectal dysplasia or rectal cancer, many clinicians advocate mucosectomy, although definitive data regarding reduction in cancer risk are lacking.

The stapled IPAA leaves the distal anal mucosa and requires less manipulation of the sphincter complex, with less risk of postoperative incontinence. The Cleveland Clinic reported outcomes of the two different approaches in 119 patients treated by IPAA. Patients who underwent mucosectomy and hand-sewn anastomosis had worse seepage, higher incontinence rates, and more frequently used undergarment pads to protect against drainage [38]. The worse functional outcomes were tempered against less neoplasia. Fourteen percent of patients in the mucosectomy group developed adenomas in the anal transition zone, which was half of the rate of neoplasia in the non-mucosectomy, stapled anastomosis group. A meta-analysis by Lovegrove et al. included over 4000 patients from 21 studies comparing the two approaches. Worse nocturnal incontinence in the mucosectomy group correlated with anorectal physiology studies that demonstrate reduced and resting and squeeze pressures [39].

Duodenal Adenomas

Duodenal adenomas can progress to cancer, but this rate is relatively low and, as such, the lesions can usually be managed endoscopically. Burke et al. reported progression from adenoma to carcinoma in duodenal adenomas in 11 % of cases at 7-year follow-up [40]. Adenomas greater than 1 cm or those that contain high-grade dysplasia should be removed endoscopically [41]. If smaller polyps are not completely removed, representative biopsies need to be taken for accurate Spigelman staging which guides surveillance and treatment algorithms [42]. The Spigelman staging system estimates duodenal cancer risk based on several factors as given in Table 23-2. Early-stage lesions may safely be surveyed with low risk of cancer. However, those with Spigelman stage IV disease have a 36 % risk of adenocarcinoma [43]. Adenocarcinoma, persistent or recurrent high-grade dysplasia, or Spigelman stage IV disease warrants the consideration of surgery. Surgical options include pancreaticoduodenectomy or pancreas-preserving duodenectomy.

Desmoid Disease

Desmoid disease can be clinically devastating and is the second cause of death in FAP. Clinically, presentation ranges from asymptomatic to severe pain, obstruction, or fistulization. Treatment depends on symptoms, desmoid location, size, and extent of disease. Church has proposed a staging system for abdominal desmoids (Table 23-3) [44]. The Cleveland Clinic uses this staging system to guide medical management. Stage I desmoids are either observed or treated with a nonsteroidal anti-inflammatory drug such as sulindac (150–200 mg twice daily) [45]. Stage II desmoid treatment includes sulindac and antiestrogen therapy, such as raloxi-

Table 23-3. Proposed intra-abdominal desmoid disease clinical staging system

Disease stage	Clinical characteristics
I	Asymptomatic disease and not growing and <10 cm in maximum diameter
II	Minimally symptomatic and not growing or >10 cm in maximum diameter
III	Symptomatic disease or slowly growing or obstructive complications
IV	Symptomatic disease and rapidly growing or severe complications (e.g., fistula)

fene (60 mg twice daily) [46]. Stage III desmoids are usually treated with chemotherapy agents such as methotrexate and vinorelbine or Doxil [47, 48]. Stage IV desmoids are difficult to control and are treated with more aggressive anti-sarcoma chemotherapy such as Doxil or Adriamycin [49]. Although desmoid tumors are radiosensitive, the close proximity to the small bowel limits its use due to toxicity.

Surgery for abdominal desmoids is usually reserved for the treatment of disease complications such as bowel obstruction, enterocutaneous fistula, and ureteric obstruction. If possible, resection to negative margins is the goal. Intra-abdominal tumors are frequently located at the root of the small bowel mesentery and are often not resectable due to the proximity to critical small bowel blood supply. Enteroenteric or enterocolic bypass may provide a palliative option in these situations. Small bowel and multivisceral transplant have been described as treatment for desmoid disease and its complications. Intestinal transplantation for desmoid disease is a growing field, and there have been reports of success [50, 51].

Surgery is usually the first-line treatment for symptomatic abdominal wall desmoids. Due to the location, these tumors are usually able to be safely resected with minimal complications. The defect in the abdominal wall may need to be closed with tissue flaps or mesh.

Thyroid Neoplasia

Thyroid disease may be detected in FAP by evaluation of symptoms or routine ultrasound screening. Nodules larger than 1 cm should undergo fine-needle aspiration. Since cancers tend to be multifocal, thyroid cancer should be treated by total thyroidectomy and radioiodine ablation [52, 53].

Evaluation of At-Risk Relatives

As FAP is autosomal dominantly inherited, all first-degree relatives of an FAP patient have a 50 % chance of also having the disease. Therefore, all first-degree relatives in an FAP family should be evaluated. Due to the implications of both positive and negative results, pretest counseling, preferably with a genetic counselor, should be done. Potentially affected family members should be evaluated at the time of diagnosis or, for children, when they reach the age of 12. Evaluating a

potentially affected family member depends on the family situation. If there is a known APC mutation in the family, then germline DNA testing is appropriate. Importantly, if no mutation is detected, genetic testing for APC mutations in the family is not indicated. The clinical diagnosis of FAP guides surveillance and treatment recommendations. At-risk relatives in a family without a genetic diagnosis should undergo screening by flexible sigmoidoscopy at age 12 years or colonoscopy if the initial screening is done as an adult. Subsequent testing intervals for children depend on findings at the initial proctosigmoidoscopy. If polyps are seen, a full colonoscopy is warranted. If no polyps are identified, the exam should be repeated every 1–2 years or earlier if symptoms develop. For those without a genetic diagnosis, first-degree relatives who are not found to have any polyps by age 40 can safely be transitioned to screening guidelines for the general population.

MUTYH-Associated Polyposis

Clinical Presentation

Approximately 0.3 % of CRC patients have MAP. The clinical presentation is not distinct from other patients with colorectal polyps or cancer. Bleeding or obstruction may occur, but the disease is suspected on findings from a screening colonoscopy. The syndrome is primarily characterized by multiple colorectal adenomas and an increased risk for CRC at a younger age (40–50s), but the colorectal polyp phenotype is highly variable. Moderate polyposis (less than 100 adenomas) is the most common phenotype and occurs in 11–42 % of reported cases [54–56]. Biallelic MUTYH mutations are rare among patients with profuse adenomatous polyposis [57].

Polyposis is not necessary for an MAP diagnosis, and as many as 20 % of patients present with colorectal cancer without a history of colorectal polyps or synchronous polyps [58]. Some authors have proposed calling the syndrome MYH-associated neoplasia (MAN) instead of MAP to avoid diagnostic confusion given the lack of polyposis in a significant amount of patients [59]. MAP is the only hereditary CRC syndrome with an autosomal recessive inheritance pattern, and thus family history may help guide counseling and testing in patients who are suspected of having MAP.

Despite the similar colorectal phenotype to FAP, patients with MAP are less likely to have the extracolonic manifestations that are commonly seen in FAP. Approximately 20 % of patients with MAP will have duodenal polyposis, and gastric fundic polyps are rare. Osteomas, desmoids, and CHRPE are not associated with MAP.

Underlying Genetics

MAP is caused by inherited biallelic mutations in the MUTYH gene, which codes for a base excision repair protein. Approximately 1–2 % of the general population carries a

MUTYH mutation. Mutations at Y179C (previously referred to as Y165C) and G396D (previously referred to as G382D) cause approximately 80 % of MAP in persons who are of Northern European descent [60]. *MUTYH* is located on the short arm of chromosome 1 and encodes MYH glycosylase, a DNA base excision repair protein. Specifically MYH glycosylase repairs DNA G:C to T:A transversions and thus corrects potential mutations [61, 62]. A *MUTYH* causes defective base excision repair function and subsequently the accumulation of unrepaired G:C to T:A transversions caused by oxidative damage. Importantly, the phenotype of MAP is related to the gene that is affected by the unrepaired transversions. For example, *APC* contains an abundance of guanine nucleotides, and in the absence of MYH function, these transversions go unrepaired and the phenotype appears as if APC is defective. This explains why the phenotype of MAP is similar to that of FAP. When G:C to T:A transversions occur and remain uncorrected in a DNA mismatch repair gene, the mutator phenotype and microsatellite-unstable neoplasia ensue [63]. If a gene involved in control of methylation is predominantly affected by the transversions and a mutated MYH protein does not repair the errors, a methylated tumor may develop [64, 65].

Diagnosis

MAP diagnosis is confirmed by genetic testing for mutations in the *MUTYH* gene. Germline *MUTYH* testing should be offered to patients who have a recessive pattern of family history of colorectal cancer or polyposis, who have a clinical phenotype of FAP or attenuated FAP but test negative for an *APC* mutation, or who have a personal history of >10 colorectal adenomas. Nearly 30 % patients with a clinical phenotype of FAP without an identified *APC* mutation have biallelic *MUTYH* mutations [66, 67].

CRC Risk

The cumulative lifetime risk of developing colorectal cancer for patients with biallelic *MUTYH* mutations is estimated at 75 % for males and 72 % for females by age 70 [68]. Onset of cancer is earlier than sporadic colorectal cancer, with the mean age of diagnosis reported between 45 and 56 years old [54, 67, 69, 70]. The risk of CRC for monoallelic *MUTYH* carriers continues to be defined. Data from the Colon Cancer Family Registry estimate the cumulative lifetime risk of developing CRC for people with monoallelic *MUTYH* mutations at 7.2 % for males and 5.6 % for females by age 70 [68].

Extracolonic Cancer Risk

The spectrum of extracolonic neoplasia in MAP continues to be defined. An increased risk of upper gastrointestinal polyps and cancers is consistently reported [67, 71]. About 17 % of cases have duodenal adenomas with a lifetime duodenal cancer risk of 4 %. The overall incidence of malignancy outside the gastrointestinal tract is 38 %, almost double that of the general population. The most common extraintestinal cancers found in a study of 276 international cases from Germany, the United Kingdom, and the Netherlands were bladder, ovarian, and skin cancers with standard incidence ratios of 7.2, 5.7, and 2.8, respectively [71]. Some studies report an increased risk of thyroid cancer to approximately double that of the general population, at an average age at diagnosis of 25–33 years [71, 72]. Benign and malignant sebaceous gland tumors have also been reported in MAP.

Management

Screening

Screening and surveillance are difficult as most cases of MAP are diagnosed at the time of CRC detection. In the rare cases when an individual is diagnosed with biallelic *MUTYH* mutations (as may be done with appropriate genetic counseling and testing) but does not have an indication for colectomy, colonoscopy screening should begin at age 25–30 years. If no neoplasia is identified on the exam, it should be repeated every 3–5 years with consideration for decreasing the interval with advancing age [73, 74]. Any polyps found on colonoscopy should be removed and examined histologically. When polyps are present, the interval is shortened to 1–2 years depending on the findings. Patients with a polyp burden that cannot be controlled endoscopically should be referred for consideration of colectomy.

Esophagogastroduodenoscopy with side-viewing gastroscope should be performed to evaluate for duodenal adenomatous neoplasia. This screening should start at age 30 years and repeated every 3–5 years if the exam is normal. For patients with duodenal adenomas, management is similar to the recommendations for FAP patients with duodenal adenomas [74]. The American College of Gastroenterology also recommends annual thyroid ultrasound screening in patients with MAP. Despite the increased risk, the incidence is not high enough to warrant routine screening for the cancers outside the intestine [71].

As stated above, the risk of colorectal cancer development in monoallelic carriers is uncertain but most likely elevated. There is no consensus if routine screening should be done for these patients. Some clinicians have suggested screening these people by colonoscopy every 5 years, beginning 10 years earlier than the youngest patient afflicted with CRC in the family [74].

Treatment

The phenotype dictates treatment in MAP. Polyps should be removed endoscopically as able with follow-up colonoscopy at least annually. Indications for surgery include CRC, high-grade dysplasia in an adenoma that cannot be removed endoscopically, or a polyp burden that cannot be safely managed by colonoscopy. Surgical options include total abdominal colectomy, subtotal colectomy, or proctocolectomy. A segmental colectomy may be considered in certain circumstances such as metastatic cancer or medical comorbidities that preclude extended resection. Since the entire colon is at risk, a total colectomy and ileorectal anastomosis are recommended for otherwise healthy patients with curable disease. Patients with rectal cancer in MAP should be considered for proctocolectomy and ileal pouch-anal anastomosis. Any remaining colorectum should be surveyed annually, with the removal of subsequent polyps. Despite this rationale, there are no prospective data that show extended resection reduces the risk of subsequent colorectal cancers. One small study retrospectively reviewed 11 patients with biallelic *MUTYH* mutations and polyposis who underwent total abdominal colectomy and ileorectal anastomosis. Endoscopic findings of the remaining rectum using a yearly surveillance regimen were reported. At a median follow-up of 5 years using an annual surveillance regimen, no patient developed rectal cancer [75].

Evaluation of At-Risk Relatives

As this syndrome is autosomal recessive, patients must have two abnormal alleles to manifest the disease. Each sibling of an affected individual has a 25 % chance of also having the disease. Different from other inherited colorectal cancer syndromes, it is the siblings of patients with MAP that are at greatest risk, rather than the parents or children. Genetic counseling and testing for specific *MUTYH* mutation in the family should be offered at the age of 18 years to reduce morbidity and mortality through early diagnosis and treatment. Children of biallelic patients will be at least a monoallelic carrier. Approximately 1 % of the general population is a monoallelic carrier. If the spouse of the affected patient is a carrier, then each offspring has a 50 % chance of having MAP. Therefore, the partner of the affected patient should be tested to evaluate risk to the offspring.

Polymerase Proofreading-Associated Polyposis

A new syndrome has recently been reported as polymerase proofreading-associated polyposis (PPAP). This syndrome continues to be defined and has only been characterized in a few families [76, 77]. It is inherited in an autosomally dominant fashion and caused by a germline mutation in proofreading regions of one of two DNA polymerases, POLE and POLD1. The resulting cancers are microsatellite stable and have chromosomal instability. The clinical phenotype is one of oligo-adenomatous polyposis and early-age CRC and endometrial cancer. Guidelines are in evolution, but expert opinions support surveillance via colonoscopy every 1–2 years starting at age 20–25 and EGD every 3 years. For females with a POLD1 mutation, endometrial cancer screening by ultrasound is recommended starting at age 40 years.

Hamartomatous Polyposis Syndromes

Hamartomas are nonneoplastic growths of an abnormal mixture of tissue that is normally found at that anatomic site. Juvenile polyps and Peutz-Jeghers polyps are hamartomatous polyps in the small bowel and colorectum. Although these lesions are generally not considered neoplastic, they can be the hallmark of inherited hamartomatous polyposis syndromes such as juvenile polyposis syndrome (JPS), Peutz-Jeghers syndrome (PJS), and the PTEN hamartoma tumor syndrome (PHTS). These syndromes are rare but clinically important as they predispose to colorectal and other cancers. Less than 1 % of all CRC is associated with hamartomatous polyposis syndromes. Recognition of these syndromes is important so that appropriate genetic counseling and testing may be performed and cancer risk can be accurately assigned and appropriate surveillance done.

Juvenile Polyposis Syndrome

Clinical Presentation

Juvenile polyps are usually round, smooth, cherry-red lesions that are often pedunculated on a long stalk. An abundance and overgrowth of the lamina propria with mucin-filled spaces are the characteristic histologic features. Chronic inflammatory cells are often seen which can lead to an inaccurate diagnosis of inflammatory polyp. Juvenile polyps occur throughout the gastrointestinal tract including the stomach, small bowel, colon, and rectum, starting in the first or second decade of life. The number of polyps varies from a few to hundreds. Symptoms are related to the polyps and most commonly include acute or chronic gastrointestinal bleeding, iron-deficiency anemia, prolapsed rectal polyps, abdominal pain, or diarrhea [78, 79]. JPS is also associated with extracolonic congenital malformations such as cardiac and cranial abnormalities, duplication of the renal pelvis, cleft palate, gut malrotation, and polydactyly [78, 80]. JPS along with a *SMAD4* mutation may present as hereditary hemorrhagic telangiectasia (HHT) [81]. HHT may manifest with skin and mucosal telangiectasias; cerebral, pulmonary, and hepatic arteriovenous malformations; and an increased risk of associated hemorrhage [82, 83].

Underlying Genetics

JPS is an autosomal dominantly inherited disease caused by germline mutations in *BMPR1A* or *SMAD4*. Approximately 20 % of JPS cases have detectable SMAD4 mutations whose normal function is as a tumor suppressor in the transforming growth factor beta (TGF-β) signal transduction pathway [84]. Another 25 % of JPS cases will have an alteration in *BMPR1A* [84–86]. This gene is also involved in the TGF-β superfamily by regulating BMP intracellular signaling through SMAD4. ENG1 mutations have also recently been described to cause JPS [87]. About 60 % of JPS cases of JPS are familial, while the remaining 40 % occur sporadically [88].

Diagnosis

JPS diagnosis is based on clinical criteria which include the following: (1) more than five juvenile polyps of the colon or rectum, (2) juvenile polyps in the extracolonic gastrointestinal tract, or (3) any number of juvenile polyps and a positive family history [80]. Patients that satisfy any of these criteria should be offered genetic counseling and genetic testing. A causative germline mutation is identified in approximately 50 % of cases.

CRC and Extracolonic Risk

JPS patients have an approximately 50 % lifetime CRC risk, with reports of varying incidence between 17 and 68 % [89–91]. The mean age of CRC diagnosis is 43 years [92], but CRC may develop at a young age and there is a case report of CRC in a 15-year-old patient [80]. The stomach, duodenum, pancreas, and jejunum are at increased risk for cancer in JPS. The risk of gastric or duodenal cancer is 15–21 % [90, 93]. *SMAD4* mutations are associated with a higher risk of extracolonic cancer compared to patients with *BMPR1A* mutations [94].

Management

Screening

Screening by colonoscopy should begin at age 12–15 or earlier if symptoms are present [74, 95]. The interval between colonoscopies depends on the exam findings. If there are no polyps, colonoscopy should be repeated in 2–3 years. Any polyps seen should be removed at colonoscopy and examined histologically. When polyps are present and removed, colonoscopy should be done annually until an exam is clear, after which the interval may be extended to every 2–3 years. Upper gastrointestinal screening should begin between ages 15 and 25 or earlier if symptoms develop. Endoscopic management principles follow those as given for adenomas of the upper GI tract.

Treatment

Surgical indications include the presence of high-grade dysplasia or cancer or if the polyp burden cannot be effectively managed endoscopically. Prophylactic colectomy may be considered for patients with poor surveillance compliance or those with a family history of CRC. For colorectal disease, surgical options include colectomy and ileorectal anastomosis, subtotal colectomy with ileosigmoid anastomosis, or total proctocolectomy. The authors favor abdominal colectomy with ileorectal anastomosis unless there is rectal cancer or symptoms referred to rectal disease. Risk of proctectomy after colectomy is approximately 50 % at 9 years, with a range of 6–34 years in one small retrospective study [96].

Surgery for the upper gastrointestinal tract is indicated for significant symptoms, malignancy, or development of protein-losing gastropathy or enteropathy. For gastric disease, subtotal gastrectomy is usually done. For small bowel disease, treatment is segmental resection.

Evaluation of At-Risk Relatives

If a specific mutation is identified in an individual, all at-risk family members should be counseled and tested for that mutation. Approximately 75 % of patients will have an affected parent. If a parent carries the mutation, then siblings of the parent as well as siblings of the proband should be tested as they have a 50 % chance of also having the mutation. Children of the proband should also be tested after counseling and testing in the early teenage years. If a mutation is not found in the family, at-risk individuals should be initially screened for gastrointestinal polyps and followed accordingly based on results.

Peutz-Jeghers Syndrome

Clinical Presentation

Nearly 90 % of PJS patients will develop hamartomatous polyps [97], most commonly in the small bowel, followed by the colon, stomach, and rectum in decreasing frequency. Polyps vary in size from a few millimeters to several centimeters and tend to become pedunculated as they grow larger. Peutz-Jeghers polyps differ histologically from juvenile polyps in that they arise due to an overgrowth of the muscularis mucosa, rather than the lamina propria. They have less inflammatory infiltrate and less mucin than juvenile polyps. Multiple branching of the muscularis mucosa gives the histologic appearance of a tree under the microscope. Although the polyp burden is usually low (<20), the larger size of the polyp often cause symptoms of obstruction, pain, gastrointestinal bleeding, polyp prolapse per anus, or small bowel intussusception. Symptoms usually develop by the teen years or early twenties.

The classical extraintestinal lesion seen in PJS is benign mucocutaneous pigmentation, which is present in approximately 95 % of cases. The pigmentation is usually a small, dark-brown or blue-brown macule that is obvious in infancy but may fade in adolescence. The most common locations are the vermillion border of the lips (94 %), buccal mucosa (66 %), hands (74 %), and feet (62 %) [98, 99].

Underlying Genetics

PJS is autosomal dominantly inherited and caused by germ-line mutations in *STK11* [100]. This gene encodes a member of the serine/threonine kinase family, which functions as a tumor suppressor.

Diagnosis

PJS is a clinical diagnosis based on meeting any one of the following World Health Organization criteria: (1) three or more histologically confirmed Peutz-Jeghers polyps; (2) any number of Peutz-Jeghers polyps with a family history of PJS; (3) characteristic, prominent, mucocutaneous pigmentation with a family history of PJS; or (4) any number of Peutz-Jeghers polyps and characteristic prominent, mucocutaneous pigmentation [98]. An individual meeting any of the above criteria should be offered genetic counseling and testing.

CRC and Extracolonic Risk

Patients with PJS have an increased risk of developing colorectal and extracolonic cancers. PJS patients have more than 90 % estimated lifetime risk of developing cancer of some type [101]. The risk for developing breast, colon, pancreatic, and gastric cancer is 54, 39, 36, and 29 %, respectively. In addition, males are at risk for Sertoli cell testicular tumors and women for sex cord tumors with annular tubules of the ovary and adenoma malignum of the cervix.

Management

Surveillance

Given the broad spectrum of disease in PJS, surveillance is complex and includes multiple organs. Randomized controlled trials have not been performed to evaluate the efficacy of cancer surveillance protocols, and published recommendations are based on expert opinion. Specific testing depends on the patient's age and gender. The NCCN recommends starting screening at age 8–10 years via evaluation of the small bowel, with the interval exam based on findings. If initial exam is normal, then the repeat evaluation is recommended at age 18 years and then at 2–3-year intervals [73]. Males should undergo annual testicular physical examination starting at age 10 years, and females should undergo annual pelvic examination and Papanicolaou stain starting at age 18–20 years. Women should have breast physical examinations every 6 months and yearly mammogram and breast MRI starting at age 25 years. Colonoscopy and upper endoscopy should in the late teens be repeated every 2–3 years for both genders. Pancreatic cancer screening involves endoscopic ultrasound or MRCP along with serum CA19-9 every 1–2 years starting at age 25–30 years. Other screening regimens have been proposed by other authors [95, 98, 99].

Polypectomy

Endoscopic intervention plays a key role in the management of PJS. Polypectomy treats polyp-related symptoms and prophylactically prevents development of symptoms. As with the surveillance guidelines, intervention recommendations are based on expert opinion. Asymptomatic gastric or colonic polyps larger than 1 cm should be removed endoscopically. Small bowel polyps larger than 1–1.5 cm or those that are have grown rapidly from prior exam should be removed to decrease future complications such as bleeding and intussusception. Some symptomatic polyps may be beyond the reach of conventional endoscopy, and intervention may require push enteroscopy or combined laparoscopy/laparotomy with endoscopy in the operating room, which allows guidance of the endoscope further distally into the small bowel.

Surgery

Surgery is most commonly reserved for symptoms, the most common being obstruction and bleeding in the small bowel. Obstruction is often caused by intussusception. Most cases resolve spontaneously, but if the obstruction persists more than a few hours, surgery is required. The goal of surgery is to remove the affected segment, preserving as much bowel as possible. If surgery is required, a "clean sweep" at surgery is recommended to reduce the need for future operations [102]. This technique involves evaluating the entire small bowel and removing all polyps. An endoscope may be placed through the open resection ends of the bowel or via an enterotomy.

As in the other syndromes, development of high-grade dysplasia, colorectal cancer, or an uncontrolled colorectal polyp burden is indication for colorectal surgery. Total abdominal colectomy and ileorectal anastomosis are the preferred operation unless the pathology is in the rectum.

Evaluation of At-Risk Relatives

For individuals with a specific known mutation, at-risk family members should be tested for that mutation. Approximately 50 % of individuals will have an affected parent, and parents should be evaluated for PJS traits. If one of the parents is affected, then testing should be offered to the siblings of the proband. Additionally, all children of the proband have a 50 % risk of inheriting the mutation and should be tested accordingly. Genetic testing for at-risk family members may be performed at age 8 after appropriate genetic counseling and informed consent [98]. If a specific mutation is not identified in the affected individual, at-risk family members are surveyed as if they potentially have the disease. This includes surveillance of the colon, stomach, small bowel, pancreas, breast, ovary, uterus, cervix, and testes as described above.

PTEN Hamartoma Tumor Syndrome (PHTS)

PHTS is a spectrum of extremely rare hereditary syndromes that are characterized by hamartomatous polyps in the gastrointestinal tract and abnormalities of the skull, skeleton, and skin. The two main syndromes are Cowden syndrome and Bannayan-Riley-Ruvalcaba syndrome (BRRS).

Clinical Presentation

About 95 % of Cowden syndrome patients have colorectal polyps, ranging from few to hundreds in number and are distributed throughout the colorectum [103, 104]. The most common polyps are hamartomas, accounting for about 30 % of all polyps [103, 223]. Other types of polyps include adenomas, juvenile polyps, inflammatory polyps, leiomyomas, lipomas, fibromas, neurofibromas, and ganglioneuromas. Any of these polyps may present with obstruction or bleeding. The majority of patients have multiple histologic types of polyps. About 30 % of Cowden syndrome patients have macrocephaly. Trichilemmomas are considered to be pathognomonic. Other benign and malignant lesions of the breast, thyroid, uterus, and skin are seen in Cowden syndrome.

Underlying Genetics

Cowden syndrome and BRRS are both autosomally dominant inherited disorders associated with a *PTEN* mutation. *PTEN* is a tumor suppressor gene that encodes a phosphatase that is involved in the PI3K/AKT signaling pathway. It plays a key role in apoptosis. Approximately 80 % of patients who meet the diagnostic criteria for Cowden syndrome, and 60 % of patients with BRRS, have PTEN mutations [105, 106].

Diagnosis

The International Cowden Consortium developed clinical diagnostic criteria for Cowden syndrome, including both major and minor criteria [99, 107]. Major criteria include breast cancer, thyroid cancer (especially follicular), macrocephaly, endometrial cancer, and Lhermitte-Duclos disease. Minor features include benign thyroid changes (such as a goiter), mental retardation, hamartomatous intestinal polyps, fibrocystic changes in the breast, lipomas, fibromas, genitourinary tumors (such as kidney cancer or uterine fibroids), or malformations. Cowden syndrome is diagnosed if a patient has either macrocephaly or Lhermitte-Duclos disease and one other major feature. A diagnosis of Cowden is also made when a person has one major feature and three minor features or at least four minor features. Definitive diagnosis is based on a *PTEN* mutation.

Specific diagnostic criteria for BRRS are not established, but patients with macrocephaly, hamartomatous colonic polyposis, lipomas, and pigmented macules of the glans penis should be considered for genetic testing [108].

CRC and Extracolonic Risk

A recent study reported CRC in 13 % of *PTEN* mutation carriers in Cowden syndrome with early age of onset, all before the age of 50 years. The adjusted standardized incidence ratio was 224 (95 % confidence interval, 109.3–411.3; $P<0.0001$) [103]. Other groups have supported a 9–16 % lifetime risk for CRC cancer [104, 109, 110]. It is uncertain if the cancers develop from the hamartomatous or adenomatous polyps in PHTS. Most of PHTS cancer risk is extracolonic. Women have a 50 % lifetime risk of developing breast cancer and a 5–10 % lifetime risk of developing endometrial cancer. Men and women with Cowden syndrome have a 10 % lifetime risk of developing epithelial thyroid cancer.

Approximately half of the patients with BRRS will have hamartomatous polyps in the digestive tract, particularly in the ileum and colon [108] These polyps can become symptomatic but are not believed to increase the risk of colon cancer. Patients with BRRS have similar extracolonic malignancy risks as those with Cowden syndrome.

CRC Risk Management

There is debate regarding the need for colonoscopy screening in PHTS. Given the recent findings of increased CRC risk, we recommend starting colonoscopy at age 35, with repeat examinations every 1–2 years. Colectomy should be considered if the polyp burden cannot be controlled endoscopically or if cancer develops.

Evaluation of At-Risk Relatives

At-risk relatives should be counseled and tested for the presence of PTEN mutation. For families with PHTS but no detected gene mutation, at-risk individuals should be initially surveyed as if they have the disease. Screening includes the evaluation of the colorectum, stomach, small bowel, thyroid, breast, uterine, kidney, and skin [74].

Serrated Polyposis Syndrome (SPS)

Clinical Presentation

SPS is usually asymptomatic and is often detected on screening colonoscopy. Bleeding and diarrhea may be present if polyps become large or numerous. More than 90 % of SPS patients are of white European descent. It affects both men and women nearly equally with a slight female inclination. The median age at diagnosis ranges from 44 to 62 years, with extremes of age including SPS in a 10-year-old and a man in his eighties [111–114].

SPS encompasses a variety of clinical phenotypes and is likely a heterogeneous disease that has not yet been characterized genetically. It can be characterized by the presence of either multiple or large serrated colorectal polyps (see WHO diagnosis below). Serrated polyps are a family of polyps characterized by a classic serrated or sawtooth appearance of the arrangement of glands. The family consists of hyperplastic polyps, sessile serrated adenomas (SSAs) which are also called sessile serrated polyps (SSPs), SSAs or SSPs with dysplasia, and serrated adenomas. Different phenotypes have been described based on the size and number of serrated polyps. Some patients have multiple small polyps distributed throughout the colon, while others have a few large, right-sided polyps. The cancer risk is similar for both phenotypes [114]. In addition to serrated polyps, SPS patients often are prone to having adenomas [114, 115]. First-degree relatives do not have increased risk of extracolonic malignancy [116].

Underlying Genetics

A causative germline mutation has not been identified for SPS. There is no genetic testing for this syndrome.

Diagnosis

SPS is diagnosed by clinical criteria as defined by the World Health Organization as follows: (1) >20 serrated polyps of any size, distributed throughout the colon, (2) at least five serrated polyps proximal to the sigmoid colon with two or more of these being >10 mm, and (3) any number of serrated polyps proximal to the sigmoid colon in an individual who has a first-degree relative with SPS [117].

CRC Risk

Although the true incidence of CRC in SPS is yet to be defined by prospective studies, it is consistently reported as increased compared to the general population. Reports are variable from multiple relatively small series, ranging from 0 to 77 %, with an estimate of around 25 % [112–114, 118–125]. The initial SPS diagnosis is often made at the time of cancer diagnosis, and thus the natural history progression from SPS to cancer is uncertain [111, 114]. Bopari reported a 20 % CRC rate in a retrospective review of 77 SPS patients (without CRC at SPS diagnosis) who were followed for a mean of 5.6 years [111]. Cancer risk seems to be similar regardless of the polyp phenotype [114]. Identification of a genetic cause of SPS will allow for a more precise definition of cancer risk.

Management

Screening

For patients with an established SPS diagnosis, colonoscopy should be performed every 1–2 years. The goal is to diminish or eliminate the risk of CRC development by detection and timely removal of precancerous polyps (see treatment below).

Management guidelines are based on clinical experience and expert opinion [126, 127]. Although some studies suggest an association with extracolonic malignancies, the data are not strong enough to justify surveillance recommendations for extracolonic neoplasia.

Treatment

Treatment is determined by the clinical phenotype and patient's wishes. The goal of treatment for SPS patients is to decrease or eliminate CRC risk by removing polyps before they become cancer. Expert panels recommend removing any single polyp larger than 5 mm for histologic evaluation. For clusters of small (3–4 mm) left-sided polyps, which are likely benign hyperplastic polyps, representative biopsies should be performed. Screening colonoscopies should be done yearly, with consideration of the number, size, and histology of the polyps to adjust the interval. If successive colonoscopies reveal no polyps, the interval to the next examination may be extended to 2–3 years, but this should be considered on a case-by-case basis [126].

Hazewinkel et al. demonstrated effective cancer risk reduction using annual colonoscopy with polypectomy of lesions greater than 3 mm in size for 50 patients with SPS. The cumulative risks of detecting CRC, advanced adenomas, and large (≥10 mm) serrated polyps were 0 %, 9 %, and 34 %, respectively. Of note, 12 patients (24 %) underwent preventative surgery [128].

Endoscopic management alone is often difficult as polyps are large, flat, and right sided. If the polyp burden cannot successfully be controlled via colonoscopy and polypectomies, surgery should be considered. The development of CRC or adenoma with high-grade dysplasia that cannot be adequately or safely removed endoscopically is an indication for surgery. The inability to adequately examine or remove polyps on a yearly basis and rapidly changing size or number of polyps at interval screening examinations are also reasonable indications for surgical consultation. As the risk of neoplasia is not limited to the specific location of the cancer but rather the entire colorectal mucosa, extended surgery should be entertained. This includes a subtotal or total colectomy and ileosigmoid or ileorectal anastomosis, respectively. Decision-making for the extent of surgery should be taken for each individual and evaluated within the context of medical comorbidities and anal sphincter function. A segmental colectomy may be considered for patients with focal disease (few large right-sided polyps) and who are not medically fit for extended resection. Any remaining colorectum should undergo annual endoscopy to prevent manage future neoplasia [126, 127].

Evaluation of At-Risk Relatives

Compared to the general population, first-degree relatives of patients with SPS have an approximately fivefold increased CRC incidence [111, 129]. As there is no genetic test to screen for SPS, colonoscopy serves as the screening mechanism. Hazelwinkel evaluated 77 asymptomatic first-degree relatives of SPS patients who underwent annual colonoscopy. They identified significant polyps (adenomas, SSP, or proximal HP) in 43 % of cases of first-degree relatives, including 8 % with advanced adenomas and 9 % with multiple polyps. No cancers were identified, but the substantial neoplasia seen led the authors to conclude that screening is warranted [130]. Expert panels recommend colonoscopy screening for first-degree relatives, particularly those older than 40 years. Endoscopic findings and polyp histology should guide the interval to the next colonoscopy. Patients with a normal colonoscopy may reasonably be evaluated every 5 years. As more information is learned, more precise definitions and intervals may be determined. First-degree relatives do not have increased risk of extracolonic malignancy [116].

Lynch Syndrome

Lynch syndrome (LS), previously used as a synonym for hereditary nonpolyposis colorectal cancer (HNPCC), accounts for 3–5 % of all CRCs and 10–19 % of CRCs diagnosed before age 50 [131–134]. The underlying genetic cause is a germline mutation in a DNA mismatch repair (MMR) gene, which results in a nonfunctioning MMR protein. As the normal function of the MMR system is to detect and correct DNA replication errors, a defective system enables accumulation of genetic errors and confers increased susceptibility to colorectal, endometrial, and other cancers. The syndrome follows an autosomal dominant inheritance pattern. As discussed in detail below, when an individual is suspected to have LS based on clinical features, every effort should be made to identify the pathogenic or disease-causing germline mutation through genetic counseling and genetic testing. This information is critical for guiding the management of the proband and for establishing the risk of transmission but also enables efficient identification of other at-risk family members who would benefit from strategies to prevent or reduce their cancer risks.

Historical Perspective, Nomenclature, and Definitions

More than 100 years have elapsed since Sir Aldred Scott Warthin first reported the remarkable pedigree of intestinal and gynecologic cancers in the original family G of a local seamstress in 1913 [135]. Over this time period, a variety of nomenclature and definitions have been developed, reflective of our evolving understanding of this disease. In 1966, Dr. Henry Lynch comprehensively described two families with extensive history of endometrial and stomach cancers and used the terms "site-specific colon cancer syndrome"

and "family cancer syndrome" [136]. In 1984, "Lynch syndrome" was coined to refer to this disorder, and Lynch I and II defined two main patterns of disease: Lynch I for families with CRC only and Lynch II for families with colorectal and other malignancies. Later, the term "hereditary nonpolyposis colorectal cancer (HNPCC)" arose to distinguish LS from the inherited polyposis syndromes that also confer CRC predisposition. In an effort to more accurately characterize the families that were being treated and studied, the International Collaborative Group on HNPCC convened in Amsterdam in 1991 and defined the Amsterdam criteria (Table 23.4). With increasing awareness that extracolonic malignancy was prevalent in the syndrome, Amsterdam II criteria (Table 23.4) were defined in 1999 to be more inclusive. While Amsterdam I criteria are highly specific for LS, they are not as sensitive as Amsterdam II criteria. Once the genetic defect underlying HNPCC was identified, a more precise characterization of the disease could be established [137]. By 2004, the revised Bethesda Guidelines (Table 23-4) were developed to identify individuals whose tumors should be evaluated for MSI and who should subsequently undergo genetic counseling and evaluation [138, 139]. At this time, it was felt that the term "HNPCC" was a misnomer because patients can develop many non-colorectal cancers, as well as one or more polyps or adenomas. The term "LS" was reintroduced, and it continues to be used today to define patients with hereditary pathogenic germline mutations in DNA MMR genes. Thus, LS is a genetic definition, independent of personal or family history.

There are several conditions that should be distinguished from LS as defined above. First, a subgroup of the HNPCC patients meeting Amsterdam criteria has microsatellite-stable, rather than microsatellite-unstable, tumors. These patients are called familial colorectal cancer type X. The CRC risk is between that of the general population, and patients with LS develop CRC at later ages compared to LS and do not have increased extracolonic malignancy risk. The exact genotype remains to be elucidated [140–142]. Second, in contrast to LS where an inherited mutation is present in one allelic copy of a MMR gene, a rare group of patients has inherited mutations of the MMR gene in both of their alleles. These patients have constitutional mismatch repair deficiency (CMMRD) syndrome. Patients exhibit a distinct phenotype with the development of CRC at very young ages (before age 20), multiple adenomatous polyps numbering between 10 and 100, café-au-lait skin lesions, hematologic malignancies, and brain tumors [143]. Finally, there are patients who present with MSI-H tumors, but subsequent germline mutation testing fails to detect a pathogenic mutation in any of the major MMR genes. The terms "Lynch-like syndrome" [144], "suspected LS" [145, 146], and "mutation-negative LS" [147] have been utilized, and the molecular characterization of these patients represents areas of active research. The remainder of this chapter will focus on LS.

TABLE 23-4. Clinical criteria defining hereditary nonpolyposis colorectal cancer (HNPCC) and the revised Bethesda Guidelines for testing colorectal tumors for microsatellite instability

Amsterdam I criteria (1991)
Three or more relatives with colorectal cancer, plus all of the following:
1. One affected patient is a first-degree relative of the other two
2. Colorectal cancer involves at least two generations
3. At least one case of colorectal cancer is diagnosed before the age of 50 years
Amsterdam II criteria (revised International Collaborative Group on Hereditary Non-Polyposis Colorectal Cancer (ICG-HNPCC) criteria 1998)
Three or more relatives with HNPCC-associated cancer (colorectal cancer or cancer of the endometrium, small bowel, ureter, or renal pelvis) plus all of the following:
1. One affected patient is a first-degree relative of the other two
2. Two or more successive generations are affected
3. Cancer in one or more affected relatives is diagnosed before the age of 50 years
4. Familial adenomatous polyposis is excluded
5. Pathologic diagnosis of cancer is verified
The revised Bethesda Guidelines for testing colorectal tumors for microsatellite instability (MSI)
Tumors from individuals in the following situations should be tested for MSI:
1. Colorectal cancer diagnosed in a patient before age 50
2. Presence of synchronous/metachronous colorectal or other HNPCC-related tumors (including: endometrial, stomach, ovarian, pancreas, ureter and renal pelvis, biliary tract, brain (usually glioblastoma), sebaceous gland adenomas and keratoacanthomas, and carcinoma of the small bowel), regardless of age
3. Colorectal cancer with the MSI-H histology (defined by: presence of tumor-infiltrating lymphocytes, Crohn's-like lymphocytic reaction, mucinous/signet-ring differentiation, or medullary growth pattern) diagnosed in a patient before age 60
4. Colorectal cancer diagnosed in at least one first-degree relative with an HNPCC-related tumor, where one cancer was diagnosed before age 50
5. Colorectal cancer diagnosed in at least two first- or second-degree relatives with HNPCC-related tumors, regardless of age

Modified from Genetic/Familial High-risk Assessment: Colorectal. Version 1.2015. www.ncc.org. and from Umar A, Boland CR, Terdiman JP, Syngal S, de la Chapelle A, Ruschoff J, et al. Revised Bethesda Guidelines for hereditary nonpolyposis colorectal cancer (Lynch syndrome) and microsatellite instability. Journal of the National Cancer Institute. 2004;96(4):261–8

Underlying Genetics and Molecular Profile

Patients with LS harbor an inherited dominant mutation in an MMR gene on one allele. This germline mutation, propagated through all somatic cells, confers susceptibility for cancer but requires a "second hit" within the specific somatic tissue for malignant transformation (Figure 23-6). The "second hit" alters the wild-type copy of the allele, leading to loss of DNA MMR activity in the somatic cell and further cancer development. Thus, malignant tumor cells in patients with LS harbor DNA MMR gene mutations in both alleles (one inherited and another acquired as a "second hit").

The four major DNA MMR genes responsible for LS are *MLH1*, *MSH2*, *MSH6*, and *PMS2*. Additionally, mutations in the gene *EPCAM* (or *TACSTD1*) upstream of *MSH2* can silence or disrupt MSH2 expression and lead to clinical features similar to LS [148, 149]. Based on data from 12,624 observations worldwide, it has been estimated that *MLH1* accounts for 39 %, *MSH2* for 34 %, *MSH6* for 20 %, and *PMS2* for 8 % of the entries in the International Society for Gastrointestinal Hereditary Tumours (InSiGHT) database (www.insight-group.org/mutations/), and up to 3 % of the cases are due to *EPCAM* mutations [150, 151].

The underlying genetic mutations and mismatch repair deficiency yield molecular changes within the tumor that can be examined as part of the screening process toward an LS diagnosis. As discussed earlier, MSI is the hallmark molecular feature of LS CRC. DNA microsatellites are tandem sequences of mono-, di-, or trinucleotide repeats that are particularly susceptible to replication errors when MMR function is impaired. These differences can be measured by the PCR-based MSI test, which assesses a standard panel of (typically five) microsatellite markers in paired tumor and normal tissue (Figure 23-6). By consensus, a tumor is considered MSI-H if 30 % or more of the markers tested show instability and microsatellite stable (MSS) if none of the markers are unstable. MSI-low connotation is reserved for tumors that have some markers that are unstable but fewer than 30 % [152, 153]. MSI low is infrequently encountered and its clinical significance has been regarded similar to that of MSS tumors.

Measuring expression of mismatch repair proteins using immunohistochemistry is the other means of determining mismatch repair proficiency or deficiency of a tumor. In vivo, the MMR protein products function as dimers, with MSH2 forming a complex with MSH6 and MLH1 with PMS2 protein (Figure 23-7). Thus, mutations in either *MSH2* or *EPCAM* genes typically result in loss of staining in both MSH2 and MSH6 protein products, while mutations that lead to loss of MLH1 protein result in the loss of staining for both MLH1 and PMS2 proteins. On the other hand, mutations in *MSH6* and *PMS2* genes typically result only in the loss of the respective single gene product [154]. While IHC is widely available, test accuracy depends on antibody fixation and other technical issues [155]. Also, lack of expression does not elucidate whether the protein loss expression is secondary to an under-

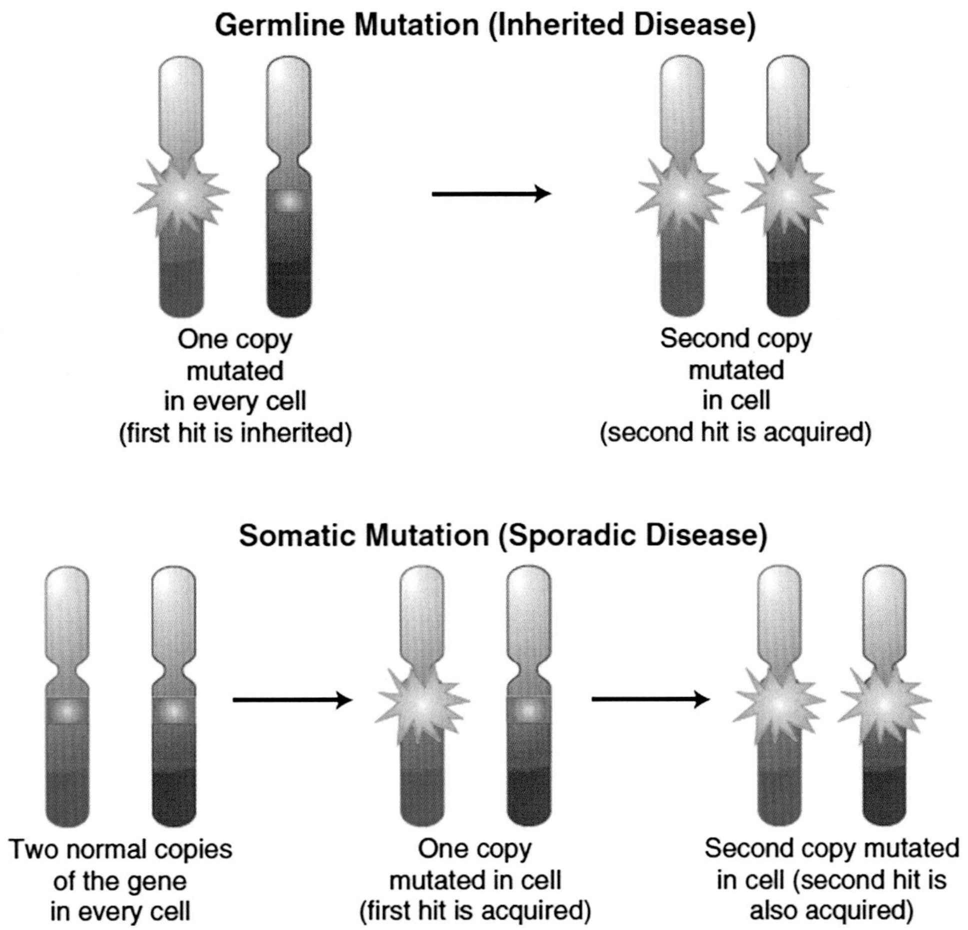

Germline Mutation (Inherited Disease)

One copy
mutated
in every cell
(first hit is inherited)

Second copy
mutated
in cell
(second hit is acquired)

Somatic Mutation (Sporadic Disease)

Two normal copies
of the gene
in every cell

One copy
mutated in cell
(first hit is acquired)

Second copy mutated
in cell (second hit is
also acquired)

FIGURE 23-6. A germline MMR gene mutation confers susceptibility for cancer but requires a "second hit" within the specific somatic tissue for it to develop into a malignancy. The "second hit" causes the wild-type copy of the allele to also become mutated, leading to loss of DNA MMR activity in the somatic cell and further cancer development.

lying germline mutation or acquired somatic loss. Nonetheless, IHC has demonstrated 92 % sensitivity for identifying dMMR in tumors from known LS patients with a germline pathogenic mutation [155]. As discussed above, the vast majority of MSI-H in CRC is caused by methylation of the *MLH1* gene promoter as seen in the methylator pathway. Mutations in the *BRAF* oncogene are strongly associated with the methylator pathway and are rare in LS-related CRC. Thus, the presence of a somatic *BRAF* mutation within a CRC is often used to rule out further screening for an LS diagnosis [156, 157]. Rarely, dMMR tumors can arise from acquired double somatic mutations in the MMR genes. In these patients, germline DNA extracted from blood or other normal tissue shows no genetic defect in the MMR genes [158].

Distinguishing Lynch from Sporadic Epigenetic Changes: Methylation of MLH1 Gene Promoter

Approximately 85 % of mismatch repair deficiency in CRC is caused by methylation of the promoter region of *MLH1* gene. This epigenetic phenomenon silences MLH1 expression in the tumor tissue [159]. These tumors characteristically arise in elderly female patients and in the right colon [159]. Identifying *MLH1* promoter methylation from tumor tissue can help eliminate the diagnosis of LS. However, should *MLH1* promoter methylation be encountered in young patients with a family history suggestive of LS, the clinicians should be aware of two rare exceptions: (1) the patient may have LS with an inherited *MLH1* mutation and *MLH1* promoter methylation may have developed as the "second hit," leading to cancer development [154]; (2) germline *MLH1* hypermethylation has been reported in rare families which exhibit characteristic cancers associated with LS [160].

Clinical Presentation and Spectrum of Disease

Genotype-Phenotype Correlations

While the clinical hallmarks of LS are CRC and extracolonic malignancies, the cancer risks are highly variable within and among families with LS. Genotype-phenotype correlation studies have shown that the lifetime risks of

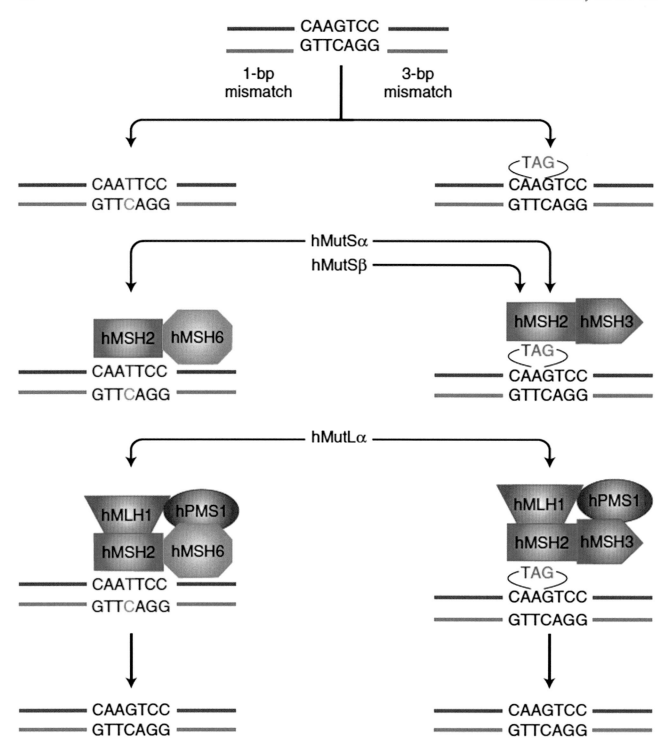

FIGURE 23-7. The DNA mismatch repair system functions to repair single base-pair mismatches or larger loops of inappropriately matched DNA. MSH2 forms a dimer complex with MSH6 which together recognizes the area of DNA mismatch. The second dimer complex of MLH1 and PMS2 is then recruited to excise and correct the mismatch area.

LS-related malignancies vary by gender and the mutated gene (Table 23-5). For example, *MSH2* mutations appear to be associated with later age of onset of malignancies and higher incidences of rectal and extracolonic cancers, when compared to *MLH1* mutations. On the other hand, the risk for endometrial cancer is highest among *MSH6* mutation carriers [161, 162]. The presence of risk-modifying genes that may modulate cancer risks conferred by the MMR genes has also been recognized. For example, two variants (rs16892766 and rs3802842) on chromosomes 8 and 11, previously shown to be associated with sporadic CRC, have been shown to elevate the risk of CRC among LS patients [163, 164]. The potential impact of risk modifiers on clinical practice needs to be further elucidated.

TABLE 23-5. Summary of reported cumulative risks of colorectal and extra-colorectal cancers by age 70 in patients with Lynch syndrome

Cancer	Mutated gene	Cumulative risk, %		Mean age at diagnosis (years)
Colorectal	MLH1/MSH2	Male:	27–74	27–46
		Female:	22–53	
	MSH6	Male:	18–22	54–63
		Female:	10–18	
	PMS2	Male:	20	47–66
		Female:	15	
Endometrial	MLH1/MSH2	14–54		48–62
	MSH6	17–71		54–57
	PMS2	15		49
Ovary		4–20		43–45
Stomach		0.2–13		49–55
Genitourinary		0.2–25		52–60
Hepatobiliary		0.02–4		54–57
Small bowel		0.4–12		46–49
Brain/central nervous system		1–4		50
Sebaceous skin neoplasms		1–9		Unknown

These reported risks and mean ages of diagnosis should not be used to exclude the possibility of Lynch syndrome in a patient who have suggestive clinical features
Modified from Giardiello FM, Allen JI, Axilbund JE, Boland CR, Burke CA, Burt RW, et al. Guidelines on genetic evaluation and management of Lynch syndrome: a consensus statement by the US Multi-society Task Force on colorectal cancer. The American Journal of Gastroenterology. 2014;109(8):1159–79. [11]

Muir-Torre Syndrome (MTS)

Muir-Torre syndrome (MTS) is a clinical variant of LS, where patients are affected by skin sebaceous gland neoplasms (sebaceous adenomas and carcinomas) and/or hair follicle neoplasms (keratoacanthomas). MTS can be associated with mutations in any of the MMR genes, but MSH2 mutation appears most common [165]. Sebaceous adenoma, especially when multiple or when arising from the trunk or extremities, is characteristic for MTS [166, 167]. Sebaceous tumors can occur before, with, or after the development of other cancers, and CRC and genitourinary tumors are the most common visceral malignancies associated with MTS. Referral for genetic counseling and for colonoscopic screening should be considered in patients with sebaceous neoplasm, especially when there is suggestive personal or family history. However, there is currently no uniform recommendation for systemic screening of sebaceous neoplasms for dMMR [166, 168].

Turcot Syndrome

Turcot syndrome describes patients with CRC and brain tumors. Turcot syndrome is not considered an independent entity, and it can be associated with two main types of germline genetic defects: mutation of the APC gene in association with anaplastic astrocytoma, ependymoma, or medulloblastoma or mutation of an MMR gene that is usually associated with glioblastoma [28]. Although excellent survival of more than 3 years has been reported in patients with Turcot syndrome, whether LS patients with these tumors have more favorable prognosis remains unestablished [169].

Colorectal Cancer Risk

The lifetime risk for CRC ranges from 30 to 74 % among MLH1 and MSH2 mutation carriers but only 15–20 % among PMS2 carriers and 10–22 % among MSH6 carriers [74, 161, 170]. The mean age of diagnosis for LS-related CRC is 44–61 years, significantly younger than the average age of CRC onset in the United States which is 72 years. The LS-associated CRCs show a predilection for the right colon when compared to sporadic CRC, but left-sided colon cancers, rectal cancers, and synchronous lesions at different sites of the colon and rectum are also common presentations. Among LS patients who have had an initial CRC treated by less than a total colectomy, the risk for metachronous CRC is 16% at 10 years, 41 % at 20 years, and 62 % at 30 years [171]. Furthermore, the adenoma-to-carcinoma sequence progresses more rapidly in LS patients secondary to more rapid accumulation of errors due to the deficiency in MMR genes. Adenoma may progress to carcinoma within 2–3 years, compared with from 4 to 10 years in the general population [161, 172]. Up to 70 % of the mutation carriers develop at least one adenoma by age 60 [173]. The adenomas tend to be larger and flat and are more likely to show high-grade dysplasia at the time of diagnosis. It has been estimated that endoscopic polypectomy can prevent one CRC for every 2.8 adenoma removed in an LS patient, compared to one CRC for every 41–119 adenomas in the general population [174]. Finally, unique histologic features have been described for MSI-H CRCs, including greater proportion of tumors showing poor differentiation, mucinous or signet-ring cell histology, tumor-infiltrating lymphocytes, and lymphoid (Crohn's-like pattern and/or peritumoral lymphocytes) host response [138]. In summary, common, but not exclusive, features of LS-associated CRC include early age of onset, right-side predominance, high rates of synchronous and metachronous lesions, rapid adenoma-to-carcinoma sequencing, and unique histologic features.

Endometrial and Ovarian Cancer Risk

Endometrial cancer is the most common extracolonic malignancy in patients with LS. It poses the highest risk in women with MSH6 and MSH2 mutations, in whom the lifetime risk can be up to 44 % (Table 23-5). The lowest risk (15 %) is observed among *PMS2* mutation carriers [175, 176]. The mean age at diagnosis ranges between 48 and 62 years. LS-associated endometrial cancers are more commonly of endometrioid histology and arise from the lower uterine segment [177, 178]. Synchronous endometrial and ovarian cancers have been reported in 7–21 % of the women with LS [179].

Other LS-Associated Cancer Risks

The spectrum of other extracolonic cancers associated with LS is wide and continues to evolve. Classically, LS is associated with increased lifetime risk of genitourinary tumors including transitional cell carcinoma of the ureter, renal pelvis, and bladder, as well as cancers of the stomach, hepatobiliary tract, and small bowel, brain cancer (glioblastoma), and sebaceous skin neoplasms (Table 23-5) [180]. More recently, studies have demonstrated that compared to the general population, patients with LS may face two- to 2.5-fold higher risk for prostate cancer [181], 8.6-fold increased risk for pancreas cancer [182], and possibly also elevated risks for breast cancer [180, 183]. The true risk of breast and prostate cancer remains an area of research and debate.

Diagnosis

LS is diagnosed by the identification of a germline mutation in one of the MMR genes as described above. Current commercial germline testing detects both sequence changes and large rearrangements in these genes. It is most commonly performed on DNA isolated from peripheral blood or buccal mucosa samples. Independent of tumor tissue, germline testing can be performed in patients who are affected or unaffected by malignancy.

Genetic testing should be preceded by genetic counseling to ensure that the patients are fully informed of the significance, advantages, and disadvantages of genetic testing. Key components of genetic counseling include: (1) assessment of genetic risk based on personal history and family pedigree; (2) education about genetic syndrome and genetic testing; (3) promoting informed choices regarding testing, including information about insurance coverage and genetic discrimination; (4) disclosing test results and recommending surveillance plans; and (5) counseling for psychosocial and emotional concerns [162]. In 2008, the Genetic Information Nondiscrimination Act (GINA) removed the finding of a pathogenic germline mutation as a preexisting condition for health insurance or employment purposes [184].

Screening and Diagnostic Strategies

Appropriately determining which patients should undergo genetic counseling and testing remains a challenge. Both clinical and cost-based strategies have been proposed ranging from screening all CRCs for MSI to only screening patients who meet strict criteria. The diagnostic approach somewhat depends on the clinical situation as discussed below.

CRC in a Patient Without Known LS

This is the most frequently encountered indication for testing in clinical practice. Over the past several decades, the approach to diagnostic testing has moved from a selective approach, where patients deemed to be at elevated risk of harboring MMR mutations by clinicopathologic criteria undergo testing, to a universal approach, where CRCs are screened using MSI or immunohistochemistry.

The selective approaches utilize clinicopathologic criteria and prediction models to select patients to undergo germline mutation testing. Amsterdam I and II criteria (Table 23-4) require knowledge about CRC age of onset and other LS-associated cancers in both the proband and first- and second-degree relatives. The reported sensitivity for diagnosing LS using these criteria is only 22 % [133, 185]. Revised Bethesda criteria (Table 23-4) consider the above information but also tumor characteristics. These criteria were intended as triggers for testing CRC for MMR deficiency by IHC or MSI. Patients with deficient MMR CRC are then referred for genetic counseling and confirmatory germline testing. When patients who meet at least one of the five revised Bethesda criteria are tested, the reported sensitivity for diagnosing LS may be as high as 82 % [186, 187]. In addition, several prediction models have recently been introduced to calculate the probability of an affected individual harboring a pathogenic MMR gene mutation. The MMRPro (http://www4.utsouthwestern.edu/breasthealth/cagene/) [188] and PREMM1,2,6 (http://premm.dfci.harvard.edu/) [189] models are most commonly used in the United States. The specific inputs of the various models differ, but personal and family history of colorectal and endometrial cancers, ages of onset of cancers, CRC tumor histology, location, and synchronous/metachronous presentation, as well as tumor IHC test result if available, are collected. Each model outputs a probability of an identifiable germline mutation in *MLH1*, *MSH2*, and *MSH6* genes. It has been shown that when a probability cutoff of 5 % was used as a criterion for undergoing germline genetic testing, the sensitivity of the models can approach 90 % [162, 185, 187, 190]. Collectively, although these selective approaches do not depend on the availability of tumor tissue and of tumor molecular tests (i.e., IHC, MSI), they are subject to the accuracy, the availability, and the recall bias of the personal and family histories obtained.

As tumor molecular testing has become increasingly available, a universal screening approach for all CRCs for MMR deficiency has been advocated as the most sensitive strategy to identify patients at risk for LS. This two-step approach involves a screening step where all CRCs are tested for evidence of MMR deficiency independent of somatic mechanisms, followed by a confirmatory step where patients undergo germline MMR mutation testing. Tumors may be testing for MSI and/or MMR protein expression. If the tumor is MSI-H and/or if one of the MMR proteins is not expressed, further exploration is warranted. Since the majority of CRC MSI is not caused by MLH1 loss secondary to hypermethylation of the *MLH1* promoter region, strategies to evaluate MSI with MLH1 IHC loss have been used before proceeding with genetic testing. CRC lacking expression of MLH1 may be further evaluated for DNA hypermethylation of the *MLH1* promoter or for *BRAF* mutations which are highly associated with sporadic MSI-H tumors. If the tumor is methylated and/or has a BRAF mutation, the likelihood of LS is less and testing does not need to be pursued unless there is a strong suspicion based on clinical or family history. If MSH2, MSH26, or PMS2 is lost, then it is highly likely to be caused by a germline mutation, and directed testing for that particular gene proceeds along those lines [191]. One algorithmic approach to screening for LS in CRC is demonstrated in Figure 23-8 [133, 150, 187, 192].

The success and effectiveness of a universal screening strategy depends on availability of tumor tissue, accuracy of tumor molecular testing, and on a significant infrastructure for navigating the patients between tumor-based and germline testing along with genetic counseling [151]. Indeed, a key determinant of the cost-effectiveness of universal testing is the participation rate of at-risk blood relatives who undergo subsequent testing for LS [193]. In other words, if more at-

risk relatives are screened and diagnosed before cancers develop, more people will be effectively enrolled in appropriate preventative surveillance programs. The Evaluation of Genomic Applications in Practice and Prevention (EGAPP) [194], the National Comprehensive Cancer Network (NCCN) [191], and the US Multi-Society Task Force on Colorectal Cancer [162] recommend universal screening of CRC. A cost-effective analysis identified that the cost per incremental life year gained was half if universal testing for CRC patients aged 70 and younger is compared to those without an age cutoff [193].

Whichever strategy is used, one must be able to interpret and take action on germline testing results. In general, germline testing yields one of three possible results: (1) a deleterious (pathogenic) mutation, (2) a variant of unknown significance, or (3) uninformative negative or no mutation found. Finding of a pathogenic mutation confirms the diagnosis of LS in the patient. The latter two findings should be considered inconclusive, in the setting of a dMMR tumor without evidence of *MLH1* promoter methylation and/or BRAF mutation. Patients with an MSI-H tumor and loss of MMR protein expression but without a confirmatory germline mutation are considered to have "Lynch-like syndrome" [146]. About 50 % of these patients can be explained by biallelic somatic alterations and do not have LS [195], although routine commercial tumor testing for biallelic somatic testing is not routinely available at this time. In the absence of

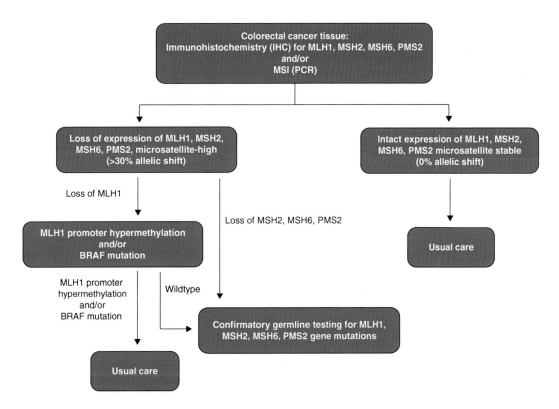

FIG. 23.8. One algorithm for testing of colorectal tumors for MMR deficiency as a first step to screen for patients with Lynch syndrome.

clearly defined cancer risks for patients with Lynch-like syndrome, it remains the most prudent today to clinically manage these patient and families in the same way as LS patients [145, 172]. One caveat is that strategies that involve only germline testing (i.e., based on Amsterdam criteria or predictive models) without accompanying tumor MMR status testing are thus at risk for missing patients who might have "Lynch-like syndrome."

The proportions of patients with pathogenic mutations vs. inconclusive results vary inversely with the sensitivity of the selective approach to testing [147]. A variant of unknown significance is a variation in genetic sequence whose clinical consequence and associated disease risk are unknown. Variant reclassification is an extensive process that involves accumulation of clinical and pedigree data, functional studies, and in silico predictions [147]. Therefore, patients who have an inconclusive result on initial germline testing should be encouraged to undergo periodic repeat assessments as new genetic data emerge. Patients with a VUS should be managed based on family history and clinical suspicion for LS.

Individual with a Family Diagnosis of LS

Once a pathogenic mutation is identified in a proband, all at-risk blood relatives should undergo site-specific germline testing for the known family mutation. In these cases of site-specific testing (for affected relatives) or predictive testing (for unaffected relatives), there are two possible results: (1) true positive, when the specific mutation is identified and the individual is confirmed to have LS, and (2) true negative, when it is a conclusive negative result and effectively rules out LS in the individual, who carries only general population risks for malignancies [151, 162].

Individual Whose Family Meets Amsterdam Criteria But Does Not Have Any Clinical Phenotype

It is not uncommon for a healthy individual from an Amsterdam criteria family to seek consult regarding his/her own screening recommendations. The initial evaluation should begin with a detailed personal and family cancer history. The most informative individual to evaluate would be a

relative with an LS-associated cancer, particularly at a young age. If tumor is available, screening may be conducted as discussed above. If a pathogenic mutation is found, then directed germline testing can be performed for at-risk relatives. If tumor screening is not feasible, germline testing of an affected individual within the context of appropriate genetic counseling is an option. We do not recommend broad germline genetic testing for an unaffected individual as the yield is low and inconclusive results such as variant of unknown significance or uninformative negative would be clinically difficult to interpret in an unaffected individual [162]. More recently, panels that include multiple genes that confer a range of CRC risks have emerged and may be most efficient in differentiating patients with pedigrees that could be consistent with LS, attenuated polyposis syndromes, or other syndromes [196]. Involvement of a certified genetic counselor is recommended in these cases.

Clinical Management

Screening

For patients with LS, key elements of their lifelong care include screening for cancers in unaffected individuals and surveillance for recurrent, metachronous, or other syndromic cancers in affected individuals (Table 23-6). For CRC, young age of disease onset, accelerated progression from adenoma to carcinoma, and right-sided dominance have led to the recommendation that patients with LS undergo colonoscopy every 1–2 years starting at age 20–25 years [161, 162, 191]. Surveillance colonoscopy has been shown to reduce CRC incidence (62 % reduction), disease stage at diagnosis, and CRC-related mortality (72 % reduction) in LS patients who undergo colonoscopy compared to those who do not [197]. Recent guidelines have suggested varying the age to initiate colonoscopy depending on family history (at least 2–5 years younger than the earliest affected age in the family).

LS patients are also at increased risk for developing extracolonic malignancies that can potentially benefit from screening of asymptomatic individuals. A definitive survival benefit has not been proven by prospective studies, and management is based on expert opinion and published

TABLE 23-6. Summary of possible surveillance regimen for Lynch syndrome patients

Cancer	Test	Frequency (years)	Age to commence (years)
Colorectal	Colonoscopy	1–2	20–25 or 2–5 years prior to earliest colon cancer before age 25
Endometrial and ovarian	Transvaginal ultrasound with endometrial sampling; consideration for serum CA-125	1–2 years	30–35
Gastric/small bowel	Consideration for extended esophagogastroduodenoscopy	3–5	30–35
Urinary tract	Consideration for urinalysis	1	25–30
Sebaceous neoplasms	Physical examination	1	25–30
Brain/central nervous system	Physical/neurologic examination	1	25–30

Modified from the National Comprehensive Cancer Network Guideline on Genetic/Familial High-risk Assessment: Colorectal. Version 1.2015. www.ncc.org

guidelines. Women with LS should be educated regarding symptoms of endometrial cancer, including abnormal uterine bleeding and pain. There is no established evidence for annual screening, but pelvic examination, CA-125, transvaginal ultrasound, and endometrial biopsy (performed under sedation in coordination with colonoscopy) have been commonly performed [191]. Upper endoscopy and small bowel X-ray and/or upper endoscopy can be utilized to screen for gastric and small bowel cancers, while urinalysis and cytology have been considered for urothelial cancers [198]. Finally, annual or biannual dermatologic patients with LS can be considered too for the detection of sebaceous skin neoplasms [161, 162]. An example of screening strategies is listed in Table 23-6.

Modifiers of Risk for Colorectal and Other Cancers

Lifestyle and environmental factors may influence the risk for adenoma and CRC in patients with LS. The GeoLynch study prospectively analyzed 486 subjects with LS for their modifiable lifestyle factors. Dietary patterns particularly those with high meat and high snack contents are associated 1.7 and 2.2 times risks for developing colorectal adenomas [199]. Active smoking [200] and obesity (with body mass index ≥ 25 kg/m^2) [201] also increase the risk of developing colorectal neoplasia when compared to nonsmokers or normal weight men, respectively.

Resistant starch and aspirin are two chemoprevention agents studied in patients with LS. The Colorectal Adenoma/Carcinoma Prevention Programme 2 (CAPP2) randomized 727 participants to resistant starch (30 g per day) or placebo and 693 participants to aspirin (600 mg per day) and placebo in a 2×2 design. After a median follow-up of 52.7 months, resistant starch did not impact on CRC development [202]. However, after a mean follow-up of 55.7 months, 18 vs. 30 participants developed CRC (63 % fewer CRCs) after 4 years of aspirin use [203]. An intention-to-treat analysis of all LS cancers (i.e., colorectal, endometrial, ovarian, pancreatic, small bowel, gallbladder, ureter, stomach, kidney, and brain) also showed a benefit of aspirin vs. placebo (hazard ratio 0.65; $p=0.005$). Although the incidence of adverse events did not differ between the aspirin and placebo groups during treatment, whether the high dose is necessary for benefit remains to be elucidated in the proposed CAPP 3 study [204]. Currently the evidence is not sufficiently mature to recommend routine use of high-dose aspirin in LS patients [161, 162, 191].

Surgery for Colorectal Cancer

Surgical treatment of LS-associated colon cancer starts with the same oncologic principles as those for sporadic colon cancer. Colectomy should be performed with adequate proximal, distal, and radial resection margin, regional lymphadenectomy, and R0 and en bloc resection of all malignant tissue [205]. The extent of resection (segmental colectomy or total abdominal colectomy with ileorectal anastomosis) depends on balancing surgical morbidity, patient comorbidities and wishes, and risk of future malignancy in the remaining colorectum. Factors to consider include the presence of synchronous pathology, age of the patient, disease prognosis and life expectancy, risk of metachronous CRC, expected compliance with surveillance, morbidity of reoperation, bowel function, and patient preferences. The American Society of Colon and Rectal Surgeons recommends extended colectomy for patients with colon cancer and LS, based mainly on metachronous cancer risk. Multiple retrospective studies have demonstrated a higher rate of metachronous colorectal cancer following segmental colectomy compared to extended colectomy [195, 206–209]. In a large international study from the Colon Cancer Family Registry, 332 LS patients with colon cancer treated with segmental colectomy were compared to 50 LS patients treated with extended colectomy. The cumulative risk of metachronous CRC after segmental colectomy was 16, 41, and 62 % at 10, 20, and 30 years, respectively [171]. These risks may vary further depending on the compliance with endoscopic surveillance and feasibility of endoscopic removal of premalignant polyps. There have not been prospective studies to prove that extended colectomy improves survival in LS patients. In a Markov model, the calculated gain in life expectancy from extended compared to segmental colectomy was 2.3 years if surgery were performed at age 27 years, 1 year at age 47 years, and 0.3 years at age 67 years, and these numbers became 3.4 years at age 27 years, 1.5 years at age 47 years, and 0.4 year at age 67 years if the colon cancer were stage I [210]. Therefore, extended colectomy may have the most benefit in young patients with early-stage disease only. Advanced CRC stage, significant medical comorbidities, and other LS-associated malignancies that pose competing risks to the patient's life expectancy should also be considered.

Functional expectations of each operation should be discussed with patients. In a retrospective review of bowel function for 201 patients undergoing total colectomy and ileorectal anastomosis, 56 % reported dietary restrictions and 20 % used daily medications, and compared to preoperative levels, patients reported restricted social activity (32 %), housework (20 %), recreation (32 %), and travel (43 %) [211]. Another study of 52 LS patients treated with extended colectomy reported increased stool frequency, decreased social life, and more defecation difficulties compared to 51 patients who had segmental colectomy [212]. Despite the bowel function reports, no measurable differences in quality of life have been reported after either procedure, suggesting that most patients adapt to their choice of the operation over time. Current guidelines suggest that extended colectomy is preferred treatment for LS-associated colon cancer, but segmental colectomy might be an option in older patients [161, 162, 191].

Management of rectal cancer in LS involves complex decision-making. The cancer should be managed like any other rectal cancer in terms of indications for multimodality therapy and oncologic principles. However, just as in colon cancer in LS, the extent of the resection is determined by many factors. The surgeon and patient must decide between a proctectomy and total proctocolectomy (TPC) with or without sphincter preservation as determined by the tumor location. Compared to TPC with an ileal pouch reconstruction, proctectomy alone results in less frequent bowel movements and less incontinence [213]. However, proctectomy without colectomy leaves the entire colon in situ and at risk for subsequent cancer. There are a few retrospective studies that have reported the risk of colon cancer after proctectomy in LS to be between 15 and 54 %, although the inclusion criteria of the study cohorts were heterogeneous [37, 214–217].

Data from the Colon Cancer Family Registry reported the cumulative risk of metachronous colon cancer after proctectomy in 79 LS patients to be 19 % at 10 years, 47 % at 20 years, and 69 % at 30 years [214].

The need for pelvic radiation should be considered when an ileal pouch is to be done. A recent analysis of 157 IPAA patients who received preoperative pelvic radiation showed no significant elevation of 30-day morbidity rate compared to patients who did not receive pelvic radiation [218]. However, little data exists regarding the long-term functional outcome of an IPAA performed after pelvic radiation, but there is general reluctance to perform this based on perceived risks for radiation enteritis, pelvic fibrosis, and pouch dysfunction.

Given the high risk of metachronous neoplasia after a segmental proctectomy, the risks and benefits of TPC with IPAA should be discussed with all Lynch syndrome patients presenting with non-stage IV rectal cancer. Total proctocolectomy for rectal cancer in LS remains debated, and several factors including the patient's age, medical comorbidities, rectal cancer stage, the need for pelvic radiation, sphincter function, and compliance with surveillance regimens should be evaluated with the patient in the larger clinical picture.

Prophylactic Surgery for Endometrial and Ovarian Cancer

In women undergoing surgical treatment of CRC, concomitant prophylactic gynecologic surgery may be considered and discussed with the patient. In a case-matched study of LS women who underwent prophylactic total abdominal hysterectomy and salpingo-oophorectomy, the procedure successfully eliminated the risks of endometrial and ovary cancers [219]. When several risk-reducing strategies were compared in a cost-effectiveness model, annual gynecologic screening (with CA-125, transvaginal ultrasound, and endo-metrial biopsy) and prophylactic surgery at 40 years were the most cost-effective strategies, with the former being favored where the cost of screening is low [220]. Thus, the age of the patient and the availability and expected compliance with screening are key factors to consider in decision-making regarding prophylactic gynecologic surgery for LS.

Evaluation of At-Risk Relatives

When an LS or an MMR pathogenic mutation has been identified in an individual, genetic counseling and site-specific testing for the pathogenic mutation should be offered to all first-degree relatives (parents, siblings, and children). Due to the considerable psychosocial issues associated with germline testing, it is usually not recommended for at-risk individuals younger than age 18 years. Surveillance of asymptomatic at-risk relatives for premalignant lesions or early manifestations of cancer is appropriate and has been recommended to commence 5–10 years younger than the youngest age of onset of cancer in the family or between age 20 and 25 [161, 191]. A major reason to identify individuals with LS is to optimize the care of their at-risk relatives, with the goal of ultimately minimizing the morbidity and mortality of LS.

Probands and their at-risk relatives with LS greatly benefit from enrollment in a hereditary CRC registry. Such a registry is typically associated with an established institutional infrastructure and with access to expert clinical care, innovative research, patient education, and support networks. Multidisciplinary care teams including gastroenterologists, surgeons, medical oncologists, and genetic counselors are coordinated to provide lifelong and multi-organ cancer screening or surveillance. Families often gain access to research protocols investigating novel diagnostic, screening, treatment, or chemoprevention strategies. Finally, registry provides a support network for families and a basis for knowledge and experience exchange [221]. Registration and screening reduce CRC incidence and mortality in LS patients [222]. Surgeons play an integral role in the care of the patients with LS, from clinical recognition and genetic diagnosis to cancer treatment and guidance of family and long-term care.

References

1. Ogino S, Goel A. Molecular classification and correlates in colorectal cancer. J Mol Diagn. 2008;10(1):13–27.
2. Vogelstein B, Fearon ER, Hamilton SR, Kern SE, Preisinger AC, Leppert M, et al. Genetic alterations during colorectal-tumor development. N Engl J Med. 1988;319(9):525–32.
3. Dahabreh IJ, Terasawa T, Castaldi PJ, Trikalinos TA. Systematic review: anti-epidermal growth factor receptor treatment effect modification by KRAS mutations in advanced colorectal cancer. Ann Intern Med. 2011;154(1):37–49.

4. Cancer Genome Atlas N. Comprehensive molecular characterization of human colon and rectal cancer. Nature. 2012;487(7407):330–7.

5. Bahnassy AA, Zekri AR, Salem SE, Abou-Bakr AA, Sakr MA, Abdel-Samiaa AG, et al. Differential expression of p53 family proteins in colorectal adenomas and carcinomas: Prognostic and predictive values. Histol Histopathol. 2014;29(2):207–16.

6. Weisenberger DJ, Siegmund KD, Campan M, Young J, Long TI, Faasse MA, et al. CpG island methylator phenotype underlies sporadic microsatellite instability and is tightly associated with BRAF mutation in colorectal cancer. Nat Genet. 2006;38(7):787–93. see comment.

7. Kambara T, Simms LA, Whitehall VL, Spring KJ, Wynter CV, Walsh MD, et al. BRAF mutation is associated with DNA methylation in serrated polyps and cancers of the colorectum. Gut. 2004;53(8):1137–44.

8. Bettington M, Walker N, Clouston A, Brown I, Leggett B, Whitehall V. The serrated pathway to colorectal carcinoma: current concepts and challenges. Histopathology. 2013;62(3):367–86.

9. Sanchez JA, Krumroy L, Plummer S, Aung P, Merkulova A, Skacel M, et al. Genetic and epigenetic classifications define clinical phenotypes and determine patient outcomes in colorectal cancer. Br J Surg. 2009;96(10):1196–204.

10. Jass JR. Hereditary non-polyposis colorectal cancer: the rise and fall of a confusing term. World J Gastroenterol. 2006;12(31):4943–50.

11. Giardiello FM, Allen JI, Axilbund JE, Boland CR, Burke CA, Burt RW, et al. Guidelines on genetic evaluation and management of Lynch syndrome: a consensus statement by the US Multi-Society Task Force on colorectal cancer. Gastroenterology. 2014;147(2):502–26.

12. Sener SF, Miller HH, DeCosse JJ. The spectrum of polyposis. Surg Gynecol Obstet. 1984;159(6):525–32.

13. Itoh H, Hirata K, Ohsato K. Turcot's syndrome and familial adenomatous polyposis associated with brain tumor: review of related literature. Int J Colorectal Dis. 1993;8(2):87–94.

14. Knudsen AL, Bisgaard ML, Bulow S. Attenuated familial adenomatous polyposis (AFAP). A review of the literature. Fam Cancer. 2003;2(1):43–55.

15. de Vos tot Nederveen Cappel WH, Jarvinen HJ, Bjork J, Berk T, Griffioen G, Vasen HF. Worldwide survey among polyposis registries of surgical management of severe duodenal adenomatosis in familial adenomatous polyposis. Br J Surg. 2003;90(6):705–10.

16. Wallace MH, Phillips RK. Upper gastrointestinal disease in patients with familial adenomatous polyposis. Br J Surg. 1998;85(6):742–50.

17. Clark SK, Neale KF, Landgrebe JC, Phillips RK. Desmoid tumours complicating familial adenomatous polyposis. Br J Surg. 1999;86(9):1185–9.

18. Soravia C, Berk T, McLeod RS, Cohen Z. Desmoid disease in patients with familial adenomatous polyposis. Dis Colon Rectum. 2000;43(3):363–9.

19. Elayi E, Manilich E, Church J. Polishing the crystal ball: knowing genotype improves ability to predict desmoid disease in patients with familial adenomatous polyposis. Dis Colon Rectum. 2009;52(10):1762–6.

20. Church J, Xhaja X, LaGuardia L, O'Malley M, Burke C, Kalady M. Desmoids and genotype in familial adenomatous polyposis. Dis Colon Rectum. 2015;58(4):444–8.

21. Feng X, Milas M, O'Malley M, LaGuardia L, Berber E, Jin J, et al. Characteristics of benign and malignant thyroid disease in familial adenomatous polyposis patients and recommendations for disease surveillance. Thyroid. 2015;25(3):325–32.

22. Donnellan KA, Bigler SA, Wein RO. Papillary thyroid carcinoma and familial adenomatous polyposis of the colon. Am J Otolaryngol. 2009;30(1):58–60.

23. Herraiz M, Barbesino G, Faquin W, Chan-Smutko G, Patel D, Shannon KM, et al. Prevalence of thyroid cancer in familial adenomatous polyposis syndrome and the role of screening ultrasound examinations. Clin Gastroenterol Hepatol. 2007;5(3):367–73.

24. Jarrar AM, Milas M, Mitchell J, Laguardia L, O'Malley M, Berber E, et al. Screening for thyroid cancer in patients with familial adenomatous polyposis. Ann Surg. 2011;253(3):515–21.

25. Giardiello FM, Offerhaus GJ, Lee DH, Krush AJ, Tersmette AC, Booker SV, et al. Increased risk of thyroid and pancreatic carcinoma in familial adenomatous polyposis. Gut. 1993;34(10):1394–6.

26. Giardiello FM, Offerhaus GJ, Krush AJ, Booker SV, Tersmette AC, Mulder JW, et al. Risk of hepatoblastoma in familial adenomatous polyposis. J Pediatr. 1991;119(5):766–8.

27. Hughes LJ, Michels VV. Risk of hepatoblastoma in familial adenomatous polyposis. Am J Med Genet. 1992;43(6):1023–5.

28. Hamilton SR, Liu B, Parsons RE, Papadopoulos N, Jen J, Powell SM, et al. The molecular basis of Turcot's syndrome. N Engl J Med. 1995;332(13):839–47.

29. Valanzano R, Cama A, Volpe R, Curia MC, Mencucci R, Palmirotta R, et al. Congenital hypertrophy of the retinal pigment epithelium in familial adenomatous polyposis. Novel criteria of assessment and correlations with constitutional adenomatous polyposis coli gene mutations. Cancer. 1996;78(11):2400–10.

30. Olsen KO, Juul S, Bulow S, Jarvinen HJ, Bakka A, Bjork J, et al. Female fecundity before and after operation for familial adenomatous polyposis. Br J Surg. 2003;90(2):227–31.

31. Bulow S, Bulow C, Vasen H, Jarvinen H, Bjork J, Christensen IJ. Colectomy and ileorectal anastomosis is still an option for selected patients with familial adenomatous polyposis. Dis Colon Rectum. 2008;51(9):1318–23.

32. Slors FJ, van Zuijlen PP, van Dijk GJ. Sexual and bladder dysfunction after total mesorectal excision for benign diseases. Scand J Gastroenterol Suppl. 2000;232:48–51.

33. Gunther K, Braunrieder G, Bittorf BR, Hohenberger W, Matzel KE. Patients with familial adenomatous polyposis experience better bowel function and quality of life after ileorectal anastomosis than after ileoanal pouch. Colorectal Dis. 2003;5(1):38–44.

34. Church J, Burke C, McGannon E, Pastean O, Clark B. Risk of rectal cancer in patients after colectomy and ileorectal anastomosis for familial adenomatous polyposis: a function of available surgical options. Dis Colon Rectum. 2003;46(9):1175–81.

35. Wu JS, Paul P, McGannon EA, Church JM. APC genotype, polyp number, and surgical options in familial adenomatous polyposis. Ann Surg. 1998;227(1):57–62.

36. Church J. Ileoanal pouch neoplasia in familial adenomatous polyposis: an underestimated threat. Dis Colon Rectum. 2005;48(9):1708–13.

37. O'Connell PR, Pemberton JH, Weiland LH, Beart Jr RW, Dozois RR, Wolff BG, et al. Does rectal mucosa regenerate after ileoanal anastomosis? Dis Colon Rectum. 1987;30(1):1–5.

38. Remzi FH, Church JM, Bast J, Lavery IC, Strong SA, Hull TL, et al. Mucosectomy vs. stapled ileal pouch-anal anastomosis in patients with familial adenomatous polyposis: functional outcome and neoplasia control. Dis Colon Rectum. 2001;44(11):1590–6.

39. Lovegrove RE, Constantinides VA, Heriot AG, Athanasiou T, Darzi A, Remzi FH, et al. A comparison of hand-sewn versus stapled ileal pouch anal anastomosis (IPAA) following procto-colectomy: a meta-analysis of 4183 patients. Ann Surg. 2006;244(1):18–26.

40. Burke CA, Beck GJ, Church JM, van Stolk RU. The natural history of untreated duodenal and ampullary adenomas in patients with familial adenomatous polyposis followed in an endoscopic surveillance program. Gastrointest Endosc. 1999;49(3 Pt 1):358–64.

41. Church J, Simmang C. Practice parameters for the treatment of patients with dominantly inherited colorectal cancer (familial adenomatous polyposis and hereditary nonpolyposis colorectal cancer). Dis Colon Rectum. 2003;46(8):1001–12.

42. Spigelman AD, Williams CB, Talbot IC, Domizio P, Phillips RK. Upper gastrointestinal cancer in patients with familial adenomatous polyposis. Lancet. 1989;2(8666):783–5.

43. Groves CJ, Saunders BP, Spigelman AD, Phillips RKS. Duodenal cancer in patients with familial adenomatous polyposis (FAP): results of a 10 year prospective study. Gut. 2002;50(5):636–41.

44. Church J, Berk T, Boman BM, Guillem J, Lynch C, Lynch P, et al. Staging intra-abdominal desmoid tumors in familial adenomatous polyposis: a search for a uniform approach to a troubling disease. Dis Colon Rectum. 2005;48(8):1528–34.

45. Tsukada K, Church JM, Jagelman DG, Fazio VW, McGannon E, George CR, et al. Noncytotoxic drug therapy for intra-abdominal desmoid tumor in patients with familial adenomatous polyposis. Dis Colon Rectum. 1992;35(1):29–33.

46. Tonelli F, Ficari F, Valanzano R, Brandi ML. Treatment of desmoids and mesenteric fibromatosis in familial adenomatous polyposis with raloxifene. Tumori. 2003;89(4):391–6.

47. Azzarelli A, Gronchi A, Bertulli R, Tesoro JD, Baratti D, Pennacchioli E, et al. Low-dose chemotherapy with methotrexate and vinblastine for patients with advanced aggressive fibromatosis. Cancer. 2001;92(5):1259–64.

48. Bertagnolli MM, Morgan JA, Fletcher CDM, Raut CP, Dileo P, Gill RR, et al. Multimodality treatment of mesenteric desmoid tumours. Eur J Cancer. 2008;44(16):2404–10.

49. Poritz LS, Blackstein M, Berk T, Gallinger S, McLeod RS, Cohen Z. Extended follow-up of patients treated with cytotoxic chemotherapy for intra-abdominal desmoid tumors. Dis Colon Rectum. 2001;44(9):1268–73.

50. Chatzipetrou MA, Tzakis AG, Pinna AD, Kato T, Misiakos EP, Tsaroucha AK, et al. Intestinal transplantation for the treatment of desmoid tumors associated with familial adenomatous polyposis. Surgery. 2001;129(3):277–81.

51. Nikeghbalian S, Aliakbarian M, Shamsaeefar A, Kazemi K, Bahreini A, Malekhosseini SA. Multivisceral transplantation for the treatment of intra-abdominal tumors. Transplant Proc. 2013;45(10):3528–30.

52. Bell B, Mazzaferri EL. Familial adenomatous polyposis (Gardner's syndrome) and thyroid carcinoma. A case report and review of the literature. Dig Dis Sci. 1993;38(1):185–90.

53. Bulow C, Bulow S. Is screening for thyroid carcinoma indicated in familial adenomatous polyposis? The Leeds Castle Polyposis Group. Int J Colorectal Dis. 1997;12(4):240–2.

54. Sampson JR, Dolwani S, Jones S, Eccles D, Ellis A, Evans DG, et al. Autosomal recessive colorectal adenomatous polyposis due to inherited mutations of MYH. Lancet. 2003;362(9377):39–41.

55. Nielsen M, Franken PF, Reinards TH, Weiss MM, Wagner A, van der Klift H, et al. Multiplicity in polyp count and extracolonic manifestations in 40 Dutch patients with MYH associated polyposis coli (MAP). J Med Genet. 2005;42(9):e54.

56. Croitoru ME, Cleary SP, Berk T, Di Nicola N, Kopolovic I, Bapat B, et al. Germline MYH mutations in a clinic-based series of Canadian multiple colorectal adenoma patients. J Surg Oncol. 2007;95(6):499–506.

57. Grover S, Kastrinos F, Steyerberg EW, Cook EF, Dewanwala A, Burbidge LA, et al. Prevalence and phenotypes of APC and MUTYH mutations in patients with multiple colorectal adenomas. JAMA. 2012;308(5):485–92.

58. Cleary SP, Cotterchio M, Jenkins MA, Kim H, Bristow R, Green R, et al. Germline MutY human homologue mutations and colorectal cancer: a multisite case-control study. Gastroenterology. 2009;136(4):1251–60.

59. Church J, Heald B, Burke C, Kalady M. Understanding MYH-associated neoplasia. Dis Colon Rectum. 2012;55(3):359–62.

60. Tenesa A, Campbell H, Barnetson R, Porteous M, Dunlop M, Farrington SM. Association of MUTYH and colorectal cancer. Br J Cancer. 2006;95(2):239–42.

61. Jones S, Emmerson P, Maynard J, Best JM, Jordan S, Williams GT, et al. Biallelic germline mutations in MYH predispose to multiple colorectal adenoma and somatic G:C → T:A mutations. Hum Mol Genet. 2002;11(23):2961–7.

62. Parker AR, Eshleman JR. Human MutY: gene structure, protein functions and interactions, and role in carcinogenesis. Cell Mol Life Sci. 2003;60(10):2064–83.

63. Guillen-Ponce C, Castillejo A, Barbera VM, Pascual-Ramirez JC, Andrada E, Castillejo MI, et al. Biallelic MYH germline mutations as cause of Muir-Torre syndrome. Fam Cancer. 2010;9(2):151–4.

64. Boparai KS, Dekker E, Van Eeden S, Polak MM, Bartelsman JF, Mathus-Vliegen EM, et al. Hyperplastic polyps and sessile serrated adenomas as a phenotypic expression of MYH-associated polyposis. Gastroenterology. 2008;135(6):2014–8.

65. Castells A. MYH-associated polyposis: adenomas and hyperplastic polyps, partners in crime? Gastroenterology. 2008;135(6):1857–9.

66. Gismondi V, Meta M, Bonelli L, Radice P, Sala P, Bertario L, et al. Prevalence of the Y165C, G382D and 1395delGGA germline mutations of the MYH gene in Italian patients with adenomatous polyposis coli and colorectal adenomas. Int J Cancer. 2004;109(5):680–4.

67. Sieber OM, Lipton L, Crabtree M, Heinimann K, Fidalgo P, Phillips RK, et al. Multiple colorectal adenomas, classic adenomatous polyposis, and germ-line mutations in MYH. N Engl J Med. 2003;348(9):791–9.

68. Win AK, Dowty JG, Cleary SP, Kim H, Buchanan DD, Young JP, et al. Risk of colorectal cancer for carriers of mutations in

MUTYH, with and without a family history of cancer. Gastroenterology. 2014;146(5):1208–11.e1–5.

69. Goodenberger M, Lindor NM. Lynch syndrome and MYH-associated polyposis: review and testing strategy. J Clin Gastroenterol. 2011;45(6):488–500.

70. Wang L, Baudhuin LM, Boardman LA, Steenblock KJ, Petersen GM, Halling KC, et al. MYH mutations in patients with attenuated and classic polyposis and with young-onset colorectal cancer without polyps. Gastroenterology. 2004;127(1):9–16.

71. Vogt S, Jones N, Christian D, Engel C, Nielsen M, Kaufmann A, et al. Expanded extracolonic tumor spectrum in MUTYH-associated polyposis. Gastroenterology. 2009;137(6):1976–85.e1–10.

72. Ponti G, Ponz de Leon M, Maffei S, Pedroni M, Losi L, Di Gregorio C, et al. Attenuated familial adenomatous polyposis and Muir-Torre syndrome linked to compound biallelic constitutional MYH gene mutations. Clin Genet. 2005;68(5):442–7.

73. National Comprehensive Cancer Network Practice Guidelines in Oncology 2015. version 2.

74. Syngal S, Brand RE, Church JM, Giardiello FM, Hampel HL, Burt RW, et al. ACG clinical guideline: genetic testing and management of hereditary gastrointestinal cancer syndromes. Am J Gastroenterol. 2015;110(2):223–62. quiz 63.

75. Nascimbeni R, Pucciarelli S, Di Lorenzo D, Urso E, Casella C, Agostini M, et al. Rectum-sparing surgery may be appropriate for biallelic MutYH-associated polyposis. Dis Colon Rectum. 2010;53(12):1670–5.

76. Palles C, Cazier JB, Howarth KM, Domingo E, Jones AM, Broderick P, et al. Germline mutations affecting the proofreading domains of POLE and POLD1 predispose to colorectal adenomas and carcinomas. Nat Genet. 2013;45(2):136–44.

77. Briggs S, Tomlinson I. Germline and somatic polymerase epsilon and delta mutations define a new class of hypermutated colorectal and endometrial cancers. J Pathol. 2013;230(2):148–53.

78. Desai DC, Neale KF, Talbot IC, Hodgson SV, Phillips RK. Juvenile polyposis. Br J Surg. 1995;82(1):14–7.

79. Merg A, Howe JR. Genetic conditions associated with intestinal juvenile polyps. Am J Med Genet C Semin Med Genet. 2004;129(1):44–55.

80. Jass JR, Williams CB, Bussey HJ, Morson BC. Juvenile polyposis – a precancerous condition. Histopathology. 1988;13(6):619–30.

81. O'Malley M, LaGuardia L, Kalady MF, Parambil J, Heald B, Eng C, et al. The prevalence of hereditary hemorrhagic telangiectasia in juvenile polyposis syndrome. Dis Colon Rectum. 2012;55(8):886–92.

82. Gallione CJ, Repetto GM, Legius E, Rustgi AK, Schelley SL, Tejpar S, et al. A combined syndrome of juvenile polyposis and hereditary haemorrhagic telangiectasia associated with mutations in MADH4 (SMAD4). Lancet. 2004;363(9412):852–9.

83. Iyer NK, Burke CA, Leach BH, Parambil JG. SMAD4 mutation and the combined syndrome of juvenile polyposis syndrome and hereditary haemorrhagic telangiectasia. Thorax. 2010;65(8):745–6.

84. Howe JR, Sayed MG, Ahmed AF, Ringold J, Larsen-Haidle J, Merg A, et al. The prevalence of MADH4 and BMPR1A muta-tions in juvenile polyposis and absence of BMPR2, BMPR1B, and ACVR1 mutations. J Med Genet. 2004;41(7):484–91.

85. Aretz S, Stienen D, Uhlhaas S, Stolte M, Entius MM, Loff S, et al. High proportion of large genomic deletions and a genotype phenotype update in 80 unrelated families with juvenile polyposis syndrome. J Med Genet. 2007;44(11):702–9.

86. van Hattem WA, Brosens LA, de Leng WW, Morsink FH, Lens S, Carvalho R, et al. Large genomic deletions of SMAD4, BMPR1A and PTEN in juvenile polyposis. Gut. 2008;57(5):623–7.

87. Sweet K, Willis J, Zhou XP, Gallione C, Sawada T, Alhopuro P, et al. Molecular classification of patients with unexplained hamartomatous and hyperplastic polyposis. JAMA. 2005;294(19):2465–73.

88. Sayed MG, Ahmed AF, Ringold JR, Anderson ME, Bair JL, Mitros FA, et al. Germline SMAD4 or BMPR1A mutations and phenotype of juvenile polyposis. Ann Surg Oncol. 2002;9(9):901–6.

89. Agnifili A, Verzaro R, Gola P, Marino M, Mancini E, Carducci G, et al. Juvenile polyposis: case report and assessment of the neoplastic risk in 271 patients reported in the literature. Dig Surg. 1999;16(2):161–6.

90. Howe JR, Mitros FA, Summers RW. The risk of gastrointestinal carcinoma in familial juvenile polyposis. Ann Surg Oncol. 1998;5(8):751–6.

91. Jass J. Juvenile polyposis. 1st ed. In: Spiegelman RPaA, editor. London: Edward Arnold; 1994. 203–14 p.

92. Brosens LA, van Hattem A, Hylind LM, Iacobuzio-Donahue C, Romans KE, Axilbund J, et al. Risk of colorectal cancer in juvenile polyposis. Gut. 2007;56(7):965–7.

93. Scott-Conner CE, Hausmann M, Hall TJ, Skelton DS, Anglin BL, Subramony C. Familial juvenile polyposis: patterns of recurrence and implications for surgical management. J Am Coll Surg. 1995;181(5):407–13.

94. Aytac E, Sulu B, Heald B, O'Malley M, LaGuardia L, Remzi FH, et al. Genotype-defined cancer risk in juvenile polyposis syndrome. Br J Surg. 2015;102(1):114–8.

95. Calva D, Howe JR. Hamartomatous polyposis syndromes. Surg Clin North Am. 2008;88(4):779–817. vii.

96. Oncel M, Church JM, Remzi FH, Fazio VW. Colonic surgery in patients with juvenile polyposis syndrome: a case series. Dis Colon Rectum. 2005;48(1):49–55. discussion 6.

97. Utsunomiya J, Gocho H, Miyanaga T, Hamaguchi E, Kashimure A. Peutz-Jeghers syndrome: its natural course and management. Johns Hopkins Med J. 1975;136(2):71–82.

98. Giardiello FM, Trimbath JD. Peutz-Jeghers syndrome and management recommendations. Clin Gastroenterol Hepatol. 2006;4(4):408–15.

99. Zbuk KM, Eng C. Hamartomatous polyposis syndromes. Nat Clin Pract Gastroenterol Hepatol. 2007;4(9):492–502.

100. Hemminki A, Markie D, Tomlinson I, Avizienyte E, Roth S, Loukola A, et al. A serine/threonine kinase gene defective in Peutz-Jeghers syndrome. Nature. 1998;391(6663):184–7.

101. Giardiello FM, Brensinger JD, Tersmette AC, Goodman SN, Petersen GM, Booker SV, et al. Very high risk of cancer in familial Peutz-Jeghers syndrome. Gastroenterology. 2000;119(6):1447–53.

102. Oncel M, Remzi FH, Church JM, Connor JT, Fazio VW. Benefits of "clean sweep" in Peutz-Jeghers patients. Colorectal Dis. 2004;6(5):332–5.

103. Heald B, Mester J, Rybicki L, Orloff MS, Burke CA, Eng C. Frequent gastrointestinal polyps and colorectal adenocarcinomas in a prospective series of PTEN mutation carriers. Gastroenterology. 2010;139(6):1927–33.

104. Stanich PP, Owens VL, Sweetser S, Khambatta S, Smyrk TC, Richardson RL, et al. Colonic polyposis and neoplasia in Cowden syndrome. Mayo Clin Proc. 2011;86(6):489–92.

105. Marsh DJ, Dahia PL, Caron S, Kum JB, Frayling IM, Tomlinson IP, et al. Germline PTEN mutations in Cowden syndrome-like families. J Med Genet. 1998;35(11):881–5.

106. Marsh DJ, Dahia PL, Coulon V, Zheng Z, Dorion-Bonnet F, Call KM, et al. Allelic imbalance, including deletion of PTEN/MMAC1, at the Cowden disease locus on 10q22-23, in hamartomas from patients with Cowden syndrome and germline PTEN mutation. Genes Chromosomes Cancer. 1998;21(1):61–9.

107. Gustafson S, Zbuk KM, Scacheri C, Eng C. Cowden syndrome. Semin Oncol. 2007;34(5):428–34.

108. Gorlin RJ, Cohen Jr MM, Condon LM, Burke BA. Bannayan-Riley-Ruvalcaba syndrome. Am J Med Genet. 1992;44(3):307–14.

109. Tan MH, Mester JL, Ngeow J, Rybicki LA, Orloff MS, Eng C. Lifetime cancer risks in individuals with germline PTEN mutations. Clin Cancer Res. 2012;18(2):400–7.

110. Riegert-Johnson DL, Gleeson FC, Roberts M, Tholen K, Youngborg L, Bullock M, et al. Cancer and Lhermitte-Duclos disease are common in Cowden syndrome patients. Hered Cancer Clin Pract. 2010;8(1):6.

111. Boparai KS, Mathus-Vliegen EM, Koornstra JJ, Nagengast FM, van Leerdam M, van Noesel CJ, et al. Increased colorectal cancer risk during follow-up in patients with hyperplastic polyposis syndrome: a multicentre cohort study. Gut. 2010;59(8):1094–100.

112. Carvajal-Carmona LG, Howarth KM, Lockett M, Polanco-Echeverry GM, Volikos E, Gorman M, et al. Molecular classification and genetic pathways in hyperplastic polyposis syndrome. J Pathol. 2007;212(4):378–85.

113. Chow E, Lipton L, Lynch E, D'Souza R, Aragona C, Hodgkin L, et al. Hyperplastic polyposis syndrome: phenotypic presentations and the role of MBD4 and MYH. Gastroenterology. 2006;131(1):30–9.

114. Kalady MF, Jarrar A, Leach B, LaGuardia L, O'Malley M, Eng C, et al. Defining phenotypes and cancer risk in hyperplastic polyposis syndrome. Dis Colon Rectum. 2011;54(2):164–70.

115. Rosty C, Buchanan DD, Walsh MD, Pearson SA, Pavluk E, Walters RJ, et al. Phenotype and polyp landscape in serrated polyposis syndrome: a series of 100 patients from genetics clinics. Am J Surg Pathol. 2012;36(6):876–82.

116. Hazewinkel Y, Reitsma JB, Nagengast FM, Vasen HF, van Os TA, van Leerdam ME, et al. Extracolonic cancer risk in patients with serrated polyposis syndrome and their first-degree relatives. Fam Cancer. 2013;12(4):669–73.

117. Snover D, Ahnen D, Burt R, Odze RD. Serrated polyps of the colon and rectum and serrated polyposis. In: Bosman FT, Carneiro F, Hruban RH, editors. WHO classification of tumours of the digestive system. 4th ed. Lyon, France: IARC; 2010.

118. Ferrandez A, Samowitz W, DiSario JA, Burt RW. Phenotypic characteristics and risk of cancer development in hyperplastic polyposis: case series and literature review. Am J Gastroenterol. 2004;99(10):2012–8.

119. Hyman NH, Anderson P, Blasyk H. Hyperplastic polyposis and the risk of colorectal cancer. Dis Colon Rectum. 2004;47(12):2101–4.

120. Leggett BA, Devereaux B, Biden K, Searle J, Young J, Jass J. Hyperplastic polyposis: association with colorectal cancer. Am J Surg Pathol. 2001;25(2):177–84.

121. Rubio CA, Stemme S, Jaramillo E, Lindblom A. Hyperplastic polyposis coli syndrome and colorectal carcinoma. Endoscopy. 2006;38(3):266–70.

122. Yeoman A, Young J, Arnold J, Jass J, Parry S. Hyperplastic polyposis in the New Zealand population: a condition associated with increased colorectal cancer risk and European ancestry. N Z Med J. 2007;120(1266):U2827.

123. Lage P, Cravo M, Sousa R, Chaves P, Salazar M, Fonseca R, et al. Management of Portuguese patients with hyperplastic polyposis and screening of at-risk first-degree relatives: a contribution for future guidelines based on a clinical study. Am J Gastroenterol. 2004;99(9):1779–84.

124. Rashid A, Houlihan PS, Booker S, Petersen GM, Giardiello FM, Hamilton SR. Phenotypic and molecular characteristics of hyperplastic polyposis. Gastroenterology. 2000;119(2):323–32.

125. Jasperson KW, Kanth P, Kirchhoff AC, Huismann D, Gammon A, Kohlmann W, et al. Serrated polyposis: colonic phenotype, extracolonic features, and familial risk in a large cohort. Dis Colon Rectum. 2013;56(11):1211–6.

126. Rex DK, Ahnen DJ, Baron JA, Batts KP, Burke CA, Burt RW, et al. Serrated lesions of the colorectum: review and recommendations from an expert panel. Am J Gastroenterol. 2012;107(9):1315–29. quiz 4, 30.

127. Kalady MF. Sessile serrated polyps: an important route to colorectal cancer. J Natl Compr Canc Netw. 2013;11(12):1585–94.

128. Hazewinkel Y, Tytgat KM, van Eeden S, Bastiaansen B, Tanis PJ, Boparai KS, et al. Incidence of colonic neoplasia in patients with serrated polyposis syndrome who undergo annual endoscopic surveillance. Gastroenterology. 2014;147(1):88–95.

129. Win AK, Walters RJ, Buchanan DD, Jenkins MA, Sweet K, Frankel WL, et al. Cancer risks for relatives of patients with serrated polyposis. Am J Gastroenterol. 2012;107(5):770–8.

130. Hazewinkel Y, Koornstra JJ, Boparai KS, van Os TA, Tytgat KM, Van Eeden S, et al. Yield of screening colonoscopy in first-degree relatives of patients with serrated polyposis syndrome. J Clin Gastroenterol. 2015;49(5):407–12.

131. Aaltonen LA, Sankila R, Mecklin JP, Jarvinen H, Pukkala E, Peltomaki P, et al. A novel approach to estimate the proportion of hereditary nonpolyposis colorectal cancer of total colorectal cancer burden. Cancer Detect Prev. 1994;18(1):57–63.

132. de la Chapelle A. The incidence of Lynch syndrome. Fam Cancer. 2005;4(3):233–7.

133. Hampel H, Frankel WL, Martin E, Arnold M, Khanduja K, Kuebler P, et al. Screening for the Lynch syndrome (hereditary nonpolyposis colorectal cancer). N Engl J Med. 2005;352(18):1851–60.

134. Salovaara R, Loukola A, Kristo P, Kaariainen H, Ahtola H, Eskelinen M, et al. Population-based molecular detection of hereditary nonpolyposis colorectal cancer. J Clin Oncol. 2000;18(11):2193–200.

135. Lynch HT, Smyrk T, Lynch J. An update of HNPCC (Lynch syndrome). Cancer Genet Cytogenet. 1997;93(1):84–99.

136. Lynch HT, Shaw MW, Magnuson CW, Larsen AL, Krush AJ. Hereditary factors in cancer. Study of two large midwestern kindreds. Arch Intern Med. 1966;117(2):206–12.

137. Ionov Y, Peinado MA, Malkhosyan S, Shibata D, Perucho M. Ubiquitous somatic mutations in simple repeated sequences reveal a new mechanism for colonic carcinogenesis. Nature. 1993;363(6429):558–61.

138. Umar A, Boland CR, Terdiman JP, Syngal S, de la Chapelle A, Ruschoff J, et al. Revised Bethesda Guidelines for hereditary nonpolyposis colorectal cancer (Lynch syndrome) and microsatellite instability. J Natl Cancer Inst. 2004;96(4):261–8.

139. Rodriguez-Bigas MA, Boland CR, Hamilton SR, Henson DE, Jass JR, Khan PM, et al. A National Cancer Institute Workshop on Hereditary Nonpolyposis Colorectal Cancer Syndrome: meeting highlights and Bethesda guidelines. J Natl Cancer Inst. 1997;89(23):1758–62.

140. Lindor NM. Familial colorectal cancer type X: the other half of hereditary nonpolyposis colon cancer syndrome. Surg Oncol Clin N Am. 2009;18(4):637–45.

141. Shiovitz S, Copeland WK, Passarelli MN, Burnett-Hartman AN, Grady WM, Potter JD, et al. Characterisation of familial colorectal cancer Type X, Lynch syndrome, and non-familial colorectal cancer. Br J Cancer. 2014;111(3):598–602.

142. Lindor NM, Rabe K, Petersen GM, Haile R, Casey G, Baron J, et al. Lower cancer incidence in Amsterdam-I criteria families without mismatch repair deficiency: familial colorectal cancer type X. JAMA. 2005;293(16):1979–85.

143. Durno CA, Holter S, Sherman PM, Gallinger S. The gastrointestinal phenotype of germline biallelic mismatch repair gene mutations. Am J Gastroenterol. 2010;105(11):2449–56.

144. Boland CR. The mystery of mismatch repair deficiency: lynch or lynch-like? Gastroenterology. 2013;144(5):868–70.

145. Buchanan DD, Rosty C, Clendenning M, Spurdle AB, Win AK. Clinical problems of colorectal cancer and endometrial cancer cases with unknown cause of tumor mismatch repair deficiency (suspected Lynch syndrome). Appl Clin Genet. 2014;7:183–93.

146. Rodriguez-Soler M, Perez-Carbonell L, Guarinos C, Zapater P, Castillejo A, Barbera VM, et al. Risk of cancer in cases of suspected lynch syndrome without germline mutation. Gastroenterology. 2013;144(5):926–32.e1. quiz e13–4.

147. You YN, Vilar E. Classifying MMR variants: time for revised nomenclature in Lynch syndrome. Clin Cancer Res. 2013;19(9):2280–2.

148. Lynch HT, Riegert-Johnson DL, Snyder C, Lynch JF, Hagenkord J, Boland CR, et al. Lynch syndrome-associated extracolonic tumors are rare in two extended families with the same EPCAM deletion. Am J Gastroenterol. 2011;106(10):1829–36.

149. Kovacs ME, Papp J, Szentirmay Z, Otto S, Olah E. Deletions removing the last exon of TACSTD1 constitute a distinct class of mutations predisposing to Lynch syndrome. Hum Mutat. 2009;30(2):197–203.

150. Palomaki GE, McClain MR, Melillo S, Hampel HL, Thibodeau SN. EGAPP supplementary evidence review: DNA testing strategies aimed at reducing morbidity and mortality from Lynch syndrome. Genet Med. 2009;11(1):42–65.

151. Weissman SM, Burt R, Church J, Erdman S, Hampel H, Holter S, et al. Identification of individuals at risk for Lynch syndrome using targeted evaluations and genetic testing: National Society of Genetic Counselors and the Collaborative Group of the Americas on Inherited Colorectal Cancer joint practice guideline. J Genet Couns. 2012;21(4):484–93.

152. Boland CR, Thibodeau SN, Hamilton SR, Sidransky D, Eshleman JR, Burt RW, et al. A National Cancer Institute Workshop on Microsatellite Instability for cancer detection and familial predisposition: development of international criteria for the determination of microsatellite instability in colorectal cancer. Cancer Res. 1998;58(22):5248–57.

153. Hegde M, Ferber M, Mao R, Samowitz W, Ganguly A, Working Group of the American College of Medical Genetics, et al. ACMG technical standards and guidelines for genetic testing for inherited colorectal cancer (Lynch syndrome, familial adenomatous polyposis, and MYH-associated polyposis). Genet Med. 2014;16(1):101–16.

154. Bellizzi AM, Frankel WL. Colorectal cancer due to deficiency in DNA mismatch repair function: a review. Adv Anat Pathol. 2009;16(6):405–17.

155. Shia J. Immunohistochemistry versus microsatellite instability testing for screening colorectal cancer patients at risk for hereditary nonpolyposis colorectal cancer syndrome. Part I. The utility of immunohistochemistry. J Mol Diagn. 2008;10(4):293–300.

156. Domingo E, Niessen RC, Oliveira C, Alhopuro P, Moutinho C, Espin E, et al. BRAF-V600E is not involved in the colorectal tumorigenesis of HNPCC in patients with functional MLH1 and MSH2 genes. Oncogene. 2005;24(24):3995–8.

157. Nakagawa H, Nagasaka T, Cullings HM, Notohara K, Hoshijima N, Young J, et al. Efficient molecular screening of Lynch syndrome by specific 3' promoter methylation of the MLH1 or BRAF mutation in colorectal cancer with high-frequency microsatellite instability. Oncol Rep. 2009;21(6):1577–83.

158. Sourrouille I, Coulet F, Lefevre JH, Colas C, Eyries M, Svrcek M, et al. Somatic mosaicism and double somatic hits can lead to MSI colorectal tumors. Fam Cancer. 2013;12(1):27–33.

159. Poynter JN, Siegmund KD, Weisenberger DJ, Long TI, Thibodeau SN, Lindor N, et al. Molecular characterization of MSI-H colorectal cancer by MLHI promoter methylation, immunohistochemistry, and mismatch repair germline mutation screening. Cancer Epidemiol Biomarkers Prev. 2008;17(11):3208–15.

160. Niessen RC, Hofstra RM, Westers H, Ligtenberg MJ, Kooi K, Jager PO, et al. Germline hypermethylation of MLH1 and EPCAM deletions are a frequent cause of Lynch syndrome. Genes Chromosomes Cancer. 2009;48(8):737–44.

161. Vasen HF, Blanco I, Aktan-Collan K, Gopie JP, Alonso A, Aretz S, et al. Revised guidelines for the clinical management of Lynch syndrome (HNPCC): recommendations by a group of European experts. Gut. 2013;62(6):812–23.

162. Giardiello FM, Allen JI, Axilbund JE, Boland CR, Burke CA, Burt RW, et al. Guidelines on genetic evaluation and management of Lynch syndrome: a consensus statement by the US Multi-society Task Force on colorectal cancer. Am J Gastroenterol. 2014;109(8):1159–79.

163. Wijnen JT, Brohet RM, van Eijk R, Jagmohan-Changur S, Middeldorp A, Tops CM, et al. Chromosome 8q23.3 and 11q23.1 variants modify colorectal cancer risk in Lynch syndrome. Gastroenterology. 2009;136(1):131–7.

164. Talseth-Palmer BA, Scott RJ, Vasen HF, Wijnen JT. 8q23.3 and 11q23.1 as modifying loci influencing the risk for CRC in

Lynch syndrome. Eur J Hum Genet. 2012;20(5):487–8. author reply 8.

165. Lazar AJ, Lyle S, Calonje E. Sebaceous neoplasia and Torre-Muir syndrome. Curr Diagn Pathol. 2007;13(4):301–19.

166. Roberts ME, Riegert-Johnson DL, Thomas BC, Thomas CS, Heckman MG, Krishna M, et al. Screening for Muir-Torre syndrome using mismatch repair protein immunohistochemistry of sebaceous neoplasms. J Genet Couns. 2013;22(3): 393–405.

167. Cesinaro AM, Ubiali A, Sighinolfi P, Trentini GP, Gentili F, Facchetti F. Mismatch repair proteins expression and microsatellite instability in skin lesions with sebaceous differentiation: a study in different clinical subgroups with and without extracutaneous cancer. Am J Dermatopathol. 2007;29(4): 351–8.

168. Lee BA, Yu L, Ma L, Lind AC, Lu D. Sebaceous neoplasms with mismatch repair protein expressions and the frequency of co-existing visceral tumors. J Am Acad Dermatol. 2012;67(6):1228–34.

169. Merlo A, Rochlitz C, Scott R. Survival of patients with Turcot's syndrome and glioblastoma. N Engl J Med. 1996;334(11):736–7.

170. Barrow E, Hill J, Evans DG. Cancer risk in Lynch syndrome. Fam Cancer. 2013;12(2):229–40.

171. Parry S, Win AK, Parry B, Macrae FA, Gurrin LC, Church JM, et al. Metachronous colorectal cancer risk for mismatch repair gene mutation carriers: the advantage of more extensive colon surgery. Gut. 2011;60(7):950–7.

172. Vasen HF, Tomlinson I, Castells A. Clinical management of hereditary colorectal cancer syndromes. Nat Rev Gastroenterol Hepatol. 2015;12(2):88–97.

173. Lanspa SJ, Lynch HT, Smyrk TC, Strayhorn P, Watson P, Lynch JF, et al. Colorectal adenomas in the Lynch syndromes. Results of a colonoscopy screening program. Gastroenterology. 1990;98(5 Pt 1):1117–22.

174. Winawer SJ, Zauber AG, Ho MN, O'Brien MJ, Gottlieb LS, Sternberg SS, et al. Prevention of colorectal cancer by colonoscopic polypectomy. The National Polyp Study Workgroup. N Engl J Med. 1993;329(27):1977–81.

175. Stoffel E, Mukherjee B, Raymond VM, Tayob N, Kastrinos F, Sparr J, et al. Calculation of risk of colorectal and endometrial cancer among patients with Lynch syndrome. Gastroenterology. 2009;137(5):1621–7.

176. Baglietto L, Lindor NM, Dowty JG, White DM, Wagner A, Gomez Garcia EB, et al. Risks of Lynch syndrome cancers for MSH6 mutation carriers. J Natl Cancer Inst. 2010; 102(3):193–201.

177. Lu KH, Broaddus RR. Gynecologic cancers in Lynch syndrome/HNPCC. Fam Cancer. 2005;4(3):249–54.

178. Westin SN, Lacour RA, Urbauer DL, Luthra R, Bodurka DC, Lu KH, et al. Carcinoma of the lower uterine segment: a newly described association with Lynch syndrome. J Clin Oncol. 2008;26(36):5965–71.

179. Pal T, Permuth-Wey J, Sellers TA. A review of the clinical relevance of mismatch-repair deficiency in ovarian cancer. Cancer. 2008;113(4):733–42.

180. Win AK, Young JP, Lindor NM, Tucker KM, Ahnen DJ, Young GP, et al. Colorectal and other cancer risks for carriers and non-carriers from families with a DNA mismatch repair gene mutation: a prospective cohort study. J Clin Oncol. 2012;30(9): 958–64.

181. Raymond VM, Mukherjee B, Wang F, Huang SC, Stoffel EM, Kastrinos F, et al. Elevated risk of prostate cancer among men with Lynch syndrome. J Clin Oncol. 2013;31(14):1713–8.

182. Kastrinos F, Mukherjee B, Tayob N, Wang F, Sparr J, Raymond VM, et al. Risk of pancreatic cancer in families with Lynch syndrome. JAMA. 2009;302(16):1790–5.

183. Buerki N, Gautier L, Kovac M, Marra G, Buser M, Mueller H, et al. Evidence for breast cancer as an integral part of Lynch syndrome. Genes Chromosomes Cancer. 2012;51(1):83–91.

184. Prince AE, Roche MI. Genetic information, non-discrimination, and privacy protections in genetic counseling practice. J Genet Couns. 2014;23(6):891–902.

185. Balmana J, Balaguer F, Castellvi-Bel S, Steyerberg EW, Andreu M, Llor X, et al. Comparison of predictive models, clinical criteria and molecular tumour screening for the identification of patients with Lynch syndrome in a population-based cohort of colorectal cancer patients. J Med Genet. 2008;45(9):557–63.

186. Pinol V, Castells A, Andreu M, Castellvi-Bel S, Alenda C, Llor X, et al. Accuracy of revised Bethesda guidelines, microsatellite instability, and immunohistochemistry for the identification of patients with hereditary nonpolyposis colorectal cancer. JAMA. 2005;293(16):1986–94.

187. Green RC, Parfrey PS, Woods MO, Younghusband HB. Prediction of Lynch syndrome in consecutive patients with colorectal cancer. J Natl Cancer Inst. 2009;101(5): 331–40.

188. Terespolsky D. The MMRpro model accurately predicted the probability of carrying a cancer-susceptibility gene mutation for the Lynch syndrome. ACP J Club. 2007;146(2):53.

189. Kastrinos F, Steyerberg EW, Mercado R, Balmana J, Holter S, Gallinger S, et al. The PREMM(1,2,6) model predicts risk of MLH1, MSH2, and MSH6 germline mutations based on cancer history. Gastroenterology. 2011;140(1):73–81.

190. Barzi A, Sadeghi S, Kattan MW, Meropol NJ. Comparative effectiveness of screening strategies for Lynch syndrome. J Natl Cancer Inst. 2015;107(4), djv005.

191. The National Comprehensive Cancer Network Guideline on Genetic/Familial High-risk Assessment: Colorectal. Version 1.2015. www.ncc.org.

192. Moreira L, Balaguer F, Lindor N, de la Chapelle A, Hampel H, Aaltonen LA, et al. Identification of Lynch syndrome among patients with colorectal cancer. JAMA. 2012;308(15): 1555–65.

193. Ladabaum U, Wang G, Terdiman J, Blanco A, Kuppermann M, Boland CR, et al. Strategies to identify the Lynch syndrome among patients with colorectal cancer: a cost-effectiveness analysis. Ann Intern Med. 2011;155(2):69–79.

194. Evaluation of Genomic Applications in Practice and Prevention (EGAPP) Working Group. Recommendations from the EGAPP Working Group: can UGT1A1 genotyping reduce morbidity and mortality in patients with metastatic colorectal cancer treated with irinotecan? Genet Med. 2009;11(1): 15–20.

195. Mensenkamp AR, Vogelaar IP, van Zelst-Stams WA, Goossens M, Ouchene H, Hendriks-Cornelissen SJ, et al. Somatic mutations in MLH1 and MSH2 are a frequent cause of mismatch-repair deficiency in Lynch syndrome-like tumors. Gastroenterology. 2014;146(3):643–6. e8.

196. Yurgelun MB, Allen B, Kaldate RR, Bowles KR, Judkins T, Kaushik P, et al. Identification of a variety of mutations in

cancer-predisposition genes in patients with suspected Lynch syndrome. Gastroenterology. 2015;149(3):604–613.e20.

197. Jarvinen HJ, Aarnio M, Mustonen H, Aktan-Collan K, Aaltonen LA, Peltomaki P, et al. Controlled 15-year trial on screening for colorectal cancer in families with hereditary nonpolyposis colorectal cancer. Gastroenterology. 2000;118(5):829–34.

198. Mork M, Hubosky SG, Roupret M, Margulis V, Raman J, Lotan Y, et al. Lynch syndrome: a primer for urologists and panel recommendations. J Urol. 2015;194(1):21–9.

199. Botma A, Vasen HF, van Duijnhoven FJ, Kleibeuker JH, Nagengast FM, Kampman E. Dietary patterns and colorectal adenomas in Lynch syndrome: the GEOLynch cohort study. Cancer. 2013;119(3):512–21.

200. Winkels RM, Botma A, Van Duijnhoven FJ, Nagengast FM, Kleibeuker JH, Vasen HF, et al. Smoking increases the risk for colorectal adenomas in patients with Lynch syndrome. Gastroenterology. 2012;142(2):241–7.

201. Botma A, Nagengast FM, Braem MG, Hendriks JC, Kleibeuker JH, Vasen HF, et al. Body mass index increases risk of colorectal adenomas in men with Lynch syndrome: the GEOLynch cohort study. J Clin Oncol. 2010;28(28):4346–53.

202. Mathers JC, Movahedi M, Macrae F, Mecklin JP, Moeslein G, Olschwang S, et al. Long-term effect of resistant starch on cancer risk in carriers of hereditary colorectal cancer: an analysis from the CAPP2 randomised controlled trial. Lancet Oncol. 2012;13(12):1242–9.

203. Burn J, Gerdes AM, Macrae F, Mecklin JP, Moeslein G, Olschwang S, et al. Long-term effect of aspirin on cancer risk in carriers of hereditary colorectal cancer: an analysis from the CAPP2 randomised controlled trial. Lancet. 2011;378(9809):2081–7.

204. Burn J, Mathers JC, Bishop DT. Chemoprevention in Lynch syndrome. Fam Cancer. 2013;12(4):707–18.

205. Smith AJ, Driman DK, Spithoff K, Hunter A, McLeod RS, Simunovic M, et al. Guideline for optimization of colorectal cancer surgery and pathology. J Surg Oncol. 2010;101(1):5–12.

206. Fitzgibbons Jr RJ, Lynch HT, Stanislav GV, Watson PA, Lanspa SJ, Marcus JN, et al. Recognition and treatment of patients with hereditary nonpolyposis colon cancer (Lynch syndromes I and II). Ann Surg. 1987;206(3):289–95.

207. Natarajan N, Watson P, Silva-Lopez E, Lynch HT. Comparison of extended colectomy and limited resection in patients with Lynch syndrome. Dis Colon Rectum. 2010;53(1):77–82.

208. Vasen HF, Mecklin JP, Watson P, Utsunomiya J, Bertario L, Lynch P, et al. Surveillance in hereditary nonpolyposis colorectal cancer: an international cooperative study of 165 families. The International Collaborative Group on HNPCC. Dis Colon Rectum. 1993;36(1):1–4.

209. Kalady MF, McGannon E, Vogel JD, Manilich E, Fazio VW, Church JM. Risk of colorectal adenoma and carcinoma after colectomy for colorectal cancer in patients meeting Amsterdam criteria. Ann Surg. 2010;252(3):507–11. discussion 11–3.

210. de Vos Tot Nederveen Cappel WH, Buskens E, van Duijvendijk P, Cats A, Menko FH, Griffioen G, et al. Decision analysis in the surgical treatment of colorectal cancer due to a mismatch repair gene defect. Gut. 2003;52(12):1752–5.

211. You YN, Chua HK, Nelson H, Hassan I, Barnes SA, Harrington J. Segmental vs. extended colectomy: measurable differences in morbidity, function, and quality of life. Dis Colon Rectum. 2008;51(7):1036–43.

212. Haanstra JF, de Vos Tot Nederveen Cappel WH, Gopie JP, Vecht J, Vanhoutvin SA, Cats A, et al. Quality of life after surgery for colon cancer in patients with Lynch syndrome: partial versus subtotal colectomy. Dis Colon Rectum. 2012;55(6):653–9.

213. Fazio VW, Kiran RP, Remzi FH, Coffey JC, Heneghan HM, Kirat HT, et al. Ileal pouch anal anastomosis: analysis of outcome and quality of life in 3707 patients. Ann Surg. 2013;257(4):679–85.

214. Win AK, Parry S, Parry B, Kalady MF, Macrae FA, Ahnen DJ, et al. Risk of metachronous colon cancer following surgery for rectal cancer in mismatch repair gene mutation carriers. Ann Surg Oncol. 2013;20(6):1829–36.

215. Kalady MF, Lipman J, McGannon E, Church JM. Risk of colonic neoplasia after proctectomy for rectal cancer in hereditary nonpolyposis colorectal cancer. Ann Surg. 2012;255(6):1121–5.

216. Lee JS, Petrelli NJ, Rodriguez-Bigas MA. Rectal cancer in hereditary nonpolyposis colorectal cancer. Am J Surg. 2001;181(3):207–10.

217. Cirillo L, Urso ED, Parrinello G, Pucciarelli S, Moneghini D, Agostini M, et al. High risk of rectal cancer and of metachronous colorectal cancer in probands of families fulfilling the Amsterdam criteria. Ann Surg. 2013;257(5):900–4.

218. Wertzberger BE, Sherman SK, Byrn JC. Differences in short-term outcomes among patients undergoing IPAA with or without preoperative radiation: a National Surgical Quality Improvement Program analysis. Dis Colon Rectum. 2014;57(10):1188–94.

219. Schmeler KM, Lynch HT, Chen LM, Munsell MF, Soliman PT, Clark MB, et al. Prophylactic surgery to reduce the risk of gynecologic cancers in the Lynch syndrome. N Engl J Med. 2006;354(3):261–9.

220. Kwon JS, Sun CC, Peterson SK, White KG, Daniels MS, Boyd-Rogers SG, et al. Cost-effectiveness analysis of prevention strategies for gynecologic cancers in Lynch syndrome. Cancer. 2008;113(2):326–35.

221. Bannon SA, Mork M, Vilar E, Peterson SK, Lu K, Lynch PM, et al. Patient-reported disease knowledge and educational needs in Lynch syndrome: findings of an interactive multidisciplinary patient conference. Hered Cancer Clin Pract. 2014;12(1):1.

222. Barrow P, Khan M, Lalloo F, Evans DG, Hill J. Systematic review of the impact of registration and screening on colorectal cancer incidence and mortality in familial adenomatous polyposis and Lynch syndrome. Br J Surg. 2013;100(13):1719–31.

223. Kalady MF, Heald B. Diagnostic approach to hereditary colorectal cancer syndromes. Clin Colon Rectal Surg. 2015;28:205–214.

24

Colorectal Neoplasms: Screening and Surveillance After Polypectomy

Evie H. Carchman and Charles P. Heise

Key Concepts

- Screening can reduce colorectal mortality.
- Screening recommendations are based upon risk for polyp/cancer development (family history of cancer or polyps, personal history cancer/polyps, genetic syndromes (FAP, MYH, and HNPCC), and inflammatory bowel disease).
- Surveillance after polypectomy depends on the histology of polyp and the completeness of its resection.
- The decision to perform colectomy for a polyp that contains cancer depends on the extent of invasion (Haggitt staging for pedunculated polyp and Kikuchi classification for sessile polyp).

Introduction

Colorectal cancer is the second leading cause of cancer-related deaths in the United States in men and women combined [1]. In 2014, the National Cancer Institute (NCI) estimated 96,000 new colon cancer and 40,000 new rectal cancer cases, and the estimated number of deaths for both colon and rectal cancer combined was 50,310. The fortunate news is that the death rate from colorectal cancer has been decreasing over the last 20 years. This reduction in the number of new cancer cases and cancer-related deaths is a consequence of current screening programs [2, 3]. The rationale for the above is that adenomatous polyps are considered precursors to cancer, and through their early endoscopic removal, carcinoma can be prevented. In addition to the therapeutic roles of colonoscopy, it also allows for the identification of individuals at higher risk for accelerated carcinogenesis (e.g., multiple polyps, unfavorable histology, dysplasia, and large polyps ($\geq$1.0 cm)), who may benefit from more frequent screening.

Of further interest and consideration is that upon following current routine screening recommendations, the potential to identify large groups of patients with adenomatous polyps

also exists. This creates a huge burden on the healthcare system (costs, risks, and resources) in terms of surveillance of these patients.

Recommended Screening Guidelines

Guidelines from the American Cancer Society (ACS), the American Society of Colon and Rectal Surgeons (ASCRS), and the American Gastroenterological Association (AGA) all recommend that colorectal cancer screening begin at the age of 50 for both men and women with average risk (i.e., no family history of colorectal cancer, no personal history of inflammatory bowel disease, and asymptomatic) [4–6]. These accepted guidelines are based on joint efforts set forth in 2008 by the ACS, the US Multi-Society Task Force on Colorectal Cancer, and the American College of Radiology (ACR) [7]. Screening regimens can be divided into two categories: fecal testing and structural examinations. While structural examinations are designed to detect both polyps and cancer, fecal testing primarily detects already established cancers or possibly advanced adenomas. It is the opinion of the above organizations that the goal of colorectal cancer screening should be that of prevention. There are various screening options for asymptomatic individuals. The recommended time intervals are listed below and will be further evaluated in this section [7].

Screening Options and Timing for Average-Risk Individuals

- Colonoscopy every 10 years
- CT colonography (virtual colonoscopy) every 5 years
- Flexible sigmoidoscopy every 5 years
- Double-contrast barium enema every 5 years
- Guaiac-based fecal occult blood test (gFOBT) every year
- Fecal immunochemical test (FIT) every year
- Stool DNA (sDNA) test every 3 years

© Springer International Publishing 2016
S.R. Steele et al. (eds.), *The ASCRS Textbook of Colon and Rectal Surgery*, DOI 10.1007/978-3-319-25970-3_24

It is important to note that in order for the above to be effective, each of these screening regimens should be performed at regular intervals. In addition, if any of the non-colonoscopy screening tests listed are abnormal, a full colonoscopy is warranted, and the patient should be made aware of this possibility prior to initiation of screening.

Screening Guidelines for Individuals at an Increased Risk Based on Family History

1. If there is a history of colorectal cancer or adenomatous polyps in a first-degree relative before age 60, or in two or more first-degree relatives at any age (non-hereditary syndrome), then screening should begin at age 40 or 10 years prior to the youngest case, whichever is earlier. A colonoscopy is the recommended test in this instance, with screening every 5 years.
2. If there is a history of colorectal cancer or adenomatous polyps in a first-degree relative aged 60 or older, or in at least two or more second-degree relatives at any age, then screening should begin at age 40. Any of the screening options for average-risk individuals may be recommended along with the same screening intervals [8].

Screening Guidelines for Individuals Considered at High Risk Based on Genetics

1. If there is positive genetic testing for familial adenomatous polyposis (FAP) or suspected FAP without testing, then screening should begin at age 10–12 years. Screening should include yearly flexible sigmoidoscopy and consideration for genetic testing if not yet performed. Consideration for colectomy is recommended when testing is positive.
2. If there is a genetic or clinical diagnosis of Lynch syndrome or an individual at increased risk for Lynch, screening should begin at age 20–25 years or 10 years prior to the youngest case. This should include colonoscopy every 1–2 years and genetic testing if not yet performed. In addition, genetic testing should be offered to all first-degree relatives if a Lynch mutation is identified.
3. Individuals with inflammatory bowel disease (chronic ulcerative colitis or Crohn's disease) should begin screening 8 years after the onset of pan colitis or 12–15 years after the onset of left-sided colitis. Screening should be performed by colonoscopy every 1–2 years with biopsies assessing for dysplasia [8].

Screening Cessation

The US Preventive Services Task Force recommends screening up to the age of 75. Screening should be discontinued in individuals aged 76–85 years, if they have had routine screening. However, screening may be considered in this age group if never screened previously and according to each individual's health status and risk. Screening should not be performed in individuals after the age of 85 years [9].

Methods of Screening

Colonoscopy

The use of colonoscopy as a screening and therapeutic modality has become widespread since its initial undertaking by Wolf and Shinya in 1969 [10]. In 2009, there were 11.5 million colonoscopies performed in the United States [11]. In fact, colonoscopy has become one of the most commonly performed medical procedures performed today. The major advantages for colonoscopy as a screening regimen are that it allows visualization of the entire colon, along with the identification, biopsy, or removal of encountered polyps or cancer. Although colonoscopy is widely utilized in the United States for colorectal cancer screening, there are no prospective, randomized trials demonstrating a reduction in the incidence of, or the mortality from, colorectal cancer as a result of colonoscopy. However, as other screening modalities result in subsequent therapeutic colonoscopy after polyp detection, there is indirect evidence suggesting that colonoscopy is beneficial in reducing cancer incidence. This is evident from the Minnesota Colon Cancer Control Study, a randomized, controlled trial which demonstrated a 20 % reduction in colon cancer incidence after subsequent colonoscopy and follow-up based on FOBT screening [12]. Furthermore, studies evaluating cancer incidence after initial complete colonoscopy with polypectomy also demonstrate significant reductions in the incidence of colorectal cancer, ranging from 76 to 90 % depending on the reference population [2, 13]. More recently, subsequent follow-up of the National Polyp Study with a median surveillance period of 15.8 years after colonoscopic polypectomy also demonstrated a 53 % reduction in colorectal cancer-related mortality [14]. It is therefore evident that colonoscopy has the ability to effectively screen and remove adenomatous polyps, thereby reducing the risk of colorectal cancer development and mortality.

Although the use of colonoscopy as a screening modality has major benefits in risk reduction, there are also associated drawbacks with this procedure. Colonoscopy is usually done with sedation and thus requires a chaperone to accompany the patient for transportation. In addition, a complete bowel preparation is required and is often the most difficult part of the process for the patient. However, it is also one of the most important components to completing the procedure successfully and is critical in terms of quality. Rex et al. published an update of several quality indicators set forth by the American Society for Gastrointestinal Endoscopy (ASGE) and American College of Gastroenterology (ACG) Task Force on Quality in Endoscopy [15]. In this update, proposed quality indicators and performance targets are summarized for colonoscopy examinations in the pre-procedure, intra-procedure, and post-procedure periods (Table 24-1). It is imperative that each individual endoscopist be familiar with these targets and utilize them for guidance when screening.

TABLE 24-1. Proposed quality indicators in colonoscopy

Quality indicator	Grade of recommendation	Measure type	Performance target (%)
Pre-procedure			
1. Frequency with colonoscopy is performed for an indication that is included in a published standard list of appropriate indications, and the indication is documented	IC+	Process	>80
2. Frequency with which informed consent is obtained, including specific discussion of risks associated with colonoscopy, and fully documented	IC	Process	>98
3. Frequency with which colonoscopies follow recommended post-polypectomy and post-cancer resection surveillance intervals and 10-year intervals between screening colonoscopies in average-risk patients who have negative examination results and adequate bowel cleansing (priority indicator)	IA	Process	≥90
4. Frequency with which ulcerative colitis and Crohn's colitis surveillance is recommended with proper intervals	2C	Process	≥90
Intraprocedure			
5. Frequency with which the procedure note documents the quality of preparation	3	Process	>98
6. Frequency with which bowel preparation is adequate to allow the use of recommended surveillance or screening intervals	3	Process	≥85 of outpatient exams
7. Frequency with which visualization of the cecum by notation of landmarks and photodocumentation of landmarks is documented in every procedure (priority indicator)	1C	Process	
Cecal intubation rate with photography (all examinations)			≥90
Cecal intubation rate with photography (screening)			≥95
8. Frequency with which adenomas are detected in asymptomatic average-risk individuals (screening) (priority indicator)	1C	Outcome	
Adenoma detection rate for male/female population			≥25
Adenoma detection rate for male patients			≥30
Adenoma detection rate for female patients			≥20
9a. Frequency with which withdrawal time is measured	2C	Process	>98
9b. Average withdrawal time in negative-result screening colonoscopies	2C	Process	≥6 min
10. Frequency with which biopsy specimens are obtained when colonoscopy is performed for indication of chronic diarrhea	2C	Process	>98
11. Frequency of recommended tissue sampling when colonoscopy is performed for surveillance in ulcerative colitis and Crohn's colitis	1C	Process	>98
12. Frequency with which endoscopic removal of pedunculated polyps and sessile polyps <2 cm is attempted before surgical referral	3	Outcome	>98
13. Indication of perforation by procedure type (all indications vs. colorectal cancer screening/polyp surveillance) and post-polypectomy bleeding	1C	Outcome	
Incidence of perforation—all examinations			<1:500
Incidence of perforation—screening			<1:10,000
Incidence of post-polypectomy bleeding			<1 %
14. Frequency with which post-polypectomy bleeding is managed without surgery	1C	Outcome	≥90
15. Frequency with which appropriate recommendation for timing of repeat colonoscopy is documented and provided to the patient after histologic findings are reviewed	1A	Process	≥90

This list of potential quality indicators is meant to be a comprehensive listing of measurable end points. It is not the intention of the task force that all end points be measured in every practice setting. In most cases, validation may be required before a given end point may be adopted universally
With permission from Rex DK, Schoenfeld PS, Cohen J, Pike IM, Adler DG, Fennerty MB, et al. Quality indicators for colonoscopy. Am J Gastroenterol. 2015;110(1):72–90. ©Nature Publishing Group (15)

Selected important target areas include: (1) cecal intubation rates for screening with photodocumentation of ≥95 %, (2) an overall adenoma detection rate of ≥25 % (≥30 % for males, ≥20 % for females), (3) average scope withdrawal time of ≥6 min, (4) incidence of perforation during screening of <1:1000, (5) incidence of post-polypectomy bleeding of <1 %, and (6) the frequency with which appropriate recommendations for timing of repeat colonoscopy are documented and provided to the patient of ≥90 %. Furthermore, an adequate bowel preparation is also necessary in this context and is also listed as a pre-procedure quality indicator.

The target recommendation for the frequency for which bowel preparation is adequate should be ≥85 %. Sherer et al. reported that in cases where poor bowel preparation was recorded, the detection rate of advanced histology was significantly affected as compared with adequate preparation [16].

Unfortunately, despite best efforts, there are reported miss rates for both polyps and cancers with the use of colonoscopy. A systematic review evaluating miss rates by same-day colonoscopy revealed a miss of 2.1 % for polyps ≥10 mm and 13 % for polyps 5–10 mm in size [17]. Higher miss rates were noted when concomitant CT colonography was utilized rather than tandem colonoscopy. With this approach, a miss rate of 11.8 % was noted for polyps ≥10 mm in size [18]. Similarly, potential miss rates for cancer are reported to be 3.4 %, especially lesions within the proximal colon (5.9 %), based upon evaluation of patients who have received a screening colonoscopy within 3 years of diagnosis [19]. While there may be several reasons for failure of neoplasia detection, it only further stresses the importance of adequate bowel preparation and adherence to evaluation guidelines in order to minimize miss rates.

It also appears that miss rates may be somewhat dependent on location within the colon in that the proximal colon may not be as reliably or consistently evaluated. Again, Bressler et al. noted that most cancer misses occurred within the right colon compared to the left side (5.9 % vs. 2.3 % in the sigmoid or rectum) [19]. Similarly, Baxter et al. revealed that colonoscopy screening reduced the number of deaths due to left-sided colorectal cancer, but not right-sided, suggesting that screening colonoscopy for right-sided lesions may be less effective [20]. This finding was not evident with the use of CT colonography; however, Pickhardt et al. revealed that misses can occur throughout the colon, usually behind the proximal aspect of a fold and even within 10 cm of the anal verge [18]. In any event, it is apparent that even with our best screening modality, the ability to screen reliably is not without error.

Incomplete Colonoscopy

As noted in Table 24-1, recommended rates of incomplete colonoscopy (without cecal intubation) should be <5 % during screening and <10 % overall. Unfortunately, there are no apparent guidelines or consensus as to the best management strategies in cases of incomplete colonoscopy. Advanced neoplasia is noted in 4 % of these cases within the non-visualized portion of the colon [21]. When colonoscopy is incomplete, options include repeat colonoscopy, use of other endoscopic modalities (i.e., smaller endoscope, double balloon endoscopy), CT colonography, or barium enema. The decision of which modality is best suited is dependent on both the reasons for the incomplete exam and the institution-specific resources available [22].

Adjuncts to Colonoscopy

In an effort to improve colonoscopy screening, more recent technical developments in colonoscopic imaging have targeted advancements in polyp detection. These advances have included (1) techniques applied to current colonoscopy methods, including high-definition monitors, chromoendoscopy, or cap-assisted colonoscopy (CAC), and (2) colonoscope enhancements to current imaging, such as narrow band imaging (NBI), autofluorescence imaging (AFI), and Fujinon intelligent color enhancement (FICE).

The addition of high-definition white light (HDWL) and high-definition monitors to standard colonoscopy may optimize mucosal visualization. A meta-analysis evaluating five studies comparing high-definition to conventional colonoscopy revealed a slight improvement (3.5 %) in adenoma detection rates [23].

Pan-colonic chromoendoscopy (PCC) involves the topical spray application of a dye, usually 0.4 % indigo carmine via the colonoscope. The dye is not absorbed but rather highlights irregular, flat, or small lesions that may be less obvious. Possible advantages to this technology are noted in two prospective, randomized trials comparing chromoendoscopy to either standard or HDWL colonoscopy. While a marginal, though not significant, improvement in overall adenoma detection rate was noted when compared to HDWL, there were improvements in flat adenoma detection [24]. In contrast, compared to standard colonoscopy, Pohl et al. found improvements in both flat and overall adenoma detection rates. However, PCC required more time to complete the procedure as well [25].

CAC attaches a clear cap to the tip of the colonoscope. This allows for deflection of mucosal folds without obscuring visualization, potentially improving detection in these locations. However, the findings of randomized, controlled trials are mixed as to whether CAC offers improvements in adenoma detection rates over conventional colonoscopy [26, 27].

A virtual chromoendoscopy technique, NBI, involves the placement of narrow band filters behind the light source to remove red light and thus increase blue and green wavelengths. This enhances mucosal surface vascularity and therefore polyp visualization. A meta-analysis comparing NBI with standard colonoscopy demonstrated no improvements in adenoma detection with the addition of NBI [28]. Similarly, systematic comparisons between high-definition NBI and HDWL colonoscopy also failed to show improvements in adenoma detection [29]. However, there is a suggestion that high-definition NBI may have an advantage over standard colonoscopy with respect to minimizing polyp and adenoma miss rates [30].

Other virtual techniques include AFI which utilizes a blue filter to create an autofluorescent image from the tissue. Neoplastic tissue will take on a red-green fluorescence in contrast to surrounding normal mucosa [31]. Similarly, FICE utilizes a computed spectral estimation technology that narrows light bandwidth without the use of filters and allows for visualization at various wavelengths. In particular, this allows for enhancement of mucosal vascular and pit patterns [32]. In a randomized study of over 1600 subjects, neither NBI nor FICE increased the adenoma detection rate when compared with standard colonoscopy [33]. A meta-analysis of 42 studies assessed each of the previously discussed colonoscopy enhancement modalities, including each of the virtual capabilities in their ability to improve adenoma detection rates over standard high-definition/white light colonoscopy. In doing so, only chromoendoscopy with indigo carmine demonstrated potential improvement [34].

Complications

Complications related to colonoscopy have included cardiopulmonary events, bleeding, perforation, diverticulitis, and post-polypectomy syndrome. The risk of unplanned cardiopulmonary events after colonoscopy is 1.1 % and is usually related to the effects of conscious sedation [35]. In a review by Rutter et al., the overall 30-day risk of serious adverse events after colonoscopy was 4.7 per 1000 screening colonoscopies and 6.8 per 1000 follow-up colonoscopies. The risk of perforation was 0.04 % for screening (0.07 % with polypectomy) and 0.12 % after follow-up. Most related bleeding occurs after polypectomy, with a rate of 0.27 % for screening and 0.50 % after polypectomy. Post-polypectomy bleeding can be immediate or delayed. Older age was associated with higher rates of perforation or bleeding [36]. Post-polypectomy syndrome is related to an electrocautery full-thickness burn resulting in localized peritonitis. In a review by Ko et al., the risk of post-polypectomy syndrome ranged from 0.003 to 0.1 %, while the risk of diverticulitis ranged from 0.04 to 0.08 % and the overall risk of death from 0 to 0.09 % [37]. Overall, there is a 1.17 % admission rate after colonoscopy for the above complications.

CT Colonography or Virtual Colonoscopy

CT colonography (CTC) or virtual colonoscopy is a minimally invasive, radiographic option for colorectal cancer screening. It utilizes computed tomography to generate two-dimensional (2D) images that allow for further three-dimensional (3D) reconstruction with the assistance of software technology. Together, evaluation of both 2D and 3D images allows for accurate neoplasia detection. Figure 24-1a–d demonstrates 2D and 3D imaging of a pedunculated sigmoid polyp and subsequent colonoscopic identification.

CTC still requires adequate bowel preparation and must have gaseous distension of the colon to allow for adequate examination. This entails insertion of a rectal catheter to allow for manual or automated inflation with carbon dioxide, infused continuously as images are acquired. Tagging of residual stool contents with an oral delivery of dilute barium (2 %) and residual fluid tagging with water-soluble iodinated contrast (diatrizoate) have further increased sensitivity [38]. As with optical colonoscopy, meeting appropriate quality parameters is also important in CTC. These parameters as recommended by the ACR should include (1) adequate colon cleansing and distension, (2) complete anatomic coverage of the colon and rectum, (3) visualization of each colonic segment in at least one position, (4) appropriate physician training for CTC performance and interpretation, and (5) proper documentation and communication of clinical findings [39].

CTC does not require sedation, and the exam can be performed rather quickly. However, in cases where polyps are detected, subsequent therapeutic colonoscopy is required. Ideally, this should be performed on the same day since bowel preparation is already complete. This requires program coordination between gastroenterology and radiology departments. In cases where polyps are detected, findings of one or more polyps ≥10 mm or three or more polyps ≥6 mm should be referred for subsequent colonoscopy and polypectomy. Though somewhat controversial, isolated polyps in the 6–9 mm range may also be referred for therapeutic intervention [38, 40]. Since very small polyps (≤5 mm) carry low clinical risk, reporting and referral for these isolated lesions are currently not recommended [39, 41]. A further advantage of CTC is that it allows for a limited evaluation for extracolonic findings as well [42]. Of these potential findings, it was noted that 7.4 % were clinically relevant with 2.1 % gaining clinical benefit from detection [43].

Complications related to CTC are very rare. A survey of a virtual colonoscopy working group reported no perforations in more than 11,000 CTC screening examinations, and two perforations in more than 10,000 exams for diagnostic indications (0.02 %), only one of which was symptomatic [44]. Although often discussed, the radiation exposure associated with CTC is also quite low, reportedly around 5 mSv for screening purposes [45]. This is well below the 100 mSv threshold often considered when attempting to address associated health risk [46].

In an early assessment of over 1200 asymptomatic subjects undergoing same-day CTC and optical colonoscopy, a 94 % sensitivity for the detection of adenomas greater than 1 cm was noted and 89 % for adenomas ≥6 mm [47]. More recently, the American College of Radiology Imaging Network (ACRIN) national, multicenter CTC trial assessed over 2500 patients. The per-patient sensitivity for the detection of polyps or cancer ≥10 mm was 90 % and 78 % for polyps ≥6 mm [48]. Furthermore, when considering detection rates for cancer only, meta-analysis conferred a 96 % sensitivity for the detection by CTC with a prevalence of 3.6 % [49]. These findings compare favorably to optical colonoscopy. In a parallel screening program utilizing both colonoscopy and CTC in over 3100 patients, similar detection rates for advanced neoplasia (polyps and cancer) were noted (3.4 % and 3.2 %, respectively). There were many more polypectomies performed in the optical colonoscopy group and also more procedure-related complications [50]. Upon assessing the outcomes in over 1000 cases where screening CTC exams were negative, one interval cancer and 11 large adenomas were noted after a mean follow-up of 4.7 years [51]. Together, these studies suggest that CTC is an

FIGURE 24-1. CT colonography images demonstrate both (**a**) 2D and (**b**) 3D imaging of a pedunculated sigmoid polyp, and subsequent (**c**) colonoscopic identification (**d**) demonstrates the virtual location of the polyp by CT imaging.

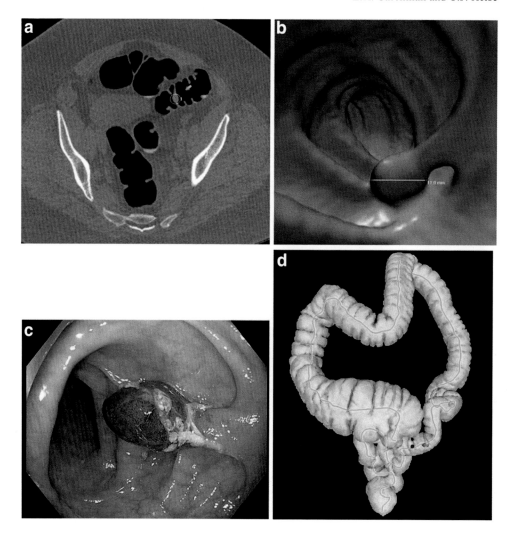

acceptable alternative to optical colonoscopy and that current 5-year screening intervals are appropriate.

Flexible Sigmoidoscopy

Flexible sigmoidoscopy may be useful as a component of the screening regimen for colorectal cancer. The standard sigmoidoscope is 60 cm in length. To be effective as a screening modality, the quality of the evaluation must be adequate. Therefore, it has been recommended that the scope be advanced to a minimum of 40 cm in order to minimize the risk of missing a distal colorectal cancer [52]. In addition, if distal pathology is identified, it must be properly biopsied in order to best determine the need for further evaluation. With adenoma detection, the risk of harboring concomitant disease more proximally is at least twofold and thus requires formal colonoscopy [53]. The advantages of flexible sigmoidoscopy lie in the ability to perform the procedure without sedation (although with some potential patient discomfort), by a variety of healthcare professionals and after only minimal bowel preparation.

The major problem with sigmoidoscopy lies in its inability to evaluate the more proximal colon. Despite this, meta-analyses have demonstrated a beneficial reduction in the incidence of colorectal cancer and long-term mortality when compared with no screening [54]. When considering only intention to treat analyses, a reduction in the incidence of distal colorectal cancer and mortality was reported as 31 % and 46 %, respectively [55]. Results of a large randomized, clinical trial demonstrated a 21 % reduction in colorectal cancer incidence and a 26 % reduction in mortality. However, mortality from proximal colorectal cancer was not affected, with a mortality reduction of 50 % when considering only distal colorectal cancer [56]. Finally, a more recently published randomized, controlled trial compared the use of flexible sigmoidoscopy alone or in combination with fecal occult blood testing (FOBT) as a one-time screening regimen in age groups beginning at both 50 and 55 years of age. Patients with positive findings with either test were then offered a colonoscopy. This study revealed a 63 % rate of adherence to screening and a 28 % reduction in the incidence of colorectal cancer and a 12 % reduction in mortality. Interestingly, there was no difference noted between groups receiving flexible sigmoidoscopy alone or in combination with FOBT [57].

Complications

The risk of GI complications including perforation with flexible sigmoidoscopy is extremely low, reported to be 0.02 % [58]. Gatto et al. reported an incidence of perforation after flexible sigmoidoscopy of 0.88 per 1000 procedures for patients aged 65 or older [59].

Fecal Occult Blood Testing/Fecal Immunochemical Testing

FOBT is aimed at detecting subtle blood loss in the gastrointestinal tract. Based on randomized, controlled trials, annual screening for FOB is recommended for detecting cancer and precancerous polyps in average-risked patients starting at the age of 50. There are two general types of FOBT based on the analyte detected: guaiac versus immunochemical. With positive testing, the patient will then need to undergo appropriate diagnostic testing (colonoscopy or flexible sigmoidoscopy) within a year of the abnormal result. Previous reports demonstrated that only 25–59 % of patients with a positive FOBT receive diagnostic evaluation after a positive test [60].

A stool guaiac test (gFOBT) is done by smearing feces onto an absorbent paper that has been chemically treated. Hydrogen peroxide is then placed onto the paper, and if a trace amount of blood is present, the color will change. The color change is due to the fact that heme has peroxidase-like activities that breakdown hydrogen peroxide. Optimal use depends on following strict dietary adjustments prior to collecting the stool sample. This test requires at least 2 mL of blood loss a day to become positive. There have been several randomized, controlled trials that demonstrate a benefit of FOBT in reducing mortality from CRC (about 15 % reduction) [61, 62].

FIT utilizes specific antibodies to detect globin. FIT has replaced most gFOBT tests in that it is both cheap and quantitative. There is evidence that FIT has higher sensitivity and specificity over gFOBT (13–25 % vs. 81 %). FIT can pick up as little as 0.3 mL of blood in the stool, and patients are not required to follow any dietary restrictions prior to testing. A recent systematic review demonstrated an overall accuracy of 95 % for CRC detection with 79 % sensitivity and 94 % specificity [63]. However, it does have a lower sensitivity in terms of adenoma detection (only 28 %) [64].

Stool DNA Testing

Perhaps the most recent advancement in colorectal cancer screening involves the use of DNA testing of stool samples. Tumor cells and their associated DNA are continuously passed into the stool. Tumor DNA constitutes a very small amount of the fecal content; therefore, a large stool sample is needed for analysis. This assay tests for DNA mutations and methylations of common genes associated with colorectal cancer (i.e., KRAS mutations). These tests also assay for human hemoglobin similar to FIT. This test concomitantly tests for beta-actin to allow for an estimation of the total amount of human DNA present. The results of the assay allow for a composite score that is compared to a standardized value in order to determine a positive or negative test result. There are no dietary restrictions with this test. In a recent study in asymptomatic patients, stool DNA testing detected significantly more cancers than did FIT but also had more false positives [65]. In screening and surveillance, polyps greater than 1 cm can be detected with stool DNA testing, unlike FIT testing [66]. Its sensitivity for polyps greater than 1 cm is 57 %, for greater than 2 cm is 73 %, and for greater than 3 cm is 83 % (the same rate for detecting polyps with high-grade dysplasia) [67].

Double-Contrast Barium Enema

With the more widespread use of the previously described screening entities, the use of contrast enema has diminished as a screening modality. However, it may still be utilized in regions where other screening modalities are not available. Double-contrast barium enema (DCBE) involves coating the colonic mucosal surface with barium followed by distension with air through a rectally placed catheter. Fluoroscopic and standard radiographic imaging is utilized during various positional changes to assess the entire colon. Prior bowel preparation is also required to allow for removal of adherent fecal content.

A small number of studies utilized both colonoscopy and DCBE to assess neoplasia detection. Winawer et al. reported the sensitivity of DCBE to detect polyps ≤5 mm, 6–10 mm, and >10 mm as 32 %, 53 %, and 48 %, respectively [68]. Similarly, Rockey et al. noted sensitivities of 48 % for lesions ≥10 mm and 35 % for lesions 6–9 mm [69]. Furthermore, a meta-analysis comparing DCBE and CTC demonstrated lower sensitivities for detecting polyps ≥6 mm with DCBE [70]. When considering only colorectal cancer detection, the sensitivity of DCBE increases to 85 % [71]; however, the rate of new or missed cancers following DCBE has also been reported as high as 22 % [72]. These findings suggest that DCBE may be inferior to other methods of screening. In addition, the use of DCBE may be less attractive to both patient and radiologist, due to the nature and labor intensiveness of the exam [7].

Screening Reality

Although there are several modalities available for colorectal cancer screening, the ACS reports that in 2012 only 59 % of Americans over the age of 50 were screened according to current guidelines. Furthermore, there appears to be a wide variability in screening patterns by state of residence [73].

Surveillance

Guidelines for Surveillance After Polypectomy

History

In the 1970s, the follow-up recommendations for post-polypectomy included a repeat colonoscopy on an annual basis. In 1997, guidelines were published by the gastrointestinal consortium, based on the results of the 1993 National Polyp Study [2], which recommended that the first follow-up examination after polypectomy occur at 3 years. These guidelines were then updated in 2003 based on risk stratification into low-risk and higher-risk adenomas, the goal of which was to identify predictors of future advanced adenomas and cancers to create risk stratification for patients. Higher-risk patients are categorized as those with ≥3 adenomas, high-grade dysplasia, villous features, or an adenoma ≥1 cm. Lower-risk patients are those with 1–2 adenomas with no high-grade dysplasia. With this stratification system, the secondary goals were to decrease the surveillance burden on the system and to decrease the risks to the patients by tailoring follow-up based on risk. It is important to note that the current guidelines for surveillance are to be applied only after high-quality baseline colonoscopy with complete removal of all detected lesions. If either of these two criteria is not met, then repeat examination should be planned. Also, discontinuation of surveillance should be considered in patients with serious comorbidities with less than a 10-year life expectancy. Finally, these guidelines apply only to asymptomatic individuals; new symptoms need diagnostic workup.

Surveillance Based on Pathology of Polyp

Hyperplastic and Serrated Polyps

Serrated lesions of the colon and rectum are classified by the World Health Organization (WHO) into three general categories based on cytological features, architectural features, and location. The categories include hyperplastic polyps, sessile serrated adenoma/polyps, and traditional serrated adenomas (Figure 24-2a, b). These lesions are usually located proximally, sessile or flat in morphology, and pale in color, with indistinct borders, and usually have a mucus cap. Due to their indistinct appearance, there is a high rate of incomplete resection. NBI and chromoendoscopy techniques can be used to facilitate identification and delineation of borders. Given that incomplete resection rates are high in serrated adenomas greater than 1 cm, it seems reasonable to tattoo these lesions so that they can be identified on repeat endoscopy in 3–6 months [74].

Most international post-polypectomy surveillance guidelines do not recommend surveillance for serrated polyps. However, there is increasing awareness that these lesions may be major precursor lesions to cancer development in about 1/3 of colorectal cancer cases. The US Multi-Society Task Force guidelines for post-polypectomy surveillance are 1–5 years depending on the number, size, and presence of dysplasia. Recent reviews on the management of serrated lesions recommended complete removal of all lesions except for ≤5 mm in the sigmoid or rectum. Those small lesions should be randomly biopsied for histology.

Those patients with small rectal hyperplastic polyps are considered to have normal colonoscopies and therefore should be screened every 10 years. The exceptions to this are those patients who have hyperplastic polyposis syndromes (HPS). HPS is a rare syndrome characterized by multiple hyperplastic and/or serrated adenomas. Patients with this syndrome have a lifetime risk of colorectal cancer of up to 50 % [75]. The WHO criteria for HPS are defined as meeting one of the following criteria: having five or greater serrated lesions proximal to the sigmoid colon (with two being greater than 1.0 cm) or more than 30 serrated lesions throughout the colon. There are no evidence-based guidelines for surveillance for these patients, but most physicians are screening them annually or biennially [76]. First-degree relatives of patients with HPS should undergo colonoscopy at the age of 40 or 10 years before the age of diagnosis of HPS. With regard to patients with serrated adenomas that do not have HPS, there are limited observational studies to make strong recommendations for surveillance. However, there are consensus recommenda-

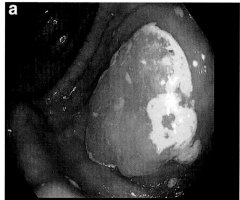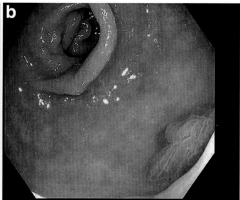

FIGURE 24-2. Endoscopic views of two different types of serrated polyps. (**a**) Sessile serrated adenoma/polyp in the cecum and (**b**) a traditional serrated adenoma of the rectum.

TABLE 24-2. Recommendations for screening intervals based on consensus guidelines for patients with serrated polyps based on histology, number, location, and size[a]

Histology	Size (mm)	Number	Location	Interval in years
HP	<10	Any number[b,c]	Rectosigmoid	10
HP	≤5	≤3	Proximal to sigmoid	10
HP	Any	≥4	Proximal to sigmoid	5
HP	>5	≥1	Proximal to sigmoid	5
SSA/P or TSA	<10	<3	Any	5
SSA/P or TSA	≥10	1	Any	3
SSA/P or TSA	<10	≥3	Any	3
SSA/P	≥10	≤2	Any	1–3[d]
SSA/P w/dysplasia	Any	Any		1–3[e]

[a]The interval recommendations presented here represent consensus opinion based on low-quality or very low-quality evidence. They are likely to change as higher quality evidence becomes available, and alternatives may be equally reasonable

[b]Patients with >20 HPs in the rectosigmoid meet the World Health Organization definition of serrated polyposis if there are additional serrated lesions proximal to the sigmoid

[c]Some panel members follow a policy of 5 years if there are multiple HPs 6–9 mm in size in the rectosigmoid

[d]Patients with two or more serrated polyps ≥10 mm in the proximal colon meet the World Health Organization criteria for serrated polyps if three additional serrated lesions of any size are proximal to the sigmoid are identified

[e]SSA/P with cytological dysplasia is a more advanced lesion than SSA/P. Depending on the size of the lesion, the confidence in complete endoscopic resection and other associated lesions, intervals shorter than 3 years may be appropriate

Note 1: Patients with both significant serrated findings and concurrent adenomas may be at a more advanced stage in the progression toward cancer. Closer follow-up may be indicated in some cases based on clinical judgment

Note 2: In general, these recommendations for surveillance are for the first follow-up. For findings with short follow-up recommendations, a longer subsequent follow-up interval may be appropriately applied when a follow-up exam shows improvement in findings, i.e., reduction in the number, size, and/or histologic severity of lesions

Note 3: Because of interobserver variation in the pathologic differentiation of HP from SSA/P, proximal colon serrated lesions >10 mm in size that are designated HP may be considered to be SSA/P by clinicians

With permission from Rex DK, Ahnen DJ, Baron JA, Batts KP, Burke CA, Burt RW, et al. Serrated lesions of the colorectum: review and recommendations from an expert panel. Am J Gastroenterol. 2012;107(9):1315–29; quiz 4, 3 Reproduced with permission. ©Nature Publishing Group [77]

tions that were made in 2012 where surveillance intervals were made based on histology (HP, SSA/P, or TSA), size, number, and location (Table 24-2) [77].

Adenoma

Adenomas can be classified histologically as tubular, villous, or tubulovillous. According to the World Health Organization criteria, tubular adenomas have less than 25 % villous component, tubulovillous 25–75 %, and villous greater than 75 % [78]. Tubular adenomas are the most common type of adenoma found followed by tubulovillous and then villous. Tubular adenomas have <5 % of harboring cancer, while the risk of tubulovillous is 20–25 % and villous adenomas is 35–40 % [79]. Screening series have reported an adenoma prevalence rate of 15–30 %. With the addition of high-definition colonoscopy, this number has been quoted as high as 50 % [80].

The recommendations for post-polypectomy surveillance in patients with one or two small polyps that are less than 1 cm in size range from 3 to 10 years post-polypectomy, depending on which recommendation is followed. The ASGE and the Polyp Guidelines from the ACG recommend follow-up in 5 years. The ACS recommends follow-up in 3–6 years. The Multi-Society Task Force and the Joint ACS and Multi-Society Task Force recommend follow-up in 5–10 years [81]. If low-grade dysplasia is identified on pathology for these patients, the surveillance guidelines do not change.

Patients with 3–10 adenomas, any adenoma ≥1 cm, any adenoma with villous features, or high-grade dysplasia should have their next colonoscopy in 3 years provided the entire polyp was removed in a non-piecemeal fashion (Figure 24-3).

Those patients with sessile adenomas that were removed in piecemeal should be reexamined in 2–6 months to confirm complete removal. If on follow-up colonoscopy there are only 1–2 tubular adenomas, the interval to screening is increased to 5 years. A meta-analysis evaluated the safety and efficacy of endoscopic resection specifically for large polyps (greater than 2 cm). They found a recurrence rate of 14 % with the majority of recurrences being amenable to further endoscopic therapy. It was noted that endoscopic submucosal dissection appeared to reduce the risk of recurrence, while invasive cancer on histology was the main reason for endoscopic failure [82].

Those patients with >10 adenomas at one examination should have follow-up in less than 3 years and should be referred for consultation with a genetic counselor.

FIGURE 24-3. Endoscopic view of a cecal ulceration which pathology after biopsy demonstrated colonic mucosa with adenomatous change and focal high-grade dysplasia.

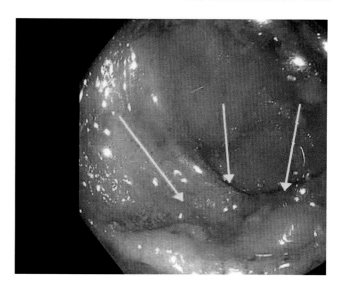

Inflammatory Polyps

Inflammatory polyps include benign lymphoid polyps and pseudopolyps (such as those seen in ulcerative colitis). Benign lymphoid polyps are composed of the normal lymphoid tissue and therefore do not require any surveillance if this is seen on pathology. Pseudopolyps are discussed below in the inflammatory disease section.

Hamartomatous Polyps

Hamartomatous of the colon and rectum include juvenile polyps and polyps seen in Peutz-Jeghers disease. Juvenile polyps, as the name suggests, occur in children. These are not frequently seen after 15 years of age. In 70 % of cases, there is only one polyp identified. Juvenile polyposis syndrome (JPS) is a disorder of multiple juvenile polyps. These polyps may cause bleeding, abdominal pain, or obstruction. The diagnosis is made when there is any one of the following: (1) more than five juvenile polyps of the colon or rectum, (2) juvenile polyps in other parts of the gastrointestinal tract, and (3) any number of juvenile polyps and one or more affected family members. Three different types of JPS have been described based on the signs and symptoms of the disease. Most juvenile polyps are benign. It is estimated that people with JPS have a 10–50 % risk of developing cancer of the gastrointestinal tract (most commonly colon and rectal cancer). This disorder is associated with mutations in the BMPR1A and SMAD4 genes. It is inherited in an autosomal dominant fashion. Treatment depends on size and number of polyps found. When there are only a few polyps identified and the polyps are small enough, they can be removed endoscopically. Polyps that are too large or too numerous to be removed this way may require an operative resection. If a polyp is seen on endoscopy, it should be removed, and screening should be done yearly until no polyps are found.

Thereafter, patients with juvenile polyps should be screened every 3 years if endoscopies are negative [83].

Peutz-Jeghers syndrome (PJS) is an autosomal dominant disorder characterized by intestinal hamartomatous polyps along with a distinct pattern of skin and mucosal melanin deposition. These patients have a 15-fold increased risk of developing intestinal cancers compared to the general population. The genetic mutation identified with this syndrome is in the STK11 gene (also known as LKB1). A clinical diagnosis of PJS requires the presence of one of the following: (1) two or more histologically confirmed PJ polyps, (2) any number of PJ polyps detected in a patient with a family history, (3) characteristic mucocutaneous pigmentation in an individual who has family history of PJS, and (4) any number of PJ polyps in an individual who has the characteristic mucocutaneous pigmentation. Those patients that met clinical criteria should undergo genetic testing for a germline mutation. In terms of surveillance, these patients should undergo a colonoscopy every 2–3 years starting in late adolescence. They should also have upper endoscopies every 2–3 years. Small bowel interrogation (CT enterography) should also occur every 2–3 years [84].

Inflammatory Bowel Disease

In patients with inflammatory bowel disease (IBD), the presence of chronic inflammation puts them at an increased risk for dysplasia and cancer. Polyps detected in patients with IBD are referred to as a dysplasia-associated lesion or mass (DALM). DALM lesions are then divided into three categories based on endoscopic appearance and location: (1) It is a sporadic adenoma if the polyp resembles an adenoma both endoscopically and histologically and is located outside an area of histologically proven colitis. Complete polypectomy with routine surveillance is adequate with these lesions. (2) It is an IBD-associated adenoma-like polypoid dysplasia if

FIGURE 24-4. (a) Endoscopic
view of a polyp in the sigmoid
colon of a patient with ulcerative
colitis. (b) The use of
chromoendoscopy in 4 Ballows
for better visualization of the
borders of the polyp compared
to the images without indigo
carmine in 4A.

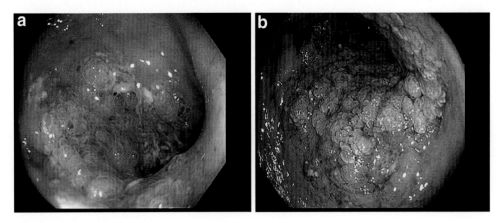

the lesion resembles an adenoma endoscopically and histologically and is located in an area of colitis. For these lesions, if they are not associated with flat dysplasia or carcinoma, polypectomy with surveillance at a shortened interval is recommended. (3) Finally, IBD-associated non-adenoma-like dysplasia, which is considered a true DALM, is a lesion that is irregular and broadly based and is located in an area of colitis. These lesions are at high risk for associated carcinoma and should be treated with colectomy after the diagnosis of dysplasia is confirmed by an experienced pathologist (Figure 24-4a, b) [85].

Surveillance with Cancer Resection

Patients who are undergoing curative resection for colon cancer are recommended to obtain a colonoscopy 1 year after resection. If the examination at 1 year is normal, then the interval should be extended to 3 years. If that subsequent one is normal, then the interval is again increased to 5 years.

For those patients who are undergoing resection for rectal cancer then there should be periodic examinations to identify early recurrence. This usually entails proctoscopic examination every 3–6 months for the first 2–3 years.

Early Cancer (T1) Within Polyp

There are two classification systems that are established for the identification of cancer within a polyp. The first is Haggitt classification which is utilized for quantifying the extent of invasion in pedunculated polyps. The second is the Kikuchi classification for sessile polyps.

Haggitt Classification

- Haggitt level 0: Noninvasive.
- Haggitt level 1: Cancer invades into the submucosa but limited to the head of the polyp.
- Haggitt level 2: Cancer invades into the neck of the polyp.

- Haggitt level 3: Cancer invades the stalk of the polyp.
- Haggitt level 4: Cancer invades the submucosa of the bowel wall below the stalk.

The risk of spread to the lymph nodes is less than 1 % for levels 1–3. For Haggitt level 4, the risk of lymph node disease ranges from 12 to 25 % [86, 87].

Kikuchi classification of the submucosa is divided into three levels:

- SM1 is invasion of the upper one-third.
- SM2 is invasion of the middle third.
- SM3 is invasion into the lower one-third.

Haggitt levels 1–3 are equivalent to SM1 and Haggitt level 4 can be SM1, SM2, or SM3. There have been several factors identified that increase the risk of lymph node metastases. These factors include lymphovascular invasion, poor differentiation, gender, extensive budding, and SM3 invasion [88].

For low-risk cancers, Haggitt levels 1–3, Kikuchi SM1, or no evidence of poor differentiation or angioinvasion, where the lesion has been completely resected in one piece with negative margins, endoscopic or local excision is regarded as adequate treatment. However, patients should be made aware that although the risk of nodal metastases is very low, it is not zero and that there is no effective surveillance that will reliably detect nodal metastases prior to distant metastatic spread. Although surveillance colonoscopy is recommended at frequent intervals (e.g., yearly), the risk of tumor growth is in the nodes, not in the lumen, calling into question the value of frequent colonoscopy. Surveillance is usually continued for 5 years. There has been some debate on this matter, however, in that there are studies that demonstrate that the risk for recurrence extends past 5 years post-polypectomy [89]. Formal surgical resection is indicated for high-risk cancers (Haggitt level 4, Kikuchi SM3, lymphovascular invasion, poor differentiation, or positive resection margin, cancer in sessile lesions removed in piecemeal fashion).

When to Tattoo an Area After Polypectomy

Current guidelines strongly recommend tattooing of suspicious lesions during colonoscopy. Given that the risk of cancer arising from a polyp in the National Bowel Cancer Screening Program increased significantly when the polyp was greater than 1 cm in size, most would recommend tattoo of all polyps greater than 1 cm (Figure 24-5a, b). In addition, when sessile lesions are removed in piecemeal fashion, the risk of recurrence is high. Tattoo at the site of polypectomy should be considered to help identify the area at subsequent colonoscopy.

Benefits of Surveillance

There have been several studies that have examined the benefits of post-polypectomy surveillance in terms of cancer prevention [90, 91]. These studies identified the risk of colorectal cancer after adenoma resection that depended not only upon the characteristics of the adenoma (advanced or non-advanced) but also colonoscopy surveillance practices. None of these studies are randomized, controlled trials, so there is no direct evidence on the exact benefit that is obtained through surveillance. Most of these studies emphasize the importance of surveillance especially in high-risk adenomas, but there is evidence of the importance of surveillance in low-risk lesions. A recent meta-analysis found that patients with low-risk adenomas had a relative risk of 1.8 (95 % CI: 1.3–2.6) for a metachronous advanced neoplasm compared to those without adenomas, though the absolute risk noted in both groups was low [92].

Reality of Surveillance

Surveys demonstrated that 50 % of endoscopists are not following the guidelines for post-polypectomy surveillance [93]. Levin indicated that failure to follow these guidelines was due to uncertainty, fear of malpractice, and financial incentives [94].

Chemoprevention

A variety of oral agents have been evaluated as possible chemopreventive strategies for both adenoma and carcinoma formation. These agents have included nonsteroidal anti-inflammatory agents, folic acid, calcium, and various antioxidants. A systematic review identified several randomized, controlled trials evaluating for the potential benefits of these agents [95]. They concluded that the use of aspirin (81–325 mg/day) in individuals with a history of adenomas or colorectal cancer (CRC) resulted in a 21 % reduction in adenoma recurrence. Though not evident until after a prolonged follow-up period (23 years), a 26 % reduction in CRC incidence was noted in the general population in studies evaluating a larger aspirin dose (300–1500 mg/day). Furthermore, nonaspirin anti-inflammatory medications such as celecoxib (400 mg/day) have also demonstrated benefit in patients with a history of adenomas, revealing a 34 % reduction in adenoma recurrence.

Though the use of folic acid failed to show benefit with respect to adenoma recurrence, calcium intake (1200–2000 mg/day) was found beneficial with an 18 % risk reduction after a history of prior adenomas. Finally, there was no significant benefit toward adenoma recurrence noted with antioxidant ingestion (vitamins A, C, and E, beta-carotene, or selenium) after a history of adenoma removal.

Conclusion

Proper screening recommendations are based on age and risk, which can be based on personal or family history. Screening for colorectal cancer now has several options, though colonoscopy currently remains most common. CT colonography, although not therapeutic, is an ideal alternative to colonoscopy. It also has the potential to reveal extracolonic lesions. Surveillance after colonoscopic polypectomy is dependent on polyp type, size, and number. When an occult cancer is encountered within a polyp after colonoscopic excision, management considerations should be based

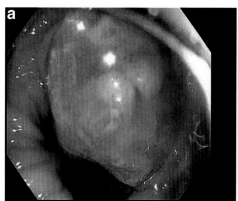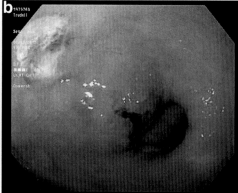

FIGURE 24-5. (a) A 2 cm rectal polyp noted endoscopically. (b) Polyp was resected and tattooed based on size criteria. Final pathology demonstrated moderately differentiated invasive colonic adenocarcinoma with mucinous features arising from tubulovillous adenoma. Carcinoma was present at cauterized margins.

on histology and polyp morphology (sessile vs. pedunculated). Adherence to recommended guidelines and monitoring of published quality indicators may improve outcomes and minimize polyp miss rates during colonoscopy.

References

1. Colorectal (Colon) Cancer Centers for Disease Control and Prevention [cited 2015]. 2015. http://www.cdc.gov/cancer/colorectal/.
2. Winawer SJ, Zauber AG, Ho MN, O'Brien MJ, Gottlieb LS, Sternberg SS, et al. Prevention of colorectal cancer by colonoscopic polypectomy. The National Polyp Study Workgroup. N Engl J Med. 1993;329(27):1977–81.
3. Kahi CJ, Imperiale TF, Juliar BE, Rex DK. Effect of screening colonoscopy on colorectal cancer incidence and mortality. Clin Gastroenterol Hepatol. 2009;7(7):770–5. quiz 11.
4. American Cancer Society Recommendations for colorectal cancer early detection. 2014. http://www.cancer.org/cancer/colonandrectumcancer/moreinformation/colonandrectumcancerearlydetection/colorectal-cancer-early-detection-acs-recommendations. Accessed 5 Feb 2015.
5. Champagne B. Rectal cancer. https://www.fascrs.org/patients/disease-condition/rectal-cancer. Accessed 27 Mar 2015.
6. Colorectal cancer prevention and treatment. 2014. http://www.gastro.org/patient-center/digestive-conditions/colorectal-cancer. Accessed 27 Mar 2015.
7. Levin B, Lieberman DA, McFarland B, Andrews KS, Brooks D, Bond J, et al. Screening and surveillance for the early detection of colorectal cancer and adenomatous polyps, 2008: a joint guideline from the American Cancer Society, the US Multi-Society Task Force on Colorectal Cancer, and the American College of Radiology. Gastroenterology. 2008;134(5):1570–95.
8. Winawer S, Fletcher R, Rex D, Bond J, Burt R, Ferrucci J, et al. Colorectal cancer screening and surveillance: clinical guidelines and rationale-update based on new evidence. Gastroenterology. 2003;124(2):544–60.
9. U.S. Preventive Services Task Force. Screening for colorectal cancer: U.S. Preventive Services Task Force recommendation statement. Ann Intern Med. 2008;149:627–37.
10. Wolff WI. Colonoscopy: history and development. Am J Gastroenterol. 1989;84(9):1017–25.
11. Peery AF, Dellon ES, Lund J, Crockett SD, McGowan CE, Bulsiewicz WJ, et al. Burden of gastrointestinal disease in the United States: 2012 update. Gastroenterology. 2012;143(5):1179–87.
12. Mandel JS, Church TR, Bond JH, Ederer F, Geisser MS, Mongin SJ, et al. The effect of fecal occult-blood screening on the incidence of colorectal cancer. N Engl J Med. 2000;343(22):1603–7.
13. Citarda F, Tomaselli G, Capocaccia R, Barcherini S, Crespi M, Group IMS. Efficacy in standard clinical practice of colonoscopic polypectomy in reducing colorectal cancer incidence. Gut. 2001;48(6):812–5.
14. Zauber AG, Winawer SJ, O'Brien MJ, Lansdorp-Vogelaar I, van Ballegooijen M, Hankey BF, et al. Colonoscopic polypectomy and long-term prevention of colorectal-cancer deaths. N Engl J Med. 2012;366(8):687–96.
15. Rex DK, Schoenfeld PS, Cohen J, Pike IM, Adler DG, Fennerty MB, et al. Quality indicators for colonoscopy. Am J Gastroenterol. 2015;110(1):72–90.
16. Sherer EA, Imler TD, Imperiale TF. The effect of colonoscopy preparation quality on adenoma detection rates. Gastrointest Endosc. 2012;75(3):545–53.
17. van Rijn JC, Reitsma JB, Stoker J, Bossuyt PM, van Deventer SJ, Dekker E. Polyp miss rate determined by tandem colonoscopy: a systematic review. Am J Gastroenterol. 2006;101(2):343–50.
18. Pickhardt PJ, Nugent PA, Mysliwiec PA, Choi JR, Schindler WR. Location of adenomas missed by optical colonoscopy. Ann Intern Med. 2004;141(5):352–9.
19. Bressler B, Paszat LF, Chen Z, Rothwell DM, Vinden C, Rabeneck L. Rates of new or missed colorectal cancers after colonoscopy and their risk factors: a population-based analysis. Gastroenterology. 2007;132(1):96–102.
20. Baxter NN, Goldwasser MA, Paszat LF, Saskin R, Urbach DR, Rabeneck L. Association of colonoscopy and death from colorectal cancer. Ann Intern Med. 2009;150(1):1–8.
21. Neerincx M, Terhaar sive Droste JS, Mulder CJ, Rakers M, Bartelsman JF, Loffeld RJ, et al. Colonic work-up after incomplete colonoscopy: significant new findings during follow-up. Endoscopy. 2010;42(9):730–5.
22. Gawron AJ, Veerappan A, McCarthy ST, Kankanala V, Keswani RN. Impact of an incomplete colonoscopy referral program on recommendations after incomplete colonoscopy. Dig Dis Sci. 2013;58(7):1849–55.
23. Subramanian V, Mannath J, Hawkey CJ, Ragunath K. High definition colonoscopy vs. standard video endoscopy for the detection of colonic polyps: a meta-analysis. Endoscopy. 2011;43(6):499–505.
24. Kahi CJ, Anderson JC, Waxman I, Kessler WR, Imperiale TF, Li X, et al. High-definition chromocolonoscopy vs. high-definition white light colonoscopy for average-risk colorectal cancer screening. Am J Gastroenterol. 2010;105(6):1301–7.
25. Pohl J, Schneider A, Vogell H, Mayer G, Kaiser G, Ell C. Pancolonic chromoendoscopy with indigo carmine versus standard colonoscopy for detection of neoplastic lesions: a randomised two-centre trial. Gut. 2011;60(4):485–90.
26. de Wijkerslooth TR, Stoop EM, Bossuyt PM, Mathus-Vliegen EM, Dees J, Tytgat KM, et al. Adenoma detection with cap-assisted colonoscopy versus regular colonoscopy: a randomised controlled trial. Gut. 2012;61(10):1426–34.
27. Rastogi A, Bansal A, Rao DS, Gupta N, Wani SB, Shipe T, et al. Higher adenoma detection rates with cap-assisted colonoscopy: a randomised controlled trial. Gut. 2012;61(3):402–8.
28. Dinesen L, Chua TJ, Kaffes AJ. Meta-analysis of narrow-band imaging versus conventional colonoscopy for adenoma detection. Gastrointest Endosc. 2012;75(3):604–11.
29. Pasha SF, Leighton JA, Das A, Harrison ME, Gurudu SR, Ramirez FC, et al. Comparison of the yield and miss rate of narrow band imaging and white light endoscopy in patients undergoing screening or surveillance colonoscopy: a meta-analysis. Am J Gastroenterol. 2012;107(3):363–70. quiz 71.
30. Gross SA, Buchner AM, Crook JE, Cangemi JR, Picco MF, Wolfsen HC, et al. A comparison of high definition-image enhanced colonoscopy and standard white-light colonoscopy

for colorectal polyp detection. Endoscopy. 2011;43(12): 1045–51.

31. Haringsma J, Tytgat GN, Yano H, Iishi H, Tatsuta M, Ogihara T, et al. Autofluorescence endoscopy: feasibility of detection of GI neoplasms unapparent to white light endoscopy with an evolving technology. Gastrointest Endosc. 2001;53(6):642–50.

32. Pohl J, May A, Rabenstein T, Pech O, Ell C. Computed virtual chromoendoscopy: a new tool for enhancing tissue surface structures. Endoscopy. 2007;39(1):80–3.

33. Chung SJ, Kim D, Song JH, Kang HY, Chung GE, Choi J, et al. Comparison of detection and miss rates of narrow band imaging, flexible spectral imaging chromoendoscopy and white light at screening colonoscopy: a randomised controlled back-to-back study. Gut. 2014;63(5):785–91.

34. Omata F, Ohde S, Deshpande GA, Kobayashi D, Masuda K, Fukui T. Image-enhanced, chromo, and cap-assisted colonoscopy for improving adenoma/neoplasia detection rate: a systematic review and meta-analysis. Scand J Gastroenterol. 2014; 49(2):222–37.

35. Sharma VK, Nguyen CC, Crowell MD, Lieberman DA, de Garmo P, Fleischer DE. A national study of cardiopulmonary unplanned events after GI endoscopy. Gastrointest Endosc. 2007;66(1):27–34.

36. Rutter CM, Johnson E, Miglioretti DL, Mandelson MT, Inadomi J, Buist DS. Adverse events after screening and follow-up colonoscopy. Cancer Causes Control. 2012;23(2):289–96.

37. Ko CW, Dominitz JA. Complications of colonoscopy: magnitude and management. Gastrointest Endosc Clin N Am. 2010;20(4): 659–71.

38. Kim DH, Pickhardt PJ, Hoff G, Kay CL. Computed tomographic colonography for colorectal screening. Endoscopy. 2007;39(6): 545–9.

39. ACR-SAR-SCBT-MR practice parameter for the performance of Computed Tomography (CT) colonography in adults. http://www.acr.org/%7E/media/ACR/Documents/PGTS/guidelines/CT_Colonography.pdf.

40. Pickhardt PJ. CT colonography for population screening: ready for prime time? Dig Dis Sci. 2015;60(3):647–59.

41. Zalis ME, Barish MA, Choi JR, Dachman AH, Fenlon HM, Ferrucci JT, et al. CT colonography reporting and data system: a consensus proposal. Radiology. 2005;236(1):3–9.

42. Pickhardt PJ, Taylor AJ. Extracolonic findings identified in asymptomatic adults at screening CT colonography. AJR Am J Roentgenol. 2006;186(3):718–28.

43. Chin M, Mendelson R, Edwards J, Foster N, Forbes G. Computed tomographic colonography: prevalence, nature, and clinical significance of extracolonic findings in a community screening program. Am J Gastroenterol. 2005;100(12):2771–6.

44. Pickhardt PJ. Incidence of colonic perforation at CT colonography: review of existing data and implications for screening of asymptomatic adults. Radiology. 2006;239(2):313–6.

45. Liedenbaum MH, Venema HW, Stoker J. Radiation dose in CT colonography–trends in time and differences between daily practice and screening protocols. Eur Radiol. 2008;18(10):2222–30.

46. On the risk to low doses (<100 mSv) of ionizing radiation during medical imaging procedures—IOMP policy statement. J Med Phys. 2013;38(2):57–8.

47. Pickhardt PJ, Choi JR, Hwang I, Butler JA, Puckett ML, Hildebrandt HA, et al. Computed tomographic virtual colonoscopy to screen for colorectal neoplasia in asymptomatic adults. N Engl J Med. 2003;349(23):2191–200.

48. Johnson CD, Chen MH, Toledano AY, Heiken JP, Dachman A, Kuo MD, et al. Accuracy of CT colonography for detection of large adenomas and cancers. N Engl J Med. 2008;359(12): 1207–17.

49. Pickhardt PJ, Hassan C, Halligan S, Marmo R. Colorectal cancer: CT colonography and colonoscopy for detection–systematic review and meta-analysis. Radiology. 2011;259(2): 393–405.

50. Kim DH, Pickhardt PJ, Taylor AJ, Leung WK, Winter TC, Hinshaw JL, et al. CT colonography versus colonoscopy for the detection of advanced neoplasia. N Engl J Med. 2007;357(14): 1403–12.

51. Kim DH, Pooler BD, Weiss JM, Pickhardt PJ. Five year colorectal cancer outcomes in a large negative CT colonography screening cohort. Eur Radiol. 2012;22(7):1488–94.

52. Doria-Rose VP, Newcomb PA, Levin TR. Incomplete screening flexible sigmoidoscopy associated with female sex, age, and increased risk of colorectal cancer. Gut. 2005;54(9):1273–8.

53. Imperiale TF, Wagner DR, Lin CY, Larkin GN, Rogge JD, Ransohoff DF. Risk of advanced proximal neoplasms in asymptomatic adults according to the distal colorectal findings. N Engl J Med. 2000;343(3):169–74.

54. Littlejohn C, Hilton S, Macfarlane GJ, Phull P. Systematic review and meta-analysis of the evidence for flexible sigmoidoscopy as a screening method for the prevention of colorectal cancer. Br J Surg. 2012;99(11):1488–500.

55. Brenner H, Stock C, Hoffmeister M. Effect of screening sigmoidoscopy and screening colonoscopy on colorectal cancer incidence and mortality: systematic review and meta-analysis of randomised controlled trials and observational studies. BMJ. 2014;348:g2467.

56. Schoen RE, Pinsky PF, Weissfeld JL, Yokochi LA, Church T, Laiyemo AO, et al. Colorectal-cancer incidence and mortality with screening flexible sigmoidoscopy. N Engl J Med. 2012; 366(25):2345–57.

57. Holme Ø, Løberg M, Kalager M, Bretthauer M, Hernán MA, Aas E, et al. Effect of flexible sigmoidoscopy screening on colorectal cancer incidence and mortality: a randomized clinical trial. JAMA. 2014;312(6):606–15.

58. Levin TR, Conell C, Shapiro JA, Chazan SG, Nadel MR, Selby JV. Complications of screening flexible sigmoidoscopy. Gastroenterology. 2002;123(6):1786–92.

59. Gatto NM, Frucht H, Sundararajan V, Jacobson JS, Grann VR, Neugut AI. Risk of perforation after colonoscopy and sigmoidoscopy: a population-based study. J Natl Cancer Inst. 2003; 95(3):230–6.

60. Miglioretti DL, Rutter CM, Bradford SC, Zauber AG, Kessler LG, Feuer EJ, et al. Improvement in the diagnostic evaluation of a positive fecal occult blood test in an integrated health care organization. Med Care. 2008;46(9 Suppl 1):S91–6.

61. Kronborg O, Fenger C, Olsen J, Jørgensen OD, Søndergaard O. Randomised study of screening for colorectal cancer with faecal-occult-blood test. Lancet. 1996;348(9040):1467–71.

62. Hardcastle JD, Chamberlain JO, Robinson MH, Moss SM, Amar SS, Balfour TW, et al. Randomised controlled trial of faecal-occult-blood screening for colorectal cancer. Lancet. 1996;348(9040):1472–7.

63. Lee JK, Liles EG, Bent S, Levin TR, Corley DA. Accuracy of fecal immunochemical tests for colorectal cancer: systematic review and meta-analysis. Ann Intern Med. 2014; 160(3):171.

64. Rennert G. Fecal occult blood screening–trial evidence, practice and beyond. Recent Results Cancer Res. 2003;163:248–53. discussion 64-6.

65. Imperiale TF, Ransohoff DF, Itzkowitz SH. Multitarget stool DNA testing for colorectal-cancer screening. N Engl J Med. 2014;371(2):187–8.

66. Heigh RI, Yab TC, Taylor WR, Hussain FT, Smyrk TC, Mahoney DW, et al. Detection of colorectal serrated polyps by stool DNA testing: comparison with fecal immunochemical testing for occult blood (FIT). PLoS One. 2014;9(1): e85659.

67. Lidgard GP, Domanico MJ, Bruinsma JJ, Light J, Gagrat ZD, Oldham-Haltom RL, et al. Clinical performance of an automated stool DNA assay for detection of colorectal neoplasia. Clin Gastroenterol Hepatol. 2013;11(10):1313–8.

68. Winawer SJ, Stewart ET, Zauber AG, Bond JH, Ansel H, Waye JD, et al. A comparison of colonoscopy and double-contrast barium enema for surveillance after polypectomy. National Polyp Study Work Group. N Engl J Med. 2000;342(24): 1766–72.

69. Rockey DC, Paulson E, Niedzwiecki D, Davis W, Bosworth HB, Sanders L, et al. Analysis of air contrast barium enema, computed tomographic colonography, and colonoscopy: prospective comparison. Lancet. 2005;365(9456):305–11.

70. Sosna J, Sella T, Sy O, Lavin PT, Eliahou R, Fraifeld S, et al. Critical analysis of the performance of double-contrast barium enema for detecting colorectal polyps > or = 6 mm in the era of CT colonography. AJR Am J Roentgenol. 2008;190(2): 374–85.

71. Rex DK, Rahmani EY, Haseman JH, Lemmel GT, Kaster S, Buckley JS. Relative sensitivity of colonoscopy and barium enema for detection of colorectal cancer in clinical practice. Gastroenterology. 1997;112(1):17–23.

72. Toma J, Paszat LF, Gunraj N, Rabeneck L. Rates of new or missed colorectal cancer after barium enema and their risk factors: a population-based study. Am J Gastroenterol. 2008; 103(12):3142–8.

73. Simon S. Achieving 80% by 2018 screening goal could prevent 200,000 colon cancer deaths in less than 2 decades. 2015. http://www.cancer.org/cancer/news/news/impact-of-achieving-80-by-2018-screening-goal. Accessed 27 Mar 2015.

74. Crockett SD, Snover DC, Ahnen DJ, Baron JA. Sessile serrated adenomas: an evidence-based guide to management. Clin Gastroenterol Hepatol. 2015;13(1):11–26.

75. Boparai KS, Mathus-Vliegen EM, Koornstra JJ, Nagengast FM, van Leerdam M, van Noesel CJ, et al. Increased colorectal cancer risk during follow-up in patients with hyperplastic polyposis syndrome: a multicentre cohort study. Gut. 2010; 59(8):1094–100.

76. Hamilton SR, Aaltonen LA, editors. World Health Organization classification of tumours. Pathology and genetics of tumours of the digestive system. Lyon: IARC Press; 2000. p. 103–44.

77. Rex DK, Ahnen DJ, Baron JA, Batts KP, Burke CA, Burt RW, et al. Serrated lesions of the colorectum: review and recommendations from an expert panel. Am J Gastroenterol. 2012; 107(9):1315–29.

78. Hamilton SR, Bofetta P, et al. Carcinoma of the Colon and Rectum. WHO Classification of tumours of the digestive system. 2010. p. 134–46.

79. Amersi F, Agustin M, Ko CY. Colorectal cancer: epidemiology, risk factors, and health services. Clin Colon Rectal Surg. 2005;18(3):133–40.

80. Hassan C, Quintero E, Dumonceau JM, Regula J, Brandão C, Chaussade S, et al. Post-polypectomy colonoscopy surveillance: European Society of Gastrointestinal Endoscopy (ESGE) Guideline. Endoscopy. 2013;45(10):842–51.

81. Ransohoff DF, Yankaskas B, Gizlice Z, Gangarosa L. Recommendations for post-polypectomy surveillance in community practice. Dig Dis Sci. 2011;56(9):2623–30.

82. Hassan C, Repici A, Sharma P, Correale L, Zullo A, Bretthauer M, et al. Efficacy and safety of endoscopic resection of large colorectal polyps: a systematic review and meta-analysis. Gut. 2015. doi:10.1136/gutjnl-2014-308481.

83. Larsen Haidle J, Howe JR. Juvenile polyposis syndrome. In: Pagon RA, Adam MP, Ardinger HH, Wallace SE, Amemiya A, Bean LJH, editors. Gene reviews (R). Seattle, WA: University of Washington, Seattle; 1993.

84. Beggs AD, Latchford AR, Vasen HF, Moslein G, Alonso A, Aretz S, et al. Peutz-Jeghers syndrome: a systematic review and recommendations for management. Gut. 2010;59(7):975–86.

85. DeRoche TC, Xiao SY, Liu X. Histological evaluation in ulcerative colitis. Gastroenterol Rep (Oxf). 2014;2(3):178–92.

86. Nascimbeni R, Burgart LJ, Nivatvongs S, Larson DR. Risk of lymph node metastasis in T1 carcinoma of the colon and rectum. Dis Colon Rectum. 2002;45(2):200–6.

87. Nivatvongs S, Rojanasakul A, Reiman HM, Dozois RR, Wolff BG, Pemberton JH, et al. The risk of lymph node metastasis in colorectal polyps with invasive adenocarcinoma. Dis Colon Rectum. 1991;34(4):323–8.

88. Resch A, Langner C. Risk assessment in early colorectal cancer: histological and molecular markers. Dig Dis. 2015;33(1): 77–85.

89. Freeman HJ. Long-term follow-up of patients with malignant pedunculated colon polyps after colonoscopic polypectomy. Can J Gastroenterol. 2013;27(1):20–4.

90. Cottet V, Jooste V, Fournel I, Bouvier AM, Faivre J, Bonithon-Kopp C. Long-term risk of colorectal cancer after adenoma removal: a population-based cohort study. Gut. 2012;61(8): 1180–6.

91. Brenner H, Chang-Claude J, Jansen L, Seiler CM, Hoffmeister M. Role of colonoscopy and polyp characteristics in colorectal cancer after colonoscopic polyp detection: a population-based case-control study. Ann Intern Med. 2012;157:225–32.

92. Hassan C, Gimeno-Garcia A, Kalager M, Spada C, Zullo A, Costamagna G, et al. Systematic review with meta-analysis: the incidence of advanced neoplasia after polypectomy in patients with and without low-risk adenomas. Aliment Pharmacol Ther. 2014;39(9):905–12.

93. Mysliwiec PA, Brown ML, Klabunde CN, Ransohoff DF. Are physicians doing too much colonoscopy? A national survey of colorectal surveillance after polypectomy. Ann Intern Med. 2004;141:264–71.

94. Levin TR. Dealing with uncertainty: surveillance colonoscopy after polypectomy. Am J Gastroenterol. 2007;102:1745–7.

95. Cooper K, Squires H, Carroll C, Papaioannou D, Booth A, Logan RF, et al. Chemoprevention of colorectal cancer: systematic review and economic evaluation. Health Technol Assess. 2010;14(32):1–206.

25

Colon Cancer: Preoperative Evaluation and Staging

Cary B. Aarons and Najjia N. Mahmoud

Key Concepts

- Total colonic evaluation is recommended prior to surgical intervention to exclude synchronous tumors that may alter surgical plan.
- Evaluation for metastatic disease by cross-sectional imaging is recommended prior to surgical intervention, as it may alter treatment decisions.
- Preoperative carcinoembryonic antigen (CEA) level should be obtained, as changes in CEA may herald tumor recurrence.
- Tumor location should be identified preoperatively.
- Tumor grade, lymphovascular invasion, margin status, and immunohistochemical assessment of mismatch repair proteins may have prognostic significance and should be routinely reported.

Background

Colorectal cancer remains a challenging clinical entity worldwide—affecting more than one million individuals annually [1–3]. Marked geographic variations exist, with industrialized countries bearing significantly higher incidences that are believed to be attributed to a mix of diet and environment [2, 3]. In the United States, it is the third leading cause of cancer-related deaths and is the third most common cancer following lung cancer and prostate and breast cancers in men and women, respectively [2–4]. In recent years, it has been estimated that annually there are roughly 100,000 new cases of colon cancer and more than 40,000 cases of rectal cancer [5–7]. Fortunately, both the incidence and mortality of colorectal cancer have declined steadily in the past three decades—largely due to more effective screening programs and improvements in treatment modalities [5–7]. However, despite these measurable gains, there remain significant disparities in incidence and mortality, particularly among African Americans [8–10]. Overall, the lifetime risk of developing colorectal cancer in the United States is approximately 5 % with a likelihood rising notably after 50 years of age. It is estimated that up to 90 % of cases occur in individuals over the age of 50 [11].

Once the diagnosis of colon cancer is made, the goal of preoperative evaluation is to establish the location of the tumor, assess for metastatic disease and adjacent organ invasion, and identify other patient and tumor factors that may affect outcome or alter the medical or surgical approach to treatment. The primary importance of staging in colon cancer is to rule out additional pathology and distant metastatic disease (stage IV), which can affect treatment approach. This differs from rectal cancer where estimates of locoregional tumor stage have a greater effect on treatment planning.

Clinical Presentation

Colon cancer presents in three common ways: an asymptomatic lesion detected during routine screening examination; manifestation of vague but suspicious symptoms such as change in bowel habits, weight loss, and fatigue that lead to further investigation; and emergently, with perforation or obstruction.

Early colon cancers are often asymptomatic, which underscores the importance of routine screening. Even so, it is estimated that about 30 % of all cancers are diagnosed by endoscopy in the absence of symptoms [12]. Routine screening detects the majority of early cancers, but the definition of "effective screening" is in flux and overall compliance with colonoscopic screening in the United States is still quite low—below 50 % for most average risk adults. Rates of screening can vary widely between states and regions. The Centers for Disease Control and Prevention estimates that when surveyed for appropriate screening which could include fecal occult blood testing alone within 1 year, flexible sigmoidoscopy within 3 years, or colonoscopy within 10 years, the highest rates recorded are in the northeast topping out at 75 % and the lowest in the west with maximal screening

© Springer International Publishing 2016
S.R. Steele et al. (eds.), *The ASCRS Textbook of Colon and Rectal Surgery*, DOI 10.1007/978-3-319-25970-3_25

compliance rates of 54 % [13]. When symptoms do occur, patients commonly present with abdominal pain, gastrointestinal bleeding, iron-deficiency anemia, change in bowel habits, or vague nonspecific symptoms such as lethargy, weight loss, and loss of appetite [4, 14, 15]. Symptoms will often manifest differently depending on tumor location and size. Late findings can include palpable abdominal mass, severe weight loss, intestinal obstruction, and, in rare cases, perforation leading to peritonitis or fistulization to adjacent organs.

Abdominal pain in the setting of colon cancer is often poorly localized and, therefore, a nonspecific finding. Patients may describe a vague visceral discomfort, which changes to crampy, colicky pain as luminal narrowing occurs—resulting in partial or complete colonic obstruction. While rectal bleeding is a common finding, its clinical manifestation can be varied; therefore, taking a careful history is imperative. Patients with distal, left-sided lesions will often present with bright red bloody stools, while more proximal lesions will cause melena or occult bleeding that results in iron-deficiency anemia [3, 14]. This anemia can ultimately result in dizziness, weakness, or generalized fatigue. Similarly, changes in bowel habits will be affected by tumor location within the colon. Typically, patients will report changes in the caliber, frequency, and consistency of their stools. This is more notable with left-sided lesions, which are more likely to cause narrowing of the colon lumen and impede passage of solid stool. Since the luminal diameter tends to be wider in the proximal colon and stool more liquid, alterations in stools generally coincide with large, exophytic lesions or cancers that obstruct the ileocecal valve.

Approximately 20–25 % of colon cancer will present with metastatic disease at the time of diagnosis; therefore, it is also critical to evaluate patients for signs and symptoms associated with metastatic disease. On the whole, widely advanced cancers can result in constitutional symptoms such as unintentional weight loss, cachexia, weakness, and anorexia [3].

Colon cancer typically spreads via lymphatic, hematogenous, or intraperitoneal extension, and the most common sites include the liver, lungs, and peritoneal surfaces. Spread to the brain or CNS and bones is less likely but possible. While symptoms of liver metastasis are uncommon, some patients may develop right upper quadrant pain, abdominal distention, anorexia, weakness, or jaundice when the burden of liver metastases is high. Direct local invasion of colon cancers into adjacent structures such as the small intestine, bladder, or abdominal wall can result to bowel obstruction, abscesses, pneumaturia, fecaluria, or enterocutaneous fistula. A Virchow node (left supraclavicular node) or Sister Mary Joseph node (umbilical nodule) is another uncommon finding that has been associated with the distant spread of colon cancer [3]. Patients who present with symptoms seem to be at much higher risk of having advanced disease at diagnosis than those for whom the primary is detected by routine screening. For example, in one study of over 1000 patients with colorectal cancer, only 217 were found during screening. Those that

came to attention via symptoms were twice as likely to have a transmural tumor, twice as likely to present with stage III disease, and over three times as likely to have distant spread at diagnosis and have double the risk of recurrence [16].

Preoperative Evaluation

The evaluation of a patient with a new diagnosis of colon cancer should begin with a complete history and physical examination [11]. The history should focus on the duration and severity of symptoms associated with the primary tumor such as intestinal obstructive symptoms, anemia, and abdominal pain, as well as those associated with metastatic disease such as weight loss and fatigue. Information should also be obtained about any family history of colorectal cancer or other cancers known to be associated with inherited colon cancer syndromes. Finally, details regarding the patient's overall health will provide initial insight into their readiness for any surgical intervention. A focused physical examination can elucidate important signs such as a palpable mass, distant adenopathy, tenderness, or distention [11].

Assessment of Inherited Risk

The vast majority of colorectal cancers are sporadic in nature. However, there are factors associated with the development of colorectal cancer. Modifiable risk factors include low-fiber, high-fat diet, obesity, smoking, and heavy alcohol consumption. The primary inherent risk factor for colorectal cancer is increasing age; however, having a personal history of colorectal cancer, polyps, or inflammatory bowel disease will substantially increase risk. Approximately 5–10 % of colorectal cancers can be linked to discrete inherited syndromes, among which familial adenomatous polyposis (FAP) and Lynch syndrome are the most common. It is important to identify these risk factors, particularly inflammatory bowel disease, personal history of colorectal neoplasia, and presence of inherited colorectal cancer syndromes, as they will guide choice of therapy, surveillance strategies, and screening of at-risk relatives. For example, a patient with long-standing ulcerative colitis who is found to have a colon cancer should be considered for total proctocolectomy. A patient with colon cancer who is suspected of having Lynch syndrome should be considered for subtotal colectomy, as well as total abdominal hysterectomy and bilateral salpingo-oophorectomy in women.

Colonoscopy

If not completed at the time of diagnosis, a thorough endoscopic examination of the entire colon is critical as it provides added information about any synchronous cancers or polyps, which may need to be removed or marked preoperatively. The rate of synchronous cancers is understood to be about 5 %, and the overall rate of synchronous neoplasia that would change operative approach is somewhat higher [17]. If a synchronous polypoid neoplasm is detected outside of the normal field of planned resection for the primary tumor, it is optimal to attempt complete endoscopic resection preoperatively. This will allow for histologic analysis—if cancer is found, then a more extensive colectomy than was originally planned may be indicated [4]. Colonoscopy allows for the localization and biopsy of the primary tumor; however, it is important to keep in mind that the flexible scope may not provide an exact measurement of distance. Therefore, it is important to assess known landmarks and whenever possible to mark the location of the cancer with an endoscopic tattoo, particularly if the cancer was contained within a polyp and therefore entirely resected. This is increasingly important for smaller lesions that may not be easily palpated at the time of surgery or if a laparoscopic approach is planned. It is not unusual for the endoscopist to resect a large polyp only to find an occult cancer within it requiring formal resection on pathology. Rapid reevaluation of the colon via colonoscopy with marking is essential. Typically, if the colon can be reevaluated within 2 weeks, a healing ulcer can be identified and tattooed.

Over time, a number of agents for endoscopic marking have been evaluated. Only India ink and SPOT (GI Supply, Camp Hill, PA) have been widely accepted. Both agents are colloid suspensions of fine carbon particles. India ink is suspended in a 0.9 % solution of saline at a 1:100 dilution and sterilized by autoclaving or being passed through a Millipore filter. SPOT is a marker composed of highly purified, fine carbon particles and is the only FDA-approved marking solution for endoscopic tattooing. Both have been tested extensively and are safe as well as durable. Identification of the endoscopic tattoo can be made well after the 1-year mark and commonly after 2 or more years. Other agents that have been used include methylene blue, hematoxylin, and toluene blue. Brevity of duration of marking and mucosal ulceration has limited use of these other agents. Technique of injection has been studied fairly extensively. Four-quadrant injection of 2–4 cm^3 of agent at or near the level of the lesion allows for accurate identification even if the lesion is on the mesenteric aspect of the colon lumen. Submucosal injection limits intraperitoneal spread that can make intraoperative identification confusing or difficult. Some advocate for placing a tattoo both proximally and distally to the tumor or polyp to help identify the extent or length of the lesion; however, this may confuse the surgeon if only one of the tattoo marks is visible. Other surgeons advocate marking only distal to the lesion. While there are no current recommendations regarding this aspect of marking, it seems clear that good documentation of technique in the report is mandatory and will limit misunderstandings or confusion [18]. Additional benefits of tattoo placement may include increased nodal harvest by virtue, most likely, of the ability to see and enumerate lymph nodes that take up the colloid carbon particles. A number of studies, both prospective as well as retrospective, have noted a significant increase in the number of specimens with >12 lymph nodes harvested when tattooing had taken place [19, 20].

An alternative to marking with tattoo is deployment of endoscopic metal clips followed by immediate plain radiograph. The colon outline is frequently visible due to retained air from colonoscopy. CT can also be obtained within a few days; the clips are usually retained and the tumor site can be clearly localized. Another strategy is to perform intraoperative colonoscopy to localize a small tumor. This can be performed immediately prior to operation or after exploration of the abdomen. The use of carbon dioxide as an insufflation gas is preferred, in order to limit bowel dilatation.

If colonoscopy cannot be completed preoperatively, then a suitable radiographic study, such as CT colonography or contrast enema, should be considered or intraoperative colonoscopy performed via the colon proximal to the tumor. For cases of obstructing cancers that preclude adequate endoscopic or radiographic assessment preoperatively, intraoperative colonic lavage and colonoscopy should be considered. If this is not possible, the proximal colon should be palpated intraoperatively, and if no obvious lesions are detected, a full colonoscopy should be performed when safe to do so after surgery [4].

Carcinoembryonic Antigen

Preoperative evaluation should also include routine laboratory studies, including a complete blood count (CBC) with focus on anemia that may need to be corrected before surgery. Another important test is the serum CEA level, which has been shown to provide some prognostic information [21]. CEA is a glycoprotein primarily involved in intercellular adhesion [22]. It is produced by columnar and goblet cells and can be found in normal colonic mucosa. Additionally, it can be found in low levels in the circulation of healthy individuals, but it is overexpressed in a variety of cancers, including colorectal cancer. Elevated serum levels may be identified in heavy smokers and in benign conditions such as pancreatitis and inflammatory bowel disease as well as malignancies outside of the gastrointestinal tract [22]; therefore, CEA is not a sensitive or specific screening tool for colorectal cancer [3, 23]. However, it is an important tool in CRC surveillance after surgical resection since its elevation may be the first indication of locally recurrent or metastatic disease [24].

Patients with preoperative serum CEA >5 ng/mL have a worse prognosis, stage for stage, than those with lower levels. Elevated preoperative CEA levels have been shown to be associated with poorer survival and increased recurrence in several studies; however, contradictory studies do exist [23, 25–29]. Therefore, there is currently insufficient evidence to support the use of elevated preoperative serum CEA levels as an absolute indication for adjuvant chemotherapy [4, 28].

Current American Society of Clinical Oncology (ASCO) guidelines recommend that serum CEA levels be obtained preoperatively in patients with demonstrated colorectal cancer for posttreatment follow-up and assessment of prognosis. Elevated preoperative CEA levels that do not normalize following surgical resection imply the presence of persistent disease. Furthermore, serial testing of CEA levels should be performed for 5 years for patients with stage II and III disease in those eligible for surgery or chemotherapy if metastatic disease is discovered. Rising CEA levels after surgical resection imply recurrent disease and should prompt consideration of radiologic and endoscopic evaluation to look for treatable disease [28].

Radiographic Evaluation

Preoperative radiographic imaging is fundamental for initial staging of newly diagnosed or recurrent colon cancers [4]. Computed tomography (CT) scans are the most widely used studies in this setting as they provide valuable preoperative information about liver or lung metastasis and are cost effective. This test should be done with both oral and intravenous contrast if there is no contraindication (anaphylaxis to contrast or renal insufficiency) to maximize accuracy of visualization of the abdominal viscera as well as highlight vascular structures and better determine the relationships between lymphatics, ureters, and vessels [30]. Additionally, cross-sectional imaging also facilitates more precise tumor location and delineates the extent of any extracolonic invasion of adjacent organs or the abdominal wall, all of which are important for operative planning [31]. In these cases, the appropriate consulting services can be mobilized if necessary for en bloc resections. CT scan has a sensitivity ranging from 75–90 % for detecting distant metastasis; however, the ability to accurately detect nodal involvement or small peritoneal metastasis is poor. The routine use of CT for imaging of the chest remains controversial for initial staging of colon cancer, as compared to rectal cancers. In asymptomatic patients in whom the suspicion of lung metastasis is low, a plain chest X-ray will suffice. Any suspicious findings on chest X-ray can be investigated with a noncontrast chest CT scan.

As imaging technology has improved, so has the sensitivity of CT scans for identifying liver metastases. However, there are studies that suggest that contrast-enhanced magnetic resonance imaging (MRI) is particularly valuable in evaluating smaller suspicious liver lesions (especially in the presence of fatty liver changes) with sensitivities up to 97 % [3, 32]. In routine clinical practice, MRI should be reserved for the evaluation of suspicious liver lesions not clearly characterized on CT scan and for operative planning prior to liver metastasectomy.

Positron emission tomography–computed tomography (PET/CT) scan has emerged as a useful imaging modality in the evaluation of many cancers. However, for initial staging of colorectal cancer, the routine use of PET/CT remains controversial. While it has been shown to be more sensitive in the detection of liver metastases as well as extrahepatic disease as compared with routine CT scan, other studies suggest that it does not add significant information [14, 33–35]. The strongest evidence for use of PET/CT in the management of colorectal cancer is in the evaluation of patients with recurrent disease [34–36]. It is often more helpful as an adjunct to conventional imaging studies in patients suspected of having metastasis, especially those with a rising CEA level [31, 37]. Additionally, in patients with potentially resectable metastatic disease, PET/CT has been shown in a randomized trial to reduce the number of unnecessary laparotomies [38].

Preoperative Evaluation of Coexisting Medical Conditions

Regardless of the operative approach, colorectal procedures carry inherent risks, which can be divided into procedure-specific risks and cardiopulmonary risks. Therefore, a thorough history and physical examination encompassing the patient's comorbidities is also vital. This is immensely important because surgical morbidity and mortality can be greatly improved by a careful assessment of organ-specific risks and, if feasible, preoperative optimization. Additionally, a detailed knowledge of the patient's prior abdominal surgery will aid in the appropriate operative planning.

Routine preoperative testing should be obtained and should include a CBC, a metabolic panel, type and screen, and a 12-lead electrocardiogram in older patients with cardiac risk factors. Liver function tests are not sensitive for liver metastasis and, therefore, are not required in the initial preoperative testing. Similarly, nutritional panels are not generally required unless there are significant concerns for underlying malnutrition. Complete optimization of nutritional parameters, either parenterally or enterally, typically takes weeks, which would delay surgery unnecessarily.

There are several classification systems that have been reported, which aim to gauge the overall risk of the surgical patient. The American Society of Anesthesiologists (ASA) classification is the simplest and most commonly used system, which highlights the patient's underlying illnesses that may impact outcomes from surgery [39, 40]:

- ASA I—a normal healthy patient
- ASA II—a patient with mild systemic disease
- ASA III—a patient with severe systemic disease
- ASA IV—a patient with severe systemic disease that is a constant threat to life
- ASA V—a moribund patient who is not expected to survive without the operation
- ASA E—emergency

The preoperative cardiac assessment should include a history of recent or remote myocardial infarction, angina, valvular disease, arrhythmias, or heart failure. Baseline functional status should also be quantified using metabolic equivalents (METs) [41]. Perioperative risk of an adverse cardiac event can then be estimated using the Goldman cardiac risk index or the revised cardiac risk index (Table 25-1), which are among the most widely used tools for cardiac risk assessment [39].

Chronic obstructive pulmonary disease (COPD), obesity, obstructive sleep apnea, pulmonary hypertension, recent respiratory infection, and smoking are some of the most important pulmonary risk factors that should be considered prior to surgery. These comorbidities can be gleaned from a thorough history and should prompt further investigation; however, this testing should be selective. The routine use of chest X-ray varies by institution and is often of limited value for the evaluation of significant pulmonary disease; therefore, this study should be reserved for patients with known cardiopulmonary disease or those older than 50 years of age as recommended by the American College of Physicians [42]. Because CXR is a part of staging of colon cancer, it is necessarily included in the preoperative evaluation. Pulmonary function testing and baseline arterial blood gases are not indicated routinely prior to abdominal surgery [43]. Complex patients with high-risk underlying pulmonary illnesses should be referred for pulmonary consultation prior to surgery for medical optimization and to outline appropriate perioperative strategies.

Smoking cessation should be emphasized but should not delay surgery, as any substantial benefits would not be realized for several weeks. However, there may be measurable gains in improving postoperative wound healing [44]. A recent meta-analysis of randomized trials demonstrated that smoking cessation was associated with a 41 % relative risk reduction in postoperative pulmonary complications [44].

In patients with renal insufficiency, care must be taken with choosing preoperative bowel preparation, and special attention must be paid to perioperative fluid balances. Additionally, diuretics, angiotensin-converting enzyme inhibitors, and angiotensin receptor blockers should be held the day prior to surgery to minimize the risk of profound hypotension during surgery.

Staging of Colon Cancer

The preferred staging system for colon and rectal cancers is the TNM staging system put forth by the American Joint Committee on Cancer and the International Union Against Cancer (UICC) [4, 36]. This system, which is summarized in Table 25-2, consists of three categories: tumor depth of invasion, nodal involvement, and distant metastasis. Based on the clinical and pathologic data, the combination of these categories forms the final stage, which correlates with the overall prognosis. Recent analysis of survival outcomes in a large group of patients with invasive colon cancer from the Surveillance, Epidemiology, and End Results (SEER) population-based database has led to the revision of the CRC TNM staging system in the 7th edition of the *AJCC Cancer Staging Manual* [45]. These changes include [6]:

- Stage II is further subdivided into IIA (T3N0), IIB (T4aN0), and IIC (T4bN0).
- Satellite tumor deposits in the pericolonic adipose tissue are classified as N1c.
- Several stage III groups have been revised based on survival outcomes.
- N1 and N2 subcategories are further subdivided according to the number of involved nodes to reflect prognosis.
- T4 lesions are subdivided as T4a (tumor penetrates the surface of the visceral peritoneum) and as T4b (tumor directly invades adjacent organs or structures).

TABLE 25-1. Revised cardiac risk index (RCRI)

Risk factors	
1. High-risk type of surgery (intraperitoneal, intrathoracic, or suprainguinal vascular procedures)	
2. Ischemic heart disease	
3. Congestive heart failure	
4. History of cerebrovascular disease	
5. Insulin therapy for diabetes	
6. Preoperative serum creatinine >2.0 mg/dL	
Risk classification (one point is assigned to each risk factor present)	*Rates of major cardiac complications*[a] *(%)*
Class I (0 points)	0.50
Class II (1 point)	1.30
Class III (2 points)	3.60
Class IV (≥3 points)	9.10

[a]Major cardiac complications include myocardial infarction, pulmonary edema, ventricular fibrillation or primary cardiac arrest, and complete heart block
Adapted from Lee, TH et al., Derivation and prospective validation of a simple index for prediction of cardiac risk of major noncardiac surgery Circulation 1999;100(10):1043–9 [63]

TABLE 25-2E. TNM classification and AJCC 7th edition staging of colon cancer

Primary tumor staging (T)		
T0		No evidence of primary tumor
Tis		Carcinoma in situ
T1		Tumor invades submucosa
T2		Tumor invades the muscularis propria
T3		Tumor invades through the muscularis propria into the pericolonic tissue
T4a		Tumor penetrates to the surface of the visceral peritoneum (serosa)
T4b		Tumor invades and/or is adherent to other organs or structures
Regional lymph node staging (N)		
N0		No regional lymph node metastasis
N1a		Metastasis in one regional lymph node
N1b		Metastasis in 2–3 regional lymph nodes
N1c		Tumor deposits in subserosa, mesentery, or nonperitonealized pericolic or perirectal tissues without regional nodal metastases
N2a		Metastasis in 4–6 regional lymph nodes
N2b		Metastasis in seven or more regional lymph nodes
Distant metastasis staging (M)		
M0		No distant metastasis
M1a		Metastasis confined to one organ or site
M1b		Metastasis in more than one organ/site or the peritoneum

Stage	T	N	M
0	Tis	N0	M0
I	1–2	N0	M0
IIA	T3	N0	M0
IIB	T4a	N0	M0
IIC	T4b	N0	M0
IIIA	T1–T2	N1–N1c	M0
	T1	N2a	M0
IIIB	T3–T4a	N1–N1c	M0
	T2–T3	N2a	M0
	T1–2	N2b	M0
IIIC	T4a	N2a	M0
	T3–T4a	N2b	M0
	T4b	N1–N2	M0
IVA	Any T	Any N	M1a
IVB	Any T	Any N	M1b

With permission from Chang GJ et al., Practice parameters for the management of colon cancer. Dis Colon Rectum 2012;55(8):834. © Wolters Kluwer [4]

- M1 is subdivided into M1a (single metastatic site) and M1b (metastasis to more than one organ or the peritoneum).

The completeness of resection should also be noted by the surgeon [4, 6, 46]:

- R0—complete tumor resection with negative margins
- R1—incomplete tumor resection with microscopic involvement of the margin
- R2—incomplete tumor resection with gross residual disease that was not resected

In addition to the aforementioned components of the TNM staging system, there are several other histologic criteria that should be reported routinely. These include histologic grade, tumor ("satellite") deposits, lymphovascular invasion, perineural invasion, and margin status (distal, proximal, and radial). Each of these features provides important prognostic information.

Histologic Grade

Histologic grade has consistently been shown to be a stage-independent prognostic factor and is determined by the degree of differentiation in the colon tumor. While most systems stratify cancers into four grades, ranging from well differentiated (grade 1) to undifferentiated (grade 4) [46], histologic assessment is often plagued by interobserver variability. Consequently, the AJCC has recommended a two-tiered system for reporting: low grade (well and moderately differentiated) and high grade (poorly differentiated and undifferentiated) [21, 46, 47].

There are histologic variants such as mucinous adenocarcinomas and signet ring cell adenocarcinomas that are also important in assessing overall prognosis. Mucinous adenocarcinomas are characterized by extracellular mucin in greater than 50 % of the tumor volume. When compared with conventional invasive adenocarcinomas, mucinous adenocarcinomas typically behave more aggressively, especially in patients without microsatellite instability (MSI). Signet ring cell adenocarcinomas are rare but when they occur in the colon, they carry a worse prognosis as compared with conventional adenocarcinomas [14]. These tumors are characterized histologically by greater than 50 % tumor cells with signet ring features—prominent intra-cytoplasmic mucin vacuole that pushes the nucleus to the periphery [47].

Lymph Node Evaluation

Other than radial margin status, lymph node status is the most important prognostic factor following resection of colon cancer [14]. The identification of at least 12 lymph nodes has been suggested as a key quality indicator in the resection of colon cancers [6]. While there are patient-related factors that influence lymph node yield, the completeness of mesenteric resection and the interest of the pathologist in obtaining the maximal number for nodes for examination are also paramount. Numerous studies have shown that increasing the number of lymph nodes examined is associated with improved survival in stage II and stage III patients [48]. Tumor deposits that are found in the pericolonic fat that do not show any evidence of residual lymph node are not counted as lymph nodes replaced by tumor and are designated as N1c. The number of these nodules should be reported as they confer a poor prognosis [6, 49].

During the past 20 years, there has been interest in improving harvest of at-risk lymph nodes and in better identification of tumor in lymph nodes. Some investigators have proposed injection of vital dye around the tumor at the time of operation as a method of identifying lymph nodes at greatest risk for metastases (sentinel node mapping).

Studies of sentinel lymph node mapping have focused on the detection of metastatic lesions in nodes that would ordinarily be missed by routine nodal retrieval and pathologic processing. However, with few exceptions, the "sentinel" nodes retrieved in these studies have been subjected to ultra-processing (microsectioning, immunohistochemical analysis, or RT-PCR), while other "nonsentinel" nodes have been examined by bivalving and hematoxylin and eosin staining only, biasing the results heavily in favor of sentinel lymph node mapping. Even with this bias, results have varied widely in the literature, with false-negative rates (patients with negative "sentinel" nodes and positive "nonsentinel" nodes/total patients with positive nodes) of 9–60 % [50–52]. Variation in reported success rates may also result from different methods of data analysis and presentation.

The ultimate goal of any protocol examining lymph nodes in nonstandard fashion is to identify patients with occult nodal metastases, to treat them with chemotherapeutic agents, and to improve survival. At present, there is no definitive evidence that treatment of patients with occult nodal metastases with chemotherapy improves survival.

Margin Status

Surgical resection with curative intent requires removal of the entire tumor as well as the associated lymphatics and nodal basin at risk, which will vary based on the location of the primary tumor. It would seem obvious that it is of critical importance to resect the entire tumor when operating for colon cancer. However, the concept that the radial margin of resection is important was largely ignored by the surgical and pathology communities until recently. Just as with rectal cancer, it is important to ink the radial margin of resection and assess it histologically, as it has profound prognostic significance and will drive some decisions regarding adjuvant treatment and can be used as an assessment of surgical quality. It should be noted that the visceral peritoneum is not considered a surgical margin. However, pathologists often have difficulty in assessing this layer in relation to margin status, making inking of the nonperitonealized radial margin all the more critical.

The proximal and distal margin of resection should also be measured and reported. Traditionally, some authors have advocated obtaining a 5 cm segment of normal bowel on the proximal and distal sides of the tumor to avoid local failure [4, 46, 53]. However, this recommendation has little to do with the primary tumor, as colon cancers do not often spread longitudinally in the wall of the bowel in occult fashion. Rather, the recommendation arises from the need to resect mesentery surrounding the tumor to ensure adequate removal of at-risk lymph nodes. Adequate resection of the mesentery, including named feeding vessels, will result in devascularization of the colon surrounding the tumor, thus mandating resection of the colon rendered ischemic.

Other Prognostic Features

The presence of lymphovascular and perineural invasion has been shown to be significantly associated with poorer prognosis [21, 46, 54–57]. Tumor budding refers to small clusters of undifferentiated cancer cells ahead of the invasive front of the lesion. While this is not a routinely examined pathologic parameter, there is increasing evidence that the quantitative assessment of tumor budding reflects clinical aggressiveness of colon cancers. This has also been shown by some to be a poor prognostic feature [46, 54].

DNA Mismatch Repair/Microsatellite Instability

A germ line mutation in one of the DNA mismatch repair (MMR) genes (*MLH1*, *MSH2*, *MSH6*, *PMS2*) is typically found in Lynch syndrome. In sporadic colon cancers, mismatch repair defects occur in approximately 20 % of cases and results from the hypermethylation of *MLH1* [3, 58]. Patients with dropout of *MLH1* on immunohistochemistry (IHC) can be accurately identified as either a sporadic or germ line mutation by staining for *BRAF*. If *BRAF* is mutated as well, then a sporadic mutation is 96 % likely in MLH1 [59]. Typically, tumors found to be lacking in MMR expression are subject to *BRAF* analysis. If *BRAF* mutation is detected, then Lynch syndrome is unlikely, and in most cases, the patient can be considered to have a sporadic cancer and genetic testing will cease. However, if *BRAF* is normal, then Lynch syndrome is likely and genetic counseling and testing should be considered.

The presence of MMR proteins in tumor tissue can be assessed by IHC and should be done routinely in patients suspected of having Lynch syndrome, based on the clinical criteria [36]. In many hospitals, IHC testing for MMR is done routinely for patients under the age of 50. Increasingly, because of the prognostic implications, many urge IHC for MMR proteins to be assessed on all patients with colorectal cancer in an effort to align pathology with prognosis and therapy.

MSI is another indicator of DNA repair defects caused by defective mismatch repair proteins. It is typically assessed by PCR amplification of repeated single nucleotide units of DNA, or microsatellites, in tumor tissue. Tumors are characterized as MSI high (MSI-H) or MSI low (MSI-L) based on the number of microsatellite sequences that appear. If the tumor has two or more mutated sequences, it is termed MSI-H, while if only one sequence is mutated, it is classified as MSI-L. Finally, if no mutation is present, then the tumor is microsatellite stable (MSS) [47, 60]. Recent studies demonstrate that stage II patients with MSI-H tumors did not have the same survival benefit from 5-FU-based adjuvant chemotherapy as compared with those that had MSI-L and MSS tumors although differences were slight [36, 50–52, 61–63].

Summary

Assessment of the patient and the tumor preoperatively is increasingly important. Today, treatment decisions are made by careful preoperative evaluation of the health of the patient, the genetics of the tumor, and the extent of disease. A sophisticated, organized, and educated approach to preoperative evaluation yields the best long-term results.

References

1. Cunningham D, Atkin W, Lenz HJ, Lynch HT, Minsky B, Nordlinger B, et al. Colorectal cancer. Lancet. 2010;375: 1030–47.
2. Haggar FA, Boushey RP. Colorectal cancer epidemiology: incidence, mortality, survival, and risk factors. Clin Colon Rectal Surg. 2009;22:191–7.
3. Cappell MS. Pathophysiology, clinical presentation, and management of colon cancer. Gastroenterol Clin North Am. 2008;37:1–24. v.
4. Chang GJ, Kaiser AM, Mills S, Rafferty JF, Buie WD. Practice parameters for the management of colon cancer. Dis Colon Rectum. 2012;55:831–43.
5. Aarons CB, Mahmoud NN. Current surgical considerations for colorectal cancer. Chin Clin Oncol. 2013;2:14.
6. Engstrom PF, Arnoletti JP, Benson 3rd AB, Chen YJ, Choti MA, Cooper HS, et al. NCCN Clinical Practice Guidelines in Oncology: colon cancer. J Natl Compr Canc Netw. 2009;7:778–831.
7. Engstrom PF, Arnoletti JP, Benson 3rd AB, Chen YJ, Choti MA, Cooper HS, et al. NCCN Clinical Practice Guidelines in Oncology: rectal cancer. J Natl Compr Canc Netw. 2009; 7:838–81.
8. Govindarajan R, Shah RV, Erkman LG, Hutchins LF. Racial differences in the outcome of patients with colorectal carcinoma. Cancer. 2003;97:493–8.
9. Tammana VS, Laiyemo AO. Colorectal cancer disparities: issues, controversies and solutions. World J Gastroenterol. 2014;20:869–76.
10. Winawer SJ, Stewart ET, Zauber AG, Bond JH, Ansel H, Waye JD, et al. A comparison of colonoscopy and double-contrast barium enema for surveillance after polypectomy. National Polyp Study Work Group. N Engl J Med. 2000;342:1766–72.
11. Lynch ML, Brand MI. Preoperative evaluation and oncologic principles of colon cancer surgery. Clin Colon Rectal Surg. 2005;18:163–73.
12. Moiel D, Thompson J. Early detection of colon cancer-the kaiser permanente northwest 30-year history: how do we measure success? Is it the test, the number of tests, the stage, or the percentage of screen-detected patients? Perm J. 2011;15:30–8.
13. Joseph DA, King JB, Miller JW, Richardson LC. Prevalence of colorectal cancer screening among adults—Behavioral Risk Factor Surveillance System, United States, 2010. MMWR Morb Mortal Wkly Rep. 2012;61(Suppl):51–6.
14. Fleshman JW, Wolff BG. The ASCRS textbook of colon and rectal surgery. New York: Springer; 2007.
15. Majumdar SR, Fletcher RH, Evans AT. How does colorectal cancer present? Symptoms, duration, and clues to location. Am J Gastroenterol. 1999;94:3039–45.
16. Amri R, Bordeianou LG, Sylla P, Berger DL. Impact of screening colonoscopy on outcomes in colon cancer surgery. JAMA Surg. 2013;148:747–54.
17. Mulder SA, Kranse R, Damhuis RA, de Wilt JH, Ouwendijk RJ, Kuipers EJ, et al. Prevalence and prognosis of synchronous colorectal cancer: a Dutch population-based study. Cancer Epidemiol. 2011;35:442–7.
18. Luigiano C, Ferrara F, Morace C, Mangiavillano B, Fabbri C, Cennamo V, et al. Endoscopic tattooing of gastrointestinal and pancreatic lesions. Adv Ther. 2012;29:864–73.

19. Dawson K, Wiebusch A, Thirlby RC. Preoperative tattooing and improved lymph node retrieval rates from colectomy specimens in patients with colorectal cancers. Arch Surg. 2010; 145:826–30.

20. Bartels SA, van der Zaag ES, Dekker E, Buskens CJ, Bemelman WA. The effect of colonoscopic tattooing on lymph node retrieval and sentinel lymph node mapping. Gastrointest Endosc. 2012;76:793–800.

21. Compton CC, Fielding LP, Burgart LJ, Conley B, Cooper HS, Hamilton SR, et al. Prognostic factors in colorectal cancer. College of American Pathologists Consensus Statement 1999. Arch Pathol Lab Med. 2000;124:979–94.

22. Au FC, Stein BS, Gennaro AR, Tyson RR. Tissue CEA in colorectal carcinoma. Dis Colon Rectum. 1984;27:16–8.

23. Fletcher RH. Carcinoembryonic antigen. Ann Intern Med. 1986;104:66–73.

24. McCall JL, Black RB, Rich CA, Harvey JR, Baker RA, Watts JM, et al. The value of serum carcinoembryonic antigen in predicting recurrent disease following curative resection of colorectal cancer. Dis Colon Rectum. 1994;37:875–81.

25. Wiratkapun S, Kraemer M, Seow-Choen F, Ho YH, Eu KW. High preoperative serum carcinoembryonic antigen predicts metastatic recurrence in potentially curative colonic cancer: results of a five-year study. Dis Colon Rectum. 2001;44:231–5.

26. Huh JW, Oh BR, Kim HR, Kim YJ. Preoperative carcinoembryonic antigen level as an independent prognostic factor in potentially curative colon cancer. J Surg Oncol. 2010;101:396–400.

27. Kirat HT, Ozturk E, Lavery IC, Kiran RP. The predictive value of preoperative carcinoembryonic antigen level in the prognosis of colon cancer. Am J Surg. 2012;204:447–52.

28. Locker GY, Hamilton S, Harris J, Jessup JM, Kemeny N, Macdonald JS, et al. ASCO 2006 update of recommendations for the use of tumor markers in gastrointestinal cancer. J Clin Oncol. 2006;24:5313–27.

29. Park IJ, Choi GS, Lim KH, Kang BM, Jun SH. Serum carcinoembryonic antigen monitoring after curative resection for colorectal cancer: clinical significance of the preoperative level. Ann Surg Oncol. 2009;16:3087–93.

30. Mauchley DC, Lynge DC, Langdale LA, Stelzner MG, Mock CN, Billingsley KG. Clinical utility and cost-effectiveness of routine preoperative computed tomography scanning in patients with colon cancer. Am J Surg. 2005;189:512–7. discussion 517.

31. Gollub MJ, Schwartz LH, Akhurst T. Update on colorectal cancer imaging. Radiol Clin North Am. 2007;45:85–118.

32. Sahani DV, Bajwa MA, Andrabi Y, Bajpai S, Cusack JC. Current status of imaging and emerging techniques to evaluate liver metastases from colorectal carcinoma. Ann Surg. 2014; 259:861–72.

33. Furukawa H, Ikuma H, Seki A, Yokoe K, Yuen S, Aramaki T, et al. Positron emission tomography scanning is not superior to whole body multidetector helical computed tomography in the preoperative staging of colorectal cancer. Gut. 2006;55:1007–11.

34. Pelosi E, Deandreis D. The role of 18F-fluoro-deoxy-glucose positron emission tomography (FDG-PET) in the management of patients with colorectal cancer. Eur J Surg Oncol. 2007;33:1–6.

35. Whiteford MH, Whiteford HM, Yee LF, Ogunbiyi OA, Dehdashti F, Siegel BA, et al. Usefulness of FDG-PET scan in the assessment of suspected metastatic or recurrent adenocarcinoma of the colon and rectum. Dis Colon Rectum. 2000;43:759–67. discussion 767–70.

36. Edge SB, Byrd DR, Compton CC, Fritz AG, Greene FL, Trotti AIII. AJCC cancer staging manual. New York: Springer; 2010.

37. Flamen P, Hoekstra OS, Homans F, Van Cutsem E, Maes A, Stroobants S, et al. Unexplained rising carcinoembryonic antigen (CEA) in the postoperative surveillance of colorectal cancer: the utility of positron emission tomography (PET). Eur J Cancer. 2001;37:862–9.

38. Ruers TJ, Wiering B, van der Sijp JR, Roumen RM, de Jong KP, Comans EF, et al. Improved selection of patients for hepatic surgery of colorectal liver metastases with (18)F-FDG PET: a randomized study. J Nucl Med. 2009;50:1036–41.

39. Parsons DP. Preoperative evaluation and risk management. Clin Colon Rectal Surg. 2009;22:5–13.

40. Menke H, Klein A, John KD, Junginger T. Predictive value of ASA classification for the assessment of the perioperative risk. Int Surg. 1993;78:266–70.

41. Fleisher LA, Fleischmann KE, Auerbach AD, Barnason SA, Beckman JA, Bozkurt B, et al. 2014 ACC/AHA guideline on perioperative cardiovascular evaluation and management of patients undergoing noncardiac surgery: a report of the American College of Cardiology/American Heart Association Task Force on Practice Guidelines. Circulation. 2014;130:e278–333.

42. Smetana GW, Lawrence VA, Cornell JE. Preoperative pulmonary risk stratification for noncardiothoracic surgery: systematic review for the American College of Physicians. Ann Intern Med. 2006;144:581–95.

43. Taylor A, DeBoard Z, Gauvin JM. Prevention of postoperative pulmonary complications. Surg Clin North Am. 2015;95(2): 237–54.

44. Mills E, Eyawo O, Lockhart I, Kelly S, Wu P, Ebbert JO. Smoking cessation reduces postoperative complications: a systematic review and meta-analysis. Am J Med. 2011;124: 144–54.

45. Gunderson LL, Jessup JM, Sargent DJ, Greene FL, Stewart AK. Revised TN categorization for colon cancer based on national survival outcomes data. J Clin Oncol. 2010;28: 264–71.

46. Compton CC. Colorectal carcinoma: diagnostic, prognostic, and molecular features. Mod Pathol. 2003;16:376–88.

47. Fleming M, Ravula S, Tatishchev SF, Wang HL. Colorectal carcinoma: pathologic aspects. J Gastrointest Oncol. 2012; 3:153–73.

48. Chang GJ, Rodriguez-Bigas MA, Skibber JM, Moyer VA. Lymph node evaluation and survival after curative resection of colon cancer: systematic review. J Natl Cancer Inst. 2007;99: 433–41.

49. Ueno H, Hashiguchi Y, Shimazaki H, Shinto E, Kajiwara Y, Nakanishi K, et al. Peritumoral deposits as an adverse prognostic indicator of colorectal cancer. Am J Surg. 2014;207:70–7.

50. Read TE, Fleshman JW, Caushaj PF. Sentinel lymph node mapping for adenocarcinoma of the colon does not improve staging accuracy. Dis Colon Rectum. 2005;48:80–5.

51. Broderick-Villa G, Ko A, O'Connell TX, Guenther JM, Danial T, DiFronzo LA. Does tumor burden limit the accuracy of lymphatic mapping and sentinel lymph node biopsy in colorectal cancer? Cancer J. 2002;8:445–50.

52. Joosten JJ, Strobbe LJ, Wauters CA, Pruszczynski M, Wobbes T, Ruers TJ. Intraoperative lymphatic mapping and the sentinel node concept in colorectal carcinoma. Br J Surg. 1999;86:482–6.

53. Nelson H, Petrelli N, Carlin A, Couture J, Fleshman J, Guillem J, et al. Guidelines 2000 for colon and rectal cancer surgery. J Natl Cancer Inst. 2001;93:583–96.

54. Aarons CB, Shanmugan S, Bleier JI. Management of malignant colon polyps: current status and controversies. World J Gastroenterol. 2014;20:16178–83.

55. Bujanda L. Malignant colorectal polyps. World J Gastroenterol. 2010;16:3103–11.

56. Hassan C, Zullo A, Risio M, Rossini FP, Morini S. Histologic risk factors and clinical outcome in colorectal malignant polyp: a pooled-data analysis. Dis Colon Rectum. 2005;48: 1588–96.

57. Tominaga K, Nakanishi Y, Nimura S, Yoshimura K, Sakai Y, Shimoda T. Predictive histopathologic factors for lymph node metastasis in patients with nonpedunculated submucosal invasive colorectal carcinoma. Dis Colon Rectum. 2005;48:92–100.

58. Coppede F, Lopomo A, Spisni R, Migliore L. Genetic and epigenetic biomarkers for diagnosis, prognosis and treatment of colorectal cancer. World J Gastroenterol. 2014;20:943–56.

59. Gausachs M, Mur P, Corral J, Pineda M, Gonzalez S, Benito L, et al. MLH1 promoter hypermethylation in the analytical algorithm of Lynch syndrome: a cost-effectiveness study. Eur J Hum Genet. 2012;20:762–8.

60. Kurzawski G, Suchy J, Debniak T, Kladny J, Lubinski J. Importance of microsatellite instability (MSI) in colorectal cancer: MSI as a diagnostic tool. Ann Oncol. 2004;15 Suppl 4:iv283–4.

61. Benatti P, Gafa R, Barana D, Marino M, Scarselli A, Pedroni M, et al. Microsatellite instability and colorectal cancer prognosis. Clin Cancer Res. 2005;11:8332–40.

62. Ribic CM, Sargent DJ, Moore MJ, Thibodeau SN, French AJ, Goldberg RM, et al. Tumor microsatellite-instability status as a predictor of benefit from fluorouracil-based adjuvant chemotherapy for colon cancer. N Engl J Med. 2003;349:247–57.

63. Lee TH, Marcantonio ER, Mangione CM, Thomas EJ, Polanczyk CA, Cook EF, et al. Derivation and prospective validation of a simple index for prediction of cardiac risk of major noncardiac surgery. Circulation. 1999;100:1043–9.

26
The Surgical Management of Colon Cancer

Matthew G. Mutch

Key Concepts

- Complete clinical staging for colon cancer includes a total colon exam; computed tomography of the chest, abdomen, and pelvis; and a serum CEA level.
- The principles of an oncologic resection include a total mesocolic resection, a ligation of the primary vessel at its origin, a wide mesenteric resection with >12 lymph nodes examined, and at least a 5 cm resection margin.
- There is no difference in cancer-related outcomes for open and laparoscopic resections.
- Anastomotic assessment for left-sided anastomosis is associated with a decreased leak rate.
- Surgical resection is the most effective therapy for patients who present with obstruction colon cancers.
- Endoscopic stenting of an obstructing colon cancer is an effective bridge to surgery within 72 h.
- Perforated cancers should be treated with an oncologic resection.
- First-line therapy for patients with metastatic colon cancer and an asymptomatic primary tumor is chemotherapy.

Introduction

Our understanding of the pathogenesis, staging, and management of adenocarcinoma of the colon has evolved greatly over the last decade. Today, it is accepted that colorectal cancers develop via one of three distinct genetic pathways: (1) chromosomal instability, (2) mismatch repair, and (3) CpG island hypermethylation. This increased understanding of the genetics of colorectal cancer development has led to the identification of several putative molecular markers to predict their biologic and clinic behavior. However, pathologic staging using the TNM system remains the most valuable prognostic tool available, with depth of invasion (T stage) and lymph node involvement (N stage) being the best markers to risk stratifying regional and distant metastatic spread,

respectively. Preoperative imaging has allowed for more accurate clinical staging and earlier detection of metastatic disease that may impact the treatment of the patient. Advances in chemotherapy have allowed for improved outcomes for patients with selected stage II and stage III and IV cancers. Despite all of these advances, surgical resection remains the cornerstone and most important facet in the management of colon cancer. An intimate understanding of the anatomy of the colon, its vasculature, and the retroperitoneum are critical to performing an appropriate oncologic resection for colon cancer. This chapter will focus on the technical aspects of the principles of an oncologic resection such as the importance of total mesocolic resection, ligation of primary vasculature at its origin, obtaining an adequate lymph node harvest to ensure an examination of >12 lymph nodes, and obtaining appropriate distal and proximal margins for open and laparoscopic resections. Special topics such as laparoscopic colectomy for cancer, management of obstructing and perforated colon cancers, treatment of the primary tumor in the setting of metastatic disease, and the short-term and long-term outcomes for colectomy for cancer will be addressed.

Preoperative Preparation

When preparing to take a patient to the operating room for resection of his/her colon cancer, it is imperative to have a complete understanding of the patient's physiologic status, tumor location, and clinical staging. Being able to provide patients with individualized risk stratification for complications after colorectal surgery is becoming more and more important because of the increasing scrutiny of patient safety and outcomes. The general population in the USA is getting older and has an increasing number of comorbidities, so surgeons will be making more and more challenging decisions regarding the management of patients with colorectal cancer.

© Springer International Publishing 2016
S.R. Steele et al. (eds.), *The ASCRS Textbook of Colon and Rectal Surgery*, DOI 10.1007/978-3-319-25970-3_26

Physiologic Assessment

A variety of scoring systems are available for stratifying a patient's risk of perioperative morbidity and mortality after undergoing major digestive system surgery. Each scoring system differs in the included parameters and the outcomes that they measure. The most widely utilized scoring system is the American Society of Anesthesia (ASA) score, but it only provides assessment of an anesthesia complication for a given patient's physiologic status. In contrast, the Physical and Operative Severity Score for the Enumeration of Mortality and Morbidity (POSSUM) and modified Portsmouth-POSSUM scoring systems provide an assessment of the risk of postoperative mortality and morbidity [1]. The scoring system includes 12 preoperative physiologic factors such as age, blood pressure, heart rate, electrocardiogram status, hemoglobin, and electrolytes. It can also be reevaluated in the postoperative period using six additional intraoperative parameters including operative procedure, estimated blood loss, peritoneal contamination, presence of malignancy, and urgency of the operative procedure. However, it has been repeatedly shown that POSSUM and P-POSSUM scores underestimate the risk of morbidity and mortality for patients undergoing major colorectal surgery. In an effort to improve the performance prediction of patients undergoing colorectal resections, a colorectal-specific POSSUM (CR-POSSUM) score was developed [2]. Multiple retrospective and prospective studies have demonstrated improved accuracy with the CR-POSSUM compared to POSSUM and P-POSSUM for predicting mortality after colorectal surgery for a variety of diseases such as cancer and diverticulitis [3, 4]. The CR-POSSUM scoring system has also been validated in multiple health-care systems around the globe such as the USA, the UK, India, Middle East, Caribbean, and Asia [5, 6]. Furthermore, the CR-POSSUM scoring system has improved accuracy in elderly patients defined as >80 years of age when compared to P-POSSUM [7]. There are also suggestions that physiologic health status of an elderly patient is more important than the type of surgery when attempting to predict mortality in this age group. The American College of Surgeons developed a surgical risk calculator using data from National Surgical Quality Improvement Program (NSQIP) to provide patient-specific postoperative risks of various complications. The scoring system is based on over 1.4 million patients with over 1500 unique Current Procedural Terminology (CPT) codes and has performed very well for predicting mortality, overall morbidity, and risk of six specific complications (pneumonia, cardiac, surgical site infection, urinary tract infection, venous thromboembolism, renal failure, and return to the operating room) [8–10]. The NSQIP risk calculator has been shown to underestimate the risk of complications for colorectal resections, and more surgeon- and patient-specific data are needed. However, it remains a useful tool to preoperatively assess morbidity and mortality risk. The risk calculator is available at http://riskcalculator.facs.org.

Tumor Localization

Accurate tumor localization is a critical component of the preoperative assessment of the patient and operative planning. Intraoperative tumor localization can be challenging from several standpoints such a small or early tumor, obese patient, adhesions, laparoscopy, or inadequate tattooing. The utilization of intraluminal anatomic markings for tumor localization is inaccurate, 12–14 % of the time, and may be higher if cecal and rectal tumors are excluded [11]. In other words, the colonoscopy will not accurately locate the tumor 1 out of 7 times. Localization with endoscopic tattooing provides the most accurate method for localization. The tattoo should be placed distal to the lesion and in three separate areas around the circumference of the lumen (Fig. 26.1). A single injection into the mesenteric border or sprayed into the peritoneal cavity may be difficult to identify. Chou et al. reported that endoscopic tattooing provided accurate localization in 94 of 97 (98 %) tumors [12]. This study also examined radiographic methods for tumor localization and found barium enema and CT colonography to be 93 % and 95 % accurate, respectively. Alternatively, endoscopic placement of metal clips at the site of the tumor with immediate plain radiograph (or CT) will localize the tumor with a high degree of accuracy. The ultimate fallback to identify a lesion is intraoperative colonoscopy, ideally using carbon dioxide as the insufflation gas to limit bowel dilatation.

Patients who present with endoscopically obstructing lesions can be effectively evaluated with CT colonography to complete their total colon exam prior to surgery. CT colonography has replaced contrast enema studies in many situations because of improved accuracy in detecting synchronous lesions and often provides better tumor localization. A study of 411 consecutive patients evaluated with CT colonography for incomplete colonoscopy due to a stenosing colorectal cancer and the preoperative CT colonography was compared to the intraoperative and pathologic findings [13]. The study demonstrated a sensitivity of 100 % for detecting

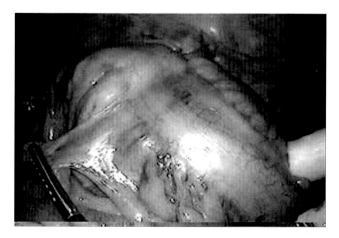

FIGURE 26-1. Tattoo localization of a sigmoid colon cancer.

proximal synchronous cancers and negative predictive value of 97 % for identifying advanced neoplastic lesions (advanced adenomas or cancers). Other studies have demonstrated similar results [14–16]. CT colonography can safely be used in the acute and subacute settings as demonstrated by Maras-Simunic et al. [17]. They examined 44 patients who presented with signs and symptoms of a large bowel obstruction, and CT colonography was able to accurately identify the cause of obstruction as a cancer in 41 and due to a benign process in nine patients. It was also able to accurately detect two synchronous cancers in this small study population. Therefore, if it is safe and feasible, patients presenting with a distally obstructing lesion (clinically or endoscopically) who have a negative CT colonography can be safely treated with a segmental resection without significant risk of missing of synchronous, proximal lesions.

Surgical Technique

Extent of Resection

The National Comprehensive Cancer Network provides the recommended principles of surgical resection for colon cancer, which include obtaining an adequate proximal margin, distal margin, and lymphadenectomy [18]. Colon cancers tend to grow circumferentially around the lumen of the colon, extend out radially and, to a lesser degree, longitudinally along the bowel. Therefore, a 5 cm proximal or distal margin has always been recommended. This is important to remove all tumors bearing mucosa but also to resect all lymph nodes with potential to drain tumor cells. A retrospective study by Rorvig et al. compared final pathologic stage in resected colon cancer specimens with a tumor margin <5 cm to those with a >5 cm margin. The node positivity rate for tumors with a margin <5 cm was 37 % versus 51 % for a margin >5 cm [19]. This highlights that even though the primary tumor does not grow in a longitudinal fashion, lymphatic drainage can extend in a longitudinal or somewhat aberrant fashion. In order to obtain an adequate lymphadenectomy, the feeding vessel to the resected segment of the colon should be taken at its origin. For example, the ileocolic pedicle should be ligated at its origin on the superior mesenteric artery, and the inferior mesenteric artery should be ligated at the level of the aorta. The goal is to clear all regional lymph nodes and provide a minimum of 12 lymph nodes for pathologic evaluation. The impact of an adequate lymph node harvest and evaluation on the accuracy of pathologic staging is well documented and is addressed in Chap. 34. The concept of high versus low ligation of the primary feeding vessel had been debated throughout the literature. Historical data and recent prospective randomized trials have demonstrated no difference in morbidity associated with high ligation [20–23]. However, the rate of positive lymph nodes along the IMA above the level of aortic bifurcation has been reported to be as high as 8 % and when resected is associated with better disease-free survival [22]. Therefore, to maximize the lymph

node harvest and to ensure complete resection of potentially metastatic lymph nodes, the mesentery should be resected with the primary vessel ligated at its origin and at least a 5 cm margin distal or proximal to the tumor.

Mesocolic Resection

The concept of total mesorectal excision (TME), which was popularized by R.J. Heald, also pertains to the resection of the colon and associated mesentery along the appropriate fascial planes. Just as the mesorectum is enveloped in a fascia, the mesocolon also has a visceral fascial plane that separates it from the retroperitoneum (parietal fascia). A serosal surface on the bowel and mesentery excludes the anterior aspect of the mesentery from the perineal cavity. Therefore, a complete mesocolic excision (CME) is the sharp dissection of the visceral fascia from the parietal fascia of the retroperitoneum and central ligation of the primary vasculature. Hohenberger et al. adopted this concept in the mid-1990s and published their results on 1329 consecutive patients [24]. They reported an improvement in 5-year local recurrence and 5-year survival from 6.5 to 3.6 % and 82.1 to 89.1 %, respectively, after adoption of CME plus central ligation of the mesenteric vessels. Subsequent studies have demonstrated several other benefits of CME such as increased lymph node harvest, longer vascular ligation, increased resection of extranodal tumor deposits, and increased upstaging, which led to no differences in morbidity but improved locoregional control and survival [25, 26]. The technical concept of sharp dissection of the colon and mesocolon off the retroperitoneum, excision of the mesentery along the lines of resection, and central ligation of the vasculature is as important to colon cancer as TME is to rectal cancer.

Right Colectomy

Tumors located anywhere from the cecum to the proximal transverse colon can safely be treated with a right colectomy. The basic tenets of resection of a right-sided tumor include full abdominal exploration, full mobilization of the right colon, and hepatic flexure with a mesenteric resection including ligation of the ileocolic and right branch of the middle colic vessels at their origin. The resection can be performed safely and effectively via either an open or laparoscopic approach. Data regarding laparoscopy and colorectal cancer is presented in detail below.

Open Approach

The peritoneal cavity can be accessed with a midline incision or as some surgeons prefer a right-sided transverse incision. Once the abdomen is open, explored, and the tumor is located, the wound should be protected with a wound protector. The first step in mobilizing the right colon is to access the retroperitoneum, which can be accomplished laterally along the white line of Toldt, inferiorly near the cecum, posteriorly under the small bowel mesentery, or superiorly through the lesser sac. Once the retroperitoneum is entered, the mesentery and hepatic flexure are mobilized. The duodenum should be identified and reflected into the retroperitoneum. The omentum associated with the resected colon should be resected as well. With the colon completely mobilized, the vascular pedicles can be ligated. Regardless of the approach used, the step is the same and only their order is different.

Lateral Approach

The surgeon stands on the patient's left side and the first assistant on the patient's right side. The right colon is grasped, and the peritoneum is incised just anterior to the white line of Toldt from the cecum to the hepatic flexure. This allows access to the retroperitoneum or the avascular plane between the visceral and parietal planes of the colon and retroperitoneum. It is important not to violate the mesenteric side of this plane in order to ensure a total mesocolic resection. Under tension, the right colon is separated sharply from the retroperitoneum. The duodenum should be identified and reflected into the retroperitoneum. The cecum is then mobilized off the retroperitoneum, and the posterior attachments of the small bowel mesentery are divided all the way up to the duodenum. This provides the mobility of the small bowel for the anastomosis. With the duodenum safely reflected posteriorly, the hepatic flexure can be mobilized. The surgeon's left hand is placed under the colon and its mesentery and brought out laterally to expose the superior attachments along the inferior edge of the liver. Eventually, the lesser sac is entered, and the lesser omentum is divided. Care must be taken so the plane between the omentum and the transverse colon mesentery is separated, and dissection into the transverse colon is avoided. These two planes are typically fused up to the midline, and beyond this point, the proper lesser sac is entered. After the right colon and hepatic flexure are completely mobilized, the cecum is put on stretch, and the ileocolic pedicle can easily be identified. Since the right colon and its mesentery have been mobilized, there should be bare areas on the cephalad and caudad aspects of the ileocolic pedicle. The peritoneum is incised along the lines of resection for both bare areas allowing isolation of the pedicle so it can be ligated at its origin on the superior mesenteric vessels. The terminal ileal mesentery is divided so that a 5 cm margin on the terminal ileum is obtained. The right branch of the middle colic vessels is identified by elevating the transverse colon mesentery. The pedicle should become evident either by it bowstringing under tension or there should be another bare area where the omentum has been dissected free during the exposure of the lesser sac. The peritoneum should be incised from the distal site of transection of the colon to the base of the pedicle and across the pedicle to the cut edge of the right colon mesentery. The pedicle can then be ligated at its origin. Ileocolic anastomotic techniques will be discussed later.

Posterior Approach

The small bowel is eviscerated and reflected toward the right upper quadrant to expose the posterior aspect of the small bowel mesentery from the ligament of Treitz to the cecum (Fig. 26.2). The peritoneum is incised along this entire length, and the retroperitoneum is entered (Fig. 26.3). The duodenum is readily identified and reflected into the retroperitoneum.

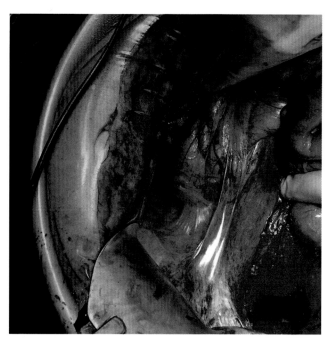

FIGURE 26-2. Exposure of the posterior aspect of the small bowel mesentery for the posterior approach to a right colon.

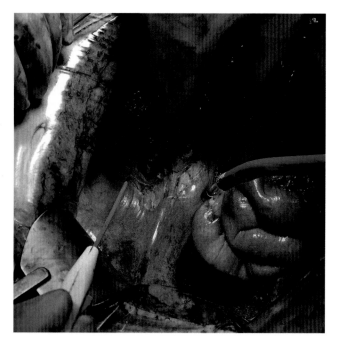

FIGURE 26-3. Entry into the retroperitoneum from the posterior approach to a right colectomy.

The right colon mesentery is elevated off the retroperitoneum out beyond the ascending colon laterally and the transverse colon superiorly. The further this dissection can be performed from a medial-to-lateral direction beyond the transverse colon, hepatic flexure, and ascending colon, the easier the lateral dissection becomes as all that remains are the lateral peritoneal and lesser omental attachments. At this point, starting at the level of the cecum, the surgeon while standing on the patient's left side places his/her left hand under the right colon mesentery and lateral to the colon to expose the lateral peritoneal attachments. These are then divided heading up toward the hepatic flexure. If the dissection is continuing easily, the lesser omentum is separated from the transverse colon mesentery in order to enter the lesser sac. If this plane is difficult to develop, the distal site of transection is identified, and the lesser sac can be entered at this point. This begins by dividing the greater omentum to the level of the colon, and the lesser omentum is bluntly separated from the colon and its mesentery to enter the lesser sac. Once the lesser sac is entered, this plane is developed toward the hepatic flexure. Eventually, the posterior retroperitoneal dissection plane is entered. With the duodenum free, the remaining attachments along the inferior liver can be safely divided. The right colon and hepatic flexure are completely mobilized so the vascular pedicles can be ligated and the mesentery can be resected as described above.

Superior Approach

This dissection begins at the distal site of transection of the transverse colon. This is accomplished by elevating the transverse colon to expose its inferior aspect of the mesentery so the right branch of the middle colon vessels can be identified. It is the first pedicle medial to the bare area of the duodenum and should bowstring under the tension of elevating the transverse colon. The greater omentum is divided up to the transverse colon, and the lesser omentum is separated from the colon and mesentery to enter the lesser sac. As this plane is developed toward the hepatic flexure, the lesser omentum is divided. The stomach superiorly and duodenum posteriorly should be identified and separated from the colon mesentery. Once the lesser omentum or hepatic attachments to the colon are divided beyond the hepatic flexure, the hepatic flexure can be elevated under tension to develop the retroperitoneal plane, identify and free the duodenum, and divide the lateral peritoneal attachments of the right colon. With the peritoneal attachments divided, the remaining colon is mobilized in the same manner as described in the lateral approach. The superior approach is very useful for big bulky or locally advanced tumors of the cecum and proximal ascending colon because it allows for complete mobilization of the colon and mesentery before addressing the site of the tumor.

Anastomosis

The anastomosis can be accomplished via handsewn or stapled techniques. For the handsewn technique, the anastomotic orientation can either be end to end or side to side, and it can be created in a single or double layer of sutures. However, an end-to-end anastomosis is often difficult given the significant size discrepancies between the lumens of the small bowel and colon, so only the side-to-side technique will be presented. For the handsewn technique, the bowel is divided with a stapler or sharply, and the cut edges are closed with an absorbable monofilament 3-0 suture. To close the enterotomy, a Connell stitch is used in a running fashion, and this suture line can be dunked with interrupted Lembert stitches using an absorbable 3-0 suture. The bowel is then oriented in a side-to-side, antiperistaltic fashion. A single-layer anastomosis can be created using an absorbable monofilament 3-0 suture in either a running or interrupted fashion. For a single-layer, interrupted anastomosis, a 6–7 cm enterotomy is created. The first two stitches are placed 180° from each other in the proximal and distal corners, which allows for the "back walls" of the anastomosis to be aligned. With the "back wall" edges of the anastomosis inverted, the next stitch is placed in a bisecting position, and the subsequent stitches are placed in the same bisecting fashion until the "back wall" is complete. For the "front wall" of the anastomosis, sutures are alternately placed at proximal and distal corners until they meet in the middle. The suture is place from an inside out of the first lumen to the outside in of the second lumen. This technique places the knot of the suture intraluminally and inverts the two edges of the bowel. The last stitch will need to be placed in an out-to-in and in-to-out fashion, so the knot is on the outside of the bowel. For a running handsewn anastomosis, two sutures are placed in the middle of the "back wall" of the anastomosis, so one suture will run the anastomosis in the proximal direction and the other suture will run in the distal direction, and after completing the "front wall," the two sutures will be tied together. For the "back wall" of the anastomosis, the suture can be run in an overlapping, baseball-type fashion as the two bowel edges are already inverted. At each corner as the "front wall" of the anastomosis is created, the stitch should be transitioned to a Connell stitch, so the front edges will be inverted as well. For a double-layered anastomosis, the first step is to place the back row of Lembert stitches along the length of the anastomosis. The enterotomies are then made parallel to the Lembert stitches, and the inner layer is created in the same fashion of the running anastomosis described above. The front outer layer of Lembert stitches are then placed once the inner layer is completed.

Stapled anastomoses are most commonly performed in a side-to-side fashion but can also be performed in a side-to-end configuration as well. The traditional side-to-side, stapled anastomosis is created by individually dividing the proximal (Fig. 26.4) and distal limbs (Fig. 26.5) of the bowel with a stapler. The antimesenteric corner of each staple line is then excised, and forks of the stapler are placed into the lumen of each limb of the intestine. The stapler is reassembled and fired with the bowel in an antiperistaltic and antimesenteric fashion (Fig. 26.6). The resulting common enterotomy is reapproximated, so the longitudinal staple lines are offset, which prevents the intersection of more than two staple lines (Fig. 26.7). This common enterotomy can be

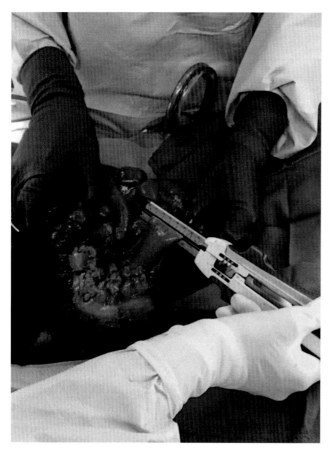

FIGURE 26-4. Division of the terminal ileum. Courtesy of Howard Ross, M.D.

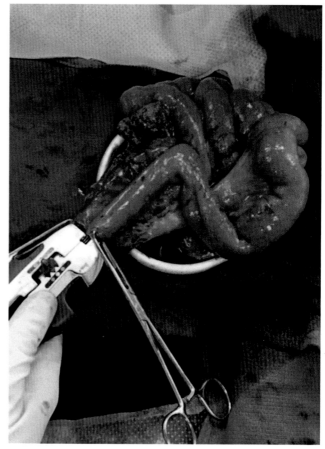

FIGURE 26-6. Firing of the linear stapler for a side-to-side stapled anastomosis. Courtesy of Howard Ross, M.D.

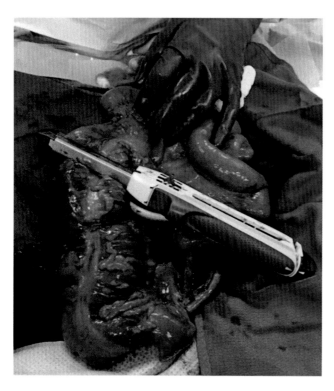

FIGURE 26-5. Division of the transverse colon. Courtesy of Howard Ross, M.D.

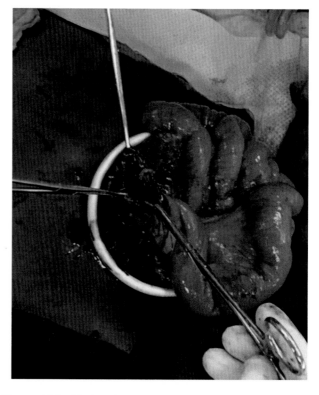

FIGURE 26-7. Closing the common enterotomy by offsetting the longitudinal staple line. Courtesy of Howard Ross, M.D.

closed with suture or staples (Figs. 26.8 and 26.9). An alternative method for creating the side-to-side anastomosis is not to divide the proximal and distal bowel. Enterotomies are then made on the antimesenteric side at the site of transection. The forks of the staple are then passed through each enterotomy where they are reassembled and fired in an antiperistaltic and antimesenteric fashion. The common enterotomy is once again reapproximated with the longitudinal staple lines offset, and then it is closed with a firing of the stapler that incorporates the proximal and distal limbs of the bowel. This technique saves the use of two stapler loads.

A stapled anastomosis can also be created in a side-to-end fashion. This anastomosis is created with an end-to-end anastomotic (EEA) stapler. The distal limb is divided sharply; a purse string is placed; and the stapler anvil, typically 28 or 29 mm, is placed inside. The proximal limb is also divided sharply, and the stapling cartridge is passed into the lumen of the proximal bowel. It is aligned for the spike to come out through the antimesenteric border. The spike should be positioned proximal enough, so the distal aspect of the circular staple line is at least 4 cm proximal to the cut edge of the bowel. This is important to ensure that the distal strip of the bowel remains viable once the enterotomy is closed. The end

enterotomy of the proximal limb is then closed with a linear stapler or can be handsewn.

Laparoscopic Approach

Proper room setup and instrumentation are critical for success. A mechanical bed is essential, so the patient can be placed in extremes of positions to maximize the use of gravity for retraction and exposure. The patient needs to be safely secured to the bed, and there are a myriad of techniques to accomplish this such as bean bags, nonskid pads, or shoulder braces. Placing the patient in stirrups has the advantage of allowing the assistant or surgeon to stand between the legs, which allows for visualization in the direction of the dissection and minimizes working against the camera angle. Instrumentation is up to the surgeon's preference, but the use of atraumatic graspers is recommended. There are several energy devices available such as monopolar cautery, bipolar vessel sealers, and ultrasonic sealers that can be used for dissection and ligation of appropriate vessels. With regard to port placement, there are no hard-set rules, and they should be based on the surgical approach and surgeon's preference (Fig. 26.10a, b). Laparoscopic colectomy is a multi-quadrant procedure, so placement of the camera port as to maximize visualization is important. The most optimal place for the

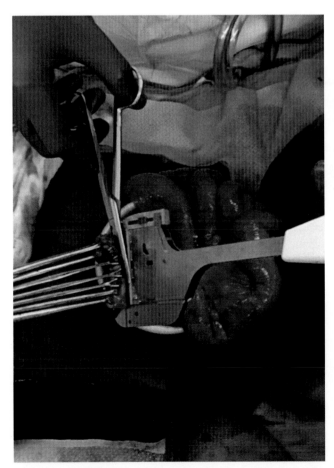

FIGURE 26-8. Closing the common enterotomy for a side-to-side anastomosis. Courtesy of Howard Ross, M.D.

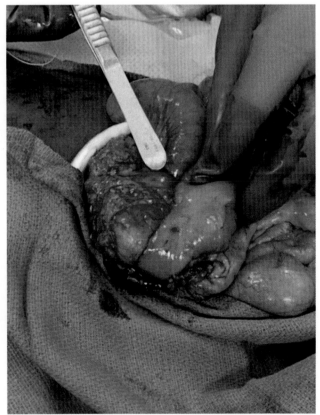

FIGURE 26-9. Complete side-to-side ileocolic anastomosis. Courtesy of Howard Ross, M.D.

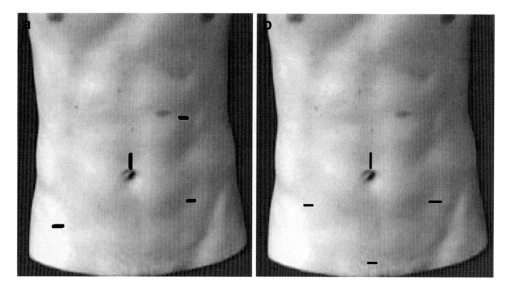

FIGURE 26-10. (a) Port placement for a laparoscopic right colectomy, (b) port placement for a laparoscopic right colectomy.

camera port is at the apex of the pneumoperitoneum. This is typically in the midline and at the midpoint between the xiphoid process and the pubic symphysis, which can either be above or below the umbilicus. Once pneumoperitoneum is established and the abdomen is adequately explored, the dissection can be carried out in a medial-to-lateral, lateral-to-medial, or posterior approach. For this chapter, the medial-to-lateral and posterior approaches will be presented.

Medial-to-Lateral Approach

Once the peritoneum is accessed, pneumoperitoneum is established and the ports are placed, the abdomen is completely examined, and the tumor is localized. The patient is then placed in steep Trendelenburg and airplaned right-side up. The omentum is placed in the upper abdomen to expose the transverse colon and the hepatic flexure. The small bowel is moved to the left side of the abdomen to fully expose the right colon mesentery. The first step of the dissection is to grab the mesentery at the junction of the terminal ileum and cecum and pull it to the right lower quadrant. This puts the ileocolic pedicle on tension and can be identified as it creates a bowstring in the mesentery. The pedicle is then grasped more proximally, and the peritoneum on the caudad aspect is incised in a direction parallel to the vessels. A wider incision in the peritoneum provides better exposure. Blunt dissection is used to get through the mesentery into the retroperitoneum. Once in the retroperitoneum, the duodenum is readily identified and reflected into the retroperitoneum. This dissection is aided by providing sufficient traction allowing tension, and 15 mmHg of CO_2 pressure aids the development of the avascular planes between the visceral and parietal fascia of the retroperitoneum. The dissection is done bluntly and carried cephalad and lateral as far as possible to safely separate the duodenum from the right colon mesentery, which

allows the ileocolic pedicle to be isolated and ligated at its origin from the superior mesenteric vessels. The pedicle can be ligated with clips, staples, or vessel-sealing devices. In order to identify and isolate the right branch of the middle colic vessels, the transverse colon mesentery is elevated under tension. The pedicle is then identified as the vessel that bowstrings just medial to the cut edge of the right colon mesentery. This will help identify the distal site of transection of the colon. The peritoneum from the colon medial to the pedicle is scored down to the base of the pedicle and across it to the mesenteric cut edge. The pedicle is isolated with gentle blunt dissection along this plane. Once through the transverse colon mesentery, the omentum may be adherent to the mesentery in the lesser sac, so it may need to be dissected free to isolate the pedicle. With the pedicle ligated, the window through the mesentery into the retroperitoneum is wider, and the right colon mesentery should be mobilized off the retroperitoneum from the mid-transverse colon, out to the hepatic flexure, and lateral to the ascending colon. Ideally, all that remains at this point is the lateral peritoneal and omental attachments. The cecum is grasped and reflected medially and cephalad, the peritoneum is incised, and the dissected retroperitoneal space is entered. The posterior peritoneal attachments of the small bowel mesentery need to be divided up to the level of duodenum, so the small bowel has enough mobilization for extraction, resection, and anastomosis. Now the lateral attachments of the right colon are divided under tension all the way up the hepatic flexure. If the dissection is proceeding well, the hepatic flexure can be mobilized in this same direction by separating the hepatocolic/lesser omentum from the transverse colon mesentery to enter the lesser sac. If it is difficult to get adequate exposure, the approach can be altered by returning the colon to its anatomic position and identifying the distal site where the colon will be divided. The greater omentum is then divided at this point, and the lesser sac is entered by separating the lesser omentum from the transverse colon and its mesentery. This is an avascular plane, so it can be separated bluntly under tension. Once this plane has been developed, the dissection progresses toward the hepatic flexure by dividing the lesser omentum. As the dissection progresses beyond the pylorus, the retroperitoneal dissection plane should be entered, and the remaining attachments along the liver can be safely divided because the duodenum has been dissected free of this tissue. The colon is now completely mobilized and can be extracted via the surgeon's site of choice. For cancer cases, the use of a wound protector for extraction is highly recommended to minimize the risk of a wound recurrence. Once the colon is extracted, it is resected, and the anastomosis can be created using one of the techniques described earlier.

Posterior Approach

The peritoneal cavity is entered, ports are placed, and the abdomen is thoroughly explored. The patient is placed in steep Trendelenburg, and the omentum is reflected over the transverse colon to expose the hepatic flexure. The small bowel is placed in the right upper quadrant to expose the posterior aspect of the small bowel mesentery. The patient should not be tilted right-side up, so the small bowel will stay in the right upper quadrant. To obtain the exposure, the terminal ileum is identified and reflected toward the right colon. This will expose the fold of where the small bowel mesentery joins the retroperitoneum. Moving the small bowel to the right upper quadrant and following this fold in a cephalad direction will expose the fourth portion of the duodenum (Fig. 26.11). An instrument in the surgeon's right hand elevates the proximal aspect of the small bowel mesentery under tension, and the first assistant via a right lower quadrant port elevates the distal aspect of the small bowel mesentery, which provides exposure of the duodenum and posterior peritoneum of the small bowel mesentery. With the use of an energy source, the

peritoneum is incised from the duodenum to the cecum allowing access to the retroperitoneum, and the right colon mesentery can be elevated off the retroperitoneum. The duodenum is reflected posteriorly, and the mesentery is elevated from the mid-transverse colon, out to the hepatic flexure, and down the ascending colon to the cecum (Fig. 26.12). The further this dissection is carried beyond the colon laterally and superiorly, the easier the lateral and hepatic flexure mobilization will be. Now the patient is airplaned right-side up, and the small bowel and omentum are pulled to the left side of the abdomen to expose the lateral aspect of the right colon. The lateral attachments are divided by grabbing the cecum and retracting it medial and cephalad toward the spleen (Fig. 26.13). The attachments are divided toward the hepatic flexure as far as possible. Just like that described in the medial-to-lateral approach, if the lesser sac can be easily developed and entered, the dissection can proceed in this direction. If this approach is too difficult, place the colon back in its anatomic position, and identify the distal site where the colon will be

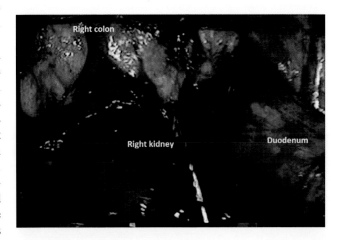

FIGURE 26-12. Posterior mobilization of the right colon mesentery off the retroperitoneum.

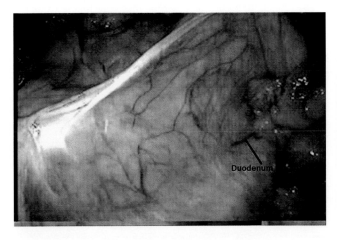

FIGURE 26-11. Exposure of posterior aspect of the small bowel mesentery for a laparoscopic posterior approach.

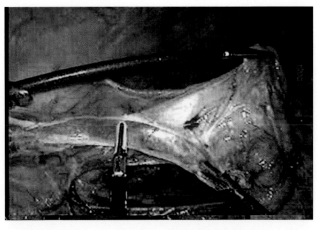

FIGURE 26-13. Exposure of the lateral attachments after the posterior dissection.

452 M.G. Mutch

divided. This is accomplished by elevating the transverse colon mesentery and putting the right branch of the middle colic vessels on stretch (Fig. 26.14). The vessel is medial to the bare area of the right colon mesentery. The greater omentum is then divided at this point, and the lesser sac is entered by separating the lesser omentum from the transverse colon and its mesentery (Fig. 26.15). This is an avascular plane, so it can be separated bluntly under tension. Once this plane has been developed, the dissection progresses toward the hepatic flexure by dividing the lesser omentum. As the dissection progresses beyond the pylorus, the retroperitoneal dissection plane can be identified by the purplish tissue planes indicative of the previous posterior dissection. This plane can be safely entered, and the remaining attachments along the liver can be safely divided because the duodenum has been dissected free of the right colon mesentery (Fig. 26.16). At this point, the right colon and hepatic flexure have been completely mobilized. The next step is to isolate and ligate the vasculature. The ileocolic pedicles are identified by grasping the mesentery on the inside of the ileocecal valve and pulling to the right lower quadrant. The pedicle will bowstring, and because

it has been mobilized off the retroperitoneum, bare areas can be seen on the caudad and cephalad (bare area over the duodenum) aspects (Fig. 26.17). The peritoneum on the caudad aspect is scored parallel to the pedicle, and blunt dissection through the mesentery will allow entry into the retroperitoneum. The duodenum can be visualized to ensure it is completely free of the pedicle. The peritoneum is then scored over the base of the pedicle toward the cephalad bare area, and the pedicle is safely isolated and ligated. The medial cut edge of the mesentery near the right branch of the middle colic vessels is grasped and reflected to the video right, allowing any remaining attachments to the duodenum, stomach, or omentum which can be seen and gently sweep free. The transverse colon mesentery is then elevated under tension, which allows for the right branch to bowstring, and, ideally, a bare area is seen medial to the vessel (Fig. 26.18). The peritoneum is then scored from the colon down to the base of the vessel and then across it to connect with the cut edge of the mesentery. Blunt dissection of the bare area will allow access into the lesser sac and for safe ligation of the pedicle. Because the omentum has been previously dissected free from entering the lesser sac, the vessel can be safely ligated without the risk of injury to

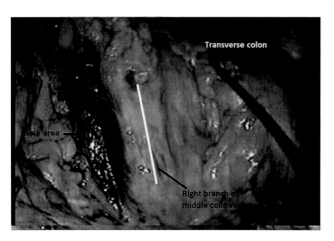

FIGURE 26-14. Exposure of the right branch of the middle colic vessels.

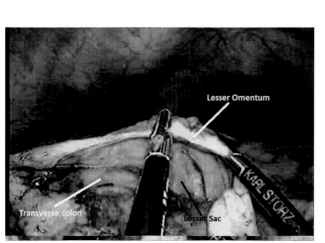

FIGURE 26-15. Entering the lesser sac by separating the lesser omentum from the transverse colon at the distal site of transection.

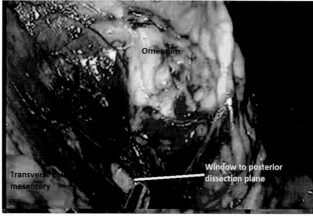

FIGURE 26-16. Exposure of posterior dissection plane from the superior approach.

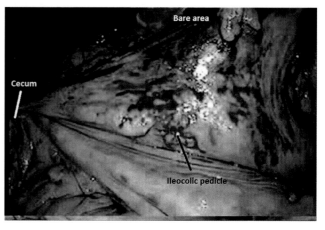

FIGURE 26-17. Identification of the ileocolic pedicle.

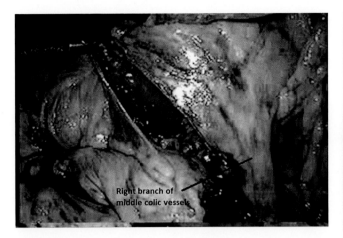

FIGURE 26-18. Identification of the right branch of the middle colic vessels.

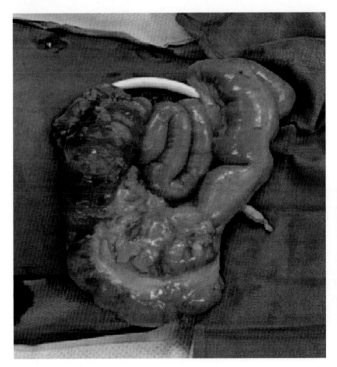

FIGURE 26-19. Extraction of the right colon.

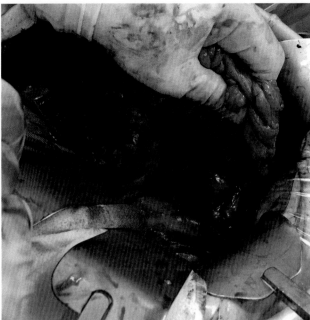

FIGURE 26-20. Medial exposure of the IMA.

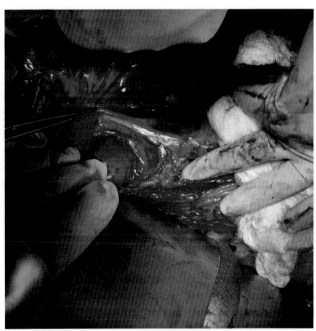

FIGURE 26-21. Medial exposure of the IMV.

surrounding structures. The colon can now be extracted and resected and the anastomosis created as described in the medial-to-lateral section (Fig. 26.19).

Left Colectomy

Open

The patient is placed in the lithotomy position to have access to the perineum for the anastomosis and anastomotic assessment. One of the patient's arms can be tucked to his/her side, and the Mayo stand for the scrub nurse can be placed over the patient's head, or the scrub nurse can stand off one of the patient's hips. The peritoneum is entered via a midline inci-

sion that allows for complete exploration and mobilization of the splenic flexure. With the abdomen open, a wound protector can be inserted, and a self-retaining retractor can be utilized. Initial exposure of the left colon anatomy is accomplished by packing the small bowel in the right upper quadrant, so the base of the left colon mesentery includes exposing the inferior mesenteric artery (IMA) at its origin (Fig. 26.20) and the inferior mesenteric vein (IMV) as it courses near the ligament of Treitz and inferior border of the pancreas (Fig. 26.21). The cecum and terminal ileum are also packed away to provide complete exposure into the pelvis and the sacral promontory. The dissection begins with division of the lateral attachments of the sigmoid colon to allow for visualization of the white line of Toldt from the upper rectum to the proximal descending colon. The sigmoid colon and descending colon are elevated and retracted medially, and a long incision is made in the peritoneum to enter the retroperitoneal plane. With adequate tension on the colon and its mesentery, the areolar plane of dissection along the retroperitoneal plane is easily identified. The dissection is facilitated by exposing and dividing the retroperitoneal attachments along a plane of dissection as long as possible. The sigmoid colon and its mesentery should be completely medialized to the midline to expose and identify the left ureter. The dissection is then carried toward the splenic flexure. Mobilization of the splenic flexure can be facilitated by dissecting the posterior aspect of the mesentery up to the inferior border of the pancreas. The anatomy of the splenic flexure can be obscured by attachments of the omentum to the descending colon or medial aspect of the transverse colon. Separating these attachments restores normal anatomy, which can make the splenic flexure mobilization much easier. The next goal is to enter the lesser sac, and this is accomplished by separating the omentum from the transverse colon. By incising the peritoneal layer along the length of the transverse colon, the lesser sac is eventually entered, and the posterior attachments of the omentum to the colon mesentery can be exposed and divided. This will allow the lesser sac to be completely exposed from the flexure to beyond midline. This will also expose the remaining lateral attachments of the flexure which can be divided by either retracting the colon medially or placing a hand into the retroperitoneum and rolling the colon medially over the hand. With the lesser sac completely open and the flexure mobilized, the posterior attachments along the inferior border of the pancreas can be divided. With the posterior mesenteric dissection carried all the way up to the inferior border of the pancreas, the surgeon's right hand is passed into the retroperitoneum in the lateral-to-medial direction. The fold of the splenic flexure mesentery can be palpated and separated from the inferior aspect of the pancreas, and the overlying peritoneum is divided to the midline. Care should be taken not to injure the IMV as the dissection is carried medially. With the left colon and splenic flexure completely mobilized, the vascular pedicles can be isolated and ligated. The sigmoid colon is elevated and retracted laterally to expose the base of the mesentery at the level of the sacral promontory. The peritoneum is incised from just below the promontory toward the attachments of the proximal jejunum and ligament of Treitz. This will allow for the superior rectal artery to be elevated off the retroperitoneum and expose the lateral plane of dissection. The surgeon can then pass his/her right hand under the superior rectal artery and divide the cephalad attachments, so the IMA can be isolated at its origin from the aorta (Fig. 26.22). The artery is isolated by creating a window on its cephalad side and medial to the IMV. It can then be ligated once the left ureter is clearly out of harm's

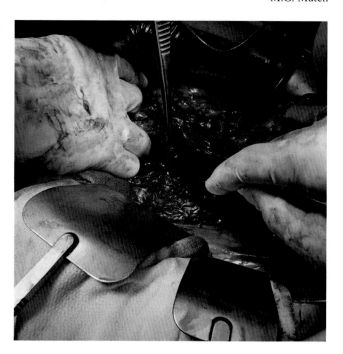

FIGURE 26-22. Isolation of the IMA.

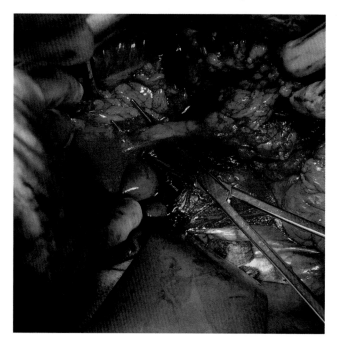

FIGURE 26-23. Isolation of the IMV.

way. The IMV is now elevated off the retroperitoneum and isolated at the inferior border of the pancreas, and its ligation will ensure adequate mobilization for a tension-free anastomosis (Fig. 26.23). This allows for complete exposure of the retroperitoneum (Fig. 26.24). The proximal site of transection is dependent upon the location of the tumor and should ensure a minimum of a 5 cm margin. The distal site of transection should be at the proximal rectum to ensure an adequate distal margin and avoid having distal sigmoid colon

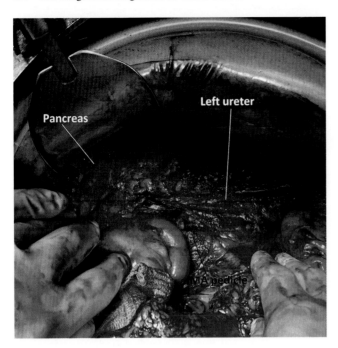

Figure 26-24. Left retroperitoneum.

included in the anastomosis. The rectum is stapled and divided with a linear stapler. The anastomosis is most easily accomplished with an end-to-end double-stapled technique (see Chap. 9). The anvil is placed in the proximal colotomy after the creation of a purse string. The purse string is tightened while ensuring that the edges of the colotomy are everted, so all edges of the colotomy are incorporated into the purse string. The stapling cartridge is passed transanally to the top of the rectal stump. The stapler head should be flushed with the transverse staple line. A rectal fold or pelvic adhesion will sometimes prevent the stapler head from sitting flush. If a rectal fold is preventing this, the rectum can be further mobilized and divided a few centimeters lower, and if it is a pelvic adhesion preventing passing of the stapling cartridge, further mobilization of the rectum will often be adequate to get the stapler up to the staple line. The spike of the stapler is deployed just anterior or posterior to the transverse staple line. The anvil is reassembled to make sure there is no twist in the left colon and its mesentery.

Anastomotic Assessment

Anastomotic assessment with either an air leak test alone or combined with endoscopic visualization is critical to ensuring a safe anastomosis. Anastomotic assessment has been shown to be associated with a decreased incidence of anastomotic leak from left-sided anastomosis. Kwon et al. audited the data from the Washington state's Surgical Care and Outcomes Assessment Program regarding the utilization and outcomes associated with routine testing of colorectal anastomosis [27]. For this study, anastomotic testing consisted of insufflation of Betadine, methylene blue, or air under pres-

sure, and an adverse event included a return to the operating room for an ostomy creation, anastomotic revision, or drainage of abscess associated with a documented leak. For hospitals where the surgeons routinely performed anastomotic leak tests (defined as occurring in >90 % of cases), there was a 75 % lower risk of anastomotic leak (adjusted OR, 0.50; 95 % CI, 0.05–0.99) compared to those hospitals that employed selective leak testing (adjusted OR, 2.68; 95 % CI, 1.14–6.26). A retrospective review by Ricciardi et al. demonstrated an overall leak rate of 4.8 % for 998 patients that underwent a left-sided colorectal anastomosis without proximal diversion [28]. Ninety percent of patients underwent air leak testing, and the associated leak rates were 7.7 % with a positive air leak test, 3.8 % with a negative air leak test, and 8.1 % when no air leak test was performed ($p<0.03$). Additionally, they examined the measures taken to address the positive air leak test and the associated outcomes. Suture repair alone resulted in a leak rate of 12.2 % versus 0 % ($p=0.19$) for either anastomotic revision or proximal diversion. The lack of statistical significance is most likely related to the small number of leaks. Despite this, it is clear that anastomotic testing is critical, and an anastomosis with a positive leak test can be safely managed with a low incidence of a clinical leak. An acceptable alternative to the above-described leak testing is an endoscopic assessment. Li et al. compared the outcomes of patients with left-sided colorectal anastomosis who underwent routine intraoperative endoscopy (107 patients) versus those who had selective intraoperative endoscopy (137 patients) [29]. The routine endoscopy group had a 0 % anastomotic leak rate, and 0.9 % of the patients had bleeding from the staple line that required intervention. Twenty-two percent of the patients in the selective group underwent endoscopic assessment with a 5 % incidence of an anastomotic complication. This was not statistically significant, but it does highlight the safety and utility to assess for and address anastomotic complications intraoperatively. A second study examining the utility of intraoperative endoscopy included 415 consecutive patients with 17 patients having an anastomotic abnormality identified [30]. Fifteen patients had an air leak from the staple line, and all were managed safely without an anastomotic leak. The data above clearly supports the routine use of anastomotic assessment for left-sided anastomosis, which can be performed with either an air leak test alone or in conjunction with endoscopic visualization. However, successful anastomotic healing is also dependent upon both ends of the bowel having adequate blood supply and the creation of a tension-free anastomosis using soft, pliable, normal bowel.

Straight Laparoscopic Medial-to-Lateral Approach

The patient is positioned and secured to the operating table in the same manner as described above for the laparoscopic right colectomy. Typically, both arms are tucked to the patient's sides, and the legs are in the lithotomy position. The abdomen is accessed via an open or closed technique in the supraumbilical position. There are various options for port placement, and the choice is dependent upon surgeon preference (Fig. 26.25). Typically, there are three working ports—two for the surgeon and one for the assistant. Once the abdomen has been thoroughly explored and the lesion located, the patient is placed in steep Trendelenburg and air-planed so the left side is up. This allows gravity to retract the small bowel to the right upper quadrant and expose the left colon mesentery. The omentum is reflected cephalad to the transverse colon to expose it and the splenic flexure. The IMV and the superior rectal artery are the vascular landmarks to be identified. At the level of the sacral promontory, the superior rectal artery is grasped and elevated with the surgeon's right hand. This will allow for the course of the artery to be seen and traced to its origin. With the energy source of choice in the left hand, the peritoneum is incised from below the sacral promontory to the IMA origin on the aorta. The wider the incision, the wider the window to the retroperitoneum will be, and this will maximize visualization of the retroperitoneum. Once the incision is made, the facial covering of the artery can be identified. Early in this dissection, the proper retroperitoneal plane is often difficult to see because it is heading up and away from the view as it follows the curve of the pelvic brim anteriorly. With a wide window to the retroperitoneum, the superior rectal artery can be elevated and pulled slightly toward the camera to visualize the proper plane. The retroperitoneum is swept posteriorly until the left ureter is identified. If the left ureter is difficult to identify, an alternative approach should be taken, and it will be described below. Once the left ureter is safely swept into the retroperitoneum, the superior rectal artery is dissected free to the origin of the IMA at the aorta. The peritoneum is then scored across the base of the IMA and medial to the IMV. The vein is then grasped and elevated off the retroperi-

toneum by scoring the peritoneum up to the ligament of Treitz. This will allow access into the retroperitoneum once again, and the plane is developed in a caudad direction to join with the original retroperitoneal dissection plane. The IMA is safely isolated, and the left ureter can be traced from the pelvic brim up to near the kidney. The IMA can be ligated with any energy source of choice. Next, the IMV can be isolated by separating the mesentery from the retroperitoneum to the inferior border of the pancreas. Once isolated, it can be safely ligated. Now there is a giant window into the retroperitoneum, and the left colon mesentery is mobilized out beyond the colon laterally. This dissection should extend from the sigmoid colon up to the splenic flexure, so all that remains are the lateral attachments. Beginning near the pelvic brim, the lateral peritoneum is incised by retracting the sigmoid colon medially and cephalad. This will allow for entry into the medial plane of dissection, and the lateral dissection continues toward the splenic flexure. As the splenic flexure is neared, there needs to be a transition from dividing the lateral peritoneal attachments to separating the omentum from the colon, and this is dependent upon the adhesions between the two structures. Mobilization of the splenic flexure usually requires a third working instrument. The omentum just above its attachment to the colon is retracted anteriorly, and the colon is retracted posteriorly, which puts the plane to be incised in a vertical position. This superficial peritoneal plane is incised toward the midline, and the lesser sac is eventually entered. Once the lesser sac is entered, the deeper attachments of the omentum and transverse colon can be divided. These deeper attachments are identified by pulling the colon down to the lower abdomen and watching for where the omentum moves or is attached. The omentum and colon are grabbed at this point, and by making the plane vertical, they are divided. The lesser sac is completely opened in this fashion so that all that remains are the peritoneal attachments to the inferior border of the pancreas. These attachments are divided by retracting the splenic flexure medially and caudad while elevating it off the retroperitoneum. This will allow for visualization along the retroperitoneal and lesser sac sides of this attachment. Division of this attachment to the midline will allow for adequate mobilization for extraction, resection, and tension-free anastomosis. The rectum can be divided either intracorporeally or in an open fashion through a suprapubic extraction site. If the rectum is divided intracorporeally, the colon can be extracted through either a left lower quadrant or suprapubic site. With either method of rectal division, the colon is extracted and resected, and the anvil is placed in the same method as described above for an end-to-end anastomosis. The proximal colon is then returned to the abdomen, and the extraction port can be closed temporarily or definitively. Under laparoscopic visualization, the stapler is passed transanally up to the top of the rectal stump, and the anvil is reassembled making sure there is no twist in the left colon and its mesentery. An air leak test or endoscopic assessment is performed under laparoscopic

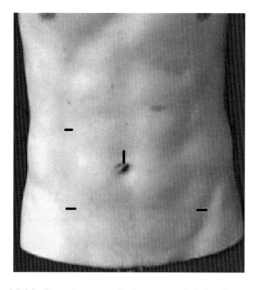

FIGURE 26-25. Port placement for laparoscopic left colectomy.

visualization. Typically, only 10–12 mm port sites need to have the fascial defect closed, and this can be accomplished open via the skin incision or laparoscopically using a trans-fascial suture passer.

Hand-Assisted Medial-to-Lateral Approach

Patient preparation and position are the same as for the straight laparoscopic approach. The hand port can be placed in the suprapubic, periumbilical, or left lower quadrant based on surgeon preference (Fig. 26.26). A suprapubic hand port has the advantage of having direct access to the pelvis to aid the pelvic dissection, divide the rectum, perform the anasto-mosis, and manage anastomotic complications. The port can be placed through a vertical midline or Pfannenstiel incision. For a suprapubic hand port, the camera port is placed in the supraumbilical position to avoid interfering with the hand port. A working port is placed on the right side, half the dis-tance between the hand and camera ports and lateral to the rectum muscle. A second working port is placed in the left lower quadrant to help with the lateral and splenic flexure mobilization. This port is placed lateral to the rectus muscle and as low as possible to minimize the time working against the camera. With the patient placed in steep Trendelenburg and left-side up, the small bowel is put in the right upper quadrant, and the omentum is reflected to the upper abdo-men. This exposes the left colon mesentery and splenic flex-ure as previously described. The surgeon stands on the patient's right side and places his/her right hand in the abdo-men. The superior rectal artery at the level of the sacral promontory is grasped and elevated (Fig. 26.27), and the peritoneum is incised as described above (Fig. 26.28). The hand acting as a retractor elevates the vessel to expose the

retroperitoneum. The identification of the left ureter and its reflection into the retroperitoneum is the same as described above (Fig. 26.29). Once the left ureter is identified and sep-arated from the mesentery, the index finger is used to elevate

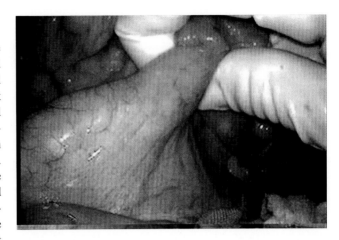

FIGURE 26-27. Isolation of the superior rectal artery at the level of the sacral promontory.

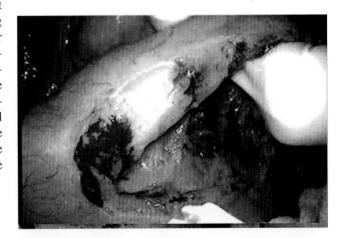

FIGURE 26-28. Accessing the retroperitoneum at the level of the sacral promontory.

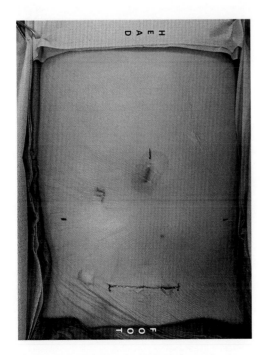

FIGURE 26-26. Port placement for HALS left colectomy.

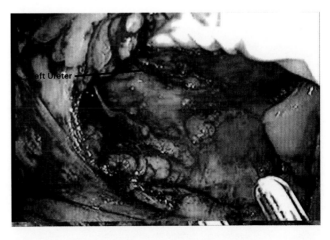

FIGURE 26–29. Identification of the left ureter from a medial-to-lateral approach.

the superior rectal artery under tension. The middle finger can then bluntly sweep down the retroperitoneum working toward the origin of the IMA (Fig. 26.30). Care should be used to sweep the retroperitoneal tissue and associated sympathetic nerves posteriorly to avoid their injury during the ligation of the vessel. This dissection is carried cephalad to the vessel to expose and elevate the window medial to the IMV. The peritoneum is incised across the IMA origin, and the retroperitoneum can be entered medial to the IMV. The hand now elevates the IMV, and the peritoneum is incised up to the ligament of Treitz (Fig. 26.31). The retroperitoneum is swept down, and the thumb elevates the IMV and mesentery to keep it on tension. Once the retroperitoneal plane is adequately developed, the index finger elevates the IMV, and the middle finger sweeps the retroperitoneum down as the IVM is elevated to isolate it at the inferior border of the pancreas (Fig. 26.32). Now that both vascular structures are safely isolated and the left ureter is safely in the retroperitoneum, both vessels can be ligated (Fig. 26.33). For ligating both the artery and vein, the index and middle fingers are placed in the retroperitoneum behind the vessel to create space, the fourth and fifth fingers lay in front of the vessel to protect the small bowel, and the thumb can help elevate any mesentery

or fat obscuring the view (Fig. 26.34). With both pedicles ligated, the hand is placed palm down under the mesentery. It elevates the mesentery under tension, so the retroperitoneal dissection can be carried out laterally beyond the colon (Fig. 26.35). The extent of the dissection should be from the

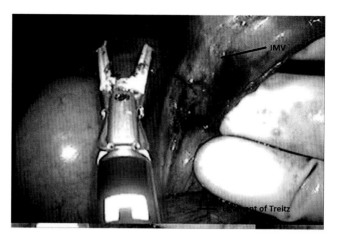

FIGURE 26-32. Isolating the IMV near the ligament of Treitz and the inferior border of the pancreas.

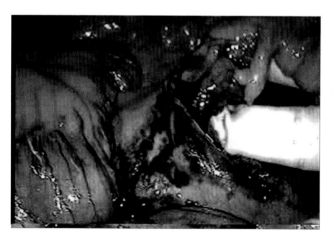

FIGURE 26-30. Isolating the IMA at its origin.

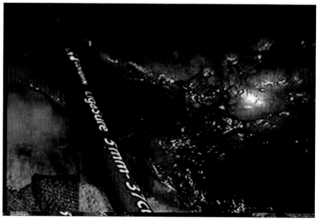

FIGURE 26-33. Safe isolation of the IMA.

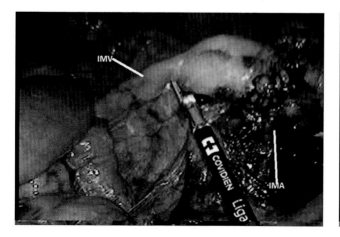

FIGURE 26-31. Accessing the retroperitoneum medial to the IMV.

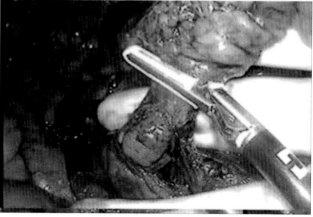

FIGURE 26-34. Hand position for ligating the IMA and IMV.

sigmoid colon caudad up to the splenic flexure cephalad and along the inferior border of the pancreas medially. The lateral dissection begins by mobilizing the sigmoid colon. Often, the hand gets in the way for this dissection, so solutions include depressing the sigmoid colon with the fingers and passing the energy device between the fingers to get the proper angle or removing the hand and placing an instrument through the hand port to begin the dissection straight laparoscopically. Once the retroperitoneal dissection plane is entered (Fig. 26.36), the hand can be passed into the retroperitoneum, and the lateral attachments can be exposed on the hand just like an open case (Fig. 26.37). The assistant stands between the legs and uses the left lower quadrant port to divide the tissue. The dissection continues toward the splenic flexure until the need to transition to the omentum. At the omental attachments, the omentum is elevated and pulled to the video right with the grasper, and the colon is retracted down with the hand (Fig. 26.38). Pulling with the grasper to the right helps to keep it out of the way of the energy device during this dissection. The peritoneum is incised along the transverse colon, and the lesser sac is eventually entered.

With the hand and instrument, the colon is pulled to the lower abdomen, and the next level of omental attachments is identified. At this point, the omentum is elevated, and the colon is depressed allowing for the attachments to be divided. This is continued until the lesser sac is wide open from the splenic flexure to the midline (Fig. 26.39). The only remain-

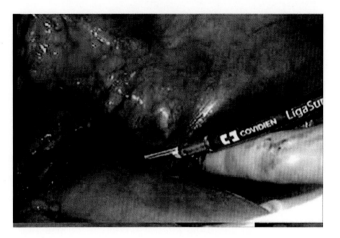

FIGURE 26-37. Lateral mobilization of the left colon.

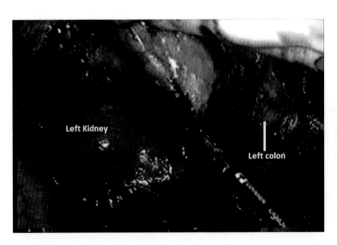

FIGURE 26-35. Medial-to-lateral mobilization of the left colon mesentery off the retroperitoneum.

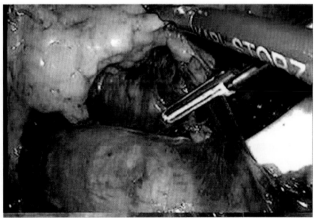

FIGURE 26-38. Entering the lesser sac by separating the omentum from the transverse colon.

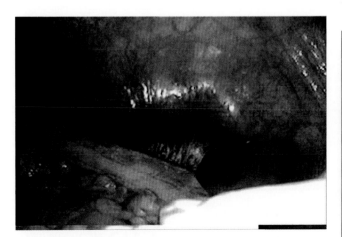

FIGURE 26-36. Incision of the lateral attachments and entry into the retroperitoneal plane.

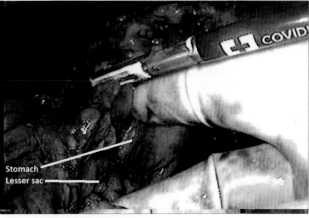

FIGURE 26-39. Completing the opening of the lesser sac.

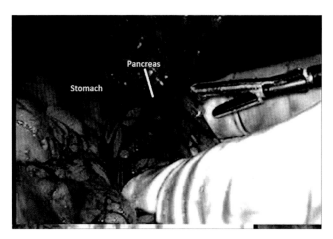

FIGURE 26-40. Division of the peritoneal attachments between the transverse colon mesentery and the inferior border of the pancreas.

ing attachments are along the inferior border of the pancreas. With the colon pulled to the lower abdomen, the lateral cut edge of the mobilization is seen. The hand is passed into the retroperitoneum along the inferior border of the pancreas. Much like the open approach, the fold of the mesentery can be palpated and separated from the pancreas allowing for safe division to the midline (Fig. 26.40). The colon is completely mobilized at this point and can be extracted for resection and anastomosis. Typically, the proximal colon is divided, the stapling anvil is placed, and the rectum is divided. This procedure has been previously described. However, this can be difficult in patients with a fat or bulky mesentery. This can be managed by dividing the rectum and the mesorectum first allowing for easier extraction of the proximal colon. The anastomosis and anastomotic assessment can be performed under direct vision via the hand port or laparoscopically.

Laparoscopic Identification of the Left Ureter

The IMA or IMV should not be ligated until the left ureter is clearly identified and safely dissected free of the left colon mesentery. There is a simple three-step algorithm that can help facilitate safe identification of the left ureter. The first approach is at the level of the superior rectal artery as the retroperitoneum is accessed at the level of the sacral promontory as described above. If the ureter is not easily identified, the approach should change to the IMV. The IMV is grasped and elevated, and the medial aspect of the peritoneum is incised. The retroperitoneum is accessed and the plane developed. This part of the retroperitoneum is flat, so identification of the proper plane is much easier. Once in the proper plane, the dissection can be directed in a caudad direction to see if the original plane started at the level of the sacral promontory can be entered to identify the ureter. If the left ureter can still not be identified, the colon can be mobilized in a lateral-to-medial direction. If unable to identify the

ureter at this point, consider conversion to an open procedure, or, if using a hand port, remove the top of the port and identify it in an open fashion through the hand port. A ureteral stent should be employed at the discretion of the surgeon.

Subtotal Colectomy

Tumors of the transverse colon often increase the complexity of the required resection because of the need to divide most or all of the branches of the middle colic vessels. An extended right colectomy can adequately treat a tumor from the hepatic flexure to the mid-transverse colon. With complete mobilization of the small bowel mesentery and widely opening the lesser sac toward the splenic flexure, there should be adequate mobilization to create an ileocolic anastomosis with proper bowel orientation and without tension from either an open or laparoscopic approach. However, distal transverse colon tumors tend be more difficult to manage. Some surgeons advocate a transverse colectomy, but challenges associated with this type of resection include obtaining an adequate mesenteric resection and mobilization of the right and left colon to create a safe, tension-free anastomosis. For patients with a redundant and mobile transverse colon, it may be feasible to perform an extended left colectomy. If the transverse colon cannot be mobilized enough to reach the top of the rectum, it may be more appropriate to perform a subtotal colectomy. This entails resection of the right and transverse colon and creation of an ileo-descending colon anastomosis.

Open Approach

The right colon mobilization begins as described above, and as the hepatic flexure is mobilized, the lesser sac is entered by separating the omentum from the transverse colon mesentery. The plane to the right of the midline tends to be fused, but it is an avascular plane so it can be developed bluntly. With careful dissection under tension, the plane can be developed, and the proper lesser sac is entered. The lesser omentum is divided toward the splenic flexure as far as possible. With the right colon and hepatic flexure mobilized and the lesser sac completely open, the mesentery can be ligated. This begins with isolation and ligation of the ileocolic pedicle and division of the terminal ileum and its mesentery as described in the open right colectomy section. The middle colic vessels are isolated by pulling the transverse colon caudad and having the surgeon, who is standing on the patient's left side, pass his/her left hand through the ileocolic mesenteric defect from the retroperitoneal to peritoneal side. The index finger is elevated against the junction of the SMA and the origins of the middle colic vessels, which allows for a safe high ligation of these vessels. Now the left colon needs to be mobilized, and the surgeon switches to the patient's right side packing the small bowel into the right upper quadrant. The sigmoid colon, left colon, and splenic flexure are mobilized as described in the open left colectomy section. The IMV is isolated by grasping and elevating it, so the peritoneum medial to it can be incised. This allows access into the retroperitoneal dissection plane, and the IMV can be isolated and ligated at the inferior border of the pancreas. The IMA is not isolated or ligated to preserve the blood supply to the distal colon. The distal bowel and mesentery are divided to provide an adequate distal margin. For the creation of a side-to-side ileocolic anastomosis, the orientation of the small bowel is very important. If the stapled end of the terminal ileum is brought over the top of the small bowel to perform a side-to-side anastomosis on the left side, this will create the potential for the small bowel to volvulize through the mesenteric defect. To avoid this complication, the small bowel needs to be rotated 180° counterclockwise, so the cut edge of the mesentery is brought underneath the remaining small bowel. This allows for the cut edge of the small bowel mesentery to pass under the small bowel and face the patient's left side in a straight line. Also, the entire small bowel from the ligament of Treitz to the anastomosis is on top of the mesenteric defect, so there is no risk of a small bowel volvulus. This will allow for a side-to-side stapled anastomosis to be performed.

Laparoscopic Approach

This extended resection can occur either straight laparoscopically or hand assisted. For the straight laparoscopic approach, the right colon is mobilized in the same fashion as described for right colectomy. Once the lesser sac is entered, the lesser omentum is divided as far as possible toward the splenic flexure. This exposes the lesser sac as much as possible and facilitates ligation of the middle colic vessels by clearing any posterior mesenteric attachments. With the ileocolic vessel ligated, the middle colic vessels are exposed. This is accomplished with the first assistant via one or two right-sided ports elevating the transverse colon in an ole-type fashion. The peritoneum from near the ligament of Treitz is scored across the base of the vessels to the cut edge of the mesentery on the right. This allows the individual branches of the middle colic vessels to be isolated and safely ligated. With the right colon and transverse colon mobilized and the mesentery ligated, attention is turned to the left colon. The patient is positioned as described for a laparoscopic left colon. The IMV is identified and elevated so the peritoneum can be incised allowing access to the retroperitoneum. The IMV is mobilized, isolated, and ligated at the inferior border of the pancreas. The mesenteric side of the IMV and the cut edge of the transverse colon mesentery are elevated, and the intervening mesentery is divided. Ideally, there should not be any remaining vessels in this remaining bit of mesentery. With the mesentery of the colon to be resected completely divided, the left colon mesentery is

mobilized out laterally beyond the colon. To ensure adequate mobilization for extraction and the anastomosis, the sigmoid colon should be mobilized. The lateral attachments starting at the sigmoid colon are incised and divided toward the splenic flexure. The splenic flexure is mobilized as described in the left colectomy section. Once the colon is completely mobilized and before it can be extracted, the IMV needs to be divided again along the line of the distal resection margin. If it is not divided before extraction, the specimen will be tethered by this vessel preventing adequate exposure. Some surgeons will divide the entire specimen intracorporeally. Prior to performing the anastomosis, the small bowel and its mesentery must be oriented as described above. The specimen can then be extracted via a midline incision.

For a hand-assisted approach, the port placement is the same as described for the left colectomy. The dissection begins with mobilization of the right colon. The posterior approach will be described here. The small bowel is placed in the right upper quadrant exposing the posterior attachments of the small bowel mesentery to the retroperitoneum. The mesentery is grasped and elevated with the middle finger and thumb of the left hand. The index finger pointing toward the head swings over the pedicle to further expose the duodenum (Fig. 26.41). The peritoneum is incised from the duodenum to the cecum. With the hand palm down, the fingers elevate this peritoneal incision, and the retroperitoneum is entered. The hand continues to elevate the right colon mesentery, and the duodenum is exposed and reflected posteriorly (Fig. 26.42). This dissection is continued superiorly and laterally beyond the transverse colon, hepatic flexure, and ascending colon. The patient is then tilted right-side up to move the small bowel to the left side of the abdomen and expose the lateral planes. The lateral dissection begins at the level of the cecum by placing the hand in the retroperitoneal plane and lateral to the cecum and right colon to expose the lateral attachments (Fig. 26.43). They are divided heading toward the hepatic flexure, which is mobilized by entering

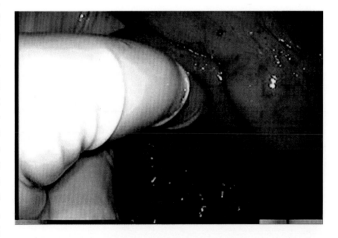

FIGURE 26-41. HALS exposure of the posterior aspect of the small bowel mesentery for the right colon dissection.

the lesser sac. The lesser sac is entered by separating the lesser omentum from the transverse colon mesentery (Fig. 26.44). Once the plane is developed, the cut edge of the lesser omentum is grasped with a grasper and elevated, so the hand can control the colon and develop the plane into the lesser sac. The lesser omentum is divided out toward the splenic flexure as far as possible. Now the right colon and transverse colon mesentery can be ligated. The ileocolic pedicle is isolated by pulling to the right lower quadrant. The peritoneum on the caudad aspect is incised, and the mesentery is dissected to expose the retroperitoneum. The index and middle fingers are passed through the mesenteric defect to expose the vessels and the bare area on their cephalad aspect (Fig. 26.45). The bare area is incised along the lines of resection to isolate and ligate the ileocolic pedicles. To isolate the middle colic vessels, the left hand is passed through the mesenteric defect into the retroperitoneum and lesser sac. The transverse colon mesentery is exposed by elevating the hand, and the first assistant via right lower quadrant port elevated the distal transverse colon (Fig. 26.46). The peritoneum is incised from the ligament of Treitz to the

cut edge of the right colon mesentery. The hand is able to palpate each middle colic vessel to facilitate its isolation and ligation. With the right and transverse colon mesentery

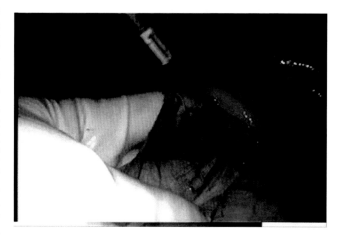

FIGURE 26-44. Mobilization of the hepatic flexure by entering the lesser sac.

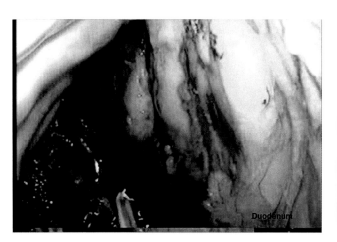

FIGURE 26-42. Accessing the retroperitoneal plane: elevating the right colon mesentery and dissecting the duodenum posteriorly.

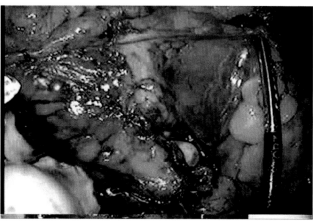

FIGURE 26-45. Isolation of the ileocolic pedicle by passing the hand through the mesenteric defect on the ileal side of the pedicle.

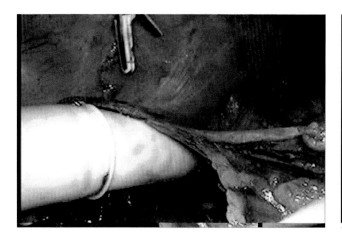

FIGURE 26-43. Division of the lateral attachments of the right colon.

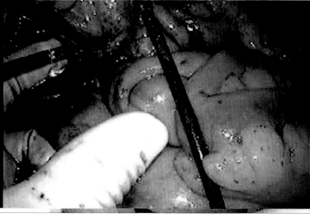

FIGURE 26-46. Exposure of the middle colic vessels.

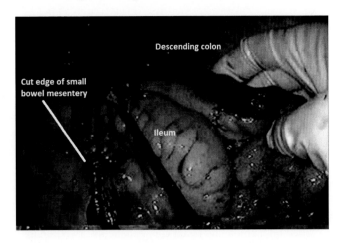

FIGURE 26-47. Orientation of the small bowel mesentery for an ileo-descending colon anastomosis.

divided, attention is turned to the left colon, and the left colon is mobilized as described in the paragraph above but using the hand-assisted technique for the left colon. The IMA is preserved to maintain blood supply to the sigmoid and descending colon. The IMV is then again divided at the distal resection margin, and the colon is then extracted through the hand port for resection. Just as described for the open approach, the small bowel and its mesentery are rotated 180° counterclockwise to allow the cut edge of the mesentery to face the patient's left side (Fig. 26.47). After the small bowel is properly oriented, a side-to-side anastomosis can be performed via the hand port.

Total Abdominal Colectomy with Ileorectal Anastomosis

Total abdominal colectomy may be indicated for patients with synchronous tumors or hereditary cancer syndromes such as hereditary nonpolyposis colorectal cancer or familial adenomatous polyposis. The entire abdominal colon is resected, and an ileorectal anastomosis can be performed in either an end-to-end, end-to-side, or isoperistaltic side-to-side fashion. Postoperative cancer surveillance can often be performed in the office, without sedation using either a rigid or flexible endoscopy.

Open Approach

The procedure begins with accessing the abdomen via a midline incision and performing a thorough exploration. The right colon and transverse colon are mobilized, and the associated mesentery is divided as described above in the open right colectomy and subtotal colectomy sections. The terminal ileal mesentery is divided up to the level of the bowel. For an end-to-end anastomosis, the bowel is divided sharply, the purse string is placed, and a 28 or 29 mm stapler anvil is placed inside the lumen. The purse string is cinched down

making sure that all of the edges of the enterotomy are everted. It is rare that 28 or 29 mm anvil will not fit into the small bowel, so the need to use a smaller circular stapler is rare. The small bowel is then packed to the right upper quadrant and the left colon, and the splenic flexure is mobilized as described in the open left colectomy section. After the IMA is ligated at its origin and the IMV divided near the inferior border of the pancreas, the entire mesentery of the colon has been divided. The top of the rectum is identified, and the upper rectum is mobilized. At the site of distal transection, the peritoneum of the mesorectum is scored, and a window is created between the posterior rectal wall and the mesorectum. The rectum is then stapled and divided. The remaining mesorectum is then ligated. With the specimen removed, the anastomosis is completed by passing the stapling cartridge that is passed transanally to the top of the rectal stump. The spike is deployed, and the anvil is reassembled making sure the small bowel mesentery is not twisted. The small bowel should be oriented, so it is on the left side of the abdomen and the cut edge of the mesentery is facing to the patient's right side. The anastomosis must be tested with either an air leak test or endoscopically.

Laparoscopic Approach

The procedure can be performed by a straight laparoscopic approach or a hand-assisted approach based on the surgeon's preference. Port placement is typically symmetrical around the camera port. In other words, the surgeon's working ports are placed in same place for a right and left colectomy, so they are mirror images of each other. For a hand-assisted approach, the hand port is typically placed in the suprapubic position. Once again, the procedure begins with mobilization of the right and transverse colon with ligation of its mesentery as described in the laparoscopic right colectomy and subtotal colectomy sections. The left colon and its mesentery are resected as described in the laparoscopic left colectomy section. For the straight laparoscopic approach, the rectum and mesorectum are divided intracorporeally, and the specimen is extracted. The extraction site for a straight laparoscopic approach can be in the midline around the umbilicus or suprapubic or a muscle-splitting incision in the right or left lower quadrant. The terminal ileal mesentery is divided, and the terminal ileum is prepared for anastomosis. For the hand-assisted approach, the colon is extracted via the hand port. During the extraction, the small bowel must be passed underneath the colon, so when exteriorized, the small bowel mesentery will be properly oriented. The terminal ileum is resected and prepared for anastomosis, and the rectum and mesorectum are divided through the hand port. For the straight laparoscopic approach, the terminal ileum is returned to the abdomen, the extraction site is closed, and the anastomosis is created and tested laparoscopically. For the hand-assisted approach, this can be performed open through the hand port.

Special Circumstances

Laparoscopy

In 2004, the laparoscopic approach began its adoption into the surgeon's armamentarium for treating colon cancer with the publishing of the results of the US multicenter prospective randomized COST trial. The results of UK's CLASICC and European COLOR trials soon followed. Collectively, these studies demonstrated that the laparoscopic approach is not inferior to the open approach for the surgical management of colon cancer. Each study had unique findings that are worth discussing.

The COST Trial

The COST trial was designed as a non-inferiority study, which means it was designed to test the hypothesis that the laparoscopic approach was as effective as and not worse than the open approach for the treatment of colon cancer [31]. It included right and left colon cancers but excluded transverse colon cancers. Forty-eight centers and 66 credentialed surgeons participated and enrolled and randomized 435 patients to the laparoscopic group and 428 patients to the open group. The initial results were published with 4.4 years of follow-up and demonstrated that short-term outcomes favored the laparoscopic group with a shorter length of stay [5.6 days vs. 6.4 days ($p<0.001$)] and fewer days of intravenous and oral analgesics [3.2 days vs. 4.0 days ($p<0.001$) and 1.9 days vs. 2.2 days ($p=0.03$), respectively] [31, 32]. However, this did not translate into any significant difference in pain or quality of life scores, except that laparoscopy had a better global quality of life at 2 weeks after surgery only. There was a 21 % conversion rate and no difference in intraoperative complications, 30-day morbidity, or hospital readmission rates. Finally, there was no difference in the 3-year recurrence or overall survival rates [16 % vs. 18 % ($p=0.32$) and 86 % vs. 85 % ($p=0.51$) in the laparoscopic versus open groups, respectively], and these outcomes were similar stage for stage [32]. The initial results of this trial demonstrated that the laparoscopic approach was not inferior to the open surgical approach for the resection of colon cancer. The 5-year results confirmed the initial results as there was no difference in the primary endpoint of time to recurrence and secondary endpoints of disease-free (laparoscopic 69.2 % vs. open 68.4 %, $p=0.94$) and overall survival (laparoscopic 76.4 % vs. open 74.6 %, $p=0.93$) [33]. The site of first recurrence was also equivalent for each group [liver (5.8 % vs. 5.5 %)>lung (4.6 % vs. 4.6 %)>wound (0.5 % vs. 0.9 %), respectively]. Patients that underwent conversion had a worse 5-year overall survival compared to those completed laparoscopically and open. However, there was no difference in 5-year disease-free survival or recurrence associated with conversion. Long-term follow-up of quality of life data demonstrated that the laparoscopic group had a small but significant improvement in total quality of life index at 18 months after surgery, and those patients with poor preoperative quality of life were at higher risk of a "difficult" postoperative course [34].

The MRC CLASICC Trial

The CLASICC trial took place in the UK and included 27 medical centers. The surgeons were credentialed similarly to the COST trial. The study design was to assess short-term endpoints such as pathologic findings, hospital course, and quality of life and long-term endpoints of survival and recurrence at 3 and 5 years [35]. Patients were randomized 2:1 to the laparoscopic and open arms. Additionally, the study included both colon and rectal cancer patients. Two hundred seventy-three patients were randomized to the laparoscopic group and 140 patients to the open arm for colon cancer. Short-term outcomes showed no statistical difference in length of stay, return of bowel function, rate of curative resection, complications, and quality of life measures. There was a 29 % conversion rate, which steadily decreased over the course of enrollment into the study. Patients who underwent conversion were more likely to have a complication and less likely to have a curative resection, which highlights the importance of patient selection. Analysis of the cost of care and resource utilization for colectomy revealed that there was no difference in overall cost as well as cost of the operating room, equipment, recovery room, intensive care, and hospitalization [36]. An interesting sidenote was that the cost of laparoscopic surgery for rectal cancer was found to be higher than for open surgery. In 2007, the 3-year survival and recurrence data was published [37]. The 3-year overall survival ($p=0.51$) and 3-year disease-free survival ($p=0.75$) rates were similar for the laparoscopic and open arms of the colon cancer group. Additionally, these outcomes were equivalent for all stages. The results held up for the 5-year outcomes as well [38, 39]. They reported a median overall survival of 105.7 months in the open arm versus 81.9 months in the laparoscopic arm (log rank$=0.87$, $p=0.352$). There was no difference between overall survival and disease-free survival. However, conversion from laparoscopy to open for patients with colon cancer was associated with a worse overall survival (HR, 2.28; 95 % CI, 1.47–3.53; $p<0.001$) and disease-free survival (HR, 2.20; 95 % CI, 1.31–3.67; $p<0.007$). Therefore, based on the long-term data of the CLASICC trial, the utilization of the laparoscopic approach for colon cancer is equivalent to the open approach, but patient selection is critical to ensure an optimal outcome.

The COLOR Trial

The COLOR trial was a European-based prospective, randomized trial of laparoscopic versus open resection of colon cancer designed as non-inferiority study to identify a 7 % difference in outcome between each arm [40]. A total of 29 hospitals throughout Europe participated. The trial's primary endpoint was a 3-year cancer-free survival. There were 534 patients in the laparoscopic arm and 542 patients in the open arm in the final analysis. The laparoscopic approach was found to have the short-term benefits of faster return of bowel function and shorter length of stay and was associated with a conversion rate of 19 % [41]. There was no difference in lymph node harvest or overall morbidity. Analysis of short-term outcomes with regard to hospital volume (high, medium, and low volume) demonstrated that operative times, conversions, and complications were lowest in the high-volume centers and were highest in the low-volume centers [42]. There was no difference in the 3-year disease-free survival at 74.2 % in the laparoscopic group and 76.2 % in the open group ($p=0.70$), which equated to a 2 % difference between the two treatment arms [43]. The final analysis was unable to rule out a difference in 3-year disease-free survival that favored the open approach because the upper limit of the 95 % confidence interval exceeds the predetermined non-inferiority boundary of 7 %. However, the authors felt the difference was small and clinically acceptable to justify that the laparoscopic approach for colon cancer is safe.

Other Trials

The Japan Clinical Oncology Group Study JCOG 0404 was a prospective randomized trial of laparoscopic versus open resection of T3 or T4 (without involvement of other organs) colon cancers [44]. It was a non-inferiority study design with 524 patients in the laparoscopic arm and 533 patients in the open arm. Short-term outcomes demonstrated shorter length of stay, faster return of bowel function, less narcotic use, and fewer complications in the laparoscopic arm. The 3-year oncologic results are pending at this point in time.

A prospective, randomized trial of laparoscopic versus open resection of colon cancer in Australia and New Zealand included a total of 587 patients [45]. The primary endpoints were 5-year overall survival, recurrence-free survival, and freedom from recurrence, and the long-term results demonstrated no difference in these outcomes between the two treatment groups.

These five prospective, randomized clinical trials all demonstrated short-term benefits for the laparoscopic approach with no associated differences in long-term overall survival, disease-free survival, and recurrence rates. Therefore, it is safe and effective to employ the laparoscopic approach for the surgical management of colon cancer.

Obstructing Colon Cancers

The management of obstructing colon cancers presents unique challenges in that the treatment of the acute or sub-acute obstructive process is dictating the oncologic management of the cancer. As a result, the overall outcome in terms of survival and recurrence is worse for patients whose initial presentation is with obstruction or obstructive symptoms. This is because by the time a tumor grows to the point of luminal obstruction, it is frequently a T3 or T4 lesion, and these tumors have a higher incidence of lymph node, peritoneal, or distant metastasis. Cortet et al. presented recurrence and survival data on 3375 colon cancers of which 8.5 % ($N=287$) presented with obstruction [46]. The 5-year risk of local recurrence [HR, 1.53; 95 % CI, 1.01–2.34 ($p=0.047$)] and distant recurrence [HR, 1.25; 95 % CI, 0.99–1.59 ($p=0.057$)] were higher for obstructing versus nonobstructing colon cancers.

The management options for obstructing colon cancers are many, and there are no well-established guidelines. For example, proximal diversion alleviates the obstruction but does not address the cancer, and resection of the primary tumor addresses both issues but carries significant morbidity and a high stoma rate. The introduction of self-expanding stents as a means for a bridge to therapy (surgery vs. chemotherapy) or as palliation in the setting of unresectable tumors is an additional option. The morbidity associated with urgent resection with ostomy creation or primary anastomosis can be as high as 60 % with wound complications, deep organ-space infections, respiratory complications, and intensive care unit admissions being some of the most common [47]. Therefore, the concept of endoscopically alleviating the obstruction, which would allow for complete colonic evaluation and elective, one-step resection, has significant appeal.

Initial single-institution reports demonstrated significant benefit of endoscopic stenting as a bridge to surgery compared to emergent surgery. These studies have reported a high incidence of technical and clinical success of greater than 90 % of cases and are associated with a stoma-free rate of 60–90 % [47–51]. The major complications associated with endoscopic stents are perforation, migration, and bleeding, which have been reported as being relatively low. It must be kept in mind that retrospective, single-institution studies suffer from many potential sources of bias such as patient selection, small numbers, and missing data. A multicenter, prospective, randomized trial of colonic stenting versus emergent surgery for acute left-sided malignant colon obstruction was undertaken in the Netherlands [49]. The study was scheduled to enroll 60 patients in each arm with the primary outcome being the mean global quality of life, and secondary outcomes were morbidity and mortality. The study was stopped after the enrollment of 47 patients in the stenting arm and 51 in the surgery arm due to six procedure-related perforations in the stent arm. The technical success rate of 70 % was felt to be too low compared to the previous published literature, and the study was stopped. Interestingly, there was no statistical difference between the two arms with regard to global quality of life, morbidity/mortality profiles, and stoma rates. There have been two subsequent meta-analysis that have examined the safety and efficacy of endoscopic stenting as a bridge to surgery. The review by Cirocchi et al. analyzed three clinical trials with a total of 97 patients in the stent arm and 100 patients in the surgery arm [52]. The clinical success rate (which was defined differently in each study) was significantly higher in the surgery group (99 % vs. 52 %, $p < 0.00001$), respectively. The stent group had a higher primary anastomosis rate (64.9 % vs. 55 %, $p = 0.003$), and the overall stoma rate (45.3 % vs. 62 %, $p = 0.02$) was lower. However, there was no difference in the overall or 30-day postoperative complication rates. A more recent meta-analysis, which included seven studies, confirmed the findings that endoscopic stenting is associated with increased rate of primary anastomosis, decreased stoma rate, and a trend toward improved complication rates [48]. Endoscopic stenting clearly has a role in the management of obstructing colon cancers, but proper patient selection is of paramount importance to its success [53]. Completely obstructing cancers, particularly when confirmed by contrast enema, have a low rate of technical success and increased likelihood of a stent-related complication. Stenting should also be avoided in patients with peritonitis, hemodynamic instability, or concern for impending perforation. Patients with obstructive symptoms but who are not completely obstructed have a normal white blood cell count and no peritonitis, and normal or correctable laboratory values are candidates for endoscopic stenting as a bridge to surgical resection 72 or more days later. Concern has been raised that endoscopic stenting can have a negative impact on the oncologic outcomes of these patients. There is limited data examining this issue, and what is available are small single-institution retrospective reviews. However, these studies have not demonstrated a deleterious effect of stenting on cancer-related outcomes [54].

Surgical intervention remains the mainstay of managing obstructed colon cancers as it provides alleviation of the obstruction and resection of the tumor in one setting. The extent of the operative procedure is highly dependent upon the condition of the patient and the extent of the obstruction. Proximal diversion alone should be performed only in selected situations such as complete obstruction with dilated small bowel that makes resection too difficult or in a setting where neoadjuvant therapy would be beneficial. The extent of resection and restoration of intestinal continuity remain to be debated and are dependent upon the physiology of the patient and the intraoperative findings. If there is evidence of impending perforation or ischemia of the proximal colon, resection of the entire colon proximal to the obstruction is recommended, and performing a primary anastomosis should be avoided. However, if the proximal colon is dilated, a healthy segmental versus extended colectomy can be performed based on the clinical situation. A recent literature review found no difference in morbidity or mortality between segmental resection and total abdominal colectomy for obstructing colon cancers. However, patients who underwent total abdominal colectomy have a significantly higher rate of bowel dysfunction. The creation of an end stoma is the technically easier procedure and eliminates the risk of anastomotic leak, but 40–60 % of the stomas created will remain permanent [55, 56]. The decision to perform a primary anastomosis is dependent upon the condition of the patient and quality of the proximal bowel. There is limited data comparing a Hartmann's resection with end colostomy or resection and primary anastomosis, but a recent review of the literature reported the anastomotic leak rate for primary anastomosis to range from 2 to 12 % [55, 56]. This appears to be comparable to the literature for elective left-sided resection and anastomosis, which ranges from 2 to 8 %. There does appear to be benefit of decreased anastomotic leaks and infectious complications when either manual disimpaction or on-table lavage of the proximal colon is performed prior to a primary anastomosis.

Perforated Colon Cancers

Perforated colon cancers present the challenge of adequately addressing the sepsis associated with a perforated colon while attempting to maintain the oncologic principles of resection for the malignant disease. The acute septic injury has the greatest impact on short-term outcomes, which in turn impacts the long-term outcome of the cancer. These patients typically present with a contained perforation much like diverticulitis or with a free perforation requiring an emergent operation. Either scenario results in a poorer outcome compared to non-perforated cancers. Cheynel et al. presented a comparison of the short- and long-term outcomes for 89 perforated colon cancers and 5462 uncomplicated colon cancers [57]. They reported that perforated cancers had higher operative mortality [20.2 % vs. 6.6 % ($p = <0.001$)] and 5-year local recurrence and peritoneal carcinomatosis rates [15.7 % vs. 7.8 % ($p = 0.021$) and 13.8 % vs. 7.8 % ($p = 0.036$), respectively] than uncomplicated colon cancers. Zielinski et al. compared 41 patients with free perforation and 45 patients with contained perforation to 85 non-perforated patients that were matched for age, stage, and resection status [58]. They found that patients with free perforation were more likely to get a stoma [79 % vs. 39 % vs. 29 % ($p = 0.008$)] and had a higher rate of metastatic disease at the time of presentation. Interestingly, in the small study size, they found no difference in the rates of R0, R1, and R2 resections between the three groups. Sixty-seven percent of patients with free perforations were able to have all gross disease resected (R0 62 % and R1 5 %). The 5-year overall survival was significantly poorer in the free perforation versus the contained perforation group (24 % vs. 62 % ($p = 0.003$)). Additionally, patients with a free perforation had a significantly higher operative morality, and their 5-year disease-free survival was significantly poorer. Interestingly, on the multivariate analysis, perforation (free or contained) was not a risk factor for adjusted survival, but residual gross disease after resection was a risk factor (HR, 1.94; 95 % CI, 1.09–3.46; $p = 0.02$). Therefore, patients that present with perforated tumors should undergo an oncologically based resection if their physiologic state will allow as this will provide them with the best cancer-related outcome.

Management of Primary Colon Cancer in the Setting of Distant Metastasis

Advances in chemotherapy have greatly impacted our management strategies of patients who present with metastatic colon cancer. Current recommendations are for patients with symptomatic (bleeding or obstructing) primary tumors to undergo resection of their primary tumor before initiating systemic therapy for their metastatic disease. However, if the tumor is asymptomatic and the patient has a good performance status, the first-line treatment should be systemic chemotherapy, the rationale being that most patients will succumb to their metastatic disease before the primary tumor causes complications. This concept has gained traction with the significant improvement in tumor response to FOLFOX-based chemotherapies and a low rate of complications associated with leaving the primary tumor in situ. In 2007, Muratore et al. reported that patients with stage IV colon cancer with asymptomatic primary tumors who received FOLFOX chemotherapy had a 43 % rate of downstaging of metastatic disease to resectability, and none of the 35 patients developed symptoms related to their primary tumor while receiving chemotherapy [59]. A subsequent review of the literature examined seven studies comparing chemotherapy as initial therapy ($N=314$ patients) versus resection of the primary followed by chemotherapy ($N=536$ patients) [60]. For the patients who received chemotherapy first, the rate of symptoms associated with the primary tumor was obstruction 13 %, bleeding 3 %, and perforation/fistula 6 %. Ultimately, greater than 40 % of patients went on to have their liver lesions resected with curative intent. For the patients that had resection of their primary tumor as first-line therapy, the pooled major complication rate was 12 %, and the pooled minor complication rate was 21 %. The survival rate for the chemotherapy-first group ranged from 8.2 to 22 months, and the surgery first group was 14–23 months. Multivariate analysis identified the extent of hepatic disease and presence of peritoneal disease, performance statuses were independent predictors of the outcome, and resection status of the primary tumor did not impact survival. The benefit of FOLFOX-based chemotherapy has on the ability to downstage a patient to the point of resectability was reported in a recent literature review by Lam et al. [61]. They examined ten studies with 1886 patients who received neoadjuvant chemotherapy for liver metastasis. Sixty-four percent of patients had regression of their tumor with 22 % of these patients undergoing resection of the liver metastasis with curative intent. This translated to a 45-month overall median survival with 15 % of the patients remaining disease-free at that time point. Therefore, the literature supports a chemotherapy-first approach to stage IV colon cancer with an asymptomatic primary as a chemotherapy that has the ability to downstage metastatic disease, minimize the progression of symptoms associated with the primary tumor, and improve overall survival.

Outcomes for Colon Cancer

Short Term

Short-term outcomes for colectomy for cancer include morbidity, mortality, length of hospital stay, and intraoperative parameters such as conversion from laparoscopy. The most recent clinical trials that have examined operative techniques and the perioperative outcomes are the major multicenter, prospective, randomized trials comparing laparoscopic versus open colectomy for cancer, and they provide some of the best data for short-term outcomes. The COST trial reported an overall complication rate of 21 % for laparoscopy and 20 % for the open approach ($p=0.64$), with only 4 and 2 % ($p=0.11$) occurring intraoperatively, respectively [32]. The 30-day morbidity was similar between the groups, but the rate of specific complications was not reported. Overall mortality was 2 and 4 % ($p=0.40$). The conversion rate was 21 % and was associated with an increased length of stay and 30-day complication rate. The CLASICC trial reported an overall complication rate of 26 % in the laparoscopic group, 27 % in the open group, and 45 % in the converted group [35]. The mortality rate of laparoscopy was 2 and 4 % for open patients. They did include specific complications for the laparoscopic, open, and converted groups, which included wound complications of 5 %, 5 %, and 8 %; pneumonia rate of 7 %, 4 %, and 10 %; anastomotic leak rate of 3 %, 3 %, and 3 %; and deep venous thrombosis rate of 2 %, 0 %, and 0 %, respectively. The COLOR trial reported a similar morbidity and mortality profile [41]. The overall complication rate was 21 % for laparoscopy and 20 % for the open approach, with a 4 % and 3 % wound infection rate, 2 % and 2 % pulmonary complication rate, 1 % and 2 % cardiac complication rate, 2 % and 2 % rate of significant bleeding, 2 % and 2 % rate of urinary tract infection, 3 % and 2 % anastomotic leak rate, and 1 % and 2 % associated mortality, respectively. The complication profiles are very similar between the three clinical trials, so it would appear that this data sets a reasonable benchmark. It must be kept in mind that there were ASA and BMI exclusions for these studies, and those factors are associated with increased rates of morbidity and mortality. As mentioned in the beginning of the chapter, the ACS-NSQIP risk calculator can provide a reasonable assessment of operative and perioperative complication risk. Results regarding length of stay, return of bowel function, narcotic use, and quality of life were discussed previously.

Long-Term Outcomes

The 5-year survival and recurrence rates for colon cancer are dependent upon the stage of disease at the time of surgery. Based on data published from 2012 by the Surveillance, Epidemiology, and End Results Program (SEERS), the

5-year overall relative survival for stage I is 90 %, stage IIA is 87 %, stage IIB is 63 %, stage IIIA is 89 %, stage IIIB is 69 %, stage IIIC is 53 %, and stage IV is 13 % [62]. The survival has improved every 5 years since 1975, which reflects improvements in detection, surgical technique, and adjuvant therapy. The aspects of these statistics that need to be noted are that patients with stage IIB (T4, N0, M0) colon cancer behave similarly to patients with stage IIIB (T3–T4a, N1, M0; T2–T3, N2a, M0; or T1–T2, N2b, M0). Therefore, it is imperative for the surgeon to understand and recognize patients with stage IIB cancers, so they can be appropriately referred for adjuvant therapy in a timely fashion. Surgeons play a critical role in the referral of cancer patients to medical oncologist, so a comprehensive knowledge of the indications for adjuvant chemotherapy is essential. The other notable observation is that patients with stage IIIA (T1–T2, N1, M0 or T1, N2a, M0) do as well as those with stage IIA (T3, N0, M0). This highlights the importance of surgical technique and the importance of resecting all potentially metastatic lymph nodes. Additionally, the addition of adjuvant chemotherapy to node-positive colon cancer with FOLFOX-based therapies improved 5-year disease-free survival from 65 to 78 % [63, 64]. This improvement is significant, but it also demonstrates that surgical quality is the most important component of care because surgical clearance of potentially metastatic lymph nodes offers the greatest chance for cure.

References

1. Teeuwen PH, Bremers AJ, Groenewoud JM, van Laarhoven CJ, Bleichrodt RP. Predictive value of POSSUM and ACPGBI scoring in mortality and morbidity of colorectal resection: a case-control study. J Gastrointest Surg. 2011;15(2):294–303.
2. Tekkis PP, Prytherch DR, Kocher HM, Senapati A, Poloniecki JD, Stamatakis JD, Windsor AC. Development of a dedicated risk-adjustment scoring system for colorectal surgery (colorectal POSSUM). Br J Surg. 2004;91(9):1174–82.
3. Oomen JL, Cuesta MA, Engel AF. Comparison of outcome of POSSUM, p-POSSUM, and cr-POSSUM scoring after elective resection of the sigmoid colon for carcinoma or complicated diverticular disease. Scand J Gastroenterol. 2007;42(7):841–7.
4. Leung E, Ferjani AM, Stellard N, Wong LS. Predicting postoperative mortality in patients undergoing colorectal surgery using P-POSSUM and CR-POSSUM scores: a prospective study. Int J Colorectal Dis. 2009;24(12):1459–64.
5. Ren L, Upadhyay AM, Wang L, Li L, Lu J, Fu W. Mortality rate prediction by Physiological and Operative Severity Score for the Enumeration of Mortality and Morbidity (POSSUM), Portsmouth POSSUM and Colorectal POSSUM and the development of new scoring systems in Chinese colorectal cancer patients. Am J Surg. 2009;198(1):31–8.
6. Hariharan S, Chen D, Ramkissoon A, Taklalsingh N, Bodkyn C, Cupidore R, Ramdin A, Ramsaroop A, Sinanan V, Teelucksingh S, Verma S. Perioperative outcome of colorectal cancer and validation of CR-POSSUM in a Caribbean country. Int J Surg. 2009;7(6):534–8.
7. Gomes A, Rocha R, Marinho R, Sousa M, Pignatelli N, Carneiro C, Nunes V. Colorectal surgical mortality and morbidity in elderly patients: comparison of POSSUM, P-POSSUM, CR-POSSUM, and CR-BHOM. Int J Colorectal Dis. 2015;30(2):173–9.
8. Cologne KG, Keller DS, Liwanag L, Devaraj B, Senagore AJ. Use of the American College of Surgeons NSQIP surgical risk calculator for laparoscopic colectomy: how good is it and how can we improve it? J Am Coll Surg. 2015;220(3):281–6.
9. Kohut AY, Liu JJ, Stein DE, Sensenig R, Poggio JL. Patient-specific risk factors are predictive for postoperative adverse events in colorectal surgery: an American College of Surgeons National Surgical Quality Improvement Program-based analysis. Am J Surg. 2015;209(2):219–29.
10. Cohen ME, Bilimoria KY, Ko CY, Hall BL. Development of an American College of Surgeons National Surgery Quality Improvement Program: morbidity and mortality risk calculator for colorectal surgery. J Am Coll Surg. 2009;208(6):1009–16.
11. Vignati P, Welch JP, Cohen JL. Endoscopic localization of colon cancers. Surg Endosc. 1994;8(9):1085–7.
12. Cho YB, Lee WY, Yun HR, Lee WS, Yun SH, Chun HK. Tumor localization for laparoscopic colorectal surgery. World J Surg. 2007;31(7):1491–5.
13. Park SH, Lee JH, Lee SS, Kim JC, Yu CS, Kim HC, Ye BD, Kim MJ, Kim AY, Ha HK. CT colonography for detection and characterization of synchronous proximal colonic lesions in patients with stenosing colorectal cancer. Gut. 2012;61(12):1716–22.
14. Morrin MM, Farrell RJ, Raptopoulos V, McGee JB, Bleday R, Kruskal JB. Role of virtual computed tomographic colonography in patients with colorectal cancers and obstructing colorectal lesions. Dis Colon Rectum. 2000;43(3):303–11.
15. Kim JH, Kim WH, Kim TI, Kim NK, Lee KY, Kim MJ, Kim KW. Incomplete colonoscopy in patients with occlusive colorectal cancer: usefulness of CT colonography according to tumor location. Yonsei Med J. 2007;48(6):934–41.
16. McArthur DR, Mehrzad H, Patel R, Dadds J, Pallan A, Karandikar SS, Roy-Choudhury S. CT colonography for synchronous colorectal lesions in patients with colorectal cancer: initial experience. Eur Radiol. 2010;20(3):621–9.
17. Maras-Simunic M, Druzijanic N, Simunic M, Roglic J, Tomic S, Perko Z. Use of modified multidetector CT colonography for the evaluation of acute and subacute colon obstruction caused by colorectal cancer: a feasibility study. Dis Colon Rectum. 2009;52(3):489–95.
18. http://www.nccn.org/professionals/physician_gls/f_guidlines. asp#site
19. Rørvig S, Schlesinger N, Mårtensson NL, Engel S, Engel U, Holck S. Is the longitudinal margin of carcinoma-bearing colon resections a neglected parameter? Clin Colorectal Cancer. 2014;13(1):68–72.
20. Read TE, Mutch MG, Chang BW, McNevin MS, Fleshman JW, Birnbaum EH, Fry RD, Caushaj PF, Kodner IJ. Locoregional recurrence and survival after curative resection of adenocarcinoma of the colon. J Am Coll Surg. 2002;195(1):33–40.
21. Matsuda K, Hotta T, Takifuji K, Yokoyama S, Oku Y, Watanabe T, Mitani Y, Ieda J, Mizumoto Y, Yamaue H. Randomized clinical trial of defaecatory function after anterior resection for rectal cancer with high versus low ligation of the inferior mesenteric artery. Br J Surg. 2015;102(5):501–8.
22. Kanemitsu Y, Hirai T, Komori K, Kato T. Survival benefit of high ligation of the inferior mesenteric artery in sigmoid colon or rectal cancer surgery. Br J Surg. 2006;93(5):609–15.

23. Chin CC, Yeh CY, Tang R, Changchien CR, Huang WS, Wang JY. The oncologic benefit of high ligation of the inferior mesenteric artery in the surgical treatment of rectal or sigmoid colon cancer. Int J Colorectal Dis. 2008;23(8):783–8.

24. Hohenberger W, Weber K, Matzel K, Papadopoulos T, Merkel S. Standardized surgery for colonic cancer: complete mesocolic excision and central ligation–technical notes and outcome. Colorectal Dis. 2009;11(4):354–64.

25. Galizia G, Lieto E, De Vita F, Ferraraccio F, Zamboli A, Mabilia A, Auricchio A, Castellano P, Napolitano V, Orditura M. Is complete mesocolic excision with central vascular ligation safe and effective in the surgical treatment of right-sided colon cancers? A prospective study. Int J Colorectal Dis. 2014;29(1):89–97.

26. West NP, Kobayashi H, Takahashi K, Perrakis A, Weber K, Hohenberger W, Sugihara K, Quirke P. Understanding optimal colonic cancer surgery: comparison of Japanese D3 resection and European complete mesocolic excision with central vascular ligation. J Clin Oncol. 2012;30(15):1763–9.

27. Kwon S, Morris A, Billingham R, Frankhouse J, Horvath K, Johnson M, McNevin S, Simons A, Symons R, Steele S, Thirlby R, Whiteford M, Flum DR, Surgical Care and Outcomes Assessment Program (SCOAP) collaborative. Routine leak testing in colorectal surgery in the Surgical Care and Outcomes Assessment Program. Arch Surg. 2012;147(4):345–51.

28. Ricciardi R, Roberts PL, Marcello PW, Hall JF, Read TE, Schoetz DJ. Anastomotic leak testing after colorectal resection: what are the data? Arch Surg. 2009;144(5):407–11.

29. Li VK, Wexner SD, Pulido N, Wang H, Jin HY, Weiss EG, Nogueras JJ, Sands DR. Use of routine intraoperative endoscopy in elective laparoscopic colorectal surgery: can it further avoid anastomotic failure? Surg Endosc. 2009;23(11):2459–65.

30. Kamal T, Pai A, Velchuru V, Zawadzki M, Park J, Marecik S, Abcarian H, Prasad L. Should anastomotic assessment with flexible sigmoidoscopy be routine following laparoscopic restorative left colorectal resection? Colorectal Dis. 2015;17(2):160–4.

31. Weeks JC, Nelson H, Gelber S, Sargent D, Schroeder G, Clinical Outcomes of Surgical Therapy (COST) Study Group. Short-term quality-of-life outcomes following laparoscopic-assisted colectomy vs. open colectomy for colon cancer: a randomized trial. JAMA. 2002;287(3):321–8.

32. Clinical Outcomes of Surgical Therapy Study Group. A comparison of laparoscopically assisted and open colectomy for colon cancer. N Engl J Med. 2004;350(20):2050–9.

33. Fleshman J, Sargent DJ, Green E, Anvari M, Stryker SJ, Beart Jr RW, Hellinger M, Flanagan Jr R, Peters W, Nelson H, Clinical Outcomes of Surgical Therapy Study Group. Laparoscopic colectomy for cancer is not inferior to open surgery based on 5-year data from the COST Study Group trial. Ann Surg. 2007;246(4):655–62.

34. Stucky CC, Pockaj BA, Novotny PJ, Sloan JA, Sargent DJ, O'Connell MJ, Beart RW, Skibber JM, Nelson H, Weeks JC. Long-term follow-up and individual item analysis of quality of life assessments related to laparoscopic-assisted colectomy in the COST trial 93-46-53 (INT 0146). Ann Surg Oncol. 2011;18(9):2422–31.

35. Guillou PJ, Quirke P, Thorpe H, Walker J, Jayne DG, Smith AM, Heath RM, Brown JM, MRC CLASICC trial group. Short-term endpoints of conventional versus laparoscopic-assisted surgery in patients with colorectal cancer (MRC CLASICC trial): multicentre, randomised controlled trial. Lancet. 2005;365(9472):1718–26.

36. Franks PJ, Bosanquet N, Thorpe H, Brown JM, Copeland J, Smith AM, Quirke P, Guillou PJ, CLASICC trial participants. Short-term costs of conventional vs. laparoscopic assisted surgery in patients with colorectal cancer (MRC CLASICC trial). Br J Cancer. 2006;95(1):6–12.

37. Jayne DG, Guillou PJ, Thorpe H, Quirke P, Copeland J, Smith AM, Heath RM, Brown JM, UK MRC CLASICC Trial Group. Randomized trial of laparoscopic-assisted resection of colorectal carcinoma: 3-year results of the UK MRC CLASICC Trial Group. J Clin Oncol. 2007;25(21):3061–8.

38. Green BL, Marshall HC, Collinson F, Quirke P, Guillou P, Jayne DG, Brown JM. Long-term follow-up of the Medical Research Council CLASICC trial of conventional versus laparoscopically assisted resection in colorectal cancer. Br J Surg. 2013;100(1):75–82.

39. Jayne DG, Thorpe HC, Copeland J, Quirke P, Brown JM, Guillou PJ. Five-year follow-up of the Medical Research Council CLASICC trial of laparoscopically assisted versus open surgery for colorectal cancer. Br J Surg. 2010;97(11):1638–45.

40. Hazebroek EJ, Color Study Group. COLOR: a randomized clinical trial comparing laparoscopic and open resection for colon cancer. Surg Endosc. 2002;16(6):949–53.

41. Veldkamp R, Kuhry E, Hop WC, Jeekel J, Kazemier G, Bonjer HJ, Haglind E, Påhlman L, Cuesta MA, Msika S, Morino M, Lacy AM, Colon cancer Laparoscopic or Open Resection Study Group (COLOR). Laparoscopic surgery versus open surgery for colon cancer: short-term outcomes of a randomised trial. Lancet Oncol. 2005;6(7):477–84.

42. Kuhry E, Bonjer HJ, Haglind E, Hop WC, Veldkamp R, Cuesta MA, Jeekel J, Påhlman L, Morino M, Lacy A, Delgado S, COLOR Study Group. Impact of hospital case volume on short-term outcome after laparoscopic operation for colonic cancer. Surg Endosc. 2005;19(5):687–92.

43. Colon Cancer Laparoscopic or Open Resection Study Group, Buunen M, Veldkamp R, Hop WC, Kuhry E, Jeekel J, Haglind E, Påhlman L, Cuesta MA, Msika S, Morino M, Lacy A, Bonjer HJ. Survival after laparoscopic surgery versus open surgery for colon cancer: long-term outcome of a randomised clinical trial. Lancet Oncol. 2009;10(1):44–52.

44. Yamamoto S, Inomata M, Katayama H, Mizusawa J, Etoh T, Konishi F, Sugihara K, Watanabe M, Moriya Y, Kitano S, Japan Clinical Oncology Group Colorectal Cancer Study Group. Short-term surgical outcomes from a randomized controlled trial to evaluate laparoscopic and open D3 dissection for stage II/III colon cancer: Japan Clinical Oncology Group Study JCOG 0404. Ann Surg. 2014;260(1):23–30.

45. Bagshaw PF, Allardyce RA, Frampton CM, Frizelle FA, Hewett PJ, McMurrick PJ, Rieger NA, Smith JS, Solomon MJ, Stevenson AR, Australasian Laparoscopic Colon Cancer Study Group. Long-term outcomes of the australasian randomized clinical trial comparing laparoscopic and conventional open surgical treatments for colon cancer: the Australasian Laparoscopic Colon Cancer Study trial. Ann Surg. 2012;256(6):915–9.

46. Cortet M, Grimault A, Cheynel N, Lepage C, Bouvier AM, Faivre J. Patterns of recurrence of obstructing colon cancers after surgery for cure: a population-based study. Colorectal Dis. 2013;15(9):1100–6.

47. Gianotti L, Tamini N, Nespoli L, Rota M, Bolzonaro E, Frego R, Redaelli A, Antolini L, Ardito A, Nespoli A, Dinelli M. A

prospective evaluation of short-term and long-term results from colonic stenting for palliation or as a bridge to elective operation versus immediate surgery for large-bowel obstruction. Surg Endosc. 2013;27(3):832–42.

48. Huang X, Lv B, Zhang S, Meng L. Preoperative colonic stents versus emergency surgery for acute left-sided malignant colonic obstruction: a meta-analysis. J Gastrointest Surg. 2014;18(3):584–91.

49. van Hooft JE, Bemelman WA, Oldenburg B, Marinelli AW, Lutke Holzik MF, Grubben MJ, Sprangers MA, Dijkgraaf MG, Fockens P, Collaborative Dutch Stent-In study group. Colonic stenting versus emergency surgery for acute left-sided malignant colonic obstruction: a multicentre randomised trial. Lancet Oncol. 2011;12(4):344–52.

50. Dastur JK, Forshaw MJ, Modarai B, Solkar MM, Raymond T, Parker MC. Comparison of short-and long-term outcomes following either insertion of self-expanding metallic stents or emergency surgery in malignant large bowel obstruction. Tech Coloproctol. 2008;12(1):51–5.

51. Kim JS, Hur H, Min BS, Sohn SK, Cho CH, Kim NK. Oncologic outcomes of self-expanding metallic stent insertion as a bridge to surgery in the management of left-sided colon cancer obstruction: comparison with nonobstructing elective surgery. World J Surg. 2009;33(6):1281–6.

52. Cirocchi R, Farinella E, Trastulli S, Desiderio J, Listorti C, Boselli C, Parisi A, Noya G, Sagar J. Safety and efficacy of endoscopic colonic stenting as a bridge to surgery in the management of intestinal obstruction due to left colon and rectal cancer: a systematic review and meta-analysis. Surg Oncol. 2013;22(1):14–21.

53. Sagar J. Colorectal stents for the management of malignant colonic obstructions. Cochrane Database Syst Rev. 2011;11, CD007378.

54. Knight AL, Trompetas V, Saunders MP, Anderson HJ. Does stenting of left-sided colorectal cancer as a "bridge to surgery" adversely affect oncological outcomes? A comparison with non-obstructing elective left-sided colonic resections. Int J Colorectal Dis. 2012;27(11):1509–14.

55. Trompetas V. Emergency management of malignant acute left-sided colonic obstruction. Ann R Coll Surg Engl. 2008;90(3):181–6.

56. Ansaloni L, Andersson RE, Bazzoli F, Catena F, Cennamo V, Di Saverio S, Fuccio L, Jeekel H, Leppäniemi A, Moore E, Pinna AD, Pisano M, Repici A, Sugarbaker PH, Tuech JJ. Guidelines in the management of obstructing cancer of the left colon: consensus conference of the world society of emergency surgery (WSES) and peritoneum and surgery (PnS) society. World J Emerg Surg. 2010;5:29.

57. Cheynel N, Cortet M, Lepage C, Ortega-Debalon P, Faivre J, Bouvier AM. Incidence, patterns of failure, and prognosis of perforated colorectal cancers in a well-defined population. Dis Colon Rectum. 2009;52(3):406–11.

58. Zielinski MD, Merchea A, Heller SF, You YN. Emergency management of perforated colon cancers: how aggressive should we be? J Gastrointest Surg. 2011;15(12):2232–8.

59. Muratore A, Zorzi D, Bouzari H, Amisano M, Massucco P, Sperti E, Capussotti L. Asymptomatic colorectal cancer with un-resectable liver metastases: immediate colorectal resection or up-front systemic chemotherapy? Ann Surg Oncol. 2007;14(2):766–70.

60. Scheer MG, Sloots CE, van der Wilt GJ, Ruers TJ. Management of patients with asymptomatic colorectal cancer and synchronous irresectable metastases. Ann Oncol. 2008;19(11):1829–35.

61. Lam VW, Spiro C, Laurence JM, Johnston E, Hollands MJ, Pleass HC, Richardson AJ. A systematic review of clinical response and survival outcomes of downsizing systemic chemotherapy and rescue liver surgery in patients with initially unresectable colorectal liver metastases. Ann Surg Oncol. 2012;19(4):1292–301.

62. http://seer.cancer.gov/statfacts/html/colorect.html

63. Kuebler JP, Wieand HS, O'Connell MJ, Smith RE, Colangelo LH, Yothers G, Petrelli NJ, Findlay MP, Seay TE, Atkins JN, Zapas JL, Goodwin JW, Fehrenbacher L, Ramanathan RK, Conley BA, Flynn PJ, Soori G, Colman LK, Levine EA, Lanier KS, Wolmark N. Oxaliplatin combined with weekly bolus fluorouracil and leucovorin as surgical adjuvant chemotherapy for stage II and III colon cancer: results from NSABP C-07. J Clin Oncol. 2007;25(16):2198–204.

64. André T, Boni C, Mounedji-Boudiaf L, Navarro M, Tabernero J, Hickish T, Topham C, Zaninelli M, Clingan P, Bridgewater J, Tabah-Fisch I, de Gramont A, Multicenter International Study of Oxaliplatin/5-Fluorouracil/Leucovorin in the Adjuvant Treatment of Colon Cancer (MOSAIC) Investigators. Oxaliplatin, fluorouracil, and leucovorin as adjuvant treatment for colon cancer. N Engl J Med. 2004;350(23):2343–51.

27

Rectal Cancer: Preoperative Evaluation and Staging

Jorge Marcet

Key Concepts

- Accurate preoperative staging of patients with rectal cancer helps identify patients at risk for local or distant metastasis and guides treatment decisions.
- Endorectal ultrasound (ERUS) is effective for staging the depth of invasion (T stage), especially for early-stage rectal tumors (uT0, uT1) that may be considered for local excision.
- Magnetic resonance (MR) has the ability to delineate the extent of locally advanced tumors and estimate the involvement of the mesorectal fascia.
- ERUS and MR use surrogate markers to estimate nodal involvement—size and node morphology—and are not particularly accurate in predicting nodal metastatic spread unless there are multiple large nodes in the mesorectum.
- The potential for understaging and overstaging of patients should be realized and taken into account when making treatment decisions.
- High-resolution computed tomography (CT) can detect distant metastatic lesions greater than 1 cm in diameter.
- Positron emission tomography (PET) scan is the most accurate assessment of total body tumor burden, especially when combined with CT (PET-CT).
- PET-CT is indicated when there are equivocal findings on CT and finding distant metastatic disease would alter therapeutic decisions.

Introduction

Careful pretreatment evaluation of the patient with rectal cancer is paramount for the successful management of their disease. By identifying the location of the tumor and its stage at the time of presentation, the surgeon is best prepared to discuss treatment options and prognosis with the patient and his or her family. As such, all healthcare providers caring for patients with rectal cancer should have a thorough understanding of the evaluation and staging of this disease.

Preoperative staging is performed according to the TNM classification of malignant tumors, estimating the depth of invasion into the rectal wall (cT), the presence or absence of lymph node metastasis (cN), and the presence of distant metastasis (cM). Also of importance is the determination of invasion of the anal sphincter and pelvic floor musculature, adjacent pelvic organs, or pelvic sidewall, all with significant consequences of planning and treatment to the patient.

The prefix "c" is used to indicate clinical staging, which is the estimate of stage based on physical examination and radiographic studies. Unfortunately, there is often confusion regarding this distinction, with some authors describing treatment recommendations for "T3N0" tumors as determined by pretreatment staging, when instead they should describe the tumor as "cT3N0." The difference at first glance appears trivial but can have significant consequences if the clinician fails to understand that estimates of tumor stage are just that, estimates, and that treatment planning must take into account the potential inaccuracy of these estimates. For example, understaging of the cancer preoperatively may result in the omission of preoperative radiotherapy/chemoradiotherapy and lead to an increased risk of local recurrence. Conversely, overstaging may lead to overtreatment, increasing the overall morbidity and cost of treatment.

Pretreatment evaluation begins with physical examination and colonoscopic evaluation. Radiographic studies may include computed tomography (CT), endorectal ultrasound (ERUS), magnetic resonance imaging (MRI), and PET. These tests are complementary, each with their own advantages and disadvantages, and may be used in combination. Laboratory evaluation includes determination of the carcinoembryonic antigen (CEA) level.

Physical Examination

When evaluating a patient diagnosed with rectal cancer, the patient's history is recorded, and an inquiry is made as to the duration of symptoms, changes in weight, bowel habits, bowel control, and presence of pain. If restorative proctectomy

© Springer International Publishing 2016
S.R. Steele et al. (eds.), *The ASCRS Textbook of Colon and Rectal Surgery*, DOI 10.1007/978-3-319-25970-3_27

or local excision is to be contemplated, a detailed assessment of anal sphincter function and prior trauma (e.g., obstetrical history, prior anal operations) should be obtained. A general physical examination is performed with special attention for signs of muscle wasting, abdominal distension, hepatomegaly, and lymphadenopathy. A careful digital rectal examination is performed, noting the distance of the tumor from the anal verge and its proximity to the anal sphincter and pelvic floor. Tumors located in the anterior portion of the rectum have the risk of invasion into the genital structures, and special attention should be made to the potential for fixation to adjacent structures (i.e., prostate, vagina, sacrum, puborectalis). In a woman with an anterior rectal cancer, a pelvic examination should be done to ensure there is no invasion of the vaginal wall that may affect treatment. When the tumor is located in the posterior or lateral rectal wall, pelvic sidewall invasion should be considered. In addition, assessment of anal sphincter bulk and tone should be performed.

The texture of the tumor also gives a clue as to the stage. Benign adenomas are soft and the tumor may occasionally be difficult to detect on digital rectal examination. When a tumor invades the rectal wall, a desmoplastic reaction occurs and the resulting fibrosis will be felt as firm tissue. Evaluating the mobility of the tumor can also give information on how deep the tumor invades. A tumor tethered to the rectal wall, but that is otherwise mobile, is likely to invade into but not through the wall. Tumors that are fixed within the pelvis and are not mobile are locally advanced, deeply invading the full thickness of the rectal wall and possibly invading surrounding pelvic structures. Using these qualities of adherence of the tumor to the rectal wall and pelvis based on the digital rectal examination, Mason proposed a clinical staging system (CS-I to CS-IV) and recommended treatment options for patients with rectal cancer [1]. The digital rectal examination may occasionally also detect peritumoral lymphadenopathy, though this is often difficult. It should be noted that digital rectal examination has limitations in that only tumors of the distal rectal rectum can be adequately assessed. Furthermore, accuracy in staging depth of invasion is better for advanced tumors than for early tumors and improves with the surgeon's experience [2].

Clearance of the proximal large bowel, preferably by complete colonoscopy, should be performed in all patients with rectal cancer to exclude synchronous lesions and to confirm the histopathology of the tumor via biopsy. Other radiological testing may occasionally be used (i.e., CT colonography, air-contrast enema), though each has inherent limitations that providers should be aware of such as the need for an adequate preparation or failure to identify small lesions. Patients that are unable to be cleared prior to surgery due to an obstructing lesion should undergo proximal evaluation within 6 months after their operation. The endoscopic appearance of a tumor also gives a clue as to the relative degree of invasion, with benign tumors being soft to manipulation with the colonoscope or endoscopic forceps and

malignant tumors being firm. Ulceration of the tumor implies invasion into the rectal wall, while deep ulceration may be a sign of transmural invasion.

Limiting pretreatment evaluation to digital rectal examination and colonoscopy prior to surgery for a rectal tumor is only appropriate for lesions that are considered benign. For patients with known or suspected rectal cancer, additional pretreatment locoregional imaging to stage depth of invasion and body scanning to detect distant metastasis should be performed prior to starting any treatment—whether with surgery, chemotherapy, or radiation.

Locoregional Imaging

Computed Tomography

Computed tomography (CT) is widely available and is one of the primary modalities used in preoperative staging of rectal cancer. CT accuracy is improved by administering oral, intravenous, and rectal contrast. CT can localize the tumor in the rectum but is not able to accurately delineate the layers of the rectal wall. For locally advanced tumors, CT may show extension beyond the rectal wall and invasion into surrounding structures. The addition of multidetector-row CT (MDCT) has improved accuracy for local staging of rectal cancer but still lacks the detail required. By including multiplanar (coronal, sagittal) images to standard axial images, this provides improved accuracy rates for higher T staging and N staging of rectal cancer than axial images alone [3].

Limitations to CT scanning for local staging of rectal cancer include the limited ability to define the mesorectal fascial layers and layers of the rectal wall. Although the mesorectal fat (MRF) surrounding a tumor can be clearly visualized on CT, perirectal fat stranding or induration secondary to rectal inflammation or peritumoral fibrosis cannot be definitively differentiated from tumor extension. In addition, the diagnosis of T4 tumors can be difficult due to lack of soft tissue resolution in the pelvis. Tumor involvement of an adjacent organ or the pelvic sidewall is also not accurate and is inferred by the loss of the fat plane between the tumor and the adjacent organ or structure.

Endorectal Ultrasound

On endorectal ultrasound (ERUS), the bowel wall is defined by five distinct sonographic layers of alternating hyper- and hypoechoic qualities [4]. Extending from the lumen outward, these layers correspond to (1) the interface between the ultrasound probe and the mucosa, (2) the interface between the mucosa and muscularis mucosa, (3) the submucosa, (4) the muscularis propria, and (5) the serosa or pericolic fat. The prefix "u" is used to describe ERUS T and N staging of rectal cancer (Figure 27-1, 27-2, 27-3, 27-4, and 27-5) [5].

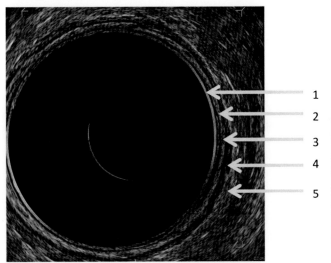

FIGURE 27-1. Endosonographic layers of the rectal wall. (1) Interphase of endoscopic balloon with mucosa. (2) Interphase of mucosa/submucosa. (3) Submucosa. (4) Muscularis propria. (5) Serosa and pericolic fat.

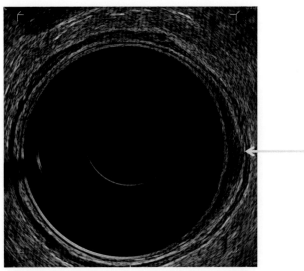

FIGURE 27-3. ERUS of uT1 tumor. Hypoechoic tumor invades into the middle hyperechoic layer (*arrow*) but does not invade the outer hypoechoic layer.

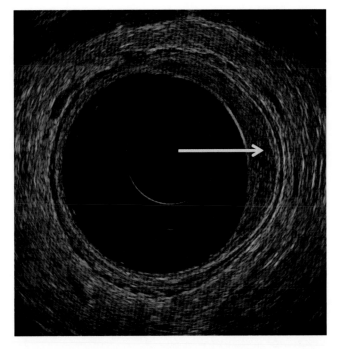

FIGURE 27-2. ERUS of uT0 tumor. Hypoechoic tumor (*arrow*) does not invade into the first hyperechoic layer. Notice that the submucosa (*white layer*) remains intact.

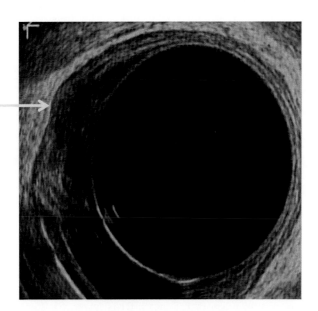

FIGURE 27-4. ERUS of uT2 tumor. Hypoechoic tumor invades through the middle hyperechoic layer and into the outer hypoechoic layer.

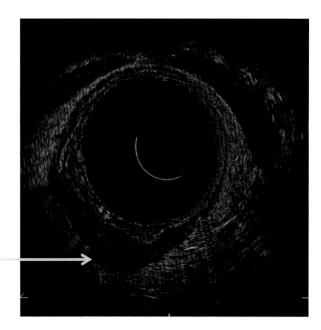

FIGURE 27-5. ERUS of uT3 tumor. Tumor extends through the second hypoechoic layer and into the outer hyperechoic layer (*arrow*).

ERUS has advantages in that it is simple to perform and inexpensive compared to CT or MR. The patient is given an enema to evacuate the rectum prior to the procedure. The procedure is often combined with a flexible or rigid procto-sigmoidoscopy. Some patients require sedation to allay discomfort or anxiety. The ultrasound probe needs to pass proximal to the tumor in order to evaluate the entire extent of the tumor, thus making it difficult or impossible with obstructing lesions. 3-D ultrasonography records the image in real time and allows for subsequent manipulation of the image for axial, coronal, and sagittal evaluation. Malignant lymph nodes appear as hypoechoic and rounded peritumoral structures, whereas benign lymph nodes are less likely to be detected as they are isoechoic with the perirectal fat.

T Staging

There is variation in the reported accuracy of ERUS in accessing the T stage of rectal cancer, with an overall accuracy of about 84 % (ranging from 63 to 96 %), while the reported accuracy of CT and MRI is lower, 65–75 % and 75–85 %, respectively [6]. The accuracy of ERUS T staging in rectal cancer was analyzed in a meta-analysis of 42 studies ($N=5039$) where ERUS T stage was compared to pathological stage (Table 27-1) [7]. The authors reported that ERUS has a sensitivity of 81–96 % and a specificity of 91–98 %, showing a higher sensitivity for locally advanced rectal cancer or LARC (95 %), compared with early cancer (88 %). The authors concluded that ERUS should be the preferred test for preoperative tumor staging rectal cancer.

As with many interpretive studies, operator experience plays a significant role in staging accuracy. In a prospective,

multicenter study conducted in 384 hospitals in Germany, investigators analyzed the diagnostic accuracy of preoperative ERUS (uT) with pathological (pT) findings in 7096 patients with rectal cancer who had not received neoadjuvant therapy [8]. The overall accuracy of uT to pT was found to be 65 %, with understaging occurring in 18 % and overstaging in 17 % of patients. The hospital volume of yearly ERUS procedures performed was found to affect the accuracy for staging, with uT-pT correlation of 63 % for hospitals undertaking ≤10 ERUS/year, 65 % for those performing 11–30 ERUS/year, and 73 % for hospitals where more than 30 ERUS/year were performed. The poorest correlation was found for T2 and T4 rectal cancers. The authors cautioned that ERUS is a useful tool for guiding the therapeutic strategy of rectal cancer only when performed by expert diagnosticians.

Several investigators have demonstrated a lower accuracy of ERUS in detecting T2 tumors compared to T1, T3, or T4 [9–11]. Reasons for this include difficulty in differentiating those tumors that have deep invasion into the muscularis propria from those with microscopic invasion into the perirectal fat and in differentiating peritumoral inflammation and edema from neoplastic infiltration. One group retrospectively subdivided patients with preoperative T2 tumors into uT2a, for tumors with focal invasion into the muscularis propria, and uT2b, for tumors with extensive invasion into the muscularis propria, and found improved weighted kappa accuracy (from 0.89 to 0.94) when the uT2b tumors were included in the enlarged uT3 group [12].

ERUS has been studied for the selection of patients with early-stage rectal cancer (T0, T1) who may benefit from transanal excision instead of traditional transabdominal rectal resection. In a study of 552 patients undergoing transanal excision of rectal tumors, investigators evaluated the accuracy of ERUS to clinical staging and found that ERUS had a sensitivity of 95 % vs. 78 % and a positive predictive value of 93 % vs. 85 % in detecting adenoma or T1 rectal carcinoma as compared to clinical staging, whereas specificity was similar in both (62 % vs. 58 %) [13]. A meta-analysis designed to evaluate the accuracy of ERUS in T0 staging of rectal cancers found 11 studies ($N=1791$) which met the inclusion criteria. The pooled sensitivity of ERUS in diagnosing T0 was 97.3 % (95 % CI: 93.7–99.1) and a pooled specificity of 96.3 % (95 % CI: 95.3–97.2) [9].

N Staging

Accuracy for detecting metastatic lymph nodes by endorectal ultrasound is less precise than for T staging, with a variable accuracy in reported studies of 63–85 % [6]. Differences in accuracy among studies may be due in part to differences in criteria used in defining nodal metastases. Hildebrandt et al. reported that hypoechoic, sharply demarcated nodes and those with heterogeneous pattern are more indicative of metastasis [14]. Katsura and associates found that nodes

TABLE 27-1. ERUS accuracy compared to histological stage.

Meta-analysis of 42 studies, $N = 5039$ patients		
T stage	Pooled sensitivity	Pooled specificity
T1	87.8 % (95 % CI 85.3–90.0 %)	98.3 % (95 % CI 97.8–98.7 %)
T2	80.5 % (95 % CI 77.9–82.9 %)	95.6 % (95 % CI 94.9–96.3 %)
T3	96.4 % (95 % CI 95.4–97.2 %)	90.6 % (95 % CI 89.5–91.7 %)
T4	95.4 % (95 % CI 92.4–97.5 %)	98 % (95% CI 97.8–98.7 %)

Adapted from Puli S, Bechtold M, Reddy J, Choudhary A, Antillon M, Brugge W. How good is endoscopic ultrasound in differentiating various T stages of rectal cancer? Meta-analysis and systematic review. Ann Surg Oncol 2009; 16:254–265 [7]

>5 mm, with well-defined boundaries and uneven and greatly hypoechoic patterns, were more likely to represent metastasis [15]. Akasu related the size of the short axis diameter of the largest lymph node to the rate of metastasis and found that for nodes <2 mm, the incidence of nodal metastases was 9.5 %, increasing to 47 % for nodes 3–5 mm in diameter and 87 % for nodes larger than 6 mm [16]. A meta-analysis of 35 studies evaluating the accuracy of EUS in diagnosing N stage in patients with rectal cancer showed a sensitivity of 73 % and specificity of 76 %. The data analyzed supported the hypothesis that ERUS is more accurate in excluding nodal involvement, rather than diagnosing it [17].

Staging accuracy for lymph node metastasis improves when the findings are associated with the T stage, with a higher risk of metastasis correlating with higher T stage. In a retrospective review of 134 patients with rectal cancer who underwent ERUS followed by radical surgery without neoadjuvant therapy, the accuracy of ERUS for N staging was 48 % for pT1 cancers, increasing to 84 % for pT3 cancers [18]. Notably, early rectal lesions are more likely to have lymph node micrometastases not detected by endorectal ultrasound. This may explain the somewhat high recurrence rates seen after local excision of early-uT-stage rectal cancer. On the other hand, CT has an accuracy of 55–65 % and MRI has an accuracy of 60–65 %. ERUS is more reliable than CT in being able to detect lymph nodes smaller than 1 cm and has comparable sensitivity and specificity to MRI [19].

Limitations to ERUS for staging rectal cancer include incomplete exams due to tumors that are bulky or stenotic. In women, these limitations may be overcome by vaginal insertion of the ultrasound probe [20]. Other causes of inadequate contact of the ultrasound probe with the tumor may be air or stool in the rectum or angulation of the tumor. Operator experience has also been shown to play a role in the accuracy of ERUS staging [21, 22].

Magnetic Resonance

High-resolution magnetic resonance (MR) with phased array pelvic coils is being increasingly used in the preoperative assessment of rectal cancer given its improved ability to evaluate the at-risk surgical circumferential resection margin. The pelvic coil is a wraparound surface coil placed around the pelvis. Patients are prepared with an enema on the morning of the examination. Thin-section (3 mm) T2-weighted fast spin-echo sequences are obtained in a plane orthogonal to the tumor [23]. Higher-resolution MRI allows improved definition of bowel and tumor infiltration [24]. MRI with endorectal coil is no longer recommended. Although endorectal MRI can show five layers of the rectal wall, the field of view is limited and the mesorectal fascia is not always visible. Additionally, the endorectal coil is more uncomfortable to the patient than the external coil and cannot be inserted in stenosing tumors [25]. Endorectal coil also has the potential to distort the tissues.

Three layers of the rectal wall are visible on a phased array external MRI. The innermost mucosa is thin and hypointense, the middle submucosa is hyperintense, and the outer muscularis propria is darkly hypointense. Below the peritoneal reflection, the rectum is surrounded by the MRF which is limited by the thin mesorectal fascia, which fuses with the rectoprostatic or rectovaginal fascia anteriorly and the presacral fascia posteriorly. The MRF surrounds the rectum completely only in the lower third and is best seen laterally as a thin hypointense line on T2W sequences. Inferiorly, the MRF thins out as it reaches the levator ani, which forms the roof of the ischiorectal fossa. MR is the best imaging modality to identify this avascular plane surrounding the mesorectum, which includes the mesorectum in its fascial envelope—the circumferential radial margin (CRM) (Figure 27-6).

In a meta-analysis of 21 studies designed to determine the accuracy of MR for T category (T1–2 vs. T3–4), lymph node metastases, and circumferential resection margin (CRM) involvement in primary rectal cancer that did not undergo preoperative chemoradiotherapy, MRI specificity was significantly higher for CRM involvement (94 %) than for T stage (75 %) or nodal metastases (71 %) [26]. Diagnostic odds ratio was significantly higher for CRM (56.1) than for nodal metastases (8.3) but did not differ significantly from T category (20.4) (Table 27-2). The authors concluded that MRI has good accuracy for both CRM and T category and should be considered for preoperative rectal cancer staging (Figure 27-7).

FIGURE 27-6. MR of cT3 tumor. Circumferential resection margin is preserved (*arrows*).

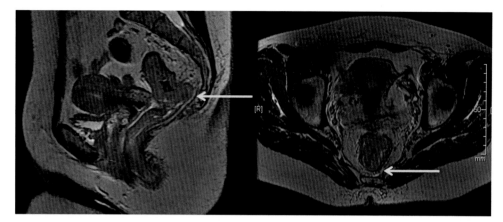

FIGURE 27-7. MR of cT4 tumor. Tumor invades the anal sphincter and levator ani (*arrows*).

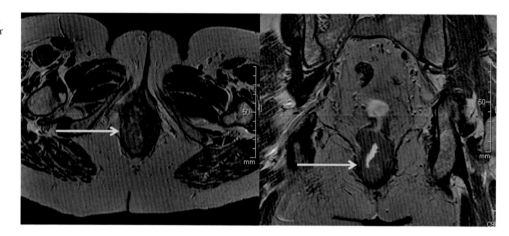

TABLE 27-2. Meta-analysis of magnetic resonance accuracy in T stage, N stage, and circumferential resection margin (CRM)

	Specificity
T stage 19 studies (*N*=1986)	75 % (95 % CI 68–80)
N stage 12 studies (*N*=1249)	71 % (95 % CI 59–81)
CRM 10 studies (*N*=986)	94 % (95 % CI 88–97)

Adapted from Al-Sukhni E, Milot L, Fruitman M, Beyene J, Victor J, Schmocker S, Brown G, McLeod R, Kennedy E. Diagnostic accuracy of MRI for assessment of T category, lymph node metastases, and circumferential resection margin involvement in patients with rectal cancer: a systematic review and meta-analysis. Ann Surge Oncol 2012; 19:2212-2223 [26]

Park et al. [27] evaluated the accuracy of preoperative MRI in predicting pN stage by doing a node-for-node matched histopathology evaluation. The overall success rate of matching between the two techniques was 91 %. Preoperative MRI revealed a node-by-node sensitivity and positive predictive value of 58.0 and 61.7 %. Of the 341 nodes harvested, 120 were too small (<3 mm) to be depicted on magnetic resonance images, and 18 of these contained metastasis (15 %).

MR limitations include foreign bodies in patients that are MR incompatible. Foreign bodies that are compatible, such as surgical clips, may also obscure images. Movement-related artifacts may preclude accurate visualization of the rectal wall. MR is not portable to the operating room and is more expensive than ERUS [28].

Many referral centers with an expertise in rectal cancer treatment are now utilizing MR as the preferred locoregional staging evaluation, especially for locally advanced tumors.

ERUS is utilized for evaluation of early-stage lesions or used in combination with MR for select patients.

Whole Body Imaging

Computed Tomography

CT of the chest, abdomen, and pelvis is indicated in patients with rectal cancer to evaluate for distant metastasis, primarily of the liver and lung (Figure 27-8) [29]. The overall sensitivity of MDCT for liver metastases ranges from 77 to 94 % [30–32]. Most lesions measuring over 1 cm in size can be reliably differentiated from benign liver lesions (such as cysts or hemangiomas). However, for lesions under 1 cm in size, sensitivities drop to as low as 41.9 % [33]. The finding of small nonspecific hypodensities measuring <1 cm (also known as "too-small-to-characterize" hypodensities) is very common, perhaps present in as many as 17 % of all patients [34]. In the majority of cases, even in those patients with a known underlying malignancy, these small hypodensities in the liver are likely to be benign (~90 %) and can be followed over time.

Evaluation of lung metastases is also an important component of MDCT distant staging. In one study of 56 patients with rectal cancer, 18 % had evidence of at least one pulmonary metastasis on MDCT, with an increasing risk of pulmonary metastasis with rising tumor grade [35].

Positron Emission Tomography

PET is a whole body nuclear medicine imaging examination utilizing 2-(^{18}F) fluoro-2-deoxy-D-glucose (FDG) that exploits the increased rate of glycolysis in tumor cells to detect tumor. FDG is a glucose analog that is taken up by cellular glucose transport mechanisms and is phosphorylated by hexokinase. Most malignant cells have an increased metabolism of glucose and thus take up the FDG at a greater rate than surrounding tissues. FDG-6-phosphate then becomes metabolically "trapped" intracellularly, because of the relative lack of glucose-6-phosphatase activity in tumor cells. PET detects the increased FDG uptake. This uptake can be assessed both qualitatively (via visual examination of the degree of uptake of a tumor relative to other tissues) and quantitatively (via an SUV value). While PET was traditionally performed as a stand-alone examination, these studies are now typically performed in conjunction with CT to allow for more precise correlation of FDG activity with anatomy [30].

Although PET has been demonstrated to be more accurate in the assessment of whole body tumor burden than a combination of conventional imaging [31], it does have limitations. There is a limit to the resolution of the scan, and lesions less than 1–2 cm may be missed. This makes accurate assessment of nodal metastases difficult. In addition, the activity of the primary tumor may interfere with detection of mesorectal lymph nodes due to the proximity of the primary rectal tumor. Lastly, mucinous adenocarcinomas may not be detected, given that the FDG uptake per unit volume of tissue is reduced as compared to non-mucinous tumor [31].

The role of PET in the management of patients with primary rectal adenocarcinoma is to investigate equivocal findings on CT, when the detection of metastatic disease would change treatment strategy. In addition, PET should also be performed prior to consideration of resection of distant metastatic disease or local pelvic recurrence, to exclude incurable occult disease that would make the operation palliative rather than curative. PET is extremely useful in the differentiation of pelvic scar from recurrent tumor in those patients who have undergone proctectomy for rectal adenocarcinoma.

In one study, PET-CT showed a diagnostic accuracy of 92 % (as opposed to 87 % for MDCT), changed the patient's stage in 13.5 % of cases, identified previously unknown disease in 19.2 % of cases, changed the patient's planned surgery in 11.5 % of cases, and changed the patient's therapy in 17.8 % of cases [32]. Another study found that PET-CT upstaged 50 % of patients, downstaged 21 % of patients, and changed the patient's treatment plan in 27 % of patients [36]. This study noted that PET-CT was particularly likely to identify "discordant" findings (i.e., findings not identified on MDCT) in patients with low rectal cancers due to the propensity of this group of lesions to metastasize to local lymph nodes in the pelvis (particularly nodes in the inguinal, femoral, or iliac chains), as PET-CT identified metastatic lymphadenopathy in 13.5 % of patients in this study which were not diagnosed on MDCT.

PET has been evaluated as a potential technique to determine histologic response to neoadjuvant chemoradiotherapy and better identify patients for local excision or nonoperative therapy, but like CT, MR and ERUS have not been found to be accurate in the assessment of residual tumor in the pelvis [37]. At present, PET is not recommended in the routine evaluation of patients presenting with primary rectal adenocarcinoma

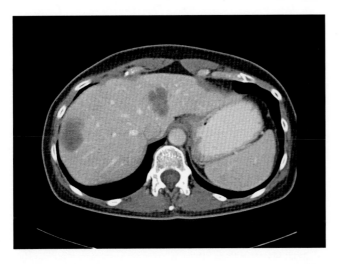

FIGURE 27-8. CT of the abdomen demonstrating two liver metastases.

[38] but is utilized to evaluate equivocal findings on CT when finding distant metastatic disease would alter management.

References

1. Mason A. President's address. Rectal cancer: the spectrum of selective surgery. Proc R Soc Med. 1976;69(4):237–44.
2. Nicholls RJ, York-Mason A, Morson BC, Dixon AK, Fry IK. The clinical staging of rectal cancer. Br J Surg. 1982;69:404–9.
3. Sinha R, Verma R, Rajesh A, Richards CJ. Diagnostic value of multidetector row CT in rectal cancer staging: comparison of multiplanar and axial images with histopathology. Clin Radiol. 2006;61(11):924–31.
4. Kumar A, Scholefield JH. Endosonography of the anal canal and rectum. World J Surg. 2000;24:208–15.
5. Hildebrandt U, Feifel G. Preoperative staging of rectal cancer by intrarectal ultrasound. Dis Colon Rectum. 1985;28:42–6.
6. Marone P, Bellis M, D'Angelo V, et al. Role of endoscopic ultrasonography in the loco-regional staging of patients with rectal cancer. World J Gastrointest Endosc. 2015;7:688–701.
7. Puli S, Bechtold M, Reddy J, Choudhary A, Antillon M, Brugge W. How good is endoscopic ultrasound in differentiating various T stages of rectal cancer? Meta-analysis and systematic review. Ann Surg Oncol. 2009;16:254–65.
8. Marusch F, Ptok H, Sahm M, Schmidt U, Ridwelski K, Gastinger I, Lippert H. Endorectal ultrasound in rectal carcinoma—do the literature results really correspond to the realities of routine clinical care? Endoscopy. 2011;43:425–31.
9. Puli SR, Bechtold ML, Reddy JB, Choudhary A, Antillon MR. Can endoscopic ultrasound predict early rectal cancers that can be resected endoscopically? A meta-analysis and systematic review. Dig Dis Sci. 2010;55:1221–9.
10. Solomon MJ, McLeod RS, Cohen EK, Simons ME, Wilson S. Reliability and validity studies of endoluminal ultrasonography for anorectal disorders. Dis Colon Rectum. 1994;37:546–51.
11. Anderson BO, Hann LE, Enker WE, Dershaw DD, Guillem JG, Cohen AM. Transrectal ultrasonography and operative selection for early carcinoma of the rectum. J Am Coll Surg. 1994;179:513–7.
12. Mackay SG, Pager CK, Joseph D, Stewart PJ, Solomon MJ. Assessment of the accuracy of transrectal ultrasonography in anorectal neoplasia. Br J Surg. 2003;90:346–50.
13. Kneist W, Terzic A, Burghardt J, Heintz A, Junginger T. Selection of patients with rectal tumors for local excision based on preoperative diagnosis. Results of a consecutive evaluation study of 552 patients. Chirurg. 2004;75:168–75.
14. Hildebrandt U, Klein T, Feilfel G, Schwarz H, Koch B, Schimtt R. Endosonography of pararectal lymph nodes: in vitro and in vivo evaluation. Dis Colon Rectum. 1990;33:863–8.
15. Katsura Y, Yamada K, Ishizawa T, Yoshinaka H, Shimazu H. Endorectal ultrasonography for the assessment of wall invasion and lymph node metastasis in rectal cancer. Dis Colon Rectum. 1992;35:362–8.
16. Akasu T, Sugihara K, Moriya Y, Fujita S. Limitations and pitfalls of transrectal ultrasonography for staging of rectal cancer. Dis Colon Rectum. 1997;40:S10–5.
17. Puli SR, Reddy JB, Bechtold ML, Choudhary A, Antillon MR, Brugge WR. Accuracy of endoscopic ultrasound to diagnose nodal invasion by rectal cancers: a meta-analysis and systematic review. Ann Surg Oncol. 2009;16:1255–65.
18. Landmann RG, Wong WD, Hoepfl J, Shia J, Guillem JG, Temple LK, Paty PB, Weiser MR. Limitations of early rectal cancer nodal staging may explain failure after local excision. Dis Colon Rectum. 2007;50:1520–5.
19. Kim NK, Kim MJ, Yun SH, Sohn SK, Min JS. Comparative study of transrectal ultrasonography, pelvic computerized tomography, and magnetic resonance imaging in preoperative staging of rectal cancer. Dis Colon Rectum. 1999;42:770–5.
20. Scialpi M, Rotondo A, Angelelli G. Water enema transvaginal ultrasound for local staging of stenotic rectal carcinoma. Abdom Imaging. 1999;24:132–6.
21. Garcia-Aguilar J, Pollack J, Lee SH, et al. Accuracy of endorectal ultrasonography in preoperative staging of rectal tumors. Dis Colon Rectum. 2002;45:10–5.
22. Marusch F, Koch A, Schmidt U, et al. Routine use of transrectal ultrasound in rectal carcinoma: results of a prospective multicenter study. Endoscopy. 2002;34:385–90.
23. Nougaret S, Reinhold C, Mikhael HW, Rouanet P, Bibeau F, Brown G. The use of MR imaging in treatment planning for patients with rectal carcinoma: have you checked the "DISTANCE"? Radiology. 2013;268:330–44.
24. Beets-Tan RG, Lambregts DM, Maas M, Bipat S, Barbaro B, Caseiro-Alves F, et al. Magnetic resonance imaging for the clinical management of rectal cancer patients: recommendations from the 2012 European Society of Gastrointestinal and Abdominal Radiology (ESGAR) consensus meeting. Eur Radiol. 2013;23:2522–31.
25. Arya S, Das D, Engineer R, Saklani A. Imaging in rectal cancer with emphasis on local staging with MRI. Indian J Radiol Imaging. 2015;25:148–61.
26. Al-Sukhni E, Milot L, Fruitman M, Beyene J, Victor J, Schmocker S, Brown G, McLeod R, Kennedy E. Diagnostic accuracy of MRI for assessment of T category, lymph node metastases, and circumferential resection margin involvement in patients with rectal cancer: a systematic review and meta-analysis. Ann Surg Oncol. 2012;19:2212–23.
27. Park J, Jang Y, Choi G, Park S, Kim H, Kang H, Cho S. Accuracy of preoperative MRI in predicting pathology stage in rectal cancers: node-for-node matched histopathology validation of MRI features. Dis Colon Rectum. 2014;57:32–8.
28. Skandarajah A, Tjandra J. Preoperative loco-regional imaging in rectal cancer. ANZ J Surg. 2006;76:497–504.
29. Dewhurst C, Rosen M, Blake M, Baker M, Cash B, Fidler J, Greene F, Hindman N, Jones B, Katz D, Lalani T, Miller F, Small W, Sudakoff G, Tulchinsky M, Yaghmai V, Yee J. ACR appropriateness criteria retreatment staging of colorectal cancer. J Am Coll Radiol. 2012;9:775–81.
30. Raman S, Chen Y, Fishman E. Evolution of imaging in rectal cancer: multimodality imaging with MDCT, MRI, and PET. J Gastrointest Oncol. 2015;6:172–84.
31. Whiteford MH, Whiteford HM, Yee LF, Ogunbiyi OA, Dehdashti F, Siegel BA, Birnbaum EH, Fleshman JW, Kodner IJ, Read TE. Usefulness of FDG-PET scan in the assessment of suspected metastatic or recurrent adenocarcinoma of the colon and rectum. Dis Colon Rectum. 2000;53:759–70.
32. Llamas-Elvira JM, Rodríguez-Fernández A, Gutiérrez-Sáinz J, et al. Fluorine-18 fluorodeoxyglucose PET in the preoperative staging of colorectal cancer. Eur J Nucl Med Mol Imaging. 2007;34:859–67.
33. Berger-Kulemann V, Schima W, Baroud S, Koelblinger C, Kaczirek K, Gruenberger T, Schindl M, Maresch J, Weber M,

Ba-Ssalamah A. Gadoxetic acid-enhanced 3.0 T MR imaging versus multidetector-row CT in the detection of colorectal metastases in fatty liver using intraoperative ultrasound and histopathology as a standard of reference. Eur J Surg Oncol. 2012;38:670–6.

34. Jones E, Chezmar J, Nelson R, Bernardino M. The frequency and significance of small (less than or equal to 15 mm) hepatic lesions detected by CT. AJR Am J Roentgenol. 1992;158:535–9.

35. Kirke R, Rajesh A, Verma R, Bankart M. Rectal cancer: incidence of pulmonary metastases on thoracic CT and correlation with T staging. J Comput Assist Tomogr. 2007;31:569–71.

36. Gearhart SL, Frassica D, Rosen R, Choti M, Schulick R, Wahl R. Improved staging with pretreatment positron emission tomography/computed tomography in low rectal cancer. Ann Surg Oncol. 2006;13:397–404.

37. Guillem JG, Ruby JA, Leibold T, Akhurst TJ, Yeung HW, Gollub MJ, Ginsberg MS, Shia J, Suriawinata AA, Riedel ER, Mazumdar M, Saltz LB, Minsky BD, Nash GM, Paty PB, Temple LK, Weiser MR, Larson SM. Neither FDG-PET Nor CT can distinguish between a pathological complete response and an incomplete response after neoadjuvant chemoradiation in locally advanced rectal cancer: a prospective study. Ann Surg. 2013;258(2):289–95.

38. Benson 3rd AB, Venook AP, Bekaii-Saab T, Chan E, Chen YJ, Cooper HS, Engstrom PF, Enzinger PC, Fenton MJ, Fuchs CS, Grem JL, Grothey A, Hochster HS, Hunt S, Kamel A, Kirilcuk N, Leong LA, Lin E, Messersmith WA, Mulcahy MF, Murphy JD, Nurkin S, Rohren E, Ryan DP, Saltz L, Sharma S, Shibata D, Skibber JM, Sofocleous CT, Stoffel EM, Stotsky-Himelfarb E, Willett CG, Gregory KM, Freedman-Cass D. NCCN guidelines for rectal cancer, version 2.2015. J Natl Compr Canc Netw. 2015;13(6):719–28.

28
Rectal Cancer: Neoadjuvant Therapy

Andrea Cercek and Julio Garcia-Aguilar

Key Concepts

- Neoadjuvant radiotherapy is associated with an improvement in local pelvic control following proctectomy for rectal cancer as compared to surgery alone.
- Neoadjuvant chemoradiotherapy is associated with an improvement in local pelvic control and has lower toxicity as compared to postoperative chemoradiotherapy.
- Short-course neoadjuvant radiotherapy has been demonstrated to have similar outcomes in terms of overall survival, disease-free survival, and local pelvic control when compared to long-course neoadjuvant chemoradiotherapy and is associated with lower cost and shorter time to multidrug systemic cytotoxic chemotherapy.
- Current research is focused on limiting the morbidity of therapy, by omitting either proctectomy or radiotherapy in select patients.

Introduction

Neoadjuvant therapy is a critical component of the multidisciplinary treatment of patients with rectal cancer. The objective of neoadjuvant therapy, either radiotherapy, combined chemoradiotherapy, or chemotherapy alone, is to reduce the risk of local recurrence in patients with locally advanced rectal cancer (LARC) undergoing surgical resection. But neoadjuvant therapy provides other potential advantages to rectal cancer patients. It allows early assessment of tumor responsiveness to therapy, which is closely correlated with long-

A. Cercek, M.D.
Department of Medicine, Memorial Sloan Kettering Cancer Center, New York, NY, USA

J. Garcia-Aguilar, M.D., Ph.D. (✉)
Department of Surgery, Memorial Sloan Kettering Cancer Center, 1233 York Avenue, New York, NY 10065, USA
e-mail: garciaaj@mskcc.org

term oncologic outcomes [1–3]. In addition, neoadjuvant therapy could potentially enable the consideration of organ preservation by allowing for more effective local excision and nonoperative management (NOM) strategies. Finally, delivering systemic chemotherapy before surgery in patients at risk for distant metastasis has the potential to improve survival by addressing micrometastatic disease earlier and improving treatment compliance. Maximizing neoadjuvant treatment response can therefore have a profound effect on both oncologic and quality-of-life outcomes.

In this chapter, we will focus primarily on neoadjuvant therapy for LARC, widely accepted to be clinical stage II (cT3–4, cN0) or stage III (any cT, cN1–2) invasive adenocarcinomas of the rectum. We will review various treatment paradigms and the data supporting each.

Historical Context

The story of neoadjuvant radiotherapy and chemoradiotherapy for patients suffering from rectal cancer is long and convoluted, and although much has been published on the topic, there is no universally agreed-upon treatment strategy. It is important for the reader to understand how we arrived at our current state of affairs so that the data from published trials can be put in the proper context.

The concept of neoadjuvant therapy for rectal cancer was first introduced by Janeway and Quick in c. 1917, who noted significant tumor response when gold filtered radon emanation seeds were implanted directly into rectal cancers [4]. In the era when the surgical mortality and morbidity for a rectal cancer operation was prohibitive, contact radiation with emanation seeds containing radium salts or radon was explored as a curative treatment. Surgery was considered a salvage procedure for patients with tumors resistant to radiation [5]. As surgery became safer and the limitations of contact radiation as the only treatment modality became apparent, radiation lost its role as a primary treatment and became an adjuvant to surgical resection. In fact, for many years, proctectomy alone became standard treatment for rectal cancer. It was eventually realized that the outcomes of surgery alone were often suboptimal, with 5-year local recurrence rates in published trials of 25–30 % [6–8]. It was demonstrated that adjuvant chemoradiotherapy improved oncologic outcomes, and in 1990 the National Institutes of Health advocated adjuvant external beam radiotherapy and chemotherapy for patients with stage II and stage III tumors [9]. In the United States, except for a few select referral centers, upfront proctectomy followed by selective postoperative chemoradiotherapy was the regimen utilized for most patients. However, postoperative radiotherapy is associated with relatively high toxicity and is poorly tolerated by many patients. Investigators in Europe and select US centers explored utilizing neoadjuvant radiotherapy and chemoradiotherapy, and eventually the benefits of administering radiotherapy in the preoperative period were demonstrated. In response to these data, many US clinicians simply moved the chemoradiotherapy package from the postoperative to the preoperative period. It is puzzling that, although much of the data demonstrating the benefits of neoadjuvant radiotherapy came from trials of short-course radiotherapy, and neoadjuvant short-course radiotherapy has been demonstrated to have similar oncologic outcomes as neoadjuvant long-course chemoradiotherapy in two prospective randomized trials [10, 11], the use of short-course radiotherapy has been limited in the United States.

At the same time that neoadjuvant radiotherapy was demonstrated to be more effective and less toxic than postoperative radiotherapy, there was a realization that oncologic outcomes following proctectomy for rectal cancer were highly technique dependent [12]. Wide variability in outcomes was seen, depending on who did the operation and how it was performed. So once again the wheel of opinion turned full circle, with some surgeons arguing that radiotherapy primarily compensated for "sloppy" surgery and that there was no need for the patient with non-fixed tumors to undergo radiotherapy if proctectomy was performed properly. Data from the Dutch Rectal Cancer trial and others, however, suggested that the oncologic benefits of neoadjuvant radiotherapy and good surgical technique were additive, not compensatory, with regard to pelvic control [13].

Clinicians are aware that therapies for rectal cancer are morbid and unfortunately the most effective treatment, proctectomy is associated witht he greatest chance of lasting morbidity. We continue to search for treatment regimens in which morbidity can be lessened while preserving the chance for cure, especially in patients with non-fixed tumors. Definitive chemoradiotherapy, or local excision +/− adjuvant chemoradiotherapy, would avoid proctectomy. Chemotherapy regimens are now more effective, and there is interest in upfront proctectomy in patients with mesorectal margins that are not threatened based on preoperative imaging followed by selective use of postoperative chemotherapy. In addition, there is interest in the use of neoadjuvant chemotherapy alone. Both of these strategies would avoid the toxicity of radiotherapy. Another approach that has been utilized extensively in Europe and in select US centers is to administer neoadjuvant short-course radiotherapy, followed by proctectomy and selective use of postoperative chemotherapy. The three aforementioned strategies allow the patient to receive effective systemic chemotherapy faster than the regimen commonly employed in the United States—long-course chemoradiotherapy (in which the patient receives only a radiosensitizing chemotherapeutic agent) followed by delayed proctectomy. This concept has intrinsic appeal, given that most patients with rectal cancer who ultimately fail treatment succumb to distant metastatic disease, not local pelvic recurrence, and that the benefit of neoadjuvant radiotherapy has primarily been to improve pelvic control without improvement in overall survival.

One of the difficulties in constructing guidelines for treatment of patients with rectal cancer is that treatment decisions must take into account multiple variables: tumor fixation, circumferential position in the rectum, relation to the pelvic floor musculature, pelvic morphology, clinical T and N stage, presence of symptoms, presence of metastases, continence status, planned operation, etc. It is virtually impossible to publish straightforward guidelines that account for all of these variables. At present, the clinician caring for the patient with rectal cancer must have a firm grasp of the rationale for, and the data supporting, any proposed treatment algorithm and be facile enough to tailor recommendations for therapy based on the characteristics of the patient and the tumor.

Postoperative Radiotherapy

Although currently out of favor, one of the advantages of the strategy of upfront proctectomy followed by selective chemoradiotherapy is that the exact stage of the tumor is known prior to initiation of radiotherapy, and radiation can be avoided in patients with early-stage tumors who may not derive benefit. A number of studies demonstrated that surgery followed by radiation, delivered in 180–200 cGy a day for a total dose of 45–50 Gy, was more effective than surgery alone in achieving local control in patients with stage II or III rectal cancer [14]. The Gastrointestinal Tumor Study Group (GITSG) trial was aimed to accrue 520 patients with rectal cancer located within 12 cm from the anal verge, extending to the perirectal fat or metastasizing to the regional lymph nodes, with no evidence of distant metastasis. After recovery from surgery, patients who had a complete resection were randomized to one of four arms: observation, postoperative radiation (40–48 Gy of total radiation in 1.8 or 2 Gy fractions), chemotherapy (bolus infusion 5-FU and semustine for 18 months), or radiation plus chemotherapy [6]. The study was terminated after 227 patients had been accrued because interim analysis showed statistical differences between treatment arms. The combined modality therapy was superior to resection alone in preventing recurrence (33 % vs. 55 %; $p=0.42$). Radiation and chemotherapy and chemotherapy were also associated with lower risk of recurrence compared to surgery alone, but the differences did not reach statistical significance [6]. A larger study from Denmark found that the probability of survival without local recurrence was higher when patients with Dukes' B or C rectal cancer received postoperative radiation, compared to surgery alone. The risk of distant metastasis was not influenced by radiation [15]. The Medical Research Council Rectal Cancer Group trial also demonstrated that postoperative radiotherapy reduced the risk of local recurrence with patients with mobile Dukes' stage B or C rectal cancer, without increasing the risk of serious late bowel complications. In this study, radiation did not affect the risk of distant metastasis or overall survival [16]. Finally, the NSABP-R02 protocol found that radiotherapy added to chemotherapy, either 5-FU/LV or 5-FU, semustine, and vincristine, reduced the risk of locoregional recurrence compared to chemotherapy alone in patients with Dukes' B or C rectal cancer [17].

Preoperative Radiotherapy

A number of prospective trials randomizing patients to preoperative radiation and surgery versus surgery alone provided mixed results [14–18]. These studies used variable total radiation doses, fractionation schemas, number of beams, portals, target volumes, radiation, and surgery. In general, only studies that use higher biologically equivalent radiation doses and a higher number of beams proved to reduce local recurrence in patients treated with preoperative radiation compared to surgery alone. The Swedish Rectal Cancer trial demonstrated that short-course preoperative radiation (25 Gy of radiation delivered in 5 equal doses in 5 consecutive days) improved not only local recurrence but also overall survival [7]. However, this study was later criticized because surgery was not standardized and the rate of local recurrence in the control arm was considered high for those years' standards. The Dutch Rectal Cancer trial (CKVO 95-04) was the first to prove that preoperative radiation also reduced the risk of local recurrence rate in patients having optimal surgery according to the principles of total mesorectal excision [13]. The study compared preoperative radiotherapy (5 Gy×5) followed by quality-controlled TME with TME alone. In this study, the rate of local recurrence in the TME-only arm was substantially lower compared with patient treated with surgery alone in previous trials. Despite the improved surgical technique in both arms, the rate of local recurrence at 5 years was reduced from 10.9 % in the surgery-only group to 5.6 % in the radiotherapy plus surgery group ($p<0.001$). While no benefit in overall survival was observed for the entire group, the 12-year updated results demonstrated that preoperative short-term radiotherapy

significantly improved 10-year survival in patients with stage III disease and negative circumferential margins, and the benefit in terms of local control persisted [19].

Radiosensitizing Agents

Further improvements in local tumor control have been achieved by adding systemic chemotherapy to radiotherapy. Numerous chemotherapeutic agents including fluoropyrimidines (5FU) and capecitabine; irinotecan, oxaliplatin, and antiepidermal growth factor agents; and cetuximab and panitumumab have been tested in the neoadjuvant setting with radiotherapy. With the exception of fluoropyrimidines, however, none have been effectively validated in prospective trials.

Fluoropyrimidines

5-Fluorouracil (5-FU) is the primary agent for radiosensitization in rectal cancer. While its potential to create a state of radiosensitivity was recognized early on, numerous studies eventually led to the understanding that 5-FU's benefit was linked to the schedule of its administration. 5-FU must be present after radiation exposure to establish the radiosensitive state, and for this reason, bolus 5-FU quickly fell out of favor and continuous venous infusion (CVI) 5-FU 225 mg/m^2 daily became the standard [18, 20].

The GITSG proved the overall benefit of combining chemotherapy with postoperative radiation in patients with Dukes' B and C rectal cancer [6]. The North Central Cancer Treatment Group (NCCTG) study compared postoperative radiotherapy with 5-FU administered either as a bolus or as CVI. Patients in the NCCTG trial also received two months of systemic chemotherapy before and after the combined chemotherapy and radiation [21]. This study showed that CVI was associated with a significant decrease in the overall rate of local tumor relapse and distant metastasis, compared to bolus infusion of 5-FU during radiation [21]. Other trials from the Intergroup consortia have shown that CVI 5-FU was associated with lower hematologic toxicity compared to bolus 5-FU [22].

The European Organization for Research and Treatment of Cancer (EORTC) protocol 22921 was developed to assess the effect of adding chemotherapy (CT) to preoperative RT and the value of postoperative chemotherapy in LARC [23]. One thousand and eleven patients were randomized across four arms: (a) preoperative radiotherapy, (b) preoperative radiotherapy plus bolus 5-FU and leucovorin, (c) preoperative radiotherapy followed by postoperative CT, and (d) preoperative radiotherapy and bolus 5-FU and leucovorin followed by postoperative chemotherapy. Five-year local recurrence was significantly lower in all three arms receiving any form of chemotherapy (pre- or postoperative) compared to radiotherapy alone, though there was no significant improvement in survival. Additional work by the Federation Francophone de la Cancerologie Digestive demonstrated that the addition of 5-FU to RT improves local control but not survival, consistent with the EORTC 22921 trial data [24]. More recently, in a randomized phase III trial, Hofheinz and colleagues were able to show non-inferiority of capecitabine, the oral prodrug of fluorouracil, when compared to 5-FU, providing us a convenient treatment alternative for reliable and motivated patients [25]. The equivalence of capecitabine and 5-FU has also been corroborated with the NSABP-R04 cohort [26].

Oxaliplatin

A number of large phase III trials have evaluated the potential role of oxaliplatin to increase radiosensitivity. The STAR-01 [27], the ACCORD 12/0405-PRODIGE2 [28], and the NSABP-R04 [26] trial each investigated the addition of oxaliplatin to a fluoropyrimidine as radiosensitizing agents. This combination, however, resulted in greater toxicity with no improvement in therapy. Conversely, the CAO/ARO/AIO-04 trial [28] found that the inclusion of oxaliplatin to a 5-FU-based CRT regimen led to a higher pCR rate, with no increase in toxicity [29]. While encouraging, their 5-FU dosing and schedule differed between the control arm and the arm with oxaliplatin, which could have affected the outcomes. At this point, oxaliplatin is not routinely included in the neoadjuvant regimens currently used for rectal cancer.

Irinotecan

This topoisomerase inhibitor has shown significant antitumor activity in metastatic colorectal cancer. While there have been small phase II trials to show that irinotecan may be effective and safe as an adjunct to traditional 5-FU and radiotherapy [30, 31], there has not yet been any trial to show its efficacy over 5-FU and radiotherapy alone.

EGFR Inhibitors

The success and efficacy of anti-EGFR agents like cetuximab and panitumumab in KRAS wild-type metastatic colorectal cancer have brought about a number of studies evaluating its use in the preoperative treatment of LARC. Response rates when EGFR inhibitors are used in the neoadjuvant setting with other agents and radiotherapy have been inconsistent, sometimes positive [32], but mostly equivocal or negative [33, 34]. Some studies have found worse response with their use, which suggests there may be mechanisms of response in tumors to these combined modality treatments that are not yet understood. EGFR inhibitors are not used in the setting of neoadjuvant chemoradiation.

Preoperative Versus Postoperative Radiation

Although there was once great debate on this subject, the preponderance of the evidence supports the use of neoadjuvant radiotherapy versus postoperative adjuvant radiotherapy. The rationale for this approach is logical: neoadjuvant radiotherapy requires less of a dose to achieve the same biologic effect, most likely due to the absence of postoperative scarring and tissue hypoxia in the pelvis. In addition the toxicity, both short term and long term, of neoadjuvant therapy is markedly reduced compared to postoperative radiotherapy, especially when the patient undergoes neorectal reconstruction. Lastly, the proportion of patients who can complete that therapy is markedly improved when radiotherapy is administered in the preoperative period. A small Scandinavian trial comparing preoperative short-course radiation (25.5 Gy in 1 week) for all rectal cancer patients with prolonged postoperative radiation (60 Gy in sever or 8 weeks) for patients with tumors that penetrated into the perirectal fat and/or involved the regional lymph nodes demonstrated that local recurrence was lower after preoperative radiation (13 % vs. 22 %), but survival was similar in both groups. Morbidity was also similar in both groups [35]. The RTOG 94-01 trial aimed to compare preoperative and postoperative CRT but closed after having accrued only 53 of the intended 770 patients. Similarly the National Surgical Adjuvant Breast and Bowel Project (NSABP R-03) also validated the role of neoadjuvant 5-FU-based chemoradiotherapy for LARC. While this study also failed to meet the accrual goal of 900 patients, the analysis of the 267 patients randomized before closure suggested that the preoperative CRT arm had better disease-free survival and probably better overall survival, but similar local recurrence compared to the postoperative arm [36].

The landmark German Rectal Cancer Study (CAO/ARO/AIO-94) compared pre- and postoperative chemoradiotherapy in 823 patients with LARC [37]. The local recurrence rate after 5 years was lower in the preoperative treatment group, 6 % vs. 13 % ($p = 0.006$), while overall survival and the frequency of distant metastases were not significantly different. Importantly, preoperative chemoradiotherapy was associated with a lower risk of grade 3 or 4 toxicities (27 %) compared to postoperative chemoradiation (40 %) [37]. Based on these studies, a commonly employed treatment paradigm for LARC is preoperative 5-FU-based chemoradiotherapy, followed by proctectomy and additional 5-FU-based adjuvant chemotherapy. Specifically, patients receive combined radiation (180 cGy/day/5 days a week for 5 weeks followed by a 540 cGy boost) and chemotherapy (either continuous infusion 5-FU or capecitabine), followed by proctectomy 6–8 weeks later, and postoperative systemic adjuvant chemotherapy, usually mFOLFOX6. In this treatment paradigm, now considered

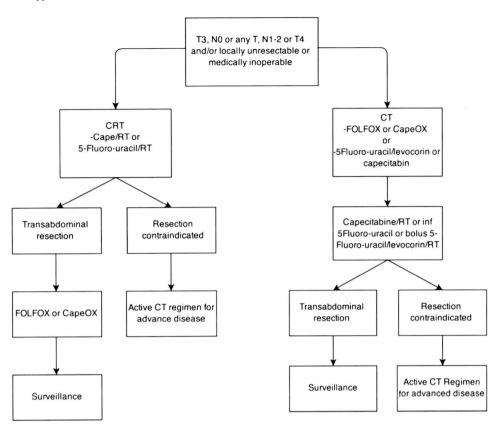

FIGURE 28-1. National Comprehensive Cancer Network guidelines for locally advanced rectal cancer. Permission from JCO/NCCN (*Cape* capecitabine, *CapeOx* capecitabine plus oxaliplatin, *CRT* chemoradiation, *CT* chemotherapy, *FLOX* fluorouracil, leucovorin, and oxaliplatin, *FOLFOX* infusional fluorouracil, leucovorin, and oxaliplatin; FU, fluorouracil, *inf.* infusional, *LR* local recurrence, *LV* leucovorin, *MRF* mesorectal fascia, *RT* radiotherapy, *TME* total mesorectal excision). With permission from Neoadjuvant chemoradiation therapy and pathological complete response in rectal cancer. Gastroenterology Report. Gastroenterol Rep 2015 doi: 10.1093/gastro/gov039. http://gastro.oxfordjournals.org/content/early/2015/08/19/gastro.gov039.full. Copyright © 2015 Oxford University Press and Digestive Science Publishing Co. Limited.

standard practice in the United States (Figure 28-1), imaging has become increasingly important for preoperative tumor staging and patient selection.

Short- Versus Long-Course Preoperative Radiotherapy

The effectiveness of radiation depends on the balance between the cytotoxicity against cancer and the preservation of adjacent normal tissues. There is now evidence of a dose-response relationship with radiotherapy, with an improved cytotoxic effect with higher total doses of radiation. However, the total dose of radiation depends on the dose per fraction and the number of fractions, the dose-fractionation schedule. But the dose per fraction and the number of fractions used in clinical practice vary widely. To compare different dose fractionation schedules, radiation therapists have introduced the concept of biologically equivalent doses. The most common dose-fractionation schedules used in rectal cancer, 1.8–2 Gy per day, 5 days per week for 5 weeks (usually in combination with a fluoropyrimidine) and 5 Gy as day for 5 consecutive days, are considered biologically equivalent. The advantages and disadvantages of each one of these regimens have been the subject of a heated debate. Proponents of long-course chemoradiotherapy point to a greater tumor

response, although this may be an artifact of the greater time delay prior to proctectomy typically utilized after long-course chemoradiotherapy (typically 6–8 weeks) as compared to after short-course radiotherapy (typically 1 week). Those in favor of short-course radiation argue that improved patient convenience, lower cost, reduced toxicity in the neoadjuvant treatment period, and faster time to effective systemic chemotherapy are important advantages. Two trials have compared these two approaches directly.

Bujko and colleagues prospectively compared the two regimens, randomizing 316 patients with clinical T3 or T4 disease to either neoadjuvant long-course chemoradiotherapy or neoadjuvant short-course radiotherapy, and found that long-course chemoradiotherapy was associated with a significantly decreased incidence of positive radial margins (4.4 % vs. 12.9 %, $p=0.017$) and a higher rate of pCR (0.7 % vs. 16.1 %), but this did not carry over into a significant difference in pelvic control, disease-free survival, or overall survival [10]. Moreover, they reported greater radiation toxicity in the long-course chemoradiotherapy group and poorer compliance to treatment schedule. Their conclusion was that short-course radiotherapy was a viable alternative to long-course chemoradiotherapy with neither holding a long-term oncologic advantage, but with short-course radiotherapy potentially benefiting from lower cost and lower morbidity associated with its use. More recently, theTrans Tasman Radiation Oncology Group 01.04 randomized 326 patients with ERUS- or MRI-staged T3, N0–2, M0 tumors to short-course radiotherapy and surgery followed by 6 months of adjuvant chemotherapy or chemoradiotherapy and surgery followed by 4 months of adjuvant chemotherapy [11]. Their study was powered to detect a 10 % difference in local recurrence at 3 years, with a 5 % level of significance. Similar to the work of Bujko et al., the Trans Tasman trial found no difference in pelvic control, disease-free survival, and overall survival between the groups. Patient imbalances between groups have been called to attention, with fewer patients with low rectal cancers in chemoradiotherapy than the short-course radiotherapy arms (which would bias the results in favor of the chemoradiotherapy group) and varying rates of APR. The quality of surgery and accuracy of MRI staging have also been criticized [38, 39]. Nevertheless, two prospective randomized trials have demonstrated no obvious oncologic differences between neoadjuvant long-course chemoradiotherapy and neoadjuvant short-course radiotherapy.

The short-course and long-course divide has remained somewhat static across national boundaries, with a Western preference for long-course chemoradiotherapy and a majority of European countries favoring short-course radiotherapy. It is puzzling that, except for a few expert centers, short-course radiotherapy has not been embraced by US physicians. One could argue that it is the best-studied neoadjuvant radiotherapy regimen, with demonstrated efficacy in prospective randomized trials of neoadjuvant radiotherapy versus surgery alone, and shortens the time to administration of full-dose adjuvant cytotoxic chemotherapy.

Because of a current trend exploring the incorporation of therapies traditionally reserved for the adjuvant period into the neoadjuvant regimen, combinations of either short-course radiotherapy or long-course chemoradiotherapy with systemic therapies are being explored and gaining greater traction. Therefore, it may never be clearly determined whether short-course or long-course RT is more effective as independent modalities.

Impact of Pelvic Radiotherapy on Quality of Life

Another advantage of preoperative radiotherapy is the potential ability to downstage tumors and to increase the potential for sphincter-sparing surgery, which can improve long-term quality of life for patients with low-lying rectal cancers [37]. The issue of sphincter salvage, however, is complicated. As one might imagine, the assessment of whether a restorative proctectomy could possibly be performed based on initial evaluation of a patient is somewhat subjective. In addition, given that radiotherapy does not kill tumor in a wave front, and that multiple studies have demonstrated residual tumor scattered throughout the bed of the initial volume of tissue involved with the tumor, many surgeons would argue that

changing the operation based on the clinically observed effect of radiotherapy is potentially dangerous. However, by improving the chances of an R0 resection and decreasing the rates of local recurrence, which can be associated with significant morbidity, radiotherapy can improve long-term quality of life. Nevertheless, pelvic radiotherapy remains associated with significant short- and long-term side effects. Overall short-term toxicity has been reported in as many as 50 % of patients [40]. Long-term side effects of pelvic radiotherapy include fibrosis and autonomic nerve injury, which can lead to bowel and bladder dysfunction, sexual dysfunction, and infertility due to hormonal effects and uterine incompetence. Moreover, because the pelvis is an active site of bone marrow function, patients who undergo pelvic irradiation can suffer from diminished hematopoiesis.

Adjuvant Systemic Chemotherapy in Patients Treated with Chemoradiotherapy and Proctectomy

Although prevention of local recurrences is important for patients' quality of life, most patients with rectal cancer succumb to metastatic disease. Consequently, similar to patients with stage III colon cancer, patients with LARC patients treated with neoadjuvant chemoradiotherapy and proctectomy are considered for postoperative adjuvant chemotherapy independent of the histologic tumor stage in the proctectomy specimen [41]. Patients with clinical stage II and III rectal cancer treated with preoperative chemoradiotherapy and proctectomy usually receive 5-FU or capecitabine plus oxaliplatin-based adjuvant chemotherapy [41]. While the use of postoperative adjuvant chemotherapy in rectal cancer is not supported unequivocally by a prospective randomized trial, a recent meta-analysis of 21 randomized controlled trials concluded that postoperative 5-FU-based chemotherapy is effective in patients with LARC [42].

In spite of these recommendations, up to 27 % of eligible LARC patients never start adjuvant chemotherapy and less than 50 % [43] receive the full prescribed treatment without interruptions or delay [23, 29] due to postoperative complications, slow recovery, interference with closure of their temporary ileostomy [44], or simply treatment refusal [45]. A systematic review of ten studies including more than 15,000 patients evaluated the effect of timing on the efficacy of postoperative adjuvant chemotherapy and demonstrated that each 4-week delay in treatment correlated with a 14 % decrease in OS [46].

It is interesting to note that, despite the common practice of administering chemotherapy, a recent meta-analysis of adjuvant chemotherapy in LARC did not demonstrate a survival benefit. In total 1196 patients with stage II or III disease and R0 resection were evaluated; 598 were observed while 598 received adjuvant chemotherapy [47]. However, of the four studies included in the analysis, only one used oxaliplatin in combination with fluorouracil, the CHRONICLE trial which contributed only 75 patients to this analysis [48]. Moreover, completion of planned chemotherapy was low in all of the studies (43–76 %). This low adherence could certainly have affected the results [47].

Due to the low rate of completion of planned adjuvant therapy, splitting adjuvant chemotherapy and delivering a limited number of cycles pre-chemoradiotherapy, then delivering the remaining cycles postsurgery, has been proposed to increase tumor response in LARC patients. A number of randomized phase II trials have reported mixed results, without clear survival advantage for the split neoadjuvant or the postoperative regimen [48–52].

Another potential approach is to deliver all chemotherapy upfront. This neoadjuvant chemotherapy has several potential advantages compared to the standard adjuvant chemotherapy; it theoretically treats occult micrometastasis several months earlier and increases treatment compliance, potentially enhancing the efficacy of chemotherapy and ultimately improving survival [53, 54]. Other benefits of neoadjuvant chemotherapy include increased response of the primary tumor, early identification of nonresponders, and earlier removal of the loop ileostomy. A recent study at Memorial Sloan Kettering Cancer Center (MSKCC) investigated the safety and efficacy of FOLFOX before CRT, demonstrating excellent treatment compliance and no evidence of serious adverse effects requiring treatment delay. All patients undergoing proctectomy had an R0 resection, and nearly half had a tumor response greater than 90 % including 30 % who had either a pCR or a clinical complete response (cCR) [55]. Induction chemotherapy before chemoradiation and proctectomy is now considered as a valid alternative to the more widely accepted neoadjuvant chemoradiation, proctectomy, and postoperative systemic chemotherapy (Figure 28-1).

Chemotherapy can also be delivered as consolidation (after chemoradiotherapy completion and before surgery). The Timing of Rectal Cancer Response to Chemoradiation Trial, which completed accrual in 2012, showed that delivering 2, 4, or 6 cycles of FOLFOX after chemoradiotherapy in LARC patients increased the pCR rates up to 25 %, 30 %, and 38 %, respectively, compared to CRT alone (18 %), without any associated increase in adverse events or surgical complications [56]. Eighty percent of patients received consolidation chemotherapy without interruption. These studies suggest that delivering systemic chemotherapy in the neoadjuvant setting, both before or after chemoradiotherapy, is well tolerated and has potential advantages for the patient. Although solid data from large prospective studies are still lacking, in the most recent edition of the NCCN guidelines, neoadjuvant chemotherapy is contemplated as an option for the treatment of LARC patients. However, none of these studies have reported long-term oncologic outcomes.

Setting the Right Limits

Chemoradiotherapy has clearly proved itself useful at improving local tumor control in patients with LARC. We find that the weight of evidence is also demonstrating that systemic chemotherapy—when applied in the neoadjuvant setting—is able to similarly control tumor progression, possibly acting on micrometastatic disease to improve distant control. But while the benefits of these intensive neoadjuvant regimens are alluring, they have also sparked a heated debate about whether all patients require such intensive treatment. The oncologic success in treating LARC has been achieved at the cost of significant morbidity and compromised quality of life [40]. The task before us is to develop treatment approaches that maximize oncological outcome while preserving quality of life by minimizing morbidity associated with this intense multimodality approach [57]. Do all patients with LARC really require chemoradiotherapy, chemotherapy, and proctectomy? The necessity of this intense multimodality approach is called into question.

The European Approach

In a number of European countries, the "right limits" have been framed around MRI-based measures of tumor aggressiveness. A risk stratification system that covers all rectal cancers and that incorporates the proximity of the primary rectal cancer to the mesorectal fascia, the depth of tumor invasion, the presence of metastatic lymph nodes, and the presence of venous invasion are used to classify LARC into "the good," "the bad," and "the ugly" [58, 59]. For the low-risk, "good" tumors, proctectomy alone is recommended; for intermediate-risk "bad" tumors, the recommendation is short-course radiotherapy followed by proctectomy; and for high-risk "ugly" tumors, chemoradiotherapy followed by proctectomy is recommended (Table 28-1). These MRI-based risk stratification schemas have been incorporated into clinical practice guidelines and clinical trial design (e.g., Expert-C and RAPIDO). However, the treatment approach guided by MRI risk categorization is based on prospective observational studies conducted in institutions with significant expertise in rectal cancer and has not been tested in prospective randomized trials.

Selected Adjuvant Systemic Chemotherapy

Many LARC patients experience variable degrees of response to chemoradiotherapy, and tumor response is now one of the most important prognosticators in LARC patients [2, 57]. The need for adjuvant chemotherapy in patients with a complete or near-complete response after chemoradiotherapy has been questioned [60–62]. Recent work from a multi-institutional, retrospective analysis of 3133 patients shows that the benefit of adjuvant therapy differs between LARC subgroups. For example, patients with ypT1-2 or ypT3-4 tumors benefitted

TABLE 28-1. European/Scandinavian model of stratification for patients with locally advanced rectal cancer based on magnetic resonance imaging and subsequent treatment decisions

Risk	Treatment
Low risk	
• T1–T3 (<5 mm) mid-/upper rectum	Total mesorectal incision (TME)
• T1–T3 (superficial) lower rectum	
• N0	
• Extramural vascular invasion: no mesorectal fascia clear	
• Risk of local recurrence <10%	
Intermediate risk	
T3 (<5 mm)	• Preoperative short course radiation
T4 (posterior vaginal wall only), or N1/2, or	• Total mesorectal excision
Extramural vascular invasion: yes	• Adjuvant chemotherapy
Mesorectal fascia clear (<1 mm)	
Risk of local recurrence: 10–20 %	
High risk	
T4 (other than posterior vaginal wall)	• Preoperative chemoradiation
N01/2	• Total mesorectal excision
Mesorectal fascia involved	• Adjuvant chemotherapy
Risk of local recurrence >20 %	

Modified from Smith JJ, Garcia-Aguilar J. Advances and challenges in treatment of locally advanced rectal cancer. J Clin Oncol 2005

the most from adjuvant therapy compared with ypT0N0 patients [63]. Some centers now use postoperative chemotherapy selectively based on tumor response to chemoradiotherapy. In the recently published ADORE phase II trial, which examined use of selective adjuvant chemotherapy, LARC patients with ypT3-4N0 or ypTanyN1-2 tumors after fluoropyrimidine-based chemoradiotherapy were randomized to adjuvant chemotherapy with either 4 cycles of 5-FU and LV or 8 cycles of FOLFOX. The administration of FOLFOX after surgery was associated with prolonged progression-free survival in stage III patients but not in stage II patients. Additionally, FOLFOX was associated with a prolonged overall survival for both stage II/III rectal cancer patients [64]. Identification of those patients who will most likely to derive benefit from adjuvant treatment will be better informed by carefully conducted correlative studies that more accurately delineate molecular, pathologic, and clinical markers of resistance.

Chemotherapy Only to Improve Local Tumor Control

The risk of local pelvic failure in LARC depends on tumor stage, but also on the distance of the tumor from the anal verge and the proximity of the tumor from the mesorectal fascia [13, 65]. Upper rectal tumors away from the mesorectal fascia have a low risk of local recurrence when treated with proctectomy. The added benefit of radiotherapy in these patients has been questioned [40, 66, 67]. A growing body of evidence suggests that radiotherapy could be safely avoided in patients with

intermediate-risk rectal cancer (e.g., rectal cancers located between 5 and 12 cm from the anal verge that do not threaten the mesorectal fascia) on MRI [68, 69]. In a pilot phase II trial conducted at MSKCC, 32 patients with resectable, clinically staged II–III rectal cancer were treated with preoperative FOLFOX/anti-VEGF and selective chemoradiotherapy, based on tumor response. The 30 patients who completed preoperative chemotherapy had tumor regression and underwent proctectomy without preoperative chemoradiotherapy. Eight (27 %) had pathologic complete responses. No local recurrences were noted at 4 years, and an 84 % disease-free survival was achieved [70]. Given these data, a large multicenter phase II/III study is currently accruing patients. In the CALGB PROSPECT Study (Preoperative Radiation Or Selective Preoperative Evaluation of Chemotherapy and TME) [71], patients are randomized to either the standard arm (chemoradiotherapy, surgery, and adjuvant FOLFOX chemotherapy) or the selective arm with FOLFOX×6 cycles, evaluation of response followed by surgery or standard therapy with chemoradiotherapy if the reduction in the primary tumor is <20 % (Figure 28-2). Eligible patients must have biopsy-proven adenocarcinoma with the primary tumor located 5–12 cm from the anal verge. They must be candidates for sphincter-sparing surgery. The primary outcomes of the phase II component are R0 resection rate and time to local recurrence. The primary endpoints of the phase III components are time to local recurrence and disease-free survival. The selective chemoradiation arm will be favored if either the disease-free survival is superior compared to the standard arm or if it is non-inferior to the standard arm for both disease-free survival and local recurrence. In addition to this study, there is currently an ongoing study, the GEMCAD study, on induction chemotherapy with or without chemoradiation in intermediate-risk rectal cancer defined by MRI. This study was presented in abstract form in the 2010 annual ASCO meeting; the final data have not yet been presented [72]. In this study which is no longer accruing patients, patients with T3 or T1–2N1 tumors based on MRI were treated with bevacizumab and CapeOX (capecitabine and oxaliplatin) for three cycles followed by repeat MRI evaluation. Those patients with response went on to proctectomy, while nonresponders received standard chemoradiotherapy. A third study is a phase II randomized study of neoadjuvant FOLFOX/bevacizumab versus FOLFOXIRI/bevacizumab in patients with high-risk rectal cancer as defined by MRI. This study is not yet open to accrual but will also add insight into the response of the primary rectal tumor to chemotherapy alone [73]. These studies will provide important insight into the potential for a more individualized treatment approach through selective use of radiation in LARC.

Selective Nonoperative Management

Proctectomy is the cornerstone of the treatment algorithm for LARC patients. However, up to 33 % of LARC patients treated with neoadjuvant chemoradiotherapy exhibit

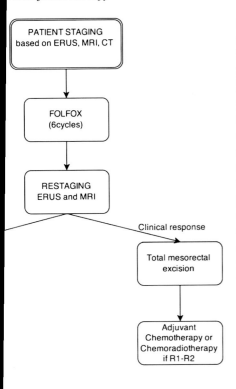

PATIENT STAGING
based on ERUS, MRI, CT

↓

FOLFOX
(6cycles)

↓

RESTAGING
ERUS and MRI

Clinical response

Total mesorectal
excision

↓

Adjuvant
Chemotherapy or
Chemoradiotherapy
if R1-R2

PECT (Chemotherapy Alone or Chemotherapy
apy in Treating Patients with Locally Advanced
Surgery) trial schema. A phase II/III randomized
aluate the impact of selective use of radiotherapy
selective use of chemoradiation for patients with
tal cancer. (*FOLFOX* infusional fluorouracil, leu-
atin, *LAR* low anterior resection, *FUCMT* fluo-
abine plus radiotherapy, *TME* total mesorectal
mission from Neoadjuvant chemoradiation ther-
gical complete response in rectal cancer.
eport. Gastroenterol Rep 2015 doi: 10.1093/
   http://gastro.oxfordjournals.org/content/early/
ov039.full. Copyright © 2015 Oxford University
Science Publishing Co. Limited.

plete response (pCR) at the time of surgical
]. Patients with a pCR have improved onco-
ith local recurrence rates of less than 1 % and
rate of over 90 % [3, 76], leading us to ques-
enefit of proctectomy for these patients. The
f avoiding proctectomy—reduced morbidity,
quality of life, and potential reduction of
ses—could be significant. The current chal-
ccurately identifying which patients have
and could safely avoid proctectomy [77].
es not always correlate with pCR, and cur-
odalities cannot distinguish with certainty
from tissue fibrosis [78, 79], a number of
reported their experience with the selective

use of an organ-preserving or NOM approach in patients with
a complete clinical response after chemoradiotherapy (Table
28-2) [80–84]. The largest experience with the NOM approach
to rectal cancer comes from Habr-Gama's group in Sao Paulo,
Brazil [80–82]. Patients with persistent tumor underwent
proctectomy; those with a complete clinical response were
enrolled in a strict follow-up protocol. Patients with evidence
of tumor relapse were directed to surgery, while patients with
a sustained complete clinical response after 1 year continued
surveillance every 3 months for an additional year and every 6
months thereafter. Twenty-seven percent of rectal cancer
patients treated according to this protocol had a sustained
complete clinical response and were spared from proctectomy.
Of the patients who survived 1 year following treatment and
did not show any evidence of tumor progression, local recurrence during follow-up developed in 10 %, but all had proctectomy with curative intent. The oncologic results in this NOM
group were equivalent to those of patients who had a pathologic complete response after proctectomy. However, the
authors did not evaluate patients on an intention-to-treat basis.
By excluding those patients who failed treatment during the
first year, results were heavily biased in favor of the NOM
group. A group from Maastricht University in the Netherlands
reported their NOM experience in 21 patients with complete
clinical response as determined by clinical exam, MRI, and
endoscopic biopsy among 192 patients treated with chemoradiotherapy between 2004 and 2010 [83]. After a mean follow-
up of 25 ± 19 months, 1 patient developed LR, but was able to
undergo curative salvage surgery. The other 20 patients are
alive without disease. Outcomes in patients with complete
clinical response treated according to the NOM protocol were
similar to outcomes of patients with a pathologic complete
response after proctectomy. At MSKCC, rectal cancer patients
with a complete clinical response have been managed under
an NOM strategy since 2006. Of the 32 patients starting treatment before 2010 who were followed for a median of 23
months, 6 patients developed relapse, and all underwent salvage surgery with curative intent; additionally, 3 of these
patients also developed distant metastases [84]. The combined
experience of these series suggests that NOM may be an
alternative approach to proctectomy in highly select patients
with distal rectal cancer who achieve a complete clinical
response to neoadjuvant therapy (Table 28-2). However, the
safety and efficacy of the NOM approach outside of centers
specializing in the treatment of rectal cancer is controversial.
It is now clear that even with strict complete clinical response
definitions, some patients will later develop local recurrence,
emphasizing the importance of close surveillance, because the
success of this approach relies on the early diagnosis of recurrences and timely salvage therapy. In addition, the risk of distant metastases in patients with an apparent complete clinical
response that develop local tumor regrowth and subsequent
outcomes is unknown. Therefore, at the present time, the
NOM of rectal cancer should be considered experimental.

The design of large, prospective randomized trials investigating the efficacy of the NOM approach is challenging,

TABLE 28-2. Summary of the most representative series, nonoperative vs. operative management of LARC after CRT

Series	# cCRs	%	Mean interval to LR	# Patients	OS NOM Survival	%	OS Operative arm Survival	%	DFS NOM Survival	%
Habr-Gama et al. [80]	71	27	60	2	5 years	100	5 years	88	5 years	92
Habr-Gama et al. [81]	90	49	17	28	5 years	91	NA		5 years	68
Maas et al. [83]	21	11	22	1	2 years	100	2 years	91	2 years	89
Smith et al. [84]	32	NA	11	6	2 years	97	2 years	88	2 years	100
Dalton [90]	12	24	24[a]	6	26 months	100	26 months	100	26 months	100

cCR clinical complete response, CRT chemoradiotherapy, DFS disease-free survival, LARC locally advanced rectal cancer, LR lo
available, NOM nonoperative management, OS overall survival, RT radiotherapy, pCR pathological complete response
[a]Mean time to surgery
[b]All six with pCR

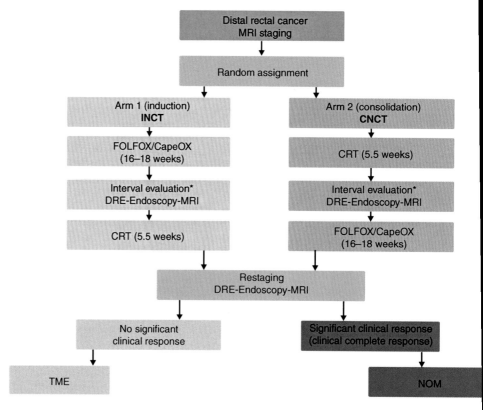

FIGURE 28-3. Memorial Sloan Kettering Cancer Center phase II trial schema that is underway to test the feasibility of incorporating a nonoperative management (NOM) to the multimodality treatment of rectal cancer in a multi-institutional setting. (*Cape* capecitabine, *CapeOx* capecitabine plus oxaliplatin, *CNCT* chemotherapy plus consolidation CRT, *CRT* chemoradiation, *DRE* digital rectal examination, *FOLFOX* infusional fluorouracil, leucov
tin, *FU* fluorouracil, *FUCMT* fluorouracil or
radiotherapy, *INCT* induction chemotherapy, *M*
nance imaging, *RT* radiotherapy, *TME* total me
Courtesy of Julio Garcia-Aguilar.

given the relatively small proportion of patients with a complete clinical response to standard neoadjuvant chemoradiotherapy and the disparity of the treatment arms—observation versus proctectomy. However, a number of prospective observational studies [85–87] and phase II trials, including our own (Figure 28-3), are underway to test the feasibility of incorporating an NOM approach to the multimodality treatment of rectal cancer in a multi-institutional setting [88, 89].

Summary

Decades of clinical research have resulted
multimodality treatment paradigms for recta
providing unprecedented local tumor control
vival. Although this represents a significant
oncologic outcome, multimodality therapy c
with significant morbidity and long-term se
impair quality of life permanently. Identificat

different risk levels for tumor recurrence and survival based on baseline tumor characteristics and response or resistance to therapy should enable us to tailor treatments accordingly and in certain cases omit radiation or surgery to decrease morbidity without compromising outcomes.

References

1. De Campos-Lobato LF, Stocchi L, da Luz Moreira A, et al. Pathologic complete response after neoadjuvant treatment for rectal cancer decreases distant recurrence and could eradicate local recurrence. Ann Surg Oncol. 2011;18:1590–8.

2. Maas M, Nelemans PJ, Valentini V, et al. Long-term outcome in patients with a pathological complete response after chemoradiation for rectal cancer: a pooled analysis of individual patient data. Lancet Oncol. 2010;11:835–44.

3. Martin ST, Heneghan HM, Winter DC. Systematic review and meta-analysis of outcomes following pathological complete response to neoadjuvant chemoradiotherapy for rectal cancer. Br J Surg. 2012;99:918–28.

4. Janeway HH. Treatment of cancer, particularly of the tongue, tonsil and rectum, by buried emanation. Read at the Third Annual Meeting of the American Radium Society. 1919 June 5; Atlantic City, NJ.

5. Binkley GE. Radiation in the treatment of cancer of the rectum. Ann Surg. 1929;90(6):1000–14.

6. Prolongation of the disease-free interval in surgically treated rectal carcinoma. Gastrointestinal Tumor Study Group. N Engl J Med. 1985;312:1465–72.

7. Improved survival with preoperative radiotherapy in resectable rectal cancer. Swedish Rectal Cancer Trial. N Engl J Med. 1997;336(14):980–7. Erratum in: N Engl J Med. 1997;336(21): 1539.

8. Gerard A, Buyse M, Nodingler B, et al. Preoperative radiotherapy as adjuvant treatment in rectal cancer. Final results of a randomized study of the European Organization for Research and Treatment of Cancer (EORTC). Ann Surg. 1988;208(5):606–14.

9. Adjuvant therapy for patients with colon and rectum cancer. Consens Statement. 1990;8(4):1–25.

10. Bujko K, Nowacki MP, Nasierowska-Guttmejer A, et al. Long-term results of a randomized trial comparing preoperative short-course radiotherapy with preoperative conventionally fractionated chemoradiation for rectal cancer. Br J Surg. 2006;93:1215–23.

11. Ngan SY, Burmeister B, Fisher RJ, et al. Randomized trial of short-course radiotherapy versus long-course chemoradiation comparing rates of local recurrence in patients with T3 rectal cancer: Trans-Tasman Radiation Oncology Group trial 01.04. J Clin Oncol. 2012;30:3827–33.

12. Heald RJ, Ryall RD. Recurrence and survival after total mesorectal excision for rectal cancer. Lancet. 1986;1:1479–82.

13. Kapiteijn E, Marijnen CA, Nagtegaal ID, et al. Preoperative radiotherapy combined with total mesorectal excision for resectable rectal cancer. N Engl J Med. 2001;345:638–46.

14. Colorectal Cancer Collaborative Group. Adjuvant radiotherapy for rectal cancer: a systematic overview of 8,507 patients from 22 randomised trials. Lancet. 2001;358:1291–304.

15. Balslev I, Pedersen M, Teglbjaerg PS, Hanberg-Soerensen F, Bone J, Jacobsen NO, Overgaard J, Sell A, Bertelsen K, Hage E, et al. Postoperative radiotherapy in Dukes' B and C carcinoma of the rectum and rectosigmoid. A randomized multicenter study. Cancer. 1986;58(1):22–8.

16. Randomised trial of surgery alone versus surgery followed by radiotherapy for mobile cancer of the rectum. Medical Research Council Rectal Cancer Working Party. Lancet. 1996;348(9042): 1610–4.

17. Wolmark N, Wieand HS, Hyams DM, Colangelo L, Dimitrov NV, Romond EH, Wexler M, Prager D, Cruz Jr AB, Gordon PH, Petrelli NJ, Deutsch M, Mamounas E, Wickerham DL, Fisher ER, Rockette H, Fisher B. Randomized trial of postoperative adjuvant chemotherapy with or without radiotherapy for carcinoma of the rectum: National Surgical Adjuvant Breast and Bowel Project Protocol R-02. J Natl Cancer Inst. 2000;92(5):388–96.

18. Cammà C, Giunta M, Fiorica F, et al. Preoperative radiotherapy for resectable rectal cancer: a meta-analysis. JAMA. 2000;284:1008–15.

19. van Gijn W, Marijnen CA, Nagtegaal ID, Kranenbarg EM, Putter H, Wiggers T, Rutten HJ, Påhlman L, Glimelius B, van de Velde CJ, Dutch Colorectal Cancer Group. Preoperative radiotherapy combined with total mesorectal excision for resectable rectal cancer: 12-year follow-up of the multicentre, randomised controlled TME trial. Lancet Oncol. 2011; 12(6):575–82.

20. Byfield JE. 5-Fluorouracil radiation sensitization—a brief review. Invest New Drugs. 1989;7:111–6.

21. O'Connell MJ, Martenson JA, Wieand HS, et al. Improving adjuvant therapy for rectal cancer by combining protracted-infusion fluorouracil with radiation therapy after curative surgery. N Engl J Med. 1994;331:502–7.

22. Smalley SR, Benedetti JK, Williamson SK, et al. Phase III trial of fluorouracil-based chemotherapy regimens plus radiotherapy in postoperative adjuvant rectal cancer: GI INT 0144. J Clin Oncol. 2006;24:3542–7.

23. Bosset J-F, Calais G, Mineur L, et al. Enhanced tumoricidal effect of chemotherapy with preoperative radiotherapy for rectal cancer: preliminary results—EORTC 22921. J Clin Oncol. 2005;23:5620–7.

24. Gerard JP, Conroy T, Bonnetain F, et al. Preoperative radiotherapy with or without concurrent fluorouracil and leucovorin in T3-4 rectal cancers: results of FFCD 9203. J Clin Oncol. 2006;24:4620–5.

25. Hofheinz R-D, Wenz F, Post S, et al. Chemoradiotherapy with capecitabine versus fluorouracil for locally advanced rectal cancer: a randomised, multicentre, non-inferiority, phase 3 trial. Lancet Oncol. 2012;13:579–88.

26. O'Connell MJ, Colangelo LH, Beart RW, Petrelli NJ, Allegra CJ, Sharif S, Pitot HC, Shields AF, Landry JC, Ryan DP, Parda DS, Mohiuddin M, Arora A, Evans LS, Bahary N, Soori GS, Eakle J, Robertson JM, Moore Jr DF, Mullane MR, Marchello BT, Ward PJ, Wozniak TF, Roh MS, Yothers G, Wolmark N. Capecitabine and oxaliplatin in the preoperative multimodality treatment of rectal cancer: surgical end points from National Surgical Adjuvant Breast and Bowel Project trial R-04. J Clin Oncol. 2014;32(18):1927–34.

27. Aschele C, Cionini L, Lonardi S, et al. Primary tumor response to preoperative chemoradiation with or without oxaliplatin in locally advanced rectal cancer: pathologic results of the STAR-01 randomized phase III trial. J Clin Oncol. 2011;29:2773–80.

28. Gérard J-P, Azria D, Gourgou-Bourgade S, et al. Comparison of two neoadjuvant chemoradiotherapy regimens for locally advanced rectal cancer: results of the phase III trial ACCORD 12/0405-Prodige 2. J Clin Oncol. 2010;28:1638–44.

29. Rödel C, Liersch T, Becker H, et al. Preoperative chemoradiotherapy and postoperative chemotherapy with fluorouracil and oxaliplatin versus fluorouracil alone in locally advanced rectal cancer: initial results of the German CAO/ARO/AIO-04 randomised phase 3 trial. Lancet Oncol. 2012;13:679–87.

30. Navarro M, Dotor E, Rivera F, et al. A phase II study of preoperative radiotherapy and concomitant weekly irinotecan in combination with protracted venous infusion 5-fluorouracil, for resectable locally advanced rectal cancer. Int J Radiat Oncol Biol Phys. 2006;66(1):201–5.

31. Willeke F, Horisberger K, Kraus-Tiefenbacher U, et al. A phase II study of capecitabine and irinotecan in combination with concurrent pelvic radiotherapy (CapIri-RT) as neoadjuvant treatment of locally advanced rectal cancer. Br J Cancer. 2007; 96(6):912–7.

32. Velenik V, Ocvirk J, Oblak I, et al. A phase II study of cetuximab, capecitabine and radiotherapy in neoadjuvant treatment of patients with locally advanced resectable rectal cancer. Eur J SurgOncol. 2010;36(3):244–50. doi:10.1016/j.ejso.2009.12.002.

33. Horisberger K, Treschl A, Mai S, et al. Cetuximab in combination with capecitabine, irinotecan, and radiotherapy for patients with locally advanced rectal cancer: results of a Phase II MARGIT trial. Int J Radiat Oncol Biol Phys. 2009;74(5):1487–93. doi:10.1016/j.ijrobp.2008.10.014.

34. Dewdney A, Cunningham D, Tabernero J, et al. Multicenter randomized phase II clinical trial comparing neoadjuvant oxaliplatin, capecitabine, and preoperative radiotherapy with or without cetuximab followed by total mesorectal excision in patients with high-risk rectal cancer (EXPERT-C). J Clin Oncol. 2012;30(14):1620–7. doi:10.1200/JCO.2011.39.6036.

35. Pahlman L, Glimelius B. Pre- or postoperative radiation in rectal and rectosigmoid carcinoma. Ann Surg. 1990;21:187–94.

36. Roh MS, Colangelo LH, O'Connell MJ, Yothers G, Deutsch M, Allegra CJ, Kahlenberg MS, Baez-Diaz L, Ursiny CS, Petrelli NJ, Wolmark N. Preoperative multimodality therapy improves disease-free survival in patients with carcinoma of the rectum: NSABP R-03. J Clin Oncol. 2009;27(31):5124–30.

37. Sauer R, Becker H, Hohenberger W, et al. Preoperative versus postoperative chemoradiotherapy for rectal cancer. N Engl J Med. 2004;351:1731–40.

38. Tan D, Glynne-Jones R. But some neoadjuvant schedules are more equal than others. J Clin Oncol. 2013;31:1799–800.

39. Bujko K. Short-course preoperative radiotherapy for low rectal cancer. J Clin Oncol. 2013;31:1799.

40. Peeters KC, van de Velde CJ, Leer JW, et al. Late side effects of short-course preoperative radiotherapy combined with total mesorectal excision for rectal cancer: increased bowel dysfunction in irradiated patients—a Dutch colorectal cancer group study. J Clin Oncol. 2005;23:6199–206.

41. Benson AB, Bekaii-Saab T, Chan E, et al. Rectal cancer [Internet]. J Natl Compr Canc Netw. 2012;10:1528–64. http://www.ncbi.nlm.nih.gov/pubmed/23221790. Accessed 25 Oct 2014.

42. Petersen SH, Harling H, Kirkeby LT, et al. Postoperative adjuvant chemotherapy in rectal cancer operated for cure. Cochrane database Syst Rev. 2012;3, CD004078. http://www.ncbi.nlm.nih.gov/pubmed/22419291. Accessed 6 Nov 2014.

43. Bosset JF, Calais G, Mineur L, Maingon P, Stojanovic-Rundic S, Bensadoun RJ, Bardet E, Beny A, Ollier JC, Bolla M, Marchal D, Van Laethem JL, Klein V, Giralt J, Clavère P, Glanzmann C, Cellier P, Collette L, EORTC Radiation Oncology Group. Fluorouracil-based adjuvant chemotherapy after preoperative chemoradiotherapy in rectal cancer: long-term results of the EORTC 22921 randomised study. Lancet Oncol. 2014;15(2): 184–90.

44. Hayden DM, Pinzon MC, Francescatti AB, et al. Hospital readmission for fluid and electrolyte abnormalities following ileostomy construction: preventable or unpredictable? J Gastrointest Surg. 2013;17:298–303. http://www.ncbi.nlm.nih.gov/pubmed/23192425. Accessed 10 Sep 2014.

45. Khrizman P, Niland JC, ter Veer A, et al. Postoperative adjuvant chemotherapy use in patients with stage II/III rectal cancer treated with Neoadjuvant therapy, LARC: a national comprehensive cancer network analysis. J Clin Oncol. 2013;31:30–8. http://www.ncbi.nlm.nih.gov/pubmed/23169502. Accessed 21 Oct 2014.

46. Biagi JJ, Raphael MJ, Mackillop W, et al. Association between time to initiation of adjuvant chemotherapy and survival in colorectal cancer: a systematic review and meta-analysis. JAMA. 2011;305:2335–42. http://www.ncbi.nlm.nih.gov/pubmed/21642686. Accessed 25 Oct 2014.

47. Breugom AJ, Swets M, Bosset JF, et al. Adjuvant chemotherapy after preoperative (chemo)radiotherapy and surgery for patients with rectal cancer: a systematic review and meta-analysis of individual patient data. Lancet Oncol. 2015;16:200–7.

48. Glynne-Jones R, Counsell N, Quirke P, et al. Chronicle: results of a randomised phase III trial in locally advanced rectal cancer after neoadjuvant chemoradiation randomising postoperative adjuvant capecitabine plus oxaliplatin (XELOX) versus control. Ann Oncol. 2014;25:1356–62.

49. Calvo FA, Serrano FJ, Diaz-González JA, et al. Improved incidence of pT0 downstaged surgical specimens in locally advanced rectal cancer (LARC) treated with induction oxaliplatin plus 5-fluorouracil and preoperative chemoradiation. Ann Oncol. 2006;17:1103–10. http://www.ncbi.nlm.nih.gov/pubmed/16670204. Accessed 22 Sep 2014.

50. Chau I, Brown G, Cunningham D, et al. Neoadjuvant capecitabine and oxaliplatin followed by synchronous chemoradiation and total mesorectal excision in magnetic resonance imaging-defined poor-risk rectal cancer. J Clin Oncol. 2006;24:668–74. http://www.ncbi.nlm.nih.gov/pubmed/16446339. Accessed 22 Sep 2014.

51. Fernández-Martos C, Pericay C, Aparicio J, et al. Phase II, randomized study of concomitant chemoradiotherapy followed by surgery and adjuvant capecitabine plus oxaliplatin (CAPOX) compared with induction CAPOX followed by concomitant chemoradiotherapy and surgery in magnetic resonance imaging-defined, l. J Clin Oncol. 2010;28:859–65. http://www.ncbi.nlm.nih.gov/pubmed/20065174. Accessed 22 Sep 2014.

52. Maréchal R, Vos B, Polus M, et al. Short course chemotherapy followed by concomitant chemoradiotherapy and surgery in locally advanced rectal cancer: a randomized multicentric phase II study. Ann Oncol. 2012;23:1525–30. http://www.ncbi.nlm.nih.gov/pubmed/22039087. Accessed 6 Oct 2014.

53. Schou JV, Larsen FO, Rasch L, et al. Induction chemotherapy with capecitabine and oxaliplatin followed by chemoradiotherapy before total mesorectal excision in patients with locally advanced rectal cancer. Ann Oncol. 2012;23:2627–33. http://

www.ncbi.nlm.nih.gov/pubmed/22473488. Accessed 4 Sep 2014.

54. Glynne-Jones R, Grainger J, Harrison M, et al. Neoadjuvant chemotherapy prior to preoperative chemoradiation or radiation in rectal cancer: should we be more cautious? Br J Cancer. 2006;94:363–71. http://www.pubmedcentral.nih.gov/articlerender.fcgi?artid=2361136&tool=pmcentrez&rendertype=abstract. Accessed 21 Oct 2014.

55. Cercek A, Goodman KA, Hajj C, et al. Neoadjuvant chemotherapy first, followed by chemoradiation and then surgery, in the management of locally advanced rectal cancer. J Natl Compr Canc Netw. 2014;12(4):513–9.

56. Garcia-Aguilar J, Chow OS, Smith DD, et al. Effect of adding mFOLFOX6 after neoadjuvant chemoradiation in locally advanced rectal cancer: a multicentre, phase 2 trial. Lancet Oncol. 2015;16(8):957–66. doi:10.1016/S1470-2045(15)00004-2.

57. Glynne-Jones R, Harrison M, Hughes R. Challenges in the neoadjuvant treatment of rectal cancer: balancing the risk of recurrence and quality of life. Cancer Radiother. 2013;17:675–85. http://www.ncbi.nlm.nih.gov/pubmed/24183502. Accessed 5 Sep 2014.

58. Glimelius B, Tiret E, Cervantes A, et al. Rectal cancer: ESMO Clinical Practice Guidelines for diagnosis, treatment and follow-up. Ann Oncol. 2013;24:vi81–8.

59. Smith N, Brown G. Preoperative staging of rectal cancer. Acta Oncol. 2008;47:20–31.

60. Chang GJ, Park IJ, Eng C, et al. Exploratory analysis of adjuvant chemotherapy benefits after preoperative chemoradiotherapy and radical resection for rectal cancer. ASCO Meet Abstr. 2012;30:3556. http://hwmaint.meeting.ascopubs.org.proxy.library.vanderbilt.edu/cgi/content/abstract/30/15_suppl/3556. Accessed 7 Nov 2014.

61. Fietkau R, Barten M, Klautke G, et al. Postoperative chemotherapy may not be necessary for patients with ypN0-category after neoadjuvant chemoradiotherapy of rectal cancer. Dis Colon Rectum. 2006;49:1284–92. http://www.ncbi.nlm.nih.gov/pubmed/16758130. Accessed 7 Nov 2014.

62. Nelson VM, Benson AB. Pathological complete response after neoadjuvant therapy for rectal cancer and the role of adjuvant therapy. Curr Oncol Rep. 2013;15:152–61. http://www.ncbi.nlm.nih.gov/pubmed/23381584. Accessed 19 Nov 2014.

63. Maas M, Nelemans PJ, Valentini V, et al. Adjuvant chemotherapy in rectal cancer: defining subgroups who may benefit after neoadjuvant chemoradiation and resection: a pooled analysis of 3,313 patients. Int J Cancer. 2015;137(1):212–20. doi:10.1002/ijc.29355.

64. Hong YS, Nam B-H, Kim K-P, et al. Oxaliplatin, fluorouracil, and leucovorin versus fluorouracil and leucovorin as adjuvant chemotherapy for locally advanced rectal cancer after preoperative chemoradiotherapy (ADORE): an open-label, multicentre, phase 2, randomised controlled trial. Lancet Oncol. 2014;15:1245–53. http://www.ncbi.nlm.nih.gov/pubmed/25201358. Accessed 12 Sep 2014.

65. Taylor FG, Quirke P, Heald RJ, et al. Preoperative high-resolution magnetic resonance imaging can identify good prognosis stage I, II, and III rectal cancer best managed by surgery alone: a prospective, multicenter, European study. Ann Surg. 2011;253:711–9. http://www.ncbi.nlm.nih.gov/pubmed/21475011. Accessed 27 Oct 2014.

66. Birgisson H, Påhlman L, Gunnarsson U, et al. Adverse effects of preoperative radiation therapy for rectal cancer: long-term follow-up of the Swedish Rectal Cancer Trial. J Clin Oncol. 2005;23:8697–705. http://www.ncbi.nlm.nih.gov/pubmed/16314629. Accessed 27 Oct 2014.

67. Joye I, Haustermans K. Early and late toxicity of radiotherapy for rectal cancer. Recent Results Cancer Res. 2014;203:189–201. http://www.ncbi.nlm.nih.gov/pubmed/25103006. Accessed 7 Nov 2014.

68. Gunderson LL, Sargent DJ, Tepper JE, et al. Impact of T and N stage and treatment on survival and relapse in adjuvant rectal cancer: a pooled analysis. J Clin Oncol. 2004;22:1785–96. http://www.ncbi.nlm.nih.gov/pubmed/15067027. Accessed 13 Oct 2014.

69. Schrag D. Evolving role of neoadjuvant therapy in rectal cancer. Curr Treat Options Oncol. 2013;14:350–64. http://www.ncbi.nlm.nih.gov/pubmed/23828092. Accessed 13 Oct 2014.

70. Schrag D, Weiser MR, Goodman KA, et al. Neoadjuvant chemotherapy without routine use of radiation therapy for patients with locally advanced rectal cancer: a pilot trial. J Clin Oncol. 2014;32:513–8. http://www.ncbi.nlm.nih.gov/pubmed/24419115. Accessed 4 Sep 2014.

71. Alliance for clinical trials in oncology: PROSPECT Trial. http://clinicaltrials.gov/sho/NCT01515787

72. Fernandez-Martos C, Safont M, Feliu J, et al. Induction chemotherapy with or without chemoradiation in intermediate-risk rectal cancer patients defined by magnetic resonance imaging (MRI): a GEMCAD study. J Clin Oncol (Meeting Abstracts). 2010;28:15. Suppl TPS 196.

73. Bevacizumab And Combination Chemotherapy in Rectal Cancer Until Surgery (BACCHUS). www.clinicaltrials.gov. Accessed 9 Sep 2015.

74. Francois Y, Nemoz CJ, Baulieux J, et al. Influence of the interval between preoperative radiation therapy and surgery on downstaging and on the rate of sphincter-sparing surgery for rectal cancer: the Lyon R90-01 randomized trial. J Clin Oncol. 1999;17:2396. http://www.ncbi.nlm.nih.gov/pubmed/10561302. Accessed 9 Nov 2014.

75. Park IJ, You YN, Agarwal A, et al. Neoadjuvant treatment response as an early response indicator for patients with rectal cancer. J Clin Oncol. 2012;30:1770–6. http://www.pubmedcentral.nih.gov/articlerender.fcgi?artid=3383178&tool=pmcentrez&rendertype=abstract. Accessed 6 Nov 2014.

76. Zorcolo L, Rosman AS, Restivo A, et al. Complete pathologic response after combined modality treatment for rectal cancer and long-term survival: a meta-analysis. Ann Surg Oncol. 2012;19(9):2822–32. doi:10.1245/s10434-011-2209-y.

77. Guillem JG, Chessin DB, Shia J, et al. Clinical examination following preoperative chemoradiation for rectal cancer is not a reliable surrogate end point. J Clin Oncol. 2005;23:3475–9. http://www.ncbi.nlm.nih.gov/pubmed/15908656. Accessed 23 Sep 2014.

78. Pastor C, Subtil JC, Sola J, et al. Accuracy of endoscopic ultrasound to assess tumor response after neoadjuvant treatment in rectal cancer: can we trust the findings? Dis Colon Rectum. 2011;54:1141–6. http://www.ncbi.nlm.nih.gov/pubmed/21825895. Accessed 3 Nov 2014.

79. Guillem JG, Ruby JA, Leibold T, et al. Neither FDG-PET nor CT can distinguish between a pathological complete response and an incomplete response after neoadjuvant chemoradiation

in locally advanced rectal cancer: a prospective study. Ann Surg. 2013;258:289–95. http://www.ncbi.nlm.nih.gov/pubmed/23187748. Accessed 4 Nov 2014.

80. Habr-Gama A, Perez RO, Nadalin W, et al. Operative versus nonoperative treatment for stage 0 distal rectal cancer following chemoradiation therapy: long-term results. Ann Surg. 2004;240:711–7. http://www.pubmedcentral.nih.gov/articlerender.fcgi?artid=1356472&tool=pmcentrez&rendertype=abstract. Accessed 22 Sep 2014.

81. Habr-Gama A, Perez RO, Proscurshim I, et al. Patterns of failure and survival for nonoperative treatment of stage c0 distal rectal cancer following neoadjuvant chemoradiation therapy. J Gastrointest Surg. 2006;10:1319–28. http://www.ncbi.nlm.nih.gov/pubmed/17175450. Accessed 4 Nov 2014.

82. Habr-Gama A, Gama-Rodrigues J, São Julião GP, et al. Local recurrence after complete clinical response and watch and wait in rectal cancer after neoadjuvant chemoradiation: impact of salvage therapy on local disease control. Int J Radiat Oncol Biol Phys. 2014;88:822–8. http://www.ncbi.nlm.nih.gov/pubmed/24495589. Accessed 2 Nov 2014.

83. Maas M, Beets-Tan RG, Lambregts DM, et al. Wait-and-see policy for clinical complete responders after chemoradiation for rectal cancer. J Clin Oncol. 2011;29:4633–40. http://www.ncbi.nlm.nih.gov/pubmed/22067400. Accessed 19 Sep 2014.

84. Smith JD, Ruby JA, Goodman KA, et al. Nonoperative management of rectal cancer with complete clinical response after neoadjuvant therapy. Ann Surg. 2012;256:965–72. http://www.ncbi.nlm.nih.gov/pubmed/23154394. Accessed 18 Sep 2014.

85. Vejle Hospital. Watchful waiting. An observational study of patients with rectal cancer after concomitant radiation and chemotherapy. http://clinicaltrials.gov/show/NCT00952926.

86. Maria Sklodowska-Curie Memorial Cancer Center I of O: organ preservation in elderly patients with rectal cancer. http://clinicaltrials.gov/show/NCT01863862.

87. Paulo I do C do E de S. Observation versus surgical resection in patients with rectal cancer who achieved complete clinical response after neoadjuvant chemoradiotherapy. http://clinicaltrials.gov/show/NCT02052921

88. Hospital RM. Timing and deferral of rectal surgery following a continued response to pre-operative chemoradiotherapy. http://public.ukcrn.org.uk/search/StudyDetail.aspx

89. Garcia Aguilar J and collaborators. Trial evaluating 3-year DFS in patients with locally advanced rectal cancer treated with chemoradiation plus induction or consolidation chemotherapy and TME or NOM. 2014. http://clinicaltrials.gov/show/NCT02008656.

90. Dalton RS, Velineni R, Osborne ME, Thomas R, Harries S, Gee AS, Daniels IR. A single-centre experience of chemoradiotherapy for rectal cancer: is there potential for nonoperative management? Colorectal Dis. 2012;14(5):567–71.

29

Local Excision of Rectal Neoplasia

Mark H. Whiteford

Key Concepts

- When anatomically appropriate, local excision is the preferred over proctectomy for benign rectal polyps due to high success rates and lower morbidity.
- If local excision is to be utilized as definitive surgical therapy for rectal cancer, the depth of dissection should be full thickness of the rectal wall.
- Histologic predictors of lymph node metastasis in early rectal cancers include tumor depth, lymphatic and vascular invasion, poor differentiation, and tumor budding.
- Five-year disease-free survival after local excision of rectal cancer is lower than after proctectomy, although it is unclear whether overall survival is different.
- Survival and local recurrence rates for T2 rectal cancers treated with neoadjuvant chemoradiation and local excision appear to be similar to those of T1 cancers treated with local excision alone.
- Transanal endoscopic surgery may be associated with improved outcomes as compared to conventional transanal excision, although the quality of comparative studies is suboptimal.

Transanal Surgery, a Historical Perspective

The initial report of transanal excision (TAE) of a rectal tumor is attributed to Dr. Jacques Lisfranc in the early 1800s whereby a protruding and painful rectal tumor was excised via a prolapsing and incising technique [1]. There was no mention of anesthesia, no defect closure was attempted, and hemostasis was eventually maintained with serial intrarectal packing. Sir Alan Parks popularized the era of modern TAE in the 1960s [2]. This more familiar technique employed anesthesia, a self-retaining rectal retractor, epinephrine injection, a submucosal resection plane, use of stay sutures,

and primary closure of the defect [2]. The appeal and benefits of TAE are obvious: direct endoluminal approach to the target pathology via the natural orifice; avoidance of a stoma; and avoidance of the morbidity associated with abdominal or transacral operations.

The goal of local excision is to completely remove the target pathology en bloc with negative margins. When applied to benign rectal polyps, this should be curative. When applied to rectal cancer, this has the potential to be curative if the tumor has not spread beyond the rectal wall. Due to technical limitations of the anus, rectum, and surgical instrumentation, conventional TAE has been limited to lesions within 8 cm from the anal verge, at or below the first rectal valve, ≤ 3 cm in size, and occupying $\leq 40\%$ of the rectal circumference. Lesions that exceed these parameters are technically more challenging to remove.

In the early 1980s, Prof. Gerhard Buess, inspired by the poor visibility and limited reach of conventional TAE, ushered in the era of transanal endoscopic surgery (TES) when he invented a new technique and series of instruments for removal of rectal tumors [3]. His technique and instruments were termed transanal endoscopic microsurgery (TEM, Richard Wolf, GmbH, Knittlingen, Germany). TEM involves a 4×12 (or 20) cm cylindrical metal reusable operating rectoscope mounted to the operating table. The rectoscope has a sealed faceplate with multiple access ports that permit simultaneous pneumodistention of the rectum along with passage of a stereoscopic camera and modified laparoscopic instruments into the rectum. Stable pneumorectum is maintained with a dedicated TEM suction-CO_2 insufflation pump. TEM instruments could now remove larger lesions as well as lesions up to the rectosigmoid junction (~17 cm from the anal verge).

TEM proved to produce a specimen with less fragmentation and more negative margins and lead to a lower local recurrence than conventional TAE. Larger lesions and lesions up to the upper rectum could now be removed without the need for radical surgery. A similar reusable rigid proctoscopic transanal endoscopic operations (TEO®) system is also commercially

© Springer International Publishing 2016
S.R. Steele et al. (eds.), *The ASCRS Textbook of Colon and Rectal Surgery*, DOI 10.1007/978-3-319-25970-3_29

available (Karl Storz, GmbH, Tuttlingen, Germany). The acceptance of TEM and TEO, however, was very slow due to the high capital cost of the equipment, requirement for specialized training, and complexity and technically challenging nature of the instrumentation and procedure. An additional obstacle was the lack of a category 1 CPT code for the procedure in the United States that made reimbursement problematic.

In 2010, Atallah first described the use of a commercially available single port laparoscopic platform placed transanally in conjunction with standard laparoscopic instruments and insufflators to perform transanal surgery [4]. This technique has been coined transanal minimally invasive surgery (TAMIS) and appears to show similar benefits as TEM [5]. This technique offers the promise of instrument simplicity and low upfront cost. Due to the similarities of the techniques and clinical results, TEM, TEO, and TAMIS are collectively termed TES.

Techniques

Technique for Conventional TAE

Patients undergo routine surgical history and physical examination with including evaluation of comorbidities, bowel function, and continence [6]. Examination should include digital rectal examination with proctoscopy to determine and document the longitudinal and circumferential location, extent of the lesion, and its proximity to the sphincter. Repeat or deeper biopsy can also be performed if colonoscopic biopsy was nondiagnostic. When concern for malignancy exists, then additional imaging studies such as endoscopic ultrasound, MRI, or CT scan may be considered.

The patient receives a full mechanical bowel prep and perioperative antibiotics. General anesthesia is the most common mode of anesthesia, but spinal anesthesia an acceptable option. Patient positioning is chosen such that the target pathology is placed dependently: lithotomy position for posterior lesions, prone jack knife for anterior and lateral lesions. Exposure is obtained via the surgeons preferred method of self-retaining anal retractor, lighted anoscope, operating proctoscope, Lone Star® retractor (Cooper Surgical, Inc, Trumbull, CT). A headlight provides ideal illumination in the tight confined operating field. Electrocautery is then utilized to demarcate a 5–10 mm margin around the lesion. Stay sutures may be placed laterally for retraction and improved visibility. Dissection progresses distally, laterally, then proximally with sharp or electrocautery dissection. Depth of dissection is in the submucosal plane for benign appearing lesions or to avoid sphincter injury, and full thickness dissection for biopsy-proven malignant lesions or lesions with gross features of malignancy. Additional stay sutures may be placed as one progresses proximally in order to maintain control of the proximal edge. Most authors advocate for primary transverse closure as longitudinal closure is thought

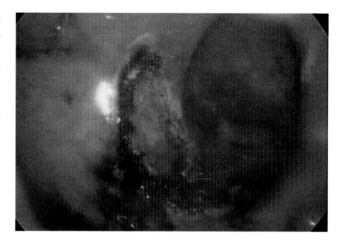

FIGURE 29-1. Open wound following local excision.

to predispose to stricture. At times, there may be too much tension to close the defect. These can then either be partially closed or left open to heal by secondary intention if the defect is extraperitoneal (Figure 29-1).

Technique for TEM and TEO [7]

Bowel preparation, anesthetic choice, and positioning are the same as TAE. Gentle digital dilation is performed to accommodate the 4 cm diameter proctoscope, which is then inserted and attached to the table mount. Both 12 and 20 cm lengths are available. The faceplate attached and tubing connected to the suction insufflator unit. Pneumorectum is established and the proctoscope adjusted to view the target lesion through the stereoscopic microscope or the laparoscopic video monitor. Three 5–9 mm instrument ports are available for use of the modified angled TEM laparoscopic instruments. Needle tip electrocautery is utilized to demarcate a 5–10 mm margin around the lesion. Submucosal or full thickness dissection is then initiated. This is most easily started in the distal right corner of the lesion with progression towards the proximal left corner. Partial en bloc resection of the mesorectum has also been described for deeper malignant lesions [8]. Continuous suction functions to clear the cautery smoke during the procedure. The integrated suction-insufflation unit prevents loss of pneumorectum from the suctioning. Following specimen removal, the defect is closed transversely using a running absorbable suture. A metal clip is locked at each end of the suture in lieu of intracorporeal knot tying. With the increased proximal reach of TEM, intraperitoneal entry occasionally occurs, and in experience hands, can safely be closed via the TEM instrumentation [9, 10]. TEM does suffer from technical limitations of the rigid proctoscope causing significant instrument conflict and has a longer learning curve for both technique and instrument troubleshooting than compared to other transanal techniques (Figures 29-2, 29-3, and 29-4).

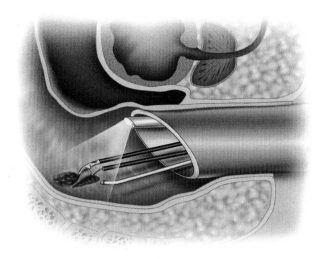

FIGURE 29-2. Transanal endoscopic microsurgery.

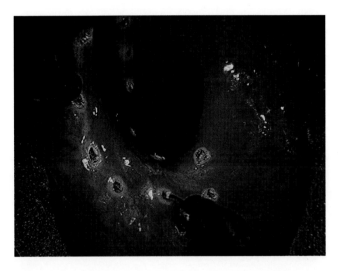

FIGURE 29-3. Margin around sessile polyp demarcated with monopolar cautery during TEM. *Courtesy Mark Whiteford, MD.*

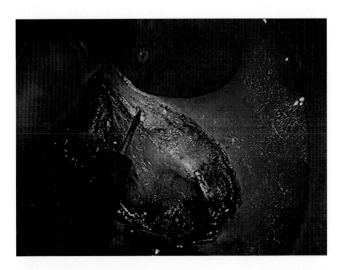

FIGURE 29-4. Full thickness depth of excision during TEM. *Courtesy Mark Whiteford, MD.*

Technique for TAMIS

TAMIS is a modification of TEM whereby the reusable rigid 4 cm diameter operating proctoscope is replaced by a flexible, disposable single port laparoscopic platform. Standard laparoscopic insufflators, camera, instruments, and vessel sealing devices are also utilized. Patient selection and preparation is similar to TAE and TEM. The shorter length and flexible platform of the TAMIS technique more easily permits operating on the non-dependent (downward) wall of the rectum, as is required with TAE and TEM. For this reason the majority of cases can be done in the lithotomy position. Dissection is performed in a similar fashion as with TEM. Laparoscopic suctioning must be done judiciously as not to lose pneumorectum and exposure. A more liberal use of laparoscopic vessel sealing devices provides improved hemostasis over that of monopolar cautery, thereby reducing the need for suctioning. Defect closure techniques vary among authors and include use of different laparoscopic suturing devices or barbed sutures [5]. Intraperitoneal entry during TAMIS is more likely to require laparoscopic assistance for defect closure due to loss of rectum and visualization of the defect via the transanal device [11]. Since the TAMIS devices rely on radial fixation to the top of the sphincter complex, low-lying rectal polyps become partially obscured by the transanal device and require a hybrid TAMIS and TAE resection technique. This involves dissection of the proximal portion of the lesion utilizing the TAMIS technique, and then removal of the TAMIS device followed by the conventional TAE technique to complete the distal dissection and defect closure.

All forms of TAE techniques have limitations such as the potential for incomplete resection or the requirement for conversion to an alternate technique, such as staged transanal procedures or need for an abdominal approach to complete the resection or defect closure. These events are more likely when the tumor is too bulky to permit adequate working space, the proximal extent of tumor cannot be visualized around a fold or sigmoid bend, uncontrolled bleeding is encountered, or there is an inadequate bowel preparation. Fortunately these situations are uncommon and or can be avoided with proper preoperative patient selection and preparation.

Transcoccygeal (Kraske) and transsphincteric (York-Mason) approaches to locally excise rectal neoplasia have largely been supplanted by these purely transanal techniques. If interested, the reader is directed to the previous addition of ASCRS textbook for an excellent overview of these topics [12].

TAE of Benign Rectal Polyps

The ideal indication for TAE is for the complete removal of benign lesions in the rectum. Radical surgery, in the form of proctectomy, which includes a complete regional lymphadenectomy, provides no clinical benefit over TAE in the setting of benign disease, yet subjects the patient to considerable perioperative morbidity and significant long-term risk of urinary, sexual, and defecatory dysfunction. Local excision has the advantage of acting as a "total biopsy" to assess for completeness of resection and presence of otherwise occult cancer.

Most rectal polyps are detected on screening colonoscopy in asymptomatic patients. Occasionally rectal polyps produce symptoms such as rectal bleeding, blood or mucus on the stool, change in stool caliber, or tissue prolapse symptoms. While most small polyps are readily removed using colonoscopic polypectomy, larger polyps that would generally require piecemeal snare polypectomy are better served with TAE which provides a higher chance of complete polyp removal and a resultant lower chance of polyp recurrence.

Larger rectal polyps, particularly villous adenomas, have a higher incidence of harboring an occult cancer despite benign appearance and biopsies. For this reason preoperative assessment with endoscopic ultrasound is always reasonable to further assess tumor and nodal staging. Interpretation of endoscopic ultrasound performed soon after a full-thickness excision may be more challenging due to scar tissue, cautery artifact, and difficulty in differentiating between reactive and potentially malignant lymphadenopathy. These factors may result in overstaging of patients.

Benign polyps can be removed using either a partial thickness (submucosal plane) or full-thickness technique (deep to muscularis propria). Partial thickness dissection is facilitated through the use of submucosal injection of saline with or without epinephrine to help raise the polyp and mucosa off the muscularis propria. A non-lifting sign is worrisome for invasive cancer and is an indication for consideration of conversion to full-thickness excision for complete histologic assessment. A true submucosal dissection does not require defect closure provided there is no concern for full-thickness intraperitoneal entry. Alternatively, the mucosa is usually fairly mobile, and most defects can be closed primarily.

It should be noted that the submucosal plane is much more likely to be scarred or obliterated if the patient has undergone prior piecemeal hot snare polypectomy or multiple attempts at endoscopic excision. Full-thickness excision may be required in this situation if the layers of the rectal wall are fused by scar [7].

Results

Local excision with TAE, TEM, and TAMIS is typically performed in the outpatient setting. The goal of TAE is complete en bloc removal of the target pathology with minimal morbidity and mortality. Numerous case series and several comparison trials demonstrate a low perioperative complication rate (10–17%) and a less than 1% mortality rate following TAE and TEM [13–15]. There are some non-randomized studies that suggest that the quality of TEM excision, however, is better than TAE with the incidence of specimen fragmentation (1–6% vs. 24–35%), positive margins (10–12% vs. 29–50%), and local recurrence (5–6% vs. 27–29%) favoring TEM [14, 15]. Long-term recurrence data following TAMIS is not yet available.

Unfortunately, the quality of the studies of outcomes following local excision is distressingly suboptimal. Heterogeneous study populations (mixing benign and malignant pathology of various T stage), lack of appropriate time-to-event analysis, retrospective study design, and selection bias plague much of the published literature on the topic. It should also be remembered that, as of this writing, there have been no prospective, randomized comparisons of local excision techniques. Thus, although a few non-randomized retrospective analyses favor transanal endoscopic microsurgery vs. traditional local excision [16], it is unclear whether any surgical technique is truly superior to any other, especially for lesions in the distal rectum.

Some newer advanced colonoscopic techniques, endoscopic mucosal resection (EMR) and endoscopic submucosal dissection (ESD), are being utilized for excision of benign colorectal polyps. EMR is usually a piecemeal resection whereas ESD attempts a single en bloc resection. These techniques are primarily utilized in Asia with limited North American and European experience. In early comparisons between TES and EMR, EMR shows a slightly lower complication rate (3.8% vs. 13%) but a higher local recurrence rate (11.2% vs. 5.4%) [17]. In comparisons between TES and ESD, TES shows higher percentage of en bloc excision (99% vs. 88%) and negative margins (89% vs. 74%) while maintaining similar rate of complications (8.0% vs. 8.0%) [18].

While there are no guidelines that mandate a recommended follow-up strategy following TES for benign rectal polyps, many institutions performed endoscopy every 6–12 months for 2–3 years. Routine endoscopic ultrasound and imaging are not recommended for benign disease.

TES for Rectal Cancer

Curative surgery for rectal cancer aims to maximize the oncologic clearance of the primary tumor as well as the mesorectal lymph nodes. Proctectomy is the accepted gold standard surgical procedure for rectal cancer with 5-year local recurrence rates in the 5–10% range. The procedure, however, comes with significant risk of perioperative complications, long-term defecatory, urinary, and sexual dysfunction, and frequent need for temporary or permanent ostomies [19–21].

Local excision has long been an appealing option for rectal cancer because of its low risk of morbidity and mortality, relative paucity of long-term functional sequelae and the potential for curative treatment of disease limited to the bowel wall. The ideal candidate for local excision is a patient who has no lymph node metastasis and has a primary tumor can be excised with negative margins. In such a situation local excision should be curative. The great controversy, however, is that our ability to predict lymph node metastases are disappointingly poor and local recurrence following TAE remains much higher than with radical surgery.

Local excision can be utilized as a tool to gain additional information regarding tumor biology and risk of lymph node metastasis. This may help guide clinical judgment in deciding whether or not a patient can be spared radical surgery. It is wise to clarify this concept with the patient preoperatively. The local excision will be utilized as a "total biopsy" to help guide treatment recommendations and that if this total biopsy reveals high risk histologic features then a recommendation for subsequent radical surgery will be made. However, if no high-risk features are identified and the priorities and values of a patient are such that they accept a potentially higher risk of local recurrence than with proctectomy, local excision may be considered acceptable treatment. Local excision remains most appealing in patients who are unfit or unwilling to undergo radical surgery.

Lymph node status dramatically effects patient prognosis as well as our treatment decisions and recommendations. Current efforts to predict lymph node status consist of identifying high-risk histopathologic features from biopsy specimens. This is complemented with selected imaging modalities. When considering patients for local excision, it is imperative to choose those with the lowest risk of harboring locoregional metastatic disease.

Predicting Risk of Lymph Node Metastasis

Prediction of lymph node metastasis for rectal cancer is an imprecise science. No single histologic feature can solely predict risk of lymph node metastasis nor is there any currently available genetic or molecular marker that is predictive. Through a combination of histopathologic characteristics and imaging modalities the surgeon and the patient try to roughly generate a risk-benefit calculation to guide clinical strategies related to local excision vs. radical surgery. Colonoscopic biopsies alone sample but a small portion of the tumor, whereas an excisional full-thickness biopsy allows the fullest examination of the tumor histology, death of invasion, and margin status. Unfavorable histologic features are not only independently predictive of lymph node metastasis, but multiple unfavorable features also have an additive risk [22].

Depth of Invasion

Depth of tumor invasion into the wall of the bowel has traditionally been one of the best predictors of lymph node metastasis and is assessable variable in nearly all complete excisions. T1 tumors, which are limited to the submucosa, are associated with a 10–15% incidence of occult lymph node metastases detected at the time of radical surgery. T2 tumors, which invade into but not through the muscularis propria, are associated with a 20–26% risk of lymph node metastasis [22–25]. Kikuchi further identified the importance of depth of submucosal invasion on lymph node metastases and local recurrence amongst T1 cancers. They analyzed a large series of patients subdivided by the cancer depth of invasion into the upper, middle, and lower thirds of the submucosa (SM1, SM2, SM3) and demonstrated an incremental increase in risk of lymph node metastasis or local recurrences with deeper depth of invasion. Tumors invading to the SM3 level were shown to have a similar risk of lymph node metastasis and local recurrence as T2 cancers [26].

Lymphovascular Invasion

Lymphovascular invasion is found in 12–32% of T1 rectal cancers [22, 27] and is a strong predictor of lymph node metastasis with an odds ratio between 3.0 and 11.5 reported on multivariate analysis [22, 24, 28]. Bach reviewed 487 rectal cancer subjects tracked prospectively in a national proctectomy database. The incidence of local recurrence based on depth of invasion, lymphatic invasion, and tumor diameter is shown in Table 29-1 [28].

TABLE 29-1. Local recurrence rates (percentage) at 36 months following TEM excision of rectal cancer

Depth of invasion	Lymphatic invasion	Maximum tumor diameter (cm)					
		≤1	1.1–2	2.1–3	3.1–4	4.1–5	≥5.1
pT1 sm1	No	3.0	3.6	4.4	5.4	6.6	8.1
	Yes	5.2	6.4	7.7	9.4	11.4	13.7
pT1 sm2–3	No	10.5	12.7	15.3	18.5	22.1	26.4
	Yes	17.8	21.4	25.5	30.3	35.7	41.8
pT2	No	9.8	11.9	14.3	17.3	20.7	24.7
	Yes	16.7	20.0	23.9	28.5	33.7	39.5
pT3	No	19.7	23.6	28.0	33.2	39.0	45.4
	Yes	32.2	37.9	44.1	51.0	58.3	65.7

pT = pathological tumor stage; sm1 and sm2–3 = Kikuchi submucosal stage
With permission from Bach SP, Hill J, Monson JR, Simson JN, Lane L, Merrie A, Warren B, Mortensen NJ. Transanal Endoscopic Microsurgery (TEM) Collaboration. A predictive model for local recurrence after transanal endoscopic microsurgery for rectal cancer. Br J Surg. 2009;96(3):280–90. Copyright © 2009 John Wiley & Sons, Inc. [29]

Poor Differentiation

Poorly differentiated histology also predicts for lymph node metastases in rectal cancer [22–24, 29]; however, this trait is seen infrequently, present in only 2–4% of early rectal cancers [22, 28, 30]. Odds ratio for probably of poorly differentiated tumors having lymph node metastasis is 4.8–6.1 [31, 32].

Tumor Budding

Tumor budding, defined as small nests of five or more, usually poorly differentiated, cancer cells along the invasive front, is a histologic trait not routinely mentioned on biopsy reports in the North America, but has been extensively reported in the Asian gastroenterology literature [27, 30, 32] as a strong predictor of lymph node metastasis in colon and rectal cancer. Tumor budding is present in 16–25% [27, 33] of T1 cancers and multivariate analysis has demonstrated an odds ratio of 5.1–5.8 in predicting lymph node metastasis [31, 32].

Location of the cancer within the rectum may also be a risk factor for lymph node metastasis. Nascimbeni reported 8 and 11% risk of lymph node metastasis for high and mid rectal cancers, and 34% for low rectal tumors [29]. Mucinous histology and gender have not consistently been associated with increased risk of lymph node metastasis [29]. Molecular markers are not yet able to reliably predict nodal status (Figure 29-5) [31].

Imaging for Early Rectal Cancer Staging

Imaging is a standard recommendation for the staging of rectal cancer [34]. Despite innumerable technological advances in medicine, however, imaging remains an unreliable and inadequate measure of lymph node metastasis for rectal cancer. At present, endoscopic rectal ultrasound (EUS) is the imaging modality of choice to distinguish between T1 and T2 rectal cancers. CT scan and MRI do not have adequate

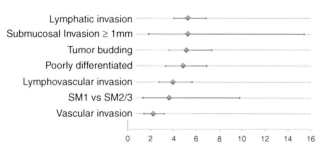

FIGURE 29-5. Relative risk (95% confidence intervals) of lymph node metastases in pT1 rectal cancers. (SM1 = invasion into superficial third of submucosa. SM2/3 = invasion into middle and deep third of submucosa. *With permission from Bosch SL, Teerenstra S, de Wilt JH, Cunningham C, Nagtegaal ID. Predicting lymph node metastasis in pT1 colorectal cancer: a systematic review of risk factors providing rationale for therapy decisions. Endoscopy. 2013 Oct; 45(10):827–34* [30].

resolution to differentiate between layers of the bowel wall in T1 and T2 rectal cancers, but are better than EUS at determining deeper T3 and T4 tumors.

Imaging features that are suspicious for malignant lymph nodes include presence of a round shape, internal heterogeneity, irregular border, and to a lesser extent, size. Lymph node size alone is not a reliable indicator of node positivity, but nodes greater than 8 mm are considered highly suspicious on EUS, CT, and MRI. MRI and EUS are the more reliable modalities for assessing lymph node metastasis in early rectal cancer [35, 37]. CT and MRI are more accurate than EUS in the setting of locally advanced and metastatic disease. There is some promise for improved lymph node accuracy through the use of gadofosveset-enhanced MRI [38].

Oncologic Results Following Local Excision of Rectal Cancer

As noted above, the methodology of many reported series of local excision for rectal neoplasia is suspect. In addition to the problems noted above, trials of local excision for rectal cancer suffer from additional issues. One is inclusion of patients who have cancer in a polyp that is completely or mostly removed by endoscopic polypectomy, and local excision is performed for unclear margins. Many of these patients will have no residual tumor in the local excision specimen and have an extremely low risk of local pelvic failure, biasing the results of the series in favor of local excision. Another is retrospective subgroup analysis, in which patients are only included in the analysis after review of the histology. This allows for exclusion of patients who have positive margins of resection, greater than T1 stage, or other unfavorable histologic features. This obviously biases the analysis in favor of local excision, but fails to replicate the true clinical situation in which margins and T stage cannot be known with certainty preoperatively. Nonrandomized comparative trials of local excision vs. proctectomy suffer from lack of information regarding mesorectal nodal status in the local excision group, which would most likely favor proctectomy. Although this bias can be mitigated by inclusion of patients in each group based on T stage alone, it cannot be completely eliminated as there may be hidden selection bias. It is thus difficult to make firm conclusions regarding the optimal place for local excision in our armamentarium of therapies for patients suffering from rectal cancer.

Local Excision for T1 Cancer

Local excision of T1 rectal cancer is a widely available and technically feasible procedure with low risk of short-term morbidity and mortality. Approximately 15% of all rectal cancers present at stage 1 with no metastatic lymph nodes and tumor confined to the bowel wall. In theory, these patients will gain no clinical benefit from the lymphadenectomy associated with a low anterior or abdominoperineal resection. Therefore there is great controversy over whether the decrease in short-term morbidity is worth the long-term oncologic compromise. As discussed in the previous section, the unmet challenge is the inability to predict with high reliability, which patients have no cancer in their regional lymphatics. The reported rate of local recurrence following TAE varies considerably in the literature, but is universally higher than for proctectomy. For these reasons, proctectomy remains the oncologic gold standard for rectal cancer surgery.

The CALGB 8984 study reported a phase 2 trial in patients with adenocarcinoma of the low rectum less than 10 cm proximal to the dentate line and less than 4 cm in diameter who underwent local excision. Fifty-nine patients with T1 rectal cancers were followed for median a 48 months. Local recurrence occurred in three patients, two local only, one local and distant recurrence. Six-year disease-free survival was 83% [38]. However, approximately one-third of the patients initially enrolled were excluded from analysis, most for positive margins of resection. Several subsequent single institution case series within the United States demonstrated local recurrence rates from 7 to 18%, cancer-specific survival rates ranging from 89 to 92%, and overall survival 72–75% [39–42]. You reported the largest cohort study comparing TAE ($n=601$) and proctectomy ($n=493$) for excision of T1 rectal cancers tracked in the National Cancer Database with a median follow-up of 3.7 years [43]. Local recurrence rates were higher for TAE compared to proctectomy (12.5% vs. 6.9%, $p=0.003$) with concomitant lower 5 year disease-specific survival (93.2% vs. 97.2%, $p=0.004$) but similar 5 year overall survival (77.4% vs. 81.7%, $p=0.09$).

A meta-analysis by Kidane reviewed 1 randomized controlled trial and 12 observational studies comparing local to radical resection in adults with T1N0M0 rectal adenocarcinoma [44]. This showed a significantly lower 5-year overall survival with local excision as compared to radical resection (relative risk (RR) 1.46, 95% CI 1.19–1.77). This difference was not present in the TEM excision subgroup. Five year local recurrence was significantly higher for local excision (RR 2.36, 95% CI 1.64–3.39) including both the TAE and TEM subgroups. With regards to postoperative complications, local excision is associated with significantly lower perioperative mortality (RR, 0.31:95% CI, 0.14–0.71), postoperative complications (RR 0.16:95% CI, 0.08–0.30), and lower need for permanent ostomy (RR 0.17:95% CI, 0.09–0.30) when compared to radical surgery. Meta-regression analysis showed that when local resection and radical resection were compared only in distal rectal cancer, then there was no significant difference in between overall survival (RR 1.13, 95% CI 0.93–1.37). This supports the observation that distal rectal cancers have a higher risk of local recurrence than mid and upper rectal cancers [29]. The authors of this meta-analysis concluded that based on low to moderate qual-

ity evidence, TEM is the preferred surgery for T1N0M0 rectal cancer because of its low risk of complications, mortality, and permanent stoma compared to radical resection without sacrificing 5 year overall survival. However, as noted above, it is impossible to know whether a patient is truly "T1N0" prior to embarking on local excision.

There exists a concern that performing local excision for cancer may oncologically contaminate the embryonic surgery planes and make subsequent restorative radical proctectomy prohibitively difficult or result in a high incidence of local recurrence. This concern did not appear to be founded in a study of 63 local excision patients identified as having high-risk histology who soon thereafter underwent radical proctectomy. Fifty-three (84%) had restorative procedures. Local recurrence occurred in 1 patient whom had a T3 tumor found following TEM. No local recurrences were seen in the T1 or T2 patients [45]. No data exists to determine if immediate proctectomy results in a higher rate of permanent colostomy.

Local Excision for T2NX Cancer

The deeper T2 rectal cancers invade into the muscularis propria permitting them greater access to the lymphatics. As a consequence, the incidence of lymph node metastasis and local recurrence is double that of T1 cancers. Even more so than for T1 cancers, proctectomy is the oncologic procedure of choice. That said, as with T1 cancers, organ sparing options have been explored but in conjunction with the supplemental use of radiation therapy. The CALGB 8984 trial included 51 patients with T2 rectal cancer whom underwent post-op chemoradiation (5400 cGy with 5-fluorouracil). Local recurrence occurred in seven patients. Six year overall survival and failure-free survival was 85 and 71%, similar to historical data for radical surgery from the National Cancer Database [38].

Neoadjuvant chemoradiation prior to radical resection of locally advanced rectal cancer has been shown to downsize and downstage rectal cancers. Read et al. reviewed 649 consecutive rectal cancer patients and found a robust pathological response of the primary tumor to chemoradiation (ypT0-1) in 87 (23%) patients. Lymph node metastasis were identified in only 3% (3 of 87) of these patients indicating that response to neoadjuvant therapy may help predict low risk of lymph node metastasis in rectal cancer [46]. Rullier reviewed data from nine studies of preoperative radiotherapy followed by local excision in cT2-T3N0 rectal cancer. Local and distant recurrence occurred in 28/365 and 24/302, respectively. Complete responders had an 87% disease-free recurrence compared with that of 64% for partial or incomplete responders [47]. These data suggest that a robust primary tumor response to neoadjuvant chemoradiation can be utilized as a surrogate marker for a patient to have low risk lymph node metastasis and, hence, a candidate for organ sparing local excision. This selection factor was included in the GRECCAR 2 multicenter, phase 3, randomized controlled trial for uT2-3 N0 low rectal cancers. Patients underwent neoadjuvant chemoradiation and the clinical response was reassessed. Good responders ($n = 120$) were randomized to local excision or radical proctectomy surgery. Poor responders were not randomized and went directly to radical proctectomy as they were considered high risk for nodal metastasis. Study endpoints include operative mortality, recurrence, major morbidity, and severe side effects after randomization. This trial has completed accrual and its follow-up and data collection phase [48].

The ACOSOG Z6041 trial was a phase 2 trial of 84 patients treated by neoadjuvant 5400 cGy radiation with capecitabine and oxaliplatin followed by local excision of uT2N0 rectal cancers in the low rectum (≤ 8 cm from the anal verge). Complete pathologic response was seen in 44% of patients and down staging to ypT0-1 was seen in 64% of patients. Thirty-nine percent of patients experienced grade 3 toxicity, high enough for the capecitabine and radiation doses to be reduced mid trial [49]. After an average 4.2-year follow-up in 72 patients who underwent local excision for ypT0-2 cancers, local recurrence developed in 2 patients, distant metastasis in 5 patients. Disease-free and overall survival was 87 and 96% at 3 years and 97% of patients had rectal preservation [50]. While this study and other studies are encouraging, inadequate evidence exists to demonstrate the equivalence of neoadjuvant chemoradiation followed by local excision for uT2N0 rectal cancers. A single center, randomized control trial compared radical surgery to TEM following neoadjuvant chemoradiation in 70 patients with clinical T2N0 low rectal cancer [51]. Forty-nine percent of patients in each arm were down staged to ypT0-1. After a median follow-up of 84 months, the local recurrence rate was 6% in the TEM group, and 3% in the radical surgery group. Five-year survival was 94% in both groups. At present, this combination therapy should be reserved for patients unfit or unwilling to undergo the accepted standard therapy of proctectomy.

Surveillance and Salvage Following Local Excision of Rectal Cancer

Surveillance following local excision is recommended to assess for early identification of local recurrence. No formal guidelines are in place but a summary of several retrospective series suggests a follow-up strategy of proctoscopy or flexible sigmoidoscopy with high resolution rectal MRI or endorectal ultrasound every 3–6 months for 3 years, then q 6–12 months through year 5, colonoscopy at years 1, 4, and 9, and CT of abdomen and chest annually.

Median time to recurrence ranges from 13 to 47 months with most occurring between 12 and 24 months. The addition of radiation therapy often delays identification of local recurrence an additional 1–2 years [28, 52–55]. Despite close follow-up, recurrences have a relatively poor prognosis. Patients with local only recurrences who were candidates for resection had an R0 resection in 79–96% of cases resulting in a 53–58% disease-free survival [53, 54, 56]. These poor results of salvage therapy should provide a sobering reminder that the best chance of curing a patient suffering from rectal cancer is with initial treatment. Trying to "mop up" after local pelvic or distant failure has occurred is often futile. In addition, it should be remembered that patients undergoing local excision are typically those with the smallest, early stage lesions, those most easily cured by proctectomy.

Complications of TAE

Complications following local excision of rectal polyps and cancers occur in 5–25% with mortality rates in the 0.3–0.6% range [16, 57, 58]. Major intraoperative bleeding is a rare event. Bleeding is usually addressed with monopolar cautery, sutures, injection of epinephrine solution, or laparoscopic vessel sealing devices. Intraperitoneal entry during TEM was initially discouraged due to the concern for intraabdominal injury or leakage at the closure site. Gavagan reported their small case series that demonstrated the safety of intraperitoneal entry and closure during TEM [9], results that have been confirmed by other groups [10, 59]. The current TAMIS platforms do not have the rigid TEM operating proctoscope which stents open the operative field during the loss of pneumorectum into the peritoneal cavity during intraperitoneal entry. In this instance, closure of the full thickness defect is more likely to require combined transanal and laparoscopic assistance or conversion to open [11].

The most common complication with local excision is postoperative urinary retention. This occurs in up to 11% of patients and is thought to be due to a combination of direct pressure on the urethra, anal stretch, local edema, and pain. This is almost always self-limiting and can be treated by intermittent straight catheterization or short-term indwelling catheter placement. Postoperative bleeding is rare and tends to occur several days post-op corresponding to a suture line dehiscence, sloughing of a scab, or reinstitution of anticoagulant medication. Minor episodes are often self-limiting but frank hemorrhage warrants evaluation with volume assessment and resuscitation followed by endoscopic evaluation and treatment. Suture line dehiscence is more common in lower rectal excisions and in irradiated fields. The patient may report feeling well for a few days post-op followed by a constellation of dark blood and mucous with bowel movements, throbbing rectal pain, fevers, and night sweats. In the absence of sepsis, treatment is usually non-operative and based on symptom control. Symptoms should slowly resolve over 2–3 months.

The concern over potential sphincter damage during TES has been raised. While mild fecal incontinence has been reported immediately post-op, return to preoperative baseline function and quality of life typically occurs within 6 weeks of surgery [60, 61].

Conclusion

Local excision of benign rectal polyps and highly selected early rectal cancers is technically feasible and is associated with a markedly reduced morbidity and mortality when compared to radical surgery. Local excision techniques include conventional TAE and TES. Local excision of early rectal cancers does not remove or adequately sample the regional mesorectal lymph nodes. Preoperative prediction of lymph node positivity is an imprecise science. Increased risk factors for lymph node metastasis and local recurrence include depth of invasion, lymphatic or vascular invasion, poor differentiation, tumor budding, and abnormal lymph nodes identified on imaging. Because of imprecise staging and possibly greater chance of positive resection margins, local excision results in a higher incidence of local recurrence when compared to radical surgery. Patients who are unfit or unwilling to undergo radical surgery may choose an oncologically less sound local excision option in order to avoid the increased short- and long-term complications related to radical surgery. The decision to perform local excision must be individualized, the patient's values and personal preferences regarding cure vs. quality of life.

References

1. Corman ML. Jacques Lisfranc 1790–1847. Dis Colon Rectum. 1983;26(10):694–5.
2. Parks AG. A technique for excising extensive villous papillomatous change in the lower rectum. Proc R Soc Med. 1968; 61(5):441–2.
3. Buess G, Hutterer F, Theiss J, Böbel M, Isselhard W, Pichlmaier H. A system for a transanal endoscopic rectum operation. Chirurg. 1984;55(10):677–80.
4. Atallah S, Albert M, Larach S. Transanal minimally invasive surgery: a giant leap forward. Surg Endosc. 2010;24(9):2200–5.
5. Albert MR, Atallah SB, deBeche-Adams TC, Izfar S, Larach SW. Transanal minimally invasive surgery (TAMIS) for local excision of benign neoplasms and early-stage rectal cancer: efficacy and outcomes in the first 50 patients. Dis Colon Rectum. 2013;56(3):301–7.
6. Salehomoum NM, Nogueras JJ. Conventional transanal excision: current status and role in the era of transanal endoscopic surgery. Sem Colon Rectal Surg. 2015;26(1):9–14.
7. Buess G, Whiteford MH, Swantsrom LL. Transanal endoscopic microsurgery procedure for low rectal tumors. In: Asbun HJ, Young-Fadok TM, editors. American College of Surgeons Multimedia Atlas of Surgery. Woodbury: Ciné-Med Inc.; 2008.
8. Lezoche E, Guerrieri M, Paganini AM, D'Ambrosio G, Baldarelli M, Lezoche G, Feliciotti F, De Sanctis A. Transanal endoscopic versus total mesorectal laparoscopic resections of T2-N0 low rectal cancers after neoadjuvant treatment: a prospective randomized trial with a 3-years minimum follow-up period. Surg Endosc. 2005;19(6):751–6.
9. Gavagan JA, Whiteford MH, Swanstrom LL. Full-thickness intraperitoneal excision by transanal endoscopic microsurgery does not increase short-term complications. Am J Surg. 2004; 187(5):630–4.
10. Morino M, Allaix ME, Famiglietti F, Caldart M, Arezzo A. Does peritoneal perforation affect short- and long-term outcomes after transanal endoscopic microsurgery? Surg Endosc. 2013;27(1):181–8.
11. Hahnloser D, Cantero R, Salgado G, Dindo D, Rega D, Delrio P. Transanal minimal invasive surgery for rectal lesions: should the defect be closed? Colorectal Dis. 2015;17(5): 397–402.
12. Cataldo PA. Local excison of rectal cancer. In: Beck DE et al., editors. The ASCRS textbook of colon and rectal surgery. 2nd ed. New York: Springer; 2011.
13. Middleton PF, Sutherland LM, Maddern GJ. Transanal endoscopic microsurgery: a systematic review. Dis Colon Rectum. 2005;48(2):270–84.
14. Moore JS, Cataldo PA, Osler T, Hyman NH. Transanal endoscopic microsurgery is more effective than traditional transanal excision for resection of rectal masses. Dis Colon Rectum. 2008;51(7):1026–30. discussion 1030-1.
15. de Graaf EJ, Burger JW, van Ijsseldijk AL, Tetteroo GW, Dawson I, Hop WC. Transanal endoscopic microsurgery is superior to transanal excision of rectal adenomas. Colorectal Dis. 2011;13(7):762–7.
16. Clancy C, Burke JP, Albert MR, O'Connell PR, Winter DC. Transanal endoscopic microsurgery versus standard transanal excision for the removal of rectal neoplasms: a systematic review and meta-analysis. Dis Colon Rectum. 2015; 58(2):254–61.
17. Barendse RM, van den Broek FJ, Dekker E, Bemelman WA, de Graaf EJ, Fockens P, Reitsma JB. Systematic review of endoscopic mucosal resection versus transanal endoscopic microsurgery for large rectal adenomas. Endoscopy. 2011; 43(11):941–9.
18. Arezzo A, Passera R, Saito Y, Sakamoto T, Kobayashi N, Sakamoto N, Yoshida N, Naito Y, Fujishiro M, Niimi K, Ohya T, Ohata K, Okamura S, Iizuka S, Takeuchi Y, Uedo N, Fusaroli P, Bonino MA, Verra M, Morino M. Systematic review and meta-analysis of endoscopic submucosal dissection versus transanal endoscopic microsurgery for large noninvasive rectal lesions. Surg Endosc. 2014;28(2):427–38.
19. Swellengrebel HA, Marijnen CA, Verwaal VJ, Vincent A, Heuff G, Gerhards MF, van Geloven AA, van Tets WF, Verheij M, Cats A. Toxicity and complications of preoperative chemoradiotherapy for locally advanced rectal cancer. Br J Surg. 2011;98(3):418–26.
20. van der Pas MH, Haglind E, Cuesta MA, Fürst A, Lacy AM, Hop WC, Bonjer HJ, COlorectal cancer Laparoscopic or Open Resection II (COLOR II) Study Group. Laparoscopic versus open surgery for rectal cancer (COLOR II): short-term outcomes of a randomised, phase 3 trial. Lancet Oncol. 2013; 14(3):210–8.

21. Paun BC, Cassie S, MacLean AR, Dixon E, Buie WD. Postoperative complications following surgery for rectal cancer. Ann Surg. 2010;251(5):807–18.

22. Chang HC, Huang SC, Chen JS, Tang R, Changchien CR, Chiang JM, Yeh CY, Hsieh PS, Tsai WS, Hung HY, You JF. Risk factors for lymph node metastasis in pT1 and pT2 rectal cancer: a single-institute experience in 943 patients and literature review. Ann Surg Oncol. 2012;19(8):2477–84.

23. Rasheed S, Bowley DM, Aziz O, Tekkis PP, Sadat AE, Guenther T, Boello ML, McDonald PJ, Talbot IC, Northover JM. Can depth of tumour invasion predict lymph node positivity in patients undergoing resection for early rectal cancer? A comparative study between T1 and T2 cancers. Colorectal Dis. 2008;10(3):231–8.

24. Kobayashi H, Mochizuki H, Kato T, Mori T, Kameoka S, Shirouzu K, Saito Y, Watanabe M, Morita T, Hida J, Ueno M, Ono M, Yasuno M, Sugihara K. Is total mesorectal excision always necessary for T1-T2 lower rectal cancer? Ann Surg Oncol. 2010;17(4):973–80.

25. Salinas HM, Dursun A, Klos CL, Shellito P, Sylla P, Berger D, Bordeianou L. Determining the need for radical surgery in patients with T1 rectal cancer. Arch Surg. 2011;146(5):540–4.

26. Kikuchi R, Takano M, Takagi K, Fujimoto N, Nozaki R, Fujiyoshi T, Uchida Y. Management of early invasive colorectal cancer. Risk of recurrence and clinical guidelines. Dis Colon Rectum. 1995;38(12):1286–95.

27. Okuyama T, Oya M, Ishikawa H. Budding as a risk factor for lymph node metastasis in pT1 or pT2 well-differentiated colorectal adenocarcinoma. Dis Colon Rectum. 2002; 45(5):628–34.

28. Bach SP, Hill J, Monson JR, Simson JN, Lane L, Merrie A, Warren B, Mortensen NJ, Association of Coloproctology of Great Britain and Ireland Transanal Endoscopic Microsurgery (TEM) Collaboration. A predictive model for local recurrence after transanal endoscopic microsurgery for rectal cancer. Br J Surg. 2009;96(3):280–90.

29. Nascimbeni R, Burgart LJ, Nivatvongs S, Larson DR. Risk of lymph node metastasis in T1 carcinoma of the colon and rectum. Dis Colon Rectum. 2002;45(2):200–6.

30. Masaki T, Sugiyama M, Atomi Y, Matsuoka H, Abe N, Watanabe T, Nagawa H, Muto T. The indication of local excision for T2 rectal carcinomas. Am J Surg. 2001;181(2):133–7.

31. Bosch SL, Teerenstra S, de Wilt JH, Cunningham C, Nagtegaal ID. Predicting lymph node metastasis in pT1 colorectal cancer: a systematic review of risk factors providing rationale for therapy decisions. Endoscopy. 2013;45(10):827–34.

32. Glasgow SC, Bleier JI, Burgart LJ, Finne CO, Lowry AC. Meta-analysis of histopathological features of primary colorectal cancers that predict lymph node metastases. J Gastrointest Surg. 2012;16(5):1019–28.

33. Wang HS, Liang WY, Lin TC, Chen WS, Jiang JK, Yang SH, Chang SC, Lin JK. Curative resection of T1 colorectal carcinoma: risk of lymph node metastasis and long-term prognosis. Dis Colon Rectum. 2005;48(6):1182–92.

34. Benson III AB, Venook AP, Bekaii-Saab T, Chan E, Chen YJ, Cooper HS, Engstrom PF, Enzinger PC, Fenton MJ, Fuchs CS, Grem JL, Grothey A, Hochster HS, Hunt S, Kamel A, Kirilcuk N, Leong LA, Lin E, Messersmith WA, Mulcahy MF, Murphy JD, Nurkin S, Rohren E, Ryan DP, Saltz L, Sharma S, Shibata D, Skibber JM, Sofocleous CT, Stoffel EM, Stotsky-Himelfarb E, Willett CG, Gregory KM, Freedman-Cass D. Rectal cancer, version 2.2015. J Natl Compr Canc Netw. 2015;13(6):719–28.

35. Beets-Tan RG, Lambregts DM, Maas M, Bipat S, Barbaro B, Caseiro-Alves F, Curvo-Semedo L, Fenlon HM, Gollub MJ, Gourtsoyianni S, Halligan S, Hoeffel C, Kim SH, Laghi A, Maier A, Rafaelsen SR, Stoker J, Taylor SA, Torkzad MR, Blomqvist L. Magnetic resonance imaging for the clinical management of rectal cancer patients: recommendations from the 2012 European Society of Gastrointestinal and Abdominal Radiology (ESGAR) consensus meeting. Eur Radiol. 2013;23(9):2522–31.

36. van de Velde CJ, Boelens PG, Tanis PJ, Espin E, Mroczkowski P, Naredi P, Pahlman L, Ortiz H, Rutten HJ, Breugom AJ, Smith JJ, Wibe A, Wiggers T, Valentini V. Experts reviews of the multidisciplinary consensus conference colon and rectal cancer 2012: science, opinions and experiences from the experts of surgery. Eur J Surg Oncol. 2014;40(4):454–68.

37. Lambregts DM, Beets GL, Maas M, Kessels AG, Bakers FC, Cappendijk VC, Engelen SM, Lahaye MJ, de Bruïne AP, Lammering G, Leiner T, Verwoerd JL, Wildberger JE, Beets-Tan RG. Accuracy of gadofosveset-enhanced MRI for nodal staging and restaging in rectal cancer. Ann Surg. 2011; 253(3):539–45.

38. Steele Jr GD, Herndon JE, Bleday R, Russell A, Benson III A, Hussain M, Burgess A, Tepper JE, Mayer RJ. Sphincter-sparing treatment for distal rectal adenocarcinoma. Ann Surg Oncol. 1999;6(5):433–41.

39. Mellgren A, Sirivongs P, Rothenberger DA, Madoff RD, García-Aguilar J. Is local excision adequate therapy for early rectal cancer? Dis Colon Rectum. 2000;43:1064–71. discussion 1071–4.

40. Paty PB, Nash GM, Baron P, Zakowski M, Minsky BD, Blumberg D, Nathanson DR, Guillem JG, Enker WE, Cohen AM, Wong WD. Long-term results of local excision for rectal cancer. Ann Surg. 2002;236(4):522–9. discussion 529-30.

41. Nascimbeni R, Nivatvongs S, Larson DR, Burgart LJ. Long-term survival after local excision for T1 carcinoma of the rectum. Dis Colon Rectum. 2004;47:1773–9.

42. Madbouly KM, Remzi FH, Erkek BA, Senagore AJ, Baeslach CM, Khandwala F, Fazio VW, Lavery IC. Recurrence after transanal excision of T1 rectal cancer: should we be concerned? Dis Colon Rectum. 2005;48(4):711–9. discussion 719-21.

43. You YN, Baxter NN, Stewart A, Nelson H. Is the increasing rate of local excision for stage I rectal cancer in the United States justified? A nationwide cohort study from the National Cancer Database. Ann Surg. 2007;245(5):726–33.

44. Kidane B, Chadi SA, Kanters S, Colquhoun PH, Ott MC. Local resection compared with radical resection in the treatment of T1N0M0 rectal adenocarcinoma: a systematic review and meta-analysis. Dis Colon Rectum. 2015;58(1):122–40.

45. Hahnloser D, Wolff BG, Larson DW, Ping J, Nivatvongs S. Immediate radical resection after local excision of rectal cancer: an oncologic compromise? Dis Colon Rectum. 2005;48(3): 429–37.

46. Read TE, Andujar JE, Caushaj PF, Johnston DR, Dietz DW, Myerson RJ, Fleshman JW, Birnbaum EH, Mutch MG, Kodner

IJ. Neoadjuvant therapy for rectal cancer: histologic response of the primary tumor predicts nodal status. Dis Colon Rectum. 2004;47(6):825–31.

47. Rullier E, Denost Q. Transanal surgery for cT2T3 rectal cancer: patient selection, adjuvant therapy, and outcomes. Sem Colon Rectal Surg. 2015;26(1):26–31.

48. Rullier E, Vendrely V. Can mesorectal lymph node excision be avoided in rectal cancer surgery? Colorectal Dis. 2011;13 Suppl 7:37–42.

49. Garcia-Aguilar J, Shi Q, Thomas Jr CR, Chan E, Cataldo P, Marcet J, Medich D, Pigazzi A, Oommen S, Posner MC. A phase II trial of neoadjuvant chemoradiation and local excision for T2N0 rectal cancer: preliminary results of the ACOSOG Z6041 trial. Ann Surg Oncol. 2012;19(2):384–91.

50. Garcia-Aguilar J, Renfro LA, Chow OS, Shi Q, Carrero XW, Lynn PB, Thomas CR Jr, Chan E, Cataldo PA, Marcet JE, Medich DS, Johnson CS, Oommen SC, Wolff BG, Pigazzi A, McNevin SM, Pons RK, Bleday R. Organ preservation for clinical T2N0 distal rectal cancer using neoadjuvant chemoradiotherapy and local excision (ACOSOG Z6041): results of an open-label, single-arm, multi-institutional, phase 2 trial. Lancet Oncol. 2015;16(15):1537–46.

51. Lezoche G, Baldarelli M, Guerrieri M, Paganini AM, De Sanctis A, Bartolacci S, Lezoche E. A prospective randomized study with a 5-year minimum follow-up evaluation of transanal endoscopic microsurgery versus laparoscopic total mesorectal excision after neoadjuvant therapy. Surg Endosc. 2008;22(2):352–8.

52. Chakravarti A, Compton CC, Shellito PC, Wood WC, Landry J, Machuta SR, Kaufman D, Ancukiewicz M, Willett CG. Long-term follow-up of patients with rectal cancer managed by local excision with and without adjuvant irradiation. Ann Surg. 1999;230(1):49–54.

53. Friel CM, Cromwell JW, Marra C, Madoff RD, Rothenberger DA, Garcia-Aguílar J. Salvage radical surgery after failed local excision for early rectal cancer. Dis Colon Rectum. 2002; 45:875–9.

54. Weiser MR, Landmann RG, Wong WD, Shia J, Guillem JG, Temple LK, Minsky BD, Cohen AM, Paty PB. Surgical salvage of recurrent rectal cancer after transanal excision. Dis Colon Rectum. 2005;48(6):1169–75.

55. Greenberg JA, Shibata D, Herndon II JE, Steele Jr GD, Mayer R, Bleday R. Local excision of distal rectal cancer: an update of cancer and leukemia group B 8984. Dis Colon Rectum. 2008; 51(8):1185–91.

56. Doornebosch PG, Ferenschild FT, de Wilt JH, Dawson I, Tetteroo GW, de Graaf EJ. Treatment of recurrence after transanal endoscopic microsurgery (TEM) for T1 rectal cancer. Dis Colon Rectum. 2010;53(9):1234–9.

57. de Graaf EJ, Doornebosch PG, Tetteroo GW, Geldof H, Hop WC. Transanal endoscopic microsurgery is feasible for adenomas throughout the entire rectum: a prospective study. Dis Colon Rectum. 2009;52(6):1107–13.

58. Kumar AS, Coralic J, Kelleher DC, Sidani S, Kolli K, Smith LE. Complications of transanal endoscopic microsurgery are rare and minor: a single institution's analysis and comparison to existing data. Dis Colon Rectum. 2013;56(3):295–300.

59. Ramwell A, Evans J, Bignell M, Mathias J, Simson J. The creation of a peritoneal defect in transanal endoscopic microsurgery does not increase complications. Colorectal Dis. 2009; 11(9):964–6.

60. Cataldo PA, O'Brien S, Osler T. Transanal endoscopic microsurgery: a prospective evaluation of functional results. Dis Colon Rectum. 2005;48(7):1366–71.

61. Fenech DS, Takahashi T, Liu M, Spencer L, Swallow CJ, Cohen Z, Macrae HM, McLeod RS. Function and quality of life after transanal excision of rectal polyps and cancers. Dis Colon Rectum. 2007;50(5):598–603.

30

Rectal Cancer: Watch and Wait

George J. Chang

Key Concepts

- Pathologic complete treatment response following neoadjuvant chemoradiation therapy and surgery for rectal cancer is associated with favorable prognosis.
- Pathologic complete treatment response is observed in approximately 15–20% of rectal cancer patients following chemoradiation therapy.
- Clinical and radiographic assessment of neoadjuvant therapy treatment response is suboptimal, and remains a primary challenge for safe implementation of watch and wait strategies.
- Approximately one in three patients exhibiting clinical complete response will develop tumor regrowth.
- At present, watch and wait should be offered to patients only in the context of a clinical trial.
- Local excision following neoadjuvant chemoradiation therapy is associated with significant risk for pain and poor wound healing.

Introduction

Over the past few decades, the management of rectal cancer has become increasingly complex. What was once a disease with high mortality and limited treatment options that typically necessitated a permanent colostomy has become a model for multidisciplinary evaluation and treatment and surgical advancement. For over a century, surgical resection has remained the cornerstone of curative treatment of rectal cancer. The principles of treatment include complete *en bloc* resection of the tumor-bearing rectum and mesorectum with clear margins along with clearance of pelvic lymphadenopathy and, when possible, restoration of intestinal continuity [1]. However, because of the historically high risk of local failure after surgery alone, clinicians have utilized neoadjuvant radiotherapy or chemoradiation therapy (nCRT) which has improved the rate of local tumor control [2]. Now the oncologic outcomes following treatment of rectal cancer in the modern era can equal outcomes following treatment of colon cancer [3]. Despite these advances, the multimodal treatment for rectal cancer is associated with a significant impact on long-term functional and quality of life outcomes including risks for bowel, bladder, and sexual dysfunction, pain, and potential need for permanent colostomy. Therefore there is great interest in strategies to decrease the toxicity of treatment, including strategies that employ the selective use of radiation, chemotherapy, or even surgery.

The modern concept of selective use of surgery following chemoradiation therapy for patients with rectal cancer are based on the fact that pathologic complete response (pCR) is observed in approximately 10–20% of patients following long course chemoradiation therapy. In 2004, Habr-Gama and her group first reported outcomes for selective surgery with a nonoperative (a.k.a. "watch and wait" or "wait and see") strategy in select patients who achieved a clinical complete response (cCR) following chemoradiation therapy [4]. In the decade since that initial report, a number of other investigators have attempted to bring further light to understanding the potential for a selective surgical approach. They have also highlighted a need for considering a number of important factors including assessing and improving the effectiveness of neoadjuvant therapy, predicting pCR prior to pathologic evaluation, determining the true risk for locoregional failure following a watch-and-wait approach, and understanding the potential for salvage surgical treatment and subsequent long-term survival outcome following treatment failure. While definitive surgical resection remains the standard of care for all patients with non-metastatic rectal cancer, a growing number of studies are providing supportive evidence for a watch and wait, organ-preserving approach in highly selected patients with rectal cancer.

© Springer International Publishing 2016
S.R. Steele et al. (eds.), *The ASCRS Textbook of Colon and Rectal Surgery*, DOI 10.1007/978-3-319-25970-3_30

Neoadjuvant Chemoradiation Therapy

For patients with locally advanced rectal cancers, tradition-ally considered as clinical stage II and III, neoadjuvant ther-apy has been administered to improve local control. Building upon the demonstrated oncologic benefit of total mesorectal excision (TME) surgery by Heald, the Dutch Colorectal Cancer Group randomized patients to preoperative radiother-apy (5×5 Gy) followed by immediate TME surgery to TME surgery alone [5, 6]. This demonstrated that preoperative radiotherapy, when compared to TME surgery alone, was associated with a significant reduction in local recurrence although no improvement in overall survival could be demon-strated [7]. Meanwhile, the EORTC 22921 and FCCD 9203 studies demonstrated that addition of concurrent chemother-apy administered over a 5–6 week duration followed by delayed surgery demonstrated improvement in local recur-rence free survival when compared to preoperative radiother-apy alone [8, 9]. However, the landmark study of the German Rectal Cancer Study Group definitively established the supe-riority of preoperative (neoadjuvant) vs. postoperative chemo-radiation therapy, followed by surgery 6–8 weeks later, with improved local control and sphincter preservation [2].

Preoperative chemoradiotherapy is typically administered in "long course" fashion, with radiotherapy and a radiosensi-tizing chemotherapeutic agent administered over a 5–6 week period with a 6–10 week treatment break prior to proctectomy. This extended period of time allows for tumor regression, if the tumor is sensitive to the therapy [10]. This may facilitate more optimal surgery, including sphincter preservation, by reducing the tumor bulk and permitting surgery to be safely conducted in previously uninvolved but inaccessible adjacent tissue planes [11]. It also provides potential clearance of microscopic tumor spread, safely permitting a closer distal margin at resection with subsequent restoration of intestinal continuity [12, 13]. The surgeon should be cautious, however, not to leave tissue in situ that was previously involved with tumor, as radiotherapy does not induce tumor kill in a "wave front," and residual nests of tumor cells can be found spread throughout the initial volume of tissue involved by the tumor. Lastly, studies demonstrating improved sphincter preservation

must be taken with a grain of salt, as estimation of whether a surgeon will be able to perform restorative proctectomy or not based on initial clinical examination is subjective.

As one would expect, similar responses to pelvic short-course preoperative therapy were previously not observed, as proctectomy was typically performed within a week or 2 of short-course radiotherapy, prior to the development of radia-tion induced inflammation, and too short a time to allow for significant tumor regression [14]. More recent trials in which proctectomy was delayed 4–8 weeks after short course radio-therapy reveal that tumor regression and relatively high rates of complete pathologic response do occur [15]. In addition, oncologic outcomes following short course radiotherapy and long course chemoradiotherapy for patients with locally advanced rectal cancer have been demonstrated to be similar in prospective randomized trials [14, 16]. Thus, it is likely that significant tumorcidal effect can be achieved with either regimen, but the added time delay prior to proctectomy with long course chemoradiotherapy results in more tumor involu-tion seen on histologic evaluation of the proctectomy speci-men. Furthermore, the potential systemic effects of the concurrent chemotherapy are not well understood.

Response to treatment has been an important observation, and following completion of CRT up to 50% of patients will experience a cCR as defined by replacement of the tumor bed by scar or normal appearing mucosa on clinical and endo-scopic examination [17]. Pathologic complete response (specimen without evidence of residual tumor cells) or pathologic near-complete response (specimen with only sin-gle or small groups of tumor cells) can be observed in 10–40% of patients following neoadjuvant chemoradiation therapy (nCRT) [18, 19]. Complete clinical response, how-ever, is not necessarily predictive of pathologic response. It is now widely recognized that tumor regression in response to neoadjuvant treatment is an important prognostic indicator of long-term outcome. It can be associated with tumor vol-ume reduction, down-staging and nodal sterilization and a number of pathologic grading systems now exist to describe the extent of response (Table 30-1). It is a pathologic biomarker of the effectiveness of local and systemic tumor control and major response with complete or near complete resolution is

TABLE 30-1. Tumor Regression Grading Systems

TRG	Mandard [22]	Dworak [23]	Rödel [10]	Ryan [24]	CAP [25]
0		No regression	No regression		No residual tumor cells
1	No residual cancer cells	Dominant tumor mass with obvious fibrosis and/or vasculopathy	Fibrosis <25% of tumor mass	No residual cancer cells or single cells	Single or small groups of cancer cells
2	Rare residual cancer cells	Dominantly fibrotic changes with few tumor cells or groups	Fibrosis 25–50% of tumor mass	Residual cancer outgrown by fibrosis	Residual cancer outgrown by fibrosis
3	Fibrosis greater than residual cancer	Very few (difficult to find microscopically) tumor cells in fibrotic tissue with or without mucous substance	Fibrosis >50% of tumor mass	Significant cancer outgrown by cancer or no fibrosis with extensive residual cancer	Minimal evidence of fibrosis
4	Residual cancer greater than fibrosis	Complete regression	Complete regression		
5	No regression				

highly associated with a favorable prognosis [20]. In a large study of 725 patients treated with neoadjuvant chemoradiation and total mesorectal excision for locally advanced rectal cancer at The University of Texas, MD, Anderson Cancer Center, local recurrences were virtually absent and systemic recurrences occurred in fewer than 10% of patients exhibiting complete response or major downstaging to ypT0-2 N0 disease [21]. In fact in the modern era of TME surgery, distant, rather than local, disease recurrence has emerged as the primary concern.

Surgery for Rectal Cancer

The principles for surgical curative treatment for rectal cancer have been established since the beginning of the twentieth century with Ernest Miles' description of abdominoperineal excision (APE) with end colostomy for carcinomas of the rectum and pelvic colon [26]. Since then, a number of surgical and multidisciplinary advances as outlined above have improved treatment outcomes, reduced operative mortality, and offered the potential for sphincter preservation. However, for patients with distal rectal cancer, the excellent oncologic outcomes of nCRT and surgery can be associated with the need for permanent colostomy or with significant risk for bowel dysfunction including fecal incontinence and soiling following coloanal reconstruction.

Quality of life among rectal cancer patients undergoing surgical resection with or without a permanent colostomy was compared in a systematic review of 5127 patients from 35 non-randomized studies. Fourteen of the studies reported that APE was not associated with poorer quality of life measures than low anterior resection among patients with rectal cancer. The remaining studies found some difference, although it was not always in favor of non-stoma patients. These results may in part reflect underlying bowel dysfunction among patients undergoing TME surgery with sphincter preservation, so-called low anterior resection syndrome (LARS) [27]. In a long-term follow-up study at 14 years of patients randomized to preoperative radiotherapy followed by proctectomy with TME to proctectomy with TME alone in the Dutch trial, 56% of the patients randomized to preoperative radiotherapy followed by proctectomy and 35% of the patients randomized to proctectomy alone reported major LARS [28].

Finally the prevalence of male and female sexual dysfunction is high after surgery for rectal cancer and up to one-half of the patients undergoing surgery with rectal cancer will report a deterioration in sexual function, and a third of patients will report the development of urinary dysfunction [29, 30]. While some of these effects may be attributed to pelvic autonomic injury from radiation therapy, the majority of the effect is caused by nerve injury at surgery. This is a particular concern among distal rectal cancer patients undergoing APE. While the case can be made that these effects are exacerbated when surgery is performed by less experienced surgeons, these issues remain significant problems that impact quality of life following even among patients undergoing sphincter preserving rectal cancer surgery. Thus there is a need for approaches to treating rectal cancer that can also safely preserve functional and quality of life outcomes.

The Watch and Wait Approach

Based on these concerns, the appeal of a watch and wait, organ preserving, nonoperative approach is obvious. If radical surgery to resect rectal cancer could be avoided, then patients would not be subject to the associated surgical morbidity and potential long-term effects on quality of life. However before such a strategy can be more broadly applied, it is important to ensure that oncologic outcomes are not being compromised, particular for this group of patients who are expected to have excellent outcomes, with an extremely low risk for either local or distant disease recurrence, with proctectomy. What is also unknown is if response to chemoradiotherapy is just a biologic response indicator of favorable tumor biology, or if similarly good outcomes can be achieved by increasing the rate of pCR. In light of the fact that nCRT has been associated with improvement in pelvic control, but not overall survival suggests that the former may be true. However, the body of evidence regarding the prognostic value of even an intermediate response indicates that tumor behavior is a continuum from favorable to poor. Moreover, it is now recognized that the interval from the completion of chemoradiation therapy to clinical or pathologic assessment can impact the rate of complete response as ongoing regression can be observed well beyond the traditional 6–8 week interval to assessment.

Following Habr-Gama's original report, other investigators initially reported a wide range of success with an initially nonoperative approach, including a locoregional treatment failure rate of up to 50–60%, much higher than the 3% failure rate initially reported by Habr-Gama [31, 32]. While not fully explained, the reasons for this discrepancy may have included differences in initial tumor burden, selection of patients for a watch and wait approach following neoadjuvant therapy, method and timing of assessment, or the neoadjuvant treatment regimen. In addition the method of selection of patients for nonoperative therapy in Habr-Gama's initial report may have played a major role [4]. Specifically, patients were not included in the study (observation) group until they had been followed for 12 months following chemoradiotherapy. Put another way, patients initially selected for nonoperative therapy who failed in the first 12 months were excluded from analysis. This has the potential to bias the results heavily in favor of the observation group.

Recent data, including from an updated report by Habr-Gama, indicates that the true risk for locoregional treatment failure is approximately 30% [17, 33]. This suggests that a

TABLE 30-2. Comparison of selected modern studies

Series	Number of patients observed	Number of patients operated	Median follow-up (months)	cCR	Local regrowth	Outcome
Mass 2011 [36]	21	20	15 (observed)	100%	1 patient	2-year OS 100%
			35 (operated)			2-year DFS 89%
Dalton 2012 [31]	12	37	25.5 (mean)	24%	50%	Disease free at follow-up
Habr-Gama 2014 [17]	93	90	60	49%	31%	5-year OS 91%
						5-year LRFS 69%
						5-year DFS 68%
Smith 2015 [34]	73	72			26%	4-year OS 91% (obs) vs. 95% (surg)
						4-year DSS 91% (obs) vs. 96% (surg)
Smith 2015 [37]	18	30	68.4 (mean)		1 patient	Alive with pelvic disease at 54 months

number of patients initially thought to have a pCR based on clinical assessment of complete response actually had undetected viable tumor, highlighting one of the major challenges and pitfalls of the watch and wait approach. One potential solution to the challenge of clinically identifying patients with a pCR is to ensure a close follow-up strategy. This will only be effective, however, if salvage treatment is proven to be effective. We recommend that patients be monitored with digital rectal and endoluminal examination every 3 months along with carcinoembryonic antigen level determination and biopsy of any suspicious lesions. The majority of tumor regrowth will be detected within the first 12 months, in which case patients may be eligible for curative resection with the possibility for coloanal reconstruction for tumors without anal canal involvement precluding partial sphincter resection with anastomosis. There is concern that a longer delay to surgery will result in making the salvage resection more difficult. Although it has been reported that salvage surgical resection after nonoperative management is feasible, longer delays in identification of regrowth has been associated with more than a 50% decrease in the ability to perform sphincter preserving salvage surgery [17, 33]. Tumor regrowth occurring deep to the mucosa may be difficult to identify before more extensive sphincter involvement and the addition of radiation-induced posttreatment fibrosis along the pelvic floor or anal sphincter complex may also preclude subsequent sphincter-preserving resection.

Thus when tumor regrowth occurs, subsequent sphincter preservation cannot be assured. In fact this is quite understandable and reasonable if patients are indeed selected for a watch and wait approach based on distally located tumors. Finally, what remains to be settled is if leaving the rectum containing residual viable tumor in patients with cCR but not pCR increases the risk for distant failure. Recent data regarding 73 patients from Memorial Sloan Kettering suggest that there is the potential for increased risk of distant metastasis among patients undergoing watch and wait when compared to those with pCR, but the sample size was relatively small and the difference did not achieve statistical significance ($p = 0.09$) [34].

Despite these concerns the evidence in support of a watch and wait approach is growing. A limited number of prospective series have reported on nCRT followed by observation (Table 30-2). A review of the wait and see approach published in 2012 identified 30 publications from 9 series including 650 patients. While demonstrating proof of principle, significant heterogeneity of the studies in staging, inclusion criteria, study design, and follow-up rigor limit our ability to draw firm conclusions [35].

Clinical Assessment of Treatment Response

The clinical assessment of treatment response is difficult and is perhaps the greatest challenge and limiting factor for safe implementation of the watch and wait approach. A number of different strategies have been considered including clinical assessment, full-thickness local excision, metabolic imaging, and high-resolution pelvic MRI imaging.

The concordance between clinical and pathologic evaluation has traditionally been poor both in terms of sensitivity (~25%) for detecting pCR, and specificity (~60–90%) for excluding residual disease [38, 39]. Moreover, there has not existed a standard method for the clinical evaluation of complete response. Investigators have advocated for a combination of digital rectal examination and endoluminal visualization to identify residual mass, ulceration, nodularity, or stenosis, all of which may suggest persistent tumor [40]. Findings in support of a complete response include regular and smooth mucosa, and changes such as whitening or presence of telangiectasias. However, in a recent study, the false-positive rate for pCR based on preoperative clinical assessment was 27% [41]. Improvement in the clinical detection of pCR may be possible with a higher pretest probability of complete response, as demonstrated by the ACoSOG Z6041 trial of nCRT with concurrent capecitabine and oxaliplatin followed by local excision for cT2N0 rectal cancers that observed a sensitivity of 85% for detection of pCR based on digital rectal examination and proctoscopy. However even in the setting of a prospective trial with a primary endpoint of pCR, the false positive rate was 33% [42]. These data suggest that while the detection of pCR can be improved, the risk for false-positivity remains a significant concern.

Given the challenges for clinical assessment of residual disease within the bowel wall, a number of investigators have considered local excision of the tumor bed as both a diagnostic test to assess pathologic treatment response and a therapeutic maneuver to excise any residual tumor cells residing within the bowel wall. Endoscopic biopsy alone has the obvious limitation of being able to provide only a superficial sampling of the tumor bed that can miss residual disease that may be present more deeply within the bowel wall or away from the site of biopsy. Among 39 patients exhibiting clinical response to nCRT but not meeting clinical criteria for pCR, endoluminal biopsies were associated with a negative predictive value of only 11% [43].

Full thickness excision of the entire tumor bed may be performed through a variety of approaches including transanal excision, transanal endoscopic microsurgery (TEM), or transanal minimally invasive surgery (TAMIS). However, while complete pathologic assessment of the bowel wall can be performed, it still cannot provide information regarding the status of the unresected lymph nodes, which may contain viable tumor in up to 9.1% of patients who achieve ypT0 status and 17.1% of patients with ypT1 disease [18, 44, 45]. However, the presence of ypN+ status may be influenced by pretreatment patient selection and ypT0 status among patients with earlier stage initial disease may be associated with a relatively low risk for ypN+ disease [46]. Another major limitation of full-thickness excision following nCRT is that it is associated with significant treatment associated toxicity including poor healing and pain. In fact the risk for wound dehiscence has been reported to be 26–70% following nCRT [47, 48]. Consistent with these single institutional findings, the multi-centered ACoSOG Z6041 study reported a 54% overall rate of perioperative complications following local excision [42]. Moreover, local excision following nCRT is still associated with a significant risk for anorectal and sexual dysfunction. In a study of 44 patients, 51% and 46% reported incontinence of flatus and loose stool, respectively, and 59% reported clustering and 49% reported urgency. In addition, 19% of men and 20% of women reported negative impacts on sexual quality of life [49]. Finally, the watch and wait strategy may perhaps have the greatest appeal for patients whose tumors involve the anal sphincter for whom sphincter preservation would be impossible. Full-thickness excision in this circumstance would necessitate at least partial resection of the internal sphincter. Thus the role for full-thickness excision in a watch and wait approach remains limited.

Two primary approaches to radiologic imaging for the assessment of treatment response have been investigated. Despite its utility in signaling response to systemic therapy for a variety of malignant diseases, metabolic imaging with

Table 30-3. MRI tumor regression grade (mrTRG) [54]

mrTRG	Description
1	Tumor bed with low signal intensity signaling fibrosis with no residual intermediate tumor signal
2	Tumor bed with predominance of fibrosis with minimal residual intermediate tumor signal
3	Substantial intermediate intensity tumor signal present, but does not predominate over low intensity fibrosis
4	Minimal fibrosis
5	No change from baseline

^{18}fluorodeoxyglucose positron emission computed tomography (PET) has not been shown to be reliable for the identification of complete responders (AUC 0.57–0.73) [50]. Although comparing the change in baseline with 12-week posttreatment standardized ^{18}FDG uptake values may provide some improvement in test performance [51].

Perhaps one of the most useful imaging tests is high-resolution MRI. Areas of treatment response and fibrosis are characterized by low signal intensity on T2 weighted imaging. The presence of uniform low signal intensity with the absence of areas of intermediate signal intensity within it is suggestive of a pCR. Based on these findings and a comparison to pretreatment MRI, a tumor regression grade has been proposed by the Mercury Study investigators (Table 30-3) [52]. The so-called mrTRG of 1–3 correlated with better survival outcomes when compared to mrTRG 4–5, comparable to the difference in survival observed when comparing ypT0-3a vs. ypT3b or greater [52]. There is currently great interest in the potential for the addition of diffusion weighting or functional dynamic contrast enhanced MRI to improve the detection of response, and other technologies may still be on the horizon [53]. In the meantime, MRI may play an important role in identifying patients with significant treatment response and more favorable prognosis who may be eligible for a watch and wait approach. Such a strategy was employed by a group from Maastricht University in the Netherlands to identify 21 patients for a wait and see approach that were compared to 20 matched control patients exhibiting pCR treated with surgery. They utilized strict selection criteria requiring evidence of cCR, including by posttreatment high-resolution magnetic resonance imaging (MRI) and then MRI-based follow-up every 3 months for the 1st year and biannually thereafter. With their approach, 75% of the pCR patients who had undergone resection were classified by MRI incomplete responders. After a median follow-up of 15 months (vs. 35 months in the surgery group), only 1 patient experienced a local recurrence in the study arm [36]. The TRIGGER trial lead by investigators at the Royal Marsden and the Pelican Cancer Foundation in the United Kingdom will randomize patients to deferral of surgery with watch and wait for good (mrTRG 1–2) and systemic therapy for poor (mrTRG 3–5) responders based on MRI with an opportunity for the poor responders to be converted to complete response vs. immediate surgery in the control arm.

Increasing the Rate of Complete Response

Based on the presumption that patients with pCR are eligible for an organ-preserving watch and wait approach, a number of investigators have tried to improve the rate of PCR with neoadjuvant therapy. These can broadly be categorized as (1) radiotherapy dose intensification including contact radiation; (2) utilization of more active chemotherapeutic regimens; (3) increase in the time interval from chemoradiotherapy to surgery; and (4) a combination of these approaches.

Perhaps the most common strategy for radiotherapy dose escalation is local boost therapy to the tumor volume. This approach has the advantage of increasing the delivered dose to the tumor volume without increasing toxicity to uninvolved surrounded bowel and can be achieved through IMRT or contact therapy [55]. In a randomized trial of external beam radiotherapy to 39 Gy in three fractions with endocavitary boost to 85 Gy compared to external beam radiotherapy alone, there was significant increase in complete or near-complete sterilization (57% vs. 34%, respectively) [56]. Unfortunately, while boost therapy to the primary tumor bed can increase the rate of response within the bowel wall, the lymph nodes may remain unaddressed; however these strategies appear to be well tolerated and remain the subject of further investigation.

A number of studies have attempted to increase the treatment response by incorporating more highly active concurrent chemotherapy regimens. Indeed, it has been reported that systemic chemotherapy alone may be associated with pCR in up to 25% of patients with relatively early rectal cancers [57]. Unfortunately, after several randomized studies of concurrent fluoropyrimidine-based oxaliplatin containing regimens, an increase in pCR has been observed only in the German CAO/ARO/AIO-04 randomized trial at the cost of increased toxicity as demonstrated in NASBP R-04 and STAR-01 [58–61].

The time interval between nCRT and surgery is another important factor associated with pCR. The Lyon R90-01 trial randomized patients to an interval of 6–8 weeks vs. <2 weeks and found a higher rate of complete response (26% vs. 10.3% $p = 0.005$) following the longer interval [62]. However, subsequent long-term follow-up after a median 6.3 months demonstrates no difference in local recurrence or survival [63]. Thus while it is well recognized that a longer treatment interval is associated with a higher rate of pCR, it has not been demonstrated that patients exhibiting pCR after a longer treatment interval have the same good prognosis of those who were more rapidly sterilized. Thus tumor cell death is initiated immediately (during neoadjuvant therapy), but the pCR rate can be manipulated by changing the duration of delay prior to proctectomy. Therefore, one cannot assume that one neoadjuvant therapy regimen is superior to another based on

pCR rate if proctectomy occurs at different intervals following neoadjuvant therapy.

Additional strategies for improving treatment response while providing systemically active therapy include induction and consolidation chemotherapy. Induction chemotherapy has the potential to improve survival outcomes by improving tumor regression and the ability to deliver systemic chemotherapy with a lower rate of associated toxicity. The EXPERT and EXPERT-C phase II studies of pretreatment capecitabine with oxaliplatin and with cetuximab in patients with high-risk rectal cancers showed that a high rate of R0 resection could be achieved although there was not a remarkable increase in the rate of pCR [64]. The addition of the EGFR inhibitor resulted in greater rates of radiographic response, although not in the rate of pCR [65].

Capitalizing on the potential for improved tumor regression with increased time interval to surgery, the Timing of Rectal Cancer Response to Chemoradiation trial, delivering up to six cycles of mFOLFOX6 after standard CRT was associated with an increase in pCR to 38% vs. 18% with standard nCRT alone [66]. The rate of surgical complications was not increased and no increased risk for progression was observed. Others have reported have provided supportive evidence for consolidation chemotherapy, but its potential role in improving durability of treatment response for patients undergoing a watch and wait strategy is unknown [67]. And the Rectal cAncer and Preoperative Induction therapy followed by Dedicated Operation (RAPIDO) trial is currently randomizing patients to short-course (5×5 Gy) pelvic radiation followed by six cycles of capecitabine and oxaliplatin and TME vs. standard nCRT and TME with the goal of improving disease-free and overall survival without compromising local control [68]. There is also an ongoing randomized study of induction vs. consolidative chemotherapy for patients with rectal cancer undergoing nCRT that is intended to improve disease-free survival when compared to standard CRT (NCT02008656). While these studies are not designed to investigate a strategy of watch and wait, it may shed new light on the role of consolidative chemotherapy in patients with high-risk rectal cancer.

Finding the Way Forward

The management of rectal cancer has become increasingly complex. While currently most patients with clinical stage II or III disease are treated with neoadjuvant chemoradiotherapy or short course radiotherapy followed by proctectomy, there is increasing recognition of the potential to avoid radiation therapy associated toxicity, as excellent results can be achieved with high-quality resection in appropriately selected patients without high-risk features on initial evaluation [69]. We also continue to learn about the role of neoadjuvant chemotherapy alone for treatment of intermediate-risk mid-rectal cancers [57]. Patients with intermediate-risk distal rectal cancers in whom a permanent colostomy will be required may be the optimal candidates in whom to study a watch and wait approach. These patients with small tumors close to or involving the sphincters are most likely to both require permanent colostomy at surgery and to achieve a complete response to chemoradiation therapy.

However a number of unresolved questions remain. The long-term oncologic efficacy of the watch and wait approach still requires validation, especially given the high cure potential associated with definitive surgery in this patient population. While it appears that surgical salvage for tumor regrowth is feasible, it is unknown if the delay can lead to lost window of opportunity for patients with distal cancers who were otherwise candidates for coloanal reconstruction. The potential that the risk for distant recurrence may be increased with a nonoperative approach must also be examined. Finally, there exists no reliable method for identifying patients with pCR who may then be eligible for a watch and wait approach and local tumor excision still carries significant morbidity risk without providing complete information regarding the status of the regional lymph nodes. Currently, the most objective method for identifying potential candidates for a watch and wait approach seems to be comparison of pre- and posttreatment high-resolution MRI imaging to assess response. Using MRI response to clinical response criteria with a strict protocol for follow-up may be the most reliable way of implementing a watch and wait strategy but it is far from a perfect test. Systemic chemotherapy, either as induction or consolidation, is another approach to increasing the likely of achieving pCR and identifying the low-risk in whom selective surgery can be considered and may play a role in reducing the risk for distant recurrence [66]. Finally, while there is great interest in molecular analysis that should be incorporated into all future trials, as of yet there are no molecular signatures that can predict the likelihood of achieving a pCR.

Until recently, most surgeons would have been reluctant to consider a nonoperative approach for rectal cancer, but the increasing emergence of data may have turned the tide on opinion [70]. As of yet there is no evidence from randomized controlled trials to support nonoperative strategies for patients with rectal cancer. Questions regarding patient selection, optimal method for inducing pCR, methods for assessing treatment response, and adequacy of follow-up remain unanswered.

Given the infrequent primary outcome of recurrence in this patient population, a randomized non-inferiority study is likely not feasible. But there is a critical need for evidence, perhaps through well-conducted prospective cohort studies, so that the watch and wait strategy can be safely incorporated into the overall management strategy for patients with rectal cancer. For now, radical surgery should remain standard treatment for rectal cancer, and watch and wait should only be performed in the context of clinical trials.

References

1. Monson JR, Weiser MR, Buie WD, Chang GJ, Rafferty JF, Buie WD, et al. Practice parameters for the management of rectal cancer (revised). Dis Colon Rectum. 2013;56(5):535–50.
2. Sauer R, Becker H, Hohenberger W, Rodel C, Wittekind C, Fietkau R, et al. Preoperative versus postoperative chemoradiotherapy for rectal cancer. N Engl J Med. 2004;351(17):1731–40.
3. Nedrebo BS, Soreide K, Eriksen MT, Dorum LM, Kvaloy JT, Soreide JA, et al. Survival effect of implementing national treatment strategies for curatively resected colonic and rectal cancer. Br J Surg. 2011;98(5):716–23.
4. Habr-Gama A, Perez RO, Nadalin W, Sabbaga J, Ribeiro Jr U, Silva e Sousa Jr AH, et al. Operative versus nonoperative treatment for stage 0 distal rectal cancer following chemoradiation therapy: long-term results. Ann Surg. 2004;240(4):711–7. discussion 7-8.
5. Heald RJ, Ryall RD. Recurrence and survival after total mesorectal excision for rectal cancer. Lancet. 1986;1(8496):1479–82.
6. Kapiteijn E, Marijnen CA, Nagtegaal ID, Putter H, Steup WH, Wiggers T, et al. Preoperative radiotherapy combined with total mesorectal excision for resectable rectal cancer. N Engl J Med. 2001;345(9):638–46.
7. van Gijn W, Marijnen CA, Nagtegaal ID, Kranenbarg EM, Putter H, Wiggers T, et al. Preoperative radiotherapy combined with total mesorectal excision for resectable rectal cancer: 12-year follow-up of the multicentre, randomised controlled TME trial. Lancet Oncol. 2011;12(6):575–82.
8. Bosset JF, Collette L, Calais G, Mineur L, Maingon P, Radosevic-Jelic L, et al. Chemotherapy with preoperative radiotherapy in rectal cancer. N Engl J Med. 2006;355(11):1114–23.
9. Gerard JP, Conroy T, Bonnetain F, Bouche O, Chapet O, Closon-Dejardin MT, et al. Preoperative radiotherapy with or without concurrent fluorouracil and leucovorin in T3-4 rectal cancers: results of FFCD 9203. J Clin Oncol. 2006;24(28):4620–5.
10. Rodel C, Martus P, Papadoupolos T, Fuzesi L, Klimpfinger M, Fietkau R, et al. Prognostic significance of tumor regression after preoperative chemoradiotherapy for rectal cancer. J Clin Oncol. 2005;23(34):8688–96.
11. Crane CH, Skibber JM, Feig BW, Vauthey JN, Thames HD, Curley SA, et al. Response to preoperative chemoradiation increases the use of sphincter-preserving surgery in patients with locally advanced low rectal carcinoma. Cancer. 2003;97(2):517–24.
12. Bujko K, Rutkowski A, Chang GJ, Michalski W, Chmielik E, Kusnierz J. Is the 1-cm rule of distal bowel resection margin in rectal cancer based on clinical evidence? A systematic review. Ann Surg Oncol. 2012;19(3):801–8.
13. Silberfein EJ, Kattepogu KM, Hu CY, Skibber JM, Rodriguez-Bigas MA, Feig B, et al. Long-term survival and recurrence outcomes following surgery for distal rectal cancer. Ann Surg Oncol. 2010;17(11):2863–9.
14. Ngan SY, Burmeister B, Fisher RJ, Solomon M, Goldstein D, Joseph D, et al. Randomized trial of short-course radiotherapy versus long-course chemoradiation comparing rates of local

recurrence in patients with T3 rectal cancer: Trans-Tasman Radiation Oncology Group trial 01.04. J Clin Oncol. 2012;30(31):3827–33.

15. Pettersson D, Lorinc E, Holm T, Iversen H, Cedermark B, Glimelius B, et al. Tumour regression in the randomized Stockholm III Trial of radiotherapy regimens for rectal cancer. Br J Surg. 2015;102(8):972–8. discussion 8.

16. Bujko K, Nowacki MP, Nasierowska-Guttmejer A, Michalski W, Bebenek M, Kryj M. Long-term results of a randomized trial comparing preoperative short-course radiotherapy with preoperative conventionally fractionated chemoradiation for rectal cancer. Br J Surg. 2006;93(10):1215–23.

17. Habr-Gama A, Gama-Rodrigues J, Sao Juliao GP, Proscurshim I, Sabbagh C, Lynn PB, et al. Local recurrence after complete clinical response and watch and wait in rectal cancer after neoadjuvant chemoradiation: impact of salvage therapy on local disease control. Int J Radiat Oncol Biol Phys. 2014;88(4):822–8.

18. Maas M, Nelemans PJ, Valentini V, Das P, Rodel C, Kuo LJ, et al. Long-term outcome in patients with a pathological complete response after chemoradiation for rectal cancer: a pooled analysis of individual patient data. Lancet Oncol. 2010;11(9):835–44.

19. Agarwal A, Chang GJ, Hu CY, Taggart M, Rashid A, Park IJ, et al. Quantified pathologic response assessed as residual tumor burden is a predictor of recurrence-free survival in patients with rectal cancer who undergo resection after neoadjuvant chemoradiotherapy. Cancer. 2013;119:4231–41.

20. Martin ST, Heneghan HM, Winter DC. Systematic review and meta-analysis of outcomes following pathological complete response to neoadjuvant chemoradiotherapy for rectal cancer. Br J Surg. 2012;99(7):918–28.

21. Park IJ, You YN, Agarwal A, Skibber JM, Rodriguez-Bigas MA, Eng C, et al. Neoadjuvant treatment response as an early response indicator for patients with rectal cancer. J Clin Oncol. 2012;30(15):1770–6.

22. Mandard AM, Dalibard F, Mandard JC, Marnay J, Henry-Amar M, Petiot JF, et al. Pathologic assessment of tumor regression after preoperative chemoradiotherapy of esophageal carcinoma. Clinicopathologic correlations. Cancer. 1994;73(11):2680–6.

23. Dworak O, Keilholz L, Hoffmann A. Pathological features of rectal cancer after preoperative radiochemotherapy. Int J Colorectal Dis. 1997;12(1):19–23.

24. Ryan R, Gibbons D, Hyland JM, Treanor D, White A, Mulcahy HE, et al. Pathological response following long-course neoadjuvant chemoradiotherapy for locally advanced rectal cancer. Histopathology. 2005;47(2):141–6.

25. Washington MK, Berlin J, Branton P, Burgart LJ, Carter DK, Fitzgibbons PL, et al. Protocol for the examination of specimens from patients with primary carcinoma of the colon and rectum. Arch Pathol Lab Med. 2009;133(10):1539–51.

26. Miles WE. A method of performing abdomino-perineal excision for carcinoma of the rectum and of the terminal portion of the pelvic colon (1908). Lancet. 1908;2:1812–3.

27. Juul T, Ahlberg M, Biondo S, Emmertsen KJ, Espin E, Jimenez LM, et al. International validation of the low anterior resection syndrome score. Ann Surg. 2014;259(4):728–34.

28. Chen TY, Wiltink LM, Nout RA, Meershoek-Klein Kranenbarg E, Laurberg S, Marijnen CA, et al. Bowel function 14 years after preoperative short-course radiotherapy and total mesorectal excision for rectal cancer: report of a multicenter randomized trial. Clin Colorectal Cancer. 2015;14(2):106–14.

29. Lange MM, van de Velde CJ. Urinary and sexual dysfunction after rectal cancer treatment. Nat Rev Urol. 2011;8(1):51–7.

30. Hendren SK, O'Connor BI, Liu M, Asano T, Cohen Z, Swallow CJ, et al. Prevalence of male and female sexual dysfunction is high following surgery for rectal cancer. Ann Surg. 2005;242(2):212–23.

31. Dalton RS, Velineni R, Osborne ME, Thomas R, Harries S, Gee AS, et al. A single-centre experience of chemoradiotherapy for rectal cancer: is there potential for nonoperative management? Colorectal Dis. 2012;14(5):567–71.

32. Nakagawa WT, Rossi BM, de O Ferreira F, Ferrigno R, David Filho WJ, Nishimoto IN, et al. Chemoradiation instead of surgery to treat mid and low rectal tumors: is it safe? Ann Surg Oncol. 2002;9(6):568–73.

33. Smith JD, Ruby JA, Goodman KA, Saltz LB, Guillem JG, Weiser MR, et al. Nonoperative management of rectal cancer with complete clinical response after neoadjuvant therapy. Ann Surg. 2012;256(6):965–72.

34. Smith JJ, Chow OS, Eaton A, Widmar M, Nash GM, Temple L, et al. Organ preservation in rectal cancer patients with clinical complete response after neoadjuvant therapy. Society of Surgical Oncology, 68th Cancer Symposium; March 25, 2015; Houston, 2015; p. 8.

35. Glynne-Jones R, Hughes R. Critical appraisal of the 'wait and see' approach in rectal cancer for clinical complete responders after chemoradiation. Br J Surg. 2012;99(7):897–909.

36. Maas M, Beets-Tan RG, Lambregts DM, Lammering G, Nelemans PJ, Engelen SM, et al. Wait-and-see policy for clinical complete responders after chemoradiation for rectal cancer. J Clin Oncol. 2011;29(35):4633–40.

37. Smith RK, Fry RD, Mahmoud NN, Paulson EC. Surveillance after neoadjuvant therapy in advanced rectal cancer with complete clinical response can have comparable outcomes to total mesorectal excision. Int J Colorectal Dis. 2015;30(6):769–74.

38. Glynne-Jones R, Wallace M, Livingstone JI, Meyrick-Thomas J. Complete clinical response after preoperative chemoradiation in rectal cancer: is a "wait and see" policy justified? Dis Colon Rectum. 2008;51(1):10–9. discussion 9-20.

39. Guillem JG, Chessin DB, Shia J, Moore HG, Mazumdar M, Bernard B, et al. Clinical examination following preoperative chemoradiation for rectal cancer is not a reliable surrogate end point. J Clin Oncol. 2005;23(15):3475–9.

40. Habr-Gama A, Perez RO, Wynn G, Marks J, Kessler H, Gama-Rodrigues J. Complete clinical response after neoadjuvant chemoradiation therapy for distal rectal cancer: characterization of clinical and endoscopic findings for standardization. Dis Colon Rectum. 2010;53(12):1692–8.

41. Smith FM, Wiland H, Mace A, Pai RK, Kalady MF. Clinical criteria underestimate complete pathological response in rectal cancer treated with neoadjuvant chemoradiotherapy. Dis Colon Rectum. 2014;57(3):311–5.

42. Garcia-Aguilar J, Shi Q, Thomas Jr CR, Chan E, Cataldo P, Marcet J, et al. A phase II trial of neoadjuvant chemoradiation and local excision for T2N0 rectal cancer: preliminary results of the ACOSOG Z6041 trial. Ann Surg Oncol. 2012;19(2):384–91.

43. Perez RO, Habr-Gama A, Pereira GV, Lynn PB, Alves PA, Proscurshim I, et al. Role of biopsies in patients with residual rectal cancer following neoadjuvant chemoradiation after downsizing: can they rule out persisting cancer? Colorectal Dis. 2012;14(6):714–20.

44. Park IJ, You YN, Skibber JM, Rodriguez-Bigas MA, Feig B, Nguyen S, et al. Comparative analysis of lymph node metastases in patients with ypT0-2 rectal cancers after neoadjuvant chemoradiotherapy. Dis Colon Rectum. 2013;56(2):135–41.

45. Pucciarelli S, Capirci C, Emanuele U, Toppan P, Friso ML, Pennelli GM, et al. Relationship between pathologic T-stage and nodal metastasis after preoperative chemoradiotherapy for locally advanced rectal cancer. Ann Surg Oncol. 2005;12(2):111–6.

46. Chang GJ, You YN, Park IJ, Kaur H, Hu CY, Rodriguez-Bigas MA, et al. Pretreatment high-resolution rectal MRI and treatment response to neoadjuvant chemoradiation. Dis Colon Rectum. 2012;55(4):371–7.

47. Marks JH, Valsdottir EB, DeNittis A, Yarandi SS, Newman DA, Nweze I, et al. Transanal endoscopic microsurgery for the treatment of rectal cancer: comparison of wound complication rates with and without neoadjuvant radiation therapy. Surg Endosc. 2009;23(5):1081–7.

48. Perez RO, Habr-Gama A, Sao Juliao GP, Proscurshim I, Scanavini Neto A, Gama-Rodrigues J. Transanal endoscopic microsurgery for residual rectal cancer after neoadjuvant chemoradiation therapy is associated with significant immediate pain and hospital readmission rates. Dis Colon Rectum. 2011;54(5):545–51.

49. Gornicki A, Richter P, Polkowski W, Szczepkowski M, Pietrzak L, Kepka L, et al. Anorectal and sexual functions after preoperative radiotherapy and full-thickness local excision of rectal cancer. Eur J Surg Oncol. 2014;40(6):723–30.

50. Guillem JG, Ruby JA, Leibold T, Akhurst TJ, Yeung HW, Gollub MJ, et al. Neither FDG-PET Nor CT can distinguish between a pathological complete response and an incomplete response after neoadjuvant chemoradiation in locally advanced rectal cancer: a prospective study. Ann Surg. 2013;258(2):289–95.

51. Perez RO, Habr-Gama A, Sao Juliao GP, Lynn PB, Sabbagh C, Proscurshim I, et al. Predicting complete response to neoadjuvant CRT for distal rectal cancer using sequential PET/CT imaging. Tech Coloproctol. 2014;18(8):699–708.

52. Patel UB, Blomqvist LK, Taylor F, George C, Guthrie A, Bees N, et al. MRI after treatment of locally advanced rectal cancer: how to report tumor response—the MERCURY experience. Am J Roentgenol. 2012;199(4):W486–95.

53. Beets-Tan RG, Beets GL. MRI for assessing and predicting response to neoadjuvant treatment in rectal cancer. Nat Rev Gastroenterol Hepatol. 2014;11(8):480–8.

54. Patel UB, Taylor F, Blomqvist L, George C, Evans H, Tekkis P, et al. Magnetic resonance imaging-detected tumor response for locally advanced rectal cancer predicts survival outcomes: MERCURY experience. J Clin Oncol. 2011;29(28):3753–60.

55. Engels B, Platteaux N, Van den Begin R, Gevaert T, Sermeus A, Storme G, et al. Preoperative intensity-modulated and image-guided radiotherapy with a simultaneous integrated boost in locally advanced rectal cancer: report on late toxicity and outcome. Radiother Oncol. 2014;110(1):155–9.

56. Gerard JP, Chapet O, Nemoz C, Hartweig J, Romestaing P, Coquard R, et al. Improved sphincter preservation in low rectal cancer with high-dose preoperative radiotherapy: the lyon R96-02 randomized trial. J Clin Oncol. 2004;22(12):2404–9.

57. Schrag D, Weiser MR, Goodman KA, Gonen M, Hollywood E, Cercek A, et al. Neoadjuvant chemotherapy without routine use of radiation therapy for patients with locally advanced rectal cancer: a pilot trial. J Clin Oncol. 2014;32(6):513–8.

58. Aschele C, Cionini L, Lonardi S, Pinto C, Cordio S, Rosati G, et al. Primary tumor response to preoperative chemoradiation with or without oxaliplatin in locally advanced rectal cancer: pathologic results of the STAR-01 randomized phase III trial. J Clin Oncol. 2011;29(20):2773–80.

59. O'Connell MJ, Colangelo LH, Beart RW, Petrelli NJ, Allegra CJ, Sharif S, et al. Capecitabine and oxaliplatin in the preoperative multimodality treatment of rectal cancer: surgical end points from National Surgical Adjuvant Breast and Bowel Project trial R-04. J Clin Oncol. 2014;32(18):1927–34.

60. Rodel C, Liersch T, Becker H, Fietkau R, Hohenberger W, Hothorn T, et al. Preoperative chemoradiotherapy and postoperative chemotherapy with fluorouracil and oxaliplatin versus fluorouracil alone in locally advanced rectal cancer: initial results of the German CAO/ARO/AIO-04 randomised phase 3 trial. Lancet Oncol. 2012;13(7):679–87.

61. Gerard JP, Azria D, Gourgou-Bourgade S, Martel-Laffay I, Hennequin C, Etienne PL, et al. Comparison of two neoadjuvant chemoradiotherapy regimens for locally advanced rectal cancer: results of the phase III trial ACCORD 12/0405-Prodige 2. J Clin Oncol. 2010;28(10):1638–44.

62. Francois Y, Nemoz CJ, Baulieux J, Vignal J, Grandjean JP, Partensky C, et al. Influence of the interval between preoperative radiation therapy and surgery on downstaging and on the rate of sphincter-sparing surgery for rectal cancer: the Lyon R90-01 randomized trial. J Clin Oncol. 1999;17(8):2396.

63. Glehen O, Chapet O, Adham M, Nemoz JC, Gerard JP, Lyons Oncology Group. Long-term results of the Lyons R90-01 randomized trial of preoperative radiotherapy with delayed surgery and its effect on sphincter-saving surgery in rectal cancer. Br J Surg. 2003;90(8):996–8.

64. Chau I, Brown G, Cunningham D, Tait D, Wotherspoon A, Norman AR, et al. Neoadjuvant capecitabine and oxaliplatin followed by synchronous chemoradiation and total mesorectal excision in magnetic resonance imaging-defined poor-risk rectal cancer. J Clin Oncol. 2006;24(4):668–74.

65. Dewdney A, Cunningham D, Tabernero J, Capdevila J, Glimelius B, Cervantes A, et al. Multicenter randomized phase II clinical trial comparing neoadjuvant oxaliplatin, capecitabine, and preoperative radiotherapy with or without cetuximab followed by total mesorectal excision in patients with high-risk rectal cancer (EXPERT-C). J Clin Oncol. 2012;30(14):1620–7.

66. Garcia-Aguilar J, Chow OS, Smith DD, Marcet JE, Cataldo PA, Varma MG, et al. Effect of adding mFOLFOX6 after neoadjuvant chemoradiation in locally advanced rectal cancer: a multicentre, phase 2 trial. Lancet Oncol. 2015;16(8):957–66.

67. Habr-Gama A, Perez RO, Sabbaga J, Nadalin W, Sao Juliao GP, Gama-Rodrigues J. Increasing the rates of complete response to neoadjuvant chemoradiotherapy for distal rectal cancer: results of a prospective study using additional chemotherapy during the resting period. Dis Colon Rectum. 2009;52(12):1927–34.

68. Nilsson PJ, van Etten B, Hospers GA, Pahlman L, van de Velde CJ, Beets-Tan RG, et al. Short-course radiotherapy followed by neo-adjuvant chemotherapy in locally advanced rectal cancer—the RAPIDO trial. BMC Cancer. 2013;13:279.

69. Taylor FG, Quirke P, Heald RJ, Moran B, Blomqvist L, Swift I, et al. Preoperative high-resolution magnetic resonance imaging can identify good prognosis stage I, II, and III rectal cancer best managed by surgery alone: a prospective, multicenter, European study. Ann Surg. 2011;253(4):711–9.

70. Sao Juliao GP, Smith FM, Macklin CP, George ML, Wynn GR. Opinions have changed on the management of rectal cancer with a complete clinical response to neoadjuvant chemoradiotherapy. Colorectal Dis. 2014;16(5):392–4.

31
Proctectomy

Emmanouil P. Pappou and Martin R. Weiser

Key Concepts

- A proper proctectomy with sharp dissection along the visceral and parietal layers of the endopelvic fascia facilitates margin-negative resection, reduces local recurrence, and limits nerve injury associated with sexual dysfunction.
- Precise understanding of pelvic anatomy including fascial planes, autonomic nerves, and pelvic floor musculature is critical in performing a proper proctectomy.
- The quality of mesorectal excision and the distance of the circumferential radial margin are associated with local pelvic control.
- Proctectomy can be performed using open, laparoscopic, and robot-assisted techniques.

Background and History

At the beginning of the twentieth century, the majority of patients diagnosed with rectal cancer in Europe and the United States underwent perineal proctectomy—the preferred operation of the day. While this operation was an improvement over previous surgeries, it was highly morbid, with poor oncologic results. In 1908, William Ernest Miles of St. Mark's Hospital in London recognized that nearly all of his patients suffering from rectal cancer died of recurrent disease within 3 years after perineal proctectomy. On autopsy, he noted that most recurrences were identified in the part of the mesorectum that had been left in place and/or within lymph nodes situated near the left common iliac artery. Miles termed these areas the "zone of upward spread." He concluded that perineal proctectomy was inadequate because it failed to address the ultimate cause of local recurrence: incomplete excision of the mesorectum, including its lymphovascular supply.

Based on his observations, Miles devised a different procedure, which he described as abdominal perineal excision (APE) or, as it came to be called, abdominoperineal resection (APR). APR soon became the surgical procedure of choice for treatment of carcinoma of the rectum [1]. As Miles described it, APR actually comprised two procedures performed during the same operation: an abdominal operation and a perineal operation. The abdominal part of the APR includes dissection of the rectum and mesorectum and creation of a colostomy; the perineal part includes detachment of the rectum, anus, and levator muscles from the genital/urinary organs and the ischiorectal fat. Describing the perineal approach in 1910, Miles stressed that the levator muscles should be "divided as far outwards as their origin from the white line so as to include the lateral zone of spread" [2]. Compared with perineal proctectomy, long-term outcomes following this new operation improved considerably.

Miles' emphasis on the necessity of removing the mesorectum in its entirety would become the guiding principle of what is now known as total mesorectal excision (TME). Today, TME remains the gold standard in rectal cancer surgery. TME entails sharp—rather than blunt—dissection of the visceral and parietal layers of the endopelvic fascia, resulting in intact removal of the rectum and mesorectum [3]. In Miles' time, however, most surgeons continued to perform traditional blunt dissection, limiting the benefits of APR and resulting in a 25% rate of positive resection margins, with high rates of recurrence and mortality.

The absolute necessity of sharp dissection in every rectal cancer operation—i.e., meticulous removal of the entire mesorectum along the areolar plane outside of the rectal fascia propria—was reemphasized in 1982 by Bill Heald. Heald defined TME as an "optimal dissection plane around the cancer which must clear all forms of extension and circumscribe predictably uninvolved tissue," in other words, sharp mesorectal excision along definable tissue planes. He described this as the "holy plane" of rectal cancer surgery [4]. The aims of TME are to excise the rectum and surrounding mesorectum, including its blood vessels and pararectal lymph nodes, within an intact visceral fascial "envelope"; to complete en

© Springer International Publishing 2016
S.R. Steele et al. (eds.), *The ASCRS Textbook of Colon and Rectal Surgery*, DOI 10.1007/978-3-319-25970-3_31

bloc resection of the lymph nodes along the superior rectal and inferior mesenteric arteries; and to achieve clear resection margins.

Advocates of "total mesorectal excision" have focused attention on two critical components of oncologic proctectomy: the lateral (radial) margin and the distal margin of mesorectal excision. Sharp dissection in the avascular plane surrounding the mesorectum, so as to remove the mesorectum in its fascial envelope and achieve a wide circumferential radial margin (CRM), has been demonstrated to be essential in avoiding local recurrence of tumor in the pelvis [5–7]. Although this concept is not novel [8, 9], it has served to refocus attention on surgical technique during proctectomy, which is warranted, given the widely divergent local recurrence rates reported in the literature [10]. In 1985, Quirke and colleagues showed that pelvic relapse was the result of residual tumor at the CRM, and they were among the first to describe a systematic assessment of the CRM [7]. Since the original publication of this paper, numerous studies (including prospective trials) have confirmed that CRM involvement is a strong predictor of local recurrence, as well as distant metastasis and poor survival [11].

The second component of TME, as advocated initially by Heald et al., is the removal of the entire mesorectum distal to the tumor. However, the necessity of removing mesorectum more than 4–5 cm distal to a proximal rectal tumor is not supported by pathologic studies of lymph node involvement in the mesorectum [9, 10, 12–16]. Furthermore, it may have contributed to a high anastomotic leak rate (17%) in early series [17] and has not been shown to be of benefit in a large clinical review [18]. At present, many advocates of "total mesorectal excision" limit mesorectal resection to 4–5 cm distal to proximal rectal tumors [6, 19–21], although some authors still refer to this technique as "total" mesorectal excision [19–22], which has caused confusion. Other groups have termed the concept of tailoring the mesorectal excision to the position of the tumor "tumor-specific mesorectal excision" [6], which may be more accurate.

In summary, for all patients with rectal cancer, it is critical that the primary tumor is removed in its entirety. In addition, mesenteric tissue at greatest risk for nodal metastases should also be resected. For patients with mid and distal rectal cancers, appropriate proctectomy technique will involve removing the entire mesorectum. For patients with proximal rectal cancers, it is important to remove the mesorectum for a distance of approximately 4–5 cm distal to the tumor, although resecting the mesorectum distal to that point does not appear to confer benefit.

Anatomy of the Mesorectum/Rectal Fascia

Chapter 1 has an in-depth look at the anatomy of the colon, rectum, and anus; however, surgical anatomy as it relates to proctectomy will be covered here. The proctectomy technique is based on an understanding of the anatomy of the rectum and the mesorectal fascia. The rectum is located at the end of the large intestine, where the taeniae coalesce to form a complete lineal muscular layer. This is surrounded by a recognizable annular envelope: the rectal fascia (or mesorectum, as it is better known to surgeons). The mesorectum contains the lymphovascular supply of the rectum and upper anal canal. It encloses the branches of the superior rectal artery and the perirectal lymph nodes, which drain in a caudal direction toward the inferior mesenteric artery. Around the rectum is an avascular plane, surgically recognizable as a cobweb of areolar tissue.

The mesorectum is asymmetrically distributed. The bulk of it sits posterior to the rectum, identified by two protruding bulges (the "mesorectal cheeks"); anteriorly and laterally, the perirectal tissue is thinner. Similarly, the mesorectal fascia is most developed on the posterior aspect. Anteriorly, the mesorectum is thinner and bordered by the recto-genital septum known as Denonvilliers' fascia. In men, Denonvilliers' fascia separates the rectum and mesorectum from the prostate and seminal vesicles. In women, the thinner rectovaginal fascia separates the rectum from the vagina. Ligaments below and lateral to the peritoneal reflection connect to the parietal fascia on the pelvic sidewall.

An extensive autonomic nervous system of sympathetic and parasympathetic fibers supplies the rectum and genitourinary tract, controlling continence and sexual function. The sympathetic autonomous system is responsible for urinary continence and ejaculation, whereas the parasympathetic system controls micturition, as well as genital erection and lubrication. Precise knowledge of the anatomy of this pelvic autonomic network is essential in rectal surgery, as injury to these nerves during proctectomy can lead to sexual dysfunction and incontinence. The sympathetic autonomic plexus arises from lumbar sympathetic nerves originating in the T12–L2 spinal junction, which pass anterior to the aorta and form a network in close proximity to the origin of the inferior mesenteric artery. This is known as the superior hypogastric plexus. The superior hypogastric plexus enters the pelvic cavity anterior to the sacral promontory and splits into fairly well-defined left and right hypogastric nerves (Figure 31-1). Damage to this sympathetic plexus during ligation of the inferior mesenteric artery, or damage to the hypogastric nerve trunks during mesorectal mobilization, can lead to urinary incontinence and retrograde ejaculation. The hypogastric nerves course posterolateral to the mesorectum and ultimately join parasympathetic nerves—also known as the pelvic plexus, pelvic splanchnic nerves, or nervi erigentes—to form the inferior hypogastric plexus. The parasympathetic nerves that join the sympathetic system originate from the S2–S4 sacral spinal nerve roots, lying posterolaterally along the mesorectal fascia. Preservation of the pelvic splanchnic nerves and the inferior hypogastric plexus, and careful separation of these from the rectum, is one of the most challenging aspects of proctectomy. The inferior hypogastric plexus forms an extensive network of interlocking fibers of the sympathetic

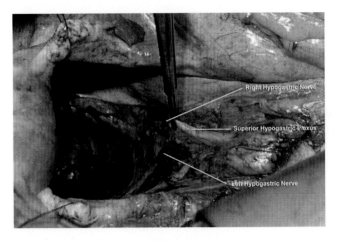

FIGURE 31-1. The superior hypogastric plexus splits into the *right* and *left* hypogastric nerves as it enters the pelvic cavity. Parasympathetic pelvic splanchnic nerves, also known as nervi erigentes, arise from sacral spinal nerves S2–S4 and pierce the presacral fascia on the *left* and *right side* to join the hypogastric nerves, forming the inferior hypogastric plexus (not shown). *With permission from Lee-Kong et al.: Autonomic nerve preservation during rectal cancer resection. J Gastrointest Surg 2010;14:416–422.* © *Springer* [104].

left and right hypogastric nerves, and parasympathetic pelvic splanchnic nerves are situated on the pelvic sidewall. Various nerves leave the inferior hypogastric plexus to enter the rectal wall, while the remaining neurovascular bundles extend anterolaterally to the seminal vesicles, distal ureters, vasa deferentia, urinary bladder, prostate and cavernous bodies in men, and in the similar anatomic area in women, for whom the lower portion of the inferior hypogastric plexus runs along the lower lateral wall of the vagina.

Laterally, the mesorectum is sometimes not completely covered by a layer of fascia and is penetrated by the middle rectal vessels (coming from the internal iliac vessels, present in about 10–20% of patients) and autonomic nerves from the inferior hypogastric plexus. The mesorectum is tethered inferolaterally to the inferior hypogastric plexus, necessitating a more challenging dissection that is best achieved with precise monopolar diathermy and subtle traction and countertraction, in order to draw the autonomic nerve fibers controlling urinary continence and sexual function carefully away from the surface of the mesorectum.

Posterior to the mesorectum is the presacral fascia, which follows the concavity of the sacrum. The presacral fascia is a thickened parietal fascia that covers the presacral veins and fat, extending laterally to join Denonvilliers' fascia anteriorly. Inferiorly, between the levels of the third and fourth sacral vertebra, the mesorectum and the presacral fascia fuse. The thick connective tissue bridging these two separate fascias is also known as the rectosacral fascia or Waldeyer's fascia. Waldeyer's fascia is an important surgical landmark during posterior rectal mobilization, because of its close relationship to the sympathetic hypogastric nerves and the

inferior hypogastric plexus. Inaccurate dissection at this level can lead anteriorly to breach of the mesorectum and posteriorly to tearing of the fascia, resulting in considerable bleeding from the presacral veins. At the most distal part of the rectum, the mesorectum thins out as a recognizable structure so that it is virtually absent over the final 1 cm of the rectum. Distal rectal cancers are thus at greater risk of invading surrounding structures than proximal rectal cancers, particularly the pelvic floor/external anal sphincter, vagina, or prostate, because of the relative paucity of mesorectum at this level.

Surgical Principles of Proctectomy for Rectal Cancer

The basic principles of proctectomy are as follows [23]:

1. Sharp dissection circumferentially around the mesorectum in an avascular areolar plane between the visceral and parietal layers of the endopelvic fascia (Figure 31-2a)
2. Identification and preservation of the autonomic nerve plexus that controls bladder and sexual function (Figure 31-2b)
3. Achievement of a circumferential margin that is macroscopically and microscopically clear of tumor
4. Preservation of the anal sphincter complex and pelvic floor, with restoration of gastrointestinal continuity when appropriate

Pathological Assessment

In addition to assessment of proximal, distal, and CRMs, pathologists can grade the quality of the mesorectal specimen. This has been demonstrated to have prognostic significance. Quirke et al. described a grading system which classifies rectal cancer specimens according to whether the surgeon has dissected outside the mesorectal fascia, in the correct plane (the mesorectal excision plane), or has violated the mesorectum, leaving mesorectal tissue behind in the pelvis by following a plane within the mesorectum (intramesorectal plane) or directly on the muscularis propria (muscularis propria plane) [24]. This mesorectal grading system has been evaluated in subsequent studies and has been found to be an independent predictor of local pelvic control [25, 26]. One study reported a significant association between plane of surgery and survival—even in patients with an uninvolved CRM [27]. However, these studies also showed that the surgical plane was related to CRM positivity rates, with the lowest rates of positive CRM in surgery that achieved sharp dissection along the mesorectal plane.

Pathological analysis of the excised proctectomy specimen provides important prognostic information on the stage and biology of the tumor. It is also a means of assessing the

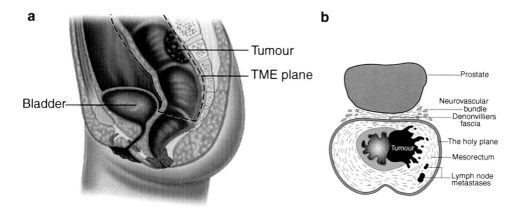

FIGURE 31-2. Total mesorectal excision. (**a**) Dissection follows the *dotted line*. Tumor deposits are often present within the lymphovascular tissue surrounding the rectum (mesorectum). Incomplete resection leaves residual deposits which are most likely the origin of local treatment failure. *With permission from Janjua AZ, Moran B, Heald RJ. Open surgical management of rectal cancer. Patel HRH, Mould T, Joseph JV, Delaney CP. (Eds). Pelvic Cancer* *Surgery: Modern Breakthroughs and Future Advances. Springer, New York, 2015: pp: 531. © Springer 2015* [105]. (**b**) The plane of total mesorectal excision allows complete removal of regional lymph nodes while sparing the neurovascular bundles. *With permission from Heald RJ et al.: Embryology and anatomy of the rectum. Semin Surg Oncol. 1998 Sep; 15(2):66–71. © John Wiley and Sons* [106].

quality of surgery, because margin status and quality of mesorectal excision can be used as surrogates for oncologic outcome assessment. The College of American Pathologists (CAP) has implemented standardized assessment of rectal cancer specimens [28]. The surgeon or pathologist should ink the non-peritonealized radial margin of the fresh resection specimen to help guide this analysis. A standardized synoptic report should include a subjective assessment of mesorectal grade and quantitative measurement of CRM in millimeters. A margin is considered positive if the primary tumor or involved lymph node extends to within 1 mm of the resection margin.

Preoperative Preparation

All patients undergoing rectal cancer surgery require preoperative preparation aimed at optimizing the technical success of the procedure and avoiding perioperative complications. Oral mechanical bowel preparation with polyethylene glycol, to reduce the bacterial load and risk of intraoperative fecal spillage, has been considered an axiom in colon and rectal surgery. However, a number of prospective trials have failed to demonstrate any benefit from mechanical bowel cleansing in preventing surgical site infections (SSIs) [29, 30]. These results were confirmed by a Cochrane systematic review of 5805 patients, in which the authors concluded that there is no statistically significant benefit from mechanical bowel preparation or the use of rectal enemas [31]. Another recent systematic review by the Agency for Healthcare Research and Quality reached similar conclusions [32]. Oral mechanical bowel preparation appeared to be protective,

compared to no preparation, for peritonitis or intra-abdominal abscess, but the evidence was weak. The study could not draw any conclusion on potential harms, such as dehydration and electrolyte imbalances, related to use of oral mechanical bowel preparation.

Despite the lack of solid data regarding the impact of bowel preparation on wound infection, there are other valid reasons for preoperative cathartic bowel preparation prior to proctectomy. It is preferable to have the rectosigmoid cleared of stool, in order to accurately assess the position of the tumor intraoperatively. In addition, division of the colon and rectum is more easily accomplished if the lumen is free of stool. Lastly, if the patient is to undergo a temporary diverting proximal stoma, it is preferable to have the intervening colon free of stool, in case of anastomotic leak. Although it is theoretically possible to have patients clear stool from the rectosigmoid with preoperative enemas, in practice this is often difficult to accomplish due to the rectal tumor itself and physical disabilities associated with the advanced age of many patients. In addition, enemas do not clear the proximal colon of stool, mitigating the benefit of proximal fecal diversion if anastomosis is performed.

High-quality evidence indicates that preoperative antibiotics covering aerobic and anaerobic bacteria, delivered orally, intravenously, or both, reduce the risk of postoperative surgical wound infection by as much as 66% in elective colorectal surgery [33]. Oral neomycin- and erythromycin-based antibiotics are typically administered the day before surgery, in combination with oral mechanical bowel preparation. For patients without penicillin allergy, a second-generation cephalosporin (cefotetan or cefoxitin) is administered intravenously within 60 min of the surgical incision, with re-dosing during the procedure as required, according to the half-life of the drug and the duration of surgery. For penicillin-allergic patients, metronidazole or clindamycin combined with either ciprofloxacin or gentamicin is acceptable, as are aztreonam and fluoroquinolones [34]. Ertapenem, a long-acting carbapenem active against gram-negative anaerobe, is an accepted alternative to second-generation cephalosporins for prophylaxis. Other measures that prevent SSI include tight glucose control in diabetic patients, smoking cessation, clipping rather than shaving the skin of the abdominal wall, and maintaining normothermia and adequate oxygenation during anesthesia [35]. Patients undergoing rectal cancer surgery are also at risk of deep venous thrombosis and pulmonary embolism and should have thromboembolic prophylaxis with unfractionated heparin or low molecular weight heparin during the perioperative and postoperative period [36].

As the incidence of rectal cancer increases with age, many patients also have cardiovascular or respiratory conditions requiring medical clearance before surgery. While technical advances have made rectal cancer operations safer, optimal outcomes require special effort to ensure that the patient's overall health is acceptable at the time of surgery. Many patients with other comorbid conditions such as diabetes, hypertension, and coronary artery disease require medical evaluation before undergoing surgery. Comorbidities can impact decision-making and affect short- and long-term outcomes. Patient's clinical and performance status should be optimized to reduce the risk of perioperative complications. Fertility options should be discussed with all individuals of childbearing potential. In the setting of Lynch syndrome, discussion regarding oophorectomy and hysterectomy is appropriate. Patients who may require a stoma should be seen before surgery by an enterostomal therapist. Adequate marking of the stoma site improves outcomes. Preoperative teaching shortens the time required by patients to gain proficiency in managing their stoma and reduces length of hospital stay [37].

The enhanced recovery after surgery (ERAS) protocols were introduced in open colorectal surgery in the 1990s, with the aim of speeding patient recovery, improving patient outcomes and satisfaction, shortening hospitalization, and reducing healthcare costs [38]. ERAS protocols span the entire perioperative period and attempt to minimize surgical stress and postoperative ileus through patient education, preoperative hydration and carbohydrate loading, goal-directed intraoperative fluid management, narcotic sparing for intraoperative and postoperative pain control, and early mobilization and oral feeding in the postoperative period. A number of prospective trials and reviews have indicated that the implementation of ERAS protocols reduces length of hospital stay, compared to conventional recovery in patients undergoing open or minimally invasive surgery for CRC [39, 40].

Operative Approaches

Optimal resection of rectal cancer according to the oncologic principles of TME can be achieved by open or minimally invasive (laparoscopic or robotic) surgical techniques. Herein, we describe methods for both open and minimally invasive approaches. General concepts such as nerve preservation are detailed in the "open" section but apply to minimally invasive approaches as well.

Open Low Anterior Resection

The patient is placed in a modified lithotomy or supine split-leg position. A variety of incisions can be utilized; however, it is important to keep the incision line away from the area of potential stoma and stoma appliance, so as to not interfere with management of the stoma postoperatively. The abdominal cavity is explored thoroughly, especially the liver and the peritoneum, to identify signs of distant metastatic disease. If unresectable distant metastatic disease is encountered, then the surgeon should carefully consider whether low pelvic anastomosis is warranted. Patients with unresectable distant metastatic spread often undergo prolonged treatment with chemotherapy, and the presence of a temporary diverting ileostomy may increase the severity of chemotherapy-induced enteritis. In addition, the added risk of colorectal or coloanal anastomotic leak may not be warranted because, if leak occurs, systemic chemotherapy may be delayed. In addition, chemotherapy must be stopped temporarily to close the ileostomy; if complications ensue from this second procedure, systemic chemotherapy may again be delayed. Lastly, the functional derangements associated with low pelvic anastomosis will only be exacerbated if the patient receives cytotoxic chemotherapy, which may produce enteritis. In sum, it may be preferable to simply perform a Hartmann's resection for mid and distal rectal adenocarcinoma that does not invade the pelvic floor or anal sphincter, in patients with unresectable distant metastatic disease. For patients with proximal rectal cancer who may not require temporary fecal diversion and are at low risk for anastomotic complications, it is reasonable to perform anterior resection with primary anastomosis, even in the setting of unresectable distant metastatic disease (if this was the original plan).

Our preferences regarding the technical aspects of restorative proctectomy are described as follows: The small bowel is carefully packed and retracted to the right, providing access to the pelvis. The sigmoid and left colon is mobilized by dissection laterally to medially along the white line of Toldt. The sigmoid colon is retracted medially. In this loose connective tissue plane, first the gonadal vessels and then, more medially, the left ureter are encountered. Dissection is continued in this plane, and the left colon is dissected away from Gerota's fascia. At the base of the sigmoid mesocolon, the retrorectal avascular plane is entered. While the sigmoid colon is elevated from the left lateral side, gonadal vessels, the left ureter, and the left hypogastric nerve are preserved in the embryologic avascular plane, and the mesorectal dissection plane is reached. The sigmoid is retracted in the right lateral direction. Then, from the right side, the sigmoid mesocolon is entered through a window over the surgeon's hand at the pelvic brim. Through this window, the inferior mesenteric artery is liberated, and separate ligations of the artery and vein are performed. The superior rectal artery (just distal to the left colic artery) or inferior mesenteric artery, at its origin 1–2 cm from the aorta, is ligated and divided to preserve the sympathetic plexus. High ligation of the IMA is useful when bulky adenopathy is present at the base of the vessel or when a coloanal anastomosis is necessary and maximal length of the left colon is required. When the inferior mesenteric artery is ligated, care must be taken to preserve the marginal artery, which provides the blood supply from the middle colic vessels to the left colon and anastomosis.

The inferior mesenteric vein is ligated at the paraduodenal (ligament of Treitz) location just inferior to the pancreas and again adjacent to the ligation site of the inferior mesenteric artery. Dividing the vein at the ligament of Treitz is critical in order to accommodate full mobilization of the splenic flexure, which is then allowed to rotate into the pelvis for maximal length. Splenic flexure mobilization is performed by continuing the lateral dissection of the descending colon superiorly, retracting and dissecting the descending colon off Gerota's fascia. Colonic attachments to the pancreas are then taken down, and care is taken to avoid aggressive retraction on the colon, which can tear the splenic capsule. Omental attachments are then taken down from the distal transverse colon to complete the mobilization.

The sigmoid mesentery is divided to the bowel wall, which is stapled and divided. The left colon is packed superiorly, facilitating visualization of the pelvis. The stapled sigmoid is

retracted anteriorly, which opens the perimesorectal planes. A sharp dissection is carried out under direct vision, circumferentially around the mesorectum. The presence of the superior hypogastric plexus posteriorly must be kept in mind throughout the dissection (Figure 31-3a). Starting the dissection in the posterior and then the lateral plane, in a stepwise manner, facilitates identification of the correct mesorectal plane (Figure 31-3b). If bleeding is encountered in one area, it is reasonable to proceed to the opposite circumference, so that pressure is applied while progress continues. The key to this phase is the recognition of the areolar tissue on the back of the mesorectum, through which the dissection should proceed when the areolar tissue is on stretch. Once there is sufficient space, a St. Mark's Pelvic Retractor is introduced behind the specimen. Traction and countertraction are critical to the pelvic dissection and are optimized by use of the retractor. The lateral dissection is carried out by extending the posterior plane of dissection anteriorly and around the sidewalls of the pelvis. At this point in the dissection, the inferior hypogastric plexuses curve around the surface of the mesorectum and are vulnerable to inadvertent injury. While retracting the divided rectosigmoid forward, the tangentially running hypogastric and pelvic parasympathetic nerves are carefully identified and dissected away from the mesorectal surface on each side (Figure 31-4a). This area of adherence between the nerves and the mesorectum is one of the most challenging and critical in proctectomy. As the lateral dissection moves deeper into the pelvis, one or two middle rectal arteries may be encountered. Middle rectal arteries are present in less than 20 % of patients and, if encountered, can be easily divided with cautery. Dissection anteriorly progresses along Denonvilliers' fascia down to the pelvic floor (Figure 31-4b). Forward retraction with the help of the St. Mark's Retractor facilitates the development of the space anteriorly. Anterior tumors require resection of Denonvilliers' fascia, which puts the parasympathetic nerves at risk, as they extend anteriorly toward the prostate. For posterior tumors, dissection can pro-

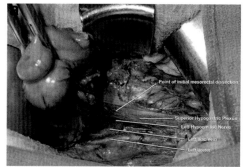
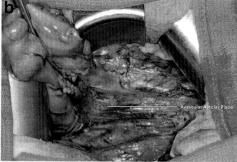
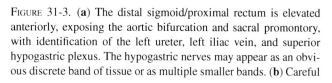

FIGURE 31-3. (a) The distal sigmoid/proximal rectum is elevated anteriorly, exposing the aortic bifurcation and sacral promontory, with identification of the left ureter, left iliac vein, and superior hypogastric plexus. The hypogastric nerves may appear as an obvious discrete band of tissue or as multiple smaller bands. (b) Careful dissection of the sigmoid mesentery distally results in an avascular, areolar plane separating the mesorectal fascia propria from the presacral fascia. *With permission from Lee-Kong et al.: Autonomic nerve preservation during rectal cancer resection. J Gastrointest Surg 2010;14:416–422. © Springer* [104].

FIGURE 31-4. (**a**) Caudal dissection in the posterior midline, while lifting the rectum "toward the ceiling" may cause the hypogastric nerves to "tent up," as they often adhere to the mesorectal fascia. (**b**) Anterior dissection during TME. *With permission from Lee Kong et al.: Autonomic nerve preservation during rectal cancer resection. J Gastrointest Surg 2010;14: 416–422.* © *Springer* [104].

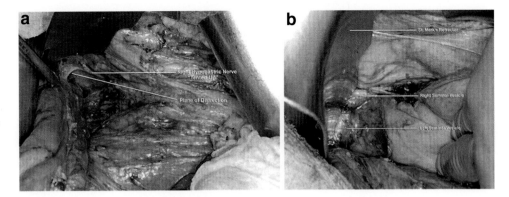

ceed below Denonvilliers' fascia. Adequacy of the dissection distal to the lower edge of the tumor is examined by palpation and/or endoscopy to ensure a proper distal margin. When mesorectal mobilization down to the pelvic floor is considered complete on both anterior and posterior sides, the rectum is elevated above the pelvic floor and cross-clamped. At this point, washout of the anorectal stump can be performed with saline solution or water. Following this, the rectum is transected with a linear stapler (TA-45), and the specimen is removed. The anastomosis between the colon conduit and the rectal stump is constructed with a circular EEA™ Stapler (Figure 31-5a). The serosa and mucosa are visually evaluated for adequate vascular supply. Intraoperative anastomotic air testing of the colorectal anastomosis is performed by filling the pelvis with saline solution and insufflating the rectum with air through a sigmoidoscope. A handsewn coloanal anastomosis is shown in Figure 31-5b and is discussed separately below.

Laparoscopic Low Anterior Resection

The patient is placed in a modified lithotomy position. A 5-trocar technique is generally utilized, with an umbilical camera port, two left-sided and two right-sided working (Figure 31-6). This allows the surgeon and second assistant to stand on the patient's right, with the first assistant standing on the left. The dissection is performed in a medial-to-lateral fashion, first dissecting the vessels, followed by takedown of the splenic flexure, and then the lateral colonic attachments before entering the pelvis for rectal resection. With the patient in head-down and right-sided tilt, enabling the surgeon to move the small bowel mesentery out of the pelvis and away from the colonic mesentery, dissection begins at the sacral promontory. The superior rectal vessels are lifted ventrally, and a plane is developed beneath the sigmoid mesentery. Dissection is carried out just beneath the vessels, in order to sweep the sympathetic nerves toward the retroperitoneum. Dissection proceeds medial to lateral beneath the mesentery and along Toldt's fascia, preserving the ureter and gonadal vessels. The root of the IMA is exposed by creating an additional window on the superior border of the IMA. The IMA is ligated, taking care not to injure the aortic nerve plexus, either just below the left colic branch or at the origin of the vessel. The IMV is subsequently divided along with the sigmoid mesentery. The left mesocolon is further mobilized along with the splenic flexure. The IMV is divided adjacent to the pancreas to allow full mobilization and rotation of the left colon, so as to reach the pelvis for a tension-free anastomosis. Again, in a medial-to-lateral fashion, dissection continues along the ventral plane of the pancreas, with entry into the lesser sac. Often, the lateral attachments of the splenic flexure can be divided in a medial approach, exposing the spleen. The transverse colon is then retracted caudally, and the omentum is dissected off the transverse colon, meeting the prior dissection place. Lastly, the remaining lateral and splenic attachments are divided by retracting the colon medially.

For pelvic dissection, it may be necessary to position the patient in a more head-down position, often with less rotation to the right. The rectum is retracted anteriorly and the retrorectal space is identified. Sharp dissection is carried out posteriorly along the areolar plane that defines the junction of the visceral and parietal layers of the endopelvic fascia. Care must be taken to sweep the hypogastric nerves laterally, and dissection proceeds posteriorly along the mesorectum. Once posterior mobilization is completed, dissection continues in the same perimesorectal plane on the lateral sides of the pelvis. The rectum is mobilized circumferentially, applying standard open TME surgical principles. Dissection can be performed with cautery, ultrasonic dissector, or vessel-sealing devices. After TME dissection is completed, the level of rectal transection is confirmed with digital rectal and endoscopic examinations. The rectum is irrigated and then stapled and divided with endoscopic staplers. The specimen is extracted via a wound protector at the umbilical camera port or the future diverting ileostomy site. The proximal sigmoid/left colon is divided, and the anvil is secured for laparoscopic circular anastomosis. An air leak test confirms the integrity of the anastomosis, and a diverting ileostomy is fashioned selectively.

FIGURE 31-5. (**a**) Stapled end-to-end colorectal anastomosis. (**b**) Handsewn end-to-end coloanal anastomosis. *With permission from Wexner SD, Fleshman JW, editors. Colon and Rectal surgery: Abdominal Operations, Master Techniques in Surgery. Philadelphia: Lippincott Williams & Wilkins; 2012* [107].

A.

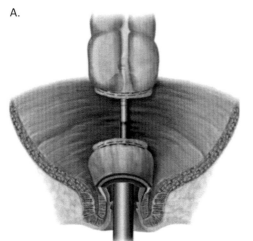

B.

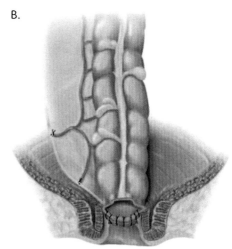

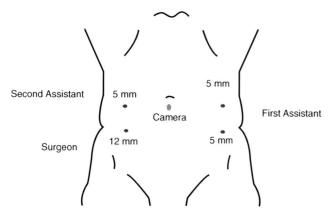

FIGURE 31-6. Preferred port placement for laparoscopic LAR with TME.

In patients with a narrow pelvis or elevated body mass index, pelvic dissection can be challenging. In such cases, a lower midline or Pfannenstiel incision may be utilized to allow open pelvic dissection, rectal division, and restoration of intestinal continuity. A combination of laparoscopic and open surgery in this manner is often referred to as a "hybrid" approach.

Robotic Low Anterior Resection

Robotics has emerged as a useful technology in pelvic dissection and may have advantages for the surgeon with respect to manual dexterity, versus standard laparoscopy. The straight laparoscopic instruments make dissection within the confines of the narrow, bony pelvis difficult and subject the surgeon to ergonomic stress. The robotic platform allows for stable retraction; enhanced three-dimensional (3D), high-definition visualization; and articulating instruments. There is some indication that use of the robot has been associated with a reduced rate of conversion to laparotomy during

proctectomy as compared to standard laparoscopic surgery (although many of the studies on this topic are plagued by selection bias) [41].

A single-docking technique using the da Vinci® Si™ robot is first described. This entails single docking of the robot for the entire procedure, from colon mobilization to pelvic dissection. The patient is placed in a modified lithotomy position. Pneumoperitoneum is established with a Hasson technique through a supraumbilical incision. The abdominal cavity is examined using the robotic camera. Four additional robotic ports are inserted, along with an assistant port, as shown in Figure 31-7a. The greater omentum and the small bowel are retracted out of the pelvis. The patient is placed in Trendelenburg position, with right-side down. The robotic cart is brought to the left lower quadrant. The robotic arms are first docked, with robot arm 1 in the right lower quadrant using monopolar curved scissors or vessel sealer, robot arm 2 in the right upper abdomen using a fenestrated bipolar forceps, and robot arm 3 in the left mid-abdomen using a ProGrasp™ or Cadiere forceps for retraction. Arm 3 begins on the left side of the robot, on the same side as arm 1. Dissection proceeds in a medial-to-lateral fashion, as in standard laparoscopic dissection. Following division of the IMA and IMV, splenic flexure mobilization, and division of the left colic mesentery, robot arm 3 is repositioned (Figure 31-7b). The robot does not need to be moved, and patient position can be maintained. On occasion, a slightly more accentuated head-down and minimal tilt is utilized for the pelvic dissection, in order to keep the small bowel out of the pelvis. This configuration ensures that all instruments can reach the pelvic floor without conflict. Proctectomy proceeds, as described above for standard laparoscopy, but with a few exceptions. Care is taken to maintain dissection along the mesorectal plane laterally and avoid dissection into the pelvic sidewall. This is facilitated by early anterior dissection, which is easily visualized with the camera setup, as described, and use of articulating instruments. We often use a tie around the rectum

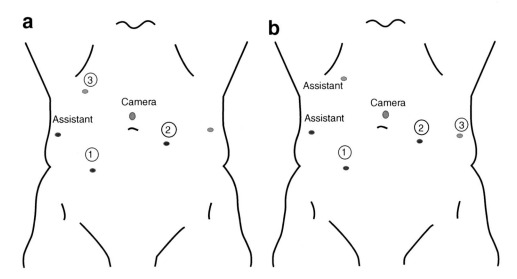

FIGURE 31-7. Trocar placement for robotic LAR using the da Vinci® Si™ robot with the two separate phases of the operation: (**a**) pedicle ligation, splenic flexure mobilization; (**b**) pelvic dissection.

(such as thin vaginal packing) to facilitate rectal retraction. During pelvic dissection, the bedside assistant utilizes the lateral assistant port and the right upper quadrant robotic port (which was used for pedicle ligation and flexure takedown). Intraoperative endoscopy, with picture-in-picture technology, allows the operating surgeon to visualize the rectal tumor at the robotic console and optimize the distal resection margin. We use cautery and the Vessel Sealer, along with the robotic stapler (EndoWrist® Stapler 45), to achieve low pelvic stapling. Superior visualization and retraction, along with articulating instruments, greatly facilitates deep pelvic dissection along the prostate and in the intersphincteric groove for colo-anal anastomosis. When the distal rectum has been divided, the robot is undocked, and the rectum is extracted via a wound protector at the umbilical port or future stoma site. The descending colon is divided, the anvil secured, and the laparoscopic anastomosis performed.

A similar setup is utilized with the da Vinci® Xi™ robot. This system has more flexibility, as the camera is 8 mm and can be used in any port. This is referred to as "port hopping" and is useful if dissection becomes difficult and a new vantage point is needed. The da Vinci® Xi™ robot instruments are longer, eliminating problems related to reaching the splenic flexure and the deep pelvis. Port setup is shown in Figure 31-8a, b.

Abdominoperineal Resection

APR is necessary for very low rectal tumors that invade the external sphincter or the levator muscles. The relative indications for APR include external sphincter involvement at any time in the patient's workup. Relative indications include patients with poor preoperative baseline bowel function who are not candidates for a Hartmann resection. Furthermore, care should be taken when planning surgery in patients with bulky low tumors that show minimal response or progression on neoadjuvant chemoradiation. This portends aggressive tumor biology with extension along lymphovascular and perineural spaces, making complete margin-negative resection more challenging. Wide resection, including APR, should be considered in such cases.

During APR, left colon/splenic flexure mobilization is not required. Dissection is generally taken down to the pelvic floor, and then the perineal phase is begun. Perineal dissection can be performed in lithotomy or prone position. Some assert that the prone dissection is more comfortable for the surgeon and facilitates anterior dissection but requires abdominal closure and stoma maturation prior to repositioning the patient facedown. When beginning the perineal phase, additional Betadine® preparation is utilized, and the anus is sutured to reduce contamination. A wide elliptical incision is created to encompass the sphincter complex, and dissection proceeds into the ischiorectal space. Care is taken to dissect just superior to the coccyx, where the pelvic floor is divided and the perineal dissection meets the anterior dissection. The lateral pelvic floor musculature is divided widely, and the anterior dissection is then performed, carefully avoiding injury to the vagina or membranous portion of the urethra. Following specimen removal and pelvic irrigation, the perineum is closed in multiple layers to eliminate the dead space. Pelvic drains are used liberally to reduce fluid buildup in the contaminated pelvis.

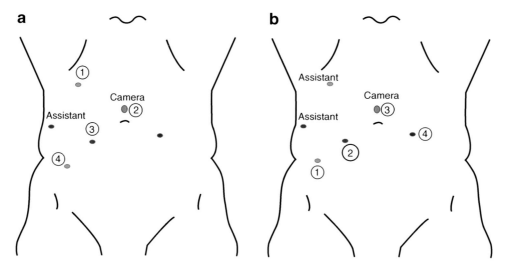

FIGURE 31-8. Trocar placement for a robotic LAR using the da Vinci® Xi™ robot. (**a**) Configuration used for pedicle ligation, splenic flexure mobilization. (**b**) Configuration used for pelvic dissection.

Extralevator or "Cylindrical" APR

In recent years, several authors have shown that oncologic outcomes after APR have not improved to the same degree as those seen after low anterior resection (LAR). In fact, compared with patients undergoing LAR during the same time period, patients undergoing APR have higher rates of local recurrence and poorer survival [42, 43]. The difference in oncologic outcomes may be explained to a substantial degree by the increased risk of tumor-involved margins (CRM) and inadvertent bowel perforations associated with APR, as both of these factors are significantly related to local control and survival. It is important to keep in mind that the distal rectum is devoid of surrounding mesorectum; therefore, tumor extension beyond the muscularis propria can invade surrounding tissues, resulting in positive CRM with standard resection. Higher rates of CRM were highlighted in a 2005 study from the UK and subsequently verified in a joint study of specimens from the Dutch trial [42, 44]. In the latter study, Nagtegaal and colleagues assessed 846 LAR and 373 APR specimens. They found that the plane of resection was within the sphincteric muscle, the submucosa, or lumen in more than one-third of the APR cases, resulting in a positive CRM rate of 30.4% in APR versus 10.7% in LAR and a perforation rate of 13.7% versus 2.5%, respectively. Others have reported improved outcomes with wide anatomic resection [45, 46].

An approach to reduce CRM involvement and specimen perforation, proposed by the Karolinska Institute in Stockholm and termed extralevator or "cylindrical" APR, involves wide resection of the levator muscles en bloc with the sphincter muscles, anal canal, and mesorectum. The abdominal component of the procedure terminates higher in the pelvis, and the levator ani muscle is divided along its attachments to the sidewall to avoid a "waist" in the specimen (Figure 31-9). The perineal phase widely resects the

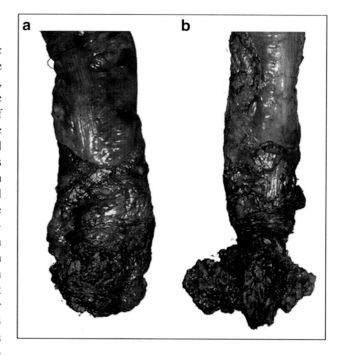

FIGURE 31-9. Abdominoperineal resection specimens. Dissections from above and below meet above the anal canal. (**a**) APR specimen with a waist. Courtesy of Eric K Johnson, MD. (**b**) Specimen with a cylindrical resection and no waist (intact mesorectum). Courtesy of Conor Delaney, MD.

ischiorectal space and completes the dissection. In a report comparing cylindrical to conventional APR specimens, Holm and colleagues demonstrated a marked reduction in CRM involvement and perforation with cylindrical APR [47]; however, flap closure is usually required, and perineal wound complications, as well as chronic pain, were significantly increased in the extralevator group [48, 49]. Many advocate "selective extralevator dissection" in areas of tumor, stressing the need for accurate preoperative imaging and examination [50]. Prone positioning for the perineal phase is not mandatory, and minimally invasive approaches are feasible [51–53]. Appropriate patient selection, methods of closing the pelvic floor to reduce wound complications and perineal hernias, and an optimal approach (open versus laparoscopic or robotic) are pertinent issues warranting further investigation in extralevator APR.

Special Considerations

Rectal Washout

It has been suggested that implantation of exfoliated malignant cells is a possible mechanism of luminal tumor recurrence in colorectal anastomoses. Intraoperative rectal washout with saline solution or water theoretically decreases the amount and viability of these cells. A study from Sweden reported a reduction in local recurrence from 10.2% with no washout to 6% with washout. However, there is no conclusive evidence regarding the effect of rectal washout on local recurrence after rectal cancer surgery. Although it may be merely a surrogate marker for attention to detail, we routinely use intraoperative rectal washout. It is a simple procedure, with minimal morbidity and with potential benefits [54].

Distal Margin

The distal resection margin is an important consideration in rectal cancer surgery. Although lymphatic drainage of the rectum generally occurs in a cephalad direction toward the major lymph node stations, pathological studies have shown distal mesorectal spread as far as 2–3 cm below the lower palpable edge of the tumor. Thus, for upper rectal cancers, mesorectal resection should include mesorectum at least 4–5 cm distal to the lower edge of the tumor, and the mesorectum is divided perpendicular to the longitudinal access of the rectum for a tumor-specific mesorectal excision. It is critical not to "cone in" and leave mesorectum behind when performing this maneuver. For mid to low rectal cancers, dissection 4–5 cm below the tumor generally ends at the pelvic floor. Thus, as long as the entire mesorectum can be removed and negative margins of resection obtained for the primary tumor, it is reasonable to consider restorative proctectomy with coloanal anastomosis for patients with distal cancers [55–58]. The exact distance that constitutes an adequate distal mural margin in this situation is the subject of debate, but an attempt to achieve 1 cm seems reasonable.

Coloanal Anastomosis

In carefully selected cases in the setting of an ultra-low rectal cancer, continued dissection along the intersphincteric plane (which is an extension of the muscularis propria of the rectum) may facilitate sphincter preservation. A handsewn anastomosis is commonly performed, with good oncologic outcomes, especially in patients with a significant response to preoperative chemoradiotherapy [53, 58]. Patient selection and counseling are critical, as patients with coloanal anastomosis have worse bowel function and potentially poorer quality of life than those with a standard stapled colorectal anastomosis [59].

Options for Reconstruction of the Gastrointestinal Tract

Following rectal resection, patients often describe frequent bowel movements, incomplete evacuation, clustering, urgency, and, at times, incontinence. In order to mitigate these symptoms, which are collectively known as LAR syndrome, various techniques have been attempted to recreate the reservoir function of the resected rectum. These are known as colonic neorectal reservoirs and include the colonic J-pouch and the end-to-side (or "Baker-type") anastomosis.

A colonic J-pouch is constructed in similar fashion to an ileal J-pouch; however, the colonic J-pouch is much smaller, about 6–8 cm in length. Randomized trials, a meta-analysis, and Cochrane review have all concluded that a colonic J-pouch results in improvement of symptoms (decreased frequency, urgency, and nocturnal bowel movements) and a better quality of life for at least 1 year after surgery, compared to an end-to-end anastomosis [60–62]. Coloplasty, longitudinal colotomy closed transversely, was proposed for patients with a narrow pelvis for whom J-pouch was not technically feasible; however, this has not been shown to be an improvement over straight anastomosis. The additional suture line has a risk of leak that can be difficult to treat, and generally coloplasty has fallen out of favor. It is difficult to interpret the results of some trials, given the variation in surgical technique: specifically, the use of either sigmoid colon or descending colon for construction of the neorectum. The use of the sigmoid colon for construction of the neorectum in patients with significant muscular hypertrophy or diverticular disease may negatively impact postoperative function.

An end-to-side or Baker anastomosis, first described in 1950, has recently been revisited as another option for improving postoperative bowel function. This side-to-end anastomosis appears to confer many of the functional advantages of the colonic J-pouch. Compared to a straight anastomosis, it is associated with significantly fewer anastomotic leaks, and overall it is safe, easier, and faster to create than the colonic J-pouch. A 2008 Cochrane review of four randomized trials comparing colonic J-pouch to the side-to-end anastomosis, as well as a more recent meta-analysis of six randomized trials, found similar functional outcomes between the two groups [63]. In many instances, there is insufficient bowel length, or the pelvis is too narrow to permit creation of a reservoir. Ensuring sufficient length of the bowel to adequately sacralize in the pelvis is crucial to healing and function. Some experts prefer to avoid the multiple staple lines associated with reservoirs and the risk of anastomotic leaks, which are difficult to remedy.

Fecal Diversion

Anastomotic leakage following proctectomy occurs in up to one-quarter of patients. Creation of a defunctioning stoma following restorative proctectomy may decrease the sequelae of anastomotic leak and pelvic sepsis. However, the value of a protective stoma has been a subject of controversy for many years. A randomized controlled trial in 2009 reported a reduction in leak rate from 28% without to 10% with a stoma [64]. A 2009 meta-analysis comparing defunctioning stoma to no stoma after rectal resection concluded that the defunctioning stoma resulted in lower rates of leak and reoperation [65]. This meta-analysis included data from four randomized controlled trials and 21 non-randomized studies, involving 11,429 patients in total. A recent meta-analysis of 13 studies published between 2004 and 2014, pooling data on 8002 patients, reported similar conclusions [66]. However, diversion does require a second operation, may result in dehydration, entails an increased risk of bowel obstruction, and is not popular with patients. Therefore, most centers divert selectively, based on anastomotic height, patient-related factors such as diabetes and previous pelvic radiation, and the results of intraoperative leak test.

Extended Resection

Up to 10% of patients with rectal cancer present with tumor invading adjacent structures, necessitating en bloc resection of the affected organ(s) [67]. En bloc resection of adjacent pelvic organs has been associated with good oncologic outcomes when pathologically negative microscopic (R0) margins can be achieved [68, 69].

Involvement of the uterus and vagina in women is best treated with en bloc resection of the rectum with the uterus and the posterior vaginal wall, in order to achieve R0 resection. Closure can be done easily after partial vaginectomy by flap reconstruction or primary closure, preserving sexual function.

Involvement of the seminal vesicles on one or both sides in men can be managed by dissection anterior to the vesicles, removing them en bloc with the rectum. The neurovascular bundles arising from the inferior hypogastric plexus, which control urinary and sexual function, are at risk during this dissection—as are the distal ureters, which should be identified and preserved. Involvement of the prostate by rectal cancer usually requires urologic consultation and is usually treated either with a partial prostatectomy or a pelvic exenteration, depending on the extent of tumor invasion. It should be noted that en bloc resection of the seminal vesicles only, with preservation of the bladder and prostate, is a challenging operation, often much more difficult than pelvic exenteration.

Involvement of the distal ureters by a locally advanced rectal tumor is rare. However, if encountered, it is best managed with en bloc resection of the ureter, with primary ureteric anastomosis over a stent or a psoas hitch, depending on the length of the ureteric defect. Rectal cancers that adhere to the urinary bladder require partial or total cystectomy, especially when the trigone is involved.

Lateral pelvic sidewall lymph node involvement has been reported in up to 20% of T3/T4 rectal cancer cases [70]. In general, pelvic sidewall lymph node involvement is associated with low-lying tumors and worse prognosis [71]. In Japanese studies, selective use of lateral pelvic lymphadenectomy has reportedly led to good outcomes. A meta-analysis of 20 studies demonstrated no improvement in survival or local recurrence when an extended lymphadenectomy was performed compared to standard proctectomy [72]. However, in selected cases where lymphatic spread is suspected clinically or radiographically, an extended lymphadenectomy is warranted in order to obtain an R0 resection.

Intraoperative Radiation Therapy

Intraoperative radiation therapy (IORT) has been used in patients with locally advanced primary rectal cancer and an involved or threatened CRM following surgical resection. The goal of IORT is to sterilize any microscopic foci of tumor, thus decreasing the risk of local recurrence. During IORT, the radiosensitive bladder and bowel can be excluded from the radiation field, allowing a higher dose to be delivered to the tumor bed. In the United States, IORT is most commonly administered by two different techniques: intraoperative electron-beam radiation therapy (IOERT) or high-dose-rate (HDR) brachytherapy. IOERT is delivered by means of a linear accelerator over the course of a few minutes; it can be used in any operating room because electrons do not penetrate the tissue as deeply as conventional radiation. The radiation is delivered through a cone, usually toward the tumor bed. HDR treatment, however, can be administered only in adequately shielded rooms. It is delivered through parallel catheters in a flexible plastic flap, which can be cut to fit the region at risk and packed onto the curving pelvic surface. HDR brachytherapy may take up to an hour.

IORT has been used in locally advanced rectal cancer for more than 30 years, yet there is no convincing evidence that it decreases local recurrence or improves survival. The only multicenter randomized trial to date included 142 patients with locally advanced rectal cancer, who had received preoperative chemoradiation and were randomly assigned to either surgical resection alone or surgery plus IORT [73]. After a 5-year follow-up, the trial did not demonstrate any significant improvement in local recurrence or disease-free survival. Observational studies have reported conflicting results with respect to the efficacy of IORT. A recent systematic review of 15 individual studies, including the previously mentioned randomized trial, with 1929 patients in the IORT group and 2343 in the non-IORT group, concluded that IORT resulted in no definite improvement in overall survival or rate of recurrence for patients with R0 resections or for the total group (including R0, R1, and R2 resections) [74]. In the setting of locally advanced primary rectal cancers, we recommend having IORT available for patients if a close or threatened CRM is highly suspected, based on preoperative imaging. IORT is more commonly utilized in resection of recurrent rectal cancer if tissue planes have been previously disrupted, and discontinued foci of tumor may be present.

Flap Closure Following APR

Special attention to perineal closure is required after APR. The bony confines of the pelvis prevent tissue collapse, leading to significant dead space. Pelvic infection requiring opening of the perineum, prolonged wound healing, and chronic perineal sinuses are not uncommon. Multilayered closure to reduce dead space and liberal use of drains are common. However, in some cases rotating a well-vascularized omentum [75] or a mucocutaneous flap [76] into the pelvis should be considered, in order to reduce dead space and facilitate perineal healing after APR, especially in patients who have received pelvic radiation. A properly designed omental pedicle graft can be easily devised by dividing the gastrocolic omental attachments, detaching the left omentum from the spleen, and ligating the left gastroepiploic pedicle and the short gastric vessels. Care is taken to avoid injury to the right gastroepiploic, which allows the bulk of well-vascularized left omentum to rotate into and fill the pelvis. Rotation of the right omentum, based on the left gastroepiploic, is also feasible. In cases of exenteration, sacrectomy, extensive perineal skin loss, or requirement of vaginal reconstruction, a myocutaneous (vertical rectus abdominus myocutaneous, gracilis, or gluteal) flap is utilized.

Functional Outcomes

High rates of postoperative sexual and urinary dysfunction were a well-known phenomenon in the early years of rectal cancer surgery, ranging from 20 to 40% [77]. For example, registry data from Norway demonstrate that less than 50% of sexually active male were able to achieve erection 2 years after rectal resection. The rate fell to less than 20% in the cohort undergoing pelvic radiation and surgery [78].

Along with the advent of sharp dissection and precise technique emphasized in TME came the goal of identifying and preserving the autonomic pelvic nerves. As an integral part of the procedure, autonomic nerve preservation resulted in improved functional outcomes.

In an early study of 42 men undergoing sphincter-preserving operations for treatment of rectal cancer, Enker and colleagues reported high rates of potency (87%) and

normal ejaculation (88%) after nerve-preserving proctectomy [79]. In a comprehensive study assessing sexual and urinary function in both women and men, through retrospective questionnaires, Havenga and colleagues reported the results of 136 patients undergoing nerve-sparing proctectomy [80]. They found that the ability to engage in intercourse was maintained by 86% of patients younger than 60 years and by 67% of patients 60 years and older. Eighty-seven percent of men maintained the ability to achieve orgasm. Type of surgery (APR compared to LAR) and age greater than 60 years were significantly associated with male sexual dysfunction. Women had similarly good results: 85% were able to experience arousal with vaginal lubrication, and 91% could achieve orgasm. The majority of patients had few or no complaints related to urinary function. Serious urinary dysfunction, such as neurogenic bladder, was not encountered.

The importance of autonomic nerve identification and preservation during proctectomy is also highlighted in a study by Shirouzou and colleagues, who assessed outcomes in 403 patients undergoing proctectomy, with or without autonomic nerve preservation, over a 20-year period [81]. In male patients who had proctectomy with nerve preservation, urinary function was preserved in greater than 80%, erection was preserved in 79%, and ejaculation in 65%; when proctectomy was performed without nerve preservation, urinary disorders were found in more than 90% and sexual dysfunction in virtually all patients, even those younger than age 60.

However, in patients with extensive pelvic disease, autonomic nerve preservation may not be feasible or oncologically sound. Involvement of the autonomic nerves by tumor, or lymphadenopathy in the pelvic sidewall, generally requires a resection that will affect nerve function permanently.

Despite suffering micturition and defecation problems, quality of life has consistently been shown to be better following an LAR compared an APR. This has been confirmed by comparative studies and in a meta-analysis of several studies [82–84]. Body image is consistently higher in patients undergoing an LAR versus APR, which may contribute to the inferior sexual function associated with APR.

In patients who undergo LAR, poor bowel function has been associated with the level of the anastomosis and the administration of pelvic radiotherapy. Low anastomoses (<3 cm) and coloanal anastomoses are associated with more incontinence of gas and solid stools compared to higher anastomoses [85]. Neoadjuvant radiation therapy causes fibrosis, leading to reduced compliance of the rectum and damage to the myenteric (Auerbach's) plexus, and has been associated with higher rates of urgency, frequency, and fecal incontinence [86]. Some of the most telling data emanates from the prospective Dutch rectal cancer study, in which patients were randomized to proctectomy or neoadjuvant short-course radiotherapy plus proctectomy. Daytime incontinence was noted in 38% of patients in the surgery alone group and 62% of patients in the surgery plus radiotherapy group. Of even more concern is the finding that bowel dysfunction increased over time (studied at 2 years and 5 years after proctectomy) in the radiation cohort [87].

Oncologic Outcomes

Attention to detail during proctectomy, especially with regard to appropriate mesorectal excision, has been associated with improved local control and survival rates. Local pelvic failure rates following proctectomy at centers of excellence are now in the single digits [19, 21, 22, 88–91]. This is a substantial improvement compared to the local pelvic failure rates following proctectomy in the past, which were 3–5 times higher.

The importance of proper proctectomy technique is also reflected in a study from the Karolinska Institute reporting that in more than half of local recurrences in Sweden, evidence of residual mesorectal fat was identified on cross-sectional imaging, suggesting that incomplete mesorectal excision was the principal cause of local recurrence [92]. The same study claimed that extra-mesorectal lateral lymph node involvement accounted for only 6% of all locoregional recurrences.

The impact of training in proper proctectomy technique has been well documented. Surgical TME educational programs in Sweden, Norway, and the Netherlands have been shown to markedly reduce local recurrence, improve survival, and reduce the rate of permanent stomas [93–96]. In an observational national cohort study of 3319 patients in Norway, implementation of TME resulted in a decrease in local recurrence from 12 to 6% [96]. Survival rates were 73% after TME and 60% after conventional surgery—an overall improvement of 10–14%. In the Netherlands, the widespread adoption of TME led to a reduction in local recurrence of 16–9% [93]. In Sweden, implementation of specialized proctectomy training, utilization of neoadjuvant short-course radiotherapy, and referral of patients with rectal cancer to specialists has led to a fall in local recurrence rates: from 15% in the control group of the Stockholm I trial, and 14% in the Stockholm II trial, to 6% [97]. Cancer-related deaths fell from 15% to 16–9%. During the same period, the proportion of APR procedures performed in Sweden decreased by more than 50%. Along with participation in workshops and the increase in surgeons' expertise, case volume directly influenced patient outcomes; when surgeons with high operative volume were compared to those with low volume, local recurrence was additionally reduced (from 10 to 4%), and there were fewer deaths from rectal cancer (18% vs. 11%) [94].

Another factor associated with oncologic outcome is the training and experience of the operating surgeon. Studies have shown that subspecialty training, surgeon experience, volume of cases, and treatment in high-volume tertiary care centers influence and enhance patient outcomes with respect to postoperative morbidity and mortality, local recurrence, and long-term survival [98–100].

Multidisciplinary Rectal Cancer Care

There is increasing evidence that multidisciplinary team management is associated with improved clinical decision-making, superior outcomes, and better patient experience in several types of cancer, including rectal cancer [101]. Cancer centers of excellence have been successfully established in several European countries over the past decade to address variability and disparity in the quality of rectal cancer care. Similar efforts in standardizing care to improve outcome have begun in the United States. The OSTRiCh (Optimizing the Surgical Treatment of Rectal Cancer) Consortium, founded in 2011, comprises a group of health-care institutions across the United States, dedicated to improving delivery of rectal cancer care by relying on evidence-based and standardized care [102].

Variability in care was recently demonstrated in a study analyzing data from the National Cancer Data Base, which examined adherence to neoadjuvant chemoradiotherapy in 30,994 patients with clinical stage II and III rectal cancers [103]. The use of neoadjuvant radiation therapy and chemotherapy varied significantly by type of cancer center, with the highest rates of adherence observed in high-volume centers compared with low-volume centers (78% vs. 69%; adjusted odds ratio = 1.46; $P<0.001$). This variation was mirrored by hospital geographic location, with little improvement observed over the last 5 years. These results further support the implementation of standardized care pathways for patients with rectal cancer.

Conclusion

The impact of optimal proctectomy technique in reducing the incidence of recurrence and improving long-term survival in rectal cancer is well established. The associated improvement in disease-free, recurrence-free, and overall survival, and increased improvement in bowel, bladder, and sexual function postoperatively, make proctectomy—with appropriate mesorectal excision and autonomic nerve preservation—the standard of care and a required part of colorectal surgical training. Complete surgical resection of the tumor and draining lymph nodes using sharp dissection are the basic principles of TME. Attention to preservation of the autonomic nerves can reduce the morbidity of this operation, improve functional outcomes, and provide a more acceptable quality of life. The use of multidisciplinary disease management teams, and implementation of centralization for the treatment of rectal cancer, has a strong potential to provide efficient delivery of evidence-based care.

References

1. Miles WE. A method of performing abdomino-perineal excision for carcinoma of the rectum and of the terminal portion of the pelvic colon. Lancet. 1908;2:1812–3.
2. Miles WE. The radical abdomino-perineal operation for cancer of the pelvic colon. BMJ. 1910;11:941–3.
3. Abel AL. The modern treatment of cancer of the rectum. Milwaukee Proc. March 3–5 1931; pp. 296–300.
4. Heald RJ. The 'Holy Plane' of rectal surgery. J R Soc Med. 1988;81(9):503–8.
5. Heald RJ, Ryall RD. Recurrence and survival after total mesorectal excision for rectal cancer. Lancet. 1986;1:1479–82.
6. Zaheer S, Pemberton JH, Farouk R, Dozois RR, Wolff BG, Ilstrup D. Surgical treatment of adenocarcinoma of the rectum. Ann Surg Oncol. 1998;227:800–11.
7. Quirke P, et al. Local recurrence of rectal adenocarcinoma due to inadequate surgical resection. Histopathological study of lateral tumour spread and surgical excision. Lancet. 1986; 2(8514):996–9.
8. Wilson SM, Beahrs OH. The curative treatment of carcinoma of the sigmoid, rectosigmoid, and rectum. Ann Surg. 1976; 183:556–65.
9. Dukes C. The surgical pathology of rectal cancer. Proc R Soc Med. 1943;37:131.
10. McCall J, Cox MR, Wattchow DA. Analysis of local recurrence rates after surgery alone for rectal cancer. Int J Colorectal Dis. 1955;10:126–32.
11. Nagtegaal ID, Quirke P. What is the role for the circumferential margin in the modern treatment of rectal cancer? J Clin Oncol. 2008;26(2):303–12.
12. Quer EA, Dahlin DC, Mayo CW. Retrograde intramural spread of carcinoma of the rectum and rectosigmoid. Surg Gynecol Obstet. 1953;96:24–30.
13. Grinnel RS. Distal intramural spread of rectal carcinoma. Surg Gynecol Obstet. 1954;99:421–30.
14. Black WA, Waugh JM. The intramural extension of carcinoma of the descending colon, sigmoid and rectosigmoid. A pathological study. Surg Gynecol Obstet. 1948;1948:457–64.
15. Scott N, Jackson P, Al-Jaberi T, Dixon MF, Quirke P, Finan PJ. Total mesorectal excision and local recurrence: a study of tumour spread in the mesorectum distal to rectal cancer. Br J Surg. 1995;82:1031–3.
16. Williams NS, Dixon MF, Johnston D. Reappraisal of the 5 centimetre rule of distal excision for carcinoma of the rectum: a study of distal intramural spread and of patients' survival. Br J Surg. 1983;70:150–4.
17. Karanjia ND, Corder AP, Bearn P, Heald RJ. Leakage from stapled low anastomosis after total mesorectal excision for carcinoma of the rectum. Br J Surg. 1994;81:1224–6.
18. Bokey EL, Öjerskog B, Chapuis PH, Dent OF, Newland RC, Sinclair G. Local recurrence after curative excision of the rectum for cancer without adjuvant therapy: role of total anatomical dissection. Br J Surg. 1999;86:1164–70.
19. Heald RJ, et al. Rectal cancer: the Basingstoke experience of total mesorectal excision, 1978–1997. Arch Surg. 1998;133(8):894–9.
20. Arenas RB, Fichera A, Mhoon D, Michelassi F. Total mesorectal excision in the surgical treatment of rectal cancer: a prospective study. Arch Surg. 1998;133:608–11.
21. Hainsworth PJ, Egan MJ, Cunliffe WJ. Evaluation of a policy of total mesorectal excision for rectal and rectosigmoid cancers. Br J Surg. 1997;84(5):652–6.
22. Arbman G, et al. Local recurrence following total mesorectal excision for rectal cancer. Br J Surg. 1996;83(3):375–9.
23. Moran B, Heald RJ. Manual of total mesorectal excision. London: CRC; 2013.
24. Quirke P, Dixon MF. The prediction of local recurrence in rectal adenocarcinoma by histopathological examination. Int J Colorectal Dis. 1988;3(2):127–31.
25. Maslekar S, et al. Mesorectal grades predict recurrences after curative resection for rectal cancer. Dis Colon Rectum. 2007;50(2):168–75.
26. Quirke P, et al. Effect of the plane of surgery achieved on local recurrence in patients with operable rectal cancer: a prospective study using data from the MRC CR07 and NCIC-CTG CO16 randomised clinical trial. Lancet. 2009;373(9666): 821–8.
27. Nagtegaal ID, et al. Macroscopic evaluation of rectal cancer resection specimen: clinical significance of the pathologist in quality control. J Clin Oncol. 2002;20(7):1729–34.
28. College of American Pathologists. Protocol for the examination of specimens from patients with primary carcinoma of the colon and rectum. 2013 [cited 2015 July 17]. http://www.cap.org/ShowProperty?nodePath=/UCMCon/Contribution%20Folders/WebContent/pdf/colon-13protocol-3300.pdf.
29. Contant CM, et al. Mechanical bowel preparation for elective colorectal surgery: a multicentre randomised trial. Lancet. 2007;370(9605):2112–7.
30. Jung B, et al. Multicentre randomized clinical trial of mechanical bowel preparation in elective colonic resection. Br J Surg. 2007;94(6):689–95.
31. Guenaga KF, Matos D, Wille-Jorgensen P. Mechanical bowel preparation for elective colorectal surgery. Cochrane Database Syst Rev. 2011(9):p. CD001544.
32. Dahabreh IJ, Steele DW, Shah N, Trikalinos TA (2014) Agency for healthcare research and quality. Comparative effectiveness review. Number 128. Oral Mechanical Bowel Preparation for Colorectal Surgery. 2014 [cited 2015 July 17]. http://effectivehealthcare.ahrq.gov/ehc/products/458/1900/colorectal-surgery-preparation-report-140428.pdf.
33. Nelson RL, Gladman E, Barbateskovic M. Antimicrobial prophylaxis for colorectal surgery. Cochrane Database Syst Rev. 2014;5: p. CD001181.
34. Bratzler DW, et al. Clinical practice guidelines for antimicrobial prophylaxis in surgery. Am J Health Syst Pharm. 2013;70(3):195–283.
35. Poggio JL. Perioperative strategies to prevent surgical-site infection. Clin Colon Rectal Surg. 2013;26(3):168–73.
36. Kakkos SK, et al. Combined intermittent pneumatic leg compression and pharmacological prophylaxis for prevention of venous thromboembolism in high-risk patients. Cochrane Database Syst Rev. 2008(4): p. CD005258.
37. Danielsen AK, Burcharth J, Rosenberg J. Patient education has a positive effect in patients with a stoma: a systematic review. Colorectal Dis. 2013;15(6):e276–83.
38. Bardram L, et al. Recovery after laparoscopic colonic surgery with epidural analgesia, and early oral nutrition and mobilisation. Lancet. 1995;345(8952):763–4.

39. Serclova Z, et al. Fast-track in open intestinal surgery: prospective randomized study (Clinical Trials Gov Identifier no. NCT00123456). Clin Nutr. 2009;28(6):618–24.

40. Spanjersberg WR, et al. Fast track surgery versus conventional recovery strategies for colorectal surgery. Cochrane Database Syst Rev. 2011(2): p. CD007635.

41. Lin S, et al. Meta-analysis of robotic and laparoscopic surgery for treatment of rectal cancer. World J Gastroenterol. 2011;17(47):5214–20.

42. Marr R, et al. The modern abdominoperineal excision: the next challenge after total mesorectal excision. Ann Surg. 2005;242(1):74–82.

43. den Dulk M, et al. The abdominoperineal resection itself is associated with an adverse outcome: the European experience based on a pooled analysis of five European randomised clinical trials on rectal cancer. Eur J Cancer. 2009;45(7):1175–83.

44. Nagtegaal ID, et al. Low rectal cancer: a call for a change of approach in abdominoperineal resection. J Clin Oncol. 2005;23(36):9257–64.

45. Enker WE, Levi GS. Macroscopic assessment of mesorectal excision. Cancer. 2009;115(21):4890–4.

46. Enker WE, et al. Abdominoperineal resection via total mesorectal excision and autonomic nerve preservation for low rectal cancer. World J Surg. 1997;21(7):715–20.

47. Holm T, et al. Extended abdominoperineal resection with gluteus maximus flap reconstruction of the pelvic floor for rectal cancer. Br J Surg. 2007;94(2):232–8.

48. West NP, et al. Multicentre experience with extralevator abdominoperineal excision for low rectal cancer. Br J Surg. 2010;97(4):588–99.

49. Han JG, et al. A prospective multicenter clinical study of extralevator abdominoperineal resection for locally advanced low rectal cancer. Dis Colon Rectum. 2014;57(12):1333–40.

50. Prytz M, et al. Extralevator abdominoperineal excision (ELAPE) for rectal cancer—short-term results from the Swedish Colorectal Cancer Registry. Selective use of ELAPE warranted. Int J Colorectal Dis. 2014;29(8):981–7.

51. Kang CY, et al. Robotic-assisted extralevator abdominoperineal resection in the lithotomy position: technique and early outcomes. Am Surg. 2012;78(10):1033–7.

52. Marecik SJ, et al. Robotic cylindrical abdominoperineal resection with transabdominal levator transection. Dis Colon Rectum. 2011;54(10):1320–5.

53. Weiser MR, et al. Sphincter preservation in low rectal cancer is facilitated by preoperative chemoradiation and intersphincteric dissection. Ann Surg. 2009;249(2):236–42.

54. Kodeda K, et al. Rectal washout and local recurrence of cancer after anterior resection. Br J Surg. 2010;97(10):1589–97.

55. Karanjia ND, et al. 'Close shave' in anterior resection. Br J Surg. 1990;77(5):510–2.

56. Pollett WG, Nicholls RJ. The relationship between the extent of distal clearance and survival and local recurrence rates after curative anterior resection for carcinoma of the rectum. Ann Surg. 1983;198(2):159–63.

57. Vernava III AM, et al. A prospective evaluation of distal margins in carcinoma of the rectum. Surg Gynecol Obstet. 1992;175(4):333–6.

58. Paty PB, et al. Treatment of rectal cancer by low anterior resection with coloanal anastomosis. Ann Surg. 1994;219(4):365–73.

59. Paty PB, et al. Long-term functional results of coloanal anastomosis for rectal cancer. Am J Surg. 1994;167(1):90–4. discussion 94-5.

60. Brown CJ, Fenech DS, McLeod RS. Reconstructive techniques after rectal resection for rectal cancer. Cochrane Database Syst Rev. 2008(2): p. CD006040.

61. Hallbook O, et al. Randomized comparison of straight and colonic J pouch anastomosis after low anterior resection. Ann Surg. 1996;224(1):58–65.

62. Heriot AG, et al. Meta-analysis of colonic reservoirs versus straight coloanal anastomosis after anterior resection. Br J Surg. 2006;93(1):19–32.

63. Si C, Zhang Y, Sun P. Colonic J-pouch versus Baker type for rectal reconstruction after anterior resection of rectal cancer. Scand J Gastroenterol. 2013;48(12):1428–35.

64. Matthiessen P, et al. Defunctioning stoma reduces symptomatic anastomotic leakage after low anterior resection of the rectum for cancer: a randomized multicenter trial. Ann Surg. 2007;246(2):207–14.

65. Tan WS, et al. Meta-analysis of defunctioning stomas in low anterior resection for rectal cancer. Br J Surg. 2009;96(5):462–72.

66. Gu WL, Wu SW. Meta-analysis of defunctioning stoma in low anterior resection with total mesorectal excision for rectal cancer: evidence based on thirteen studies. World J Surg Oncol. 2015;13(1):9.

67. Gunderson LL, et al. Revised TN categorization for colon cancer based on national survival outcomes data. J Clin Oncol. 2010;28(2):264–71.

68. Derici H, et al. Multivisceral resections for locally advanced rectal cancer. Colorectal Dis. 2008;10(5):453–9.

69. Smith JD, et al. Multivisceral resections for rectal cancer. Br J Surg. 2012;99(8):1137–43.

70. Sugihara K, et al. Indication and benefit of pelvic sidewall dissection for rectal cancer. Dis Colon Rectum. 2006;49(11):1663–72.

71. Yano H, Moran BJ. The incidence of lateral pelvic side-wall nodal involvement in low rectal cancer may be similar in Japan and the West. Br J Surg. 2008;95(1):33–49.

72. Georgiou P, et al. Extended lymphadenectomy versus conventional surgery for rectal cancer: a meta-analysis. Lancet Oncol. 2009;10(11):1053–62.

73. Dubois JB, et al. Intra-operative radiotherapy of rectal cancer: results of the French multi-institutional randomized study. Radiother Oncol. 2011;98(3):298–303.

74. Wiig JN, Giercksky KE, Tveit KM. Intraoperative radiotherapy for locally advanced or locally recurrent rectal cancer: does it work at all? Acta Oncol. 2014;53(7):865–76.

75. Killeen S, Devaney A, Mannion M, Martin ST, Winter DC. Omental pedicle flaps following proctectomy: a systematic review. Colorectal Dis. 2013;15(11):e634–45.

76. Chessin DB, Hartley J, Cohen AM, Mazumdar M, Cordeiro P, Disa J, Mehrara B, Minsky BD, Paty P, Weiser M, Wong WD, Guillem JG. Rectus flap reconstruction decreases perineal wound complications after pelvic chemoradiation and surgery: a cohort study. Ann Surg Oncol. 2005;12(2):104–10.

77. Camilleri-Brennan J, Steele RJ. Quality of life after treatment for rectal cancer. Br J Surg. 1998;85(8):1036–43.

78. Bruheim K, et al. Late side effects and quality of life after radiotherapy for rectal cancer. Int J Radiat Oncol Biol Phys. 2010;76(4):1005–11.

79. Enker WE. Potency, cure, and local control in the operative treatment of rectal cancer. Arch Surg. 1992;127(12):1396–401. discussion 1402.

80. Havenga K, et al. Male and female sexual and urinary function after total mesorectal excision with autonomic nerve preservation for carcinoma of the rectum. J Am Coll Surg. 1996; 182(6):495–502.

81. Shirouzu K, Ogata Y, Araki Y. Oncologic and functional results of total mesorectal excision and autonomic nerve-preserving operation for advanced lower rectal cancer. Dis Colon Rectum. 2004;47(9):1442–7.

82. Cornish JA, et al. A meta-analysis of quality of life for abdominoperineal excision of rectum versus anterior resection for rectal cancer. Ann Surg Oncol. 2007;14(7):2056–68.

83. Engel J, et al. Quality of life in rectal cancer patients: a four-year prospective study. Ann Surg. 2003;238(2):203–13.

84. Kasparek MS, et al. Quality of life after coloanal anastomosis and abdominoperineal resection for distal rectal cancers: sphincter preservation vs quality of life. Colorectal Dis. 2011; 13(8):872–7.

85. Guren MG, et al. Quality of life and functional outcome following anterior or abdominoperineal resection for rectal cancer. Eur J Surg Oncol. 2005;31(7):735–42.

86. Birgisson H, et al. Late adverse effects of radiation therapy for rectal cancer—a systematic overview. Acta Oncol. 2007; 46(4):504–16.

87. Lange MM, et al. Risk factors for faecal incontinence after rectal cancer treatment. Br J Surg. 2007;94(10):1278–84.

88. MacFarlane JK, Ryall RD, Heald RJ. Mesorectal excision for rectal cancer. Lancet. 1993;341(8843):457–60.

89. Enker WE, et al. Total mesorectal excision in the operative treatment of carcinoma of the rectum. J Am Coll Surg. 1995;181(4):335–46.

90. Bjerkeset T, Edna TH. Rectal cancer: the influence of type of operation on local recurrence and survival. Eur J Surg. 1996;162(8):643–8.

91. Kockerling F, et al. Influence of surgery on metachronous distant metastases and survival in rectal cancer. J Clin Oncol. 1998;16(1):324–9.

92. Syk E, et al. Local recurrence in rectal cancer: anatomic localization and effect on radiation target. Int J Radiat Oncol Biol Phys. 2008;72(3):658–64.

93. Kapiteijn E, Putter H, van de Velde CJ. Impact of the introduction and training of total mesorectal excision on recurrence and survival in rectal cancer in The Netherlands. Br J Surg. 2002;89(9):1142–9.

94. Martling A, et al. The surgeon as a prognostic factor after the introduction of total mesorectal excision in the treatment of rectal cancer. Br J Surg. 2002;89(8):1008–13.

95. Wibe A, et al. Total mesorectal excision for rectal cancer—what can be achieved by a national audit? Colorectal Dis. 2003;5(5):471–7.

96. Wibe A, et al. A national strategic change in treatment policy for rectal cancer—implementation of total mesorectal excision as routine treatment in Norway. A national audit. Dis Colon Rectum. 2002;45(7):857–66.

97. Martling AL, et al. Effect of a surgical training programme on outcome of rectal cancer in the County of Stockholm. Stockholm Colorectal Cancer Study Group, Basingstoke Bowel Cancer Research Project. Lancet. 2000;356(9224): 93–6.

98. Helsper JT. Impact of the surgeon on cancer management outcomes. J Surg Oncol. 2003;82(1):1–2.

99. Luna-Perez P, et al. The surgeon as prognostic factor for local recurrence and survival in the anal sphincter preservation for mid-rectal cancer. Rev Invest Clin. 1999;51(4):205–13.

100. Renzulli P, Laffer UT. Learning curve: the surgeon as a prognostic factor in colorectal cancer surgery. Recent Results Cancer Res. 2005;165:86–104.

101. Dietz DW. Multidisciplinary management of rectal cancer: the OSTRICH. J Gastrointest Surg. 2013;17(10):1863–8.

102. The Consortium for Optimizing the Treatment of Rectal Cancer (OSTRiCh). 2014 [cited 2015 July 17]. http://www.ostrichconsortium.org/index.html.

103. Monson JR, et al. Failure of evidence-based cancer care in the United States: the association between rectal cancer treatment, cancer center volume, and geography. Ann Surg. 2014; 260(4):625–31. discussion 631-2.

104. Guillem JG, Lee-Kong SA. Autonomic nerve preservation during rectal cancer resection. J Gastrointest Surg. 2010; 14:416–22.

105. Janjua AZ, Moran B, Heald RJ. Open surgical management of rectal cancer. In: Patel HRH, Mould T, Joseph JV, Delaney CP, editors. Pelvic cancer surgery: modern breakthroughs and future advances. New York: Springer; 2015. p. 531.

106. Heald RJ, et al. Embryology and anatomy of the rectum. Semin Surg Oncol. 1998;15(2):66–71.

107. Hockel M. Laterally extended endopelvic resection for the treatment of locally advanced and recurrent cervical cancer. In: Patel HRH, Mould T, Joseph JV, Delaney CP, editors. Pelvic cancer surgery: modern breakthroughs and future advances. New York: Springer; 2005.

32
Rectal Cancer Decision-Making

W. Donald Buie and Anthony R. MacLean

Key Concepts

- Sound decision-making requires a full assessment of the primary lesion, the presence of metastatic disease, the patient's surgical risk, and goals of care.
- A submucosal excision may be used as a radical biopsy to assess a polyp for adverse features without compromising future radical excision.
- Following endoscopic excision of a malignant polyp, the pathology should be rereviewed and strict criteria adhered to regarding the need for radical surgery.
- While cT2 (clinical stage T2) lesions can be treated with radical excision alone, neoadjuvant treatment can be selectively given to patients with cT3 lesions, based on preoperative staging by MRI and multidisciplinary discussion.
- Pretreatment staging can be inaccurate, especially with regard to mesorectal nodal status. Treatment planning should include a discussion of what will be recommended if stage changes based on histologic analysis. This is especially true if patients are assumed to be node negative, undergo up-front proctectomy, and are found to be node positive or if patients undergo local excision and are found to have higher T stage than anticipated.
- Most operative decisions should be made prior to entering the operating room. The patient and the surgeon must be prepared for all eventualities. In some situations the ultimate surgical decision may depend on intraoperative findings.
- Patients with potentially curable Stage IV disease require multidisciplinary discussion with early involvement of hepatobiliary surgeons and medical oncologists to determine the optimal sequence of treatment.

By three methods we may learn wisdom: First, by reflection, which is noblest; Second, by imitation, which is easiest; and third by experience, which is the bitterest.
Confucius

Introduction

While a comprehensive knowledge base and consummate operative skill are required for optimal management of rectal cancer, sound decision-making is essential. Poor decisions whether preoperative, intraoperative, or postoperative may have a profound and irreversible affect on both short- and long-term patient outcomes. Thus, it is important to understand not only what you can do but what you should do.

The aim of this chapter is to examine common clinical situations encountered by the colorectal surgeon who treats rectal cancer and analyze the decision points. This includes identification of the variables that affect treatment decisions, the potential treatment options including the advantages and disadvantages of each, and finally the logic behind specific treatment decisions. The chapter is organized to include early rectal cancer, endoscopically removed cancers, locally advanced lesions, synchronous metastatic lesions, and special situations. While no chapter can cover all clinical situations, it is hoped that the principles outlined below can also be used as a guide in more unusual circumstances.

Assessment

Each situation like each patient is unique. Knowledge and a comprehensive understanding are paramount to making good surgical decisions. When first encountering a patient with a rectal neoplasm, our first step is to gather information. We assess the lesion in terms of size, location (distance from anal verge, distance from the superior aspect of the anorectal muscular ring, and circumferential position—anterior/posterior/lateral), morphology, fixation (fixed, tethered, mobile), and general appearance. Additional information is needed with respect to the presence of metastatic disease [1, 2]. Finally we assess the patient for surgical risk including anesthetic risk, procedural risk, and patient risk [3, 4]. As the surgeon you are responsible for ensuring that each patient is

© Springer International Publishing 2016
S.R. Steele et al. (eds.), *The ASCRS Textbook of Colon and Rectal Surgery*, DOI 10.1007/978-3-319-25970-3_32

fully evaluated and optimized for the required treatment; the right procedure at the right time as safely as possible [5].

An important part of assessment includes goals of care. Oncologic surgery is a balance of cure versus morbidity, mortality, and quality of life. Patients with significant comorbidity or those who are elderly may place greater emphasis on quality rather than quantity of life and make decisions accordingly. You must facilitate this discussion and provide information to help each patient make a decision (s)he is comfortable with. The risk-benefit profile of each potential treatment should be outlined and discussed thoroughly.

The final part of assessment is a firm understanding of your own strengths, skills, and limitations. Utilizing senior colleagues for a second opinion or as an intraoperative assist is a sign of good judgment. The management of rectal cancer is multidisciplinary, and you must cultivate strong relationships with your colleagues in the associated disciplines of diagnostic radiology, radiation oncology, medical oncology, pathology, and hepatobiliary surgery to provide optimal patient care. Ideally rectal cancer patients should be discussed at regular multidisciplinary conferences which have been shown to enhance care and outcomes. In a study by Snelgrove et al., multidisciplinary conference resulted in a change in management plan in 29 % of patients, due in a large proportion to reinterpretation of the MRI [6].

Early Rectal Cancer

Local Excision

For rectal lesions that appear early (benign or cT1 cancers), we would typically arrange for local staging, most commonly with endorectal ultrasound to examine the depth of invasion as well as a pelvic MRI, for staging regional nodes, and to document the baseline appearance of the pelvis going forward [7–10]. If the lesion has a malignant appearance or is a proven cancer on biopsy, we also arrange systemic staging with a CT scan of the chest, abdomen, and pelvis.

As long as there are no features on biopsy or imaging that are high risk for nodal disease, we would offer local excision as a "radical biopsy." We typically use the transanal endoscopic microsurgery (TEM) technique for most lesions, although TAMIS is a good alternative [11–13]. For distal lesions below 7 cm from the anal verge, conventional transanal excision can be considered, though there are data suggesting a higher rate of specimen fragmentation and subsequent local recurrence [14].

We believe it is critical to have a thorough discussion with the patient prior to performing a local excision. While the prevailing opinion described in most textbooks advocates for full-thickness excision in all cases, we tend to be more selective in our approach.

For lesions that appear benign on biopsy and imaging or at worst T1, we try to gauge the patient's thoughts on what their wishes would be in response to the biopsy results. If the patient decides that he or she would want a radical excision for anything other than the most early, most favorable cancer, we feel that a partial thickness excision is a very reasonable option, as it provides definitive histology and allows assessment of high-risk features, including differentiation, lymphovascular invasion, tumor budding, and depth of invasion in microns (Table 32-1). For lesions invading to <1000 μm with no adverse pathologic features, particularly with no evidence of high-grade budding, local excision alone is felt to be an acceptable treatment, with close follow-up [16–18]. Additional reasons to consider a partial thickness excision also include less perioperative risk and no significant change in the perirectal fat that can affect the difficulty of (and complications from) subsequent radical excision in cases with unfavorable histologic features. Importantly, if the lesion is proven to be benign, then excision in the submucosal plane should be curative and will avoid the added morbidity of full-thickness excision.

TABLE 32-1. Risk of nodal involvement

	# Tumors	Nodal involvement (%)	Odds ratio	P-value
Tumor grade				
Favorable	176	5.7		
Unfavorable	75	29.2	2.9	0.023
Vascular invasion				
Absent	176	5.7		
Present	75	30.7	2.7	0.039
Cribriform pattern				
Absent	192	7.3		
Present	59	32.2	3.9	0.002
Tumor budding				
Negative	213	8		
Positive	38	42.1	3.7	0.008

With permission from Ueno H, Mochizuki H, Hasiguchi Y, et al. Risk factors for an adverse outcome in early invasive colorectal carcinoma. Gastroenterology 2004; 127:385–394 © Elsevier 2004 [15]

On the other hand, if the patient is more strongly in favor of avoiding radical surgery and would tolerate a slightly higher risk of local recurrence, we feel that a full-thickness excision is warranted for lesions that are proven on biopsy to be adenocarcinoma preoperatively or have gross features of malignancy, which again allows for histologic evaluation but also provides a wider deep margin for more significant lesions.

Once the histologic information is available (for which we also typically request a second opinion from an experienced GI pathologist), we have a thorough discussion with the patient about the results and define their risk of lymph node disease. For patients with T1 adenocarcinoma with high-risk features and/or depth of invasion greater than 1000 μm (or Kikuchi level SM2) [15, 18, 19], we recommend radical excision. However, in situations where the patient understands the risks and prefers to avoid radical excision, close follow-up is an acceptable alternative. For patients who are frail or have significant comorbidity that would preclude a radical excision, we consider extending our indications for local excision to more significant lesions.

Our follow-up depends somewhat on the characteristics of the lesion excised and the patient's age and comorbidity but, in general, would include sigmoidoscopic examination at 3–4 month intervals for the first 2 years when the risk of recurrence appears to be highest, then at 6-month intervals for an additional 2 years with colonoscopic evaluation as indicated for surveillance at year 1 and year 4. Additionally, we survey the pelvis with pelvic MRI scans at 6-month intervals for the first 2 years to look for nodal recurrence. Lastly, we typically arrange yearly CT scans of the chest, abdomen, and pelvis for the first 3 years to look for metastatic disease.

Endoscopically Excised Malignant Polyps

Occasionally we will be referred a patient who has had endoscopic excision of a malignant rectal polyp. In these situations, we obtain a pathologic review and then try to determine the risk of intraluminal recurrence as well as the risk of nodal disease and systemic recurrence. We examine the polypectomy site with sigmoidoscopy and, if not already done, mark it with a tattoo especially if completely excised. The patient is staged as in the early rectal cancer section above. However, it is important to remember that imaging can be affected by the thermal injury to the bowel wall from a large polypectomy. Occasionally lymphadenopathy related to local inflammation will be seen, that can be confused for nodal metastases. The risk of intraluminal recurrence is dependent on the margin of excision—while many textbooks advocate a 2 mm minimal margin, current evidence suggests that in the absence of other high-risk histologic features, a 1 mm margin is adequate [15, 20]. In terms of the risk of nodal disease, important factors include differentiation, lymphovascular invasion, tumor budding, and depth of invasion (see

Table 32-1). When all histologic features are favorable and the margin is greater than 1 mm, close follow-up is recommended. When all histologic features are favorable, but the margin is <1 mm, we discuss re-excision transanally versus radical excision. When high-risk features for nodal metastases are present, we typically recommend radical excision assuming the patient is a suitable candidate. In high-risk patients where radical excision is not an option, we extend our indications for observation.

Operable and Locally Advanced Lesions

For lesions that are not amenable to local excision, our approach is to again assess the lesion as described above but also perform local staging with pelvic MRI and systemic staging with a CT of the chest abdomen and pelvis. We do not routinely advocate the use of PET scan in the preoperative staging of rectal cancer, except to help resolve an indeterminate lesion identified on CT or MRI.

For lesions that are T2 on imaging, we typically advocate a radical excision. We do not currently feel that there is sufficient evidence to recommend local excision in association with neoadjuvant [21] or adjuvant chemoradiation [22], though there is ongoing interest in this approach and further evidence could possibly change that opinion in the future.

The current standard of care for all clinical stage 2 and stage 3 rectal cancers is to receive neoadjuvant therapy followed by radical surgery when diagnosed on preoperative imaging and to receive postoperative chemoradiotherapy when final pathology unexpectedly demonstrates stage 2 or 3 disease [23]. However, it has become clear that some of these patients derive very little benefit from chemoradiotherapy and do suffer potential long-term complications from the administration of postoperative radiotherapy, including fibrosis/stricture of the anorectum and other issues with bowel, bladder, and sexual function [24–26]. It is also clear that receiving postoperative radiotherapy is less effective than neoadjuvant radiotherapy. Thus identifying those who are likely to derive the most benefit is important [27].

Current staging modalities are very accurate at determining T stage and distance to the expected mesorectal margin but are much less accurate in determining N-stage. TRUS, CT, and MR all suffer from a lack of sensitivity and specificity when queried to predict mesorectal nodal status [7, 28–31]. All the techniques suffer from the inherent limitation that they do not detect tumor but rather the size and morphology of the node. Tumor deposits in lymph nodes do not reliably produce lymphadenopathy greater than 1 cm; in fact more than 50 % of all positive nodes will be less than 5 mm in size. In addition, the inflammatory reaction from previous biopsies, or from the tumor itself, can result in nodal enlargement without tumor involvement, resulting in false positives. Metabolic imaging with 18-fluorodeoxyglucose positron emission tomography (FDG-PET) may not be effective in detecting mesorectal nodal status because emission from the primary tumor may obscure adjacent nodal signal or because of the small size of some of the nodal metastases.

Given the limitations of preoperative staging, locally advanced lesions require a considerable amount of careful thought when deciding on the most appropriate course of treatment. One can decide that all patients with stage 2 or 3 disease require chemoradiotherapy and mandate that all patients with clinical stage 2 and 3 tumors receive neoadjuvant therapy and that all unsuspected stage 2 and 3 tumors receive postoperative chemoradiotherapy. An alternative strategy is to be more selective, trying to select those patients who are more likely to derive benefit from chemoradiotherapy, while avoiding the negative consequences of radiation in more favorable patients. We generally use the Mercury study group criteria [32, 33] to help decide which patients should be referred for neoadjuvant therapy. cT3a tumors with less than 5 mm of intrusion into the perirectal fat and predicted negative resection margins generally behave more as T2 lesions and thus can be spared the negative consequences of radiation therapy (Figure 32-1) [34]. For cT3 lesions with a close but predicted negative (>2 mm) margin based on staging MRI, neoadjuvant therapy is warranted. In this situation, both short-course radiation and long-course chemoradiation can be considered. For cT3 lesions with a predicted positive margin and for cT4 lesions, long-course neoadjuvant chemoradiation is required for tumor downstaging.

However, preoperative staging alone should not drive all treatment decisions with regard to neoadjuvant therapy. Pelvic morphology and tumor position may have a significant effect on decision-making. For example, a proctectomy in an obese man with a narrow pelvis and an anteriorly based

tumor of the mid or distal rectum can be very challenging. Such a patient should be considered for neoadjuvant therapy and should be discussed in a multidisciplinary setting, ideally with radiologic review. Alternatively, proctectomy in a thin woman with a wide pelvis and a posteriorly based tumor should be relatively straightforward with little chance of positive margin if the tumor does not extend beyond the mesorectal fascia on preoperative imaging.

The inability to predict nodal status before embarking on a treatment course is of particular concern for the subset of patients staged as cN0 who undergo proctectomy as a first step in treatment and are upstaged to pN1+(2) following histologic review of the operative specimen. Prior to simply recommending postoperative radiotherapy because of N+ status, it should be remembered that postoperative radiotherapy is not as effective as preoperative radiotherapy, must be administered at a higher dose with concurrent chemotherapy to achieve similar oncologic benefit, and has the downside of higher toxicity [35].

One strategy to avoid the issue of radiating patients postoperatively who are found unexpectedly to have node positive disease at proctectomy is to radiate all patients preoperatively regardless of pretreatment imaging results. Short-course radiotherapy is probably the best regimen for patients with non-fixed tumors if this strategy is adopted, as the oncologic results are equivalent to long-course chemoradiotherapy. In addition, short-course radiotherapy can be administered more quickly (shortening the time to full-dose cytotoxic chemotherapy in appropriate patients), is less costly, and is associated with less toxicity in the neoadjuvant period. The main downside of this approach is the large number of patients who would be treated and exposed to the

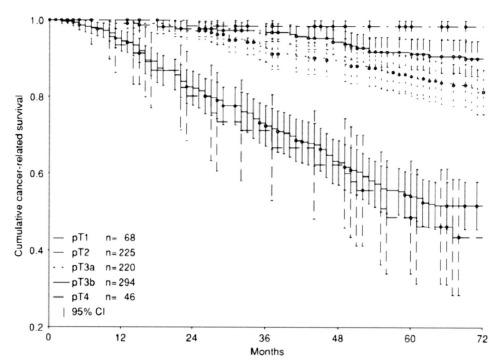

FIGURE 32-1. Cancer-related survival in relation to extended pT classification based on depth of invasion: pT1 submucosa, pT2 muscularis propria, pT3a<5 mm extramural disease, pT3b>5 mm extramural disease, and pT4 other organs. *With permission from Merkel S, Mansmann U, Siassi M, Papadopoulos T, et al. The prognostic inhomogeneity in pT3 rectal carcinomas. Int J Colorectal Dis 2001:16:298–304 © Springer 2001* [34].

long-term consequences of radiotherapy without deriving any significant benefit.

Another approach is to agree at the initial multidisciplinary conference that patients recommended for up-front proctectomy will not be considered for postoperative radiotherapy unless margins of resection are positive, and will be treated with chemotherapy alone if they are found to be node positive and resection margin negative. This strategy will also shorten the time to full-dose cytotoxic chemotherapy and avoid the toxicity of postoperative radiotherapy, which can be substantial. The argument that this is not "standard of care" is based on recommendations from decades past, when trials were conducted without surgery or pathology quality control, radial margins were not assessed, and chemotherapeutic agents were less effective. This is our current treatment approach for patients who are upstaged on pathologic review following proctectomy.

Lastly, there is continued interest in a "watch and wait" approach following neoadjuvant therapy with complete clinical response [36–38]. The issue remains that complete clinical response does not always equate with complete pathologic response. Except in situations of compromise due to patient frailty or comorbidity, we feel that this approach should be relegated to participation in a clinical trial [39]. This opinion may change as additional information becomes available.

As one may see from the above discussion, decision-making for patients with rectal cancer is complex and nuanced. Unfortunately, this complexity cannot be easily transformed into simple treatment guidelines.

Surgical Considerations

Intraoperative Decisions

Most operative decisions should be made prior to entering the operating room. There is no substitute for advance preparation having thought through the potential problems and solutions away from the OR when planning and reflection can occur without distraction and emotion. In difficult situations we will seek the advice of a colleague and plan to have a second surgeon available intraoperatively should the decision have far-reaching consequences or should the unexpected arise.

Despite the surgeon's best intentions, there are occasions where the final decision can only be made at the time of surgery. The surgeon must be flexible and have very precisely articulated goals of care; know why you are there and what you are trying to accomplish. In exceptional cases, this may include backing out if the situation requires more than what has been planned for. It is better to return on another day when the patient and surgeon are emotionally and physically prepared for the operation that is required.

Midrectal Cancers

As mesorectal spread can extend up to 3–4 cm distal to the gross tumor margin, a 5 cm mesorectal margin is required to ensure complete removal of at-risk nodal tissue [40, 41]. We advocate a tumor-specific mesorectal excision for tumors in the upper third of the rectum, preserving rectal length and function without compromising cure. When the tumor is located in the distal third of the rectum, 5 cm or less from the end of the mesorectum, we advocate a total mesorectal excision (TME) to remove all nodal tissue [40–43].

For tumors in the middle third especially in obese patients, it may be very difficult to perform a tumor-specific mesorectal excision and save 2–3 cm of viable rectum above the pelvic floor. We feel it is often technically easier and safer for the patient to extend the resection for an additional 2 or 3 cm to complete a TME. The decision is based primarily on the technical feasibility of dissecting through the distal mesorectum at that level while preserving the viability of the rectal stump.

Low Rectal Cancers

Surgical decision-making in low rectal cancer is complex balancing cure with function. In most situations, the decision to proceed with a sphincter-preserving procedure rather than an abdominoperineal resection is made preoperatively based on history, physical examination, imaging studies, response to chemoradiation, and the ability to obtain clear surgical margins. In addition patient factors including age, comorbidities, body habitus, continence, and patient wishes must be considered [44]. Good quality MRI with careful interpretation is important to identify any absolute indications for APR including involvement of the levators or external sphincter [45].

On rare occasions due to body habitus, tumor size, or pelvic shape, it may be difficult to predict preoperatively whether a tumor can be successfully resected with sphincter-preserving techniques. In this situation the patient must be fully informed and all options discussed in detail including the reasoning behind the decision, the expected outcomes, and potential complications. We consent the patient for "a low anterior resection-possible abdominoperineal resection" and emphasize that we are operating for local control and will proceed with sphincter preservation provided that cure is not compromised. The patient should be counseled and marked for both a colostomy and a loop ileostomy.

Preoperatively, all approaches that enhance distal dissection should be considered including a stapled coloanal anastomosis and a hand-sewn coloanal anastomosis with or without intersphincteric resection. Although a stapled anastomosis results in better function and less morbidity, an intersphincteric dissection provides additional distal margin length [46–48]. We restrict this technique to very low tumors that are contained within the rectal wall, that do not invade the pelvic floor or anal sphincters, in patients who can tolerate and accept the functional compromise [44]. The functional results depend on preoperative sphincter function, the effect of neoadjuvant radiation, and the variable amount of residual internal sphincter left below the dentate line [49–52]. We feel it is critical that the surgeon carefully reviews and correlates the preoperative imaging and the findings on physical examination prior to considering an intersphincteric dissection, as it is essential that the tumor is well clear of the intersphincteric plane, to prevent a positive margin and consequently a high risk of local recurrence.

Generally speaking we will accept a 1 cm distal margin although a margin less than 1 cm may be acceptable following chemoradiation [53, 54]. Every effort should be made prior to rectal division to ascertain if the margin will be adequate. Once the rectum is divided and the specimen has been removed, it should be examined off table and if possible in concert with the pathologist. If the distal mural margin is inadequate, we would proceed directly with a completion proctectomy after repositioning in prone jack-knife position.

In the obese male with a bulky tumor and relatively small pelvis, distal mesorectal dissection under direct vision and thus sphincter preservation may be impossible using standard open or laparoscopic techniques such that an APR may be required to obtain clear margins. We discuss this situation with the patient preoperatively to ensure they are aware of the surgical limitations and the potential consequences. Transanal TME (taTME) with either TEM or TAMIS is a promising new technique to augment a technically difficult distal dissection. The distal margin and lower mesorectum are dissected transanally under direct vision and when combined with a laparoscopic or open TME extends the distal limits of dissection in these patients. While the initial case series are promising, this technique is not ready for universal adoption as the oncologic results are not mature, indications and contraindications remain to be refined, and the learning curve has yet to be established [55–57].

A clear circumferential margin is also critical to local control. Every effort should be made preoperatively in conjunction with your radiologist to identify potentially difficult areas of dissection where the margin may be compromised with steps taken to extend resection to an uninvolved plane as necessary. If, the decision to proceed with an APR is made intraoperatively, it should be made as soon as possible to maximize the circumferential tumor margin with a cylindrical dissection. The mesorectal plane leads the surgeon through the levator hiatus onto the bare area of the rectum with potential compromise to the circumferential margin in an ultralow tumor [58, 59]. All options need to be considered prior to entering this area of dissection. Intraoperatively, as we proceed distally, we frequently don an extra glove and bimanually palpate the tumor changing gloves prior to reentry into the operative field. If we feel that sphincter preservation will compromise the circumferential margin, we stop

and proceed with a proctectomy in prone jack-knife position. We will often make this decision with a second surgeon present to ensure optimal care.

Low Hartmann's vs. APR

Patients with poor preoperative anal sphincter function who would normally have a low anterior resection with a coloanal anastomosis may also be treated with a low Hartmann resection. While this obviates the need for a perineal wound with its attendant risks of nonhealing and chronically draining sinus tract, a low Hartmann's is occasionally complicated by blowout of the stump and chronic pelvic sepsis [60]. We use this option primarily in the elderly in situations without preoperative radiation.

Special Situations

Obstructing Rectal Cancer

Obstructing rectal cancers present a challenging situation and require careful thought and planning to ensure that the patient's oncologic outcome is optimized. In the case of widely metastatic disease that is clearly not resectable, endoluminal stenting is a reasonable consideration provided that the bottom of the stent will lie clearly above the anorectal ring, to avoid causing pain and tenesmus [61, 62]. The tumor should be quite tight to ensure that the stent is held in place.

Alternatively, in patients with partial obstructive symptoms and without evidence of proximal colonic dilatation, administration of chemoradiotherapy will usually relieve the obstructive symptoms if instituted without delay.

In the case of curable disease, several scenarios can present themselves.

In cases requiring fecal diversion where an abdominoperineal resection will ultimately be required, we recommend using a loop colostomy for fecal diversion. At the time of the APR, the distal limb of the stoma can be divided, leaving the colostomy in situ if it is functioning well, or it can be revised to an end colostomy if needed. These patients are not good candidates for endoluminal stenting, because the stent will lie in contact with the anal canal and become symptomatic.

In cases requiring fecal diversion where an eventual reconstructive surgery is anticipated, decision-making can be more complex. In the "near-obstructing" but not clinically obstructed situation, and in situations where significant patient symptoms are a relative indication for fecal diversion, we select the type of stoma based primarily on the degree of stenosis. If the lesion can be passed by a colonoscope or gastroscope and the proximal bowel can be visualized, we would in general select a diverting loop ileostomy, which can be left in situ following the low anterior resection if needed. If the lesion cannot be passed with a colonoscope or gastroscope, then we would generally construct a diverting loop colostomy. This prevents the possibility of a "closed loop" developing between the tumor and a competent ileocecal valve should the lesion swell and obstruct during neoadjuvant therapy. It also allows us to perform a colonoscopy preoperatively through the stoma to clear the rest of the colon. If fecal diversion is required following the reconstructive procedure, a loop ileostomy can still be brought through the previous left-sided loop colostomy site. A transverse loop colostomy is another option in these situations but is a more difficult stoma to manage for the patient and in general we avoid using them.

In cases presenting with a complete obstruction requiring emergency treatment, endoluminal stenting can be considered to relieve the obstruction and allow for semi-elective treatment of the cancer. The benefits of this approach include a rapid recovery from the procedure, that allows for prompt initiation of neoadjuvant chemoradiation if required, or to proceed on to radical surgery in the less common situation where neoadjuvant therapy is not indicated. The potential downsides of stenting include the risk of perforation and stent migration. The other main treatment option in the case of complete obstruction is a diverting loop colostomy. This strategy also provides relief of the obstruction and will reliably allow the patient to get through their neoadjuvant therapy, in addition to allowing for a preoperative colonoscopy prior to radical excision. The downsides include the fact that these cases do not always lend themselves to a laparoscopic approach (e.g., if there is loss of domain because of the distended colon) and therefore might require a longer period of recovery prior to initiation of neoadjuvant therapy. The open approach can also cause adhesions and make the future radical excision slightly more difficult. Our approach for these situations in general is to consider endoluminal stenting followed by semi-urgent radical excision (tumor-specific mesorectal excision) for the proximal rectal cancers and to use a diverting colostomy for most mid and distal rectal cancers, followed by neoadjuvant therapy, and radical excision.

Perforated Rectal Cancer

We tend to think of perforated rectal cancer in two ways: intraperitoneal perforations and extraperitoneal perforations.

For free intraperitoneal perforations, urgent surgery is generally required. The operation ideally should include an oncologic resection of the primary tumor. The decision on whether to perform a primary anastomosis (with or without and proximal diverting stoma) or a Hartmann procedure depends on several factors, including the overall health of the patient, their perioperative stability, the duration and extent of fecal contamination, and the anticipated intraoperative technical difficulties. Rarely should one simply divert these patients, as they risk having ongoing intraperitoneal tumor dissemination.

For contained intraperitoneal perforations, for example, those presenting with an abscess, we typically arrange percutaneous drainage, ensure that the patient is stable and fully staged, and then typically proceed with radical excision with or without an anastomosis.

For contained extraperitoneal perforations, we typically advocate proximal fecal diversion, drainage of sepsis, neoadjuvant chemoradiation, followed by radical excision, to include all tissues felt to have been contaminated by the perforation. This can require an exenterative procedure and/or an extrafascial dissection.

In the situation where a rectal cancer presents with perianal sepsis and fistulas, we generally ensure that the sepsis is well controlled, strongly consider fecal diversion with a laparoscopic loop sigmoid colostomy, and then arrange for neoadjuvant chemoradiotherapy. This is then followed by an APR with wide pelvic and perineal excision. These patients typically have large perineal wounds, and many benefit from a rectus abdominis myocutaneous flap for perineal reconstruction.

Synchronous Hepatic Metastases

Advancements in liver surgery and systemic chemotherapy have made it possible to consider alternative approaches to traditional primary tumor resection (PTR) in stage IV rectal cancer with synchronous hepatic metastases. These include synchronous resection (SR) and primary liver resection (PLR) [63]. No all-encompassing protocol exists for resectable stage IV rectal cancer as each alternative targets a different subpopulation [64]. SR and PLR should be used selectively and require multidisciplinary discussion with group ownership of the patients and the decisions.

Assuming that the patient is a surgical candidate, there are three overriding questions that need to be answered: is the primary resectable, is the metastatic liver disease resectable, and is there extrahepatic metastatic disease?

Prior to considering liver resection, the primary tumor must be staged and determined to be resectable, either primarily or following neoadjuvant therapy. We involve the hepatobiliary (HPB) surgeon very early to determine if the liver lesions are either resectable, potentially resectable with downstaging, or unresectable. It has been shown that resectability is best judged by an HPB surgeon [65].

Provided both the primary and hepatic metastases are resectable, then the decision is made to perform the rectal and liver resections either sequentially or in low-risk situations synchronously. We would typically consider PTR followed by liver resection for most patients [66]. Synchronous resection is offered to very selected patients to take advantage of a shorter overall recovery time accepting the increased risk of morbidity [67–69]. Generally speaking the magnitude of the two surgeries, the experience of the operating teams, the level of perioperative support and patient comorbidities/operative risk determines whether or not synchronous resections can

TABLE 32-2. Ideal criteria for liver-first protocol

1. Local regional control does not require downstaging with neoadjuvant therapy
2. Liver metastases are very clearly resectable for cure with adequate residual liver
3. Good overall operative risk patient with normal physiologic status and no known risk factors for perioperative infectious complications and major morbidity
4. Surgery can be performed in a high-volume liver unit with low-operative mortality and acceptable morbidity
5. Delays due to unexpected postoperative complications will not jeopardize local control or cure

and should be performed [70, 71]. For example, a high anterior resection can be combined with a nonanatomic resection in a low-risk patient with expected good results. On the other hand, an extended right hepatectomy and an extended low anterior resection should be done sequentially. The volume of resected liver is an important risk factor for postoperative complications. In a recent retrospective study, patients with postoperative complications averaged 350 g of resected liver tissue vs. patients in the non-complication group who averaged only 150 g [72].

When the rectal lesion is clearly resectable and the liver lesion is borderline or requires an extended resection, a PLR may be the best option [73]. In this situation the liver disease is the major determinant of survival. Because PLR is associated with a considerable increase in morbidity without the application of stringent selection criteria, it should be limited to very specific situations (Table 32-2) as a significant complication following liver resection may delay treatment of the primary [74–76]. Although it is tempting to push these limits, it is important to remember that it is the patient who takes on all the risk.

Patients with liver metastases and locally advanced primaries requiring neoadjuvant therapy are much more complicated. Most liver-first protocols exclude locally advanced rectal cancer patients due to the radiotherapy requirements of neoadjuvant therapy. In addition, the chemotherapy in long-course neoadjuvant therapy is relatively low dose; consequently liver metastases run the risk of growing and becoming unresectable. The presence of a borderline liver lesion further complicates the decision. In this situation, we typically use full-dose chemotherapy to downstage both lesions [77]. If there is a favorable response to several cycles of chemotherapy, then the patient may be treated with neoadjuvant chemoradiotherapy followed by either SR, PTR or PLR as determined by multidisciplinary discussion weighing the risks and benefits of each treatment course [77].

A promising new technique for this situation is the use of short-course radiotherapy to control margins followed by full-dose chemotherapy to allow time for tumor downstaging and systemic treatment for liver metastases. Prospective trials are currently underway to assess the efficacy of this pathway [78].

The presence of extrahepatic disease is generally a contraindication to hepatic resection for cure in stage IV disease. However, in select situations, in a good risk highly motivated patient, we will consider a lung resection following curative resection of the primary and all liver lesions. Surgery should

be done sequentially at a reasonable time interval after recovery from the previous resections to ensure that the disease remains localized and the patient is fully optimized.

Conclusion

Nowhere in colorectal surgery are therapeutic decisions more complex or more important to long-term patient outcomes than in the treatment of rectal cancer.

As a young surgeon, decisions are made primarily by imitating our mentors. With experience we find that not all situations fit cleanly into algorithms, and we are forced to make decisions without a complete data set or in situations where there may not be a single correct answer only a best answer given the available information and the specific circumstances.

The treatment of rectal cancer is ever changing as new information is brought forward into practice. The surgeon must keep abreast of new developments, with a fundamental knowledge of all potential treatment options including the risks, benefits and alternatives. In addition to application of this knowledge set, each patient requires a full assessment of the primary lesion, the presence of metastatic disease, the patients' operative risk, and goals of care.

While skills and knowledge are important for optimal patient care, it is often a surgical decision that ultimately determines patient outcomes. Much like surgical skills, decision-making requires practice with continuous analysis and reflection for improvement to ensure the right care, at the right time as safely as possible for each patient.

References

1. Valentini V, Beets-Tan R, Borras JM, Krivokapic Z, Leer JW, Pahlman L, Rodel C, Schmoll HJ, Scott N, Velde CV, Verfaillie C. Evidence and research in rectal cancer. Radiother Oncol. 2008;87:449–74.
2. Muthusamy VR, Chang KJ. Optimal methods for staging rectal cancer. Clin Cancer Res. 2007;13:6877s–84s.
3. Lee TH, Marcantonio ER, Mangione CM, Thomas EJ, Polanczyk CA, Cook EF, Sugarbaker DJ, Donaldson MC, Poss R, Ho KK, Ludwig LE, Pedan A, Goldman L. Derivation and prospective validation of a simple index for prediction of cardiac risk of major noncardiac surgery. Circulation. 1999;100:1043–9.
4. Cohen ME, Bilimoria KY, Ko CY, Hall BL. Development of an American College of Surgeons National Surgery Quality

Improvement Program: morbidity and mortality risk calculator for colorectal surgery. J Am Coll Surg. 2009;208:1009–16.

5. Buie WD, MacLean AR. Perioperative risk assessment. In: Steele S, Maykel J, Champagne BJ, Orangio GR, editors. Complexities in colorectal surgery. New York: Springer; 2014. p. 17–28.

6. Snelgrove RC, Subendran J, Jhaveri K, Thippavong S, Cummings B, Brierly J, Kirsch R, Kennedy ED. Effect of multidisciplinary cancer conference on treatment plan for patients with primary rectal cancer. Dis Colon Rectum. 2015;58(7):653–8.

7. Bipat S, Glas AS, Slors FJ, Zwinderman AH, Bossuyt PM, Stoker J. Rectal cancer: local staging and assessment of lymph node involvement with endoluminal US, CT, and MR imaging—a meta-analysis. Radiology. 2004;232:773–83.

8. Lahaye MJ, Engelen SM, Nelemans PJ, Beets GL, van de Velde CJ, van Engelshoven JM, Beets-Tan RG. Imaging for predicting the risk factors—the circumferential resection margin and nodal disease—of local recurrence in rectal cancer: a meta-analysis. Semin Ultrasound CT MR. 2005;26:259–68.

9. Mercury Study Group. Diagnostic accuracy of preoperative magnetic resonance imaging in predicting curative resection of rectal cancer: prospective observational study. Br Med J. 2006;333:779.

10. Brown G, Daniels IR, Richardson C, et al. Techniques and trouble shooting in high spatial resolution thin slice MRI for Rectal cancer. Br J Radiol. 2005;78:245–51.

11. Langer C, Liersch T, Suss M, Siemer A, Markus P, Ghadimi BM, Fuzesi L, Becker H. Surgical cure for early rectal carcinoma and large adenoma: transanal endoscopic microsurgery (using ultrasound or electrosurgery) compared to conventional local and radical resection. Int J Colorectal Dis. 2003;18:222–9.

12. Doornebosch PG, Tollenaar RA, De Graaf EJ. Is the increasing role of Transanal Endoscopic Microsurgery in curation for T1 rectal cancer justified? A systematic review. Acta Oncol. 2009;48:343–53.

13. Neary P, Makin GB, White TJ, White E, Hartley J, MacDonald A, Lee PW, Monson JR. Transanal endoscopic microsurgery: a viable operative alternative in selected patients with rectal lesions. Ann Surg Oncol. 2003;10:1106–11.

14. Christoforidis D, Cho HM, Dixon MR, Mellgren AF, Madoff RD, Finne CO. Transanal endoscopic microsurgery versus conventional transanal excision for patients with early rectal cancer. Ann Surg. 2009;249:776–82.

15. Ueno H, Mochizuki H, Hasiguchi Y, et al. Risk factors for an adverse outcome in early invasive colorectal carcinoma. Gastroenterology. 2004;127:385–94.

16. Ueno H, Hase K, Hashiguchi Y, Shimasake H, Shinji Y, et al. Novel risk factors for lymph node metastasis in early invasive colorectal cancer: a multi-institution pathology review. J Gastroenterol. 2014;49:1314–23.

17. Choi JY, Jung SA, Cho WY, Keum B, et al. Meta-analysis of predictive clinicopathologic factors for lymph node metastases in patients with early rectal colorectal carcinoma. J Korean Med Sci. 2015;30:398–406.

18. Kawachi H, Eishi Y, Ueno H, Nemoto T, et al. A three-tier classification system based on the depth of submucosal invasion and budding/sprouting can improve the treatment strategy for T1 colorectal cancer: a retrospective multicenter study. Mod Pathol. 2015;28:872–9.

19. Kikuchi R, Takano M, Takaguchi K, et al. Management of early invasive colorectal cancer. Risk of recurrence and clinical guidelines. Dis Colon Rectum. 1995;38(12):1286–95.

20. Butte JM, Tang P, Gonen M, et al. Rate of residual disease after complete endoscopic resection of malignant colonic polyp. Dis Colon Rectum. 2012;55:122–7.

21. Garcia-Aguilar J, Shi Q, Thomas Jr CR, et al. A phase II trial of neoadjuvant chemoradiation and local excision for T2N0 rectal cancer: preliminary results of the ACOSOG Z6041 trial. Ann Surg Oncol. 2012;19(2):384–91.

22. Russell AH, Harris J, Rosenberg PJ, et al. Anal sphincter conservation for patients with adenocarcinoma of the distal rectum: long-term results of radiation therapy oncology group protocol 89-02. Int J Radiat Oncol Biol Phys. 2000;46(2):313–22.

23. NCCN Clinical practice guidelines in oncology (NCCN Guidelines) Rectal cancer Version 2.2015. http://www.tri-kobe.org/nccn/guideline/colorectal/english/rectal.pdf. Accessed 28 Aug 2015.

24. Peeters KC, vande Velde CJ, Leer JW, et al. Late side effects of short-course preoperative radiotherapy combined with total mesorectal excision for rectal cancer: increased bowel dysfunction in irradiated patients—a Dutch colorectal cancer group study. J Clin Oncol. 2005;23:6199–206.

25. Birgisson H, Pahlman L, Gunnarsson U, et al. Adverse effects of preoperative radiation therapy for rectal cancer: long-term follow-up of the Swedish rectal cancer trial. J Clin Oncol. 2005;23:8697–705.

26. Joye I, Hautermans K. Early and late toxicity of radiotherapy for rectal cancer. Recent Results Cancer Res. 2014;203:189–201.

27. Smith JJ, Garcia-Aguilar JG. Advances and challenges in treatment for locally advanced rectal cancer. J Clin Oncol. 2015;33:1797–808.

28. Costa-Silva L, Brown G. Magnetic resonance imaging of rectal cancer. Magn Reson Imaging Clin N Am. 2013;21:385–408.

29. Kwok H, Bissett IP, Hill GL. Preoperative staging of rectal cancer. Int J Colorectal Dis. 2000;15:9–20.

30. Brown G, Davies S, Williams GT, et al. Effectiveness of preoperative staging in rectal cancer: digital rectal examination, endoluminal ultrasound or magnetic resonance imaging? Br J Cancer. 2004;91:23–9.

31. Beets-Tan RG, Beets GL. Local staging of rectal cancer: a review of imaging. J Magn Reson Imaging. 2011;33:1012–9.

32. Burton S, Brown G, Daniels IR, Norman AR, Mason B, Cunningham D. MRI directed multidisciplinary team preoperative treatment strategy: the way to eliminate positive circumferential margins? Br J Cancer. 2006;94(3):351–7.

33. Taylor FG, Quirke P, Heald RJ, on behalf of the mercury study group, et al. Preoperative high-resolution magnetic resonance imaging can identify good prognosis stage i, ii, and iii rectal cancer best managed by surgery alone: a prospective, multicenter, European study. Ann Surg. 2011;253:711–19.

34. Merkel S, Mansmann U, siassi M, Papadopoulos T, et al. The prognostic inhomogeneity in pT3 rectal carcinomas. Int J Colorectal Dis. 2001;16:298–304.

35. Sauer R, Becker H, Hohenberger W, Rodel C, Wittekind C, Fietkau R, Martus P, Tschmelitsch J, Hager E, Hess CF, Karstens JH, Liersch T, Schmidberger H, Raab R. Preoperative versus

postoperative chemoradiotherapy for rectal cancer. N Engl J Med. 2004;351:1731–40.

36. Habr-Gama A, Perez RO, Nadalin W, et al. Operative versus nonoperative treatment for stage 0 distal rectal cancer following chemoradiation therapy: long-term results. Ann Surg. 2004; 240:711–7.

37. Habr-Gama A, Perez RO, Proscurshim I, et al. Patterns of failure and survival for nonoperative treatment of stage c0 distal rectal cancer following neoadjuvant chemoradiation therapy. J Gastrointest Surg. 2006;10:1319–28.

38. Habr-Gama A, Gama-Rodrigues J, São Julião GP, et al. Local recurrence after complete clinical response and watch and wait in rectal cancer after neoadjuvant chemoradiation: impact of salvage therapy on local disease control. Int J Radiat Oncol Biol Phys. 2014;88:822–8.

39. Glynne-Jones R, Hughes R. Critical appraisal of the 'wait and see' approach in rectal cancer for clinical complete responders after chemoradiation. Br J Surg. 2012;99:897–909.

40. Quirke P, Durdey P, Dixon MF, Williams NS. Local recurrence of rectal adenocarcinoma due to inadequate surgical resection. Histopathological study of lateral tumour spread and surgical excision. Lancet. 1986;2:996–9.

41. Adam IJ, Mohamdee MO, Martin IG, Scott N, Finan PJ, Johnston D, Dixon MF, Quirke P. Role of circumferential margin involvement in the local recurrence of rectal cancer. Lancet. 1994;344:707–11.

42. Scott N, Jackson P, al-Jaberi T, Dixon MF, Quirke P, Finan PJ. Total mesorectal excision and local recurrence: a study of tumour spread in the mesorectum distal to rectal cancer. Br J Surg. 1995;82:1031–3.

43. Hida J, Yasutomi M, Maruyama T, Fujimoto K, Uchida T, Okuno K. Lymph node metastases detected in the mesorectum distal to carcinoma of the rectum by the clearing method: justification of total mesorectal excision. J Am Coll Surg. 1997; 184:584–8.

44. Weiser MR, Quah HM, Shia J, Guillem JG, et al. Sphincter preservation in low rectal cancer is facilitated by preoperative chemoradiation and intersphincteric dissection. Ann Surg. 2009;249:236–42.

45. Mercury Study Group. Extramural depth of tumor invasion at thin-section MR in patients with rectal cancer: results of the Mercury study. Radiology. 2007;243:132–9.

46. Schiessel R, Novi G, Holzer B, et al. Technique and long-term results of intersphincteric resection for low rectal cancer. Dis Colon Rectum. 2005;48:1858–65. discussion 1865–1867.

47. Hohenberger W, Merkel S, Matzel K, et al. The influence of abdominoperianal (intersphincteric) resection of lower third rectal carcinoma on the rates of sphincter preservation and locoregional recurrence. Colorectal Dis. 2006;8:23–33.

48. Portier G, Ghouti L, Kirzin S, et al. Oncological outcome of ultra-low coloanal anastomosis with and without intersphincteric resection for low rectal adenocarcinoma. Br J Surg. 2007;94:341–5.

49. Rullier E, Zerbib F, Laurent C, et al. Intersphincteric resection with excision of internal anal sphincter for conservative treatment of very low rectal cancer. Dis Colon Rectum. 1999; 42:1168–75.

50. Gamagami R, Istvan G, Cabarrot P, et al. Fecal continence following partial resection of the anal canal in distal rectal cancer:

long-term results after coloanal anastomoses. Surgery. 2000; 127:291–5.

51. Bittorf B, Stadelmaier U, Gohl J, et al. Functional outcome after intersphincteric resection of the rectum with coloanal anastomosis in low rectal cancer. Eur J Surg Oncol. 2004;30:260–5.

52. Bretagnol F, Rullier E, Laurent C, et al. Comparison of functional results and quality of life between intersphincteric resection and conventional coloanal anastomosis for low rectal cancer. Dis Colon Rectum. 2004;47(6):832–8.

53. Rullier E, Laurent C, Bretagnol F, et al. Sphincter-saving resection for all rectal carcinomas: the end of the 2-cm distal rule. Ann Surg. 2005;241:465–9.

54. Moore HG, Riedel E, Minsky BD, et al. Adequacy of 1-cm distal margin after restorative rectal cancer resection with sharp mesorectal excision and preoperative combined-modality therapy. Ann Surg Oncol. 2003;10:80–5.

55. Attalah S, Martin-Perez B, Albert M, et al. Transanal minimally invasive surgery for total mesorectal excision (TAMIS-TME): results and experience with the first 20 patients undergoing curative-intent rectal cancer surgery at a single institution. Tech Coloproctol. 2014;18:473–80.

56. Fernandez-Hevia M, Delgado S, Castells A, et al. Transanal total mesorectal excision in rectal cancer: short-term outcomes in comparison with laparoscopic surgery. Ann Surg. 2015; 261:221–7.

57. Denost Q, Adam JP, Rullier A, Buscail E, et al. Perineal transanal approach: a new standard for laparoscopic sphincter-saving resection in low rectal cancer, a randomized trial. Ann Surg. 2014;260:993–9.

58. Holm T, Hjung A, Haggnak T. Extended abdominoperineal resection with gluteus maximus flap reconstruction of the pelvic floor for rectal cancer. Br J Surg. 2007;94:232–8.

59. West NP, Finana PJ, Anderin C, et al. Evidence of the oncologic superiority of cylindrical abdominoperineal excision for low rectal cancer. J Clin Oncol. 2008;26:3517–22.

60. Molina Rodríguez JL, Flor-Lorente B, Frasson M, et al. Low rectal cancer: abdominoperineal resection or low Hartmann resection? A postoperative outcome analysis. Dis Colon Rectum. 2011;54:958–62.

61. Hunerbein M, Krause M, Moesta KT, Rau B, Schlag PM. Palliation of malignant rectal obstruction with self-expanding metal stents. Surgery. 2005;137:42–7.

62. Watson AJ, Shanmugam V, Mackay I, Chaturvedi S, Loudon MA, Duddalwar V, Hussey JK. Outcomes after placement of colorectal stents. Colorectal Dis. 2005;7:70–3.

63. Kelly ME, Spolverato G, Le GN, Mavros MN, Doyle F, Pawlik TM, et al. Synchronous colorectal liver metastasis: a network meta-analysis review comparing classical, combined, and liver-first surgical strategies. J Surg Oncol. 2015;111(3):341–51.

64. Lykoudis PM, O'Reilly D, Nastos K, Fusai G. Systematic review of surgical management of synchronous colorectal liver metastases. Br J Surg. 2014;101:605–12.

65. D'Angelica MI, Kemeny NE. Metastatic colorectal cancer to the liver: involve the surgeon early and often. Ann Surg Oncol. 2015;22:2104–6.

66. Slesser AAP, Simillis C, Goldin R, Brown G, Mudan S, Tekkis PP. A meta-analysis comparing simultaneous versus delayed resections in patients with synchronous colorectal liver metastases. Surgical Oncol. 2013;22:36–47.

67. Weber JC, Bachellier P, Oussoultzoglou E, Jaeck D. Simultaneous resection of colorectal primary tumour and synchronous liver metastases. Br J Surg. 2003;90:956–62.
68. Ejaz A, Semenov E, Spolverato G, Kim Y, Tanner D, Hundt J, et al. Synchronous primary colorectal and liver metastasis: impact of operative approach on clinical outcomes and hospital charges. HPB (Oxford). 2014;16:1117–26.
69. Thelen A, Jonas S, Benckert C, Spinelli A, et al. Simultaneous versus staged liver resection of synchronous liver metastases from colorectal cancer. Int J Colorectal Dis. 2007;22(10):1269–76.
70. Silberhumer GR, Paty PB, Temple LK, Araujo RLC, Dentond B, et al. Simultaneous resection for rectal cancer with synchronous liver metastasis is a safe procedure. Am J Surg. 2015;209:935–42.
71. McKenzie SP, Vargas HD, Evers BM, Davenport DL. Selection criteria for combined resection of synchronous colorectal cancer hepatic metastases: a cautionary note. Int J Colorectal Dis. 2014;29:729–35.
72. Tanaka K, Shimada H, Matsuo K, et al. Outcome after simultaneous colorectal and hepatic resection for colorectal cancer with synchronous metastases. Surgery. 2004;136:650–9.
73. Lam VW, Laurence JM, Pang T, et al. A systematic review of a liver-first approach in patients with colorectal cancer and synchronous colorectal liver metastases. HPB. 2014;16:101–8.
74. Brouquet A, Mortenson MM, Vauthey JN, Rodriguez-Bigas MA, Overman MJ, Chang GJ, et al. Surgical strategies for synchronous colorectal liver metastases in 156 consecutive patients: classic, combined or reverse strategy? J Am Coll Surg. 2010;210:934–41.
75. Andres A, Toso C, Adam R, Barroso E, Hubert C, Capussotti L, et al. A survival analysis of the liver-first reversed management of advanced simultaneous colorectal liver metastases: a LiverMetSurvey-based study. Ann Surg. 2012;256:772–8. discussion 778-9.
76. Mayo SC, Pulitano C, Marques H, Lamelas J, Wolfgang CL, de Saussure W, et al. Surgical management of patients with synchronous colorectal liver metastasis: a multicenter international analysis. J Am Coll Surg. 2013;216:707–16. discussion 16-18.
77. Mentha G, Majno P, Terraz S, Rubbia-Brandt L, et al. Treatment strategies for the management of advanced colorectal liver metastases detected synchronously with the primary tumour. Eur J Surg Oncol. 2007;33 Suppl 2:S76–83.
78. Nilsson PJ, van Etten B, Hospers GA, Påhlman L, van de Velde CJ, et al. Short-course radiotherapy followed by neo-adjuvant chemotherapy in locally advanced rectal cancer—the RAPIDO trial. BMC Cancer. 2013;13:279.

33

Colorectal Cancer: Postoperative Adjuvant Therapy

Stephen M. Sentovich and Marwan Fakih

Key Concepts

- Patients with stage III colon cancer should be considered for adjuvant chemotherapy.
- Oxaliplatin-based adjuvant chemotherapy regimens improve survival of stage III colon cancer patients by an absolute 20–25 % at 5 years versus no chemotherapy.
- Adjuvant chemotherapy has not been demonstrated to have significant impact on survival for stage II colon cancer patients, but it can be considered for patients whose tumors have high-risk features.
- In colon cancer patients, radiotherapy should be considered when tumors penetrate other fixed structures (T4) and can be guided by placing surgical clips at the time of operation.
- Patients with clinical stage II and III rectal cancers who undergo neoadjuvant chemoradiotherapy should be considered for postoperative adjuvant chemotherapy, regardless of the final pathologic staging, although the efficacy of adjuvant chemotherapy in this setting has not been firmly established.

While surgery remains the primary treatment for patients with colon and rectal cancer, adjuvant treatment with chemotherapy and radiotherapy plays an increasingly important role. For patients with stage III colon cancer, adjuvant chemotherapy has been recommended since 1990 [1]. More recently the National Quality Forum has endorsed metrics related to the administration of chemotherapy in stage III colon cancer patients in order to ensure that patients with stage III colon cancer not only are considered for chemotherapy but are given chemotherapy in a timely fashion [2]. For patients with stage I colon cancer, surgery alone is highly successful, and thus no adjuvant therapy is currently recommended. On the other hand, patients with stage II colon cancer may benefit from adjuvant treatment, although this is controversial and remains the focus of clinical trials. Finally, stage IV colon cancer patients are usually primarily treated with chemotherapy—this is the subject of a later chapter (see Chap. 36).

For patients with rectal cancer, adjuvant treatment has been recommended for both stage II and stage III disease. This treatment involves both chemotherapy and radiotherapy and usually begins preoperatively (see Chap. 28). After surgery, clinical stage II and stage III rectal cancer patients are recommend to undergo adjuvant postoperative chemotherapy regardless of the final surgical pathology. As with stage I colon cancer, surgery alone is highly successful for patients with stage I rectal cancer. This chapter will present the current recommendations regarding the use of postoperative adjuvant therapy for stage II and stage III colon and rectal cancer.

Colon Cancer

Stage III Colon Cancer

Adjuvant chemotherapy is recommended for all stage III colon cancer patients because it decreases recurrence and increases survival when compared to surgery alone [3, 4]. After surgery alone for stage III colon cancer, overall 5-year survival is 40–60 % [5]. Current chemotherapeutic regimens improve overall survival to 70–80 % [6]. Thus, 5-year overall survival of stage III colon cancer patients improves by an absolute 20–25 % with adjuvant chemotherapy. Table 33-1 summarizes the results of key clinical trials establishing the efficacy of adjuvant chemotherapy for nonmetastatic colon cancer [4, 6–11]. If all patients with stage III colon cancer receive adjuvant chemotherapy, roughly 1/3 to 1/2 of disease recurrences would be prevented.

Given the significant survival benefit of adjuvant chemotherapy, colon and rectal surgeons need to ensure that their stage III colon cancer patients are evaluated for chemotherapy after surgery. The National Quality Forum has endorsed two metrics regarding the treatment of stage III colon cancer patients [2]. The first metric estimates how many stage III patients are referred or treated with chemotherapy whereas the second metric looks at the timeliness of the administration

© Springer International Publishing 2016
S.R. Steele et al. (eds.), *The ASCRS Textbook of Colon and Rectal Surgery*, DOI 10.1007/978-3-319-25970-3_33

TABLE 33-1. Key clinical trials establishing the efficacy of adjuvant chemotherapy for colon cancer

Trial	Tumor stage	Comparison	Results	Conclusion
INT 0035 1990	Stage III	Surgery alone vs. 5-FU/levamisole	3 Years survival 5-FU/levamisole 71 % Surgery alone 55 %	Postop adjuvant chemo improves survival for stage III colon cancer
IMPACT 1995	Stage III	Surgery alone vs. 5-FU/leucovorin	3 Years survival 5-FU/leucovorin 71 % Surgery alone 62 %	Postop adjuvant chemo improves survival for stage III colon cancer
QUASAR 2000	Stage III	5-FU/levamisole vs. 5-FU/folinic acid vs. 5-FU/placebo	Decreased survival and increased recurrence with levamisole compared with placebo	Postop adjuvant chemo with levamisole inferior to placebo
IMPACT 1999	Stage II	Surgery alone vs. 5-FU/leucovorin	5 Years survival = no difference 5-FU/leucovorin 82 % Surgery alone 80 %	Postop adjuvant chemo does not improve survival for stage II colon cancer
NSABP (CO-1, CO-2, CO-3, and CO-4) 1999	Stage II	Surgery alone vs. 5-FU +	5-Year survival improved with adjuvant treatment 30 % Mortality reduction with adjuvant treatment	Postop adjuvant chemo improves survival for stage II colon cancer
MOSAIC 2009	Stage II and III	FOLFOX vs. 5-FU/leucovorin	6-Year survival in stage III only FOLFOX 73 % 5-FU/Leucovorin 68 %	FOLFOX superior to 5-FU/LV for stage III colon cancer
XELOXA 2011	Stage III	XELOX vs. 5-FU/leucovorin	3 Year disease-free survival: XELOX 71 % 5-FU/Leucovorin 67 %	Capecitabine plus oxaliplatin superior to 5-FU/leucovorin

of chemotherapy. Specifically, the first metric (measure 0385) determines the percentage of patients ≥18 years old who are either referred for adjuvant chemotherapy, prescribed adjuvant chemotherapy, or have previously received adjuvant chemotherapy in the last 12 months. The other metric (measure 0223) determines the percentage of patients under the age of 80 for whom adjuvant chemotherapy is considered or administered within 4 months of the *diagnosis*. Thus, it is important for colon and rectal surgeons to promptly refer all stage III colon cancer patients for adjuvant chemotherapy.

For patients with stage III colon cancer, the National Comprehensive Cancer Network (NCCN) guidelines recommend adjuvant treatment with FOLFOX or CapeOx for 6 months [12]. FOLFOX has been found to be superior to 5-FU/leucovorin [6, 13], and CapeOx is superior to bolus 5-FU/leucovorin [14, 15]. While used frequently in patients with metastatic disease, biologic therapy with antibodies directed at VEGF-A (bevacizumab) and EGFR antibody (panitumumab, cetuximab) is not recommended for adjuvant therapy of stage III disease [16–19]. The current FOLFOX regimen, mFOLFOX6, and the CapeOx regimen are outlined in Table 33-2. These agents act in different ways on colon cancer cells. 5-Fluorouracil is a pyrimidine analog that incorporates into DNA to stop DNA synthesis. Capecitabine is an oral 5-FU prolog and thus works in the same way as 5-FU. Folinic acid (leucovorin) is a vitamin B derivative that increases the cytotoxicity of 5-FU. Oxaliplatin inhibits DNA synthesis by forming inter- and intra-strand cross-links in DNA preventing replication and transcription. Using FOLFOX, the survival benefit of adding oxaliplatin to 5-FU does come at a price, the added side effect of peripheral sensory neuropathy (PSN). While 40–50 % of patients given oxaliplatin will develop PSN,

only 10–20 % of patients will have grade 3 PSN which is defined as severe symptoms limiting activities of daily living [20]. Fortunately only 1 % of patients will have grade 3 PSN at 12 months after treatment [6]. Since the benefit of the addition of oxaliplatin to 5-FU/leucovorin is unproven in patients over the age of 70, capecitabine alone or 5-FU/leucovorin should be considered in elderly patients with stage III colon cancer [12]. Capecitabine-based regimens can be particularly complicated by palmar-plantar erythrodyskinesia (hand-foot syndrome), but this side effect can be limited by symptomatic treatment and resolves after treatment is concluded [21].

Stage II Colon Cancer

The 5-year overall survival of patients with stage II colon cancer is 65–85 % with surgery alone [22]. Unlike stage III disease, the role of adjuvant chemotherapy in stage II disease remains controversial, with some studies showing a benefit [10] and others showing no benefit [23]. If there is a benefit to adjuvant chemotherapy in stage II colon cancer patients, the benefit does not improve survival by more than 5 % unlike the 25–30 % improvement for stage III patients receiving adjuvant chemotherapy [12].

Following surgery for stage II colon cancer, the current NCCN guidelines (February 2015) recommend observation (surgery alone), enrollment in a clinical trial or adjuvant chemotherapy [12]. To sort out these options, a detailed discussion with the patient is recommended to highlight the potential benefits and risks of chemotherapy. Any high-risk features should be identified and discussed (Table 33-3). Patients with or without high-risk features should consider observation,

TABLE 33-2. Current recommended adjuvant chemotherapy regimens for stage III colon cancer

Regimen	Agents and dosage	Frequency
mFOLFOX6	Oxaliplatin 85 mg/m^2 IV over 2 h, day 1	Every 2 weeks
	Leucovorin 400 mg/m^2 IV over 2 h, day 1	
	5-FU 400 mg/m^2 IV bolus on day 1, then 1200 mg/m^2/day×2 days IV continuous infusion	
CapeOx	Oxaliplatin 130 mg/m^2 IV over 2 h, day 1	Every 3 weeks
	Capecitabine 850–1000 mg/m^2 PO twice daily for 14 days	

TABLE 33-3. High-risk factors for recurrence

- Poorly differentiated histology (exclusive of those that are MSI-H)
- Lymphatic/vascular invasion
- Perineural invasion
- Close, indeterminate, or positive margins
- Bowel obstruction
- Localized perforation
- Less than 12 lymph nodes examined

clinical trial or chemotherapy with capecitabine or 5-FU/leucovorin. Only those patients with high-risk features should be considered candidates for FOLFOX or CapeOx. It is important to remember that the addition of oxaliplatin has not been shown to improve survival in stage II colon cancer patients [6]. Finally, decision-making regarding the use of adjuvant chemotherapy for stage II disease may be aided by performing genetic testing of the tumor after surgical resection.

Genetic testing of stage II tumors has been shown to be independently predictive of prognosis. High microsatellite instability (MSI-H) or defective mismatch repair (dMMR) status has been shown to be associated with a lower recurrence rate (11 % vs. 26 %) after surgical resection alone [24]. In addition, MSI-H tumors do not benefit from 5-FU adjuvant therapy [24]. Thus, MSI/MMR testing is recommended in all patients with stage II disease in order to avoid giving adjuvant chemotherapy in patients who will derive no benefit from it. In addition to MSI/MMR testing, multigene colon cancer assays such as Oncotype Dx, ColoPrint, and ColDx are now available that can also predict prognosis and risk of recurrence. All three of these multigene assays predict recurrence independent from other factors such as TNM stage, MMR status, tumor grade, and nodes [25–31]. While these assays provide additional information regarding prognosis and recurrence risk, they are not predictive of the potential benefit of chemotherapy, and consequently are, to date, of limited clinical value.

Radiotherapy for Colon Cancer

Radiotherapy plays a limited role in patients with colon cancer. A few retrospective, single institution studies have shown that adjuvant radiotherapy improves local control for colon cancer patients at high risk of recurrence after surgery [32–34]. Unfortunately, the single randomized prospective trial comparing chemotherapy alone with combined chemotherapy and radiotherapy lacks sufficient power to draw valid conclusions [35]. Current NCCN guidelines recommend that radiotherapy for colon cancer be considered in patients with

T4 tumors with penetration to a fixed structure [12]. The radiation field should include the tumor bed as defined by preoperative imaging and the placement of surgical clips at the time of operation. A dose of 45–50 Gy in 25–28 fractions is recommended and should be delivered with concomitant 5-FU chemotherapy [12]. Thus, the colorectal surgeon should always be ready to place clips in and around the tumor bed during operations involving the resection of a fixed T4 colon tumor in order to help direct postoperative radiotherapy. Neoadjuvant chemoradiotherapy can be considered for select patients with bulky tumors invading other structures.

Rectal Cancer

Treatment of patients suffering from rectal cancer is far more complex than treatment of patients with colon cancer, due to the multitude of therapeutic options and timing of those therapies. In addition, pretreatment staging is not always accurate, and this imprecision must be taken into account when planning treatment. Initial staging, neoadjuvant therapy, and surgical treatment are covered in other chapters, and thus we will focus on postoperative therapy.

Decisions regarding postoperative adjuvant treatment for rectal cancer are based primarily on tumor location, clinical stage, histologic stage, and history of neoadjuvant therapy. Proximal rectal/rectosigmoid tumors are located at least 12 cm proximal to the anal verge and are above the peritoneal reflection. Although somewhat controversial, non-advanced proximal rectal/rectosigmoid tumors are treated in the same fashion as tumors elsewhere in the colon, with surgical resection followed by postoperative chemotherapy for stage III and select stage II tumors. Tumors of the middle/lower rectum are located from 0 to 12 cm from the anal verge as measured by rigid proctoscopy [36]. They typically have a worse prognosis, stage for stage, when compared to more proximal tumors and thus treatment recommendations are slightly different.

Patients Who Did not Undergo Neoadjuvant Therapy

Like stage I colon cancer, 5-year survival after surgery alone for stage I rectal cancer exceeds 90 % [37]. Thus, no adjuvant treatment is recommended for patients undergoing proctectomy alone who are found to have T1-2N0M0 disease, assuming that margins of resection are negative for tumor. For those found to have stage II or III disease after proctectomy, decision-making is more complex. Postoperative chemotherapy is indicated for patients with stage III disease, but the benefit for stage II disease is less certain. Postoperative radiotherapy should be considered for patients with stage II and III disease, but this recommendation is primarily based on data from the past, when there was little emphasis on surgical quality or assessment of circumferential radial margins. Postoperative radiotherapy is also associated with substantial long-term toxicity, most notable in patients undergoing restorative proctectomy. The recommendation for routine postoperative radiotherapy for patients with T3N0 disease with negative circumferential margins has thus been questioned, including in the most recent iteration of the ASCRS Practice Parameters for the Management of Rectal Cancer [38]. Even for patients with N+ disease, it is unclear whether the small benefit of postoperative radiotherapy in terms of local control is worth the risk of toxicity, which can be substantial.

If patients are to be treated with postoperative chemoradiotherapy, it is usually administered using a sandwich technique. This involves giving chemotherapy (FOLFOX or CapeOx) followed by chemoradiotherapy (Capecitabine + radiation or infusional 5FU + radiation) followed by more chemotherapy (FOLFOX or CapeOx). The radiotherapy dose is usually 45–50 Gy in 25–28 fractions using 3 or 4 fields. External iliac nodes should be included for T4 tumors involving anterior structures, and inclusion of the inguinal nodes should be considered for tumors invading the distal anal canal. In stage II and III rectal cancer patients, postoperative chemotherapy should be administered as soon as the patient has recovered from surgery as each 4 week delay in chemotherapy results in a 14 % decrease in overall survival [39].

Patients Who Underwent Neoadjuvant Radiotherapy/Chemoradiotherapy

After neoadjuvant radiotherapy/chemoradiotherapy, decisions regarding postoperative chemotherapy are more complex. Although a recent Cochrane review concluded that postoperative adjuvant chemotherapy after resection of rectal cancer was associated with improved survival regardless of stage [40], the data come from trials as old as 1975. Thus, it is difficult to draw any firm conclusions from this meta-analysis, given that some data are derived from trials in which patients were not given neoadjuvant therapy, nor was there surgical quality control or measurement of circumferential margins. Overall, there is a paucity of data on which to rely when making decisions regarding postoperative chemotherapy for patients with rectal cancer because neoadjuvant therapy regimens, surgical quality control, and pathologic processing have evolved so rapidly in the past 30 years. This evolution is ongoing, with different neoadjuvant regimens currently under investigation.

Traditionally, patients with ypT3 or ypN+ disease have been recommended to undergo postoperative chemotherapy [36]. However, a recent meta-analysis of published data found that adjuvant fluorouracil-based chemotherapy did not improve overall survival, disease-free survival, or distant recurrences, calling these recommendations into question [41]. If chemotherapy is utilized, it is also controversial as to which regimen to utilize. Two randomized clinical trials have reported a disease-free survival advantage to FOLFOX vs. fluoropyrimidine monotherapy in patients previously treated with neoadjuvant chemoradiotherapy followed by rectal surgery [42–44]. A summary of several key clinical trials regarding chemoradiotherapy for rectal cancer is shown in Table 33-4 [40, 42–44, 48–52].

Clinicians should be aware that current NCCN guidelines for clinical stage II and III rectal cancer recommend either (1) preoperative chemoradiotherapy, surgery then postoperative chemotherapy or (2) preoperative chemotherapy followed by preoperative chemoradiotherapy then surgery (see Table 33-5) [36, 45, 46]. The total duration of perioperative therapy (preoperative chemoradiotherapy and chemotherapy) should not exceed 6 months [36]. However, as noted above, these recommendations are based on incomplete and sometimes conflicting data.

Patients Undergoing Local Excision

Due to the oncologically inferior results of local excision as compared to proctectomy, even in highly select patients, many authors have recommended treatment with adjuvant chemoradiotherapy, either in the preoperative or postoperative period. The advantage of utilizing chemoradiotherapy in the postoperative period is that T stage can be known with certainty, and one can ensure healing of the wound prior to institution of radiotherapy. The advantage of utilizing neoadjuvant chemoradiotherapy is that ypT stage correlates more closely with ypN stage than T stage correlates with N stage [53] and there may be downsizing of the tumor prior to excision. The major downside of neoadjuvant therapy combined with local excision is that wound healing may be impaired, and patients may suffer substantial morbidity as a result.

For patients treated with neoadjuvant chemoradiotherapy followed by local excision, standard radiotherapy of 50.4 Gy over 28 fractions is typically given with either 5-FU or capecitabine chemotherapy. For clinical stage T2 tumors these standard neoadjuvant regimens result in complete pathologic response rates as high as 40–60 % [54, 55]. While overall 5-year survival data are insufficient, the current data suggests that there is a 90 % 5-year survival after a complete pathologic response but only a 75 % 5-year survival if there is residual disease (ypT1 or ypT2) [55]. Thus, in select stage I patients and patients with significant comorbidities that preclude an abdominal procedure, a nonstandard approach using neoadjuvant treatment with or without subsequent transanal excision may be considered (see Chap. 28).

TABLE 33-4. Key clinical trials establishing the efficacy of chemoradiotherapy for rectal cancer

Trial	Tumor stage	Comparison	Results	Conclusion
Swedish rectal cancer trial 1993	Stage II and III	Surgery alone vs. preop short course XRT	Local recurrence: 27 % vs. 12 %	Preop XRT decreases local recurrence, improves survival (?)
			5 Years survival: 48 % vs. 58 %	
Dutch TME rectal cancer trial 2001	Stage II and III	TME alone vs. preop XRT + TME	Local recurrence: 11.4 % vs. 5.6 %	Preop XRT improves local recurrence even with TME
			Survival: no difference	Preop XRT no effect on survival
German CAO/ARO/AIO-94 2003/2004	Stage II and III	Preop chemo XRT vs. postop chemo XRT	Local recurrence: 13 % vs. 6 %	Decreased toxicity and local recurrence with preop chemo XRT
			Toxicity: 40 % vs. 27 %	Pre vs. post: no effect on survival
			Survival: no difference	
EORTC 22921 2006	Stage II and III	XRT vs. chemo XRT	Survival benefit for ypT0-2 responders	Chemo in addition to XRT can improve survival in the subgroup of responders
Cochran review: postop chemo 2012	Stage II and III	No postop chemo vs. postop chemo after neoadjuvant	Recurrence reduced 25 %	Postop chemo reduces recurrence and death rate after neoadjuvant
			Deaths reduced 17 %	
ADORE 2014	Stage II and III	FOLFOX vs. 5-FU/leucovorin after neoadjuvant	3 Year disease-free survival: 72 % vs. 62 %	Postop FOLFOX superior to 5-FU after neoadjuvant
German CAO/ARO/AIO-04 2012/2014	Stage II and III	Neoadjuvant and adjuvant FOLFOX vs. 5-FU/leucovorin	Complete pathologic response: 17 % vs. 13 %	Preop and postop addition of oxaliplatin improves survival and pathologic response
			3 Years survival: 76 % vs. 71 %	

XRT Radiation therapy, *TME* Total mesorectal excision, *preop* Preoperative, *postop* Postoperative, *chemoxrt* Combined chemoradiation therapy

TABLE 33-5. Neoadjuvant and adjuvant treatment of stage II and III rectal cancer

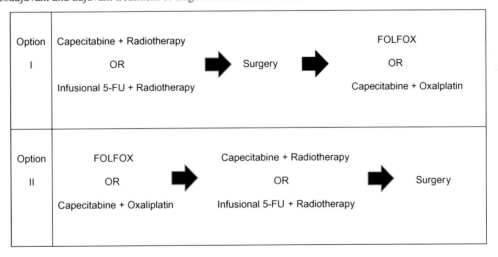

Future of Adjuvant Treatment of Colorectal Cancer

While significant progress has been made in defining optimal cytotoxic regimens in the adjuvant treatment of colorectal cancer, several questions remain regarding the optimal duration of chemotherapy treatment, the role of radiotherapy in rectal cancer, the possibility of nonsurgical interventions for rectal cancer, and the emerging role of immunotherapy.

Clinical Trials in Stage II–III Colon Cancer

Prior studies have shown no benefit from extending adjuvant therapy beyond 6 months in patients with stage III colon cancer [56]. However, a shorter duration of chemotherapy has not been adequately investigated. CALGB 80702 is currently investigating 6 cycles (3 months) vs. 12 cycles (6 months) of FOLFOX chemotherapy in patients with resected stage III colon cancer (NCT01150045). This will be one of 6 ongoing clinical trials evaluating 3 vs. 6 months of adjuvant oxaliplatin-based chemotherapy. A meta-analysis of these studies (IDEA) will test the non-inferiority of 3 months to a 6 months strategy. In addition to the investigation of the duration of adjuvant treatment in colon cancer, efforts are ongoing to define the role of COX inhibition on disease recurrence. Analysis of the Nurses' Health Study (NHS) and Health Professional Follow-up Study (HPFS) has shown a decreased recurrence rate in patients with a diagnosis of colon cancer with regular aspirin intake [57]. The benefit appeared to be limited to patient with COX-2 overexpressing tumors [58]. These analyses were limited by their retrospective nature and require further support from prospectively conducted trials. CALGB 80702 randomizes all enrolled subjects to celecoxib vs. placebo in order to investigate the role of COX-2 inhibition in the adjuvant treatment of colon cancer. Similarly, the ASCOLT clinical trial (NCT00565708) is randomizing patients with stage II or III disease to 3 years of aspirin vs. placebo to address the role of aspirin in preventing colorectal cancer recurrence. Finally, several studies are investigating immunotherapy as an adjuvant form of treatment in colon cancer. An ongoing phase III clinical trial is evaluating the role of cytokine-induced killer cell immunotherapy for stage III colon cancer following surgery and completion of adjuvant therapy (NCT02280278).

Clinical Trials in Stage II–III Rectal Cancer (Table 33-5)

Recent phase II and retrospective trials have investigated the role of FOLFOX as a neoadjuvant treatment for rectal cancer. These series have been associated with a remarkable complete pathological response rates and were associated with a low risk of local recurrence, questioning the role of adjuvant or neoadjuvant therapy in the era of effective combination therapy [59]. To test this question, the Alliance PROSPECT clinical trial (NCT01515787) is currently randomizing patients to neoadjuvant FOLFOX chemotherapy with selective use of chemoradiotherapy (in poor responders) vs. the standard approach of neoadjuvant chemoradiotherapy. Other studies are sequencing intense chemotherapeutic regimens followed by chemoradiotherapy in order to improve on DFS and OS. The NEOFIRINOX trial (NCT01804790) is randomizing patients with rectal cancer to intensive chemotherapy with irinotecan, oxaliplatin, and 5-FU (FOLFIRINOX) followed by chemoradiotherapy, surgery, and further adjuvant chemotherapy (capecitabine or FOLFOX) vs. a control arm of chemoradiotherapy followed by surgery and adjuvant chemotherapy (capecitabine or FOLFOX).

In order to maximize systemic therapy exposure, clinical trials are evaluating the administration of the all systemic chemotherapy prior to surgical resection. For example, the RAPIDO clinical trial (NCT01558921) is randomizing rectal cancer patients to 5×5 Gy of radiotherapy followed by 6 cycles of CAPOX and then surgery vs. standard chemoradiotherapy and further adjuvant therapy (at the treating physician's discretion). Finally, several studies are investigating nonsurgical approaches to patients with rectal cancer who have a complete clinical response to chemoradiotherapy. The Cancer Institute of San Paulo is leading a randomized clinical trial (NCT02052921) that randomizes rectal cancer patients with complete clinical response following neoadjuvant chemoradiotherapy to observation vs. surgical resection with a primary end point of 3 year DFS.

References

1. Conference NC. Adjuvant therapy for patients with colon and rectal cancer. JAMA. 1990;264:1444–50.
2. National Quality Forum. Endorsement summary: Cancer measures. 2012. http://www.qualityforum.org.
3. Laurie JA, Moertel CG, Fleming TR, Wieand HS, Leigh JE, Rubin J, et al. Surgical adjuvant therapy of large-bowel carcinoma: an evaluation of levamisole and the combination of levamisole and fluorouracil. The North Central Cancer Treatment Group and the Mayo Clinic. J Clin Oncol. 1989;7(10):1447–56.
4. Moertel CG, Fleming TR, Macdonald JS, Haller DG, Laurie JA, Goodman PJ, et al. Levamisole and fluorouracil for adjuvant therapy of resected colon carcinoma. N Engl J Med. 1990;322(6):352–8.
5. Jemal A, Siegel R, Ward E, Murray T, Xu J, Smigal C, et al. Cancer statistics, 2006. CA Cancer J Clin. 2006;56(2):106–30.
6. André T, Boni C, Navarro M, Tabernero J, Hickish T, Topham C, et al. Improved overall survival with oxaliplatin, fluorouracil, and leucovorin as adjuvant treatment in stage II or III colon cancer in the MOSAIC trial. J Clin Oncol. 2009;27(19):3109–16.
7. Efficacy of adjuvant fluorouracil and folinic acid in colon cancer. International Multicentre Pooled Analysis of Colon Cancer Trials (IMPACT) investigators. Lancet. 1995;345(8955):939–44.
8. Comparison of fluorouracil with additional levamisole, higher-dose folinic acid, or both, as adjuvant chemotherapy for colorectal cancer: a randomised trial. QUASAR Collaborative Group. Lancet. 2000;355(9215):1588–96.
9. Efficacy of adjuvant fluorouracil and folinic acid in B2 colon cancer. International Multicentre Pooled Analysis of B2 Colon Cancer Trials (IMPACT B2) investigators. J Clin Oncol. 1999;17(5):1356–63.
10. Mamounas E, Wieand S, Wolmark N, Bear HD, Atkins JN, Song K, et al. Comparative efficacy of adjuvant chemotherapy in patients with Dukes' B versus Dukes' C Colon cancer: results from four National Surgical Adjuvant Breast and Bowel Project adjuvant studies (C-01, C-02, C-03, and C-04). J Clin Oncol. 1999;17(5):1349–55.
11. Haller DG, Tabernero J, Maroun J, de Braud F, Price T, Van Cutsem E, et al. Capecitabine plus oxaliplatin compared with fluorouracil and folinic acid as adjuvant therapy for stage III colon cancer. J Clin Oncol. 2011;29(11):1465–71.
12. National Comprehensive Cancer Network. Colon Cancer version 2.2015. 2015. http://www.nccn.org.

13. André T, Boni C, Mounedji-Boudiaf L, Navarro M, Tabernero J, Hickish T, et al. Oxaliplatin, fluorouracil, and leucovorin as adjuvant treatment for colon cancer. N Engl J Med. 2004; 350(23):2343–51.

14. Kuebler JP, Wieand HS, O'Connell MJ, Smith RE, Colangelo LH, Yothers G, et al. Oxaliplatin combined with weekly bolus fluorouracil and leucovorin as surgical adjuvant chemotherapy for stage II and III Colon cancer: results from NSABP C-07. J Clin Oncol. 2007;25(16):2198–204.

15. Twelves C, Wong A, Nowacki MP, Abt M, Burris 3rd H, Carrato A, et al. Capecitabine as adjuvant treatment for stage III colon cancer. N Engl J Med. 2005;352(26):2696–704.

16. Alberts SR, Sargent DJ, Nair S, Mahoney MR, Mooney M, Thibodeau SN, et al. Effect of oxaliplatin, fluorouracil, and leucovorin with or without cetuximab on survival among patients with resected stage III Colon cancer: a randomized trial. JAMA. 2012;307(13):1383–93.

17. Taieb J, Tabernero J, Mini E, Subtil F, Folprecht G, Van Laethem JL, et al. Oxaliplatin, fluorouracil, and leucovorin with or without cetuximab in patients with resected stage III colon cancer (PETACC-8): an open-label, randomised phase 3 trial. Lancet Oncol. 2014;15(8):862–73.

18. Allegra CJ, Yothers G, O'Connell MJ, Sharif S, Petrelli NJ, Lopa SH, et al. Bevacizumab in stage II-III Colon cancer: 5-year update of the National Surgical Adjuvant Breast and Bowel Project C-08 trial. J Clin Oncol. 2013;31(3):359–64.

19. de Gramont A, Van Cutsem E, Schmoll HJ, Tabernero J, Clarke S, Moore MJ, et al. Bevacizumab plus oxaliplatin-based chemotherapy as adjuvant treatment for colon cancer (AVANT): a phase 3 randomised controlled trial. Lancet Oncol. 2012;13(12):1225–33.

20. Zedan AH, Hansen TF, Fex Svenningsen A, Vilholm OJ. Oxaliplatin-induced neuropathy in colorectal cancer: many questions with few answers. Clin Colorectal Cancer. 2014; 13(2):73–80.

21. Nagore E, Insa A, Sanmartín O. Antineoplastic therapy-induced palmar plantar erythrodysesthesia ('hand-foot') syndrome. Incidence, recognition and management. Am J Clin Dermatol. 2000;1(4):225–34.

22. Parkin DM, Bray F, Ferlay J, Pisani P. Global cancer statistics, 2002. CA Cancer J Clin. 2005;55(2):74–108.

23. Schrag D, Gelfand S, Bach P, et al. Adjuvant chemotherapy for stage II Colon cancer: insight from a SEER-Medicare cohort. Proc Am Soc Clin Oncol. 2001;20:488.

24. Sargent DJ, Marsoni S, Monges G, Thibodeau SN, Labianca R, Hamilton SR, et al. Defective mismatch repair as a predictive marker for lack of efficacy of fluorouracil-based adjuvant therapy in colon cancer. J Clin Oncol. 2010;28(20):3219–26.

25. O'Connell MJ, Lavery I, Yothers G, Paik S, Clark-Langone KM, Lopatin M, et al. Relationship between tumor gene expression and recurrence in four independent studies of patients with stage II/III colon cancer treated with surgery alone or surgery plus adjuvant fluorouracil plus leucovorin. J Clin Oncol. 2010;28(25):3937–44.

26. Gray RG, Quirke P, Handley K, Lopatin M, Magill L, Baehner FL, et al. Validation study of a quantitative multigene reverse transcriptase-polymerase chain reaction assay for assessment of recurrence risk in patients with stage II colon cancer. J Clin Oncol. 2011;29(35):4611–9.

27. Venook AP, Niedzwiecki D, Lopatin M, Ye X, Lee M, Friedman PN, et al. Biologic determinants of tumor recurrence in stage II Colon cancer: validation study of the 12-gene recurrence score in cancer and leukemia group B (CALGB) 9581. J Clin Oncol. 2013;31(14):1775–81.

28. Yothers G, O'Connell MJ, Lee M, Lopatin M, Clark-Langone KM, Millward C, et al. Validation of the 12-gene colon cancer recurrence score in NSABP C-07 as a predictor of recurrence in patients with stage II and III colon cancer treated with fluorouracil and leucovorin (FU/LV) and FU/LV plus oxaliplatin. J Clin Oncol. 2013;31(36):4512–9.

29. Salazar R, Roepman P, Capella G, Moreno V, Simon I, Dreezen C, et al. Gene expression signature to improve prognosis prediction of stage II and III colorectal cancer. J Clin Oncol. 2011;29(1):17–24.

30. Kopetz S, Tabernero J, Rosenberg R, Jiang ZQ, Moreno V, Bachleitner-Hofmann T, et al. Genomic classifier ColoPrint predicts recurrence in stage II colorectal cancer patients more accurately than clinical factors. Oncologist. 2015;20(2):127–33.

31. Kennedy RD, Bylesjo M, Kerr P, Davison T, Black JM, Kay EW, et al. Development and independent validation of a prognostic assay for stage II colon cancer using formalin-fixed paraffin-embedded tissue. J Clin Oncol. 2011;29(35):4620–6.

32. Willett CG, Fung CY, Kaufman DS, Efird J, Shellito PC. Postoperative radiation therapy for high-risk colon carcinoma. J Clin Oncol. 1993;11(6):1112–7.

33. Schild SE, Gunderson LL, Haddock MG, Wong WW, Nelson H, et al. The treatment of locally advanced colon cancer. Int J Radiat Oncol Biol Phys. 1997;37(1):51–8.

34. Amos EH, Mendenhall WM, McCarty PJ, Gage JO, Emlet JL, Lowrey GC, et al. Postoperative radiotherapy for locally advanced colon cancer. Ann Surg Oncol. 1996;3(5):431–6.

35. Martenson Jr JA, Willett CG, Sargent DJ, Mailliard JA, Donohue JH, Gunderson LL, et al. Phase III study of adjuvant chemotherapy and radiation therapy compared with chemotherapy alone in the surgical adjuvant treatment of Colon cancer: results of intergroup protocol 0130. J Clin Oncol. 2004;22(16):3277–83.

36. National Comprehensive Cancer Network. Rectal Cancer version 2.2015. 2015. http://www.nccn.org.

37. Gunderson LL, et al. Impact of T and N substage on survival and disease relapse in adjuvant rectal cancer: a pooled analysis. Int J Radiat Oncol Biol Phys. 2002;54(2):386–96.

38. Monson JR, Weiser MR, Buie WD, Chang GJ, Rafferty JF, et al. Practice parameters for the management of rectal cancer (revised). Dis Colon Rectum. 2013;56(5):535–50.

39. Biagi JJ, Raphael MJ, Mackillop WJ, Kong W, King WD, Booth CM. Association between time to initiation of adjuvant chemotherapy and survival in colorectal cancer: a systematic review and meta-analysis. JAMA. 2011;305(22):2335–42.

40. Petersen SH, Harling H, Kirkeby LT, Wille-Jørgensen P, Mocellin S. Postoperative adjuvant chemotherapy in rectal cancer operated for cure. Cochrane Database Syst Rev. 2012;3, CD004078.

41. Breugom AJ, Swets M, Bosset JF, Collette L, Sainato A, Cionini L, et al. Adjuvant chemotherapy after preoperative (chemo) radiotherapy and surgery for patients with rectal cancer: a systematic review and meta-analysis of individual patient data. Lancet Oncol. 2015;16(2):200–7.

42. Hong YS, Nam BH, Kim KP, Kim JE, Park SJ, Park YS, et al. Oxaliplatin, fluorouracil, and leucovorin versus fluorouracil and leucovorin as adjuvant chemotherapy for locally advanced rectal cancer after preoperative chemoradiotherapy (ADORE): an open-label, multicentre, phase 2, randomised controlled trial. Lancet Oncol. 2014;15(11):1245–53.

43. Rödel C, Liersch T, Becker H, Fietkau R, Hohenberger W, Hothorn T, et al. Preoperative chemoradiotherapy and postoperative chemotherapy with fluorouracil and oxaliplatin versus fluorouracil alone in locally advanced rectal cancer: initial results of the German CAO/ARO/AIO-04 randomised phase 3 trial. Lancet Oncol. 2012;13(7):679–87.

44. Rodel C, et al. Preoperative chemoradiotherapy and postoperative chemotherapy with 5-fluorouracil and oxaliplatin versus 5-fluorouracil alone in locally advanced rectal cancer: results of the German CAO/ARO/AIO-04 randomized phase III trial. J Clin Oncol. 2014;32:5s. (suppl; abstr 3500).

45. Fernández-Martos C, Pericay C, Aparicio J, Salud A, Safont M, Massuti B, et al. Phase II, randomized study of concomitant chemoradiotherapy followed by surgery and adjuvant capecitabine plus oxaliplatin (CAPOX) compared with induction CAPOX followed by concomitant chemoradiotherapy and surgery in magnetic resonance imaging-defined, locally advanced rectal cancer: Grupo cancer de recto 3 study. J Clin Oncol. 2010;28(5):859–65.

46. Cercek A, Goodman KA, Hajj C, Weisberger E, Segal NH, Reidy-Lagunes DL, et al. Neoadjuvant chemotherapy first, followed by chemoradiation and then surgery, in the management of locally advanced rectal cancer. J Natl Compr Canc Netw. 2014;12(4):513–9.

47. Kapiteijn E, Marijnen CA, Nagtegaal ID, Putter H, Steup WH, Wiggers T, et al. Preoperative radiotherapy combined with total mesorectal excision for resectable rectal cancer. N Engl J Med. 2001;345(9):638–46.

48. Initial report from a Swedish multicentre study examining the role of preoperative irradiation in the treatment of patients with resectable rectal carcinoma. Swedish Rectal Cancer Trial. Br J Surg. 1993;80(10):1333–6.

49. Sauer R, Fietkau R, Wittekind C, Rödel C, Martus P, Hohenberger W, et al. Adjuvant vs. neoadjuvant radiochemotherapy for locally advanced rectal cancer: the German trial CAO/ARO/AIO-94. Colorectal Dis. 2003;5(5):406–15.

50. Sauer R, Liersch T, Merkel S, Fietkau R, Hohenberger W, Hess C, et al. Preoperative versus postoperative chemoradiotherapy for locally advanced rectal cancer: results of the German CAO/ARO/AIO-94 randomized phase III trial after a median follow-up of 11 years. J Clin Oncol. 2012;30(16):1926–33.

51. Bosset JF, Collette L, Calais G, Mineur L, Maingon P, Radosevic-Jelic L, et al. Chemotherapy with preoperative radiotherapy in rectal cancer. N Engl J Med. 2006;355(11):1114–23.

52. Collette L, Bosset JF, den Dulk M, Nguyen F, Mineur L, Maingon P, et al. Patients with curative resection of cT3-4 rectal cancer after preoperative radiotherapy or radiochemotherapy: does anybody benefit from adjuvant fluorouracil-based chemotherapy? A trial of the European Organisation for Research and Treatment of Cancer Radiation Oncology Group. J Clin Oncol. 2007;25(28):4379–86.

53. Read TE, Andujar JE, Caushaj PF, Johnston DR, Dietz DW, Myerson RJ, et al. Neoadjuvant therapy for rectal cancer: histologic response of the primary tumor predicts nodal status. Dis Colon Rectum. 2004;47(6):825–31.

54. Garcia-Aguilar J, Shi Q, Thomas Jr CR, Chan E, Cataldo P, Marcet J, et al. A phase II trial of neoadjuvant chemoradiation and local excision for T2N0 rectal cancer: preliminary results of the ACOSOG Z6041 trial. Ann Surg Oncol. 2012;19(2):384–91.

55. Noh JM, Park W, Kim JS, Koom WS, Kim JH, Choi DH, et al. Outcome of local excision following preoperative chemoradiotherapy for clinically t2 distal rectal cancer: a multicenter retrospective study (KROG 12-06). Cancer Res Treat. 2014;46(3):243–9.

56. Haller DG, Catalano PJ, Macdonald JS, O'Rourke MA, Frontiera MS, Jackson DV, et al. Phase III study of fluorouracil, leucovorin, and levamisole in high-risk stage II and III Colon cancer: final report of Intergroup 0089. J Clin Oncol. 2005;23(34):8671–8.

57. Chan AT, Ogino S, Fuchs CS. Aspirin and the risk of colorectal cancer in relation to the expression of COX-2. N Engl J Med. 2007;356(21):2131–42.

58. Chan AT, Ogino S, Fuchs CS. Aspirin use and survival after diagnosis of colorectal cancer. JAMA. 2009;302(6):649–58.

59. Schrag D, Weiser MR, Goodman KA, Gonen M, Hollywood E, Cercek A, et al. Neoadjuvant chemotherapy without routine use of radiation therapy for patients with locally advanced rectal cancer: a pilot trial. J Clin Oncol. 2014;32(6):513–8.

34

Colorectal Cancer: Surveillance After Curative-Intent Therapy

Scott E. Regenbogen and Karin M. Hardiman

Key Concepts

- Liver metastases and locoregional recurrence are more likely to be amenable to curative-intent salvage resection when detected in asymptomatic patients. Therefore, active surveillance is indicated for patients who are candidates for liver and/or intestinal resection.
- Use of carcinoembryonic antigen testing and computed tomography (CT) scans is associated with increased detection of asymptomatic recurrence after curative resection for colorectal cancer. There is no evidence to support the use of any other laboratory testing or positron emission tomography (PET) scans in routine surveillance.
- Patients with advanced age and comorbidity, who would not be fit to undergo therapy for recurrence, should not be subjected to active surveillance. They should, however, receive evaluation and treatment for symptoms suggestive of recurrence.
- Patients with resected rectal cancers are at greater risk for locoregional recurrence. This risk is increased by omission of chemoradiotherapy for locally advanced tumors, close or positive margins, T4 and N2 histology. Consideration should therefore be given to local pelvic surveillance both endoluminally and extraluminally in these patients at highest risk.
- Surveillance after resection of Stage I colorectal cancer remains controversial. While the recurrence rates are low, in general, there are markers of relatively greater risk, including margin positivity, unknown lymph node status (e.g., local excision), inadequate lymph node sampling, lymphovascular invasion, poorly differentiated histology, and/or T2 disease. Active surveillance may be considered for patients with one or more of these risk factors.

Introduction

With improvements in screening, diagnosis, surgical technique, and adjuvant therapy for colon and rectal cancers, nearly two-thirds of patients who undergo surgical resection survive 5 years or more [1]. As a result, there is a rapidly growing population of colorectal cancer survivors, exceeding 1.2 million in the United States alone [2]. These individuals face varying risk for subsequent colorectal cancer throughout their lifetime, yet there is little consensus on optimal regimens for surveillance and survivorship care [3, 4].

The primary goal of colorectal cancer surveillance is to detect treatable recurrent, metastatic or metachronous colorectal malignancy and optimize the opportunities for potentially curative intervention. Thus, surveillance strategies must include not only evaluation for local recurrence and distant metastasis from the treated cancer, but also the increased personal risk for subsequent primary colorectal cancers. For patients with suspected or known genetic colorectal cancer syndromes, these strategies must also take into account the risk of other associated cancers, and the screening needs of potentially affected family members [5]. Ultimately, the success of colorectal cancer surveillance may be measured by improvements in overall survival, cancer-specific survival, disability or quality of life. Some studies have evaluated proxy measures, such as the rate of curative-intent metastasectomy or resection of colorectal neoplasia, but it is not clear to what degree these additional interventions benefit colorectal cancer survivors more broadly.

In order to demonstrate benefits from active surveillance, there must be evidence of improved detection of recurrence in patients amenable to curative-intent salvage therapy that itself is efficacious in improving outcome after recurrence. It has proven challenging to support with real data each of the steps in this chain of logic [6]. In addition, interpretation and synthesis of

© Springer International Publishing 2016
S.R. Steele et al. (eds.), *The ASCRS Textbook of Colon and Rectal Surgery*, DOI 10.1007/978-3-319-25970-3_34

findings of published studies are complicated by the heterogeneity of the interventions and comparisons—the surveillance intervention in one trial may be no more intensive than the control group regimen of another—and the challenges of obtaining adequate power to detect meaningful differences in survival and other objective oncologic outcomes in such studies.

It is also important to consider the appropriateness of surveillance for patients who might not be eligible for, or willing to undergo, treatment for recurrence. Recognizing that older adults account for the majority of colorectal cancer patients [7], patient preferences, age, comorbidities, and functional status must all contribute to the decision to pursue active surveillance. There is little need, for example, to conduct surveillance for asymptomatic liver metastases for a patient unwilling or unable to undergo hepatic resection and/or chemotherapy. For such patients, symptom-driven evaluations may suffice.

At the same time, the landscape around both the detection and treatment of recurrence continues to evolve. Compared with two decades ago, when some of the first randomized trials of intensive surveillance were conducted, the sensitivity of radiographic surveillance has increased severalfold, allowing detection of earlier metastatic disease in the liver and lungs. The advent of pelvic and liver MRI, endorectal ultrasound, and PET scanning offers new modalities for the detection of recurrent disease. Meanwhile, second- and third-line chemotherapeutic regimens, and ablative techniques for liver and lung metastases, have increased the options for both curative-intent and palliative-intent therapy for recurrent disease. More than a third of patients with recurrence undergo salvage resection, with median survival among these highly selected patients in excess of 3–5 years [8–11].

Timing and Choice of Surveillance Modalities

Intensity of Surveillance

There are various clinical, laboratory, radiographic, and endoscopic methods available for surveillance after treatment of colorectal cancer. Recommendations regarding their application and frequency of use vary between agencies involved in scripting guidelines for colorectal cancer care, and are summarized in Table 34-1. Most guidelines include more intensive early surveillance, with diminishing frequency after 2–5 years, due to the recognition that 80% of recurrences are detected within 3 years after initial curative-intent surgical therapy, and at least 95% are evident within 5 years [10, 12–14]. After 3 years without evidence of disease, cancer-specific mortality declines significantly and conditional survival thereafter is very high [15].

There have been eight prospective randomized trials addressing outcomes of surveillance after curative resection [16–23]. Overall, there is a lack of high-level evidence to support specific choices among surveillance regimens [24], but their interpretation is complicated by the heterogeneity of surveillance regimens, changes in diagnostic and therapeutic technologies available at the times they were conducted, and limitations of sample size and duration of follow-up [25].

Older trials, without intensive radiographic surveillance, have tended to show less benefit. For example, Ohlsson et al. [16] randomized 107 patients from 1983 to 1986 to either no follow-up or a surveillance regimen including CEA, colonoscopy, and chest X-rays, and found no meaningful differences in survival or recurrence patterns. Makela et al. [17] randomized 54 patients from 1988 to 1990 to yearly barium enema versus endoscopic surveillance plus liver ultrasonography and annual CT, with both groups receiving CEA testing and chest X-rays. In the intervention group, recurrences were found earlier (median 10 vs. 15 months, $p=0.002$), but patients were not significantly more likely to undergo salvage resection (19% vs. 14%, $p=0.67$) and 5-year overall survival was not significantly different (54% vs. 59%, $p=0.50$). In study of nearly 600 patients from 1983 to 1994, Kjeldsen et al. [18] applied the same modalities (clinical examination, colonoscopy, chest X-ray, hemoglobin, sedimentation rate, and liver enzymes) to the treatment and control arms, but varied the frequency of exams (every 6 months versus every 5 years). Recurrences in the every 6 months group were more likely to be asymptomatic (50% vs. 16%, $p=0.02$), and were subjected to more salvage resections (22% vs. 7%, $p=0.15$), but there was no difference in overall survival (70% vs. 68%, $p=0.48$) or cancer-specific survival (79% vs. 79%, $p=0.9$) between groups. And Schoemaker [19] et al. randomized 325 patients to clinical evaluation only versus additional chest X-ray, liver CT, and colonoscopy annually, and found only three resectable, asymptomatic recurrences (one each in the colon, liver and lung), without significant improvement in 5-year survival ($p=0.20$).

In contrast, more recent trials, incorporating more frequent endoscopy and modern imaging techniques, have been more likely to demonstrate benefit. In a study of 259 patients between 1997 and 2001, Rodriguez-Moranta et al. [20] compared routine clinical examination, colonoscopy, and CEA alone versus intensive surveillance with the addition of semi-annual abdominal CT or ultrasound, annual chest X-ray, and annual colonoscopy. They found improved survival for patients with Stage II cancers and rectal lesions, primarily due to the detection of resectable metachronous and locally-recurrent tumors. Pietra et al. [21] compared a regimen of annual CEA, ultrasound, chest X-ray, and colonoscopy against more frequent CEA and ultrasound, annual chest X-ray and colonoscopy, and the addition of annual abdominal CT. They found no difference in recurrence rates, but a significantly higher rate of salvage resection in the intensive surveillance group (65% vs. 10%, $p<0.01$), which translated into improved survival at 5 years (73% vs. 58%, $p=0.02$), particularly among those with recurrence (38% vs. 0%, $p<0.01$). Secco et al. [22] stratified patients into high and low risk of recurrence (based on primary tumor location, T stage, differentiation histology, and preoperative CEA level) then randomized to minimal surveillance versus active surveillance, with frequency of abdominopelvic ultrasound,

Table 34-1. Summary of surveillance guidelines

Modality	American Society of Colon and Rectal Surgeons [37]	National Comprehensive Cancer Network [48, 49]	American Cancer Society, US Multisociety Task Force on Colorectal Cancer [70]	American Society of Clinical Oncology [55]	Cancer Care Ontario [51]	European Society of Medical Oncology [52, 79]	British Society of Gastroenterology, Association of Coloproctology for Great Britain and Ireland [72, 73]
History and physical exam	Every 3–6 months for 2 years, then every 6 months to 5 years	Every 3–6 months for 2 years, then every 6 months to 5 years	Not addressed	Every 3–6 months for 5 years	Every 6 months for 5 years	Every 3–6 months for 3 years, then every 6 months to 5 years	Not addressed
CEA	Every 3–6 months for 2 years, then every 6 months to 5 years	Every 3–6 months for 2 years, then every 6 months to 5 years	Not addressed	Every 3–6 months for 5 years	Every 6 months for 5 years	Every 3–6 months for 3 years, then every 6 months to 5 years	"Role of CEA is uncertain"
Other laboratory testing	Not recommended	Not recommended	Not addressed	Not recommended	Not recommended	Not recommended	Not recommended
Abdominal Imaging	CT scan annually for 5 years. Consider more frequent for highest risk[a]	CT scan annually for 5 years	Not addressed	CT scan annually for 3 years. Consider 6–12 months for high risk	CT scan annually for 3 years. US every 6–12 months may be substituted	CT scan or contrast-enhanced ultrasound every 6–12 months for 3 years for patients at higher risk of recurrence	"Reasonable to offer" CT of the liver within 2 years of resection
Pelvic imaging	CT scan annually for 5 years. Consider more frequent for highest risk[a]	CT scan annually for 5 years	Not addressed	CT scans every 6–12 months for 2–3 years, then annually up to 5 years	CT scan annually for 3 years for rectal cancers only	Not specifically recommended	Not specifically recommended
Chest imaging	CT scan annually for 5 years. Consider more frequent for highest risk[a]	CT scan annually for 5 years	Not addressed	CT scan annually for 3 years. Consider 6–12 months for high risk	CT scan annually for 3 years. CXR every 6–12 months may be substituted	CT scan every 6–12 months for 3 years for patients at higher risk of recurrence	Not specifically recommended
PET scan	Not recommended for routine surveillance	Not recommended for routine surveillance	Not addressed	Not recommended for routine surveillance	Not recommended for routine surveillance	Not recommended for routine surveillance	Not recommended
Colonoscopy	1 Year after resection (or within 6 months if previously incomplete). If normal, repeat in 3 years. If adenomas, repeat in 1 year. Annual colonoscopy for patients with suspected familial syndromes who have not undergone proctocolectomy	1 Year after resection (or within 6 months if previously incomplete). If normal, repeat in 3 years, then 5 years. If advanced adenoma, repeat in 1 year. Annual colonoscopy for patients with suspected familial syndromes who have not undergone proctocolectomy	1 Year after resection (or 1 year after colonoscopy that cleared synchronous disease before primary treatment). If normal, repeat in 3 years, then 5 years. More frequent if high-risk adenoma(s) or suspicion for Lynch syndrome	1 Year after resection, or upon completion of adjuvant therapy if previously incomplete. If normal, repeat in 5 years. Otherwise, according to endoscopic findings	1 Year after resection (or within 6 months if previously incomplete). If normal, repeat in 5 years	1 Year after resection, then every 3–5 years thereafter	Every 5 years after resection, until benefits outweighed by comorbidity

(continued)

TABLE 34-1. (continued)

Modality	American Society of Colon and Rectal Surgeons [37]	National Comprehensive Cancer Network [48, 49]	American Cancer Society, US Multisociety Task Force on Colorectal Cancer [70]	American Society of Clinical Oncology [55]	Cancer Care Ontario [51]	European Society of Medical Oncology [52, 79]	British Society of Gastroenterology, Association of Coloproctology for Great Britain and Ireland [72, 73]
Stage-specific recommendations	Stage 1: high risk only[b] Stage 2: all Stage 3: all Stage 4: when metastases are resected for cure	Stage 1: colonoscopic surveillance only Stage 2: all Stage 3: all Stage 4: when metastases are resected for cure, CT scan every 3–6 months for 2 years, then every 6–12 months to 5 years	Not addressed	Recommendations apply to Stage II and III disease only. Insufficient data to make recommendations for Stage I	Recommendations apply to Stage II and III disease only	Not addressed	Not addressed
Rectal surveillance	Proctoscopy every 6–12 months for patients with anastomosis, every 6 months after local excision, for 3–5 years. Endorectal ultrasound for high risk[c]	No additional testing specifically recommended	Proctoscopy, flexible sigmoidoscopy or endorectal ultrasound every 3–6 months for patients with anastomosis	Proctosigmoidoscopy every 6 months for 2–5 years for patients who did not receive radiotherapy, those with T4 or N2 tumors. Pelvic imaging for rectal tumors only	Proctosigmoidoscopy every 6 months for 2–5 years for patients who did not receive radiotherapy. Pelvic imaging for rectal tumors only	No additional testing specifically recommended	Not addressed

CEA Carcinoembryonic antigen, CT Computed tomography, PET Positron emission tomography

[a]Highest risk for systemic recurrence includes patients with N2 disease or after curative-intent metastasectomy

[b]High risk of recurrence in Stage I disease is to be defined by provider(s) according to features such as margin positivity, unknown lymph node status (e.g., local excision), inadequate lymph node sampling, lymphovascular invasion, poorly differentiated histology, and/or T2 disease

[c]High risk for local recurrence include local excisions with poor histology (T2+, poorly differentiated), positive margins, T4 or N2 disease

chest X-ray, and proctoscopy (for rectal cancers only) adapted to risk class. Recurrence rates were similar between regimens, but the likelihood of salvage reoperation for recurrence was higher with active surveillance among the high-risk (34% vs. 12%, $p < 0.01$) but not low-risk (22% vs. 24%) patients. Survival at 5 years was improved with surveillance in both risk groups (both $p < 0.01$, proportions were not presented in the manuscript).

In the Follow-up After Colorectal Surgery (FACS) trial, the only factorial-design randomized study to evaluate the role of CT scans of the chest, abdomen, and pelvis, Primrose et al. [23] compared four groups: minimum follow-up, CEA only (every 3 months for 2 years, then semiannually to 5 years), CT only (every 6 months for 2 years, then annually to 5 years), and both CEA and CT. Colonoscopy was performed at 5 years in the non-CT groups, and at 2 and 5 years in the CT groups. Between 2003 and 2009, they randomized over 1200 patients in 39 hospitals in the United Kingdom. Again, more curative-intent salvage operations were performed in the active surveillance groups (6.7% CEA alone, 8.0% CT alone, 6.6% CEA + CT) than the minimal follow-up group (2.3%, $p = 0.02$), but there was no difference in survival (82% active vs. 84% minimal), and the addition of CT to CEA did not increase the detection of resectable recurrences.

Several meta-analyses have attempted to synthesize these and other non-randomized trials and have generally corroborated the findings of the trials described above. Tjandra and Chan [26] analyzed the seven pre-FACS studies above [16–20, 22, 27] and interim data from an ongoing study [4] and found that intensive surveillance resulted in more frequent and earlier detection of asymptomatic, resectable recurrence, with a small but statistically significant improvement in survival during follow-up (78% vs. 74%, $p = 0.01$). Pita-Fernández et al. [28] evaluated 11 trials, including more than 4000 patients, randomized according to a variety of different protocols and regimens, and found a small improvement in overall survival with more intensive surveillance (74% vs. 71%, p value not reported). Survival was significantly improved among patients subjected to colonoscopy, chest X-ray, liver ultrasonography, CT, and clinical assessment. There was also improvement in survival associated with increased frequency of CEA testing, liver ultrasonography, and clinical assessment. Findings and conclusions were similar in a meta-analysis by Renehan et al. [29]. Further, a Cochrane Collaborative meta-analysis of the pre-FACS trials found that intensive surveillance more than doubled the odds of salvage surgery and was associated with approximately 27% reduced odds of mortality. Particular benefit was found in trails that increased frequency of testing and use liver imaging [25].

There are two ongoing randomized trials whose results have not yet been reported. The COLOFOL trial [30] in Denmark, Sweden, Poland, Ireland, and Uruguay is comparing semiannual CT or MRI against imaging performed at 12 and 36 months after resection. And the GILDA trial [4], in Italy, Spain, and the United States, evaluates increased frequency of colonoscopy, chest X-ray, liver ultrasound, and abdominopelvic CT (for rectal cancers only). As of 2004, GILDA had enrolled nearly 1000 patients and interim results demonstrated no improvement in mortality (7% in the intensive arms, 5% in the minimal surveillance arm).

Ultimately, high-level evidence to support each component of any of the guidelines included herein is lacking. Nevertheless, we can likely conclude that more frequent testing and the use of advanced imaging will result in more potentially curative surgery for recurrence and a measurable, but small, improvement in survival.

Physical Examination

Most of the major societies' guidelines include periodic clinical evaluation, including assessment of symptoms and physical examination. Findings suggestive of disease recurrence may include weight loss, fatigue, anemia, cough, abdominal pain, rectal bleeding, or changes in bowel habits. Physical examination should focus on the abdomen, including evaluation for wound implants, lymph nodes, and rectal exam (or perineal wound exam after abdominoperineal resection).

In addition to their role in colorectal cancer surveillance, these visits also serve an important survivorship role in overall health maintenance and management of physical and psychosocial function after colorectal resections. More than half of rectal cancer patients who undergo low anterior resection suffer bowel dysfunction [31, 32]. And high rates of depression persist among colorectal cancer survivors even more than 5 years beyond their diagnosis [33]. Additionally, health behavior promotion can improve cancer outcomes as well. High intake of red meat and saturated fat has been associated with worse survival after treatment of colorectal cancer [34, 35], whereas regular weekly exercise is associated with significantly increased disease-free survival [36]. Interventions to improve these preventive health-related behaviors may thus improve outcomes from both the cancer and comorbid disease.

American Society of Colon and Rectal Surgeons (ASCRS) recommends visits every 3–6 months for 2 years, followed by every 6 months until 5 years [37]. Recognizing that many patients who present with recurrence are symptomatic [18, 38], a detailed history and physical examination may be sufficient to detect recurrent disease in many instances. Symptomatic recurrences, however, are far less likely to be amenable to curative-intent therapy [38, 39].

Laboratory Testing

None of the major guidelines currently endorse the routine evaluation of complete blood count, liver function tests, fecal occult blood testing, or blood chemistries. However, most recommend checking levels of carcinoembryonic antigen (CEA), an oncofetal protein that may be elevated in patients with recurrent colorectal cancer. CEA detects only about 30–60% of recurrences [10, 38, 40–43], the positive predictive value of CEA is only about 65% [44], and more than 15% of patients in surveillance have falsely elevated CEA in the absence of recurrence [40]. Yet, elevations in CEA may precede symptomatic presentation of metastasis [45], and the trials showing greatest benefit to intensive surveillance [21, 23] have included regular CEA evaluations. CEA elevations identify disease in the absence of abnormal imaging in up to 23% of patients with recurrent colorectal cancer [46], but may be more commonly elevated with metachronous liver metastases than with pulmonary metastases, luminal or locoregional recurrences [40, 42]. About a third of colorectal cancers do not produce CEA [47], but the significance of CEA elevation during surveillance seems to be independent of the preoperative CEA level [45]. Still, no studies have formally addressed the accuracy of surveillance CEA testing among patients with normal CEA at time of diagnosis.

Recommendations for management of asymptomatic CEA elevation are outlined in guidelines from both NCCN [48, 49] and ASCRS [37]. After confirmation of serial elevation in CEA level, a complete physical examination, endoscopy, and CT imaging of the chest, abdomen, and pelvis are performed. If these are all negative, consideration is given to PET-CT and/or repeat imaging every 3 months until levels decline or recurrence is detected.

Abdominal Imaging

The most common site of metachronous metastatic colorectal cancer is the liver [50]. Recommendations for routine imaging to detect liver metastases have, therefore, broadened substantially in the past decade. The Cochrane Collaborative meta-analysis [25] concluded that there was a survival benefit associated with liver imaging, with hazard ratio for mortality of 0.64 (95% confidence interval 0.49–0.85). This conclusion was derived from the results of five randomized trials [16, 17, 19–21], which used varying combinations of liver ultrasonography, abdominal CT, or both.

Observational studies have strongly supported the use of more frequent advanced liver imaging due to increased detection of resectable metastases. In a single-institution study, Fora et al. [14] reported results from their practice of CEA testing plus chest and abdominopelvic CTs every 6 months for the first 2 years, then annually to 5 years for patients with resected Stage II and III colorectal cancer. Among the 44 of 177 (25%) patients diagnosed with recurrence, CT detected the recurrence in 30 (68%). Half of patients diagnosed with recurrence had elevated CEA, but CEA was responsible for the diagnosis in only 8 (18%), and symptoms preceded diagnosis in only 3 patients (7%). Curative-intent salvage surgery was undertaken for 25 of the

44 recurrences (57%). Likewise, Arriola et al. [9] found that recurrences diagnosed by CT were far more likely to undergo curative-intent resection than those detected by CEA alone. In a meta-analysis of five surveillance trials, Renehan et al. [29] concluded that the regimens most consistently associated with improved survival included both CT scanning and frequent CEA testing.

Canadian [51] and European [52] guidelines provide the option of either CT or ultrasound, and as recently as 2004, ASCRS practice parameters for colorectal cancer [53] surveillance did not recommend routine liver imaging, because of the unclear survival benefit associated with salvage resection, the lack of evidence for incremental benefit of imaging in patients undergoing CEA testing, and the cost of CT. Since then, however, improvements in the detection and management of hepatic and pulmonary metastases have altered this calculus [54], and the current ASCRS practice parameter [37] and recommendations from other US-based agencies [48, 49, 55] recommend routine CT imaging, due to increased sensitivity for identifying early liver lesions, and the opportunity to evaluate the remainder of the abdomen and pelvis for other sites of metastasis (such as retroperitoneal lymph nodes and ovaries), and to identify local recurrence in the resection bed [37]. Despite a lack of controlled studies comparing different imaging intervals, the ASCRS guideline suggests consideration of semiannual imaging for patients at highest risk of recurrence, including those with resected N2 or Stage IV disease.

There is currently no organization that endorses routine use of PET-CT scans or liver MRI. One randomized trial compared addition of PET to a surveillance regimen including CTs at 9 and 15 months after surgery, and found shorter time to diagnosis (12.1 vs. 15.4 months, $p=0.01$) and a higher rate of resection for recurrence (44% vs. 10%, $p<0.01$) in the PET+CT group [56]. Nevertheless, a meta-analysis of the use of PET in surveillance regimens noted inadequate evidence to support its use in routine surveillance [57]. In the evaluation of unexplained CEA elevation, observational studies find that PET and PET-CT have sensitivity for detecting metastasis in excess of 90% despite somewhat lower specificity, from 70 to 80%, due to false positive findings [58–63]. In routine surveillance, however, PET does not improve sensitivity over CT due to its lower spatial resolution and the use of non-diagnostic quality CT imaging without contrast enhancement in combined PET-CT exams.

Chest Imaging

Whereas plain radiography was the mainstay of surveillance for pulmonary metastasis in the past, most of the major guidelines now recommend the use of cross-sectional thoracic imaging at least annually. This change has come with the recognition that pulmonary metastasis may present as a solitary site of disease recurrence [8, 50, 64, 65], and may even represent the most common site of distant metastasis for distal rectal cancers [66, 67]. Unfortunately, among the published randomized studies, only the FACS trial [23] has included chest CT scans in the regimen, and this study did not find a statistically significant incremental benefit to CT scan over CEA alone (though the study was not powered to examine this comparison). In an observational study of 530 patients with resected Stage II or III colorectal cancers, Chau et al. [38] found that chest CT was responsible for 35% of the diagnosed metastases, and 73% of patients found to have isolated pulmonary recurrence underwent curative-intent resection. Thus, for now, chest imaging is recommended in spite of a lack of high-level evidence to support its effectiveness in practice.

Colonoscopy

Surveillance endoscopy after colorectal cancer resection can serve three important purposes: clearance of remaining colon when preoperative colonoscopy was incomplete, anastomotic surveillance for detection of local luminal recurrence, and detection of metachronous neoplasia. For patients who did not have complete colonoscopy before resection of the primary tumor (because of an obstructing tumor for example) complete colonoscopy should be performed within 3–6 months after surgery [37], because the estimated incidence of synchronous neoplasia exceeds 30% [68–70]. Anastomotic recurrence after resection of colon cancers is rare [29, 71], representing only about 4% of recurrences [65]. On the other hand, local recurrence is a common concern after low anterior rectal resections—local surveillance for rectal cancer is discussed in more detail below.

For patients who had complete colon evaluation before their primary resection, the primary goal of surveillance colonoscopy is the detection of metachronous neoplasia, or polyps that were missed on the preoperative evaluation. The BSG/ACPGBI guidelines suggest waiting until 5 years after resection [72, 73], whereas all of the other guidelines include a complete colonoscopy at 1 year, though the rate of clinically significant findings may be quite low. In a meta-analysis of 17 studies including nearly 8000 patients followed after curative colorectal cancer resections, there were only 57 metachronous cancers found with the first 2 years—an incidence of 0.7% [70], consistent with the incidence in other studies [74–76]. In a recent single-institution study, Cone et al. [71] found that 15% of patients had polyps on their 1-year colonoscopy, but only 3% of these were greater than 1 cm in diameter. Nevertheless, these detection rates, both for malignancy and for high-risk adenomas, are at least as high as those of average-risk screening exams. Combined with the recognition that more than half of metachronous cancers are detected in the first 2 years after resection [77, 78],

these data have been considered reasonable justification for the recommendation for colonoscopy at 1 year in most guidelines [37, 48, 51, 52, 55, 70, 79, 80].

In a randomized trial, Wang et al. [75] evaluated even more frequent colonoscopy, comparing a regimen of exams every 3 months for 1 year, then every 6 months for 2 more years, then yearly to 5 years versus colonoscopy at 6, 30, and 60 months only. The overall incidence of anastomotic recurrence was 6.9% and metachronous cancers were found in 2.8%. There was a higher rate of asymptomatic recurrences and curative-intent salvage operations in the more frequent group, but no statistically significant difference in 5-year survival (77% vs. 72%, $p=0.25$). Likewise, in their meta-analysis of surveillance trials, Tjandra and Chan [26] concluded that there was an increase in the curative reoperation rate among studies with increased frequency of colonoscopy, but a mortality benefit to colonoscopy only when compared against no surveillance at all.

After the initial 1-year colonoscopy, patients with a personal history of colorectal cancer remain at increased risk for metachronous neoplasia for the rest of their lives. The annual incidence of a second primary colorectal cancer is about 0.3%, resulting in an incidence of 1.5–3.1% within 5–10 years [74, 78, 81, 82]. Up to half of patients develop metachronous polyps after resection of a primary colorectal cancer [83]. Thus, even after the first year, patients with a personal history of colorectal cancer still require more frequent endoscopic surveillance than average-risk individuals or those with a history of adenomas alone. The ASCRS guideline [37] recommends that the subsequent colonoscopy schedule be tailored to the findings at the 1-year examination, and to other patient specific risk factors and circumstances. Patients with high-risk adenomas (high-grade dysplasia, size greater than 1 cm or more than three adenomas) and those with a diagnosed or suspected hereditary colorectal cancer syndrome may require annual colonoscopy for more intensive surveillance [5]. On the other hand, patients with limited life expectancy are unlikely to benefit from the detection of an asymptomatic cancer, and may be selected for less frequent, or no, endoscopic surveillance [84–86].

Other methods of luminal surveillance are not formally recommended at this time. Air-contrast barium enema is a less effective means of surveillance after colonoscopic polypectomy [87], and would be expected to compare similarly among patients after cancer resections. CT colonography has been advocated elsewhere as a technique for simultaneous assessment of both luminal and distant disease [88, 89], but it has not been satisfactorily evaluated in the setting of colorectal cancer surveillance, and its sensitivity has not been satisfactory to replace optical colonoscopy in this setting [70, 90].

Stage I Disease

Most of the major guidelines for and studies of colorectal cancer surveillance pertain primarily to Stage II–III disease, and to Stage IV tumors that have been resected with curative intent. Stage I patients have been largely excluded from many of the randomized trials. As a result, there remains controversy regarding approaches to the surveillance of resected Stage I colon cancers (see Table 34-1). Several of the guidelines specifically recommend against routine imaging. For example, NCCN [48] and ASCO [55] recommend only endoscopic surveillance for anastomotic recurrence or metachronous cancers. Further, there is presumed to be low incidence of systemic recurrence, as 5-year colon cancer survival rates exceed 90%, and very few operations for metachronous metastatic recurrence occur in patients who initially presented with a Stage I tumor [91]. Thus, there is concern that surveillance will identify more incidental findings than treatable recurrences. Chao and Gibbs [92] estimated it would take nearly 200 patients with Stage I disease in surveillance to detect each curable metastasis, and cautioned against over-testing in this setting.

On the other hand, in a secondary analysis [8] of the Clinical Outcomes of Surgical Therapy trial [93], which compared laparoscopic and open colectomy for colon cancer, the 5-year recurrence rate was 9.5% for early stage patients (including Stage I and IIa), occurring at a median of 1.8 years after primary resection. More than a third of patients with recurrence underwent salvage resection, with no difference in salvage rates between initially early and late stage patients. Median survival after salvage surgery for early stage patients was 51 months. Finding equivalent rates of salvage and better survival for recurrences after resection of early stage disease, Tsikitis et al. [8] recommended active survival for these patients, though they did not distinguish between Stage I (T1-2, N0) and Stage 2a (T3N0) in the study. Accordingly, the most recent ASCRS [37] Practice Guideline recommends consideration of active surveillance for Stage I patients, but limits the recommendation to those designated at higher risk—for example, close or positive margins, unknown lymph node status (e.g., local or endoscopic excision), inadequate lymph node sampling, lymphovascular invasion, poorly differentiated histology, and/or T2 disease.

Local Surveillance for Rectal Cancer

Additional surveillance recommendations for rectal cancer are predicated on the greater risk of locoregional recurrence, compared with colon cancers [70], due to both anatomic and biologic differences between the tumors [94–96]. Locoregional recurrence of rectal cancer can occur either intraluminally, typically at the site of anastomosis, or extraluminally, likely associated with residual lymphatic disease, close radial margins, or tumor shed during resection. Although the use of total mesorectal excision (TME) and chemoradiotherapy for locally advanced rectal cancers have substantially reduced local failure after primary resection [97–100], between 4 and 22% of patients still experience local recurrence [98, 99, 101–103]. The resulting downstaging that may occur with the use of preoperative therapy for rectal cancer also may creates confusion about how to classify future risk of recurrence. In the ASCRS practice guidelines, it is recommended that pretreatment clinical staging be used to guide surveillance intensity unless the pathologic staging exceeds the preoperative assessment [37].

Early identification of local recurrence may offer the opportunity for curative-intent salvage resection. Therefore, surveillance of colorectal anastomoses and pelvic imaging are recommended beyond what is performed for colon cancer surveillance. Physical assessment including meticulous pelvic and groin examinations should be performed every 6 months. For patients with a low anastomosis or distal tumor with local excision or non-operative management, digital exam of the anastomosis or tumor site should be included. For patients who have undergone abdominoperineal resection (APR), careful palpation of the perineum and, in women, the posterior wall of the vagina is recommended. Special attention should be paid to areas of nodularity or changes over time. Any suspicious lesions should undergo biopsy as local recurrences after APR are frequently perineal or pre-sacral [100].

Proctosigmoidoscopy is recommended in the most recent ASCRS practice parameters [37] every 6–12 months for 3–5 years for those who have undergone a low anterior resection with anastomosis, and more frequently for those considered to be at higher risk of local recurrence. These higher risk patients and tumors might include men, distal lesions, close margins, incomplete TME, positive lymph nodes, lack of treatment response, lymphovascular invasion, and/or poor differentiation [98, 103–108]. On the other hand, in recognition of the substantially lower recurrence rate associated with TME and chemoradiotherapy, some guidelines have suggested limiting additional endoscopic surveillance only to patients who did not receive guideline-concordant multimodality therapy [51, 55]. To date, however, there have been no high-quality trials evaluating the effect of proctosigmoidoscopy on detection of recurrence, salvage resection, or survival after low anterior resection.

Recognizing that proctosigmoidoscopy only evaluates endoluminal surfaces, and thus may not detect early disease in residual mesorectum or other extraluminal tissues, the most recent ASCRS [37] and ACS/MSTF [70] guidelines also suggest consideration of endorectal ultrasonography (ERUS) for patients considered to be at high-risk for local recurrence. In three studies, ERUS identified asymptomatic rectal cancer recurrence that was otherwise undetected by digital exam, endoscopy, CT, or CEA in about 30% of cases [109–111]. Surgically resectable recurrences were more common in the ERUS-detected group, suggesting it may identify earlier recurrent disease [111]. Further, ERUS-guided biopsy may provide the best opportunity to obtain histologic evaluation of extraluminal abnormalities [112–114]. Extraluminal pelvic disease may otherwise be evaluated by cross-sectional imaging. ASCO [55] and CCO [51] both recommend pelvic CT imaging for rectal cancers only, as a means of detection of local recurrence. MRI of the pelvis can also be used and is highly accurate for the diagnosis of pelvic recurrence [115], but its use in routine surveillance did not improve the detection of resectable recurrence in a single trial [116], and its cost-effectiveness has not been evaluated.

For rectal cancers treated by local excision, rather than radical resection, particular attention must be paid to both endoluminal and mesorectal surveillance. Even among the best candidates—those with T1 cancers and no high-risk histologic features—there is a significantly higher risk of local recurrence compared with resection with TME, ranging from 4 to 33% [117–119]. Outcomes of local excision for higher stage tumors are even worse [120]. Thus, at least semiannual endoscopic surveillance after local excision is highly recommended, and consideration may be given to the use of ERUS for these patients, especially.

As there is increasing interest in and application of non-operative approaches for patients who experience complete clinical response after chemoradiotherapy [121, 122], surveillance regimens for these patients will need to be defined as well. Because non-operative treatment is currently limited to clinical trials [123], none of the guidelines include formal recommendations for such patients. However, the non-operative trials reported to date have employed remarkably intensive surveillance, including very frequent physical examination, endoscopy, and imaging, often with pelvic MRI [122–125].

Compliance with Guidelines

Despite published recommendations for surveillance after resection for colorectal cancer, compliance with surveillance remains challenging both for patients and their physicians. There is evidence that patients who adhere to recommended surveillance have a greater likelihood of curative-intent reoperation for recurrence and improved overall and disease-specific 5-year survival [126, 127]. Yet anywhere from 25 to 42% of patients have poor completion of recommended surveillance, and 11–21% have no surveillance at all [126–129]. Studies in Canada [130], the Netherlands [131, 132], and Norway [133] have found substantial differences in the surveillance patterns between providers, and noted that routines are commonly inconsistent with published guidelines. Among US Medicare beneficiaries, there is substantial geographic variation in the intensity of surveillance, with about 60% of patients failing to complete recommended testing, while 23% undergo testing more intensive than recommended by guidelines [134]. Similarly, a survey of ASCRS membership

revealed that colon and rectal surgeons employ a wide variety of surveillance approaches, and only 30% performed surveillance in accordance with a formal national or local guideline [135].

There is also little consensus regarding who should manage cancer surveillance—the operating surgeon, medical oncologist, gastroenterologist, or primary care doctor. This ambiguity may contribute to nonadherence in many patients, as responsibility for ordering and managing testing can be undefined [136]. In a survey of Canadian colorectal cancer specialists, Earle et al. found high levels of endorsement of recommended surveillance, and a belief that specialty physicians are more capable of effective surveillance. Similarly, in a Texas study, patients who saw a medical oncologist as part of surveillance were significantly more likely to exhibit compliance with minimal recommendations for office visits, CEA testing, and colonoscopy [128]. Two randomized trials have compared surveillance by general practitioners and surgeons. In both studies, surveillance by surgeons was associated with more costly and intensive diagnostic testing, but no difference in recurrence rates, time to diagnosis, survival, or quality of life [137, 138] Patients seeing general practitioners received more fecal occult blood testing, whereas those followed by surgeons had more ultrasounds and colonoscopies [137]. Patients followed by primary care doctors report that greater attention is paid to preventive health maintenance for comorbidities [139].

In a single-institution study, Standeven et al. [140] found that, compared with community-based primary care follow-up, the establishment of a formal surveillance program in a referral center improved adherence to surveillance guidelines. Strand et al. [141] trained specialty nurses to conduct surveillance and found similar patient satisfaction and detection of recurrence among patients randomized patients to visits with either the nurse or a surgeon. It remains unclear, however, whether such a model—a multidisciplinary team with a clinic dedicated to colorectal cancer surveillance—could be replicated more widely.

Quality of Life

Apart from the cancer-specific outcomes of surveillance, an essential question is the effect of intensive surveillance on psychological health and quality of life. While reassuring surveillance examinations may allay fears of cancer recurrence for some patients, there could be others for whom surveillance examinations create additional unwarranted worry and result in investigations for false positive or incidental findings.

Most patients in surveillance report, however, that these anxieties and inconveniences are outweighed by the reassurance and optimism imparted by negative results [142]. In the randomized trial by Kjeldsen et al. [143] patients randomized to more frequent evaluations reported greater confidence in the surveillance process, and somewhat less worry about test results, even in this trial which showed no effect of surveillance intensity on survival. Likewise, Stiggelbout et al. [144] interviewed more than 212 patients undergoing surveillance for colorectal cancer and found generally positive attitudes toward surveillance, with relatively little worry regarding testing. Even when asked to consider the possibility that testing would not improve the detection of recurrence, 64% of patients in that study still expressed a preference for active surveillance.

Cost

As recommendations for surveillance imaging have expanded in recent guidelines, another important consideration will be the costs of surveillance. Total costs of the surveillance regimens in published studies vary 28-fold [145], without a clear correlation between cost and efficacy. Meanwhile, between 1999 and 2006, the use of CT and MRI scans in the follow-up of patients with colorectal cancer increased at an annual rate of more than 5%, and the use of PET scans more than tripled [146].

Among a cohort of Italian patients undergoing surveillance with clinical examination, CEA, abdominal ultrasonography, chest X-ray, and colonoscopy, the 5-year cost of surveillance averaged $5400 per patient, but more than $100,000 per case of potentially curable recurrence [147]. Similarly, in a meta-analysis of five randomized trials [16–19, 21], Renehan et al. [148] estimated the average costs of surveillance at almost £2500 per patient, or about £3000 per year of life saved—within the range of acceptable cost-effectiveness for the UK's National Health Service. And a comparative study in France estimated that intensive surveillance cost an additional 3144€ per quality-adjusted life year gained over a minimal surveillance strategy [149].

We can conclude from these limited data that the cost-effectiveness of colorectal cancer surveillance is likely to be within the range of other interventions considered acceptably costly. Caution must be taken, however, if an increase in the cost, complexity, and frequency of recommended testing is contemplated.

Conclusions

There continues to be substantial uncertainty about the magnitude of benefits from active surveillance and the content of optimal surveillance regimens after curative resection for colorectal cancer. With improved imaging technology and a growing array of management options for recurrence, however, active surveillance is recommended for patients eligible for treatment of recurrent disease. Although there is likely great value to standardization of surveillance regimens, optimal approaches will require tailoring of surveillance

strategies to individual patient risk factors. Perhaps the introduction of biomarkers [150] or simulation models [151, 152] to estimate individual risk will inform choices about surveillance modalities in the future [153]. In coming years, the GILDA [4, 154] and COLOFOL [30] trials should contribute important data on the cancer-related outcomes of surveillance and will also report on health-related quality of life and the cost-effectiveness of intensive surveillance. For now, however, decisions must be based largely on clinicopathologic risk factors, preferences for intensity of testing, and willingness to pursue further investigation and active treatment for abnormalities detected by testing.

References

1. Siegel R, Naishadham D, Jemal A. Cancer statistics, 2013. CA Cancer J Clin. 2013;63(1):11–30. http://www.ncbi.nlm.nih.gov/pubmed/23335087.
2. DeSantis CE, Lin CC, Mariotto AB, Siegel RL, Stein KD, Kramer JL, et al. Cancer treatment and survivorship statistics, 2014. CA Cancer J Clin. 2014;64(4):252–71. http://www.ncbi.nlm.nih.gov/pubmed/24890451.
3. Vernava III A, Longo W, Virgo K, Coplin M, Wade T, Johnson F. Current follow-up strategies after resection of colon cancer. Dis Colon Rectum. 1994;37(6):573–83. doi:10.1007/BF02050993.
4. Grossmann EM, Johnson FE, Virgo KS, Longo WE, Fossati R. Follow-up of colorectal cancer patients after resection with curative intent—the GILDA trial. Surg Oncol. 2004;13(2–3):119–24.
5. NCCN Clinical Practice Guidelines in Oncology—Genetic/familial high-risk assessment: colorectal, Version 2.2014. 2014. http://www.nccn.org/professionals/physician_gls/pdf/genetics_colon.pdf. Accessed 24 Apr 2015.
6. Fahy BN. Follow-up after curative resection of colorectal cancer. Ann Surg Oncol. 2014;21(3):738–46. http://www.ncbi.nlm.nih.gov/pubmed/24271157.
7. Cancer of the colon and rectum—SEER stat fact sheets. http://seer.cancer.gov/statfacts/html/colorect.html. Accessed 2 Apr 2015.
8. Tsikitis VL, Malireddy K, Green EA, Christensen B, Whelan R, Hyder J, et al. Postoperative surveillance recommendations for early stage colon cancer based on results from the clinical outcomes of surgical therapy trial. J Clin Oncol. 2009;27(22):3671–6. http://jco.ascopubs.org/content/27/22/3671.abstract.
9. Arriola E, Navarro M, Parés D, Muñoz M, Pareja L, Figueras J, et al. Imaging techniques contribute to increased surgical rescue of relapse in the follow-up of colorectal cancer. Dis Colon Rectum. 2006;49(4):478–84. doi:10.1007/s10350-005-0280-9.
10. Kobayashi H, Mochizuki H, Sugihara K, Morita T, Kotake K, Teramoto T, et al. Characteristics of recurrence and surveillance tools after curative resection for colorectal cancer: a multicenter study. Surgery. 2007;141(1):67–75.
11. Fong Y, Fortner J, Sun RL, Brennan MF, Blumgart LH. Clinical score for predicting recurrence after hepatic resection for metastatic colorectal cancer: analysis of 1001 consecutive cases. Ann Surg. 1999;230(3):309–18. discussion 318–21.

12. Sargent D, Sobrero A, Grothey A, O'Connell MJ, Buyse M, Andre T, et al. Evidence for cure by adjuvant therapy in colon cancer: observations based on individual patient data from 20,898 patients on 18 randomized trials. J Clin Oncol. 2009;27(6):872–7. http://www.ncbi.nlm.nih.gov/pmc/articles/PMC2738431/.

13. Seo SI, Lim S-B, Yoon YS, Kim CW, Yu CS, Kim TW, et al. Comparison of recurrence patterns between ≤5 years and >5 years after curative operations in colorectal cancer patients. J Surg Oncol. 2013;108(1):9–13. http://www.ncbi.nlm.nih.gov/pubmed/23754582.

14. Fora A, Patta A, Attwood K, Wilding G, Fakih M. Intensive radiographic and biomarker surveillance in stage II and III colorectal cancer. Oncology. 2012;82(1):41–7.

15. Sargent DJ, Patiyil S, Yothers G, Haller DG, Gray R, Benedetti J, et al. End points for colon cancer adjuvant trials: observations and recommendations based on individual patient data from 20,898 patients enrolled onto 18 randomized trials from the ACCENT group. J Clin Oncol. 2007;25(29):4569–74.

16. Ohlsson B, Breland U, Ekberg H, Graffner H, Tranberg KG. Follow-up after curative surgery for colorectal carcinoma. Randomized comparison with no follow-up. Dis Colon Rectum. 1995;38(6):619–26.

17. Makela JT, Laitinen SO, Kairaluoma MI. Five-year follow-up after radical surgery for colorectal cancer. Results of a prospective randomized trial. Arch Surg. 1995;130(10):1062–7.

18. Kjeldsen BJ, Kronborg O, Fenger C, Jorgensen OD. A prospective randomized study of follow-up after radical surgery for colorectal cancer. Br J Surg. 1997;84(5):666–9. http://www.ncbi.nlm.nih.gov/pubmed/9171758.

19. Schoemaker D, Black R, Giles L, Toouli J. Yearly colonoscopy, liver CT, and chest radiography do not influence 5-year survival of colorectal cancer patients. Gastroenterology. 1998;114(1):7–14. http://www.sciencedirect.com/science/article/pii/S0016508598706262.

20. Rodríguez-Moranta F, Saló J, Arcusa A, Boadas J, Piñol V, Bessa X, et al. Postoperative surveillance in patients with colorectal cancer who have undergone curative resection: a prospective, multicenter, randomized, controlled trial. J Clin Oncol. 2006;24(3):386–93.

21. Pietra N, Sarli L, Costi R, Ouchemi C, Grattarola M, Peracchia A. Role of follow-up in management of local recurrences of colorectal cancer. Dis Colon Rectum. 1998;41(9):1127–33. doi:10.1007/BF02239434.

22. Secco GB, Fardelli R, Gianquinto D, Bonfante P, Baldi E, Ravera G, et al. Efficacy and cost of risk-adapted follow-up in patients after colorectal cancer surgery: a prospective, randomized and controlled trial. Eur J Surg Oncol. 2002;28(4):418–23. http://www.sciencedirect.com/science/article/pii/S0748798301912508.

23. Primrose JN, Perera R, Gray A, Rose P, Fuller A, Corkhill A, et al. Effect of 3 to 5 years of scheduled CEA and CT follow-up to detect recurrence of colorectal cancer: the FACS randomized clinical trial. JAMA. 2014;311(3):263–70. http://www.ncbi.nlm.nih.gov/pubmed/24430319.

24. Baca B, Beart RW, Etzioni DA. Surveillance after colorectal cancer resection: a systematic review. Dis Colon Rectum. 2011;54(8):1036–48.

25. Jeffery M, Hickey B, Hider P. Follow up strategies for patients treated for non-metastatic colorectal cancer. Cochrane Database Syst Rev. 2007;1, CD002200. http://espace.library.uq.edu.au/view/UQ:137177.

26. Tjandra J, Chan MY. Follow-up after curative resection of colorectal cancer: a meta-analysis. Dis Colon Rectum. 2007;50(11):1783–99. doi:10.1007/s10350-007-9030-5.

27. Jain N, Pietrobon R, Hocker S, Guller U, Shankar A, Higgins LD. The relationship between surgeon and hospital volume and outcomes for shoulder arthroplasty. J Bone Joint Surg Am. 2004;86-A(3):496–505.

28. Pita-Fernandez S, Alhayek-Ai M, Gonzalez-Martin C, Lopez-Calvino B, Seoane-Pillado T, Pertega-Diaz S. Intensive follow-up strategies improve outcomes in nonmetastatic colorectal cancer patients after curative surgery: a systematic review and meta-analysis. Ann Oncol. 2015;26(4):644–56. doi:10.1093/annonc/mdu543.

29. Renehan AG, Egger M, Saunders MP, O'Dwyer ST. Impact on survival of intensive follow up after curative resection for colorectal cancer: systematic review and meta-analysis of randomised trials. BMJ. 2002;324(7341):1–8.

30. Colofol—evaluation of the frequency of a surveillance program. http://www.colofol.com. Accessed 17 Apr 2015.

31. Juul T, Ahlberg M, Biondo S, Emmertsen KJ, Espin E, Jimenez LM, et al. International validation of the low anterior resection syndrome score. Ann Surg. 2014;259(4):728–34. http://www.ncbi.nlm.nih.gov/pubmed/23598379.

32. Peeters KCMJ, van de Velde CJH, Leer JWH, Martijn H, Junggeburt JMC, Kranenbarg EK, et al. Late side effects of short-course preoperative radiotherapy combined with total mesorectal excision for rectal cancer: increased bowel dysfunction in irradiated patients—a Dutch colorectal cancer group study. J Clin Oncol. 2005;23(25):6199–206.

33. Ramsey SD, Berry K, Moinpour C, Giedzinska A, Andersen MR. Quality of life in long term survivors of colorectal cancer. Am J Gastroenterol. 2002;97(5):1228–34.

34. Meyerhardt JA, Niedzwiecki D, Hollis D, Saltz LB, Hu FB, Mayer RJ, et al. Association of dietary patterns with cancer recurrence and survival in patients with stage III colon cancer. JAMA. 2007;298(7):754–64.

35. McCullough ML, Gapstur SM, Shah R, Jacobs EJ, Campbell PT. Association between red and processed meat intake and mortality among colorectal cancer survivors. J Clin Oncol. 2013;31(22):2773–82.

36. Meyerhardt JA, Heseltine D, Niedzwiecki D, Hollis D, Saltz LB, Mayer RJ, et al. Impact of physical activity on cancer recurrence and survival in patients with stage III colon cancer: findings from CALGB 89803. J Clin Oncol. 2006;24(22):3535–41. http://www.ncbi.nlm.nih.gov/entrez/query.fcgi?cmd=Retrieve&db=PubMed&dopt=Citation&list_uids=16822843.

37. Steele SR, Chang G, Hendren S, Weiser MR, Irani J, Buie WD, et al. Practice guidelines for the surveillance of patients after curative treatment of colon and rectal cancer. Dis Colon Rectum. 2015;58(8):713–25.

38. Chau I, Allen MJ, Cunningham D, Norman AR, Brown G, Ford HER, et al. The value of routine serum carcino-embryonic antigen measurement and computed tomography in the surveillance of patients after adjuvant chemotherapy for colorectal cancer. J Clin Oncol. 2004;22(8):1420–9.

39. Graham RA, Wang S, Catalano PJ, Haller DG. Postsurgical surveillance of colon cancer: preliminary cost analysis of

physician examination, carcinoembryonic antigen testing, chest X-ray, and colonoscopy. Ann Surg. 1998;228(1):59–63.

40. Moertel CG, Fleming TR, Macdonald JS, Haller DG, Laurie JA, Tangen C. An evaluation of the carcinoembryonic antigen (CEA) test for monitoring patients with resected colon cancer. JAMA. 1993;270(8):943–7.

41. Glover C, Douse P, Kane P, Karani J, Meire H, Mohammadtaghi S, et al. Accuracy of investigations for asymptomatic colorectal liver metastases. Dis Colon Rectum. 2002;45(4):476–84.

42. Carriquiry LA, Piñeyro A. Should carcinoembryonic antigen be used in the management of patients with colorectal cancer? Dis Colon Rectum. 1999;42(7):921–9.

43. Tan E, Gouvas N, Nicholls RJ, Ziprin P, Xynos E, Tekkis PP. Diagnostic precision of carcinoembryonic antigen in the detection of recurrence of colorectal cancer. Surg Oncol. 2009;18(1):15–24.

44. Metser U, You J, McSweeney S, Freeman M, Hendler A. Assessment of tumor recurrence in patients with colorectal cancer and elevated carcinoembryonic antigen level: FDG PET/CT versus contrast-enhanced 64-MDCT of the chest and abdomen. Am J Roentgenol. 2010;194(3):766–71.

45. Irvine T, Scott M, Clark CI. A small rise in CEA is sensitive for recurrence after surgery for colorectal cancer. Colorectal Dis. 2007;9(6):527–31.

46. Verberne C, Wiggers T, Vermeulen KM, de Jong KP. Detection of recurrences during follow-up after liver surgery for colorectal metastases: both Carcino-Embryonic Antigen (CEA) and imaging are important. Ann Surg Oncol. 2013;20:457–63.

47. Goslin R, O'Brien MJ, Steele G, Mayer R, Wilson R, Corson JM, et al. Correlation of plasma CEA and CEA tissue staining in poorly differentiated colorectal cancer. Am J Med. 1981;71(2):246–53.

48. NCCN Clinical Practice Guidelines in Oncology: colon cancer. http://www.nccn.org/professionals/physician_gls/pdf/colon.pdf. Accessed 14 Apr 2015.

49. NCCN Clinical Practice Guidelines in Oncology: rectal cancer. http://www.nccn.org/professionals/physician_gls/pdf/rectal.pdf. Accessed 14 Apr 2015.

50. Kjeldsen BJ, Kronborg O, Fenger C, Jørgensen OD. The pattern of recurrent colorectal cancer in a prospective randomised study and the characteristics of diagnostic tests. Int J Color Dis. 1997;12(6):329–34.

51. Earle C, Annis R, Sussman J, Haynes AE, Vafaei A. Follow-up care, surveillance protocol, and secondary prevention measures for survivors of colorectal cancer. Toronto, ON; 2012. https://www.cancercare.on.ca/common/pages/UserFile.aspx?fileId=124839.

52. Labianca R, Nordlinger B, Beretta GD, Mosconi S, Mandalà M, Cervantes A, et al. Early colon cancer: ESMO Clinical Practice Guidelines for diagnosis, treatment and follow-up. Ann Oncol. 2013;24 suppl 6:vi64–72. http://annonc.oxfordjournals.org/content/24/suppl_6/vi64.short.

53. Anthony T, Simmang C, Hyman N, Buie D, Kim D, Cataldo P, et al. Practice parameters for the surveillance and follow-up of patients with colon and rectal cancer. Dis Colon Rectum. 2004;47(6):807–17. http://www.ncbi.nlm.nih.gov/entrez/query.fcgi?cmd=Retrieve&db=PubMed&dopt=Citation&list_uids=15108028.

54. Cummings LC, Payes JD, Cooper GS. Survival after hepatic resection in metastatic colorectal cancer: a population-based study. Cancer. 2007;109(4):718–26.

55. Meyerhardt JA, Mangu PB, Flynn PJ, Korde L, Loprinzi CL, Minsky BD, et al. Follow-up care, surveillance protocol, and secondary prevention measures for survivors of colorectal cancer: American Society of Clinical Oncology clinical practice guideline endorsement. J Clin Oncol. 2013;31(35):4465–70. http://www.ncbi.nlm.nih.gov/pubmed/24220554.

56. Sobhani I, Tiret E, Lebtahi R, Aparicio T, Itti E, Montravers F, et al. Early detection of recurrence by 18FDG-PET in the follow-up of patients with colorectal cancer. Br J Cancer. 2008;98(5):875–80.

57. Patel K, Hadar N, Lee J, Siegel BA, Hillner BE, Lau J. The lack of evidence for PET or PET/CT surveillance of patients with treated lymphoma, colorectal cancer, and head and neck cancer: a systematic review. J Nucl Med. 2013;54(9):1518–27. http://www.pubmedcentral.nih.gov/articlerender.fcgi?artid=3980728&tool=pmcentrez&rendertype=abstract.

58. Flanagan FL, Dehdashti F, Ogunbiyi OA, Kodner IJ, Siegel BA. Utility of FDG-PET for investigating unexplained plasma CEA elevation in patients with colorectal cancer. Ann Surg. 1998;227(3):319–23.

59. Flamen P, Hoekstra OS, Homans F, Van Cutsem E, Maes A, Stroobants S, et al. Unexplained rising carcinoembryonic antigen (CEA) in the postoperative surveillance of colorectal cancer: the utility of positron emission tomography (PET). Eur J Cancer. 2001;37(7):862–9.

60. Shen Y-Y, Liang J-A, Chen Y-K, Tsai C-Y, Kao C-H. Clinical impact of 18F-FDG-PET in the suspicion of recurrent colorectal cancer based on asymptomatically elevated serum level of carcinoembryonic antigen (CEA) in Taiwan. Hepatogastroenterology. 2006;53(69):348–50.

61. Kyoto Y, Momose M, Kondo C, Itabashi M, Kameoka S, Kusakabe K. Ability of 18F-FDG PET/CT to diagnose recurrent colorectal cancer in patients with elevated CEA concentrations. Ann Nucl Med. 2010;24(5):395–401.

62. Lu YY, Chen JH, Chien CR, Chen WTL, Tsai SC, Lin WY, et al. Use of FDG-PET or PET/CT to detect recurrent colorectal cancer in patients with elevated CEA: a systematic review and meta-analysis. Int J Colorectal Dis. 2013;28(8):1039–47.

63. Huebner RH, Park KC, Shepherd JE, Schwimmer J, Czernin J, Phelps ME, et al. A meta-analysis of the literature for whole-body FDG PET detection of recurrent colorectal cancer. J Nucl Med. 2000;41:1177–89. http://www.ncbi.nlm.nih.gov/pubmed/10914907.

64. Grossmann I, Doornbos PM, Klaase JM, de Bock GH, Wiggers T. Changing patterns of recurrent disease in colorectal cancer. Eur J Surg Oncol. 2014;40:234–9.

65. Ohlsson B, Pålsson B. Follow-up after colorectal cancer surgery. ActaOncol.2003;42(8):816–26.doi:10.1080/02841860310019016.

66. Ding P, Liska D, Tang P, Shia J, Saltz L, Goodman K, et al. Pulmonary recurrence predominates after combined modality therapy for rectal cancer. Ann Surg. 2012;256(1):111–6.

67. Nordholm-Carstensen A, Krarup P-M, Jorgensen LN, Wille-Jorgensen PA, Harling H. Occurrence and survival of synchronous pulmonary metastases in colorectal cancer: a nationwide cohort study. Eur J Cancer. 2014;50(2):447–56.

68. Piñol V, Andreu M, Castells A, Payá A, Bessa X, Jover R. Synchronous colorectal neoplasms in patients with colorectal cancer: predisposing individual and familial factors. Dis Colon Rectum. 2004;47(7):1192–200. doi:10.1007/s10350-004-0562-7.

69. Van Leersum NJ, Aalbers AG, Snijders HS, Henneman D, Wouters MW, Tollenaar RA, et al. Synchronous colorectal carcinoma: a risk factor in colorectal cancer surgery. Dis Colon Rectum. 2014;57(4):460–6. http://journals.lww.com/dcrjournal/Fulltext/2014/04000/Synchronous_Colorectal_Carcinoma___A_Risk_Factor.8.aspx.

70. Rex DK, Kahi CJ, Levin B, Smith RA, Bond JH, Brooks D, et al. Guidelines for colonoscopy surveillance after cancer resection: a consensus update by the American Cancer Society and the US multi-society task force on colorectal cancer. Gastroenterology. 2006;130(6):1865–71.

71. Cone MM, Beck DE, Hicks TE, Rea JD, Whitlow CB, Vargas HD, et al. Timing of colonoscopy after resection for colorectal cancer: are we looking too soon? Dis Colon Rectum. 2013;56(11):1233–6. http://journals.lww.com/dcrjournal/Fulltext/2013/11000/Timing_of_Colonoscopy_After_Resection_for.7.aspx.

72. Scholefield JH, Steele RJ. Guidelines for follow up after resection of colorectal cancer. Gut. 2002;51 suppl 5:v3–5. http://gut.bmj.com/content/51/suppl_5/v3.short.

73. Cairns SR, Scholefield JH, Steele RJ, Dunlop MG, Thomas HJW, Evans GD, et al. Guidelines for colorectal cancer screening and surveillance in moderate and high risk groups (update from 2002). Gut. 2010;59(5):666–89.

74. Cali RL, Pitsch RM, Thorson AG, Watson P, Tapia P, Blatchford GJ, et al. Cumulative incidence of metachronous colorectal cancer. Dis Colon Rectum. 1993;36(4):388–93.

75. Wang T, Cui Y, Huang W-S, Deng Y-H, Gong W, Li C, et al. The role of postoperative colonoscopic surveillance after radical surgery for colorectal cancer: a prospective, randomized clinical study. Gastrointest Endosc. 2009;69(3, Part 2):609–15. http://www.sciencedirect.com/science/article/pii/S0016510708018397.

76. Lan Y-T, Lin J-K, Li A-Y, Lin T-C, Chen W-S, Jiang J-K, et al. Metachronous colorectal cancer: necessity of post-operative colonoscopic surveillance. Int J Colorectal Dis. 2005;20(2):121–5. doi:10.1007/s00384-004-0635-z.

77. Barillari P, Ramacciato G, Manetti G, Bovino A, Sammartino P, Stipa V. Surveillance of colorectal cancer: effectiveness of early detection of intraluminal recurrences on prognosis and survival of patients treated for cure. Dis Colon Rectum. 1996;39(4):388–93. http://journals.lww.com/dcrjournal/Fulltext/1996/39040/Surveillance_of_colorectal_cancer__Effectiveness.5.aspx.

78. Green RJ, Metlay JP, Propert K, Catalano PJ, Macdonald JS, Mayer RJ, et al. Surveillance for second primary colorectal cancer after adjuvant chemotherapy: an analysis of intergroup 0089. Ann Intern Med. 2002;136(4):261–9. doi:10.7326/0003-4819-136-4-200202190-00005.

79. Glimelius B, Tiret E, Cervantes A, Arnold D, Group on behalf of the EGW. Rectal cancer: ESMO Clinical Practice Guidelines for diagnosis, treatment and follow-up. Ann Oncol. 2013;24 suppl 6:vi81–8. http://annonc.oxfordjournals.org/content/24/suppl_6/vi81.short.

80. Davila RE, Rajan E, Baron TH. ASGE guideline: colorectal cancer screening and surveillance. Gastrointest Endosc. 2006;63(4):546–57. http://www.ncbi.nlm.nih.gov/pubmed/16564851.

81. Mulder SA, Kranse R, Damhuis RA, Ouwendijk RJ, Kuipers EJ, van Leerdam ME. The incidence and risk factors of metachronous colorectal cancer: an indication for follow-up. Dis Colon Rectum. 2012;55(5):522–31. http://journals.lww.com/dcrjournal/Fulltext/2012/05000/The_Incidence_and_Risk_Factors_of_Metachronous.5.aspx.

82. Bouvier A-M, Latournerie M, Jooste V, Lepage C, Cottet V, Faivre J. The lifelong risk of metachronous colorectal cancer justifies long-term colonoscopic follow-up. Eur J Cancer. 2008;44(4):522–7. http://www.sciencedirect.com/science/article/pii/S0959804908000129.

83. Chen F, Stuart M. Colonoscopic follow-up of colorectal carcinoma. Dis Colon Rectum. 1994;37(6):568–72. doi:10.1007/BF02050992.

84. Battersby NJ, Coupland A, Bouliotis G, Mirza N, Williams JG. Metachronous colorectal cancer: a competing risks analysis with consideration for a stratified approach to surveillance colonoscopy. J Surg Oncol. 2014;109(5):445–50.

85. Day LW, Walter LC, Velayos F. Colorectal cancer screening and surveillance in the elderly patient. Am J Gastroenterol. 2011;106(7):1197–206. doi:10.1038/ajg.2011.128.

86. Tran AH, Man Ngor EW, Wu BU. Surveillance colonoscopy in elderly patients: a retrospective cohort study. JAMA. 2014;90027(10):1675–82. http://www.ncbi.nlm.nih.gov/pubmed/25111954.

87. Winawer SJ, Stewart ET, Zauber AG, Bond JH, Ansel H, Waye JD, et al. A comparison of colonoscopy and double-contrast barium enema for surveillance after polypectomy. N Engl J Med. 2000;342(24):1766–72. doi:10.1056/NEJM200006153422401.

88. Choi YJ, Park SH, Lee SS, Choi EK, Yu CS, Kim HC, et al. CT colonography for follow-up after surgery for colorectal cancer. AJR Am J Roentgenol. 2007;189(2):283–9.

89. Kim HJ, Park SH, Pickhardt PJ, Yoon SN, Lee SS, Yee J, et al. CT colonography for combined colonic and extracolonic surveillance after curative resection of colorectal cancer. Radiology. 2010;257(3):697–704.

90. Cotton PB, Durkalski VL, Pineau BC, Palesch YY, Mauldin PD, Hoffman B, et al. Computed tomographic colonography (virtual colonoscopy): a multicenter comparison with standard colonoscopy for detection of colorectal neoplasia. JAMA. 2004;291(14):1713–9.

91. Zakaria S, Donohue JH, Que FG, Farnell MB, Schleck CD, Ilstrup DM, et al. Hepatic resection for colorectal metastases: value for risk scoring systems? Ann Surg. 2007;246(2):183–91.

92. Chao M, Gibbs P. Caution is required before recommending routine carcinoembryonic antigen and imaging follow-up for patients with early-stage colon cancer. J Clin Oncol. 2009;27(36):e279–80. http://jco.ascopubs.org/content/27/36/e279.long.

93. A comparison of laparoscopically assisted and open colectomy for colon cancer. N Engl J Med. 2004;350(20):2050–9. http://www.ncbi.nlm.nih.gov/pubmed/15141043

94. Cancer Genome Atlas Network. Comprehensive molecular characterization of human colon and rectal cancer. Nature. 2012;487(7407):330–7. http://www.ncbi.nlm.nih.gov/pubmed/22810696.

95. Zhuang C-L, Ye X-Z, Zhang X-D, Chen B-C, Yu Z. Enhanced recovery after surgery programs versus traditional care for colorectal surgery: a meta-analysis of randomized controlled trials. Dis Colon Rectum. 2013;56(5):667–78. doi:10.1097/DCR.0b013e3182812842.

96. Yamauchi M, Morikawa T, Kuchiba A, Imamura Y, Qian ZR, Nishihara R, et al. Assessment of colorectal cancer molecular

features along bowel subsites challenges the conception of distinct dichotomy of proximal versus distal colorectum. Gut. 2012;61(6):847–54. http://www.ncbi.nlm.nih.gov/pubmed/22427238.

97. Sauer R, Liersch T, Merkel S, Fietkau R, Hohenberger W, Hess C, et al. Preoperative versus postoperative chemoradiotherapy for locally advanced rectal cancer: results of the German CAO/ARO/AIO-94 randomized phase III trial after a median follow-up of 11 years. J Clin Oncol. 2012;30(16):1926–33. http://www.ncbi.nlm.nih.gov/pubmed/22529255.

98. Quirke P, Steele R, Monson J, Grieve R, Khanna S, Couture J, et al. Effect of the plane of surgery achieved on local recurrence in patients with operable rectal cancer: a prospective study using data from the MRC CR07 and NCIC-CTG CO16 randomised clinical trial. Lancet. 2009;373(9666):821–8. http://www.ncbi.nlm.nih.gov/pubmed/19269520.

99. Van Gijn W, Marijnen CA, Nagtegaal ID, Kranenbarg EM, Putter H, Wiggers T, et al. Preoperative radiotherapy combined with total mesorectal excision for resectable rectal cancer: 12-year follow-up of the multicentre, randomised controlled TME trial. Lancet Oncol. 2011;12(6):575–82. http://www.ncbi.nlm.nih.gov/pubmed/21596621.

100. Kusters M, Marijnen CA, van de Velde CJ, Rutten HJ, Lahaye MJ, Kim JH, et al. Patterns of local recurrence in rectal cancer; a study of the Dutch TME trial. Eur J Surg Oncol. 2010;36(5):470–6. http://www.ncbi.nlm.nih.gov/pubmed/20096534.

101. Rasanen M, Carpelan-Holmstrom M, Mustonen H, Renkonen-Sinisalo L, Lepisto A. Pattern of rectal cancer recurrence after curative surgery. Int J Colorectal Dis. 2015;30(6):775–85. http://www.ncbi.nlm.nih.gov/pubmed/25796493.

102. MacFarlane JK, Ryall RD, Heald RJ. Mesorectal excision for rectal cancer. Lancet. 1993;341(8843):457–60. http://www.ncbi.nlm.nih.gov/pubmed/8094488.

103. Wibe A, Rendedal PR, Svensson E, Norstein J, Eide TJ, Myrvold HE, et al. Prognostic significance of the circumferential resection margin following total mesorectal excision for rectal cancer. Br J Surg. 2002;89(3):327–34. http://www.ncbi.nlm.nih.gov/entrez/query.fcgi?cmd=Retrieve&db=PubMed&dopt=Citation&list_uids=11872058.

104. Nagtegaal ID, van de Velde CJ, van der Worp E, Kapiteijn E, Quirke P, van Krieken JH. Macroscopic evaluation of rectal cancer resection specimen: clinical significance of the pathologist in quality control. J Clin Oncol. 2002;20(7):1729–34. http://www.ncbi.nlm.nih.gov/entrez/query.fcgi?cmd=Retrieve&db=PubMed&dopt=Citation&list_uids=11919228.

105. Patel SA, Chen Y-H, Hornick JL, Catalano P, Nowak JA, Zukerberg LR, et al. Early-stage rectal cancer: clinical and pathologic prognostic markers of time to local recurrence and overall survival after resection. Dis Colon Rectum. 2014;57(4):449–59. http://www.ncbi.nlm.nih.gov/pubmed/24608301.

106. Park IJ, You YN, Agarwal A, Skibber JM, Rodriguez-Bigas MA, Eng C, et al. Neoadjuvant treatment response as an early response indicator for patients with rectal cancer. J Clin Oncol. 2012;30(15):1770–6. http://www.pubmedcentral.nih.gov/articlerender.fcgi?artid=3383178&tool=pmcentrez&rendertype=abstract.

107. Trakarnsanga A, Gonen M, Shia J, Goodman KA, Nash GM, Temple LK, et al. What is the significance of the circumferential margin in locally advanced rectal cancer after neoadjuvant chemoradiotherapy? Ann Surg Oncol. 2013;20(4):1179–84. http://www.ncbi.nlm.nih.gov/pubmed/23328971.

108. Nagtegaal ID, Quirke P. What is the role for the circumferential margin in the modern treatment of rectal cancer? J Clin Oncol. 2008;26(2):303–12. http://www.ncbi.nlm.nih.gov/pubmed/18182672.

109. Lohnert MS, Doniec JM, Henne-Bruns D. Effectiveness of endoluminal sonography in the identification of occult local rectal cancer recurrences. Dis Colon Rectum. 2000;43(4):483–91. http://www.ncbi.nlm.nih.gov/pubmed/10789743.

110. De Anda EH, Lee SH, Finne CO, Rothenberger DA, Madoff RD, Garcia-Aguilar J. Endorectal ultrasound in the follow-up of rectal cancer patients treated by local excision or radical surgery. Dis Colon Rectum. 2004;47(6):818–24. http://www.ncbi.nlm.nih.gov/pubmed/15085436.

111. Ramirez JM, Mortensen NJ, Takeuchi N, Humphreys MM. Endoluminal ultrasonography in the follow-up of patients with rectal cancer. Br J Surg. 1994;81(5):692–4.

112. Morken JJ, Baxter NN, Madoff RD, Finne 3rd CO. Endorectal ultrasound-directed biopsy: a useful technique to detect local recurrence of rectal cancer. Int J Color Dis. 2006;21(3):258–64. http://www.ncbi.nlm.nih.gov/pubmed/15942740.

113. Gleeson FC, Larson DW, Dozois EJ, Boardman LA, Clain JE, Rajan E, et al. Local recurrence detection following transanal excision facilitated by EUS-FNA. Hepatogastroenterology. 2012;59(116):1102–7. http://www.ncbi.nlm.nih.gov/pubmed/22281976.

114. Maleki Z, Erozan Y, Geddes S, Li QK. Endorectal ultrasound-guided fine-needle aspiration: a useful diagnostic tool for peri-rectal and intraluminal lesions. Acta Cytol. 2013;57(1):9–18. doi:10.1159/000342919.

115. Lambregts DM, Cappendijk VC, Maas M, Beets GL, Beets-Tan RG. Value of MRI and diffusion-weighted MRI for the diagnosis of locally recurrent rectal cancer. Eur Radiol. 2011;21(6):1250–8. http://www.ncbi.nlm.nih.gov/pubmed/21240647.

116. Titu LV, Nicholson AA, Hartley JE, Breen DJ, Monson JR. Routine follow-up by magnetic resonance imaging does not improve detection of resectable local recurrences from colorectal cancer. Ann Surg. 2006;243(3):348–52. http://www.ncbi.nlm.nih.gov/pubmed/16495699.

117. Nash GM, Weiser MR, Guillem JG, Temple LK, Shia J, Gonen M, et al. Long-term survival after transanal excision of T1 rectal cancer. Dis Colon Rectum. 2009;52(4):577–82.

118. You YN, Baxter NN, Stewart A, Nelson H. Is the increasing rate of local excision for stage I rectal cancer in the United States justified? A nationwide cohort study from the National Cancer Database. Ann Surg. 2007;245(5):726–33.

119. Paty PB, Nash GM, Baron P, Zakowski M, Minsky BD, Blumberg D, et al. Long-term results of local excision for rectal cancer. Ann Surg. 2002;236(4):522–30.

120. Mellgren A, Sirivongs P, Rothenberger DA, Madoff RD, Garcia-Aguilar J. Is local excision adequate therapy for early rectal cancer? Dis Colon Rectum. 2000;43(8):1064. http://www.ncbi.nlm.nih.gov/pubmed/10950004.

121. Habr-Gama A, Perez RO, Sabbaga J, Nadalin W, São Julião GP, Gama-Rodrigues J. Increasing the rates of complete response to neoadjuvant chemoradiotherapy for distal rectal cancer: results of a prospective study using additional chemotherapy during the resting period. Dis Colon Rectum. 2009;52(12):1927–34.

122. Smith JD, Ruby JA, Goodman KA, Saltz LB, Guillem JG, Weiser MR, et al. Nonoperative management of rectal cancer with complete clinical response after neoadjuvant therapy. Ann Surg. 2012;256(6):965–72. http://www.ncbi.nlm.nih.gov/pubmed/23154394.

123. Smith JJ, Chow OS, Eaton A, Widmar M, Nash GM, Temple LKF, et al. Organ preservation in patients with rectal cancer with clinical complete response after neoadjuvant therapy. J Clin Oncol. 2015;33(supp 3):a509. http://meetinglibrary.asco.org/content/140433-158.

124. Weiser MR, Beets-Tan R, Beets G. Management of complete response after chemoradiation in rectal cancer. Surg Oncol Clin N Am. 2014;23(1):113–25. http://www.ncbi.nlm.nih.gov/pubmed/24267169.

125. Habr-Gama A, Perez RO, Proscurshim I, Campos FG, Nadalin W, Kiss D, et al. Patterns of failure and survival for nonoperative treatment of stage c0 distal rectal cancer following neoadjuvant chemoradiation therapy. J Gastrointest Surg. 2006;10(10):1319. http://www.ncbi.nlm.nih.gov/pubmed/17175450.

126. Castells A, Bessa X, Daniels M, Ascaso C, Lacy AM, García-Valdecasas JC, et al. Value of postoperative surveillance after radical surgery for colorectal cancer: results of a cohort study. Dis Colon Rectum. 1998;41(6):714–23. discussion 723–4.

127. Laubert T, Bader FG, Oevermann E, Jungbluth T, Unger L, Roblick UJ, et al. Intensified surveillance after surgery for colorectal cancer significantly improves survival. Eur J Med Res. 2010;15(1):25–30.

128. Vargas GM, Sheffield KM, Parmar AD, Han Y, Brown KM, Riall TS. Physician follow-up and observation of guidelines in the post treatment surveillance of colorectal cancer. Surgery. 2013;154(2):244–55. doi:10.1016/j.surg.2013.04.013.

129. Sisler JJ, Seo B, Katz A, Shu E, Chateau D, Czaykowski P, et al. Concordance with ASCO guidelines for surveillance after colorectal cancer treatment: a population-based analysis. J Oncol Pract. 2012;8(4):e69–79. http://jop.ascopubs.org/content/8/4/e69.abstract.

130. Cheung WY, Pond GR, Rother M, Krzyzanowska MK, Swallow C, Brierley J, et al. Adherence to surveillance guidelines after curative resection for stage II/III colorectal cancer. Clin Colorectal Cancer. 2008;7(3):191–6. http://www.sciencedirect.com/science/article/pii/S1533002811704194.

131. Grossmann I, de Bock GH, van de Velde CJH, Kievit J, Wiggers T. Results of a national survey among Dutch surgeons treating patients with colorectal carcinoma. Current opinion about follow-up, treatment of metastasis, and reasons to revise follow-up practice. Colorectal Dis. 2007;9(9):787–92.

132. Van Steenbergen LN, de Hingh IHJT, Rutten HJT, Rijk MCM, Orsini RG, Coebergh JWW, et al. Large variation between hospitals in follow-up for colorectal cancer in southern Netherlands. Int J Colorectal Dis. 2013;28(9):1257–65. doi:10.1007/s00384-013-1693-x.

133. Søreide K, Træland JH, Stokkeland PJ, Glomsaker T, Søreide JA, Kørner H. Adherence to national guidelines for surveillance after curative resection of nonmetastatic colon and rectum cancer: a survey among Norwegian gastrointestinal surgeons. Colorectal Dis. 2012;14(3):320–4. doi:10.1111/j.1463-1318.2011.02631.x.

134. Cooper GS, Kou TD, Reynolds HL. Receipt of guideline-recommended follow-up in older colorectal cancer survivors. Cancer. 2008;113(8):2029–37. doi:10.1002/cncr.23823.

135. Giordano P, Efron J, Vernava AM, Weiss EG, Nogueras JJ, Wexner SD. Strategies of follow-up for colorectal cancer: a survey of the American society of colon and rectal surgeons. Tech Coloproctol. 2006;10(3):199–207.

136. Cardella J, Coburn NG, Gagliardi A, Maier B-A, Greco E, Last L, et al. Compliance, attitudes and barriers to post-operative colorectal cancer follow-up. J Eval Clin Pract. 2008;14(3):407–15. doi:10.1111/j.1365-2753.2007.00880.x.

137. Wattchow DA, Weller DP, Esterman AJ, Pilotto L. General practice vs. surgical-based follow-up for patients with colon cancer: randomised controlled trial. Br J Cancer. 2006;94(8):1116–21.

138. Augestad KM, Norum J, Dehof S, Aspevik R, Ringberg U, Nestvold T, et al. Cost-effectiveness and quality of life in surgeon versus general practitioner-organised colon cancer surveillance: a randomised controlled trial. BMJ Open. 2013;3(4):e002391. http://bmjopen.bmj.com/content/3/4/e002391.abstract.

139. Haggstrom D, Arora N, Helft P, Clayman M, Oakley-Girvan I. Follow-up care delivery among colorectal cancer survivors most often seen by primary and subspecialty care physicians. J Gen Intern Med. 2009;24(2):472–9. doi:10.1007/s11606-009-1017-6.

140. Standeven L, Price Hiller J, Mulder K, Zhu G, Ghosh S, Spratlin JL. Impact of a dedicated cancer center surveillance program on guideline adherence for patients with stage II and III colorectal cancer. Clin Colorectal Cancer. 2013;12(2):103–12. doi:10.1016/j.clcc.2012.09.006.

141. Strand E, Nygren I, Bergkvist L, Smedh K. Nurse or surgeon follow-up after rectal cancer: a randomized trial. Colorectal Dis. 2011;13(9):999–1003. doi:10.1111/j.1463-1318.2010.02317.x.

142. Papagrigoriadis S, Heyman B. Patients' views on follow up of colorectal cancer: implications for risk communication and decision making. Postgrad Med J. 2003;79(933):403–7. http://www.ncbi.nlm.nih.gov/pmc/articles/PMC1742752/.

143. Kjeldsen BJ, Thorsen H, Whalley D, Kronborg O. Influence of follow-up on health-related quality of life after radical surgery for colorectal cancer. Scand J Gastroenterol. 1999;34(5):509–15.

144. Stiggelbout AM, de Haes JC, Vree R, van de Velde CJ, Bruijninckx CM, van Groningen K, et al. Follow-up of colorectal cancer patients: quality of life and attitudes towards follow-up. Br J Cancer. 1997;75(6):914–20. http://www.ncbi.nlm.nih.gov/pmc/articles/PMC2063387/.

145. Virgo KS, Vernava AM, Longo WE, McKirgan LW, Johnson FE. Cost of patient follow-up after potentially curative colorectal cancer treatment. JAMA. 1995;273(23):1837–41.

146. Dinan MA, Curtis LH, Hammill BG, Patz EF, Abernethy AP, Shea AM, et al. Changes in the use and costs of diagnostic imaging among Medicare beneficiaries with cancer, 1999–2006. JAMA. 2010;303(16):1625–31.

147. Audisio R, Setti-Carraro P, Segala M, Capko D, Andreoni B, Tiberio G. Follow-up in colorectal cancer patients: a cost-benefit analysis. Ann Surg Oncol. 1996;3(4):349–57. doi:10.1007/BF02305664.

148. Renehan AG, O'Dwyer ST, Whynes DK, Renehan AG, O'Dwyer ST, Whynes DK. Cost effectiveness analysis of intensive versus conventional follow up after curative resection for colorectal cancer. BMJ Br Med J. 2004;328(7431):81. http://www.ncbi.nlm.nih.gov/pmc/articles/PMC314047/.

149. Borie F, Combescure C, Daurès J-P, Trétarre B, Millat B. Cost-effectiveness of two follow-up strategies for curative resection of colorectal cancer: comparative study using a markov model. World J Surg. 2004;28(6):563–9. doi:10.1007/s00268-004-7256-0.
150. Longley DB, McDermott U, Johnston PG. Predictive markers for colorectal cancer: current status and future prospects. Clin Colorectal Cancer. 2003;2(4):223–30.
151. Rose J, Augestad K, Kong C, Meropol N, Kattan M, Hong Q, et al. A simulation model of colorectal cancer surveillance and recurrence. BMC Med Inform Decis Mak. 2014;14(1):1–13. doi:10.1186/1472-6947-14-29.
152. Radespiel-Tröger M, Hohenberger W, Reingruber B. Improved prediction of recurrence after curative resection of colon carcinoma using tree-based risk stratification. Cancer. 2004;100(5):958–67. doi:10.1002/cncr.20065.
153. Soreide K. Endoscopic surveillance after curative surgery for sporadic colorectal cancer: patient-tailored, tumor-targeted or biology-driven? Scand J Gastroenterol. 2010;45(10):1255–61.
154. Johnson FE, Virgo KS, Grossmann EM, Longo WE, Fossati R. Colorectal cancer patient follow-up following surgery with curative intent: the GILDA trial. J Clin Oncol. 2004;22 (14 suppl):3645. http://hwmaint.meeting.ascopubs.org/cgi/content/abstract/22/14_suppl/3645.

35

Colorectal Cancer: Management of Local Recurrence

Eric J. Dozois and Dorin T. Colibaseanu

Key Concepts

- Patients with colorectal cancer at the highest risk for local recurrence are those who present with obstruction or perforation, higher-stage disease, and adverse pathologic features, or undergo an operation that does not adhere to standard oncologic principles.
- The most significant predictor of survival following surgery for local recurrence is the ability to achieve a negative-margin (R0) resection.
- The probability of achieving an R0 resection is much greater in patients with recurrences involving an anastomosis or urogynecologic structures compared with those involving para-aortic tissue, sacrum, or lateral pelvic sidewall.
- A dedicated multidisciplinary team at an institution experienced in the management of patients with local colorectal cancer recurrence can facilitate complex surgical decision-making and greatly enhance patient outcomes.
- A multimodality approach that includes chemotherapy and radiotherapy improves local control and improves 5-year survival in patients with local recurrence.

Introduction

The medical and surgical management of colorectal cancer has a rich history, and treatment paradigms have evolved significantly over the last 100 years [1–6]. Major advances have been made in our understanding of tumor biology, the role of chemoradiotherapy, and most importantly, the significance of precise surgical technique. These advances have dramatically decreased local recurrence and increased 5-year survival in patients with primary colorectal cancer [1, 6–9]. Despite these advances, local recurrence following surgery remains a significant problem [4, 10–18]. In addition to its impact on survival, major morbidity from local recurrence can have a dramatic detrimental impact on quality of life [19–21].

In the United States, approximately 90,000 patients are diagnosed with colon cancer each year, and in those that undergo surgery, somewhere between 8 and 12 % will develop a local recurrence [22, 23]. Of the 40,000 patients diagnosed with rectal cancer each year, approximately 5–30 % will develop a local recurrence [24–28]. Patients with colorectal cancer at the highest risk for local recurrence are those that have higher-stage disease, high-grade tumors, and lymphovascular involvement or present with obstruction, perforation, or a locally advanced tumor at the time of presentation [29–34]. Operations done by noncolorectal-trained surgeons, or by surgeons who perform less than 20 rectal cancer resections per year, have been reported to have higher local recurrence rates [30]. Recently, the importance of a threatened or violated circumferential margin as an independent predictor of future recurrence has reinforced the importance of meticulous surgical technique [15, 35, 36]. All efforts to reduce the risk of local recurrence should be made when managing primary colorectal cancer, and the best results are achieved when patients are managed by experienced teams [37, 38].

When patients with colorectal cancer develop local recurrence, surgery offers the best opportunity for cure [15, 24, 39]. In the last 20 years, surgery for local recurrence has become safer, indications have expanded, and better results are being achieved leading to meaningful survival for many patients [17, 18, 40–42]. This chapter will review all aspects of management in patients with local recurrence as well as outcomes of surgery. Due to the complexity of medical and surgical decision-making, in addition to the surgical expertise required to perform these technically challenging operations, the treatment of patients with local recurrence should preferentially occur at centers that have a dedicated and experienced multidisciplinary team.

© Springer International Publishing 2016
S.R. Steele et al. (eds.), *The ASCRS Textbook of Colon and Rectal Surgery*, DOI 10.1007/978-3-319-25970-3_35

Preoperative Evaluation and Patient Selection

The majority of colorectal cancer relapses following surgery occur within 3 years of resection [7, 16, 26, 28, 43]. Most but not all patients will have symptoms from recurrent disease, and these will include pain, malaise, bleeding, and symptoms of partial obstruction [21]. In some patients, carcinoembryonic antigen (CEA) levels will be elevated, and this finding in the asymptomatic patient should trigger a workup for recurrence.

In patients with suspected local recurrence, every attempt should be made to obtain tissue for confirmation. Patients with luminal local recurrences can undergo endoscopy to obtain tissue. In patients with suspicious radiographic findings, obtaining tissue confirmation may be more challenging. Most patients with recurrent colon cancer will have obvious findings on imaging to confidently diagnose them with recurrence, and a transabdominal biopsy should be avoided. In contrast, every attempt should be made to obtain tissue confirmation in patients with suspected pelvic recurrence. One should be hesitant to undertake a major pelvic resection without tissue confirmation of recurrence. In our experience, computed tomography (CT)-guided percutaneous biopsy has been very useful to confirm or refute the presence of recurrence. In some cases, it may be very difficult to differentiate postoperative changes from recurrent tumor based on imaging alone. CT-guided percutaneous biopsy can confirm recurrence, but a negative result does not rule it out. In the absence of a tissue diagnosis, a rising CEA, with a notable change in the size of the lesion on serial imaging, and lesions that are positron emission tomography (PET) avid can be considered consistent with recurrent disease.

Patients with recurrent colorectal cancer being considered for curative-intent resection undergo imaging studies to assess the local-regional characteristics of the recurrence and to exclude metastatic disease [17, 18, 40]. Our protocol includes fusion PET-CT imaging of the chest, abdomen, and pelvis and magnetic resonance imaging (MRI) of the pelvis for recurrent rectal cancers. Several studies have confirmed that 18-fluorodeoxyglucose PET imaging has a high sensitivity for the detection of locoregional and distant recurrences in patients with colorectal cancer [44–46]. In the evaluation of 58 patients for advanced or recurrent colorectal cancer, Ogunbiyi et al. found that PET imaging had a sensitivity and specificity of 91 % and 100 %, respectively [47]. Chessin et al. showed that fusion imaging that combines CT and PET imaging has an enhanced sensitivity of 98 % as compared to 64 % with standard CT for the detection of rectal recurrence; in other studies, fusion imaging led to altered management in 58 % of patients [48, 49]. Moreover, PET retains its diagnostic ability even after irradiation, and because of this, we believe that all patients being considered for resection should undergo this study.

When seeing patients with local recurrence, it is important to obtain a complete history and physical examination. All records of previous treatments (surgical and chemoradiotherapy) should be reviewed. Pain and neurologic dysfunction may be a sign of advanced pelvic disease [15]. Bilateral lower extremity edema is an indicator of venous or lymphatic obstruction. A full colonoscopy should be done to rule out any synchronous lesions. If the rectum is intact, a digital rectal exam can assess the relationship of the recurrent cancer to the sphincter complex, prostate, or posterior vaginal wall. Cystoscopy may be useful to assess transmural invasion of the bladder.

Laboratory tests should be obtained by looking particularly for anemia and the nutritional state of the patient. The patient's albumin, prealbumin, and transferrin levels will give an idea of the protein reserves of the patient. If required, nutritional supplementation should be instituted to strengthen the immune system and optimize wound healing. A significantly elevated CEA should raise concern for occult metastatic disease [50].

Operations for local recurrence are often long and can be associated with significant blood loss, systemic inflammation, and tissue trauma, and the overall stress response associated with these big operations can pose significant risk to patients [51, 52]. Despite this, recent series have demonstrated a very low mortality following these major resections [17, 18, 40]. Patients with significant chronic obstructive pulmonary disease and cardiovascular conditions should be carefully evaluated and optimized preoperatively. Patients with ASA classifications of IV or V will be at the highest surgical risk and are generally not candidates for a major resection.

The decision to go ahead with a major, potentially morbid operation for local recurrence requires that the patient is fully informed regarding the risks and life-changing impact on quality of life. Ultimately, it should be the well-informed patient who decides what disability that might arise from surgery they are willing to live with. The likelihood of a stoma is high, and patients should be counseled by a stoma therapist preoperatively [53–55]. Patients undergoing multivisceral and musculoskeletal resections will require the most intense counseling regarding their postoperative recovery, limitations, and potential morbidity and mortality [14, 27, 42, 56].

The inclusion criteria for surgery in patients with recurrence have expanded significantly in the last 10 years [57]. In determining who should be offered surgery, one must consider the goals of the operation. If palliation is the goal, surgery must have a high probability of symptomatic relief and not be significantly morbid. If oncologic cure is the goal, the ability to confidently achieve a margin-negative (R0) resection must be highly probable. Based on multiple studies in patients with recurrent colorectal cancer, the number one determinant of oncologic benefit is the ability to achieve an

R0 resection. Multiple points of tumor fixation may limit the surgeon's ability to achieve an R0 resection, and this finding on evaluation has been associated with poor outcomes [15]. Patients operated for central recurrences that extend anteriorly (urogenital, gynecologic organs) have the best opportunity for an R0 resection and, therefore, good outcomes following surgery [15, 16, 58]. When a recurrence in the pelvis extends posteriorly to the sacrum or lateral to the pelvic sidewall, the ability to achieve an R0 resection becomes much less certain. In cases where there is significant lateral extension of the tumor, specifically through the sciatic notch, a positive margin is almost certain unless an extended resection such as a hemipelvectomy is done [41].

Contraindications to surgery will vary from institution to institution and from surgeon to surgeon. Local recurrences that involve major vascular structures, the high sacrum, or extensive pelvic sidewall disease were frequently listed in publications as contraindications to surgery in the past [16, 59, 60]. In the modern era, several well-recognized and respected centers have expanded their indications in light of increasing data demonstrating meaningful survival in patients undergoing extended resections [17, 18, 40, 42, 57]. In the author's view, contraindications to surgery should be based primarily on the inability to completely clear the tumor with the understanding that limited survival benefit is achieved if gross residual tumor remains.

Classification of Local Recurrence and Determining Resectability

Classification schemes for both recurrent colon cancer and rectal cancer have been proposed and are used not only to characterize patterns of recurrence but also to predict R0 resectability and oncologic outcomes [61].

Locoregional recurrence in patients with colon cancer can be classified as four distinct groups and include peri-anastomotic (mural disease), mesenteric (regional nodal disease), retroperitoneal or pelvic (drop metastases, distant nodal disease, or residual disease transmural disease), and peritoneal. In a study from the Memorial Sloan Kettering Cancer Center, Bowne et al. demonstrated that the most common site of recurrence was peri-anastomotic (36 %), followed by peritoneal (16 %), mesenteric (15 %), and retroperitoneal (12 %) [62]. In our experience, some cases of recurrence were directly attributed to inadequate mesenteric resections at the time of original surgery. However, most nodal-based relapses were found at nodal sites (iliac, para-aortic) not typically removed during standard oncologic resection [63].

Pelvic recurrences can be broadly categorized in terms of what resection would be necessary for complete tumor removal. With this in mind, the authors have generally classified recurrences as those requiring an anterior, posterior, lateral, or combined resection (Figure 35-1). In anterior resections, the rectum and urogynecologic structures are removed. A posterior resection involves removing the rectum and a portion of the sacrum. A lateral resection involves removal of the rectum and iliac vessels and/or components of the lumbosacral plexus. The term "combined resection" or "composite resection" includes any combination of anterior, posterior, or lateral structures.

For recurrent colon cancer, CT imaging is our study of choice to make decisions regarding resectability. For recurrent rectal cancer, MRI of the pelvis is our study of choice to assess neuromuscular and bony involvement and for surgical planning. We use a musculoskeletal protocol that is done with and without gadolinium and includes sagittal, axial, and coronal oblique views (Figure 35-2). MRI has highly detailed soft-tissue resolution, which is helpful in planning lines of resection as it pertains to adjacent structures. Specifically, for tumors with posterior and lateral extension, MRI can determine proximal sacral extent, involvement of lumbosacral nerves, and whether or not a margin can be obtained on the lateral pelvic sidewall. Computerized tomography or MR angiogram or venogram may add additional information regarding vascular involvement and indicate the need for a vascular surgeon to be a member of the multidisciplinary surgical team.

A major challenge from a surgical planning perspective in many cases of local recurrence is the fact that the borders of recurrences can be indiscrete and ill defined on imaging. Recurrences may be infiltrative and sheetlike and sometimes have islands of intervening normal tissue. This makes it difficult to preoperatively determine where the "true margins" are. Because of this, one must be prepared to alter the surgical plan intraoperatively as findings may differ significantly from what the preoperative imaging suggested. Intraoperative frozen section pathologic analysis can be very useful to ensure that further resection can be done if there is a persistent microscopic margin discovered at the time of surgery.

Another challenge in management of local recurrence is differentiating both postoperative and radiation-induced fibrosis from actual tumor. MRI with T2-weighted imaging can assist because fibrosis and tumor demonstrate different signal intensities [64]. Gadolinium-enhanced MRI is reported to have an 88 % and 95 % sensitivity and specificity, for the detection of pelvic recurrences in the setting of previous surgery and radiation [65].

Multimodal Therapy Including Intraoperative Radiation

Multimodal therapy in the management of locally recurrent colorectal cancer refers to a treatment approach that includes pre- and postoperative systemic chemotherapy, preoperative external beam radiotherapy (EBRT), and, in some protocols, intraoperative radiation therapy (IORT). The authors have used this approach very selectively in patients with recurrent

FIGURE 35-1. Classification of recurrence. (**a**) *Anterior*: involves structures anterior to the neorectum. (**b**) *Posterior*: involves structures posterior to the neorectum. (**c**) *Lateral*: involves pelvic sidewall and associated structures. (**d**) *Combined anterior-posterior*: tumor includes anterior and posterior structures. ©By permission of Mayo Clinic Foundation for Medical Education and Research. All rights reserved.

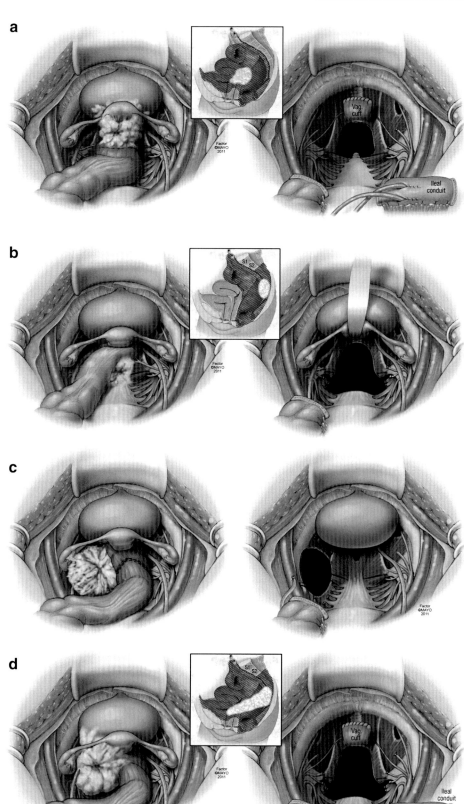

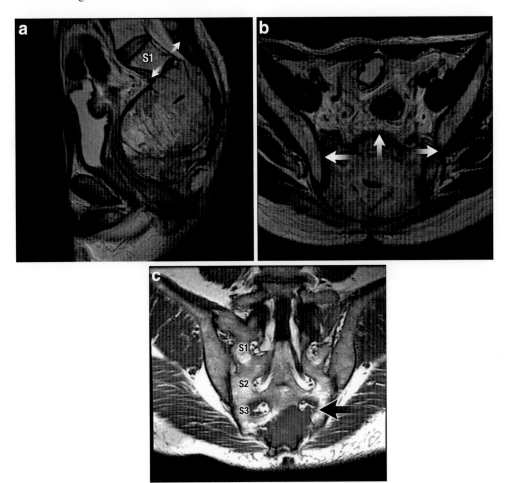

FIGURE 35-2. MRI assessing neuromuscular and bony involvement for surgical planning in recurrent rectal cancer. (**a**) Sagittal section showing cephalad and posterior extension of the recurrence to the first sacral body (S1). *White arrows* demonstrating lines of resection necessary for R0 resection; (**b**) coronal section demonstrating soft-tissue extension anteriorly and laterally, with viscera and bilateral iliac involvement (*white arrows*); (**c**) coronal/oblique view showing left nerve root involvement (*black arrow*).

colon cancer and in almost all cases of recurrent rectal cancer. In patients with locally recurrent colon cancer, there is usually less concern about the ability to get a wide surgical resection unless tumor abuts fixed critical structures (e.g., lumbar spine, aorta, vena cava). In these cases, we will employ a full multimodality approach that included IORT [63]. Since 1981, curative-intent therapy at our institution has included IORT for locally advanced and locally recurrent rectal cancer. Our protocol includes neoadjuvant chemotherapy and EBRT, IORT, and postoperative chemotherapy [13, 21, 66]. Patients who are radiation naïve receive 50.4 Gy of EBRT with concurrent five FU-based chemotherapies over 5 weeks followed by a 6–8-week recovery period before surgery. In patients who have received previous irradiation, we give 20–30 Gy with concurrent five FU-based chemotherapies, over a 3-week period followed by surgery within 7 days of the last dose of radiation. The amount of radiation given intraoperatively to the tumor resection bed depends on the margin status at the time of resection. For wide margins

(500–750 cGy), R1 (1000–1250 cGy), <2 cm of gross residual (1500 cGy) and for >2 cm gross residual (1750–2000 cGy) [66]. Given that distant relapse of disease is the most common cause of death following surgery for local recurrence, systemic chemotherapy is part of our multimodality protocol. In a series of 607 patients with locally recurrent colorectal cancer treated at our institution with a multimodality approach that included IORT, the cumulative incidence of distant relapse was 53 % at 5 years. Distant relapse was less common in patients who had R0 vs. R1 or R2 resections and in those treated with postoperative chemotherapy [66]. Significant advances in chemotherapeutic regimens over the last 20 years have likely decreased the incidence of distant failures following surgery for local recurrence, but the optimal regimen and length of treatment are still debated.

Though there is a paucity of randomized data, many authors agree that a multimodality approach can significantly decrease local relapse and improve 5-year survival in

TABLE 35-1. Survival and local recurrence after intraoperative radiation therapy in patients undergoing R0 resection (adapted with permission from Ref [66])

Study	Patients (no.)	IORT dose (Gy)	EBRT dose (Gy)	5-year survival rate (%)	5-year local control rate (%)
Vermaas et al. 2005	17	10	50	45 (3 years)	35 (3 years)
Alektiar et al. 2000	53	10–18	45–50.4	36	43
Abuchaibe et al. 1993	8	15	40–50	29	50
Dresen et al. 2008	84	10–15	50.4 or 30.6	59 (3 years)	75 (3 years)
Lindel et al. 2001	25	10–20	50.4	40	56
Eble et al. 1998	14	12	41.4	71 (4 years)	79 (4 years)
Wiig et al. 2002	18	15	46–50	60	70
Valentini et al. 1999	11	10–15	45–47	41	80
Haddock et al. 2011	226	12.5 (median)	30.0–0.4	46	72

EBRT external beam radiation therapy, *IORT* intraoperative radiation therapy. EBRT generally was delivered only to patients not previously treated with radiation, except for patients in Dresen et al. (2008) [39] and the current series. Five-year rates are shown unless otherwise indicated. Lower doses were administered in previously irradiated patients

With permission from Haddock MG, Gunderson LL, Nelson H, Cha SS, Devine RM, Dozois RR, et al. Intraoperative irradiation for locally recurrent colorectal cancer in previously irradiated patients. International journal of radiation oncology, biology, physics. 2001;49(5):1267-74. [21] ©Elsevier 2001

TABLE 35-2. Survival and local control after intraoperative radiation therapy in patients undergoing R1 and R2 resection (adapted with permission from Ref [66])

Study	Patients (no.)	Surgical margins	IORT dose (Gy)	5-year survival rate (%[a])	5-year local control rate (%)
Vermaas et al. 2005	10	R1–R2	10	21 (3 years)	21 (3 years)
Alektiar et al. 2000	21	R1	10–18	11	26
Abuchaibe et al. 1993	19	R1–R2	15	7	16
Dresen et al. 2008	34	R1	12.5	27 (3 years)	29 (3 years)
	29	R2	15–17.5	24 (3 years)	29 (3 years)
Lindel et al. 2001	9	R1	10–15	11	33
	15	R2	15–20	13	12
Eble et al. 1998	9	R1	10–20	33 (4-year RFS)	67
	8	R2	10–20	25 (4-year RFS)	63
Martinez-Mong et al. 1999	39	R1	10–15	6	26
	41	R2	15–20	7	29
Wiig et al. 2002	29	R1	15	20	50
	12	R2	17.5–20	0	–
Haddock et al. 2011	224	R1	15 (median)	27	68
	156	R2	20 (median)	16	68

IORT intraoperative radiation therapy, *RFS* relapse-free survival
Five-year rates are shown unless otherwise indicated
With permission from Haddock MG, Gunderson LL, Nelson H, Cha SS, Devine RM, Dozois RR, et al. Intraoperative irradiation for locally recurrent colorectal cancer in previously irradiated patients. International journal of radiation oncology, biology, physics. 2001;49(5):1267-74 [21]. ©Elsevier 2001

colorectal cancer patients with local recurrence [15, 67, 68]. Several centers have shown good results with the use of IORT in patients with recurrent colorectal cancer, and 5-year survival rates range from 29 to 60 % in patients undergoing R0 resection (Table 35-1). Five-year survival rates after IORT in patients having R1 or R2 resection can be as high as 16 % and 27 %, respectively (Table 35-2). In most series where IORT is not included in the management of patients who had an R2 resection, no long-term survival is seen [66].

Radiation-induced toxicity is a significant concern in patients receiving multimodality therapy that includes IORT. In many cases, it may be hard to separate IORT-related complications from surgical ones. In a published series of 607 patients from our institution with recurrent colorectal cancer treated with EBRT and IORT, we attributed radiation specifically as the cause for some septic complications (wound related, enterocutaneous fistulas), small bowel and ureteral obstructions, as well as neuropathy [66]. Both the incidence and severity of neuropathy were related to IORT dose. Doses that exceeded 12.5 Gy were associated with a higher rate and severity. In total, 15 % of patients experienced some grade of neuropathy, with only 3 % of patients suffering from grade 3 neuropathy defined as severe weakness or intractable pain.

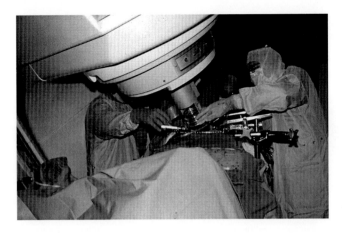

FIGURE 35-3. The IORT suite; the operating table is positioned under the linear accelerator by the radiation oncologist and the appropriate Lucite cone is affixed to direct the beam.

Technical Aspects of Surgical Resection

General Considerations

We use ureteral stents for all operations in patients with local recurrence in the pelvis. The Lloyd-Davies position is used to allow access to the perineum. Care is taken to protect the extremities from nerve injury with adequate padding of both the tucked arms and lateral lower extremities in the stirrups. An exploratory laparotomy is carried out through a midline incision to confirm absence of extra-pelvic disease and determine local resectability. Any lesions suspicious for metastatic disease are biopsied and sent for frozen section analysis. The presence of metastatic disease typically precludes resection for cure, and proceeding on to resection of the local recurrence has to be weighed carefully. All adherent tissue to the recurrence tumor should be resected en bloc. In general, the technical approach to local recurrence in the abdomen or in the pelvis is carried out by widely mobilizing normal surrounding tissues and organs in preserved embryologic planes when feasible and working toward the distorted anatomy and malignant pathology. This allows exposure of structures that are close to the recurrence but will be preserved if not invaded. In addition, vascular pedicles and collateral vasculature should be well delineated prior to ultimate mobilization of the recurrence and surrounding adherent tissue or organs, so that when significant bleeding is encountered, proximal and distal vascular control can be achieved safely.

Most cases for recurrence at our institution are done in a dedicated IORT operating room. This suite houses our linear accelerator and mobile anesthesia equipment that allows the patient to move into the optimal position for IORT (Figure 35-3). The radiation dose and field are selected based on tumor margin status. At our institution, Lucite cones are used to focus the beam of radiation delivered by the linear accelerator and protect the small bowel and other organs from radiation injury (Figure 35-4). The radiation oncologist and surgeon position the cone together for optimal radiation delivery.

Recurrent Colon Cancer

As previously stated, local recurrence in patients with colon cancer typically occurs in one of three patterns, luminal, locoregional, or para-aortic lymphatics, and in the resection bed of the previous index colectomy. Luminal and locoregional nodal recurrences are generally straightforward technically, and surgery involves resection of additional colon and adjacent mesentery. During operations in patients with retained mesentery from incomplete previous surgery, it is the author's experience that isolation and ligation of the vascular pedicles of the original tumor (that should have been removed during the index operation) is a good initial step to allow safe mobilization of the recurrence that lies within the retained mesentery. In cases where para-aortic or para-iliac nodes are involved, major vascular reconstruction may be necessary in addition to en bloc resection of surrounding structures (Figure 35-5) [69].

In cases where recurrence occurs in the previous resection bed, locoregional structures associated with the course of the colon are often involved (kidney, ureters, psoas muscle, stomach, spleen, duodenum, and pancreas). The most complex resections done for local recurrence after right colon resection are those that involve the duodenum and the head of the pancreas. When a Whipple operation is required, we involve a hepatobiliary surgeon to assist with resection and reconstruction. In cases where IORT will be used, radiation is delivered to the at-risk tumor bed just prior to closure.

Recurrent Rectal Cancer

Recurrences That Extend Anteriorly

After ruling out metastatic disease, the left colon is fully mobilized and transected at the appropriate level for subsequent end colostomy (in patients who have intestinal continuity). The entrance to the pelvis is cleared of loops of small bowel for optimal pelvic exposure. Dissection begins in the lower abdomen before entering the presacral space along the lower aorta and continues distally over the iliac vessels and ureters. Vasiloops are used to retract the ureters and vascular structures. In the re-operative pelvis, dense fibrosis and distorted anatomy require careful, meticulous dissection to avoid inadvertent injuries and major bleeding complications. In the author's experience, the most at-risk region for significant bleeding occurs during mobilization of the left common iliac vein, and this dissection should proceed with caution. Posterior lumbar branches, if not identified and injured, can lead to significant blood loss if avulsed.

The anterior and lateral lines of resection (decided upon during preoperative review of imaging) are delineated and confirmed, and the involved structures and organs are mobilized widely for subsequent en bloc resection. The presacral space is further developed, and the dissection is

FIGURE 35-4. (a) Assortment of
Lucite cones of different size
used to direct the IORT field, (b)
in situ placement of the Lucite
tube.

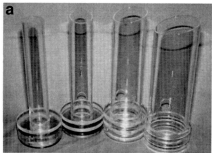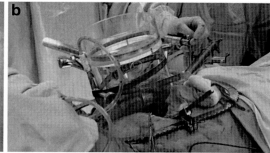

FIGURE 35-5. (a) Illustration of
a local recurrence involving the
aortic bifurcation, colon, kidney,
and ureter, (b) en bloc resection
with aortoiliac reconstruction.

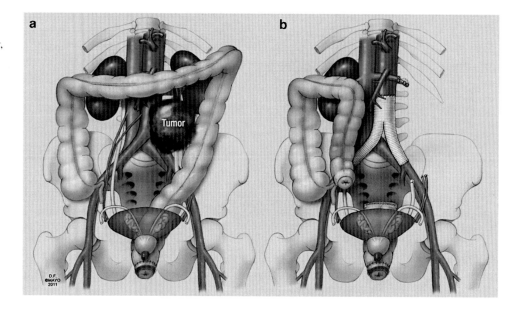

carried down along the anterior sacrum being careful to stay anterior to Waldeyer's fascia to avoid the presacral venous plexus. The dissection is then carried laterally along the pelvic sidewall on each side with careful protection of the lumbosacral plexus and internal iliac vessels. The deepest part of the pelvic dissection will be the pelvic floor musculature, which can be incised during the abdominal portion of the procedure. When the transabdominal portion reaches this point, a combined transperineal approach facilitates final tumor removal. The transperineal portion begins with purse-string closure of the anus (if present), and then a wide, elliptical incision is made to include the sphincter complex and as much pelvic floor musculature as possible. With a surgeon working above, the two dissection planes can be joined safely and with careful attention to the tumor margins.

In women, anterior involvement may require resection of the posterior wall of vagina, and this portion of the operation is approached transvaginally and transabdominally simultaneously. In men, anterior fixation often requires cystoprostatectomy due to invasion of the trigone and prostate. Partial

cystectomy may be sufficient in rare cases. When a urinary conduit is necessary, the ureters are mobilized as close to the bladder as possible to provide adequate length to reach the conduit. To mobilize the bladder, the space of Retzius is entered to fully mobilize the anterior portion of the bladder. The blood supply to the bladder (superior and inferior pedicles) is taken serially along the pelvic sidewall off the internal iliac vessels. The wings of peritoneum to the bladder are then taken down until the bilateral vasa are identified and clipped. The endopelvic fascia is opened bilaterally. The dorsal venous complex is subsequently ligated. The urethra is then delivered into the wound and transected.

Once the tumor is out, the surgeon orients the specimen for the pathologist and frozen section margins are assessed. If margins are not clear, further resection is undertaken when safe to achieve an R0 resection. At this point, IORT is given to the at-risk resection bed. Creation of end colostomy and urinary conduit completes the procedure. In women in whom a large portion of the posterior vaginal wall is removed, a vertical rectus abdominis flap (VRAM) is used for vaginal reconstruction.

Resection That Includes Sacrectomy

Stage I: Anterior Component

This dissection begins as outlined above for anterior recurrences. Once the deep pelvic portion of the operation begins, the anterior, lateral, and superior (along the spine) lines of resection are delineated, and the involved neuromuscular structures and organs are mobilized widely for subsequent en bloc resection. Frozen section biopsies are taken as needed to establish that final margins will be negative.

Vascular exposure often requires mobilization of the lower aorta and vena cava, in addition to the iliac arteries and veins. If vascular structures need to be resected en bloc with the tumor, the decision to do so is made here. If the resection does not require aortoiliac reconstruction, circumferential mobilization of the common and external iliac arteries will facilitate exposure of the veins. The internal iliac artery branches are ligated and divided first, distal to the takeoff of the posterior division superior gluteal artery branch, to preserve blood flow to the gluteal muscles and soft tissue of the perineum. Multiple internal iliac vein branches are then ligated after control of the main trunk(s) of the internal iliac vein has been achieved. The branches are ligated and divided before ligation of the main trunk to avoid venous distention of the branches, which can lead to troublesome bleeding (Figure 35-6). Lateral and middle sacral vein branches, which drain into the posterior aspect of the left common iliac vein and caval confluence, are ligated and divided. Suture ligature is preferable for short, broad-based internal iliac

vein branches. The vascular dissection is carried along both sides of the sacrum onto the pelvic floor. In general, the internal iliac vessels are taken at their confluence as part of any sacrectomy above the third sacral body. For sacrectomy at or below the third sacral body, we generally preserve the internal iliac vessels.

Once the most proximal lumbosacral level of transection is determined, unicortical anterior osteotomies are performed at the bony level of resection (Figure 35-7). Prior to closing the abdomen, a thick Silastic mesh is placed anterior to the sacrum and posterior to the ureters, aorta, iliac vessels, and soft-tissue structures to protect against injury when blind osteotomies are performed during the second stage of the procedure, at which point the patient is in prone position. A titanium screw is also placed at the level of the osteotomy site to facilitate performing the posterior osteotomies by using intraoperative fluoroscopy (Figure 35-8).

During the anterior stage of the operation, IORT may be delivered prior to final tumor resection if orientation of the Lucite cone in the prone position will not be feasible to radiate the at-risk tumor bed. A colostomy and ileal or colonic urinary conduit are fashioned as needed, and a VRAM flap is then elevated for subsequent perineal reconstruction.

Stage II: Posterior Component

The second stage of the procedure is typically carried out 2 days after the anterior portion. With the patient in the prone position, a posterior midline incision is made along the middle

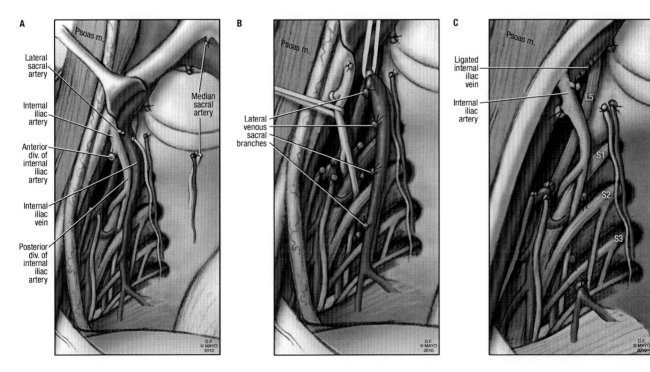

FIGURE 35-6. (a) Pelvic vascular anatomy. Ligation of anterior division of internal iliac artery, lateral sacral arteries and veins, and sacral artery and vein. (b) Ligation of lateral venous sacral branches. (c) Ligation of internal iliac vein.

580 E.J. Dozois and D.T. Colibaseanu

FIGURE 35-7. Unicortical anterior transverse osteotomy.

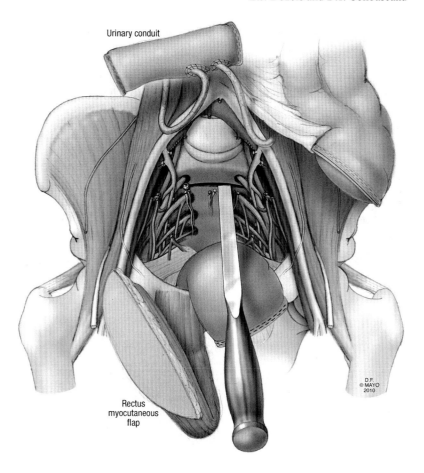

Urinary conduit

Rectus myocutaneous flap

FIGURE 35-8. Placement of Silastic mesh to protect pelvic vasculature during the posterior osteotomies. Titanium screw marks the level of the anterior osteotomy to guide fluoroscopic identification of anterior osteotomy level when performing posterior osteotomy.

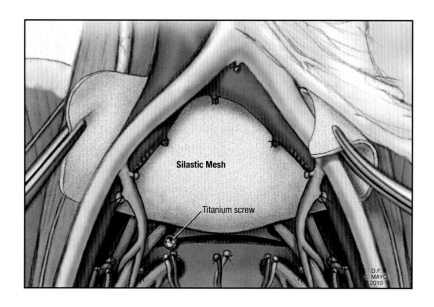

Silastic Mesh

Titanium screw

portion of the sacrum, and the gluteus maximus muscles are dissected away from the sacral attachments. The sacrospinous and sacrotuberous ligaments are divided to access the pelvic cavity posteriorly. The piriformis muscles are divided while protecting the sciatic and pudendal nerves. Laminectomy, dural sac ligation, and posterior sacral osteotomies are then carried out (Figure 35-9). Final osteotomies are performed based on the preoperative MRI imaging studies and intraoperative fluoroscopy to identify the anterior positioned titanium screw. After resection, the surgical team meets with the pathologist to accurately orient the specimen, and together they assess the completeness of resection. If frozen section analysis demonstrates an R1 or R2 margin, wider resection is undertaken as it can be done safely. Before soft-tissue wound reconstruction is done, IORT is given (if not given during stage I) and the dose is based on tumor margin status, as discussed above.

Stage III: Spinal Reconstructive Component

In cases where the lumbosacral line is transected, spinopelvic stability is compromised and patients will require instrumented reconstruction. For resections above the level of the S1 neuroforamen but below the lumbosacral junction, clinical experience and biomechanical studies have shown that in situ spinopelvic stabilization is beneficial to avoid collapse of the residual sacrum [70]. In these cases, an instrumented posterior spinopelvic fusion is made from the lower lumbar spine to the remaining pelvis.

Resections done through the lumbosacral junction, or higher, disrupt spinopelvic continuity. These patients undergo reconstruction using a combination of dual fibula grafts and instrumented stabilization from the lower lumbar spine to the remaining pelvis (Figure 35-10) [71]. The decision to use fibula allo- or autografts is individualized.

A concurrent hemipelvectomy is considered if the local extent of disease leads to sacrifice of both the femoral nerve and the lumbosacral plexus/sciatic nerve or the hip joint and the femoral or sciatic nerves. Resections of this magnitude would otherwise leave a nonfunctional limb. In addition, patients will have such a large soft-tissue defect that a pedicled quadriceps apron flap is necessary for closure. In these cases, the fibula from the amputated limb can be preserved on a pedicle at the end of the quadriceps flap for reconstruction. This is then used to restore spinopelvic continuity.

Soft-Tissue Reconstruction

Nonhealing perineal wounds following an abdominal perineal approach to complex pelvic tumors are reported to occur in 7–66 % of patients [72]. We, as well as others, have found that the use of a VRAM flap is associated with fewer perineal wound complications [72, 73]. The VRAM provides a well-vascularized, bulky tissue paddle that not only fills dead space but also can be used to reconstruct the perineal skin defect. Our technique is described elsewhere, but in essence, the VRAM is mobilized en bloc with the overlying fat and

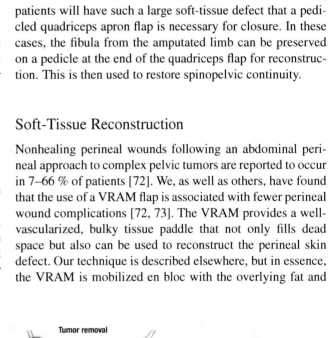

FIGURE 35-9. (**a**) Posterior transverse osteotomy (*thick dotted black line*). Sacrospinous and sacrotuberous ligament transection. The gluteus maximus muscle is reflected laterally to expose obturator vessels and the sciatic nerve. (**b**) Laminectomy to identify thecal sac, (**c**) dural sac, and sacral root ligation.

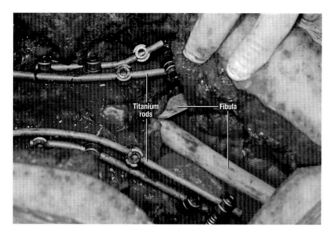

FIGURE 35-10. Intraoperative photograph of fibula grafts and instrumented spinopelvic reconstruction following total sacrectomy.

skin [74]. Particular attention is paid to the blood supply, especially the deep inferior epigastric artery and vein. Once mobilized, it is rotated transabdominally in the perineum keeping the overlying skin and fat intact, which helps bridge the significant defects that these resections leave behind. In cases where the rectus is not available, a pedicled omental flap can be a good second choice if it is robust. It can fill the pelvic dead space providing vascularized tissue and has been shown to decrease risk of pelvic sepsis following surgery [75]. Moreover, the omentum can line the raw surfaces of the pelvis, preventing the small bowel from getting trapped in the deep pelvis, which is a common cause of small bowel obstruction following exenteration.

Thigh fillet flaps are used after hindquarter amputation and are based on the superior and inferior gluteal vessels. This flap allows one to take advantage of the bulky gluteal muscle, which can cover large defects after the ipsilateral pelvis has been resected. Long anterior hemipelvectomy flaps are based on the vascular muscle distribution supplied by the superficial femoral artery. This flap includes the bulk of the quadriceps femoris and—like the posterior hemipelvectomy flap—can provide significant coverage of very large pelvic and soft-tissue defects.

Results of Surgery

Recurrent Colon Cancer

Limited data exists on surgical and oncologic outcomes in patients with locally advanced recurrent colon cancer. Few centers have published their experience, and patient groups are small and heterogeneous, making definitive conclusions regarding management difficult. In a series from the Mayo Clinic, 73 patients underwent a multimodality approach that included IORT for recurrent colon cancer [63]. In this cohort, an R0 resection was achieved in 52 % and led to a 5-year

survival of 37 %. In a series from Leeds, Harji et al. reported on 42 patients with recurrent colon cancer [76]. An R0 resection was achieved in 64 %, and mean survival did not differ between R0 vs. R1 resected patients (29 months vs. 26 months). Survival outcomes were dependent on location of recurrence, and median survival after resection was 33 months for anastomotic, 26 months for pelvic, and 19 months for abdominal recurrences. In the largest series published, Bowne et al. from the Memorial Sloan Kettering Cancer Center reported on 100 patients operated on for curative-intent resection for locally recurrent colon cancer [62]. Fourteen patients were found to have unresectable disease at the time of surgery and 65 % had an R0 resection. Multivisceral resection was common, and the best oncologic outcomes were achieved in patients undergoing R0 resection. Actuarial 5-year survival was 35 % for their entire cohort but was 58 % in those undergoing R0 resection.

In all three of these series, surgery could be performed safely, but multivisceral en bloc resection was required in many patients in attempts to reach a negative-margin resection. Margin status and location of recurrence appear to be the most important predictors of outcome in patients with recurrent colon cancer.

Recurrent Rectal Cancer

In the past, published series of surgery for locally recurrent rectal cancer were limited by small numbers and heterogeneous patient groups. In 2015, we now have robust data that confirms that an R0 resection, the ultimate goal for these operations, is achievable in 70–93 % [17, 18, 42] and overall 5-year survival can be as high as 40 %. Moreover, in series published where IORT is a component of multimodality therapy, meaningful survival can also be achieved in patients who have R1 or R2 resections [40]. Aggressive surgery that includes more lateral pelvic resections (pelvic sidewall tumors) and higher sacral resection (above the third sacral body) is increasingly reported by experienced centers with good results [17, 18, 56, 57].

In a Mayo Clinic series, Hahnloser et al. reported outcomes in 394 patients that underwent a curative-intent resection for locally recurrent cancer [15]. Operative mortality was 0.3 % (1 patient with uncontrolled hemorrhage), and significant morbidities were seen in 26 % of patients (most common was pelvic sepsis). Margin status for this cohort was R0 (45 %), R1 (9 %), and R2 (46 %). Survival was clearly impacted by margin status, 37 % for R0 and 16 % for R1/R2 patients. Other significant findings in this study were that symptomatic pain at presentation and >1 fixation point of the recurrence was associated with margin-positive resection and therefore a poor outcome. Patient demographics, factors related to the initial rectal cancer, and extended vs. limited resection did not impact overall oncologic outcomes. In a series from the Leeds General Infirmary, Boyle et al.

reviewed outcomes in 64 patients with locally recurrent rectal cancer, 57 of which underwent curative-intent resection [39]. Pelvic exenteration or sacrectomy was required in 32 %. An R0 resection was achieved in 37 %, perioperative mortality was 1.6 %, and morbidity was 40 %. Overall median survival was 34 months, and R0 resected patients had a significantly longer survival compared to R1 or R2 patients (median survival for R2 was 8 months). In a recent report from Denmark, Nielsen et al. published results on early and late outcomes of surgery for locally recurrent rectal cancer [77]. In their series, 115 patients underwent curative-intent resection. 30-day mortality was 0.8 % and an R0 resection was achieved in 61 %. The 3- and 5-year survival rates for R0 resections were 55 % and 42 %, respectively. No patients with R2 resection lived past 3 years.

Local excision for early rectal cancers has gained wider acceptance in the last 10 years [78]. The risk of local recurrence following local excision remains elevated, especially for high-risk T1 and T2 cancers. When local recurrence occurs following local excision, surgical salvage is the only treatment that has the potential to achieve meaningful survival. In a recent report, Bikhchandani et al. found that R0 resection was possible in 93 % and 5-year survival rate and DFS were 50 % and 47 %, respectively [79]. Metastatic disease following salvage surgery was the most common cause of death in this cohort. You et al. from the MD Anderson Cancer Center reported on 40 patients undergoing surgical salvage following local excision for rectal cancer [80]. A multimodality approach was used and R0 resection was achieved in 80 %. Multivisceral resection was required in 33 % and perioperative morbidity was 50 %. The 5-year overall and 3-year recurrence-free survival was 63 % and 43 %. Pathological stage at initial local excision, receipt of neoadjuvant chemoradiotherapy before local excision, pathological stage at salvage, and R0 resection at salvage significantly influenced re-recurrence-free survival.

The importance of an R0 resection in patients undergoing surgery for recurrent rectal cancer cannot be overstated. A recent meta-analysis of survival based on resection margin status following surgery for recurrent rectal cancer was published by Bhangu and colleagues [81]. In their analysis, they reviewed 22 studies that included 1460 patients and found that 57 % underwent R0 resection, 25 % R1, and 11 % R2. The range of median survival was 28–92 months for R0 resections, 12–50 months for R1, and 6–17 months for R2. Patients undergoing an R0 resection survived on average for 28 months longer than those undergoing R1 resection and 53 months longer than those undergoing R2 resection.

Surgery for Re-recurrent Disease

In the author's view, a second colorectal cancer recurrence is not a contraindication to curative resection as long as the principles of determining resectability for primary recurrence are followed. In a study by Colibaseanu et al., 47 patients underwent surgery for locally re-recurrent colorectal cancer [40]. An R0 resection was achieved in 60 % and 30-day mortality was nil. Overall 2- and 5-year survival was 83 and 33 %. Disease-free survival at 2 and 5 years was 55 and 27 %. In another study by Harji et al., 30 patients underwent resection for a second-time locally recurrent rectal cancer [82]. In their series, an R0 resection was achieved in 30 %, and they achieved a 1- and 3-year survival rate of 77 % and 27 %, respectively. It was the conclusion of both studies that in patients where R0 resection was possible, surgical resection for re-recurrent colorectal cancer had comparable oncologic outcomes than those patients undergoing surgery for first-time recurrences.

Resection That Includes the Aortoiliac Axis

The safety and feasibility of aortoiliac axis reconstruction in the course of complex tumor resections has been well described [83]. Small series have been published that specifically evaluate outcomes following resection in patients with locally recurrent colorectal cancers that involve the aortoiliac axis. In a study by Abdelsattar et al., 12 patients underwent major vessel resection that included the internal and external iliac arteries and veins and in some cases the aorta [69]. An R0 resection was achieved in 7 patients and R1 in 5. No graft complications were seen in long-term follow-up and 30-day mortality was nil. Overall survival and DFS at 4 years were 55 and 45 %. In another study by Austin et al., en bloc vascular resection was done as part of pelvic exenteration for pelvic malignancies in 36 patients (69 % were rectal cancers) [84]. An R0 resection was achieved in 60 % of the locally advanced primary and recurrent rectal cancer cases. For the overall cohort, 46 % of patients were disease-free with the average disease-free interval being 30 months. Both studies concluded that despite the complexity of the technique, the surgery can be performed safely when done by expert multidisciplinary teams, and overall survival and DFS are comparable to outcomes seen with locally advanced disease to nonvascular structures.

Sacropelvic Resections

Owing to the complex anatomical relationships of the pelvic structures, some local recurrences involve multiple fixation points and will require both multivisceral and neuromusculoskeletal resection to achieve a negative-margin resection. Operations for recurrences involving the lateral pelvic sidewall or high lumbosacral skeletal components are among the most technically challenging to perform. In the past, limited data existed regarding both the safety and the oncologic benefits of surgery in these patients. Once thought to be a common contraindication to surgery for recurrent colorectal cancer, high sacral and other complex sacropelvic resections are being done by an increasing number of centers around the world [57]. In most recent series from specialized centers, authors have shown that surgery in these complex patients can be done safely and with meaningful oncologic outcomes.

In a small series of 9 patients who had sacral resection at the level of the second sacral body or higher (up to fifth lumbar space), Dozois et al. reported an R0 rate of 100 %, no 30-day mortality, and an overall median survival of 31 months [41]. Three patients were long-term survivors at 40, 76, and 101 months. In another study from the same institution, Colibaseanu et al. reviewed 30 patients that had undergone curative-intent extended sacropelvic resections [17]. Four patients in this series underwent hindquarter amputations and over 50 % had sacral resections above the third sacral body. There were no 30-day mortalities and R0 resection was achieved in 93 %. Overall survival and DFS at 2 and 5 years were 79 and 43 %. Overall survival in this series was not different in patients undergoing high (>3rd sacral body) vs. low sacral resection.

In a study from the Royal Prince Alfred Hospital in Sydney, Australia, Milne et al. reported on 100 patients undergoing sacropelvic resection for advanced pelvic malignancies, of which 18 were primary rectal cancers and 61 were recurrent rectal cancers [18]. In the entire cohort, an R0 resection was achieved in 72 %, no 30-day mortality was seen, and overall survival and DFS were 38 % and 30 %, respectively. In a study by Sagar et al. from the Leeds General Infirmary, 40 patients underwent composite sacropelvic resection [56]. An R0 resection was achieved in 50 %, and the mean disease-free interval was 55.6 months for R0 and 32 months for R2 patients.

Postoperative Complications and Quality of Life

Despite the complex nature and magnitude of surgery for local recurrence, several recent series have demonstrated that these cases can be done with an operative mortality rate that ranges from 0 to 3 % [17, 18, 40, 42]. When it does occur, 30-day mortality is usually a result of uncontrolled sepsis. This is a dramatic improvement compared to series published 20 years ago, where operative mortality could be as high as 8.5 % [14]. Several factors are responsible for the significant decrease in operative mortality, better patient selection, improved surgical technique by experienced specialists, better anesthesia, and better postoperative ICU management.

Early and late complications following surgery for local recurrence remain a significant challenge. Most series report intra-abdominal/pelvic sepsis and wound-related complications as the most significant causes of morbidity [17, 18, 56, 60, 67, 85]. Other common complications are postoperative bleeding requiring transfusion, voiding dysfunction, prolonged ileus, delayed small bowel perforation, and late fistulas.

Universally, higher complications are associated with extended resections such a sacrectomy and exenteration [15, 17]. Urologic complications both early (ureteral obstruction, leak) and late (ureteral stricture) are reported in many series. In a study by Rahbari et al., risk factors associated with postoperative complications were analyzed [86]. In their series, 92 patients underwent curative-intent surgery for recurrent rectal cancer. To identify predictors of complications after resection, univariate and multivariate analysis was done. On univariate analysis, partial sacrectomy ($p=0.0001$), intraoperative blood loss ($p=0.005$), amount of transfusion ($p=0.02$), and operating time ($p=0.006$) were associated significantly with surgical complications. Multivariate logistic regression analysis of ASA score, BMI, partial sacrectomy (yes or no), blood loss, operating time, and the use of IORT (yes or no) revealed that partial sacrectomy is the only independent predictor of surgical morbidity. It is the author's perspective that careful surgical planning, reducing blood loss, reducing operating time, and the judicious use of soft-tissue flaps can significantly decrease postoperative morbidity.

Little information exists about the impact of major surgical intervention on quality of life in patients with recurrent colorectal cancer. While oncologic outcomes remain the most important outcome measure for patients and physicians deciding on an aggressive surgical approach, quality of life after surgery must be considered and discussed with patients so that they are well informed. In the modern era, advances in surgical technique and expertise allow surgeons to perform increasingly more complex operations, and how these operations impact quality of life is a relevant and growing area of interest to both patients and surgeons.

In a study by Austin and colleagues at the Royal Prince Alfred Hospital in Sydney, Australia, quality of life in 75 patients undergoing pelvic exenteration for advanced rectal cancer was assessed using the Short Form 36 version 2 (SF-36v2) and Functional Assessment of Cancer Therapy-Colorectal (FACT-C) instruments [87]. They found that FACT-C scores in survivors were good and comparable to those of patients who had low anterior resections or abdominal perineal resections. Though the summary scale of the SF-36v2 form was lower in exenteration patients than the general Australian population, the mental component summary scale was high and comparable. In a systematic review of health-related quality of life (HRQoL) in patients with locally recurrent rectal cancer, Harji et al. reviewed a total of 14 studies compromising 501 patients [88]. This study (the first published study to focus exclusively on HRQoL in patients with locally recurrent rectal cancer) identified several consistent themes. There are few studies of variable quality, reporting on a large number of HRQoL domains. Moreover, the heterogeneous treatment approach and patient population make study comparisons difficult. Harji and colleagues conclude that a disease-specific, validated, and reliable outcome measures are both lacking and required to provide meaningful data in patients who undergo surgery for locally recurrent rectal cancer. This tool, once developed, could then be used to prospectively measure HRQoL. This data would be very useful in assisting in surgical decision-making for both the physician and the patient.

Palliative Approach

Patients with an asymptomatic recurrence which is unresectable, either due to the presence of concurrent metastases or because of local factors, do not warrant surgical intervention [89]. In symptomatic patients, EBRT can sometimes relieve obstruction, decrease bleeding, and reduce pain [90]. Endoscopic stenting is especially helpful with malignant obstructions and can in some cases be used to palliate malignant fistulas that are inoperable [91, 92]. Patients not candidates for stents may need a colostomy for symptomatic relief.

Chemotherapy has been shown to prolong survival and palliate symptoms in patients with primary metastatic colorectal cancer, and in large, the treatment of unresectable recurrent colorectal cancer is based on extrapolations from this data. FOLFOX and FOLFIRI are the most commonly used chemotherapy protocols in patients with unresectable metastatic disease. The three most prominent trials comparing the two regimens did not distinguish which is superior, though both regimens prolong survival [93–95]. Newer agents such as bevacizumab, cetuximab, and panitumumab have and continue to be studied as monotherapy or as part of multidrug regimens [96–98].

Patients in whom a palliative approach is taken will benefit greatly by meeting with a palliative medicine team to discuss treatment goals and assist with end-of-life decisions. In addition, a cancer pain specialist can assist in reducing suffering through optimal pain management, and this should be the goal in patients undergoing a palliative approach.

References

1. Cripps H. Rectal cancer: rectal excision for cancer: the selection of suitable cases and prognosis. BMJ. 1892;10(2):1277–9.
2. Mayo CH. Cancer of the large bowel. Med Sentinel. 1904; 12:466–73.
3. Miles WE. A method of performing abdominoperineal excision for carcinoma of the rectum and the terminal portion of the pelvic colon. Lancet. 1908;2:1812–3.
4. Mayo WJ. Grafting and traumatic dissemination of carcinoma in the course of operations for malignant disease. JAMA. 1913; 60(7):512–3.
5. Sugarbaker ED. Coincident removal of additional structures in resections for carcinoma of the colon and rectum. Ann Surg. 1946;123(6):1036–46.
6. Dixon CF. Anterior resection for malignant lesions of the upper part of the rectum and lower part of the sigmoid. Ann Surg. 1948;128:425–42.
7. Heald RJ, Ryall RD. Recurrence and survival after total mesorectal excision for rectal cancer. Lancet. 1986;1(8496):1479–82.

8. Mathis KL, Larson DW, Dozois EJ, Cima RR, Huebner M, Haddock MG, et al. Outcomes following surgery without radiotherapy for rectal cancer. Br J Surg. 2012;99(1):137–43.
9. Bosset JF, Calais G, Mineur L, Maingon P, Stojanovic-Rundic S, Bensadoun RJ, et al. Fluorouracil-based adjuvant chemotherapy after preoperative chemoradiotherapy in rectal cancer: long-term results of the EORTC 22921 randomised study. Lancet Oncol. 2014;15(2):184–90.
10. Gray J. Evaluation of conservative resection with end to end anastomosis for carcinoma of the rectum and lower sigmoid colon. Arch Surg. 1948;57(3):361–72.
11. Lofgren EP, Waugh JM, Dockerty MB. Local recurrence of carcinoma after anterior resection of the rectum and the sigmoid; relationship with the length of normal mucosa excised distal to the lesion. AMA Arch Surg. 1957;74(6):825–38.
12. Pollard SG, Macfarlane R, Everett WG. Surgery for recurrent colorectal carcinoma—is it worthwhile? Ann R Coll Surg Engl. 1989;71(5):293–8.
13. Gunderson LL, Nelson H, Martenson JA, Cha S, Haddock M, Devine R, et al. Intraoperative electron and external beam irradiation with or without 5-fluorouracil and maximum surgical resection for previously unirradiated, locally recurrent colorectal cancer. Dis Colon Rectum. 1996;39(12):1379–95.
14. Wanebo HJ, Koness RJ, Vezeridis MP, Cohen SI, Wrobleski DE. Pelvic resection of recurrent rectal cancer. Ann Surg. 1994;220(4):586–95. discussion 95-7.
15. Hahnloser D, Nelson H, Gunderson LL, Hassan I, Haddock MG, O'Connell MJ, et al. Curative potential of multimodality therapy for locally recurrent rectal cancer. Ann Surg. 2003; 237(4):502–8.
16. Suzuki K, Dozois RR, Devine RM, Nelson H, Weaver AL, Gunderson LL, et al. Curative reoperations for locally recurrent rectal cancer. Dis Colon Rectum. 1996;39(7):730–6.
17. Colibaseanu DT, Dozois EJ, Mathis KL, Rose PS, Ugarte ML, Abdelsattar ZM, et al. Extended sacropelvic resection for locally recurrent rectal cancer: can it be done safely and with good oncologic outcomes? Dis Colon Rectum. 2014;57(1): 47–55.
18. Milne T, Solomon MJ, Lee P, Young JM, Stalley P, Harrison JD, et al. Sacral resection with pelvic exenteration for advanced primary and recurrent pelvic cancer: a single-institution experience of 100 sacrectomies. Dis Colon Rectum. 2014;57(10):1153–61.
19. Konski AA, Suh WW, Herman JM, Blackstock Jr AW, Hong TS, Poggi MM, et al. ACR appropriateness criteria(R)-recurrent rectal cancer. Gastrointest Cancer Res. 2012;5(1):3–12.
20. Miller AR, Cantor SB, Peoples GE, Pearlstone DB, Skibber JM. Quality of life and cost effectiveness analysis of therapy for locally recurrent rectal cancer. Dis Colon Rectum. 2000; 43(12):1695–701. discussion 701-3.
21. Haddock MG, Gunderson LL, Nelson H, Cha SS, Devine RM, Dozois RR, et al. Intraoperative irradiation for locally recurrent colorectal cancer in previously irradiated patients. Int J Radiat Oncol Biol Phys. 2001;49(5):1267–74.
22. Sjovall A, Granath F, Cedermark B, Glimelius B, Holm T. Loco-regional recurrence from colon cancer: a population-based study. Ann Surg Oncol. 2007;14(2):432–40.
23. Siegel RL, Miller KD, Jemal A. Cancer statistics, 2015. CA Cancer J Clin. 2015;65(1):5–29.
24. Bouchard P, Efron J. Management of recurrent rectal cancer. Ann Surg Oncol. 2010;17(5):1343–56.

25. Gunderson LL, Sosin H. Areas of failure found at reoperation (second or symptomatic look) following "curative surgery" for adenocarcinoma of the rectum. Clinicopathologic correlation and implications for adjuvant therapy. Cancer. 1974; 34(4):1278–92.

26. McCall JL, Cox MR, Wattchow DA. Analysis of local recurrence rates after surgery alone for rectal cancer. Int J Colorectal Dis. 1995;10(3):126–32.

27. Wanebo HJ, Antoniuk P, Koness RJ, Levy A, Vezeridis M, Cohen SI, et al. Pelvic resection of recurrent rectal cancer: technical considerations and outcomes. Dis Colon Rectum. 1999; 42(11):1438–48.

28. McDermott FT, Hughes ES, Pihl E, Johnson WR, Price AB. Local recurrence after potentially curative resection for rectal cancer in a series of 1008 patients. Br J Surg. 1985;72(1):34–7.

29. Eroglu A, Camlibel S. Risk factors for locoregional recurrence of scar carcinoma. Br J Surg. 1997;84(12):1744–6.

30. Porter GA, Soskolne CL, Yakimets WW, Newman SC. Surgeon-related factors and outcome in rectal cancer. Ann Surg. 1998; 227(2):157–67.

31. Bulow S, Christensen IJ, Iversen LH, Harling H, Danish Colorectal Cancer G. Intra-operative perforation is an important predictor of local recurrence and impaired survival after abdominoperineal resection for rectal cancer. Colorectal Dis. 2011; 13(11):1256–64.

32. Dresen RC, Peters EE, Rutten HJ, Nieuwenhuijzen GA, Demeyere TB, van den Brule AJ, et al. Local recurrence in rectal cancer can be predicted by histopathological factors. Eur J Surg Oncol. 2009;35(10):1071–7.

33. Kuru B, Camlibel M, Dinc S, Gulcelik MA, Gonullu D, Alagol H. Prognostic factors for survival in breast cancer patients who developed distant metastasis subsequent to definitive surgery. Singapore Med J. 2008;49(11):904–11.

34. Dogan L, Karaman N, Yilmaz KB, Ozaslan C, Atalay C, Altinok M. Characteristics and risk factors for colorectal cancer recurrence. J BUON. 2010;15(1):61–7.

35. Birbeck KF, Macklin CP, Tiffin NJ, Parsons W, Dixon MF, Mapstone NP, et al. Rates of circumferential resection margin involvement vary between surgeons and predict outcomes in rectal cancer surgery. Ann Surg. 2002;235(4):449–57.

36. Nagtegaal ID, Quirke P. What is the role for the circumferential margin in the modern treatment of rectal cancer? J Clin Oncol. 2008;26(2):303–12.

37. Monson JR, Weiser MR, Buie WD, Chang GJ, Rafferty JF, Buie WD, et al. Practice parameters for the management of rectal cancer (revised). Dis Colon Rectum. 2013;56(5):535–50.

38. Chang GJ, Kaiser AM, Mills S, Rafferty JF, Buie WD, Standards Practice Task Force of the American Society of C, et al. Practice parameters for the management of colon cancer. Dis Colon Rectum. 2012;55(8):831–43.

39. Boyle KM, Sagar PM, Chalmers AG, Sebag-Montefiore D, Cairns A, Eardley I. Surgery for locally recurrent rectal cancer. Dis Colon Rectum. 2005;48(5):929–37.

40. Colibaseanu DT, Mathis KL, Abdelsattar ZM, Larson DW, Haddock MG, Dozois EJ. Is curative resection and long-term survival possible for locally re-recurrent colorectal cancer in the pelvis? Dis Colon Rectum. 2013;56(1):14–9.

41. Dozois EJ, Privitera A, Holubar SD, Aldrete JF, Sim FH, Rose PS, et al. High sacrectomy for locally recurrent rectal cancer:

42. Milne T, Solomon MJ, Lee P, Young JM, Stalley P, Harrison JD. Assessing the impact of a sacral resection on morbidity and survival after extended radical surgery for locally recurrent rectal cancer. Ann Surg. 2013;258(6):1007–13.

43. Sagar PM, Pemberton JH. Surgical management of locally recurrent rectal cancer. Br J Surg. 1996;83(3):293–304.

44. Arulampalam T, Costa D, Visvikis D, Boulos P, Taylor I, Ell P. The impact of FDG-PET on the management algorithm for recurrent colorectal cancer. Eur J Nucl Med. 2001;28(12): 1758–65.

45. Moore HG, Akhurst T, Larson SM, Minsky BD, Mazumdar M, Guillem JG. A case-controlled study of 18-fluorodeoxyglucose positron emission tomography in the detection of pelvic recurrence in previously irradiated rectal cancer patients. J Am Coll Surg. 2003;197(1):22–8.

46. Whiteford MH, Whiteford HM, Yee LF, Ogunbiyi OA, Dehdashti F, Siegel BA, et al. Usefulness of FDG-PET scan in the assessment of suspected metastatic or recurrent adenocarcinoma of the colon and rectum. Dis Colon Rectum. 2000;43(6):759–67. discussion 67-70.

47. Ogunbiyi OA, Flanagan FL, Dehdashti F, Siegel BA, Trask DD, Birnbaum EH, et al. Detection of recurrent and metastatic colorectal cancer: comparison of positron emission tomography and computed tomography. Ann Surg Oncol. 1997;4(8): 613–20.

48. Chessin DB, Kiran RP, Akhurst T, Guillem JG. The emerging role of 18F-fluorodeoxyglucose positron emission tomography in the management of primary and recurrent rectal cancer. J Am Coll Surg. 2005;201(6):948–56.

49. Simo M, Lomena F, Setoain J, Perez G, Castellucci P, Costansa JM, et al. FDG-PET improves the management of patients with suspected recurrence of colorectal cancer. Nucl Med Commun. 2002;23(10):975–82.

50. Wang JY, Tang R, Chiang JM. Value of carcinoembryonic antigen in the management of colorectal cancer. Dis Colon Rectum. 1994;37(3):272–7.

51. Older P, Smith R. Experience with the preoperative invasive measurement of haemodynamic, respiratory and renal function in 100 elderly patients scheduled for major abdominal surgery. Anaesth Intensive Care. 1988;16(4):389–95.

52. Shoemaker WC, Appel PL, Kram HB, Waxman K, Lee TS. Prospective trial of supranormal values of survivors as therapeutic goals in high-risk surgical patients. Chest. 1988;94(6): 1176–86.

53. Bass EM, Del Pino A, Tan A, Pearl RK, Orsay CP, Abcarian H. Does preoperative stoma marking and education by the enterostomal therapist affect outcome? Dis Colon Rectum. 1997; 40(4):440–2.

54. Haugen V, Bliss DZ, Savik K. Perioperative factors that affect long-term adjustment to an incontinent ostomy. J Wound Ostomy Continence Nurs. 2006;33(5):525–35.

55. Nugent KP, Daniels P, Stewart B, Patankar R, Johnson CD. Quality of life in stoma patients. Dis Colon Rectum. 1999;42(12):1569–74.

56. Sagar PM, Gonsalves S, Heath RM, Phillips N, Chalmers AG. Composite abdominosacral resection for recurrent rectal cancer. Br J Surg. 2009;96(2):191–6.

57. Sagar PM. Ultraradical resection for locally recurrent rectal cancer. Dis Colon Rectum. 2014;57(1):1–2.

58. Stocchi L, Nelson H, Sargent DJ, Engen DE, Haddock MG. Is en-bloc resection of locally recurrent rectal carcinoma involving the urinary tract indicated? Ann Surg Oncol. 2006; 13(5):740–4.

59. Cima RR. Rectal cancer: locally advanced and recurrent. In: Beck ED, Roberts PL, Saclarides TJ, Senagore AJ, Stamos MJ, Wexner SD, editors. The ASCRS textbook of colon and rectal surgery. 2nd ed. New York: Springer; 2011. p. 761–72.

60. Moriya Y, Akasu T, Fujita S, Yamamoto S. Total pelvic exenteration with distal sacrectomy for fixed recurrent rectal cancer. Surg Oncol Clin N Am. 2005;14(2):225–38.

61. Beyond TMEC. Consensus statement on the multidisciplinary management of patients with recurrent and primary rectal cancer beyond total mesorectal excision planes. Br J Surg. 2013;100(8):1009–14.

62. Bowne WB, Lee B, Wong WD, Ben-Porat L, Shia J, Cohen AM, et al. Operative salvage for locoregional recurrent colon cancer after curative resection: an analysis of 100 cases. Dis Colon Rectum. 2005;48(5):897–909.

63. Taylor WE, Donohue JH, Gunderson LL, Nelson H, Nagorney DM, Devine RM, et al. The Mayo Clinic experience with multimodality treatment of locally advanced or recurrent colon cancer. Ann Surg Oncol. 2002;9(2):177–85.

64. Torricelli P, Pecchi A, Luppi G, Romagnoli R. Gadolinium-enhanced MRI with dynamic evaluation in diagnosing the local recurrence of rectal cancer. Abdom Imaging. 2003;28(1): 19–27.

65. Colosio A, Soyer P, Rousset P, Barbe C, Nguyen F, Bouche O, et al. Value of diffusion-weighted and gadolinium-enhanced MRI for the diagnosis of pelvic recurrence from colorectal cancer. J Magn Reson Imaging. 2014;40(2):306–13.

66. Haddock MG, Miller RC, Nelson H, Pemberton JH, Dozois EJ, Alberts SR, et al. Combined modality therapy including intraoperative electron irradiation for locally recurrent colorectal cancer. Int J Radiat Oncol Biol Phys. 2011;79(1):143–50.

67. Heriot AG, Byrne CM, Lee P, Dobbs B, Tilney H, Solomon MJ, et al. Extended radical resection: the choice for locally recurrent rectal cancer. Dis Colon Rectum. 2008;51(3):284–91.

68. Dresen RC, Gosens MJ, Martijn H, Nieuwenhuijzen GA, Creemers G-J, Daniels-Gooszen AW, et al. Radical resection after IORT-containing multimodality treatment is the most important determinant for outcome in patients treated for locally recurrent rectal cancer. Ann Surg Oncol. 2008;15(7):1937–47.

69. Abdelsattar ZM, Mathis KL, Colibaseanu DT, Merchea A, Bower TC, Larson DW, et al. Surgery for locally advanced recurrent colorectal cancer involving the aortoiliac axis: can we achieve R0 resection and long-term survival? Dis Colon Rectum. 2013;56(6):711–6.

70. Hugate Jr RR, Dickey ID, Phimolsarnti R, Yaszemski MJ, Sim FH. Mechanical effects of partial sacrectomy: when is reconstruction necessary? Clin Orthop Relat Res. 2006;450:82–8.

71. Dickey ID, Hugate Jr RR, Fuchs B, Yaszemski MJ, Sim FH. Reconstruction after total sacrectomy: early experience with a new surgical technique. Clin Orthop Relat Res. 2005;438: 42–50.

72. Chessin DB, Hartley J, Cohen AM, Mazumdar M, Cordeiro P, Disa J, et al. Rectus flap reconstruction decreases perineal wound complications after pelvic chemoradiation and surgery: a cohort study. Ann Surg Oncol. 2005;12(2):104–10.

73. Radice E, Nelson H, Mercill S, Farouk R, Petty P, Gunderson L. Primary myocutaneous flap closure following resection of locally advanced pelvic malignancies. Br J Surg. 1999; 86(3):349–54.

74. Sullivan PS, Dozois EJ. Exenterative surgery and reconstruction. In: Zbar AP, Madoff RD, Wexner SD, editors. Reconstructive surgery of the rectum, anus and perineum. London: Springer; 2013. p. 137–53.

75. Liebermann-Meffert D. The greater omentum. Anatomy, embryology, and surgical applications. Surg Clin North Am. 2000;80(1):275–93.

76. Harji DP, Sagar PM, Boyle K, Griffiths B, McArthur DR, Evans M. Surgical resection of recurrent colonic cancer. Br J Surg. 2013;100(7):950–8.

77. Nielsen M, Rasmussen P, Pedersen B, Hagemann-Madsen R, Lindegaard J, Laurberg S. Early and late outcomes of surgery for locally recurrent rectal cancer: a prospective 10-year study in the total mesorectal excision era. Ann Surg Oncol. 2015;22(8):2677–84.

78. You YN, Baxter NN, Stewart A, Nelson H. Is the increasing rate of local excision for stage I rectal cancer in the United States justified? A nationwide cohort study from the National Cancer Database. Ann Surg. 2007;245(5):726–33.

79. Bikhchandani J, Ong GK, Dozois EJ, Mathis KL. Outcomes of salvage surgery for cure in patients with locally recurrent disease after local excision of rectal cancer. Dis Colon Rectum. 2015;58(3):283–7.

80. You YN, Roses RE, Chang GJ, Rodriguez-Bigas MA, Feig BW, Slack R, et al. Multimodality salvage of recurrent disease after local excision for rectal cancer. Dis Colon Rectum. 2012;55(12): 1213–9.

81. Bhangu A, Ali SM, Darzi A, Brown G, Tekkis P. Meta-analysis of survival based on resection margin status following surgery for recurrent rectal cancer. Colorectal Dis. 2012;14(12): 1457–66.

82. Harji DP, Sagar PM, Boyle K, Maslekar S, Griffiths B, McArthur DR. Outcome of surgical resection of second-time locally recurrent rectal cancer. Br J Surg. 2013;100(3):403–9.

83. Carpenter SG, Stone WM, Bower TC, Fowl RJ, Money SR. Surgical management of tumors invading the aorta and major arterial structures. Ann Vasc Surg. 2011;25(8): 1026–35.

84. Austin KK, Solomon MJ. Pelvic exenteration with en bloc iliac vessel resection for lateral pelvic wall involvement. Dis Colon Rectum. 2009;52(7):1223–33.

85. Melton GB, Paty PB, Boland PJ, Healey JH, Savatta SG, Casas-Ganem JE, et al. Sacral resection for recurrent rectal cancer: analysis of morbidity and treatment results. Dis Colon Rectum. 2006;49(8):1099–107.

86. Rahbari NN, Ulrich AB, Bruckner T, Munter M, Nickles A, Contin P, et al. Surgery for locally recurrent rectal cancer in the era of total mesorectal excision: is there still a chance for cure? Ann Surg. 2011;253(3):522–33.

87. Austin KK, Young JM, Solomon MJ. Quality of life of survivors after pelvic exenteration for rectal cancer. Dis Colon Rectum. 2010;53(8):1121–6.

88. Harji DP, Griffiths B, Velikova G, Sagar PM, Brown J. Systematic review of health-related quality of life issues in locally recurrent rectal cancer. J Surg Oncol. 2015;111(4):431–8.

89. Cirocchi R, Trastulli S, Abraha I, Vettoretto N, Boselli C, Montedori A, et al. Non-resection versus resection for an asymp-

tomatic primary tumour in patients with unresectable stage IV colorectal cancer. Cochrane Database Syst Rev. 2012;8, CD008997.

90. Allum WH, Mack P, Priestman TJ, Fielding JW. Radiotherapy for pain relief in locally recurrent colorectal cancer. Ann R Coll Surg Engl. 1987;69(5):220–1.

91. Khot UP, Lang AW, Murali K, Parker MC. Systematic review of the efficacy and safety of colorectal stents. Br J Surg. 2002; 89(9):1096–102.

92. Spinelli P, Mancini A. Use of self-expanding metal stents for palliation of rectosigmoid cancer. Gastrointest Endosc. 2001; 53(2):203–6.

93. Colucci G, Gebbia V, Paoletti G, Giuliani F, Caruso M, Gebbia N, et al. Phase III randomized trial of FOLFIRI versus FOLFOX4 in the treatment of advanced colorectal cancer: a multicenter study of the Gruppo Oncologico Dell'Italia Meridionale. J Clin Oncol. 2005;23(22):4866–75.

94. Goldberg RM, Sargent DJ, Morton RF, Fuchs CS, Ramanathan RK, Williamson SK, et al. A randomized controlled trial of fluorouracil plus leucovorin, irinotecan, and oxaliplatin combinations in patients with previously untreated metastatic colorectal cancer. J Clin Oncol. 2004;22(1):23–30.

95. Tournigand C, Andre T, Achille E, Lledo G, Flesh M, Mery-Mignard D, et al. FOLFIRI followed by FOLFOX6 or the reverse sequence in advanced colorectal cancer: a randomized GERCOR study. J Clin Oncol. 2004;22(2):229–37.

96. Amado RG, Wolf M, Peeters M, Van Cutsem E, Siena S, Freeman DJ, et al. Wild-type KRAS is required for panitumumab efficacy in patients with metastatic colorectal cancer. J Clin Oncol. 2008;26(10):1626–34.

97. Cunningham D, Humblet Y, Siena S, Khayat D, Bleiberg H, Santoro A, et al. Cetuximab monotherapy and cetuximab plus irinotecan in irinotecan-refractory metastatic colorectal cancer. N Engl J Med. 2004;351(4):337–45.

98. Giantonio BJ, Catalano PJ, Meropol NJ, O'Dwyer PJ, Mitchell EP, Alberts SR, et al. Bevacizumab in combination with oxaliplatin, fluorouracil, and leucovorin (FOLFOX4) for previously treated metastatic colorectal cancer: results from the Eastern Cooperative Oncology Group Study E3200. J Clin Oncol. 2007;25(12):1539–44.

36

Colorectal Cancer: Management of Stage IV Disease

Glenn T. Ault and Kyle G. Cologne

Key Concepts

- Multidisciplinary evaluation is of paramount importance in the treatment of metastatic colorectal cancer.
- Positron emission tomography (PET) scan should be used in the evaluation of metastatic disease prior to potentially curative surgical therapy, or in cases of equivocal disease, but not for routine detection of metastatic disease.
- Patients with incurable metastatic disease and asymptomatic primary tumors should be considered for initial treatment with chemotherapy.
- For metastatic colorectal liver lesions, synchronous resection, liver-first, or colon-first strategies are all acceptable means of surgical treatment.
- Resection, ablation, or a combination of ablative and resection techniques can be used to minimize parenchymal liver resection and preserve function when treating metastatic colorectal metastases.
- Cytoreduction and hyperthermic intraperitoneal chemotherapy (HIPEC) may be considered in appropriately selected patients treated at specialized centers with expertise in this technique, although it has not been demonstrated to be superior to modern systemic chemotherapy.
- Metastases to organs other than the liver, lung, ovary, or peritoneum are uncommon and commonly occur in conjunction with widely metastatic disease. Thus, resection rarely has an impact on overall survival and should only be undertaken in select circumstances after multidisciplinary evaluation.
- Treatment of metastatic disease in the elderly requires consideration of the performance status, frailty, and impact of various treatments on quality of life.

Introduction

Despite screening protocols, approximately 20% of colorectal cancer patients present with established distant metastasis [1]. Computed tomography (CT) scan or magnetic resonance imaging (MRI) generally detects this metastasis at the time of the initial staging of the cancer. Once the diagnosis of stage IV disease is made, a multidisciplinary team should plan appropriate curative or palliative therapy. Unfortunately for the clinician, there is enormous heterogeneity with respect to sites of disease, extent of disease and symptoms, performance status, and comorbidities in these patients. Stage IV patients have a range of presentation from the asymptomatic patient with a single metastatic lesion to the rapidly deteriorating patient with colon obstruction and advanced multiorgan metastases. While treatment algorithms may exist for some forms of metastatic disease such as a solitary liver lesion, others, especially for those with multiple sites of metastases, are still being defined. This chapter aims to provide a reference source for colorectal surgeons managing patients who present with metastatic stage IV colorectal cancer.

While there has been considerable progress in the treatment of advanced colorectal cancer, the vast majority of stage IV patients are unfortunately not curable by current treatment protocols. An evaluation of data from the SEER population-based database estimates that the 5-year survival rate for stage IV patients diagnosed between 1991 and 2000 was 8% [2]. Even with this low overall cure rate, there are treatment options available to extend survival and enhance quality of life. Oncologic teams have several tools to utilize including systemic chemotherapy, radiotherapy, endoscopic treatments to palliate obstruction, surgical diversion, and surgical resection, all of which can play important roles in the treatment of these patients. Treatment approaches must be individualized based on the extent of resectability of local and distant disease, the presence or absence of bowel obstruction, performance status, and comorbidities. For patients with good performance status and minimal symptoms from the primary site of the cancer, standard treatment is systemic chemotherapy, which has been proven to prolong survival and quality of life [3, 4]. Surgical resection of the primary tumor and, if indicated, of the metastatic lesions can provide excellent palliation and in a limited number of cases can provide lasting cure.

© Springer International Publishing 2016
S.R. Steele et al. (eds.), *The ASCRS Textbook of Colon and Rectal Surgery*, DOI 10.1007/978-3-319-25970-3_36

---

590   G.T. Ault and K.G. Cologne

First-line therapy with either FOLFOX or FOLFIRI now has been shown to yield major responses in up to 50% of previously untreated patients and achieves minor responses or stable disease in an additional 20% of patients [5]. Multiple effective drug combinations are available as well, and second and third line chemotherapy is becoming more effective and more likely to impact survival. Over the past 15 years, the median survival for patients with metastatic disease who are treated with chemotherapy has improved from 9 to 12 months and is currently greater than 24 months and may be as long as 36 months [6–8]. Although cure from chemotherapy alone remains extremely rare, effective chemotherapy combined with aggressive surgery may be increasing the overall cure rate. In this setting, the care of patients with advanced disease has become quite complex. In this chapter the aim is to provide a reference source for colorectal surgeons managing patients who present with metastatic stage IV colorectal cancer.

Biology of Metastatic Disease

Metastasis is defined as the spread of malignant cells from a primary tumor to a distant organ. It is estimated that 90% of all cancer deaths are the result of metastatic spread [9]. The biologic process of metastasis is poorly understood. Numerous clinical and laboratory studies have attempted to define the complex process of metastasis formation. The process relies on properties of the tumor cells, as well as the microenvironment of the primary and secondary sites [10, 11]. A series of major events must occur (Figure 36-1).

The first step is tumorigenesis, which occurs after the initial malignant transformation. The tumor proliferates into a small mass of heterogeneous cells that are of varying metastatic or malignant potential. These tumor cells undergo multiple and sequential genetic changes, characterized by the appearance of oncogenes and a decrease in tumor suppressor genes. As a tumor grows beyond 1 mm in diameter and becomes relatively hypoxic, angiogenesis is initiated. The process of tumor angiogenesis is tightly regulated by pro- and antiangiogenic factors secreted by both the tumor and its environment. As tumors successfully grow, suppressors of angiogenesis are inhibited, and proangiogenic factors predominate, resulting in neovascularity and further growth of the tumor [12]. Some tumors may grow by utilizing other existing blood vessels in nearby tissues.

In the next step, some cells will develop an invasive phenotype. Most researchers believe that there is a selection process resulting in the clonal expansion of certain cell subpopulations with growth advantage and invasive properties. Whether this process represents a property of the whole tumor cell mass or true clonal selection of more invasive cell subpopulation is not known, and it is a subject of intense research [13]. Malignant invasion is characterized by downregulation of cell adhesion, resulting in detachment of the cell from the primary tumor mass and the extracellular matrix. Stromal invasion is accomplished through interactions with the basement membrane, including adhesion,

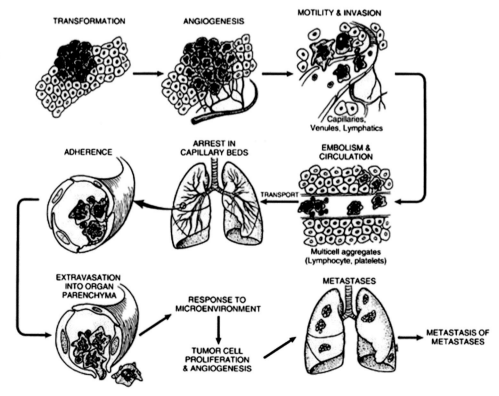

FIGURE 36-1. Schematic illustrating the multistep process involved in the development of metastasis. With permission from DeVita VT Jr., Hellman S, Rosenberg SA. Cancer: Principles and Practice of Oncology, 6th ed., Lippincott Williams and Wilkins, copyright 2001 [303].

proteolysis, and migration, ultimately resulting in detachment and invasion through the basement membrane. This invasive phenotype also enables these cells to enter thin-walled lymphatics and vasculatures, allowing access to systemic circulation [14, 15]. Once inside the vascular system, cells or cell clumps (emboli) are circulated and must survive hemodynamic filtering as well as immune surveillance. They must then arrest in distant organ. There is likely a complex interaction between the malignant cell and the endothelium or exposed basement membrane, allowing cell arrest. Once arrested in a tissue bed, the cells extravasate into the tissue, enabling formation of the metastatic focus. These metastatic cells can become dormant or proliferate; what determines this fate is not fully understood. Growth in the distant organ after deposition is a major limiting factor in the formation of metastasis. Some metastatic cells can remain dormant while others proliferate and must again go through tumor genesis, angiogenesis, and evasion of the immune system. This complex multistep process of metastasis formation is related to multiple genetic changes among malignant cells. Recent studies have shown differences in the genetic fingerprints of matched primary tumors and their lymph node metastasis suggesting that tumors may undergo continual mutagenesis. The metastatic tumor cells may genetically look very different from its parent primary cells [16]. This finding appears to confirm that there are genes specific to tumorigenesis, invasion, angiogenesis, and other steps. A number of genes have been identified that suppress metastatic potential and, by their downregulation, affect a cell's ability to metastasize without affecting tumorigenicity [16].

These discoveries provide a sense of the future challenge in elucidating the multiple, stepwise, and specific changes that regulate a cell's ability to metastasize. Advances in this field will have obvious and profound implications for the treatment of cancer.

Diagnostic Strategies

Part of the evaluation of newly diagnosed colorectal cancer includes systemic staging with cross-sectional imaging of the chest, abdomen, and pelvis. Rectal cancers will also include additional local staging with an endorectal ultrasound or pelvic MRI [17]. Twenty to thirty percentages of patients will present with evidence of metastatic disease on this staging workup [17, 18]. Increased suspicion should be given to the presence of metastatic disease when the CEA level is greater than 20 ng/mL [19].

There is the potential for some diagnostic uncertainty, as some lesions detected on staging workup may represent entities other than metastatic cancer (such as cysts, hemangiomas, granulomatous or infectious lesions, focal nodular hyperplasia, etc.). Hemangiomas have a prevalence of 7–21% and have characteristic imaging findings including a hyper-enhancing ring. Focal nodular hyperplasia is present

in up to 3% of patients [18]. There are several imaging modalities that can be used to help identify true metastatic disease from other possibilities in the differential diagnosis, and each has unique characteristics. None is infallible, and in cases of uncertainty, multiple imaging modalities or tissue biopsy may be required to confirm the diagnosis, as it dramatically changes the prognosis and perhaps the treatment strategy as well. Consultation with a radiologist specializing in these imaging techniques is also helpful.

Computed Tomography

Computed tomography has been the mainstay of distant staging workup for colorectal cancer. Technology now allows high resolution, subcentimeter slice thickness with multiplane reformatting. This allows vascular reconstruction and volumetric analysis, which can be particularly important for operative planning for large liver resections [20–22]. Triple phase scans allow improved delineation of hepatic metastases (Figure 36-2). Though enhancement characteristics differ, most metastatic lesions are hypoattenuating on portal venous phases of an abdominal CT. Numerous studies have failed to gain significant value in routine use of four-phase CT to detect hepatic metastases, and portal venous phases are the most important to detect hypoattenuating liver lesions suggestive of metastases [23–25]. Despite this, up to 25% of hepatic liver metastases may be missed on high-quality CT, due mostly either to size or confusion with other disease processes [26, 27].

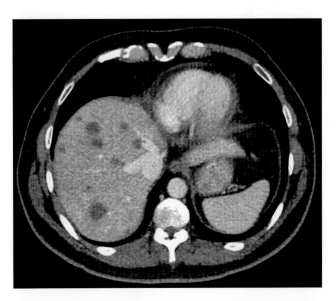

FIGURE 36-2. CT of the abdomen demonstrating liver metastases involving multiple segments of the liver. Treatment of these requires advanced planning and input in a multidisciplinary setting involving hepatobiliary, interventional radiology, oncology, and other specialties to determine planned interventions and timing.

Positron Emission Tomography

PET and PET-CT scans are a modality used both for initial staging and for follow-up imaging. The technology has dramatically improved recently and can now provide very clear pictures of tumor deposits in distant locations (Figure 36-3) [28]. Sensitivity of PET-CT for detecting metastatic lesions ranges from 87 to 100%, which compares favorably with regular CT (where sensitivities range from 52 to 69%) [29]. Specificity of PET-CT is also good and ranges from 94 to 100% (compared with 80–94% for regular CT). Limitations include a size resolution of about 1 cm and limited ability to detect mucinous tumors. Some studies suggest that the ability of PET-CT to detect subcentimeter lesions may be less than 50% [30–32]. Most protocols include a lack of intravenous contrast, which may limit the ability to evaluate some smaller lesions. National Comprehensive Cancer Network (NCCN) guidelines do not recommend routine use of PET-CT to evaluate metastatic lesions except in equivocal findings or in cases where patients are allergic to IV contrast which would otherwise limit the usefulness of regular CT [33]. In cases where patients are being considered for liver resection of metastatic tumor, there is some evidence that PET-CT can detect extrahepatic disease that is missed in up to one third of patients evaluated by CT scan alone. This changed management strategy in 8–21% of patients [34].

Magnetic Resonance Imaging

While MRI is used to perform the initial staging of rectal cancers, it can also be useful for characterizing equivocal lesions of the liver, as it is particularly good at soft tissue characteristics, especially those that fall below the resolution of PET [35, 36]. The soft tissue delineation is also better than CT scan and can help with tumor identification [34]. MRI of the liver with contrast using a liver-specific protocol can help define lesions that are potentially resectable. Sensitivity of MRI at detecting response of liver lesions to neoadjuvant treatments may be better than PET [37]. MRI cannot be used in patients with pacemakers, implantable cardiac defibrillators, cochlear implants, and other orbital foreign bodies [18]. Cost remains a significant factor that also limits routine use of MRI in the evaluation of liver lesions.

Contrast-Enhanced Ultrasound

Contrast-enhanced ultrasound (CEUS) is the newest imaging modality to gain popularity. It is highly operator dependent but highly effective (one study demonstrated 97% of lesions seen on CT were also detected on CEUS) [38]. As centers gain expertise in this modality, its use may increase in the future. Another potential limitation is that chemotherapy-induced fatty infiltration of the liver may limit diagnostic accuracy.

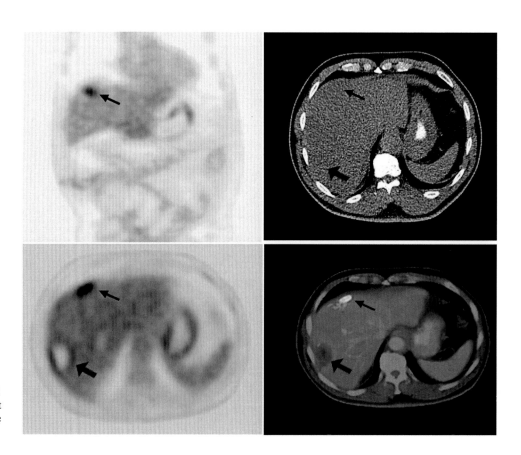

FIGURE 36-3. PET-CT scan and various phases. Lesions may not always show up or appear active on all phases of imaging.

Biopsy

In equivocal cases where imaging characteristics are not suspicious of colorectal metastases, tissue biopsy confirmation remains an option. A small percentage of patients will have a histologic process other than the primary malignancy [39, 40].

Multidisciplinary Evaluation

Multidisciplinary evaluation is of critical importance to caring for patients with metastatic disease. As there is often no one agreed-upon absolute treatment strategy, it is important to have consensus from treating oncologists, radiation oncologists, and various surgical disciplines such as colorectal, hepatobiliary, thoracic, and gynecology [41, 42]. Of particular value is whether or not an organ can be rendered disease-free. This allows surgery for cure, which has a different end point than surgery for palliation [43]. It is estimated that only 20–30% of patients with identified metastatic disease will have potentially resectable disease [44]. Goals of multidisciplinary evaluation should include relief of symptoms and quality of life improvement and determine the best means of prolonging life expectancy. In some cases, this may include chemotherapy alone. Consideration must be given to multiple variables including performance status, tumor burden, patient's expectations of treatment, and overall care goals.

If disease is determined to be resectable, common considerations are whether to perform sequential or simultaneous resections, use of chemotherapy or radiation in a neoadjuvant or adjuvant setting, and whether or not to perform an anastomosis. If the disease is not resectable, there are a few common scenarios that deserve some additional attention. A typical algorithm can be found in Figure 36-4.

Surgical Emergency

Tumors at the primary site may cause a surgical emergency, even in the setting of metastatic disease. In these cases, surgical intervention should be undertaken to relieve the immediate, life threatening issue, such as perforation with peritonitis, lower GI bleeding, or large-bowel obstruction.

If possible, and if it can be performed with limited morbidity, an oncologic surgical resection should be performed [17, 45]. A primary anastomosis can be performed in select, low risk patients, but carries the potential it may delay chemotherapy and other life-sustaining treatments if an anastomotic leak should occur [46]. This should be weighed very carefully when performing surgery in the emergent setting.

Palliative Management of Primary Cancer: Laser, Fulguration, and Stents

Incidence and Presentation

Approximately 8–29% of patients with colorectal cancer initially present with symptoms of partial or complete bowel obstruction [47]. In a review of 713 obstructing carcinomas, 77% were left-sided and 23% were right-sided cases [48]. The majority of patients with obstructing colorectal carcinomas have either stage III or stage IV disease [49]. Acute malignant colon or rectal obstruction is an indication for emergent surgical intervention. However, these emergency operations are associated with a mortality rate of 15–34% and a morbidity rate of 32–64% despite advances in perioperative care [49, 50]. Therefore, alternative palliative endoluminal strategies aimed at relieving obstruction have gained increasing popularity over the past decades.

The initial symptoms of bowel obstruction may include mild discomfort and a change in bowel habits. With disease progression and luminal narrowing, the symptoms may worsen ranging from crampy abdominal pain, abdominal distension, nausea, abdominal tenderness, and obstipation. Vomiting is a late symptom unless there is an associated small bowel obstruction. Leukocytosis is a concerning finding and may indicate near or complete obstruction. Without treatment, the process can progress to complete obstruction, ischemia, and perforation. The risk of cecal perforation is greatest in patients who have a competent ileocecal valve that does not allow decompression of the large intestine into the proximal small intestine.

In the setting of metastatic cancer, the clinician must first answer the following critical question, "is the colon or rectal obstruction a contraindication for system chemotherapy or

FIGURE 36-4. Treatment algorithm for metastatic colorectal cancer.

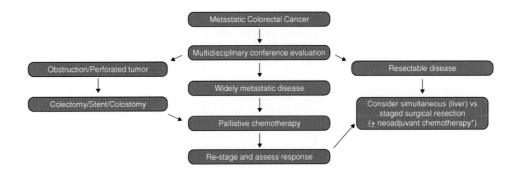

radiotherapy?" The degree of obstructive symptoms and endoscopic and radiographic findings are key elements to consider when answering this question. If the patient has minimal symptoms and there is no radiographic evidence of high-grade obstruction, many patients with partially obstructing colon and rectal cancers will tolerate aggressive chemotherapy as described previously in this chapter. In those patients with partially obstructing rectal cancers, the addition of radiation therapy is also well tolerated and can be highly effective. Patients must be instructed to monitor their symptoms closely and to report any signs of worsening obstruction immediately. A liquid diet or pureed diet with adequate protein and calorie intake taken in small portions may help reduce obstructive symptoms. For patients with advanced obstruction, nonsurgical palliative options include laser therapy, fulguration, and colonic self-expanding metal stents. If less-invasive endoluminal strategies are not successful in patients with nonresectable malignant obstruction of the colon and rectum, surgical creation of palliative proximal diverting stoma or intestinal bypass should be performed.

Laser Therapy and Fulguration

Laser therapy has been utilized for palliation of obstructing rectal cancers [51–54]. In a large series of 272 patients who underwent palliative laser therapy for rectosigmoid cancers, the immediate success rate in treating obstructive symptoms was 85% [55]. Other studies have shown similar success rates in the range of 80–90% [53, 54]. However, laser therapy is practical only for treating cancers of the distal colon and rectum and is rarely used to treat proximal lesions. In addition, multiple sessions are often required in order to achieve lasting relief of symptom. Serious complications like bleeding, perforation, and sever pain have been reported in 5–15% of patients, especially those undergoing multiple treatment sessions [52, 54–56]. While laser therapy has been shown to be practical and feasible to other palliative treatment modalities in the management of these unfortunate stage IV patients and has low morbidity and mortality [57], it does not affect overall survival of stage IV patients.

Surgical fulguration of rectal cancers is another method of opening the rectal lumen and relieving obstruction [58, 59]. Fulguration, in combination with endoluminal debulking, can remove a large volume of tumor. However, unlike laser therapy, fulguration and debulking require hospital admission and regional or general anesthesia. Both fulguration and laser therapy have given way to stenting.

Self-Expanding Metal Stents

Since their introduction in 1991, colonic stents have become an effective method of palliation for obstruction in colorectal cancer patients, especially those with unresectable metastatic disease, or used in an effort to decompress an obstructed patient preoperatively [60]. Especially in nonoperative stage IV patients or those that have significant comorbidities, these self-expanding metallic stents can potentially dilate the lumen to a near-normal diameter, providing quick relief of symptoms. Stents can be placed in patients using minimal sedation in the endoscopy suite with the aid of fluoroscopy. Moreover, these stents can be placed across relatively long lesions by overlapping stents in a "stent-within-stent" fashion. Laser therapy has also been used in certain situations, in conjunction with colonic stents, to recanalize and decompress large bowel or when tumor ingrowth occurs in patients who have had long-term stents in place. It should be noted the emergency surgery is recommended over stent placement in those patients with evidence of colonic obstruction and systemic toxicity. Presence of systemic toxicity may indicate the presence of ischemia and/or perforation which requires immediate evaluation and the potential for emergency surgery.

Stenting can achieve long-term palliation in patients who are not operative candidates. More than 75% of patients can achieve adequate palliation with stenting, although tumor ingrowth, stent migration, and perforation, especially those receiving bevacizumab, may occur [61]. If these stent-related complications occur, it may necessitate reintervention either with an additional stent or with other palliative measures such as laser or argon plasma coagulation therapy or surgery [62].

A systematic review from 1990 to 2000 of the published data on stenting of colorectal obstruction included 29 case series in the analysis [63]. The review evaluated technical and clinical success, complications, and reobstruction. Cases involving stent replacement for palliation and stent placement as a "bridge to surgery" were both assessed. Stent insertion was attempted in 598 cases. Stent deployment was technically feasible in 551 (92%) cases and clinically successful in relieving obstruction in 525 (88%) cases. Palliation of obstruction was achieved in 302 (90%) of 336 cases. Stent placement as a "bridge to surgery" was successful in 223 (88%) of 262 insertions of which 95% had a one-stage surgical procedure. There were three deaths (1%). Perforation occurred in 22 cases (4%). Stent migration was reported in 54 (1%) of the 551 technically successful cases. Stent reobstruction occurred in 52 (10%) of the 525 clinically successful cases and trended toward a higher incidence of reobstruction in the palliative treatment group. The reviewers concluded that "stent usage can avoid the need for a stoma and is associated with low rates of mortality and morbidity" [63]. A series of 52 patients with malignant obstruction secondary to either primary or recurrent colon or rectal carcinoma, who underwent stent replacement by colorectal surgeons, reported that 50 out of 52 were successfully palliated [64]. One patient had a perforation, and in another patient obstruction was not relieved because of multiple sites of obstruction. The overall complication rate in this series was 25%. Stent migration was the most common complication (15%), followed by reobstruction secondary to tumor ingrowth (4%), perforation (2%), colovesical fistula (2%), and sever tenesmus (2%). Surgical intervention was required in 17% of cases due primarily to one of the above complications or recurrent obstruction.

There are limited data evaluating stent placement proximal to the splenic flexure. In a recent publication, colonic stenting was attempted in 97 patients with malignant large-bowel obstruction [65]. Sixteen (17%) patients had lesions proximal to the splenic flexure (eight ascending, eight transverse colon). Stenting was successful in relieving obstruction in 14 (88%) of these patients. Stenting was performed for definitive palliation in nine of these patients and as a bridge to elective surgery in the other seven patients. One patient developed gastrointestinal bleeding that was managed conservatively. No perforations or stent migrations were reported [65].

Complications reported in the literature for colonic and rectal stents include stent malpositioning, perforation, stent migration, tumor ingrowth (through the stent interstices), tumor overgrowth (beyond the ends of a stent), stool impaction, bleeding, tenesmus, and postprocedure pain (Figure 36-5). Perforation and stent migration occur with the highest frequency. The rate of perforation however appears to be decreasing overall as the technique and technology have improved and in experienced hands is now approximately 5% [66]. Stent migration has been described to occur in a median of 11% of patients in a systematic review [67]. Migrations tend to occur with stents that are too narrow or too short in relation to the obstructing lesion or in the presence of tumor shrinkage following therapy [68]. Stenting of cancers in the mid to low rectum may result in urgency, pain, and incontinence. While the complications associated with stents and other less-invasive endoluminal strategies should not be taken lightly, one must keep in mind that emergency operations for malignant colon and rectal obstruction have a significant mortality rate of 15–34% and a high morbidity rate of 32–64%. Taken in the correct context, these endoluminal palliative strategies provide increasingly effective and durable relief for patients with malignant obstruction.

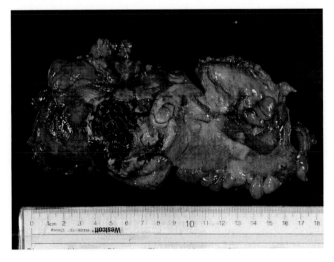

FIGURE 36-5. Perforation of the bowel in a colonic stent. Courtesy of Philip Y. Pearson, M.D.

The Challenge of Primary Tumor Management in Asymptomatic Stage IV Colorectal Cancer: To Resect or Not to Resect?

Optimal first-line therapy for patients who present initially with unresectable stage IV disease remains controversial. Some advocate initial resection of the primary, while others recommend initial chemotherapy if the primary tumor is asymptomatic.

In the era of modern chemotherapy, patients can experience increased length and quality of life with 5-FU-based multiagent chemotherapy [69]. Prophylactic resection of the primary tumor can provide long-term local control and may benefit select patients [70]. This must be weighed against the risk of surgical complications resulting in delay in chemotherapy and other palliative treatments. Particularly in rectal cancer, complications arising from surgery have been shown to delay initiation of chemotherapy beyond 8 weeks postoperatively. As these patients have worse overall survival, the risk of these complications may not be inconsequential [71]. As there are no randomized, controlled trials for this topic, some information on the natural history of the disease can aid management decisions.

Poultsides et al. [72] examined the natural history of patients receiving primary chemotherapy without surgical intervention for stage IV colorectal cancer. Left untreated, only 7% of primary lesions progressed to require emergency surgery for obstruction or perforation while receiving palliative multiagent chemotherapy. An additional 4% required a nonoperative intervention (e.g., stent or radiotherapy). The remaining 89% never required any further intervention on the primary tumor. Twenty percent responded well enough to undergo combined resection at the time of subsequent metastasectomy. Matsumoto et al. [73] reported that 75% of patients with unresectable disease could be spared primary tumor intervention. An endoscopically nontraversable primary lesion at the time of diagnosis was predictive of subsequent need for intervention (which occurred 64% of the time within the next year). Other studies suggest that 68–90.7% of patients will not require surgical intervention on the primary tumor [69, 74–76]. As there are some high-risk features that may predispose to perforation or obstruction, some oncologists will request initial surgical diversion for locally advanced, near-obstructing lesions or those that display signs of impending perforation or abscess on imaging.

Indeed, the argument for up-front primary tumor resection is based on the desire to avoid potential complications from the primary tumor during treatment. This concern may be greatest when the agent bevacizumab is utilized—which has led both surgical and medical oncologists to advocate primary tumor resection at the time of diagnosis prior to the institution of the drug [77, 78]. In fact, the majority of US patients presenting with stage IV disease will still undergo noncurative primary tumor resection, perhaps partially for this reason. However, during the past decade, several highly active systemic agents, both cytotoxic and biologic, have become available for the treatment of patients with metastatic colorectal cancer. As a result the median survival of patients with unresectable metastatic disease has increased from 9 to 12 months with fluorouracil alone to up to 24 months with sequential modern cytotoxic and biologic treatments [8]. Therefore, it may be generally accepted that, in these stage IV patients, systemic chemotherapy with or without primary resection is the essential treatment modality to prolong survival. These modern agents also have increased activity on the primary tumor and can even induce a complete response [79–81]. Thus the old question of how best to manage the primary tumor continues to be debated. It is agreed upon that resection of a lymph node basin outside the primary vascular pedicle is rarely indicated [82].

While there was some initial evidence in the literature that resection of the primary tumor was associated with a survival benefit [83], this finding was most likely the effect of selection bias. Patients with less extensive disease, or better performance status, were selected for resection [74, 84, 85]. Currently, routine surgery for the asymptomatic primary tumor in the setting of unresectable metastatic disease is not recommended. This recommendation stems in part from a Cochrane review of 798 studies involving 1086 patients that suggests there is not enough evidence to justify routine resection of primary tumors. Furthermore, survival was not consistently improved with primary tumor resection, nor was morbidity of complications from tumor complications reduced by initial resection. However, further study was recommended as there is a paucity of randomized trials on this matter [17, 86].

Investigators from the National Surgical Adjuvant Breast and Bowel Project (NSABP) have reported results of a phase II prospective single-arm study or primary systemic chemotherapy with fluorouracil, oxaliplatin (mFOLFOX6), and bevacizumab for patients with asymptomatic primary intact unresectable stage IV colorectal cancer (NSABP C-10) [87]. The investigators aimed to directly address the concerns for both primary tumor-related complications associated with first-line systemic therapy in patients with asymptomatic disease and the risk of tumor complications with the use of bevacizumab in this setting. A total of 86 patients form 29 institutions were evaluated with the primary eligibility criteria being that the treating clinician identified the patient to be asymptomatic with respect to his or her primary tumor. After a median follow-up of 20.7 months, the majority of the patients could be successfully managed nonoperatively without the need for primary tumor intervention, meeting the study's primary end point. Median overall survival was 19.9 months, and the overall rate of major morbidity related to the intact primary tumor was 16.3% (95% CI, 7.6–25.1%) at 24 months.

The investigators concluded that the first-line combination therapy with mFOLFOX6 and bevacizumab did not result in an unacceptable rate of primary tumor-related complications and that noncurative resection of the asymptomatic primary tumor in these patients could be avoided. These findings confirm prior retrospective reports demonstrating low rates of intestinal complications with either fluorouracil-based or more modern systemic chemotherapies [72, 88, 89]. In their prospective evaluation, however, the NSABP investigators [87] have further demonstrated the safety of first-line chemotherapy with bevacizumab in patients with intact but asymptomatic tumors. Indeed, 73.3% of the patients still had not required primary tumor resection at the time of death or last follow-up.

This study has moved clinical treatment decision-making forward and provides prospective evidence that routine noncurative resection may be unnecessary. This relatively small study also highlights a key question in determining which patients may be eligible for this approach. Establishing a patient as "asymptomatic" was a key eligibility criteria. In this study, asymptomatic was defined as having no bowel perforation or obstruction and no active bleeding requiring a transfusion [87]. It was at the treating physician's discretion to define whether a patient exhibited signs of obstruction. The key issue of understanding which patients are eligible for this approach can also influence the true incidence of primary tumor-related morbidity (i.e., not all patients with asymptomatic disease are the same.) Despite some limitations of the study, the results were reassuring for the safety of first-line systemic chemotherapy with bevacizumab. There will remain a group of patients who will still require subsequent primary tumor resection. The challenge of identifying these patients for planned elective resection to avoid the higher mortality and morbidity risks of emergent resection while sparing the morbidity of resection still needs to be defined.

It also needs to be acknowledged that retrospective comparative studies, even in the era of modern systemic therapies, have demonstrated survival benefits associated with resection of the primary tumor, although the individual contributions of the multiple factors of patient selection, location and extent of tumor burden, tumor biology, ability to tolerate, and availability of systemic therapy and aggressiveness of surveillance are unknown. A comparative multi-institutional study of patients with stage IV cancer at diagnosis remarkably demonstrated a median survival of 30.7 months with primary tumor resection compared with 21.9 months ($p = 0.031$), raising the question of whether primary tumor resection has the potential to further improve median survival beyond what can be achieve by even modern systemic therapy alone [90]. Perhaps there is a group of patients with putatively asymptomatic circumferential or locally advance primary tumors who might derive a survival benefit from either up-front or interval resection with the potential to avoid the need for emergent intervention or permanent ostomy. Performing a randomized study in an unselected stage IV population may indeed prove to be difficult.

The NSABP C-10 trail is the only modern prospective multi-institutional study that specifically addresses the issue of primary tumor resection in patients with asymptomatic stage IV colorectal cancer. Current treatment patterns are influenced by strong patient and provider biases but with this trial there is no additional evidence supporting the safety of systemic chemotherapy as the initial primary treatment approach for carefully selected asymptomatic patients avoiding the need for and the morbidity risk of noncurative resection. Unfortunately more questions remain and additional study is needed to help us understand how best to select patients and optimize the available treatment modalities, including surgery to improve outcomes and prevent subsequent morbidity.

Surgical Therapy of Liver Metastases

Liver metastases are a common occurrence, and surgical resection represents the best opportunity for long-term cure. Approximately 20–30% of patients have potentially resectable lesions at the time of diagnosis. With appropriate selection, 5-year survival has been reported around 30% (range 15–67%) [91–94]. Even with modern chemotherapy for colorectal cancer, surgery for metastatic cancer (if possible) has consistently been shown to improve 5-year survival and quality of life and should be considered when possible. This may require referral to a specialized center [92, 95, 96].

Untreated, potentially resectable liver lesions have a median survival of 8 months, with 5-year survival of <5% [43, 97]. With modern forms of chemotherapy, median survival can be extended to greater than 24 months and in rare cases can be up to 34 months [7, 8]. In addition, newer liver strategies may allow a staged resection, portal vein embolization, or a combination of resection, embolization, and other strategies to ablate or otherwise treat or downsize liver lesions, which may allow a greater percentage of patients to undergo some form of treatment [98]. This has allowed some centers to see overall 5-year survival rates among patients with metastatic colorectal cancer at the time of diagnosis to be as much as 19% [99]. This underscores the importance of multidisciplinary evaluation of these patients. The main reason for failure in treated patients is intrahepatic recurrence of the tumor, which occurs in 60–70% of patients, one third of whom die within 2 years of surgery for hepatic metastases [99].

For patients with resectable lesions, there are several strategies that can be utilized to treat these lesions. Each has its own merits and they will be reviewed here. Multidisciplinary evaluation and local expertise are again key to determining the appropriate strategy, as there is a paucity of data to evaluate the various treatment strategies.

Combination Liver and Colon Resection

Combination resection involves simultaneous resection of liver and colonic lesions. This allows a single operation to treat both disease foci without delay between procedures. There is evidence to suggest that this approach results in a similar long-term outcome when compared to those undergoing staged therapy. Similarly, simultaneous resection does not increase overall morbidity, though there is an inherent selection bias in trials examining this issue [92, 100–102]. This approach is typically done for relatively minor resections which can include lobectomy. Larger liver resections may result in increased morbidity when combined with other procedures and may not be appropriate candidates for this strategy [103, 104]. A meta-analysis of 2880 patients suggested that simultaneous resection was safe provided patients were less than 70 years old and did not have severe comorbidity [105, 106]. An additional meta-analysis of 18 studies including 3605 patients did not show a survival advantage to any strategy, though there is the potential for considerable selection bias toward smaller lesions in the patients undergoing a combined approach strategy [107].

Liver-First Strategy

In patients with liver metastases from colorectal cancer, it is the metastatic disease in the liver (particularly if >3 cm in size) that is the primary determinant of overall survival [108, 109]. This is a potential reason for addressing the liver disease first, particularly in the setting of larger metastatic lesions where the primary lesion is asymptomatic. As there is some evidence to suggest the primary lesion has a low chance of becoming symptomatic during follow-up, it is reasonable to proceed with treatment of the metastatic disease first [72]. This also may avoid unnecessary colorectal surgery (and its associated morbidity) in patients who go on to develop incurable metastatic disease. There is evidence to suggest that a "liver-first" strategy may still allow patients with potentially curable disease to undergo both liver and colon resection over time [109].

It is unclear whether the development of additional metastatic disease is stimulated by the liver metastases vs. the primary tumor [110–114]. This has generated considerable debate between hepatobiliary and colorectal surgeons as well as oncologists. As no randomized trials exist, this is a philosophic discussion that occurs at many tumor board interactions. The answer remains unclear, but it may affect the opinions of those involved in making recommendations.

The liver-first approach can be combined with neoadjuvant chemotherapy for borderline resectable lesions or to allow tumor biology to dictate those lesions that are likely to progress rapidly prior to surgery. While this has been recommended as standard of care by some, others have disputed this and still recommend surgical resection followed by adjuvant chemotherapy due to the effect of chemotherapy-associated steatosis that can increase surgical morbidity [115–118]. The liver-first strategy has a particular advantage in the setting or rectal cancer, where the process of neoadjuvant chemoradiotherapy can potentially take up to 3 months. This may allow surgery on the metastatic disease while treatment for the primary lesion is still ongoing. Alternatively, radiotherapy on rectal lesions can be reserved for overall disease that responds favorably to initial treatments—particularly the short course variety. The data for the liver-first approach is limited and largely based on non-randomized data, but seems to remain a viable method with good long-term results [119–125]. An international multidisciplinary consensus conference [126] suggested the liver-first strategy is as good as the conventional approach. The recommendation is to perform resection as soon as technically possible with a course of chemotherapy (if used) as short as possible in the absence of tumor progression. Furthermore age and total number of hepatic metastases should not be an absolute contraindication to surgery. The importance of a multidisciplinary approach remains crucial to ensuring long-term survival.

Colon-First Strategy

Proponents of the colon-first strategy hypothesize that the colon or rectum acts as an ongoing source of seeding metastatic disease. Additionally, the primary tumor represents a potential source of bowel-related morbidity in the form of bleeding, obstruction, or perforation. Some authors suggest the rates of this can be as high as 20%, but others suggest it is much lower than this [72, 87]. Additionally, the risk of morbidity associated with a colorectal anastomosis may be increased by addition of a liver procedure, where anesthesia and surgical techniques may include a low flow state or temporary alteration in portal blood circulation (e.g., a Pringle maneuver), which may affect blood flow to the bowel [127, 128]. Along similar lines, removal of the colon or rectum first may allow subsequent, more advanced, or aggressive strategies such as portal vein embolization to be used without compromising a future bowel procedure. Finally, resection of the colon first may allow detection of new or occult liver metastases which can then be removed with definitive surgery [129, 130].

Evidence to support each of these strategies is very limited and largely based on small, single institution series. Survival analyses across multiple studies suggest there is little difference between simultaneous, colon-, or liver-first strategies [105, 131–133]. As such, the agreed-upon treatment strategy should depend on the local expertise at an individual institution. The colon-first strategy may allow removal of the primary lesion with subsequent referral to a higher level of care or specialized center for definitive hepatectomy/metastasectomy. In counseling patients on the risk of recurrence, there have been identified factors to help determine prognosis. The Fong score is a series of five factors identified to have the greatest influence on outcome based on an analysis of 1001 patients undergoing potentially curative hepatectomy [134].

These included size >5 cm, disease-free survival less than 1 year, more than one tumor, lymph node-positive primary, and CEA >200 ng/mL.

Margin Status

Excision to negative margins in hepatic resection results in improved disease-free and overall survival. One study revealed an overall survival of 46 months was reduced to 24 months in patients with positive margins [135]. Furthermore, recurrence rates were significantly higher (28% with R1 resection vs. 17% with R0 resection, $p = 0.004$) in a study of 436 patients comparing margin status of hepatectomy specimens [136]. A consensus statement from the Society of Surgical Oncology concluded that while wide margins of >1 cm are desirable, a close margin should not preclude resection. Another study suggested that a margin <5 mm is a risk factor for local recurrence [137].

Ablation of Liver Metastases

There are a variety of techniques for ablation of liver metastases that do not require tissue resection. These include percutaneous ethanol ablation, radiofrequency ablation (RFA), microwave ablation, cryoablation, and irreversible electroporation (or NanoKnife). RFA is the most commonly employed technique, though all can be used successfully and also used in conjunction with other forms of therapy (e.g., surgical resection) [138]. As patients may develop a future recurrence, preservation of liver parenchyma may be important, especially with a larger burden of disease. This is the typical place for use of these ablative therapies. In selecting what treatment modality to use, the overarching goals of minimal morbidity with maximum treatment effect and prolongation of life remain a guiding principle during multidisciplinary evaluation. Several different treatments may be used simultaneously or in a staged approach. Recently, these combined ablation and resection (CARe) techniques have shown promising results. A four-center retrospective study showed disease-free 1- and 5-year survival rates of 87.9% and 78%, respectively [139].

RFA has been the most widely applied ablative technique, used primarily for metastatic liver tumors that are not amenable to surgical resection. Patients may not be candidates for surgery for various reasons including that the lesions are anatomically difficult for surgical resection (adjacent to the confluence of the hepatic or portal veins), the functional hepatic reserve after resection would be insufficient, there are significant comorbidities that preclude an operation, or extrahepatic metastases are present, further decreasing the likelihood of cure. RFA uses heat generated from high frequency alternating current (generally in the range of 350–500 kHz) to ablate diseased tissue. RFA can be performed with open, laparoscopic, or percutaneous approaches. Studies have reported that the approach by which RFA is performed has an impact on tumor recurrence rates, with the fewest local recurrences after open RFA, followed by laparoscopy, and finally percutaneous RFA [140–143]. However, local tumor recurrence rates overlap broadly with each technique, and physician experience as well as the type of RFA equipment is also inversely related to local recurrence rates [144, 145]. An expert panel convened by the American Society of Clinical Oncology (ASCO) to review the evidence on RFA for colorectal cancer liver metastases concluded that there is insufficient evidence to resolve the issue of optimal approach [146].

The vast majority of published data on efficacy of RFA for colorectal cancer liver metastases comes from retrospective series, many of which have limited follow-up (20 months or less), and there are few published randomized trials [140, 147–152]. A systematic review of the literature reported a wide range of 5-year survival (14–55%) and local recurrence rates (3.6–60%) [146]. However, both the retrospective series and the limited number of prospective trials consist of a variable mix of patients with potentially resectable liver-isolated disease and unresectable liver metastases with or without extrahepatic disease involvement. Finally, few series provide data on the use of chemotherapy concurrent with or following RFA, and as outcome measures differ between studies, a comparison is not always possible.

How the timing and use of RFA play into the overall treatment strategy remains an unanswered question. While many retrospective comparative series suggest RFA has higher local recurrence rates and worse progression-free survival (compared with resection), there are inherent limitations in these studies [153–159]. Given the evidence from retrospective reports that resection improves overall survival, particularly in the absence of extrahepatic disease, a systematic review of the literature by an expert panel from ASCO concluded that there is not enough evidence to support the use of RFA over resection in patients with potentially resectable colorectal cancer liver metastases [146]. A similar conclusion was reached in a 2012 Cochrane review [160].

RFA is a relatively well-tolerated technique, with a mortality rate of 0–2% and the major complication rate between 6 and 9% in most studies [146]. Complications can include liver abscess, pleural effusion, skin burns, and pneumothorax from diaphragm injury [161]. In summary, the place of RFA in the management of colorectal cancer liver metastases is still evolving, particularly in patients who have extrahepatic disease involvement. It is a potential option for patients with potentially resectable isolated liver metastases who are not surgical candidates.

Other Liver Metastasis Strategies: Hepatic Intra-arterial Chemotherapy/Chemoembolization

Regional chemotherapy through the hepatic artery is a therapeutic option for patients with isolated liver metastasis that are not amenable to surgical resection or local ablation. This method can also be combined with other forms of treatment. This mode of therapy is based upon the fact that liver macrometastases derive more than 80% of their blood supply from the hepatic arterial circulation, while normal hepatocytes are supplied primarily by the portal circulation [162]. This allows selective delivery of drug to the tumor with relative sparing of the normal hepatocytes. There is also a marked increase in the local concentration of the chemotherapy that is achieved by injection into the hepatic artery. Regional administration of agents that are rapidly metabolized in the liver by a first-pass effect leads to higher levels of drug exposure and minimizes side effects [163].

Transarterial embolization with or without chemotherapy (transarterial chemoembolization, TACE) has been investigated in patients with colorectal cancer liver metastases using both conventional techniques and drug-eluting beads. Response rates vary from 29 to 88%, which is based on limited experience. Most reported studies lack a control group, and the results from the two small-randomized controlled trials had conflicting results [164–166].

Most series of colorectal liver metastases have studied infusional hepatic artery chemotherapy without embolization. While there has been extensive clinical investigation of hepatic infusional chemotherapy in the past 30 years, there are fewer studies evaluating modern chemotherapeutic agents. A number of strategies have been explored in an attempt to overcome treatment-limiting toxicity and to maximize the safety and efficacy of HIA treatment. The majority of reports have evaluated modifications of 5-FU-based therapy, while more recent studies have explored other agents such as irinotecan and oxaliplatin. It has been shown that both oxaliplatin and irinotecan can be safely delivered and result in a high response rate in patients with unresectable disease [167–171]. A review of trials in the 1990s demonstrated that while response rates of tumors may be improved over systemic chemotherapy, the effect on survival was modest (overall survival 22.7 vs. 19.8 months). Other randomized trials have not seen any survival advantage [172, 173]. With improvements in chemotherapy, there is a paucity of high-quality data on the effectiveness of this treatment methodology. A recent review of nine studies and 1057 patients [174] did demonstrate improved 5-year disease-free survival rates (hazard ratio 0.61) when compared with systemic chemotherapy alone. A modest improvement in overall survival was also seen. This suggests it may have a role in the treatment of patients at high risk for recurrence, but this will require corroborative studies and should at present be restricted to centers with expertise in the technical aspects of its use.

Pulmonary Metastasis

Approximately 10% of patients with colorectal cancer develop pulmonary metastasis. The vast majority of patients with metastatic colorectal cancer to the lungs have advanced disease and are therefore treated with systemic chemotherapy or best supportive care. Due to differences in blood supply, pulmonary metastases may be more common after rectal (vs. colon) cancer due to the dual blood supply of the rectum (portal and systemic). A limited number of studies have reviewed the incidence of pulmonary metastases after resection of rectal cancer and have estimated that approximately 1–12% of patients develop isolated pulmonary metastases [175–178]. Of those patients with isolated pulmonary metastases, approximately 7–14% of patients would be considered as candidates for pulmonary metastasectomy [175, 178, 179].

There may be some tumor-related factors that give a predisposition to pulmonary metastasis. A recent study investigated predictive factors for pulmonary metastases after R0 resection of rectal cancer without preoperative chemoradiotherapy. Actuarial incidence of pulmonary metastases was significantly related to the number of risk factors present. Tumor depth (T2–T3), lymph node ratio >0.091, and tumor location in the anal canal were the independent risk factors for pulmonary metastases in patients with rectal cancer [180]. Another study demonstrated that adjuvant chemotherapy, extrapulmonary metastases, and prelaparotomy CEA value were independent prognostic factors for overall survival of patients with pulmonary metastases after a resection for colorectal cancer with curative intent [181].

Due to the retrospective nature of the reported information in the literature, clinical outcome data after metastasectomy for colorectal lung metastases must be interpreted with caution. Improved clinical outcome and survival data is more likely due to ideal patient selection and tumor biology rather than the surgical intervention in and of itself. In addition, there are no adequate control groups in these reports; therefore, survival statistics are difficult to interpret. However, there are patients who undergo pulmonary metastasectomy with no evidence of disease after long-term follow-up [179, 181]. In addition, long-term survival without complete resection is very rare, suggesting that select patients do occasionally benefit from pulmonary metastasectomy. Input on the

resectability of lung lesions by a thoracic surgeon at multidisciplinary evaluation is essential.

Modern series of lung resection for metastatic colorectal cancer report operative mortalities of less than 2% (Table 36-1). Five-year survival rates range from 16 to 64%, but generally cluster around 30–40%. Most studies evaluate factors associated with outcome; however, given the limited number of cases, the statistical power of these studies to detect significant factors is limited. In general, the pathology of the primary tumor (grade, location, stage) has not been shown to impact clinical outcome. The most commonly cited significant factors associated with adverse outcomes include the number and size of pulmonary metastasis, short disease-free interval, elevated CEA, and incomplete resection.

A recently published series of 94 patients from a single institution who underwent complete resection of pulmonary metastases from colorectal cancer was analyzed for survival rates as well as prognostic indicators for long-term survival. The cumulative survival rate was 45.5% after pulmonary metastasectomy [182]. Multivariate analysis revealed that an elevated preoperative CEA level was an independent prognostic indicator as shown in other studies. The study concluded that surgical resection offers a chance to prolong survival in colorectal cancer patients with resectable pulmonary metastases. However, there was a high recurrence rate (69.1%) and careful postoperative follow-up was advocated by the authors. Critiques of this study include the lack of randomization, appropiate controls, and failure to address the role of adjuvant chemotherapy.

While a majority of series have evaluated metastatic disease limited to the lungs, several series have evaluated patients with both liver and lung metastases. The majority of studies that have analyzed synchronous liver and lung metastases report a uniformly poor outcome following combined resections. Long-term survival is very uncommon in this situation [182–185]. In the setting of isolated pulmonary recurrence after partial hepatectomy, pulmonary metastasectomy appears to have more favorable outcomes similar to those for the initial hepatectomy [183, 184, 186].

TABLE 36-1. Outcome of patients undergoing pulmonary metastasectomy for colorectal cancer

Study	n	Operative mortality (%)	5-year survival (%)	Significant risk factors
Mori et al. [293]	35	–	38	None found
McCormack et al. [294]	144	0	44	Margin
McAfee et al. [185]	139	1	31	Number of lesions, CEA
Yano et al. [295]	27	–	41	Number of lesions
Saclarides et al. [296]	23	–	16	Number of lesions
van Halteren et al. [297]	38	–	43	DFI
Shirouzu et al. [298]	22	–	37	Number of lesions, size
Girard et al. [299]	86	1	24	CEA, margin
Okumura et al. [300]	159	2	41	Number of lesions, LN status
Zanella et al. [301]	22	0	62	None found
Zink [302]	110	0	33	Size, CEA
Dahabre et al. [179]	52	–	33	None found

n number of patients, yr year, LN lymph nodes, DFI disease-free interval
Source: Adapted from Rizk et al. [186]

The surgical approach to patients who are potential candidates for pulmonary metastasectomy has been somewhat controversial. Based on older studies reported in the 1980s citing a 38% yield of contralateral thoracotomy in finding radiographically occult disease, routine bilateral thoracotomy had been advocated previously [187]. With modern-day imaging, routine bilateral thoracotomy is no longer justified. The use of video-assisted thoracoscopic surgery (VATS) has increased significantly and is often used in metastasectomy when a minimal parenchymal resection is necessary. Initially, VATS was deemed substandard to thoracotomy due to the inability to palpate the lung parenchyma; a prospective study evaluating confirmatory thoracotomy after VATS showed that 22% of lesions were missed [187, 188]. However, with improvements in modern imaging and VATS techniques, a minimally invasive approach can now be employed.

Radiation therapy for colorectal cancer pulmonary metastasis has been of limited utility in the past due to radiation-induced pneumonitis, rib and spinal fractures, and skin toxicities. However, these toxicities can be minimized with the advent of robotic-assisted Gamma Knife radiotherapy or "CyberKnife" [189]. Initial reports appear to have minimal toxicity associated with single-session lung radiotherapy using robotic image-guided real-time respiratory and tumor tracking. This is an exciting field of research and may become an additional therapeutic modality in the future. However, the outcome and efficacy data is limited at this time, and the associated cost of robotic image-guided radiotherapy will be a limiting factor in widespread availability.

While it appears that certain colorectal cancer patients would benefit from pulmonary metastasectomy even in the presence of liver metastases, no randomized controlled trials have been conducted and reported, and the effectiveness of pulmonary metastasectomy has been suggested mostly by results of retrospective analyses. A randomized trial to investigate the effectiveness of pulmonary metastasectomy in colorectal cancer is currently in progress [190], and we will need to look to those results which hopefully will give clear evidences on the benefits of and to establish standard guidelines for pulmonary metastasectomy.

Peritoneal Metastasis

Peritoneal carcinomatosis represents one of the most challenging aspects of metastatic colorectal cancer. The peritoneal surface is involved in approximately 10–15% of colorectal cancer patients at time of initial presentation (synchronous metastases) and in 20–50% of patients who develop recurrence (metachronous metastases) [191–193]. As a site of colorectal cancer metastasis, the peritoneal surface ranks second only to the liver. It is characterized by intraperitoneal spread of metastatic nodules. Peritoneal metastasis occurs by direct implantation of cancer cells via one of four mechanisms: (1) spontaneous intraperitoneal

seeding from a T4 colorectal cancer that has penetrated the serosal surface of the colon, (2) extravasation of tumor cells at the time of colon perforation from an obstructing cancer, (3) iatrogenic tumor perforation through an area of serosal injury or enterotomy at the time of colon resection, and (4) leakage of tumor cells from transected lymphatics or veins at the time of colon resection [192]. The risk of peritoneal metastasis is therefore highest in the setting of locally advanced cancers, and, until recently, most oncologists viewed peritoneal carcinomatosis as a terminal condition, to be palliated only with systemic chemotherapy.

However, in a small set of cases, the peritoneal cavity is determined to be the only site of metastatic disease after a detailed workup of the lungs and liver. This has led some to hypothesize that in some cases, peritoneal carcinomatosis may represent a first site of dissemination and, therefore, not necessarily indicative of generalized disease [194–196]. This scenario appears to be rare overall. In a combined series of 2095 patients with metastatic colorectal cancer (CRC) who were enrolled in two chemotherapy trials, 364 (17%) had peritoneal carcinomatosis, but only 44 (2.1%) had peritoneal carcinomatosis as the sole presentation of metastatic disease [197].

A similar paradigm is hypothesized for appendiceal cancer, which also has a propensity to spread intraperitoneally. Radical surgical cytoreduction and intraperitoneal (IP) chemotherapy has gained acceptance for the treatment of diffuse peritoneal adenomucinosis (pseudomyxoma peritonei) and selected patients with peritoneal dissemination of an appendiceal adenocarcinoma (mucinous peritoneal carcinomatosis). This topic is covered in the chapter devoted to appendiceal neoplasms.

Peritoneal metastases are clinically important because of their frequent progression to malignant ascites and/or malignant bowel obstruction [193, 198–201]. When patients present with peritoneal metastases, the most frequent symptoms were ascites (29.7%) and bowel obstruction (19.5%). Preoperative detection of peritoneal metastases is not reliable. Noninvasive imaging frequently misses small peritoneal lesions, even when these are widely disseminated. The sensitivity of CT scanning for lesions smaller than 5 mm is only 28% as compared to 70% for lesions 2 cm or greater [202]. Thus, indirect signs such as bulky primary tumor, ascites, or bowel obstruction are important clues. The utility of MRI in diagnosis of peritoneal carcinomatosis beyond that of CT is largely unknown and PET scans are of limited value. Unfortunately, in the majority of cases, diagnosis is made at the time of primary resection [203]. There are several approaches to treatment if peritoneal involvement is discovered.

The extent of carcinomatosis is a major prognostic factor and is best assessed by either laparoscopic or open exploration. Two different peritoneal carcinomatosis staging systems (Gilly's classification and Peritoneal Cancer Index of Sugarbaker) can be used to assess the extent of carcinomatosis

[204, 205]. These staging systems have both shown utility in determining the prognosis and treatment of patients with peritoneal carcinomatosis. By Gilly's classification, carcinomatosis is classified principally by the dimensions of the peritoneal tumor implants: stage I, tumor nodules less than 5 mm in diameter localized in one part of the abdomen; stage II, tumor nodules less than 5 mm disseminated widely through the abdomen; stage III, tumor nodules 5–2 cm in diameter; and stage IV, tumor nodules greater than 2 cm. The Peritoneal Cancer Index scores the extent of carcinomatosis on the basis of tumor size and location within 13 regions of the abdomen and pelvis with the largest size in each abdominopelvic region is scored on a scale of 0–3 (0, no tumor; 1, tumor up to 0.5 cm; 2, tumor up to 5.0 cm; 3, >5 cm or confluence). The total score of the Peritoneal Cancer Index is shown to correlate with survival. Median survival and 5-year survival after surgical debulking and intraperitoneal chemotherapy were 48 months and 50% for peritoneal index <10, compared to 12 months and 0% for index >20.

Standard management of patients known to have peritoneal metastases at initial presentation (if known preoperatively) is systemic chemotherapy. Colon resection plays an important role for patients with obstructing primary cancers and also for patients with occult metastases that are first detected in the operating room. Historically, the median survival for patients with unresected peritoneal metastasis treated with 5-fluorouracil-based systemic chemotherapy was very poor (6–8 months) [194, 206, 207]. However, patient survival is highly variable, depending on the extent of metastatic disease and response to chemotherapy [194, 207]. Contemporary combination chemotherapy regimens have significantly greater efficacy and can produce long periods of disease control in certain patients.

Despite the grim prognosis for patients with peritoneal carcinomatosis from colorectal cancer, a subset of patients once thought unsalvageable are now being considered for surgery with curative intent. Pioneered by Sugarbaker, the goal of cytoreductive surgery and intraperitoneal (IP) chemotherapy is to remove all macroscopic disease with peritonectomy procedures and visceral resections followed by perioperative IP chemotherapy to destroy residual microscopic disease. IP delivery offers pharmacokinetic advantage over standard intravenous delivery by producing high regional concentrations of drug while simultaneously minimizing systemic toxicities [208–210]. For patients with isolated peritoneal carcinomatosis from colorectal cancer, radical surgery to achieve an R0 resection (if it can be accomplished) remains the mainstay of treatment. Benefit from cytoreductive surgery with heated intraperitoneal chemotherapy has been suggested in several retrospective case series, a multi-institutional registry review [211], two randomized trials, and a systematic review.

These randomized trials must be interpreted with caution as neither used modern combination chemotherapy as the control arm [212, 213]. In the first trial, 105 patients with established peritoneal carcinomatosis of colorectal (n = 87) or appendiceal (n = 18) origin were randomly assigned to (A) cytoreductive surgery and HIPEC (with intraoperative mitomycin C) followed by systemic chemotherapy (5-FU and leucovorin only) or (B) systemic 5-FU and leucovorin alone with palliative surgery as needed [212]. Despite the high postoperative mortality rate (8%), the median disease-specific survival in the IP treatment group was significantly longer (22 versus 13 months). At a median follow-up of 8 years, 45% of patients in the IP chemotherapy arm who underwent complete cytoreduction (no residual tumor nodules) were still alive [214]. It should be noted that the use of a modern systemic oxaliplatin or irinotecan containing regimens in the control arm could potentially have narrowed and even eliminated the survival difference between the groups, since median survival durations in contemporary reports approximate 20 months.

The second trial, which also randomly assigned patients following aggressive surgical cytoreduction to systemic therapy (5-FU-based) with or without hyperthermic IP chemotherapy, only accrued 35 of the planned cohort of 90 patients (30 CRC, 5 appendiceal cancers) [213]. Although the 2-year survival rate of patients undergoing IP chemotherapy was 60% (much higher than would be expected among patients treated with systemic 5-FU/leucovorin chemotherapy), the difference in survival between the experimental and control groups was not statistically significant.

A systematic review of published data of cytoreductive surgery and IP chemotherapy for peritoneal dissemination of colorectal cancer, including the two randomized trials described above [212, 213], one comparative study [215], a multi-institutional registry series (an earlier report than described above) [216], and several case series, came to the following conclusions [217]:

- Median survival varied from 13 to 29 months, and 5-year survival rates ranged from 11 to 19%.
- Patients who underwent complete surgical cytoreduction appeared to benefit the most, with median survival 28–60 months and 5-year survival from 22 to 49%.
- This survival benefit was achieved at a cost of overall treatment-related morbidity rates between 23 and 44% and mortality rates from 0 to 12%.

Although these results seem promising, many important unanswered questions remain, including which patients with colorectal cancer peritoneal carcinomatosis have a higher or considerably lower likelihood of long-term survival after cytoreductive surgery and HIPEC [218] (Figure 36-6) and whether results in any population are better than could be achieved using modern oxaliplatin and/or irinotecan-based systemic chemotherapy with or without biologic agents. These regimens have greater activity as compared with 5-FU and leucovorin alone. Median survival durations in unselected patients with metastatic disease are 22–24 months, and approximately 10% of patients remain alive at 5 years.

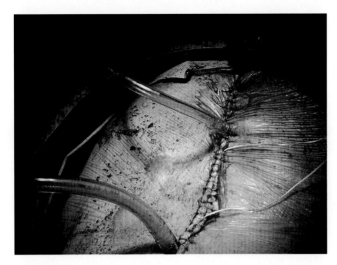

FIGURE 36-6. Hyperthermic intraperitoneal chemotherapy (HIPEC). Courtesy of Eric K. Johnson, M.D.

The only data that specifically address the efficacy of modern systemic chemotherapy in patients with isolated peritoneal carcinomatosis come from a retrospective analysis of 48 highly selected patients with peritoneal carcinomatosis from colorectal cancer who were treated with an oxaliplatin- or irinotecan-based palliative chemotherapy regimen at one of five French comprehensive cancer centers (where cytoreductive surgery and HIPEC were not available) over a 5-year period [219]. These patients were selected as the control group on the basis of their meeting clinico-pathologic criteria defined as good prognostic factors for HIPEC [213]. The 2- and 5-year survival rates were 65 and 13%, respectively, and the median survival was 24 months. In contrast, the median and 2- and 5-year survival rates for a separate group of 48 patients who underwent cytoreductive surgery and HIPEC for colorectal cancer peritoneal carcinomatosis during the same time period at the Gustave Roussy Institute were 63 months and 81 and 51%, respectively. The authors concluded that, in appropriately selected patients with isolated peritoneal carcinomatosis, results with cytoreductive surgery and HIPEC are superior to those that can be achieved with modern combination chemotherapy regimens. The retrospective nature of this analysis and the inherent bias in comparing nonrandomly assigned patients limit the confidence with which this conclusion can be judged.

While patients who undergo complete cytoreduction followed by HIPEC seem to have a more favorable prognosis than can be achieved with systemic chemotherapy alone, there remains insufficient evidence to conclude whether the survival advantage is due to treatment or to biologic features that allow these patients to undergo complete cytoreductive surgery. Furthermore, the quality of the cytoreductive surgery is dependent upon the skills and level of experience of the surgeon. The favorable results (particularly with regard to treatment-related toxicity) [211, 220] achieved by international experts in the field may not be replicated in routine

clinical practice. Finally, the independent contribution of HIPEC to the success of this approach has not been proven. Randomized trials are needed.

Based upon all of these issues, the NCCN believes [221] this approach should not be considered standard at present and only pursued in centers with demonstrated expertise [222], preferably in the context of a clinical trial. Such a trial, USMCI 8214/ACOSOG Z6091, in which patients with peritoneal carcinomatosis from colorectal cancer were randomized to standard systemic chemotherapy or surgical cytoreduction with heated intraperitoneal chemotherapy followed by systemic chemotherapy, was closed for lack of accrual. Another trial, Prodige 7, in which patients with isolated intraperitoneal metastases from colorectal cancer are randomly assigned to cytoreductive surgery with or without HIPEC, is underway in France.

In summary, the standard therapy for patients with peritoneal metastases is systemic chemotherapy. However, there is some evidence that aggressive surgical cytoreduction and IP chemotherapy may benefit highly select patients with limited peritoneal tumor burden. Additional clinical trials are needed to define optimal use of this aggressive treatment approach. As a result, if unexpected, diffuse carcinomatosis is found at the time of operative intervention, consideration should be given to referral to a specialized center prior to further operative intervention other than a possible proximal diversion or relief of any immediate surgical emergency.

Ovarian Metastases

Approximately 4–30% of ovarian neoplasms are metastatic cancers with the most common being colorectal and breast cancer [223]. A recent autopsy study demonstrated that of all women dying with colorectal cancer, between 6 and 14% were found to have ovarian metastasis at the time of death [224]. For those women with stage IV disease, the risk of developing ovarian metastases is substantially higher and approaches 90% for those with established peritoneal metastasis. Therefore, in a woman with a recent diagnosis of advanced colorectal cancer, any ovarian mass should be considered a metastasis from colorectal cancer until proven otherwise.

The pathogenesis of ovarian metastasis from colorectal cancer is multifactorial. While metastatic spread occurs primarily through the peritoneum, it can also occur by direct extension, hematogenously or lymphatically. It is imperative that careful intraoperative assessment of the ovaries is undertaken at the time of primary resection of the colon cancer. Depending on the study, synchronous metastases can occur in 0–8.6% of patients [225–228], while metachronous metastases develop in 1.4–6.8% of cases [223, 224], usually within 2 years after the primary resection [226–233]. At least half of the cases have bilateral ovarian involvement [234, 235], and 40% of these patients have associated extra-ovarian pelvic metastasis [234] and if large enough can be palpated on physical exam or with peritoneal drop metastasis known as the "Blumer's shelf." It is extremely difficult to determine a primary ovarian tumor from a metastatic colorectal tumor by gross examination alone, but through the integration of pathologic, cytogenic, and immunohistochemical features, a correct diagnosis can be generally arrived at. Most metastatic colorectal lesions are CK20+/CEA+/CK7– on immunohistochemical staining, while primary ovarian neoplasms are CK20–/CEA–/CK7+ [235–238].

The decision to perform an oophorectomy at the time of surgery requires some in-depth reasoning. Primary en bloc resection of colorectal cancer with direct extension to the ovary (T4) or resection of macroscopic metastatic disease to the ovary with prophylactic bilateral resection has been suggested to offer survival benefit and should be performed with curative intent in the absence of other significant metastatic disease. However, the removal of macroscopically normal ovaries (prophylactic oophorectomy) in women with colorectal cancer is controversial and remains the subject of much debate. Proponents of removal argue that resection improves the cure rate by removing potential microscopic "undetectable" synchronous disease, eliminates the risk of ovarian cancer, and removes the risk of future metachronous ovarian metastatic disease. Others argue that the low incidence of ovarian metastasis, the small amount of supportive data, and few clinical correlations with predictive value make the additional resection of the ovaries unnecessary [224]. Clinical studies attempting to document the benefit of ovarian metastasectomy in patients with colorectal cancer are small and retrospective [225, 239, 240]. The majority of studies to date, however, fail to show any survival benefit for prophylactic oophorectomy, and most studies demonstrate that when ovarian metastases are present, it is a very poor prognostic sign [224]. Based on available information, it is reasonable to offer prophylactic oophorectomy to all postmenopausal patients, in particular to those women who have undergone pelvic radiation as part of their treatment for rectal cancer. For premenopausal patients, only those with established peritoneal metastases, those that are proven to have an increased risk of developing ovarian carcinoma (strong family history, known carriers of breast cancer (BRCA), or those with an HNPCC mutation), or those who have already completed their families should be considered for prophylactic oophorectomy.

Most ovarian metastases are asymptomatic and are only detected at the time of surgery; however, larger metastatic lesions can compress or invade adjacent organs, rupture, and on rare occasions bleed. Larger ovarian lesions are usually visualized on initial staging imaging and should be part of the decision-making regarding surgical resection and informed consent. Survival of women with synchronous ovarian colorectal metastases is significantly worse than that of patients without such metastases [223, 241]. Ovarian

metastases are frequently resistant to systemic chemotherapy even when other sites of metastatic disease are responding, and therefore, resection of these synchronous metastases including bilateral oophorectomy and resection of gross disease should be performed at the index operation [242–245]. Reoperation for metachronous metastases should be considered in select patients with good performance status and limited tumor burden elsewhere. Discussion of these patients in a multidisciplinary fashion is imperative. To prevent local tumor progression, an aggressive surgical approach should be undertaken to achieve complete resection. The survival benefit of removing ovarian metastases had never been well documented, although complete metastasectomy is associated with significantly better outcome when compared to palliative debulking, especially in the setting of metastatic disease confined to the pelvis [246, 247]. It should be noted that complete resection is possible in 50% of these cases. The median post-resection survival for women with isolated ovarian metastases is 18 months [242]. Women with other sites have significantly shorter survival, and 5-year survival after resection of established metastasis is rare [243, 244]. In these cases, systemic chemotherapy should be strongly considered, particularly when residual disease is present. With the constant evolution and improvement of chemotherapeutic regimens, containing oxaliplatin, irinotecan, and/or bevacizumab, better survival can be expected [248–251]. See Figure 36-7 for an algorithm outlining the treatment of ovarian metastases.

Other Sites of Metastasis

Bone

Before the introduction of modern chemotherapy and targeted treatment options, bone metastases were reported in as high as 24% of cases [252, 253]. With modern therapies, bone metastases from colorectal cancer reportedly occur now in 7–9% of cases, and most often present in the context of widespread metastatic disease [254–257]. Routine diagnostic bone imaging is not indicated in colorectal cancer patients, unless there are specific bone-related symptoms. When bone metastases occur, they most commonly occur in the spine (65%), followed by hip/pelvis (34%) and long bones (17%). There are no curative modalities, but palliation of pain, fractures, or spinal cord involvement are important issues for these patients. Symptomatic relief from bony metastases can usually be accomplished with radiation, chemotherapy, as well as bisphosphonate therapy with zoledronic acid [253]. However, pathologic fractures are best treated by operative internal fixation. The systemic issues related to bone metastases are serious and include debilitation, immobility, hypercalcemia, and thromboembolic disease.

FIGURE 36-7. Treatment
algorithm for ovarian metastases.

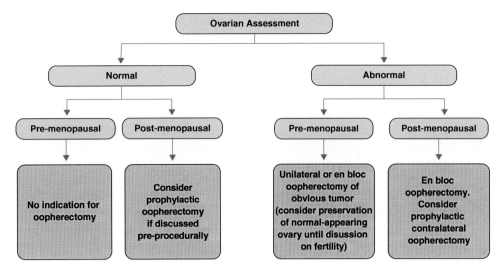

Brain

Cerebral metastases from colorectal cancer are uncommon, occurring in 1–4% of colorectal cancer cases [254–256]. Colorectal tumors account for approximately 3% of all metastatic brain tumors [257]. These are generally found in the context of widespread metastases to multiple organ sites, but on rare occasion can present as an isolated brain metastasis [258]. There is no role for routine brain imaging at primary presentation or at presentation with metastases elsewhere, unless there are specific neurologic symptoms. Once brain metastases occur, symptoms are common; palliative therapies include steroids to decrease swelling and anticonvulsants to control seizures. Definitive therapy of colorectal brain metastases usually involves surgery, radiation, or a combination of the two. For isolated, single brain metastases, resection can result in survival beyond 1–2 years; however, because brain metastases are infrequently the sole site of metastatic disease and because survival is dismal regardless of therapy chosen, craniotomy is rarely indicated [256–260]. As with pulmonary metastasis, there is increasing interest and data in the literature regarding Gamma Knife and CyberKnife radiotherapy for bone and brain metastasis [261, 262]. The outcome and efficacy data is limited at this time and the associated cost of robotic real-time image-guided radiotherapy may be a limiting factor in widespread applicability.

Pancreas

The pancreas is an uncommon location for solitary metastases from other primary cancers [263]. While the prevalence of pancreatic metastases has been described as high as 6–11% [264], reports of solitary resectable pancreatic metastases from colorectal cancer are extremely rare [265, 266]. Although long-term survival is rare, surgical resection can be performed safely in patients with isolated

pancreatic metastases from colorectal cancer and in selected patients with extrapancreatic disease [265]. As with other sites of multiorgan metastases, a multimodality approach is strongly recommended and consideration for surgical resection should be taken in context with an overall treatment plan and chances for improving survival while maintaining quality of life.

Adrenal

Adrenal metastases are uncommon with 14% found in one autopsy series [267]. Isolated adrenal metastases are even rarer. Aggressive surgical resection for isolated adrenal metastases is described in only a few case reports or small series [268–273]. In the largest series of eight patients with apparently isolated adrenal metastasis from colorectal cancer, all of whom received adjuvant chemotherapy, or remained alive and disease-free 12 months after adrenalectomy, one was lost to follow-up and six died of their malignancy. The mean survival of patients who died was 32 (range 12–60 months) [268]. In contrast to the situation with isolated adrenal metastases, the development of adrenal metastases after liver resection for colorectal cancer is associated with a poor prognosis, and adrenalectomy is not warranted [274].

Retroperitoneal Lymph Nodes

Isolated retroperitoneal nodal recurrence occurs in less than 2% of patients following a colorectal cancer resection with curative intent [275–277]. Salvage surgery has been previously avoided due to the poor prognosis; however, this concept is being challenged [278, 279]. A retrospective review of nine studies including case reports, case series, and case-control studies reported a survival benefit and no operative mortality for 110 patients undergoing a salvage retroperitoneal nodal resection. The median disease-free survival was

17–21 months, and the duration of overall survival ranged from 19 months to 18 years with a median of 34–44 months [280]. These series were collective over a time when the newer chemotherapy regimens were evolving (e.g., oxaliplatin, irinotecan, cetuximab, bevacizumab). There is no current data addressing the benefit of chemotherapy after resection of isolated retroperitoneal nodal disease. As in the case in patients with resected colorectal cancer with hepatic and pulmonary metastases, it is unclear if the addition of chemotherapy improves the observed survival statistics.

Metastatic Disease in the Elderly

Colorectal cancer remains one of the most commonly diagnosed cancers in the world with 60% of patients being over 70 years old and 43% are over 75 [281, 282]. The world's population is aging and it is estimated that the number of Americans over the age of 65 will double by the year 2030 and will account for 20% of the total population [283]. The average 65-year-old person can expect to live another 15 years and remain functionally independent for the majority of that time [284]. Thus, the number of older cancer patients is expected to increase. It is estimated that 50% of all cancer and 70% of all cancer mortality occurs in this age group [285]. Therefore, multidisciplinary teams will increasingly see older patients with colorectal cancer, and management of this distinct group deserves special mention.

When considering surgery, comorbidity, functional dependency, and older age are associated with early postoperative mortality in patients with gastrointestinal malignancies, with 30-day postoperative mortality rates underestimating postoperative mortality in older patients [286]. In regards to chemotherapy, the data available indicates that older patients derive the same benefit and have the same degree of toxicity as younger patients. The clinical trial data however may not be reflective of the average elderly patient seen in practice that is often suffering from more comorbidities and has greater functional impairment [287]. For these reasons, the International Society of Geriatric Oncology (SIOG) previously recommended that colorectal cancer patients >65 years of age requiring surgery should undergo a preoperative whole patient evaluation of the most common physiological side effects of aging, physical and mental ability, and social support. Further for those patients assessed as having physical or psychological comorbidities, it was recommended that a geriatrician was involved in the patient management [288].

Since those original recommendations, there have been multiple frailty indices proposed to detect vulnerability in elderly patients with cancer so that treatment can be adjusted accordingly. The process of these assessments, however, can be time consuming, and prescreening is often used to identify fit patients who are able to receive standard treatment versus those in whom a full comprehensive geriatric assessment should be done [289, 290]. The four most common

indices utilized appear to be the abbreviated comprehensive geriatric assessment (aCGA), the Vulnerable Elders Survey-13 (VES-13), the Groningen Frailty Indicator (GFI), and the Geriatric 8 (G8). Unfortunately, at present, there is no universal screening tool that adequately identifies frailty in at-risk older patients, and sensitivity and specificity for these indices ranged from 67 to 87% and 59 to 73%, respectively, which questions the value they may offer to the clinician [290]. There has been a study that has shown that the aCGA and G8 were the best screens for older patients with cancer that qualified for elective abdominal surgery; the G8 had the highest sensitivity and negative predictive value and the aCGA was a good overall assessment tool [291]. The American College of Surgeons NSQIP Risk Calculator (http://riskcalculator.facs.org) also uses degree of independence and other comorbidity variables that can be used to assess surgical risk in the elderly. In particular, it also gives an assessment of the risk of discharge to a long-term care facility in addition to the risk of common complications. Colorectal surgeons should be aware of the availability of these assessments and can use them as tools to aid them in evaluating the elderly population.

Because of the ever-increasing complexity and diversity of treatment options for elderly patients with colorectal cancer, SIOG reassembled their task force in 2013 to revise treatment recommendations. As a result of that group's work, it was recommended that the following outcomes need to be considered in relation to contemplating surgery in the elderly population: immediate postoperative morbidity, 30-day postoperative morbidity and mortality, length of stay, discharge to nursing home, 1-year mortality, short-term and long-term functional outcomes, quality of life, and survival. With regard to contemplating chemotherapy management in these patients, it was recommended that the following outcomes need to be considered: toxicity, completion of therapy, quality of life, functional status, progression, survival, and composite end points. Furthermore, it is important to recognize that embracing the concept of individualized treatment in a multidisciplinary setting is key to further improvements in the management of elderly patients utilizing some form of comprehensive geriatric assessment, involving patients in decision-making by providing them with tailored information and the potential for morbidities in advance of treatment, as well as the need for encouraging investigators to design trials using low-toxicity treatments that maintain efficacy of full-dose treatments and patient-centered assessments to expand the evidence base in the treatment of older patients with colorectal cancer [292].

Summary

This chapter has summarized the approach to patients with stage IV colorectal cancer. Throughout a variety of studies, the one overarching principle has been the emphasis on multidisciplinary evaluation. No one pre-scribed treatment protocol has proved more successful than others, and a combination of therapies across multiple specialties is now possible and an individualized approach to treatment is important. Available options include modern chemotherapy in the neoadjuvant or adjuvant setting, metastatic surgical resection with a variety of timing options, and nonsurgical ablative techniques. The overarching goal in the use of these treatment strategies is to improve survival and quality of life. There have been dramatic improvements in recent years, and although some patients cannot be cured, they can be effectively treated or palliated. As the approach to tumors can be highly individualized, consensus agreement with expert multidisciplinary evaluation remains of paramount importance in the care of these patients.

References

1. Siegel RL, Miller KD, Jemal A. Cancer statistics, 2015. CA Cancer J Clin. 2015;65(1):5–29.
2. O'Connell JB, Maggard MA, Ko CY. Colon cancer survival rates with the new American Joint Committee on Cancer sixth edition staging. J Natl Cancer Inst. 2004;96(19):1420–5.
3. Nordic Gastrointestinal Tumor Adjuvant Therapy Group. Expectancy or primary chemotherapy in patients with advanced asymptomatic colorectal cancer: a randomized trial. J Clin Oncol. 1992;10(6):904–11.
4. Scheithauer W, Rosen H, Kornek GV, Sebesta C, Depisch D. Randomised comparison of combination chemotherapy plus supportive care with supportive care alone in patients with metastatic colorectal cancer. BMJ. 1993;306(6880):752–5.
5. Tournigand C, André T, Achille E, Lledo G, Flesh M, Mery-Mignard D, et al. FOLFIRI followed by FOLFOX6 or the reverse sequence in advanced colorectal cancer: a randomized GERCOR study. J Clin Oncol. 2004;22(2):229–37.
6. Hurwitz H, Fehrenbacher L, Novotny W, Cartwright T, Hainsworth J, Heim W, et al. Bevacizumab plus irinotecan, fluorouracil, and leucovorin for metastatic colorectal cancer. N Engl J Med. 2004;350(23):2335–42.
7. Bokemeyer C, Bondarenko I, Makhson A, et al. Fluorouracil, leucovorin, and oxaliplatin with and without cetuximab in the first-line treatment of metastatic colorectal cancer. J Clin Oncol. 2009;27(5):663–71.
8. Grothey A, Sugrue MM, Purdie DM, Dong W, Sargent D, Hedrick E, et al. Bevacizumab beyond first progression is associated with prolonged overall survival in metastatic colorectal cancer: results from a large observational cohort study (BRiTE). J Clin Oncol. 2008;26(33):5326–34.
9. Hanahan D, Weinberg RA. The hallmarks of cancer. Cell. 2000;100(1):57–70.
10. Woodhouse EC, Chuaqui RF, Liotta LA. General mechanisms of metastasis. Cancer. 1997;80(8 Suppl):1529–37.
11. Fidler IJ. Critical factors in the biology of human cancer metastasis: twenty-eighth G.H.A. Clowes memorial award lecture. Cancer Res. 1990;50(19):6130–8.
12. Folkman J. How is blood vessel growth regulated in normal and neoplastic tissue? G.H.A. Clowes memorial Award lecture. Cancer Res. 1986;46(2):467–73.
13. Hynes RO. Metastatic potential: generic predisposition of the primary tumor or rare, metastatic variants-or both? Cell. 2003;113(7):821–3.
14. Bogenrieder T, Herlyn M. Axis of evil: molecular mechanisms of cancer metastasis. Oncogene. 2003;22(42):6524–36.
15. Chambers AF, Groom AC, MacDonald IC. Dissemination and growth of cancer cells in metastatic sites. Nat Rev Cancer. 2002;2(8):563–72.
16. Messick CA, Church JM, Liu X, Ting AH, Kalady MF. Stage III colorectal cancer: molecular disparity between primary cancers and lymph node metastases. Ann Surg Oncol. 2010;17(2):425–31.
17. Chang GJ, Kaiser AM, Mills S, Rafferty JF, Buie WD, Standards Practice Task Force of the American Society of Colon and Rectal Surgeons. Practice parameters for the management of colon cancer. Dis Colon Rectum. 2012;55(8):831–43.
18. Xu LH, Cai SJ, Cai GX, Peng WJ. Imaging diagnosis of colorectal liver metastases. World J Gastroenterol. 2011;17(42):4654–9.
19. Chen CC, Yang SH, Lin JK, Lin TC, Chen WS, Jiang JK, et al. Is it reasonable to add preoperative serum level of CEA and CA19-9 to staging for colorectal cancer? J Surg Res. 2005;124(2):169–74.
20. Johnson CD, Chen M-H, Toledano AY, Heiken JP, Dachman A, Kuo MD, et al. Accuracy of CT colonography for detection of large adenomas and cancers. N Engl J Med. 2008;359(12):1207–17.
21. Levin B, Lieberman DA, McFarland B, Smith RA, Brooks D, Andrews KS, American Cancer Society Colorectal Cancer Advisory Group, US Multi-Society Task Force, American College of Radiology Colon Cancer Committee, et al. Screening and surveillance for the early detection of colorectal cancer and adenomatous polyps, 2008: a joint guideline from the American Cancer Society, the US Multi-Society Task Force on Colorectal Cancer, and the American College of Radiology. CA Cancer J Clin. 2008;58(3):130–60.
22. Macari M, Berman P, Dicker M, Milano A, Megibow AJ. Usefulness of CT colonography in patients with incomplete colonoscopy. AJR Am J Roentgenol. 1999;173(3):561–4.
23. Ch'en IY, Katz DS, Jeffrey RB, Daniel BL, Li KC, Beaulieu CF, et al. Do arterial phase helical CT images improve detection or characterization of colorectal liver metastases? J Comput Assist Tomogr. 1997;21(3):391–7.
24. Meijerink MR, van Waesberghe JH, Golding RP, van der Weide L, van den Tol P, Meijer S, et al. Subtraction-multiphase-CT unbeneficial for early detection of colorectal liver metastases. Eur J Radiol. 2010;74(3):e132–7.
25. Wicherts DA, de Haas RJ, van Kessel CS, Bisschops RHC, Takahara T, van Hillegersberg R, et al. Incremental value of arterial and equilibrium phase compared to hepatic venous phase CT in the preoperative staging of colorectal liver metastases: an evaluation with different reference standards. Eur J Radiol. 2011;77(2):305–11.
26. Scott DJ, Guthrie JA, Arnold P, Ward J, Atchley J, Wilson D, et al. Dual phase helical CT versus portal venous phase CT for the detection of colorectal liver metastases: correlation with intra-operative sonography, surgical and pathological findings. Clin Radiol. 2001;56(3):235–42.
27. Valls C, Andía E, Sánchez A, Gumà A, Figueras J, Torras J, et al. Hepatic metastases from colorectal cancer: preoperative

detection and assessment of resectability with helical CT. Radiology. 2001;218(1):55–60.

28. Ruhlmann J, Schomburg A, Bender H, Oehr P, Robertz-Vaupel GM, Vaupel H, et al. Fluorodeoxyglucose whole-body positron emission tomography in colorectal cancer patients studied in routine daily practice. Dis Colon Rectum. 1997;40(10):1195–204.

29. Johnson K, Bakhsh A, Young D, Martin TE, Arnold M. Correlating computed tomography and positron emission tomography scan with operative findings in metastatic colorectal cancer. Dis Colon Rectum. 2001;44(3):354–7.

30. Chin BB, Wahl RL. 18F-Fluoro-2-deoxyglucose positron emission tomography in the evaluation of gastrointestinal malignancies. Gut. 2003;52 Suppl 4:iv23–9.

31. Brush J, Boyd K, Chappell F, Crawford F, Dozier M, Fenwick E, et al. The value of FDG positron emission tomography/computerised tomography (PET/CT) in pre-operative staging of colorectal cancer: a systematic review and economic evaluation. Health Technol Assess. 2011;15(35):1–192. iii–iv.

32. Jung EJ, Kim SR, Ryu CG, Paik JH, Yi JG, Hwang DY. Indeterminate pulmonary nodules in colorectal cancer. World J Gastroenterol. 2015;21(10):2967–72.

33. Tan YN, Li XF, Li JJ, Song YM, Jiang B, Yang J, et al. The accuracy of computed tomography in the pretreatment staging of colorectal cancer. Hepatogastroenterology. 2014;61(133):1207–12.

34. Potter KC, Husband JE, Houghton SL, Thomas K, Brown G. Diagnostic accuracy of serial CT/magnetic resonance imaging review vs. positron emission tomography/CT in colorectal cancer patients with suspected and known recurrence. Dis Colon Rectum. 2009;52(2):253–9.

35. Cho JY, Lee YJ, Han H-S, Yoon Y-S, Kim J, Choi Y, et al. Role of gadoxetic acid-enhanced magnetic resonance imaging in the preoperative evaluation of small hepatic lesions in patients with colorectal cancer. World J Surg. 2015;39(5):1161–6.

36. Scharitzer M, Ba-Ssalamah A, Ringl H, Kölblinger C, Grünberger T, Weber M, et al. Preoperative evaluation of colorectal liver metastases: comparison between gadoxetic acid-enhanced 3.0-T MRI and contrast-enhanced MDCT with histopathological correlation. Eur Radiol. 2013;23(8):2187–96.

37. Barabasch A, Kraemer NA, Ciritsis A, Hansen NL, Lierfeld M, Heinzel A, et al. Diagnostic accuracy of diffusion-weighted magnetic resonance imaging versus positron emission tomography/computed tomography for early response assessment of liver metastases to y90-radioembolization. Invest Radiol. 2015;50(6):409–15.

38. Bernatik T, Strobel D, Hahn EG, Becker D. Detection of liver metastases: comparison of contrast-enhanced wide-band harmonic imaging with conventional ultrasonography. J Ultrasound Med. 2001;20(5):509–15.

39. Schüle S, Altendorf-Hofmann A, Dittmar Y, Rauchfuß F, Settmacher U. Incidence of non-metastatic liver lesions in tumor patients: consequences for chemotherapy and local ablative procedures. Chirurg. 2014;85(9):806–11.

40. Sotiropoulos GC, Saner FH, Molmenti EP, Radtke A, Timm S, Baba HA, et al. Unexpected liver failure after right hemihepatectomy for colorectal liver metastasis due to chemotherapy-associated steato-hepatitis: time for routine preoperative liver biopsy? Int J Colorectal Dis. 2009;24(2):241.

41. Fahy BN, D'Angelica M, DeMatteo RP, Blumgart LH, Weiser MR, Ostrovnaya I, et al. Synchronous hepatic metastases from colon cancer: changing treatment strategies and results of surgical intervention. Ann Surg Oncol. 2009;16(2):361–70.

42. Hillingsø JG, Wille-Jørgensen P. Staged or simultaneous resection of synchronous liver metastases from colorectal cancer—a systematic review. Colorectal Dis. 2009;11(1):3–10.

43. Scheele J, Stangl R, Altendorf-Hofmann A. Hepatic metastases from colorectal carcinoma: impact of surgical resection on the natural history. Br J Surg. 1990;77(11):1241–6.

44. Nordlinger B, Sorbye H, Glimelius B, Poston GJ, Schlag PM, Rougier P, EORTC Gastro-Intestinal Tract Cancer Group, Cancer Research UK, Arbeitsgruppe Lebermetastasen und-tumoren in der Chirurgischen Arbeitsgemeinschaft Onkologie (ALM-CAO), Australasian Gastro-Intestinal Trials Group (AGITG), Fédération Francophone de Cancérologie Digestive (FFCD), et al. Perioperative chemotherapy with FOLFOX4 and surgery versus surgery alone for resectable liver metastases from colorectal cancer (EORTC Intergroup trial 40983): a randomised controlled trial. Lancet. 2008;371(9617):1007–16.

45. De Salvo GL, Gava C, Pucciarelli S, Lise M. Curative surgery for obstruction from primary left colorectal carcinoma: primary or staged resection? Cochrane Database Syst Rev. 2004;2, CD002101.

46. Smithers BM, Theile DE, Cohen JR, Evans EB, Davis NC. Emergency right hemicolectomy in colon carcinoma: a prospective study. Aust N Z J Surg. 1986;56(10):749–52.

47. Deans GT, Krukowski ZH, Irwin ST. Malignant obstruction of the left colon. Br J Surg. 1994;81(9):1270–6.

48. Phillips RK, Hittinger R, Fry JS, Fielding LP. Malignant large bowel obstruction. Br J Surg. 1985;72(4):296–302.

49. Van Hooft JE, Bemelman WA, Fockens P. A study of the value of colonic stenting as a bridge to elective surgery for the management of acute left-sided malignant colonic obstruction: the STENT-IN 2 study. Ned Tijdschr Geneeskd. 2007;151(22):1249–51.

50. Vemulapalli R, Lara LF, Sreenarasimhaiah J, Harford WV, Siddiqui AA. A comparison of palliative stenting or emergent surgery for obstructing incurable colon cancer. Dig Dis Sci. 2010;55(6):1732–7.

51. Gandrup P, Lund L, Balslev I. Surgical treatment of acute malignant large bowel obstruction. Eur J Surg. 1992;158(8):427–30.

52. Loizou LA, Grigg D, Boulos PB, Bown SG. Endoscopic Nd:YAG laser treatment of rectosigmoid cancer. Gut. 1990;31(7):812–6.

53. Daneker GW, Carlson GW, Hohn DC, Lynch P, Roubein L, Levin B. Endoscopic laser recanalization is effective for prevention and treatment of obstruction in sigmoid and rectal cancer. Arch Surg. 1991;126(11):1348–52.

54. Mandava N, Petrelli N, Herrera L, Nava H. Laser palliation for colorectal carcinoma. Am J Surg. 1991;162(3):212–4. discussion 215.

55. Brunetaud JM, Maunoury V, Cochelard D. Lasers in rectosigmoid tumors. Semin Surg Oncol. 1995;11(4):319–27.

56. Gevers AM, Macken E, Hiele M, Rutgeerts P. Endoscopic laser therapy for palliation of patients with distal colorectal carcinoma: analysis of factors influencing long-term outcome. Gastrointest Endosc. 2000;51(5):580–5.

57. Rao VS, Al-Mukhtar A, Rayan F, Stojkovic S, Moore PJ, Ahmad SM. Endoscopic laser ablation of advanced rectal carcinoma—a DGH experience. Colorectal Dis. 2005;7(1):58–60.

58. Salvati EP, Rubin RJ, Eisenstat TE, Siemons GO, Mangione JS. Electrocoagulation of selected carcinoma of the rectum. Surg Gynecol Obstet. 1988;166(5):393–6.

59. Eisenstat TE, Oliver GC. Electrocoagulation for adenocarcinoma of the low rectum. World J Surg. 1992;16(3):458–62.

60. Van Hooft JE, van Halsema EE, Vanbiervliet G, Beets-Tan RGH, DeWitt JM, Donnellan F, et al. Self-expandable metal stents for obstructing colonic and extracolonic cancer: European Society of Gastrointestinal Endoscopy (ESGE) Clinical Guideline. Endoscopy. 2014;46(11):990–1053.

61. Small AJ, Coelho-Prabhu N, Baron TH. Endoscopic placement of self-expandable metal stents for malignant colonic obstruction: long-term outcomes and complication factors. Gastrointest Endosc. 2010;71(3):560–72.

62. Lo SK. Metallic stenting for colorectal obstruction. Gastrointest Endosc Clin N Am. 1999;9(3):459–77.

63. Khot UP, Lang AW, Murali K, Parker MC. Systematic review of the efficacy and safety of colorectal stents. Br J Surg. 2002;89(9):1096–102.

64. Law WL, Choi HK, Lee YM, Chu KW. Palliation for advanced malignant colorectal obstruction by self-expanding metallic stents: prospective evaluation of outcomes. Dis Colon Rectum. 2004;47(1):39–43.

65. Dronamraju SS, Ramamurthy S, Kelly SB, Hayat M. Role of self-expanding metallic stents in the management of malignant obstruction of the proximal colon. Dis Colon Rectum. 2009;52(9):1657–61.

66. Choi JH, Lee YJ, Kim ES, Choi JH, Cho KB, Park KS, et al. Covered self-expandable metal stents are more associated with complications in the management of malignant colorectal obstruction. Surg Endosc. 2013;27(9):3220–7.

67. Watt AM, Faragher IG, Griffin TT, Rieger NA, Maddern GJ. Self-expanding metallic stents for relieving malignant colorectal obstruction: a systematic review. Ann Surg. 2007;246(1):24–30.

68. Mauro MA, Koehler RE, Baron TH. Advances in gastrointestinal intervention: the treatment of gastroduodenal and colorectal obstructions with metallic stents. Radiology. 2000;215(3):659–69.

69. Cook AD, Single R, McCahill LE. Surgical resection of primary tumors in patients who present with stage IV colorectal cancer: an analysis of surveillance, epidemiology, and end results data, 1988 to 2000. Ann Surg Oncol. 2005;12(8):637–45.

70. Rosen SA, Buell JF, Yoshida A, Kazsuba S, Hurst R, Michelassi F, et al. Initial presentation with stage IV colorectal cancer: how aggressive should we be? Arch Surg. 2000;135(5):530–4. discussion 534–5.

71. Tevis SE, Kohlnhofer BM, Stringfield S, Foley EF, Harms BA, Heise CP, et al. Postoperative complications in patients with rectal cancer are associated with delays in chemotherapy that lead to worse disease-free and overall survival. Dis Colon Rectum. 2013;56(12):1339–48.

72. Poultsides GA, Servais EL, Saltz LB, Patil S, Kemeny NE, Guillem JG, et al. Outcome of primary tumor in patients with synchronous stage IV colorectal cancer receiving combination chemotherapy without surgery as initial treatment. J Clin Oncol. 2009;27(20):3379–84.

73. Matsumoto T, Hasegawa S, Matsumoto S, Horimatsu T, Okoshi K, Yamada M, et al. Overcoming the challenges of primary tumor management in patients with metastatic colorectal cancer unresectable for cure and an asymptomatic primary tumor. Dis Colon Rectum. 2014;57(6):679–86.

74. Ruo L, Gougoutas C, Paty PB, Guillem JG, Cohen AM, Wong WD. Elective bowel resection for incurable stage IV colorectal cancer: prognostic variables for asymptomatic patients. J Am Coll Surg. 2003;196(5):722–8.

75. Scoggins CR, Meszoely IM, Blanke CD, Beauchamp RD, Leach SD. Nonoperative management of primary colorectal cancer in patients with stage IV disease. Ann Surg Oncol. 1999;6(7):651–7.

76. Liu SK, Church JM, Lavery IC, Fazio VW. Operation in patients with incurable colon cancer—is it worthwhile? Dis Colon Rectum. 1997;40(1):11–4.

77. Costi R, Mazzeo A, Di Mauro D, Veronesi L, Sansebastiano G, Violi V, et al. Palliative resection of colorectal cancer: does it prolong survival? Ann Surg Oncol. 2007;14(9):2567–76.

78. Hapani S, Chu D, Wu S. Risk of gastrointestinal perforation in patients with cancer treated with bevacizumab: a meta-analysis. Lancet Oncol. 2009;10(6):559–68.

79. Chang GJ. Challenge of primary tumor management in patients with stage IV colorectal cancer. J Clin Oncol. 2012;30(26):3165–6.

80. Karoui M, Koubaa W, Delbaldo C, Charachon A, Laurent A, Piedbois P, et al. Chemotherapy has also an effect on primary tumor in colon carcinoma. Ann Surg Oncol. 2008;15(12):3440–6.

81. Schrag D, Weiser MR, Goodman KA, Gonen M, Hollywood E, Cercek A, et al. Neoadjuvant chemotherapy without routine use of radiation therapy for patients with locally advanced rectal cancer: a pilot trial. J Clin Oncol. 2014;32(6):513–8.

82. Kawamura YJ, Umetani N, Sunami E, Watanabe T, Masaki T, Muto T. Effect of high ligation on the long-term result of patients with operable colon cancer, particularly those with limited nodal involvement. Eur J Surg. 2000;166(10):803–7.

83. Stillwell AP, Buettner PG, Ho YH. Meta-analysis of survival of patients with stage IV colorectal cancer managed with surgical resection versus chemotherapy alone. World J Surg. 2010;34(4):797–807.

84. Eisenberger A, Whelan RL, Neugut AI. Survival and symptomatic benefit from palliative primary tumor resection in patients with metastatic colorectal cancer: a review. Int J Colorectal Dis. 2008;23(6):559–68.

85. Damjanov N, Weiss J, Haller DG. Resection of the primary colorectal cancer is not necessary in nonobstructed patients with metastatic disease. Oncologist. 2009;14(10):963–9.

86. Cirocchi R, Trastulli S, Abraha I, Vettoretto N, Boselli C, Montedori A, et al. Non-resection versus resection for an asymptomatic primary tumour in patients with unresectable stage IV colorectal cancer. Cochrane Database Syst Rev. 2012;8, CD008997.

87. McCahill LE, Yothers G, Sharif S, Petrelli NJ, Lai LL, Bechar N, et al. Primary mFOLFOX6 plus bevacizumab without resection of the primary tumor for patients presenting with surgically unresectable metastatic colon cancer and an intact asymptomatic colon cancer: definitive analysis of NSABP trial C-10. J Clin Oncol. 2012;30(26):3223–8.

88. Tebbutt NC, Norman AR, Cunningham D, Hill ME, Tait D, Oates J, et al. Intestinal complications after chemotherapy for patients with unresected primary colorectal cancer and synchronous metastases. Gut. 2003;52(4):568–73.

89. Scheer MG, Sloots CE, van der Wilt GJ, Ruers TJM. Management of patients with asymptomatic colorectal cancer and synchronous irresectable metastases. Ann Oncol. 2008;19(11):1829–35.

90. Karoui M, Roudot-Thoraval F, Mesli F, Mitry E, Aparicio T, Des Guetz G, et al. Primary colectomy in patients with stage IV colon cancer and unresectable distant metastases improves overall survival: results of a multicentric study. Dis Colon Rectum. 2011;54(8):930–8.

91. Bipat S, van Leeuwen MS, Comans EFI, Pijl MEJ, Bossuyt PMM, Zwinderman AH, et al. Colorectal liver metastases: CT, MR imaging, and PET for diagnosis—meta-analysis. Radiology. 2005;237(1):123–31.

92. Simmonds PC, Primrose JN, Colquitt JL, Garden OJ, Poston GJ, Rees M. Surgical resection of hepatic metastases from colorectal cancer: a systematic review of published studies. Br J Cancer. 2006;94(7):982–99.

93. Neeff H, Hörth W, Makowiec F, Fischer E, Imdahl A, Hopt UT, et al. Outcome after resection of hepatic and pulmonary metastases of colorectal cancer. J Gastrointest Surg. 2009;13(10):1813–20.

94. Shah SA, Haddad R, Al-Sukhni W, Kim RD, Greig PD, Grant DR, et al. Surgical resection of hepatic and pulmonary metastases from colorectal carcinoma. J Am Coll Surg. 2006; 202(3):468–75.

95. Lam VWT, Laurence JM, Pang T, Johnston E, Hollands MJ, Pleass HCC, et al. A systematic review of a liver-first approach in patients with colorectal cancer and synchronous colorectal liver metastases. HPB (Oxford). 2014;16(2):101–8.

96. Pawlik TM, Choti MA. Surgical therapy for colorectal metastases to the liver. J Gastrointest Surg. 2007;11(8):1057–77.

97. Simmonds PC. Palliative chemotherapy for advanced colorectal cancer: systematic review and meta-analysis. Colorectal Cancer Collaborative Group. BMJ. 2000;321(7260):531–5.

98. Kassahun WT. Unresolved issues and controversies surrounding the management of colorectal cancer liver metastasis. World J Surg Oncol. 2015;13:61.

99. Kopetz S, Chang GJ, Overman MJ, Eng C, Sargent DJ, Larson DW, et al. Improved survival in metastatic colorectal cancer is associated with adoption of hepatic resection and improved chemotherapy. J Clin Oncol. 2009;27(22):3677–83.

100. Martin R, Paty P, Fong Y, Grace A, Cohen A, DeMatteo R, et al. Simultaneous liver and colorectal resections are safe for synchronous colorectal liver metastasis. J Am Coll Surg. 2003;197(2):233–41. discussion 241–2.

101. Capussotti L, Vigano' L, Ferrero A, Lo Tesoriere R, Ribero D, Polastri R. Timing of resection of liver metastases synchronous to colorectal tumor: proposal of prognosis-based decisional model. Ann Surg Oncol. 2007;14(3):1143–50.

102. Capussotti L, Ferrero A, Viganò L, Ribero D, Lo Tesoriere R, Polastri R. Major liver resections synchronous with colorectal surgery. Ann Surg Oncol. 2007;14(1):195–201.

103. Reddy SK, Pawlik TM, Zorzi D, Gleisner AL, Ribero D, Assumpcao L, et al. Simultaneous resections of colorectal cancer and synchronous liver metastases: a multi-institutional analysis. Ann Surg Oncol. 2007;14(12):3481–91.

104. Adam R. Colorectal cancer with synchronous liver metastases. Br J Surg. 2007;94(2):129–31.

105. Yin Z, Liu C, Chen Y, Bai Y, Shang C, Yin R, et al. Timing of hepatectomy in resectable synchronous colorectal liver metastases (SCRLM): simultaneous or delayed? Hepatology. 2013;57(6):2346–57.

106. Thelen A, Jonas S, Benckert C, Spinelli A, Lopez-Hänninen E, Rudolph B, et al. Simultaneous versus staged liver resection of synchronous liver metastases from colorectal cancer. Int J Colorectal Dis. 2007;22(10):1269–76.

107. Kelly ME, Spolverato G, Lê GN, Mavros MN, Doyle F, Pawlik TM, et al. Synchronous colorectal liver metastasis: a network meta-analysis review comparing classical, combined, and liver-first surgical strategies. J Surg Oncol. 2015;111(3): 341–51.

108. Brouquet A, Mortenson MM, Vauthey J-N, Rodriguez-Bigas MA, Overman MJ, Chang GJ, et al. Surgical strategies for synchronous colorectal liver metastases in 156 consecutive patients: classic, combined or reverse strategy? J Am Coll Surg. 2010;210(6):934–41.

109. Ayez N, Burger JWA, van der Pool AE, Eggermont AMM, Grunhagen DJ, de Wilt JH, et al. Long-term results of the "liver first" approach in patients with locally advanced rectal cancer and synchronous liver metastases. Dis Colon Rectum. 2013;56(3):281–7.

110. Van der Wal GE, Gouw AS, Kamps JA, Moorlag HE, Bulthuis ML, Molema G, et al. Angiogenesis in synchronous and metachronous colorectal liver metastases: the liver as a permissive soil. Ann Surg. 2012;255(1):86–94.

111. Jegatheeswaran S, Mason JM, Hancock HC, Siriwardena AK. The liver-first approach to the management of colorectal cancer with synchronous hepatic metastases: a systematic review. JAMA Surg. 2013;148(4):385–91.

112. Millikan KW, Staren ED, Doolas A. Invasive therapy of metastatic colorectal cancer to the liver. Surg Clin North Am. 1997;77(1):27–48.

113. Reddy SK, Barbas AS, Clary BM. Synchronous colorectal liver metastases: is it time to reconsider traditional paradigms of management? Ann Surg Oncol. 2009;16(9):2395–410.

114. Ruers TJ, Hagendoorn J. Treatment dilemmas in patients with synchronous colorectal liver metastases. Recent Results Cancer Res. 2012;196:37–49.

115. Nordlinger B, Sorbye H, Glimelius B, Poston GJ, Schlag PM, Rougier P, EORTC Gastro-Intestinal Tract Cancer Group, Cancer Research UK, Arbeitsgruppe Lebermetastasen und–tumoren in der Chirurgischen Arbeitsgemeinschaft Onkologie (ALM-CAO), Australasian Gastro-Intestinal Trials Group (AGITG), Fédération Francophone de Cancérologie Digestive (FFCD), et al. Perioperative FOLFOX4 chemotherapy and surgery versus surgery alone for resectable liver metastases from colorectal cancer (EORTC 40983): long-term results of a randomised, controlled, phase 3 trial. Lancet Oncol. 2013;14(12):1208–15.

116. Nanji S, Cleary S, Ryan P, Guindi M, Selvarajah S, Al-Ali H, et al. Up-front hepatic resection for metastatic colorectal cancer results in favorable long-term survival. Ann Surg Oncol. 2013;20(1):295–304.

117. Jones RP, Malik HZ, Fenwick SW, Poston GJ. Perioperative chemotherapy for resectable colorectal liver metastases: where now? Eur J Surg Oncol. 2013;39(8):807–11.

118. Reddy SK, Zorzi D, Lum YW, Barbas AS, Pawlik TM, Ribero D, et al. Timing of multimodality therapy for resectable synchronous colorectal liver metastases: a retrospective multi-institutional analysis. Ann Surg Oncol. 2009;16(7):1809–19.

119. Vauthey JN, Nordlinger B, Kopetz S, Poston G. Sequenced chemotherapy and surgery for potentially resectable colorectal

liver metastases: a debate over goals of research and an approach while the jury remains out. Ann Surg Oncol. 2010;17(8):1983–6.

120. Adam R, Pascal G, Castaing D, Azoulay D, Delvart V, Paule B, et al. Tumor progression while on chemotherapy: a contraindication to liver resection for multiple colorectal metastases? Ann Surg. 2004;240(6):1052–61. discussion 1061–4.

121. Mentha G, Roth AD, Terraz S, Giostra E, Gervaz P, Andres A, et al. "Liver first" approach in the treatment of colorectal cancer with synchronous liver metastases. Dig Surg. 2008; 25(6):430–5.

122. Verhoef C, van der Pool AE, Nuyttens JJ, Planting AS, Eggermont AM, de Wilt JH. The "liver-first approach" for patients with locally advanced rectal cancer and synchronous liver metastases. Dis Colon Rectum. 2009;52(1):23–30.

123. De Jong MC, van Dam RM, Maas M, Bemelmans MH, Olde Damink SW, Beets GL, et al. The liver-first approach for synchronous colorectal liver metastasis: a 5-year single-centre experience. HPB (Oxford). 2011;13(10):745–52.

124. Lehmann K, Rickenbacher A, Weber A, Pestalozzi BC, Clavien P-A. Chemotherapy before liver resection of colorectal metastases: friend or foe? Ann Surg. 2012;255(2):237–47.

125. De Rosa A, Gomez D, Brooks A, Cameron IC. "Liver-first" approach for synchronous colorectal liver metastases: is this a justifiable approach? J Hepatobiliary Pancreat Sci. 2013;20(3): 263–70.

126. Adam R, De Gramont A, Figueras J, Guthrie A, Kokudo N, Kunstlinger F, Jean-Nicolas Vauthey of the EGOSLIM (Expert Group on OncoSurgery management of LIver Metastases) group, et al. The oncosurgery approach to managing liver metastases from colorectal cancer: a multidisciplinary international consensus. Oncologist. 2012;17(10):1225–39.

127. Kimura F, Miyazaki M, Suwa T, Kakizaki S, Itoh H, Kaiho T, et al. Reduced hepatic acute-phase response after simultaneous resection for gastrointestinal cancer with synchronous liver metastases. Br J Surg. 1996;83(7):1002–6.

128. Belghiti J. Synchronous and resectable hepatic metastases of colorectal cancer: should there be a minimum delay before hepatic resection? Ann Chir. 1990;44(6):427–9. discussion 429–32.

129. Shimizu Y, Yasui K, Sano T, Hirai T, Kanemitsu Y, Komori K, et al. Validity of observation interval for synchronous hepatic metastases of colorectal cancer: changes in hepatic and extrahepatic metastatic foci. Langenbecks Arch Surg. 2008;393(2): 181–4.

130. Yoshidome H, Kimura F, Shimizu H, Ohtsuka M, Kato A, Yoshitomi H, et al. Interval period tumor progression: does delayed hepatectomy detect occult metastases in synchronous colorectal liver metastases? J Gastrointest Surg. 2008;12(8): 1391–8.

131. Fujita S, Akasu T, Moriya Y. Resection of synchronous liver metastases from colorectal cancer. Jpn J Clin Oncol. 2000; 30(1):7–11.

132. Chua HK, Sondenaa K, Tsiotos GG, Larson DR, Wolff BG, Nagorney DM. Concurrent vs. staged colectomy and hepatectomy for primary colorectal cancer with synchronous hepatic metastases. Dis Colon Rectum. 2004;47(8):1310–6.

133. Weber JC, Bachellier P, Oussoultzoglou E, Jaeck D. Simultaneous resection of colorectal primary tumour and synchronous liver metastases. Br J Surg. 2003;90(8):956–62.

134. Fong Y, Fortner J, Sun RL, Brennan MF, Blumgart LH. Clinical score for predicting recurrence after hepatic resection for metastatic colorectal cancer: analysis of 1001 consecutive cases. Ann Surg. 1999;230(3):309–18. discussion 318–21.

135. Choti MA, Sitzmann JV, Tiburi MF, Sumetchotimetha W, Rangsin R, Schulick RD, et al. Trends in long-term survival following liver resection for hepatic colorectal metastases. Ann Surg. 2002;235(6):759–66.

136. De Haas RJ, Wicherts DA, Flores E, Azoulay D, Castaing D, Adam R. R1 resection by necessity for colorectal liver metastases: is it still a contraindication to surgery? Ann Surg. 2008;248(4):626–37.

137. Nuzzo G, Giuliante F, Ardito F, Vellone M, Giovannini I, Federico B, et al. Influence of surgical margin on type of recurrence after liver resection for colorectal metastases: a single-center experience. Surgery. 2008;143(3):384–93.

138. Park J, Chen Y-J, Lu W-P, Fong Y. The evolution of liver-directed treatments for hepatic colorectal metastases. Oncology. 2014;28(11):991–1003.

139. Evrard S, Poston G, Kissmeyer-Nielsen P, Diallo A, Desolneux G, Brouste V, et al. Combined ablation and resection (CARe) as an effective parenchymal sparing treatment for extensive colorectal liver metastases. PLoS One. 2014;9(12):e114404.

140. Stang A, Fischbach R, Teichmann W, Bokemeyer C, Braumann D. A systematic review on the clinical benefit and role of radiofrequency ablation as treatment of colorectal liver metastases. Eur J Cancer. 2009;45(10):1748–56.

141. Amersi FF, McElrath-Garza A, Ahmad A, Zogakis T, Allegra DP, Krasne R, et al. Long-term survival after radiofrequency ablation of complex unresectable liver tumors. Arch Surg. 2006;141(6):581–7. discussion 587–8.

142. Kuvshinoff BW, Ota DM. Radiofrequency ablation of liver tumors: influence of technique and tumor size. Surgery. 2002;132(4):605–11. discussion 611–2.

143. Hildebrand P, Kleemann M, Roblick UJ, Mirow L, Birth M, Leibecke T, et al. Radiofrequency-ablation of unresectable primary and secondary liver tumors: results in 88 patients. Langenbecks Arch Surg. 2006;391(2):118–23.

144. Hildebrand P, Leibecke T, Kleemann M, Mirow L, Birth M, Bruch HP, et al. Influence of operator experience in radiofrequency ablation of malignant liver tumours on treatment outcome. Eur J Surg Oncol. 2006;32(4):430–4.

145. Ahmad A, Chen SL, Kavanagh MA, Allegra DP, Bilchik AJ. Radiofrequency ablation of hepatic metastases from colorectal cancer: are newer generation probes better? Am Surg. 2006;72(10):875–9.

146. Wong SL, Mangu PB, Choti MA, Crocenzi TS, Dodd GD, Dorfman GS, et al. American Society of Clinical Oncology 2009 clinical evidence review on radiofrequency ablation of hepatic metastases from colorectal cancer. J Clin Oncol. 2010;28(3):493–508.

147. Decadt B, Siriwardena AK. Radiofrequency ablation of liver tumours: systematic review. Lancet Oncol. 2004;5(9):550–60.

148. Curley SA, Izzo F, Delrio P, Ellis LM, Granchi J, Vallone P, et al. Radiofrequency ablation of unresectable primary and metastatic hepatic malignancies: results in 123 patients. Ann Surg. 1999;230(1):1–8.

149. Machi J, Oishi AJ, Sumida K, Sakamoto K, Furumoto NL, Oishi RH, et al. Long-term outcome of radiofrequency ablation for unresectable liver metastases from colorectal cancer:

evaluation of prognostic factors and effectiveness in first- and second-line management. Cancer J. 2006;12(4):318–26.

150. Siperstein AE, Berber E, Ballem N, Parikh RT. Survival after radiofrequency ablation of colorectal liver metastases: 10-year experience. Ann Surg. 2007;246(4):559–65. discussion 565–7.

151. Ruers T, Punt C, Van Coevorden F, Pierie JPEN, Borel-Rinkes I, Ledermann JA, EORTC Gastro-Intestinal Tract Cancer Group, Arbeitsgruppe Lebermetastasen und—tumoren in der Chirurgischen Arbeitsgemeinschaft Onkologie (ALM-CAO), The National Cancer Research Institute Colorectal Clinical Study Group (NCRI CCSG), et al. Radiofrequency ablation combined with systemic treatment versus systemic treatment alone in patients with non-resectable colorectal liver metastases: a randomized EORTC Intergroup phase II study (EORTC 40004). Ann Oncol. 2012;23(10):2619–26.

152. Solbiati L, Ahmed M, Cova L, Ierace T, Brioschi M, Goldberg SN. Small liver colorectal metastases treated with percutaneous radiofrequency ablation: local response rate and long-term survival with up to 10-year follow-up. Radiology. 2012;265(3):958–68.

153. Aloia TA, Vauthey J-N, Loyer EM, Ribero D, Pawlik TM, Wei SH, et al. Solitary colorectal liver metastasis: resection determines outcome. Arch Surg. 2006;141(5):460–6. discussion 466–7.

154. Abdalla EK, Vauthey J-N, Ellis LM, Ellis V, Pollock R, Broglio KR, et al. Recurrence and outcomes following hepatic resection, radiofrequency ablation, and combined resection/ablation for colorectal liver metastases. Ann Surg. 2004;239(6):818–25. discussion 825–7.

155. Ruers TJ, Joosten JJ, Wiering B, Langenhoff BS, Dekker HM, Wobbes T, et al. Comparison between local ablative therapy and chemotherapy for non-resectable colorectal liver metastases: a prospective study. Ann Surg Oncol. 2007;14(3):1161–9.

156. Otto G, Düber C, Hoppe-Lotichius M, König J, Heise M, Pitton MB. Radiofrequency ablation as first-line treatment in patients with early colorectal liver metastases amenable to surgery. Ann Surg. 2010;251(5):796–803.

157. White RR, Avital I, Sofocleous CT, Brown KT, Brody LA, Covey A, et al. Rates and patterns of recurrence for percutaneous radiofrequency ablation and open wedge resection for solitary colorectal liver metastasis. J Gastrointest Surg. 2007;11(3):256–63.

158. Lee WS, Yun SH, Chun HK, Lee WY, Kim S-J, Choi SH, et al. Clinical outcomes of hepatic resection and radiofrequency ablation in patients with solitary colorectal liver metastasis. J Clin Gastroenterol. 2008;42(8):945–9.

159. Gleisner AL, Choti MA, Assumpcao L, Nathan H, Schulick RD, Pawlik TM. Colorectal liver metastases: recurrence and survival following hepatic resection, radiofrequency ablation, and combined resection-radiofrequency ablation. Arch Surg. 2008;143(12):1204–12.

160. Cirocchi R, Trastulli S, Boselli C, Montedori A, Cavaliere D, Parisi A, et al. Radiofrequency ablation in the treatment of liver metastases from colorectal cancer. Cochrane Database Syst Rev. 2012;6, CD006317.

161. De Baère T, Risse O, Kuoch V, Dromain C, Sengel C, Smayra T, et al. Adverse events during radiofrequency treatment of 582 hepatic tumors. AJR Am J Roentgenol. 2003;181(3):695–700.

162. Breedis C, Young G. The blood supply of neoplasms in the liver. Am J Pathol. 1954;30(5):969–77.

163. Collins JM. Pharmacologic rationale for regional drug delivery. J Clin Oncol. 1984;2(5):498–504.

164. Ducreux M, Ychou M, Laplanche A, Gamelin E, Lasser P, Husseini F, gastrointestinal group of the Federation Nationale des Centres de Lutte Contre le Cancer, et al. Hepatic arterial oxaliplatin infusion plus intravenous chemotherapy in colorectal cancer with inoperable hepatic metastases: a trial of the gastrointestinal group of the Federation Nationale des Centres de Lutte Contre le Cancer. J Clin Oncol. 2005;23(22):4881–7.

165. Boige V, Malka D, Elias D, Castaing M, De Baere T, Goere D, et al. Hepatic arterial infusion of oxaliplatin and intravenous LV5FU2 in unresectable liver metastases from colorectal cancer after systemic chemotherapy failure. Ann Surg Oncol. 2008;15(1):219–26.

166. Chen Y, Wang X, Yan Z, Wang J, Luo J, Liu Q. Hepatic arterial infusion with irinotecan, oxaliplatin, and floxuridine plus systemic chemotherapy as first-line treatment of unresectable liver metastases from colorectal cancer. Onkologie. 2012;35(9):480–4.

167. Kemeny N, Jarnagin W, Paty P, Gönen M, Schwartz L, Morse M, et al. Phase I trial of systemic oxaliplatin combination chemotherapy with hepatic arterial infusion in patients with unresectable liver metastases from colorectal cancer. J Clin Oncol. 2005;23(22):4888–96.

168. Aliberti C, Tilli M, Benea G, Fiorentini G. Trans-arterial chemoembolization (TACE) of liver metastases from colorectal cancer using irinotecan-eluting beads: preliminary results. Anticancer Res. 2006;26(5B):3793–5.

169. Sanz-Altamira PM, Spence LD, Huberman MS, Posner MR, Steele G, Perry LJ, et al. Selective chemoembolization in the management of hepatic metastases in refractory colorectal carcinoma: a phase II trial. Dis Colon Rectum. 1997;40(7):770–5.

170. Martin RC, Joshi J, Robbins K, Tomalty D, Bosnjakovik P, Derner M, et al. Hepatic intra-arterial injection of drug-eluting bead, irinotecan (DEBIRI) in unresectable colorectal liver metastases refractory to systemic chemotherapy: results of multi-institutional study. Ann Surg Oncol. 2011;18(1):192–8.

171. Fiorentini G, Aliberti C, Tilli M, Mulazzani L, Graziano F, Giordani P, et al. Intra-arterial infusion of irinotecan-loaded drug-eluting beads (DEBIRI) versus intravenous therapy (FOLFIRI) for hepatic metastases from colorectal cancer: final results of a phase III study. Anticancer Res. 2012;32(4):1387–95.

172. Kemeny N, Niedzwiecki D, Hollis DR. Hepatic arterial infusion (HAI) versus systemic therapy for hepatic metastases from colorectal cancer: a CALGB randomized trial of efficacy, quality of life (QOL), cost effectiveness, and molecular markers. Proc Am Soc Clin Oncol. 2003;22:252. abstract 1010.

173. Mocellin S, Pasquali S, Nitti D. Fluoropyrimidine-HAI (hepatic arterial infusion) versus systemic chemotherapy (SCT) for unresectable liver metastases from colorectal cancer. Cochrane Database Syst Rev. 2009;3, CD007823.

174. Liu W, Song Q-K, Xing B-C. A systematic review and meta-analysis to reappraise the role of adjuvant hepatic arterial infusion for colorectal cancer liver metastases. Int J Colorectal Dis. 2015;30(8):1091–102.

175. Mitry E, Guiu B, Cosconea S, Jooste V, Faivre J, Bouvier A-M. Epidemiology, management and prognosis of colorectal cancer with lung metastases: a 30-year population-based study. Gut. 2010;59(10):1383–8.

176. Tan KK, Lopes Gde L, Sim R. How uncommon are isolated lung metastases in colorectal cancer? A review from database of 754 patients over 4 years. J Gastrointest Surg. 2009;13(4):642–8.

177. August DA, Ottow RT, Sugarbaker PH. Clinical perspective of human colorectal cancer metastasis. Cancer Metastasis Rev. 1984;3(4):303–24.

178. McCormack PM, Attiyeh FF. Resected pulmonary metastases from colorectal cancer. Dis Colon Rectum. 1979;22(8):553–6.

179. Dahabre J, Vasilaki M, Stathopoulos GP, Kondaxis A, Iliadis K, Papadopoulos G, et al. Surgical management in lung metastases from colorectal cancer. Anticancer Res. 2007;27(6C):4387–90.

180. Watanabe K, Saito N, Sugito M, Ito M, Kobayashi A, Nishizawa Y. Predictive factors for pulmonary metastases after curative resection of rectal cancer without preoperative chemoradiotherapy. Dis Colon Rectum. 2011;54(8):989–98.

181. Kim CH, Huh JW, Kim HJ, Lim SW, Song SY, Kim HR, et al. Factors influencing oncological outcomes in patients who develop pulmonary metastases after curative resection of colorectal cancer. Dis Colon Rectum. 2012;55(4):459–64.

182. Suzuki H, Kiyoshima M, Kitahara M, Asato Y, Amemiya R. Long-term outcomes after surgical resection of pulmonary metastases from colorectal cancer. Ann Thorac Surg. 2015;99(2):435–40.

183. Nagakura S, Shirai Y, Yamato Y, Yokoyama N, Suda T, Hatakeyama K. Simultaneous detection of colorectal carcinoma liver and lung metastases does not warrant resection. J Am Coll Surg. 2001;193(2):153–60.

184. Dematteo R, Minnard E, Kemeny N. Outcomes after resection of both liver and lung metastases in patients with colorectal cancer. Proc Am Soc Clin Oncol. 1999;(abstract 958).

185. McAfee MK, Allen MS, Trastek VF, Ilstrup DM, Deschamps C, Pairolero PC. Colorectal lung metastases: results of surgical excision. Ann Thorac Surg. 1992;53(5):780–5. discussion 785–6.

186. Rizk NP, Downey RJ. Resection of pulmonary metastases from colorectal cancer. Semin Thorac Cardiovasc Surg. 2002;14(1):29–34.

187. Roth JA, Pass HI, Wesley MN, White D, Putnam JB, Seipp C. Comparison of median sternotomy and thoracotomy for resection of pulmonary metastases in patients with adult soft-tissue sarcomas. Ann Thorac Surg. 1986;42(2):134–8.

188. McCormack PM, Bains MS, Begg CB, Burt ME, Downey RJ, Panicek DM, et al. Role of video-assisted thoracic surgery in the treatment of pulmonary metastases: results of a prospective trial. Ann Thorac Surg. 1996;62(1):213–6. discussion 216–7.

189. Muacevic A, Drexler C, Wowra B, Schweikard A, Schlaefer A, Hoffmann RT, et al. Technical description, phantom accuracy, and clinical feasibility for single-session lung radiosurgery using robotic image-guided real-time respiratory tumor tracking. Technol Cancer Res Treat. 2007;6(4):321–8.

190. Treasure T, Fallowfield L, Lees B, Farewell V. Pulmonary metastasectomy in colorectal cancer: the PulMiCC trial. Thorax. 2012;67(2):185–7.

191. Sugarbaker PH, Cunliffe WJ, Belliveau J, de Bruijn EA, Graves T, Mullins RE, et al. Rationale for integrating early postoperative intraperitoneal chemotherapy into the surgical treatment of gastrointestinal cancer. Semin Oncol. 1989;16(4 Suppl 6):83–97.

192. Dawson LE, Russell AH, Tong D, Wisbeck WM. Adenocarcinoma of the sigmoid colon: sites of initial dissemination and clinical patterns of recurrence following surgery alone. J Surg Oncol. 1983;22(2):95–9.

193. Russell AH, Tong D, Dawson LE, Wisbeck WM, Griffin TW, Laramore GE, et al. Adenocarcinoma of the retroperitoneal ascending and descending colon: sites of initial dissemination and clinical patterns of recurrence following surgery alone. Int J Radiat Oncol Biol Phys. 1983;9(3):361–5.

194. Jayne DG, Fook S, Loi C, Seow-Choen F. Peritoneal carcinomatosis from colorectal cancer. Br J Surg. 2002;89(12): 1545–50.

195. Sugarbaker PH. Management of peritoneal-surface malignancy: the surgeon's role. Langenbecks Arch Surg. 1999; 384(6):576–87.

196. Glehen O, Osinsky D, Beaujard AC, Gilly FN. Natural history of peritoneal carcinomatosis from nongynecologic malignancies. Surg Oncol Clin N Am. 2003;12(3):729–39.

197. Franko J, Shi Q, Goldman CD, Pockaj BA, Nelson GD, Goldberg RM, et al. Treatment of colorectal peritoneal carcinomatosis with systemic chemotherapy: a pooled analysis of north central cancer treatment group phase III trials N9741 and N9841. J Clin Oncol. 2012;30(3):263–7.

198. Chu DZ, Lang NP, Thompson C, Osteen PK, Westbrook KC. Peritoneal carcinomatosis in nongynecologic malignancy. A prospective study of prognostic factors. Cancer. 1989;63(2):364–7.

199. Willett CG, Tepper JE, Cohen AM, Orlow E, Welch CE. Failure patterns following curative resection of colonic carcinoma. Ann Surg. 1984;200(6):685–90.

200. Hansen E, Wolff N, Knuechel R, Ruschoff J, Hofstaedter F, Taeger K. Tumor cells in blood shed from the surgical field. Arch Surg. 1995;130(4):387–93.

201. Sadeghi B, Arvieux C, Glehen O, Beaujard AC, Rivoire M, Baulieux J, et al. Peritoneal carcinomatosis from non-gynecologic malignancies: results of the EVOCAPE 1 multicentric prospective study. Cancer. 2000;88(2):358–63.

202. Jacquet P, Jelinek JS, Steves MA, Sugarbaker PH. Evaluation of computed tomography in patients with peritoneal carcinomatosis. Cancer. 1993;72(5):1631–6.

203. González-Moreno S, González-Bayón L, Ortega-Pérez G, González-Hernando C. Imaging of peritoneal carcinomatosis. Cancer J. 2009;15(3):184–9.

204. Gilly FN, Beaujard A, Glehen O, Grandclement E, Caillot JL, Francois Y, et al. Peritonectomy combined with intraperitoneal chemohyperthermia in abdominal cancer with peritoneal carcinomatosis: phase I-II study. Anticancer Res. 1999;19(3B): 2317–21.

205. Jacquet P, Sugarbaker PH. Clinical research methodologies in diagnosis and staging of patients with peritoneal carcinomatosis. Cancer Treat Res. 1996;82:359–74.

206. Pestieau SR, Sugarbaker PH. Treatment of primary colon cancer with peritoneal carcinomatosis: comparison of concomitant vs. delayed management. Dis Colon Rectum. 2000; 43(10):1341–6. discussion 1347–8.

207. Machover D. A comprehensive review of 5-fluorouracil and leucovorin in patients with metastatic colorectal carcinoma. Cancer. 1997;80(7):1179–87.

208. Sugarbaker PH. Colorectal carcinomatosis: a new oncologic frontier. Curr Opin Oncol. 2005;17(4):397–9.

209. Speyer JL. The rationale behind intraperitoneal chemotherapy in gastrointestinal malignancies. Semin Oncol. 1985;12(3 Suppl 4):23–8.

210. Sugarbaker PH, Graves T, DeBruijn EA, Cunliffe WJ, Mullins RE, Hull WE, et al. Early postoperative intraperitoneal chemotherapy as an adjuvant therapy to surgery for peritoneal carcinomatosis from gastrointestinal cancer: pharmacological studies. Cancer Res. 1990;50(18):5790–4.

211. Elias D, Gilly F, Boutitie F, Quenet F, Bereder J-M, Mansvelt B, et al. Peritoneal colorectal carcinomatosis treated with surgery and perioperative intraperitoneal chemotherapy: retrospective analysis of 523 patients from a multicentric French study. J Clin Oncol. 2010;28(1):63–8.

212. Verwaal VJ, van Ruth S, de Bree E, van Sloothen GW, van Tinteren H, Boot H, et al. Randomized trial of cytoreduction and hyperthermic intraperitoneal chemotherapy versus systemic chemotherapy and palliative surgery in patients with peritoneal carcinomatosis of colorectal cancer. J Clin Oncol. 2003;21(20):3737–43.

213. Elias D, Delperro JR, Sideris L, Benhamou E, Pocard M, Baton O, et al. Treatment of peritoneal carcinomatosis from colorectal cancer: impact of complete cytoreductive surgery and difficulties in conducting randomized trials. Ann Surg Oncol. 2004;11(5):518–21.

214. Verwaal VJ, Bruin S, Boot H, van Slooten G, van Tinteren H. 8-Year follow-up of randomized trial: cytoreduction and hyperthermic intraperitoneal chemotherapy versus systemic chemotherapy in patients with peritoneal carcinomatosis of colorectal cancer. Ann Surg Oncol. 2008;15(9):2426–32.

215. Mahteme H, Hansson J, Berglund A, Påhlman L, Glimelius B, Nygren P, et al. Improved survival in patients with peritoneal metastases from colorectal cancer: a preliminary study. Br J Cancer. 2004;90(2):403–7.

216. Glehen O, Kwiatkowski F, Sugarbaker PH, Elias D, Levine EA, De Simone M, et al. Cytoreductive surgery combined with perioperative intraperitoneal chemotherapy for the management of peritoneal carcinomatosis from colorectal cancer: a multi-institutional study. J Clin Oncol. 2004;22(16):3284–92.

217. Yan TD, Black D, Savady R, Sugarbaker PH. Systematic review on the efficacy of cytoreductive surgery combined with perioperative intraperitoneal chemotherapy for peritoneal carcinomatosis from colorectal carcinoma. J Clin Oncol. 2006;24(24):4011–9.

218. Esquivel J, Lowy AM, Markman M, Chua T, Pelz J, Baratti D, et al. The American Society of Peritoneal Surface Malignancies (ASPSM) Multiinstitution Evaluation of the Peritoneal Surface Disease Severity Score (PSDSS) in 1,013 Patients with Colorectal Cancer with Peritoneal Carcinomatosis. Ann Surg Oncol. 2014;21(13):4195–201.

219. Elias D, Lefevre JH, Chevalier J, Brouquet A, Marchal F, Classe J-M, et al. Complete cytoreductive surgery plus intraperitoneal chemohyperthermia with oxaliplatin for peritoneal carcinomatosis of colorectal origin. J Clin Oncol. 2009;27(5):681–5.

220. Yan TD, Zappa L, Edwards G, Alderman R, Marquardt CE, Sugarbaker PH. Perioperative outcomes of cytoreductive surgery and perioperative intraperitoneal chemotherapy for non-appendiceal peritoneal carcinomatosis from a prospective database. J Surg Oncol. 2007;96(2):102–12.

221. National Comprehensive Cancer Network (NCCN). NCCN clinical practice guidelines in oncology. http://www.nccn.org/professionals/physician_gls/f_guidelines.asp. Accessed 19 May 2015.

222. Esquivel J, Sticca R, Sugarbaker P, Levine E, Yan TD, Alexander R, Society of Surgical Oncology Annual Meeting, et al. Cytoreductive surgery and hyperthermic intraperitoneal chemotherapy in the management of peritoneal surface malignancies of colonic origin: a consensus statement. Society of Surgical Oncology. Ann Surg Oncol. 2007;14(1):128–33.

223. Ulbright TM, Roth LM, Stehman FB. Secondary ovarian neoplasia. A clinicopathologic study of 35 cases. Cancer. 1984;53(5):1164–74.

224. Omranipour R, Abasahl A. Ovarian metastases in colorectal cancer. Int J Gynecol Cancer. 2009;19(9):1524–8.

225. Webb MJ, Decker DG, Mussey E. Cancer metastatic to the ovary: factors influencing survival. Obstet Gynecol. 1975;45(4):391–6.

226. Blamey S, McDermott F, Pihl E, Price AB, Milne BJ, Hughes E. Ovarian involvement in adenocarcinoma of the colon and rectum. Surg Gynecol Obstet. 1981;153(1):42–4.

227. Morrow M, Enker WE. Late ovarian metastases in carcinoma of the colon and rectum. Arch Surg. 1984;119(12):1385–8.

228. Cutait R, Lesser ML, Enker WE. Prophylactic oophorectomy in surgery for large-bowel cancer. Dis Colon Rectum. 1983;26(1):6–11.

229. Barr SS, Valiente MA, Bacon HE. Rationale of bilateral oophorectomy concomitant with resection for carcinoma of the rectum and colon. Dis Colon Rectum. 1962;5:450–2.

230. Young-Fadok TM, Wolff BG, Nivatvongs S, Metzger PP, Ilstrup DM. Prophylactic oophorectomy in colorectal carcinoma: preliminary results of a randomized, prospective trial. Dis Colon Rectum. 1998;41(3):277–83. discussion 83–5.

231. Burt CA. Carcinoma of the ovaries secondary to cancer of the colon and rectum. Dis Colon Rectum. 1960;3:352–7.

232. Stearns MW, Deddish MR. Five-year results of abdominopelvic lymph node dissection for carcinoma of the rectum. Dis Colon Rectum. 1959;2(2):169–72.

233. Graffner HO, Alm PO, Oscarson JE. Prophylactic oophorectomy in colorectal carcinoma. Am J Surg. 1983;146(2):233–5.

234. Koves I, Vamosi-Nagy I, Besznyak I. Ovarian metastases of colorectal tumours. Eur J Surg Oncol. 1993;19(6):633–5.

235. Harcourt KF, Dennis DL. Laparotomy for "ovarian tumors" in unsuspected carcinoma of the colon. Cancer. 1968;21(6):1244–6.

236. Lindner V, Gasser B, Debbiche A, Tomb L, Vetter JM, Walter P. Ovarian metastasis of colorectal adenocarcinomas. A clinico-pathological study of 41 cases. Ann Pathol. 1999;19(6):492–8.

237. Rayson D, Bouttell E, Whiston F, Stitt L. Outcome after ovarian/adnexal metastasectomy in metastatic colorectal carcinoma. J Surg Oncol. 2000;75(3):186–92.

238. Loy TS, Calaluce RD, Keeney GL. Cytokeratin immunostaining in differentiating primary ovarian carcinoma from metastatic colonic adenocarcinoma. Mod Pathol. 1996;9(11):1040–4.

239. DeCostanzo DC, Elias JM, Chumas JC. Necrosis in 84 ovarian carcinomas: a morphologic study of primary versus metastatic colonic carcinoma with a selective immunohistochemical analysis of cytokeratin subtypes and carcinoembryonic antigen. Int J Gynecol Pathol. 1997;16(3):245–9.

240. Wauters CC, Smedts F, Gerrits LG, Bosman FT, Ramaekers FC. Keratins 7 and 20 as diagnostic markers of carcinomas metastatic to the ovary. Hum Pathol. 1995;26(8):852–5.

241. Dionigi A, Facco C, Tibiletti MG, Bernasconi B, Riva C, Capella C. Ovarian metastases from colorectal carcinoma. Clinicopathologic profile, immunophenotype, and karyotype analysis. Am J Clin Pathol. 2000;114(1):111–22.

242. Blamey SL, McDermott FT, Pihl E, Hughes ES. Resected ovarian recurrence from colorectal adenocarcinoma: a study of 13 cases. Dis Colon Rectum. 1981;24(4):272–5.

243. Herrera-Ornelas L, Mittelman A. Results of synchronous surgical removal of primary colorectal adenocarcinoma and ovarian metastases. Oncology. 1984;41(2):96–100.

244. Huang PP, Weber TK, Mendoza C, Rodriguez-Bigas MA, Petrelli NJ. Long-term survival in patients with ovarian metastases from colorectal carcinoma. Ann Surg Oncol. 1998; 5(8):695–8.

245. Wright JD, Powell MA, Mutch DG, Rader JS, Gibb RK, Huettner PC, et al. Synchronous ovarian metastases at the time of laparotomy for colon cancer. Gynecol Oncol. 2004;92(3):851–5.

246. Miller BE, Pittman B, Wan JY, Fleming M. Colon cancer with metastasis to the ovary at time of initial diagnosis. Gynecol Oncol. 1997;66(3):368–71.

247. MacKeigan JM, Ferguson JA. Prophylactic oophorectomy and colorectal cancer in premenopausal patients. Dis Colon Rectum. 1979;22(6):401–5.

248. Ballantyne GH, Reigel MM, Wolff BG, Ilstrup DM. Oophorectomy and colon cancer. Impact on survival. Ann Surg. 1985;202(2):209–14.

249. Sielezneff I, Salle E, Antoine K, Thirion X, Brunet C, Sastre B. Simultaneous bilateral oophorectomy does not improve prognosis of postmenopausal women undergoing colorectal resection for cancer. Dis Colon Rectum. 1997;40(11):1299–302.

250. Kontoravdis A, Kalogirou D, Antoniou G, Kontoravdis N, Karakitsos P, Zourlas PA. Prophylactic oophorectomy in ovarian cancer prevention. Int J Gynaecol Obstet. 1996;54(3):257–62.

251. Barringer PL, Dockerty MB, Waugh JM, Bargen JA. Carcinoma of the large intestine; a new approach to the study of venous spread. Surg Gynecol Obstet. 1954;98(1):62–72.

252. Katoh M, Unakami M, Hara M, Fukuchi S. Bone metastasis from colorectal cancer in autopsy cases. J Gastroenterol. 1995;30(5):615–8.

253. Santini D, Tampellini M, Vincenzi B, Ibrahim T, Ortega C, Virzi V, et al. Natural history of bone metastasis in colorectal cancer: final results of a large Italian bone metastases study. Ann Oncol. 2012;23(8):2072–7.

254. Besbeas S, Stearns MW. Osseous metastases from carcinomas of the colon and rectum. Dis Colon Rectum. 1978;21(4):266–8.

255. Buckley N, Peebles Brown DA. Metastatic tumors in the hand from adenocarcinoma of the colon. Dis Colon Rectum. 1987;30(2):141–3.

256. Cascino TL, Leavengood JM, Kemeny N, Posner JB. Brain metastases from colon cancer. J Neurooncol. 1983;1(3):203–9.

257. Rovirosa A, Bodi R, Vicente P, Alastuey I, Giralt J, Salvador L. Cerebral metastases in adenocarcinoma of the colon. Rev Esp Enferm Dig. 1991;79(4):281–3.

258. Alden TD, Gianino JW, Saclarides TJ. Brain metastases from colorectal cancer. Dis Colon Rectum. 1996;39(5):541–5.

259. Zimm S, Wampler GL, Stablein D, Hazra T, Young HF. Intracerebral metastases in solid-tumor patients: natural history and results of treatment. Cancer. 1981;48(2):384–94.

260. Wroński M, Arbit E. Resection of brain metastases from colorectal carcinoma in 73 patients. Cancer. 1999;85(8):1677–85.

261. Ko FC, Liu JM, Chen WS, Chiang JK, Lin TC, Lin JK. Risk and patterns of brain metastases in colorectal cancer: 27-year experience. Dis Colon Rectum. 1999;42(11):1467–71.

262. Sio TT, Jang S, Lee S-W, Curran B, Pyakuryal AP, Sternick ES. Comparing gamma knife and cyberknife in patients with brain metastases. J Appl Clin Med Phys. 2014;15(1):4095.

263. Nakamura E, Shimizu M, Itoh T, Manabe T. Secondary tumors of the pancreas: clinicopathological study of 103 autopsy cases of Japanese patients. Pathol Int. 2001;51(9):686–90.

264. Rumancik WM, Megibow AJ, Bosniak MA, Hilton S. Metastatic disease to the pancreas: evaluation by computed tomography. J Comput Assist Tomogr. 1984;8(5):829–34.

265. Sperti C, Pasquali C, Berselli M, Frison L, Vicario G, Pedrazzoli S. Metastasis to the pancreas from colorectal cancer: is there a place for pancreatic resection? Dis Colon Rectum. 2009;52(6):1154–9.

266. Inagaki H, Nakao A, Ando N, Kotake K, Imaizumi T, Okuda N, et al. A case of solitary metastatic pancreatic cancer from rectal carcinoma: a case report. Hepatogastroenterology. 1998;45(24):2413–7.

267. Cedermark BJ, Blumenson LE, Pickren JW, Holyoke DE, Elias EG. The significance of metastases to the adrenal glands in adenocarcinoma of the colon and rectum. Surg Gynecol Obstet. 1977;144(4):537–46.

268. Mourra N, Hoeffel C, Duvillard P, Guettier C, Flejou J-F, Tiret E. Adrenalectomy for clinically isolated metastasis from colorectal carcinoma: report of eight cases. Dis Colon Rectum. 2008;51(12):1846–9.

269. Fujita K, Kameyama S, Kawamura M. Surgically removed adrenal metastasis from cancer of the rectum. Report of a case. Dis Colon Rectum. 1988;31(2):141–3.

270. Katayama A, Mafune K, Makuuchi M. Adrenalectomy for solitary adrenal metastasis from colorectal carcinoma. Jpn J Clin Oncol. 2000;30(9):414–6.

271. Watatani M, Ooshima M, Wada T, Terashita H, Matsuda T, Shindo K, et al. Adrenal metastasis from carcinoma of the colon and rectum: a report of three cases. Surg Today. 1993;23(5):444–8.

272. Kanjo T, Albertini M, Weber S. Long-term disease-free survival after adrenalectomy for isolated colorectal metastases. Asian J Surg. 2006;29(4):291–3.

273. Marangos IP, Kazaryan AM, Rosseland AR, Røsok BI, Carlsen HS, Kromann-Andersen B, et al. Should we use laparoscopic adrenalectomy for metastases? Scandinavian multicenter study. J Surg Oncol. 2009;100(1):43–7.

274. De Haas RJ, Rahy Martin AC, Wicherts DA, Azoulay D, Castaing D, Adam R. Long-term outcome in patients with adrenal metastases following resection of colorectal liver metastases. Br J Surg. 2009;96(8):935–40.

275. Choi PW, Kim HC, Kim AY, Jung SH, Yu CS, Kim JC. Extensive lymphadenectomy in colorectal cancer with isolated para-aortic lymph node metastasis below the level of renal vessels. J Surg Oncol. 2010;101(1):66–71.

276. Min BS, Kim NK, Sohn SK, Cho CH, Lee KY, Baik SH. Isolated paraaortic lymph-node recurrence after the curative resection of colorectal carcinoma. J Surg Oncol. 2008;97(2):136–40.

277. Shibata D, Paty PB, Guillem JG, Wong WD, Cohen AM. Surgical management of isolated retroperitoneal recurrences of colorectal carcinoma. Dis Colon Rectum. 2002; 45(6):795–801.

278. Biasco G, Derenzini E, Grazi G, Ercolani G, Ravaioli M, Pantaleo MA, et al. Treatment of hepatic metastases from colorectal cancer: many doubts, some certainties. Cancer Treat Rev. 2006;32(3):214–28.

279. Saltz LB. Metastatic colorectal cancer: is there one standard approach? Oncology (Williston Park). 2005;19(9):1147–54.

280. Ho TW, Mack LA, Temple WJ. Operative salvage for retroperitoneal nodal recurrence in colorectal cancer: a systematic review. Ann Surg Oncol. 2011;18(3):697–703.

281. Ferlay J, Shin H-R, Bray F, Forman D, Mathers C, Parkin DM. Estimates of worldwide burden of cancer in 2008: GLOBOCAN 2008. Int J Cancer. 2010;127(12):2893–917.

282. CancerStats Incidence 2008-UK. 2011. http://www.cancerresearchuk.org/cancer-info/cacnerstats/types/bowel/incidence/#trends. Accessed 15 May 2015.

283. Yancik R, Ries LA. Aging and cancer in America. Demographic and epidemiologic perspectives. Hematol Oncol Clin North Am. 2000;14(1):17–23.

284. Extermann M, Balducci L, Lyman GH. What threshold for adjuvant therapy in older breast cancer patients? J Clin Oncol. 2000;18(8):1709–17.

285. Lichtman SM. Therapy insight: therapeutic challenges in the treatment of elderly cancer patients. Nat Clin Pract Oncol. 2006;3(2):86–93.

286. Van Gestel YR, Lemmens VE, de Hingh IH, Steevens J, Rutten HJ, Nieuwenhuijzen GA, et al. Influence of comorbidity and age on 1-, 2-, and 3-month postoperative mortality rates in gastrointestinal cancer patients. Ann Surg Oncol. 2013;20(2):371–80.

287. Power D, Lichtman S. Adjuvant and palliative chemotherapy for colon cancer in the elderly patient. Semin Colon Rectal Surg. 2008;19:239–46.

288. Papamichael D, Audisio R, Horiot J-C, Glimelius B, Sastre J, Mitry E, et al. SIOG. Treatment of the elderly colorectal cancer patient: SIOG expert recommendations. Ann Oncol. 2009;20(1):5–16.

289. Hamaker ME, Jonker JM, de Rooij SE, Vos AG, Smorenburg CH, van Munster BC. Frailty screening methods for predicting outcome of a comprehensive geriatric assessment in elderly patients with cancer: a systematic review. Lancet Oncol. 2012;13(10):e437–44.

290. Smets IH, Kempen GI, Janssen-Heijnen ML, Deckx L, Buntinx FJ, van den Akker M. Four screening instruments for frailty in older patients with and without cancer: a diagnostic study. BMC Geriatr. 2014;14:26.

291. Kenig J, Zychiewicz B, Olszewska U, Richter P. Screening for frailty among older patients with cancer that qualify for abdominal surgery. J Geriatr Oncol. 2015;6(1):52–9.

292. Papamichael D, Audisio RA, Glimelius B, de Gramont A, Glynne-Jones R, Haller D, et al. Treatment of colorectal cancer in older patients: International Society of Geriatric Oncology (SIOG) consensus recommendations 2013. Ann Oncol. 2015;26(3):463–76.

293. Mori M, Tomoda H, Ishida T, Kido A, Shimono R, Matsushima T, et al. Surgical resection of pulmonary metastases from colorectal adenocarcinoma. Special reference to repeated pulmonary resections. Arch Surg. 1991;126(10):1297–301. discussion 1302.

294. McCormack PM, Burt ME, Bains MS, Martini N, Rusch VW, Ginsberg RJ. Lung resection for colorectal metastases. 10-year results. Arch Surg. 1992;127(12):1403–6.

295. Yano T, Hara N, Ichinose Y, Yokoyama H, Miura T, Ohta M. Results of pulmonary resection of metastatic colorectal cancer and its application. J Thorac Cardiovasc Surg. 1993;106(5):875–9.

296. Saclarides TJ, Krueger BL, Szeluga DJ, Warren WH, Faber LP, Economou SG. Thoracotomy for colon and rectal cancer metastases. Dis Colon Rectum. 1993;36(5):425–9.

297. Van Halteren HK, van Geel AN, Hart AA, Zoetmulder FA. Pulmonary resection for metastases of colorectal origin. Chest. 1995;107(6):1526–31.

298. Shirouzu K, Isomoto H, Hayashi A, Nagamatsu Y, Kakegawa T. Surgical treatment for patients with pulmonary metastases after resection of primary colorectal carcinoma. Cancer. 1995;76(3):393–8.

299. Girard P, Ducreux M, Baldeyrou P, Rougier P, Le Chevalier T, Bougaran J, et al. Surgery for lung metastases from colorectal cancer: analysis of prognostic factors. J Clin Oncol. 1996;14(7):2047–53.

300. Okumura S, Kondo H, Tsuboi M, Nakayama H, Asamura H, Tsuchiya R, et al. Pulmonary resection for metastatic colorectal cancer: experiences with 159 patients. J Thorac Cardiovasc Surg. 1996;112(4):867–74.

301. Zanella A, Marchet A, Mainente P, Nitti D, Lise M. Resection of pulmonary metastases from colorectal carcinoma. Eur J Surg Oncol. 1997;23(5):424–7.

302. Zink S, Kayser G, Gabius HJ, Kayser K. Survival, disease-free interval, and associated tumor features in patients with colon/rectal carcinomas and their resected intra-pulmonary metastases. Eur J Cardiothorac Surg. 2001;19(6):908–13.

303. DeVita VT, Hellman S, Rosenberg SA. Cancer: principles and practice of oncology. 6th ed. Philadelphia: Lippincott Williams and Wilkins; 2001.

37
Appendiceal Neoplasms

Constantine P. Spanos and Andreas M. Kaiser

Abbreviations

AJCC	American Joint Commission on Cancer
DPAM	Disseminated peritoneal adenomucinosis
ENETS	European Neuroendocrine Tumor Society
HIPEC	Hyperthermic (or heated) intraperitoneal chemotherapy
LAMN	Low grade appendiceal mucinous neoplasms
PCI	Peritoneal carcinomatosis index
PMAC	Peritoneal mucinous adenocarcinomatosis
PMCA	Peritoneal mucinous carcinomatosis
PMP	Pseudomyxoma peritonei

Key Concepts

- Although appendectomy for appendicitis is the most common emergency operation performed by general surgeons, primary neoplasms of the vermiform appendix are rare, and each individual general surgeon will have limited personal experience in the management of such lesions.
- Most primary neoplasms of the appendix are not associated with specific signs or symptoms and are incidentally diagnosed after pathological analysis of the appendectomy specimen, or detected incidentally on imaging such as computed tomography (CT) done for other indications.
- Primary neoplasms of the appendix can generally be divided into epithelial, non-epithelial, and mixed lesions. Epithelial lesions include adenoma and adenocarcinoma. Non-epithelial tumors include neuroendocrine tumors (carcinoids), lymphoma, leiomyoma, leiomyosarcoma, and other even rarer rarities. Goblet cell carcinoids are mixed lesions with features of carcinoid as well as mucinous adenocarcinoma.

- Epithelial tumors, and specifically mucinous adenocarcinomas, are the most common primary appendiceal neoplasms.
- Pseudomyxoma peritonei is the result of a perforation and peritoneal dissemination of a mucin-producing epithelial neoplasm, most commonly originating from the appendix or the ovaries. In select patients, cytoreductive surgery with HIPEC should be considered.
- A mucocele is a morphologic cystic manifestation of an epithelial appendiceal neoplasm. Perforation leads to pseudomyxoma peritonei. Therefore, intact removal en-bloc is of utmost importance.
- Appendiceal carcinoids are rarely associated with carcinoid syndrome or multicentricity.
- The newest tumor staging guidelines distinguish appendiceal tumors from colon cancer, and separate between epithelial and non-epithelial lesions.
- The extent of surgical resection depends on the cell type, preoperative staging, the ability to achieve negative resection margins, and the probability of nodal disease.
- Surgery is the primary treatment for localized disease, whereas its role in metastatic disease needs to be individually analyzed and weighed against systemic chemotherapy.

Introduction

The appendix vermiformis is commonly regarded as the organ that will introduce a surgical trainee to the art of his or her chosen specialty. Inflammation of this organ, namely appendicitis, is the disease process which will be instrumental in "teaching" the fundamentals of history taking, physical examination and differential diagnosis of the acute abdomen to medical students and surgical residents. Appendectomy is the most frequent emergency operation

© Springer International Publishing 2016
S.R. Steele et al. (eds.), *The ASCRS Textbook of Colon and Rectal Surgery*, DOI 10.1007/978-3-319-25970-3_37

TABLE 37-1. Clinical scenarios depending on type and timing of diagnosis of appendiceal neoplasms

Scenario	Acute symptoms	Presumptive preoperative diagnosis	Surgery	Pre-/intraop evidence of perforation (P) or dissemination (D)	Timing of tumor recognition	Impact/action in decision-making
1. Acute	Y	Appendicitis	N	–	N	Rely on indirect signs/risk factors for identification of affected individuals Re-imaging?
2. Acute	Y	Appendicitis	Y	P– D–	(a) Intraoperative (b) Only on final pathology (c) Not recognized at all (missed opportunity)	Primary or secondary evaluation for more extensive/oncological surgery/treatment
3. Acute	Y	Appendicitis	Y	P+ D–	(a) Intraoperative (b) Only on final pathology (c) Not recognized at all (missed opportunity)	Appropriate treatment for perforation with primary or secondary evaluation for more extensive/oncological surgery/treatment
4. Acute	Y	Appendicitis	Y	P+ D+	Intraoperative	Primary appropriate treatment for perforation Secondary assessment for more extensive surgery/treatment
5. Acute	Y	Appendicitis	Y	P– D–	Intraoperative: evidence of localized mucocele or tumor involving the appendix/cecum	Intraoperative determination of appropriate extent of resection Possible frozen section
6. Elective	Y/N	Localized mucocele/tumor involving appendix/cecum—no signs of PMP	Y	P– D+	Preoperative	Oncological resection Preparedness for HIPEC
7. Elective	Y/N	Localized mucocele/tumor of appendix/cecum AND signs of PMP	TBD	P– D+	Preoperative	PCI Systemic treatment and evaluation for CRS/HIPEC
8. Elective	Y/N	PMP, but no obvious cecal pathology	TBD	P– D+	Preoperative	Evaluation for other potential primary tumor locations PCI Systemic treatment and evaluation for CRS/HIPEC
9. Elective	Y/N	PMP+distant metastases	N	P– D+	Pre-treatment	Systemic treatment

performed by general surgeons with close to 300,000 performed in the United States annually [1, 2], of which a substantial proportion are performed laparoscopically. On comparably rare occasion, the pathology of the appendectomy specimen incidentally reveals an appendiceal neoplasm ("incidentaloma"), which sometimes is recognized even before or at least during surgery, but more often only after the patient has already been discharged from the hospital. Paradoxically and despite the fact that abdominal surgeons at all levels are very frequently involved in treating appendiceal pathology, appendiceal neoplasms are quite infrequent but may cause rather complex intellectual, management and technical challenges in subsequent surgical interventions (Table 37-1) [3].

Epidemiology

Primary neoplasms of the appendix have an incidence of 0.12 cases per 1,000,000 person years and are found in 0.9–1.4% of appendectomy specimens [3, 4]. They can be asymptomatic, be associated with appendicitis, or cause noninflammatory symptoms. Preoperative diagnosis based on symptoms, imaging, and laboratory results is extremely rare. Even intraoperatively, less than 50% appendiceal neoplasms are recognized as such. A retrospective cohort analysis of the Surveillance, Epidemiology, and End-Results database suggested that the incidence of appendiceal neoplasms has increased significantly in the past few decades from 0.63 to 0.97 per 100,000 population [5, 6]. It is unclear

TABLE 37-2. Reported incidence over time of appendiceal neoplasms in SEER database [5, 6]

Subtype	1973–2001 (N=2514)	2000–2009 (N=4765)
Mucinous adenocarcinoma (%)	38	38
Non-mucinous adenocarcinoma (%)	26	27
Carcinoid tumors (%)	17	28
Goblet cell carcinoids (%)	15	
Signet ring cell tumors (%)	4	7

TABLE 37-3. Tumor classifications and manifestations

	Localized[a]	Disseminated	Pattern of dissemination[b]
Epithelial	Adenoma (B)		L, H, P
	Adenocarcinoma (M)	Adenocarcinoma	L, H, P
	Mucocele (B)	PMP: Mucinosis peritonei	P
	Mucinous cystadenoma (IM, LAMN)	PMP: Disseminated peritoneal adenomucinosis (DPAM)	P
	Mucinous (cyst-)adenocarcinoma (M)	PMP: Peritoneal mucinous adenocarcinomatosis (PMAC)	P, L, H
		PMP: Peritoneal mucinous carcinomatosis (PMCA)	P, L, H
	Signet ring cell carcinoma (M)	Advanced/metastatic signet ring cell carcinoma	DI, P, L, H
Mixed	Goblet cell carcinoid (adenocarcinoid)	Metastatic goblet cell adenocarcinoid	P, L, H
Non-epithelial	Carcinoid	Metastatic carcinoid	L, H
	<1 cm (B)		
	1–2 cm (IM)		
	>2 cm (M)		
	Lymphoma (M)	Disseminated/multicentric lymphoma	Systemic
	Leiomyoma (B)		
	Leiomyosarcoma (M)	Metastatic leiomyosarcoma	H, L
	Kaposi sarcoma (M)	Disseminated Kaposi sarcoma	Systemic

LAMN Low grade mucinous neoplasia, *PMP* Pseudomyxoma peritonei

[a]*B* Benign, *IM* Intermediate malignant potential, *M* Malignant

[b]*P* Peritoneal, *L* Lymphatic, *H* Hematogenous, *DI* Diffuse infiltrative

though whether this is a true increase or a simple reflection of higher awareness and reclassification as a separate entity. The increase appears to have affected all histological subtypes in an equal fashion (Table 37-2) [5, 6]. Historically, carcinoid tumors were considered the most frequent neoplasms originating within the appendix, and in 1955 a systematic evaluation of 50,000 appendectomy specimens revealed only 41 epithelial neoplasms (0.082%) [7]. More recent publications, however, demonstrate that epithelial neoplasms are more frequent and represent 58% of malignant appendiceal tumors [5, 8]. At the same time, a surge was also noted for the frequency of distant metastatic disease [5]. In contrast, however, appendiceal carcinoids have an incidence of 0.15/100,000/year but the relative frequency compared to other primary sites of neuroendocrine tumors within the gastrointestinal tract has decreased to 16.7% [9, 10]. Epithelial appendiceal neoplasms—paralleling colorectal cancer—usually develop in the sixth or seventh decade of life, whereas non-epithelial pathology including neuroendocrine tumors occur at a younger age, namely the fourth to fifth decade [2, 5, 7, 8, 11]. At the time of diagnosis, a total of 74% of appendiceal cancer cases have already spread, and developed regional or distant metastases in 39% and 35%, respectively [5].

Anatomical Pathology and Staging

The literature unfortunately has for a long time shown little consistency and used a variety of nomenclatures, classification systems, and descriptive terms when referring to appendiceal neoplasms. The many synonyms for lesions of such rarity undoubtedly has led to confounding terminology. From an anatomical point of view, the appendix in essence has a smaller diameter but otherwise a similar layered wall structure as the rest of the large intestine; however there is a higher representation of immunological tissue components (GALT, gut associated lymphoid tissue). The appendix does not participate in processing of intestinal contents but produces 2–3 mL of mucin per day and may participate in immunological functions. The arterial blood supply originates from the appendicular artery which branches off the ileocolic artery; the venous drainage is via the superior mesenteric vein to the portal vein system; the lymphatic drainage follows the vascular structures and due to variability may parallel the ileocolic, right colic, and right branch of the middle colic artery.

Appendiceal neoplasms should be categorized according to the tissue of origin as well as the pattern of growth, expansion, and spreading (Table 37-3). As for the latter,

FIGURE 37-1. Appendiceal mucocele: the computed tomography shows the cystic enlargement at the base of the appendix (*asterisk*, panels (**a**) and (**b**)), as well as the moderately enlarged appendix (in-between *arrows*, panel (**c**)).

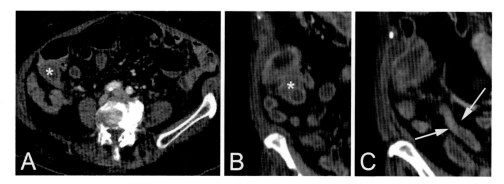

tumors may either metastasize via vascular, lymphatic, or transperitoneal route. A major distinction is made between epithelial and non-epithelial lesions, the latter of which includes among others neuroendocrine tumors such as carcinoid tumors.

Epithelial Neoplasms

Epithelial neoplasms are divided into mucinous and non-mucinous neoplasms [8]. Mucinous neoplasms of the appendix are classified according to the grade and aggressiveness of the tumor. Descriptively, these lesions characteristically can form mucoceles of the appendix, a morphologic term describing the dilation of the appendix with intraluminal accumulation of mucoid material (Figure 37-1). The obstruction can either be caused by the epithelial neoplasm itself, an independent tumor, or a benign process (retention cysts, mucosal hyperplasia). Rupture of a mucocele results in peritoneal spillage and spread of mucin and—depending on the malignant potential of the lesion—of cellular elements, which are the basis for mucinosis, pseudomyxoma peritonei, and carcinomatosis.

Low grade appendiceal mucinous neoplasms (LAMN) are well-differentiated neoplasms that morphologically resemble adenomas. LAMN has become the neutral term for a number of entities such as appendiceal villous or serrated adenoma, cystadenoma, borderline tumor of the appendix, and mucinous tumors of uncertain malignant potential. These lesions tend to grow slowly and grossly are characterized by a well-defined structure, cystic dilation, and mucinous content. The appendiceal wall is fibrotic and—as a sign of chronicity—may sometimes contain calcifications. Gross rupture (spontaneously or as a result of surgical manipulation) may be evident as mucin extruding on to the serosal surface or seeding of more distant peritoneal surfaces as evidenced by presence of mucin lakes. Histologically, the appendiceal mucosa is replaced by adenomatous proliferations of villous, papillary, serrated, or flat mucinous character. The columnar epithelial cells are mucin-rich and

may have elongated (pencil-shaped), mildly hyperchromatic nuclei with nuclear pseudostratification, rare mitoses, and apoptotic nuclear debris. It is of note that the neoplastic epithelium on occasion may herniate through the muscularis propria and form "pseudodiverticula." One might speculate that these extensions represent a route by which such lesions perforate and disseminate to the peritoneal cavity [11].

Prognosis of LAMN depends on the presence or absence of epithelial cells outside the appendix. Tumors confined to the appendix generally have an excellent prognosis. However, LAMN may proliferate outside the appendix in a malignant fashion, producing pseudomyxoma peritonei and/or distant metastases. Pseudomyxoma peritonei (PMP) derived from perforation of a LAMN is characterized by abundant extracellular mucin, hyalinized fibrotic stroma, and harboring scant strips of low-grade mucinous epithelium [8]. The term is not strictly limited to appendiceal neoplasms but the condition can result from other tumor origins such as ovaries, gallbladder, and others. The prognosis of a ruptured LAMN is dependent on the amount and cellularity of mucin deposits, and recurrence rates increase when epithelial cells are present in the mucin. Most instances of PMP resulting from LAMN remain confined to the right lower quadrant. Even if the spread of PMP goes beyond the immediate vicinity, the lesion may pursue an indolent but progressive course. The superordinate term "PMP" has been categorized into disseminated peritoneal adenomucinosis (DPAM) and peritoneal mucinous (adeno-) carcinomatosis (PMAC or PMCA) [12]. The former reflects a low-grade pseudomyxoma arising from LAMNs, whereas the latter indicates peritoneal carcinomatosis. DPAM lesions contain scarce strips of low-grade mucinous epithelium with mild atypia and no significant mitotic activity; [12] these low-grade lesions usually cover but do not infiltrate the surface of the organs to which they adhere.

Appendiceal adenocarcinoma is also divided into mucinous and non-mucinous types. Mucinous adenocarcinoma of the appendix is characterized by a destructive growth pattern with tumor invasion of the appendiceal wall beyond the muscularis mucosae; infiltrating pools of mucin harbor cytologically malignant glandular epithelium arranged in strips, clusters, and complex proliferations. Mucinous adenocarcinoma due to the increasing pressure of accumulating mucin is prone to rupture, spreading, and seeding into the peritoneal cavity, leading to formation of pseudomyxoma peritonei. Mucinous tumors spread along peritoneal surfaces, even in the absence of lymph node metastases. Peritoneal mucinous (adeno-)carcinomatosis (PMAC/PMCA) results from secondary peritoneal proliferation of appendiceal or intestinal mucinous adenocarcinoma nests that lead to invasion of parenchymal and visceral organs and the omentum, and potentially trigger secondary lymph node metastases at those sites.

Non-mucinous adenocarcinomas behave similarly to colonic adenocarcinomas, infiltrating the appendiceal wall and metastasizing to regional lymph nodes and the liver [11]. Non-mucinous adenocarcinomas show a spectrum of morphological features of the invasive component. In some cases the tumor is identical to colonic adenocarcinoma with malignant (pseudo-)glandular formations, increased stratification, and disorganization (compared to the regular columnar epithelium). In other cases, the malignant glands are tubular in shape, lined by cuboidal epithelium, associated with modest amount of extracellular mucin.

Signet-ring cell carcinoma is a rare but aggressive subentity of mucinous adenocarcinoma, characterized by dissolute growth and infiltration of mucin-containing cancer cells (signet rings); it almost never remains confined, may display an infiltrative growth below intact appearing mucosal surfaces as well as a rapid dissemination within the peritoneal cavity. Signet-ring cell carcinoma is typically associated with a poor prognosis.

Prognosis of appendiceal adenocarcinomas—similar to colon cancer—is primarily determined by the stage, but within stage IV also depends on the histological subtype and grading as well as the route of dissemination. Within each stage and histological subtype, poor differentiation is associated with unfavorable outcomes. Mucinous adenocarcinomas have a markedly worse outcome (reduced cancer-specific survival) than non-mucinous adenocarcinomas of the appendix (Table 37-4). This observation, which was based on published data analysis of the National Cancer Database (NCDB) [4], was recently implemented into the current staging guidelines by the American Joint Commission for Cancer (AJCC) [13]. Appendiceal carcinomas for the first time are classified separately from colonic adenocarcinoma, and distinction is made between mucinous and non-mucinous types; histologic grading for mucinous tumors is considered of particular importance for metastatic tumors (Table 37-5). Stage T4 is divided into T4a (penetration of visceral serosa) and T4b

TABLE 37-4. Cancer-specific survival for appendiceal adenocarcinoma stratified by stage and grade [4]

Subtype	Stages I–III (%)	Stage IV (%)
Mucinous adenocarcinoma ($N = 1375$)		
Well differentiated	82	71
Moderately differentiated	64	51
Poorly differentiated	50	0
Non-mucinous adenocarcinoma ($N = 860$)		
Well differentiated	69	48
Moderately differentiated	73	9
Poorly differentiated	55	5

TABLE 37-5. TNM staging by AJCC for appendiceal adenocarcinoma [13]

Stage T		N	M
X	Primary tumor not determined, or any T	Regional lymph nodes not determined, or any N	Metastatic disease not determined, or any M
0	No evidence of primary tumor	No regional lymph node metastasis	No distant metastasis
Is	Carcinoma in situ: intraepithelial or invasion of lamina propria	–	–
1	Tumor invades submucosa	Metastasis in 1–3 regional lymph nodes	1a: Intraperitoneal metastasis beyond the right lower quadrant, including pseudomyxoma peritonei
			1b: Non-peritoneal metastases
2	Tumor invades muscularis propria	Metastasis in four or more regional lymph nodes	
3	Tumor invades through muscularis propria into subserosa or into mesoappendix		
4	4a: Tumor penetrates visceral peritoneum, including mucinous peritoneal tumor within the right lower quadrant		
	4b: Tumor directly invades other organs or structures		

Stage I: T1–2 N0 M0; stage II: T3–4 N0 M0; stage III: Tx N1–2 M0; stage IV: Tx Nx M1 (invasion of other organs). In mucinous tumors that penetrate the visceral peritoneum and cause mucin deposits confined to the right lower quadrant are still considered a T4a (that is a stage II if no lymph nodes are involved); when mucin has dispersed beyond the right lower quadrant, it is designated M1a (stage IV) [13]. M1 is divided into M1a and M1b to distinguish pseudomyxoma peritonei (M1a) from nonperitoneal metastasis (M1b) [13].

Neuroendocrine Appendiceal Lesions/Carcinoid Tumors

The WHO classification utilizes the terms "neuroendocrine tumor" (NET), "neuroendocrine carcinoma" (NEC), and "mixed adeno-neuroendocrine carcinomas" (MANEC) [14]. Synonyms for NET include carcinoid tumors and well-differentiated endocrine tumors/carcinoma. Synonyms for NEC: poorly differentiated endocrine carcinoma and small cell/large cell endocrine carcinoma. Goblet cell carcinoids (now called carcinomas) are MANEC [14].

Carcinoids or carcinoid tumors represent NETs grade 1 and derive from a variety of dispersed neuroendocrine cells (formerly labeled as amine precursor uptake and decarboxylation cells, APUD cells). These cells and the resulting tumors are not only found in the appendix but also in the entire gastrointestinal tract and other organs and are therefore addressed more comprehensively in the next chapter. Nonetheless, appendiceal carcinoids are only extremely rarely associated with multicentricity, and there is no known association with multiple endocrine neoplasia (MEN syndrome).

Appendiceal carcinoids belong to the embryological and anatomical region of the midgut to include jejunum, ileum appendix, cecum, and right colon. More than foregut and hindgut carcinoids, these midgut carcinoid cells characteristically are hormone-active. Among other products (such as GH, GHRH, gastrin, calcitonin, substance P, insulin, and neurotensin), they produce serotonin from its precursor 5-hydroxytryptophan by means of the enzyme aromatic acid decarboxylase; serotonin is subsequently metabolized in the liver by monoamine oxidase to 5-hydroxyindoleacetic acid (5-HIAA), which is excreted in the urine.

On gross examination, carcinoid tumors of the appendix are yellow-tan firm nodules. 75% are located at the tip, 15% in the mid-appendix and 10% at the base of the organ. At the time of diagnosis, the majority (80%) is less than 1 cm, 14% measure between 1 and 2 cm, and 6% are greater than 2 cm in size [14]. Histologically, carcinoids are characterized by submucosal uniform cell conglomerates with a nested or insular pattern. The cytoplasm has a modestly eosinophilic, fine granularity, and the nuclei show the classic endocrine "salt-and-pepper" chromatin pattern. Tumors have positive reactions to silver stains (argentaffin/argyrophilic) and immunohistochemically to markers of neuroendocrine tissue, including neuron-specific enolase, synaptophysin, and chromogranin A [11]. Ki67 is used to determine the proliferative capacity of the tumor for grading according the current WHO classification [14, 15]. Under the electron microscope (which is not part of routine examinations), carcinoid tumors are typically found to contain numerous membrane-bound neurosecretory granules which store a variety of hormones and biogenic amines [16].

With increasing size of the lesion, the tumor may extend deeper into the wall and even reach the peritoneal surface or in up to 27% of cases infiltrate the mesoappendix. Hence, the AJCC staging for carcinoids is based on tumor size as it correlates with the incidence of metastases and represents the most important prognostic parameter, whereas depth of invasion, lymphatic, perineural, or serosal invasion lack prognostic power (Table 37-6). Lymph node metastases are

TABLE 37-6. TNM staging (by AJCC and ENETS) for neuroendocrine appendiceal tumors [15]

Stage	T (AJCC)	T (ENETS)	N (AJCC/ ENETS)	M (AJCC/ ENETS)
X	Primary tumor not determined, or any T	Primary tumor not determined, or any T	Lymph nodes not determined, or any N	Metastatic disease not determined, or any M
0	No evidence of primary tumor	No evidence of primary tumor	No lymph node metastasis	No distant metastasis
1	1a: Tumor ≤1 cm; 1a: Tumor 1–2 cm	T1 Tumor ≤1 cm invading submucosa and muscularis propria	Lymph node metastasis	Distant metastasis
2	Tumor 2–4 cm or with extension to the cecum	Tumor ≤2 cm with invasion of submucosa or muscularis propria, and/or minimal invasion (up to 3 mm) of subserosa/mesoappendix		
3	Tumor >4 cm or with extension to the ileum	Tumor >2 cm and/or extensive invasion (>3 mm) of subserosa/mesoappendix		
4	Tumor directly invades other adjacent organs or structures, e.g., abdominal wall and skeletal muscle[a]	Tumor invades peritoneum/other organs		

[a]Tumor adherent to other organs or structures grossly classified as cT4 but if microscopically negative adhesion as pT1–3 depending on depth of wall invasion
Stage I: T1 N0 M0; stage II: T2–3 N0 M0; stage III: T4 N0 M0 or Tx N1 M0; stage IV: Tx Nx M1

TABLE 37-7. Impact of appendiceal carcinoid size on lymph node metastasis and survival [11, 14, 18, 49]

Carcinoid size	LN metastases (%)	5-/10-Year survival rates (%)
<1 cm	<1.0–15.0	92–100
1–2 cm	3.0–47.0	81
>2 cm	20–86	31

rare for lesions of less than 10 mm diameter, but occur in 20–30% of patients with carcinoids greater than 2 cm in size (Table 37-7); distant metastases are comparably rare in appendiceal carcinoids. It should be noted that the staging system by the European Neuroendocrine Tumor Society (ENETS) differs from AJCC as it also takes into account depth of appendiceal wall and meso-appendiceal invasion with invasion greater than 3 mm representing more aggressive disease [17]. Five-year survival rates for patients with local, regional metastatic, and distant metastatic disease are 95%, 81%, and 31%, respectively [9, 15, 18].

Goblet Cell Carcinoids

This term may add confusion to the classification of appendiceal lesions. It is considered a hybrid between epithelial and NETs and is also referred to as mucinous adeno-neuroendocrine carcinoma [19–21]. These tumors have a mean age of presentation in the fifth decade and behave more like adenocarcinoma than carcinoid. Clinically, goblet cell carcinoids in the middle third of the appendix may in fact cause appendicitis [22]. At surgical exploration, 10% or more of the tumors are found to have already widespread metastatic disease; two-thirds of goblet cell carcinoids are incidental findings on appendectomy and ileocecectomy specimens. Five-year survival rates are worse than for regular carcinoids and for stages I, II, III, and IV were 100%, 76%, 22%, and 14%, respectively, i.e., range from 50 to 80% for locoregional disease to less than 20% for patients with distant metastases [19, 20].

Rare Appendiceal Neoplasms

All other neoplasms are comparably rare and often represent a more systemic disease process. Among the rarities, primary lymphoma of the appendix is seen with some frequency; it affects patients of all ages but most frequently occurs in the second to fourth decade of life. In children and young adults, Burkitt's lymphoma is the most common subtype, whereas older patients are more likely to have diffused large B-cell lymphoma. Furthermore, the appendix has been reported as the site of relapse of several subtypes of lymphoma [11]. Any of these lesions may either present with acute appendicitis or through a palpable mass, intussusception, or lower gastrointestinal bleeding as rarer manifestations. Other even less common and therefore not further detailed lesions include Kaposi sarcoma, leiomyoma or leiomyosarcoma, or leukemic infiltrates.

Clinical Features

Appendiceal epithelial neoplasms are notorious for the absence of any specific signs or symptoms, especially at early stages. Complicating factor is that they escape detection by routine screening efforts such as colonoscopy [23]. If a tumor is concentric and causes obstruction of the lumen, clinical symptomatology of appendicitis may ensue. Red flags in patients with signs of "appendicitis" should include any age above 50, family history of colorectal cancer or inflammatory bowel disease, prolonged history, or anemia. At later stages, epithelial appendiceal neoplasms may present as a localized abdominal or pelvic mass, bowel obstruction, or as progressive, painless, abdominal distention when large volumes of mucin accumulate in the peritoneal cavity (pseudomyxoma peritonei) [2–5].

Even hormone-active tumors such as carcinoids remain silent and are only incidentally detected. Since they are frequently located at the tip of the appendix, they may not even trigger appendicitis. Carcinoid syndrome or "crisis" with flushing, wheezing, diarrhea, and eventually right-sided valvular heart disease results from the release of serotonin and other vasoactive substances. From appendiceal primary carcinoids, this is extremely rare (less than 5%) and requires presence of significant metastatic disease to allow these substances to escape the hepatic first-pass effect and be released into the systemic circulation.

Given the incredible variability of clinical circumstances under which an appendiceal neoplasm may be diagnosed, clinicians will have to develop concepts and algorithms to optimize and standardize their management (Table 37-1).

Diagnostic Procedures

Clinical examination is expectedly unreliable in detecting, confirming, or ruling out an appendiceal neoplasm. Tumor markers are limited and include nonspecific carcinoembryonic antigen (CEA) for epithelial lesions, or 5-HIAA metabolites in the urine for carcinoids. Neither marker is suited for screening or as a negative predictive test. Cross-sectional imaging (CT, MRI) is of greatest value in evaluating a suspected appendiceal neoplasm. Plain radiographs or contrast small bowel follow-throughs may suggest a mass effect when adjacent loops of bowel appear to be displaced, but are rarely definitive. Similarly, contrast enemas, even though rarely done, may provide a hint of an extrinsic impression on the cecum, terminal ileum, or sigmoid colon.

Ultrasonography in skilled hands may allow for identification of appendiceal abnormalities, including appendicitis, fecoliths, mucoceles (hypoechogenic structure), or on occasion a mass in the right lower quadrant. Cystic masses may have a heterogeneous appearance due to the combination of fine cellular framework with mucin-containing chambers with synchronously liquid, gelatinous, and viscous components. A lack of appendiceal wall thickening (>6 mm) suggests

FIGURE 37-2. Pseudomyxoma peritonei: the computed tomography a coronal view (panel (**a**)) and axial view (panel (**b**)) of a patient with massive deposits of low attenuation mucin throughout the entire abdomen with scalloping of the liver contour and widening of the spaces between the compressed bowel loops.

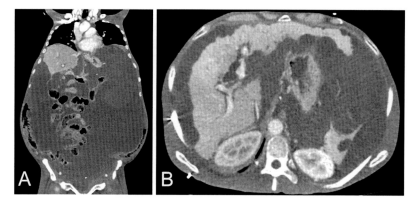

absence of inflammation (appendicitis). A target sign either implies an enlarged and edematous appendix or an intussusception. To a limited degree, mucinous ascites can be detected and even quantified, but for comprehensive assessment of pseudomyxoma, ultrasound is not well suited.

CT or, less commonly used, MRI are the cross-sectional imaging modalities of choice as they provide reproducible, complete, and quantifiable evaluation of the whole abdomen [24, 25]. They are indicated for workup of right lower quadrant symptoms, or after the fact when diagnosed tumors (epithelial and non-epithelial) require lymph node and systemic staging, treatment planning, or evaluation of treatment response. Tumors of sufficient size can be demonstrated as a moderately enhancing soft tissue mass or a cystic dilatation of the appendix beyond 15 mm, which should raise suspicion if noted as an incidental finding [26]. Bowel displacement is an indirect sign of a pathological extraluminal process and is best visualized by adequate opacification of the terminal ileum and cecum by means of intraluminal contrast and differs from an abscess by the lack of inflammatory signs. Features of a mucocele include well-encapsulated and smooth lesions in the right lower quadrant with regular wall and low attenuation that depends on the amount of mucin in the tissue and the center of the lesion [27]. Presence of punctuate, curvilinear calcifications in a right lower quadrant cystic lesion are highly suggestive of a mucocele: they develop as a dystrophic response to a chronic inflammatory process. Myxoglobulosis is an anecdotal variant of an appendiceal mucocele with formation of multiple translucent or calcified mucin globules rather than a homogenous mucin lake.

Pseudomyxoma peritonei is characterized by low attenuation ascites and serosal implants which when not obvious are best seen as scalloping of the liver contour, at peritoneal reflections, or the pouch of Douglas (Figure 37-2). For treatment strategy and prognosis, it is important to quantify areas affected by PMP. The peritoneal carcinomatosis index (PCI) is a summary score with a maximum of 39 points from nine abdominal squares and 4 small bowel segments, whereby each area is scored between 0 and 3 when deposits are >5 cm [24]. Positron emission tomography (PET scan) may have a role for detection or monitoring of systemic metastatic disease but is notoriously ineffective in assessing pseudomyxoma peritonei.

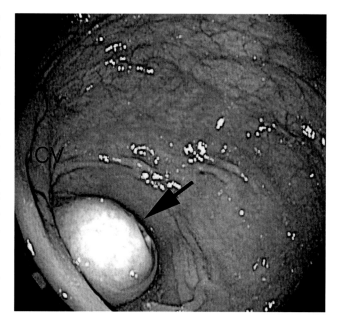

FIGURE 37-3. Colonoscopic appearance: even though appendiceal neoplasms frequently escape endoscopic detection, they occasionally lead to an extramucosal protrusion (*asterisk*) of the appendiceal orifice into the cecal lumen. ICV: ileocecal valve.

Since most carcinoids are surgical/pathological incidentalomas, most diagnostic investigations are performed after the initial operation. For the majority of incidentally diagnosed, well-differentiated appendiceal NERs of <10 mm, no postoperative diagnostic procedure is necessary [15]. After complete resection of 10–20 mm lesions, a single CT or MRI to rule out lymph node and distant metastases is recommended, but without level I evidence [15]. For lesions >20 mm, CT and or MRI of the abdomen is recommended; in addition a PET scan or a somatostatin receptor scan in combination with SPECT/CT (or Somatostatin Receptor PET with 3-phase CT scan) may be considered to detect or rule out distant tumor spread.

Appendiceal neoplasms typically evade detection by colonoscopy [23]. Occasionally, a protrusion of the appendiceal orifice or release of mucoid material may be recognized (Figure 37-3). However, colonic evaluation (colonoscopy, CT colonography) is recommended prior to any elective intervention for a suspected or proven appendiceal neoplasm, because both epithelial and NETs may be multicentric and/or be associated with a synchronous lesion in up to 10–20% [28].

Medical Management

Management of localized appendiceal neoplasms is primarily surgical. Nonsurgical modalities come into play for locally advanced or metastatic lesions as well as for primarily systemic neoplasms such as leukemia or lymphoma. Pseudomyxoma of too significant extent (high PCI) may not benefit from cytoreductive surgery and HIPEC (see later). Adjuvant and palliative systemic chemotherapy are still largely based of 5-fluorouracil and typically combined with other conventional agents (oxaliplatin and others), or biological drugs such as bevacizumab [29]. Regimens and timings before, during and after surgery remain areas of research [30, 31]. Somatostatin is being used for metastatic and particularly symptomatic carcinoid tumors. Radiation treatment is not part of routine management of any appendiceal tumor and is reserved for special circumstances on an individualized basis.

Surgical Treatment of Appendiceal Lesions

Surgery is the primary treatment for localized disease with the goal to achieve a curative R0 resection; in metastatic disease, the role of surgery needs to be individually analyzed and weighed against systemic chemotherapy or best palliative care. Surgical decision-making should therefore take five questions into consideration as also alluded to in the previously listed clinical scenarios:

1. Has the primary tumor already been removed?
2. Was the clinical situation associated with possible tumor spillage?
3. For a given tumor, what entails an adequate margin?
4. What is the probability of nodal involvement?
5. In case of locally advanced or metastatic disease, is aggressive surgical intervention superior to conservative management?

Depending on the answers, there are four possible surgical responses (Table 37-8): (a) appendectomy only, (b) hemicolectomy or completion hemicolectomy, (c) cytoreductive surgery and peritonectomy with or without HIPEC, or (d) conservative management.

Appendectomy

Appendectomy alone should be reserved for premalignant lesions, carcinoma in situ (Tis), or carcinoids of less than 1 cm diameter provided that a sufficient margin can be obtained. Carcinoids of 1–2 cm represent a grey zone but may be associated with a higher than previously reported incidence of nodal disease [18], suggesting that appendectomy may not suffice. An appendiceal mucocele requires careful dissection to avoid perforation of the lesion. If the case is approached laparoscopically, placement of the whole appendix/cecum into a specimen bag prior to starting the dissection may be a strategy to avoid rupture and spillage or conversion to a laparotomy [32].

TABLE 37-8. Operations performed for appendiceal neoplasms

Appendectomy	Right hemicolectomy	Cytoreduction + HIPEC	Nonsurgical
Intact mucocele	Invasive adenocarcinoma	PMP with PCI ≤16 (−20):[a]	PMP with PCI > (16−)20?[a]
Adenocarcinoma tis		– Diffuse mucinous adenomucinosis peritonei	Adenocarcinoma with diffuse systemic metastases
		– Peritoneal mucinous (adeno-) carcinomatosis	Adenocarcinoma with peritoneal disease AND systemic metastases
		Perforated appendiceal neoplasm without visible PMP?	
Appendiceal carcinoid <1 cm, R0	Appendiceal carcinoid 1–2 cm, R0?		Carcinoid with diffuse systemic metastases beyond one organ
	Appendiceal carcinoid >2 cm		
	Any carcinoid with insufficient margin (R1, questionable R), multifocality, invasion of mesoappendix >3 mm		
	Any carcinoid with nodal involvement		
	Any carcinoid with systemic metastases to the liver only		
	Goblet cell carcinoid	PMP from goblet cell carcinoid	Widespread systemic metastases, or PMP from goblet cell carcinoid with systemic metastases

[a]PMP Pseudomyxoma peritonei, PCI Peritoneal carcinomatosis index

Right Hemicolectomy

For non-perforated appendiceal adenocarcinoma, carcinoids larger than 2 cm and any of the previously mentioned lesions with unfavorable features or whose margins are insufficient with an appendectomy alone, an oncological right hemicolectomy with a mesocolic lymph node dissection is indicated [15, 18]. Oncological resection for adenocarcinoma achieves better 5-year survival rates than appendectomy alone [33]. The incidence of lymph node metastases in appendiceal carcinoid tumors increases with size of the tumor (Table 37-7). There is controversy regarding the surgical management of patients in which perforation of a mucinous appendiceal neoplasm has occurred resulting in pseudomyxoma peritonei. Some argue that a right hemicolectomy is not necessary in this situation as the outcome is determined by the peritoneal disease rather than the lymph nodes [32, 34].

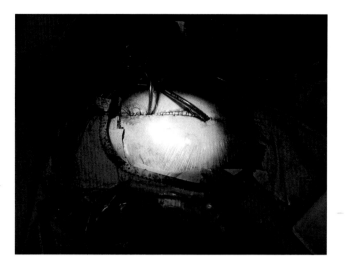

FIGURE 37-4. Hyperthermic intraperitoneal chemotherapy (HIPEC) (Courtesy of Eric K. Johnson, M.D.).

Cytoreductive Surgery and HIPEC

In cases of advanced peritoneal dissemination, cytoreductive surgery with HIPEC is performed in selected cases [15]. If pseudomyxoma peritonei is unexpectedly encountered during an operative exploration, the patient would be best served by careful retrieval and cytological analysis of any mucinous fluid present, and referral to a specialized center with expertise in cytoreductive surgery and HIPEC [35]. Minimization of surgical manipulation and mobilization of intra-abdominal viscera will facilitate the subsequent cytoreductive surgery performed later.

The mainstay of surgical treatment for disseminated peritoneal disease is the arduous operative task of cytoreductive surgery and heated intraperitoneal chemotherapy (HIPEC) (Figure 37-4). In retrospective series, this surgical modality has demonstrated favorable results in carefully selected patients [36], but at the same time was associated with a substantial morbidity and mortality; [37–41] in addition, most series note that incomplete cytoreduction was unable to achieve a relevant benefit as the recurrence rates were very high [37, 42, 43]. It seems rather obvious that the outcomes depend on the extent of the initial disease whereby a number of authors recommended to limit cytoreductive surgery and HIPEC to patients with a PCI of less than (16–)20.

In reviewing the evidence supporting the use of cytoreduction and HIPEC, it should be noted that the literature on the technique and outcomes continues to have significant limitations. On one hand, most series are retrospective and inconsistent in regards to inclusion criteria, extent of disease, concomitant treatment, protocols, and follow-up. Selection bias is inherent to their study designs. Furthermore, they are heavily dominated by Sugarbaker [44], who has advocated for the use of cytoreduction and HIPEC not only for appendiceal neoplasms, but also for peritoneal carcinomatosis arising from non-appendiceal cancers. Corroboration of his data by other groups is in process, but at the same time challenged by availability of more aggressive systemic chemotherapy

regimens, the latter of which parenthetically has been found to increase the risk of complications after HIPEC [31]. Most importantly, however, there is a lack of prospective randomized data on direct comparison of HIPEC and cytoreductive surgery with systemic chemotherapy alone. The only prospective randomized trial to date that suggested improved outcomes with HIPEC compared to systemic treatment only was limited by a chemotherapy regimen (fluorouracil-leucovorin) that many feel was not representative of modern treatment standards [43]. A heated debate continues as to whether HIPEC should be considered the standard of care or still an experimental approach [45, 46].

In preparation for cytoreductive surgery and HIPEC, adequate staging and quantitative assessment using the PCI [24], colonic clearance, aggressive hydration, and bowel cleansing are essential. Considerations include provisions for stomas, timely prophylactic vaccination for splenectomy (against pneumococcus, meningococcus, and H. Influenza) and placement of a gastrostomy tube and feeding jejunostomy tube. Cytoreductive surgery aims at removing or reducing all visible tumor implants to less than 2 mm in size as only complete cytoreduction allows for adequate drug penetration into residual tumor deposits. It typically includes omentectomy and stripping of all parietal peritoneal surfaces, including the subdiaphragmatic spaces and the paracolic recesses (peritonectomy). However, it may also involve aggressive multiorgan resection including tumor-involved bowel (colon, small bowel) or other organs (gallbladder, spleen, uterus/ovaries, and others) or the posterior rectus sheath may be removed. For the HIPEC phase of the procedure, a number of open or closed techniques have been reported. We have typically used the closed technique to minimize heat dissipation, spillage of perfusate, and safety hazard to health personnel [47, 48]. The incision is temporarily closed to the size of a gel port through which large-bore afferent and efferent cannulas are placed to the peritoneal cavity. The heated chemothera-

TABLE 37-9. Selected series on cytoreductive surgery and HIPEC for appendiceal neoplasms

Institution	Year	N	Appendiceal origin (%)	Complete CR[a] (%)	M/M[b]	RR[c]	SV[d]
Washington Cancer Institute [50]	1999	200	75	n/a	27/2	n/a	n/a
University of Cincinnati College of Medicine [51]	2004	33	67	67	27/0	>33	(49)[e] (3 years)
Wake Forest University, NC [52]	2006	110	100	28	38/4	n/a	53.4 (5 years)
Istituto dei Tumori, Milan, Italy [53]	2008	96	100	67	27/1	61	71.9 (5 years)
Washington Cancer Institute [54]	2008	472	85	100	n/a	26	n/a
Mercy Medical Center, Baltimore MD [55]	2012	77	100	65	27/0	n/a	40 (3 years)
International Multicenter [36]	2012	2298	100	51	24/2	n/a	63 (10 years)
National Cancer Centre Singapore [56]	2013	100	20	90	55/0	74	50.9 (5 years)
Mount Sinai Medical Ctr, NY [57]	2014	170	29	37	52/4	40–79	30.6 (3 years)
Basingstoke/North Hampshire Hospital, UK [58]	2015	752	100	68	46/2	50	64.5 (5 years)
Wake Forest University, NC [59]	2015	430	100	44	28/3	n/a	53.4 (5 years)

[a]CR Cytoreduction
[b]M/M 30 Day morbidity and mortality
[c]RR Recurrence rate
[d]SV Survival
[e]Number calculated from graph by weighted average

peutic drugs are circulated throughout the abdominal cavity via pumps and heat exchangers (heart-lung machine). The most frequently used drug is mitomycin-c, which is administered for a duration of 60–120 min at a temperature of 41–43 °C. Other drugs have been used and are being tested without any increased benefit. Reconstructions and anastomoses are to be performed after the hyperthermic perfusion phase. Cytoreductive surgery and HIPEC are associated with formidable morbidity that may exceed 50% (Table 37-9). Apart from myelosuppression and nephrotoxicity with intensified diuresis, complications include sepsis, respiratory failure, ileus, anastomotic leak, abscess, enterocutaneous fistula, acute renal failure, thromboembolic events, and in the long run formation of hostile adhesions. The mortality rates in initial reports were approximately 10%, but could be reduced significantly in more recent series (Table 37-9). In the majority of reports, PCI score, PMCA tumor type and completeness of cytoreduction were significant prognostic factors. Perioperative or neo-adjuvant chemotherapy is currently a matter of debate and is not routinely used.

Conclusion

Appendiceal neoplasms are rare lesions. Most individual surgeons will encounter few, if any, during their career. Nevertheless, when a diagnosis of such a lesion is made, careful investigation of the histopathology and rational analysis of the various parameters are of paramount importance in order to finalize treatment and follow-up. There are numerous areas (e.g., incidentalomas, conservatively treated "appendicitis," perforated tumor without visible implants, and others) that await clarification of guidance which should be developed on preferably prospective data.

References

1. Barrett ML, Hines AL, Andrews RM (2006) Trends in rates of perforated appendix, 2001–2010: statistical brief #159. http://www.ncbi.nlm.nih.gov/pubmed/24199256. Accessed 6 Apr 2015.
2. McCusker ME, Cote TR, Clegg LX, et al. Primary malignant neoplasms of the appendix: a population-based study from the surveillance, epidemiology and end-results program, 1973–1998. Cancer. 2002;94:3307–12.
3. Whitfield CG, Amin SN, Garner JP. Surgical management of primary appendiceal malignancy. Colorectal Dis. 2012;14:1507–11.
4. Overman MJ, Fournier K, Hu CY, et al. Improving the AJCC/TNM staging for adenocarcinomas of the appendix: the prognostic impact of histological grade. Ann Surg. 2013;257:1072–8.
5. Marmor S, Portschy PR, Tuttle TM, et al. The rise in appendiceal cancer incidence: 2000–2009. J Gastrointest Surg. 2015;19(4):743–50.
6. McGory ML, Maggard MA, Kang H, et al. Malignancies of the appendix: beyond case series reports. Dis Colon Rectum. 2005;48:2264–71.
7. Collins DC. A study of 50,000 specimens of the human vermiform appendix. Surg Gynecol Obstet. 1955;101:437–45.
8. Carr NJ, Sobin LH. Adenocarcinoma of the appendix. In: Bosman FT, Carneiro F, Hruban RH, Theise ND, editors. WHO classification of tumors of the digestive system (IARC WHO classification of tumours). 4th ed. Lyon: World Health Organization; 2010. p. 122–5.
9. Maggard MA, O'Connell JB, Ko CY. Updated population-based review of carcinoid tumors. Ann Surg. 2004;240:117–22.
10. Goede AC, Caplin ME, Winslet MC. Carcinoid tumour of the appendix. Br J Surg. 2003;90:1317–22.
11. Misdraji J. Tumors of the appendix. In: Shepherd NA, Warren BF, Williams GT, Greenson JK, Lauwers GY, Novelli MR, editors. Morson's and Dawson's gastrointestinal pathology. 5th ed. London: Wiley; 2013. p. 490–8.

12. Ronnett BM, Zahn CM, Kurman RJ, et al. Disseminated peritoneal adenomucinosis and peritoneal mucinous carcinomatosis. A clinicopathologic analysis of 109 cases with emphasis on distinguishing pathologic features, site of origin, prognosis, and relationship to "pseudomyxoma peritonei". Am J Surg Pathol. 1995;19:1390–408.

13. Appendix. In: Edge SB, Byrd DR, Compton CC, Fritz AG, Greene FL, Trotti A, editors. AJCC cancer staging manual. 7th ed. New York: Springer; 2010.

14. Komminoth P, Arnold R, Capella C, et al. Neuroendocrine neoplasms of the appendix. In: Bosman FT, Carneiro F, Hruban RH, Theise ND, editors. WHO classification of tumors of the digestive system (IARC WHO classification of tumours). 4th ed. Lyon: World Health Organization; 2010.

15. Pape UF, Perren A, Niederle B, et al. ENETS consensus guidelines for the management of patients with neuroendocrine neoplasms from the jejuno-ileum and the appendix including goblet cell carcinomas. Neuroendocrinology. 2012;95:135–56.

16. Kulke MH, Mayer RJ. Carcinoid tumors. N Engl J Med. 1999;340:858–68.

17. Rindi G, Kloppel G, Couvelard A, et al. TNM staging of midgut and hindgut (neuro) endocrine tumors: a consensus proposal including a grading system. Virchows Arch. 2007;451:757–62.

18. Mullen JT, Savarese DMF. Carcinoid tumors of the appendix: a population-based study. J Surg Oncol. 2011;104:41–4.

19. Roy P, Chetty R. Goblet cell carcinoid tumors of the appendix: an overview. World J Gastrointest Oncol. 2010;2:251–8.

20. Pham TH, Wolff B, Abraham SC, et al. Surgical and chemotherapy treatment outcomes of goblet cell carcinoid: a tertiary cancer center experience. Ann Surg Oncol. 2006;13:370–6.

21. Tang LH, Shia J, Soslow RA, et al. Pathologic classification and clinical behavior of the spectrum of goblet cell carcinoid tumors of the appendix. Am J Surg Pathol. 2008;32:1429–43.

22. Ng D, Falck V, McConnell YJ, et al. Appendiceal goblet cell carcinoid and mucinous neoplasms are closely associated tumors: lessons from their coexistence in primary tumors and concurrence in peritoneal dissemination. J Surg Oncol. 2014;109:548–55.

23. Trivedi AN, Levine EA, Mishra G. Adenocarcinoma of the appendix is rarely detected by colonoscopy. J Gastrointest Surg. 2009;13:668–75.

24. Esquivel J, Chua TC, Stojadinovic A, et al. Accuracy and clinical relevance of computed tomography scan interpretation of peritoneal cancer index in colorectal cancer peritoneal carcinomatosis: a multi-institutional study. J Surg Oncol. 2010;102:565–70.

25. Low RN, Barone RM, Lee MJ. Surveillance MR imaging is superior to serum tumor markers for detecting early tumor recurrence in patients with appendiceal cancer treated with surgical cytoreduction and HIPEC. Ann Surg Oncol. 2013;20:1074–81.

26. Madwed D, Mindelzun R, Jeffrey Jr RB. Mucocele of the appendix: imaging findings. AJR Am J Roentgenol. 1992;159:69–72.

27. Puvaneswary M, Proietto A. Mucocele of the appendix with magnetic resonance imaging findings. Australas Radiol. 2006;50:71–4.

28. Gerstle JT, Kauffman Jr GL, Koltun WA. The incidence, management, and outcome of patients with gastrointestinal carcinoids and second primary malignancies. J Am Coll Surg. 1995;180:427–32.

29. Franko J, Shi Q, Goldman CD, et al. Treatment of colorectal peritoneal carcinomatosis with systemic chemotherapy: a pooled analysis of north central cancer treatment group phase III trials N9741 and N9841. J Clin Oncol. 2012;30:263–7.

30. Bijelic L, Kumar AS, Stuart OA, et al. Systemic chemotherapy prior to cytoreductive surgery and HIPEC for carcinomatosis from appendix cancer: impact on perioperative outcomes and short-term survival. Gastroenterol Res Pract. 2012;2012:163284.

31. Eveno C, Passot G, Goere D, et al. Bevacizumab doubles the early postoperative complication rate after cytoreductive surgery with hyperthermic intraperitoneal chemotherapy (HIPEC) for peritoneal carcinomatosis of colorectal origin. Ann Surg Oncol. 2014;21:1792–800.

32. Dhage-Ivatury S, Sugarbaker PH. Update on the surgical approach to mucocele of the appendix. J Am Coll Surg. 2006;202:680–4.

33. Nitecki SS, Wolff BG, Schlinkert R, et al. The natural history of surgically treated primary adenocarcinoma of the appendix. Ann Surg. 1994;219:51–7.

34. Gonzalez-Moreno S, Sugarbaker PH. Right hemicolectomy does not confer a survival advantage in patients with mucinous carcinoma of the appendix and peritoneal seeding. Br J Surg. 2004;91:304–11.

35. Kusamura S, Moran BJ, Sugarbaker PH, et al. Multicentre study of the learning curve and surgical performance of cytoreductive surgery with intraperitoneal chemotherapy for pseudomyxoma peritonei. Br J Surg. 2014;101:1758–65.

36. Chua TC, Moran BJ, Sugarbaker PH, et al. Early- and long-term outcome data of patients with pseudomyxoma peritonei from appendiceal origin treated by a strategy of cytoreductive surgery and hyperthermic intraperitoneal chemotherapy. J Clin Oncol. 2012;30:2449–56.

37. Yan TD, Black D, Savady R, et al. A systematic review on the efficacy of cytoreductive surgery and perioperative intraperitoneal chemotherapy for pseudomyxoma peritonei. Ann Surg Oncol. 2007;14:484–92.

38. Valle M, Federici O, Carboni F, et al. Postoperative infections after cytoreductive surgery and HIPEC for peritoneal carcinomatosis: proposal and results from a prospective protocol study of prevention, surveillance and treatment. Eur J Surg Oncol. 2014;40:950–6.

39. Votanopoulos KI, Newman NA, Russell G, et al. Outcomes of Cytoreductive Surgery (CRS) with hyperthermic intraperitoneal chemotherapy (HIPEC) in patients older than 70 years; survival benefit at considerable morbidity and mortality. Ann Surg Oncol. 2013;20:3497–503.

40. Glockzin G, von Breitenbuch P, Schlitt HJ, et al. Treatment-related morbidity and toxicity of CRS and oxaliplatin-based HIPEC compared to a mitomycin and doxorubicin-based HIPEC protocol in patients with peritoneal carcinomatosis: a matched-pair analysis. J Surg Oncol. 2013;107:574–8.

41. Deraco M, Baratti D, Kusamura S. Morbidity and quality of life following cytoreduction and HIPEC. Cancer Treat Res. 2007;134:403–18.

42. Glehen O, Mohamed F, Sugarbaker PH. Incomplete cytoreduction in 174 patients with peritoneal carcinomatosis from appendiceal malignancy. Ann Surg. 2004;240:278–85.

43. Verwaal VJ, van Ruth S, de Bree E, et al. Randomized trial of cytoreduction and hyperthermic intraperitoneal chemotherapy versus systemic chemotherapy and palliative surgery in patients with peritoneal carcinomatosis of colorectal cancer. J Clin Oncol. 2003;21:3737–43.

44. Sugarbaker PH, Ryan DP. Cytoreductive surgery plus hyperthermic perioperative chemotherapy to treat peritoneal metastases

from colorectal cancer: standard of care or an experimental approach? Lancet Oncol. 2012;13:e362–9.

45. Evrard S, Maziere C, Desolneux G. HIPEC: standard of care or an experimental approach? Lancet Oncol. 2012;13:e462–3.

46. Markman M. Continued uncertainty regarding hyperthermic intraperitoneal chemotherapy in malignant peritoneal mesothelioma. J Clin Oncol. 2010;28:e418. Author reply e419.

47. Caneparo A, Massucco P, Vaira M, et al. Contamination risk for operators performing semi-closed HIPEC procedure using cisplatin. Eur J Surg Oncol. 2014;40:925–9.

48. Konate A, Poupon J, Villa A, et al. Evaluation of environmental contamination by platinum and exposure risks for healthcare workers during a heated intraperitoneal perioperative chemotherapy (HIPEC) procedure. J Surg Oncol. 2011;103:6–9.

49. Stinner B, Kisker O, Zielke A, et al. Surgical management for carcinoid tumors of small bowel, appendix, colon, and rectum. World J Surg. 1996;20:183–8.

50. Stephens AD, Alderman R, Chang D, et al. Morbidity and mortality analysis of 200 treatments with cytoreductive surgery and hyperthermic intraoperative intraperitoneal chemotherapy using the coliseum technique. Ann Surg Oncol. 1999;6:790–6.

51. Ahmad SA, Kim J, Sussman JJ, et al. Reduced morbidity following cytoreductive surgery and intraperitoneal hyperthermic chemoperfusion. Ann Surg Oncol. 2004;11:387–92.

52. Stewart JH, Shen P, Russell GB, et al. Appendiceal neoplasms with peritoneal dissemination: outcomes after cytoreductive surgery and intraperitoneal hyperthermic chemotherapy. Ann Surg Oncol. 2006;13:624–34.

53. Baratti D, Kusamura S, Nonaka D, et al. Pseudomyxoma peritonei: clinical pathological and biological prognostic factors in patients treated with cytoreductive surgery and hyperthermic intraperitoneal chemotherapy (HIPEC). Ann Surg Oncol. 2008;15:526–34.

54. Bijelic L, Yan TD, Sugarbaker PH. Treatment failure following complete cytoreductive surgery and perioperative intraperitoneal chemotherapy for peritoneal dissemination from colorectal or appendiceal mucinous neoplasms. J Surg Oncol. 2008;98:295–9.

55. El Halabi H, Gushchin V, Francis J, et al. The role of cytoreductive surgery and heated intraperitoneal chemotherapy (CRS/HIPEC) in patients with high-grade appendiceal carcinoma and extensive peritoneal carcinomatosis. Ann Surg Oncol. 2012;19:110–4.

56. Teo MCC, Tan GHC, Tham CK, et al. Cytoreductive surgery and hyperthermic intraperitoneal chemotherapy in Asian patients: 100 consecutive patients in a single institution. Ann Surg Oncol. 2013;20:2968–74.

57. Tabrizian P, Shrager B, Jibara G, et al. Cytoreductive surgery and hyperthermic intraperitoneal chemotherapy for peritoneal carcinomatosis: outcomes from a single tertiary institution. J Gastrointest Surg. 2014;18:1024–31.

58. Lord AC, Shihab O, Chandrakumaran K, et al. Recurrence and outcome after complete tumour removal and hyperthermic intraperitoneal chemotherapy in 512 patients with pseudomyxoma peritonei from perforated appendiceal mucinous tumours. Eur J Surg Oncol. 2015;41:396–9.

59. Votanopoulos KI, Russell G, Randle RW, et al. Peritoneal Surface Disease (PSD) from appendiceal cancer treated with Cytoreductive Surgery (CRS) and Hyperthermic Intraperitoneal Chemotherapy (HIPEC): overview of 481 cases. Ann Surg Oncol. 2015;22:1274–9.

38

Carcinoids, GISTs, and Lymphomas of Colon and Rectum

David J. Maron

Key Concepts

- Treatment of colonic carcinoids is segmental resection including mesenteric lymph nodes.
- Somatostatin analogues control the symptoms of carcinoid syndrome and help limit progression of disease.
- Rectal carcinoids less than 1 cm may be treated by local excision, while tumors greater than 2 cm require radical resection.
- Imatinib blocks activation of the KIT oncoprotein in gastrointestinal stromal tumors.
- Patients with colonic lymphomas that produce symptoms are best treated with surgical resection prior to chemotherapy.

The majority of neoplasms that arise in the colon and rectum are adenomas and adenocarcinomas; however, other tumors may present as well. It is important for the clinician to understand the biology of these tumors so that proper therapy may be offered. Tumors may develop from epithelial, mesenchymal, neural, vascular, or lymphoid tissue. While there are a number of rare colorectal tumors, this chapter will discuss three more commonly occurring non-adenomatous neoplasms.

Carcinoid Tumors

Carcinoid tumors were originally described in 1888 in two patients with multiple small tumors of the ileum by Otto Lubarsch, a German pathologist. In 1907, Siegfried Oberndorfer first used the term "Karzinoid," which translates as "carcinoma-like," hinting that these tumors behave differently from adenocarcinoma [1]. It was believed that although these tumors could metastasize like carcinomas, their clinical course was typically fairly benign.

Electronic supplementary material: The online version of this chapter (doi:10.1007/978-3-319-25970-3_38) contains supplementary material, which is available to authorized users.

Histology

Carcinoids are slow growing tumors of the neuroectodermal origin and belong to the amine precursor uptake and decarboxylation (APUD) system. They originate from Kulchitsky or basogranular enterochromaffin cells located in the crypts of Lieberkuhn [2]. Microscopically, these tumors are composed of monotonous sheets of small round cells with uniform nuclei and cytoplasm. The cells contain very dense neurosecretory granules that contain various secretory peptides; these granules are similar to synaptic vesicles found in neurons. The cytoplasmic features are typically benign-appearing and mitotic figures are infrequent. Five histologic patterns of carcinoid tumors include insular, trabecular, glandular, undifferentiated, and mixed. Insular and trabecular patterns are typically associated with a more favorable prognosis. Distinguishing between benign and malignant carcinoids can be difficult; however, increased cellular atypia, high mitotic activity, or necrosis is often associated with more aggressive tumors.

Carcinoid tumors have specific staining patterns related to the amines and peptides they produce as well as cytoplasmic proteins they contain. Serotonin is capable of reducing silver salts to metallic silver, and therefore carcinoid tumors that produce serotonin and stain positive with silver stains are described as "argentaffin positive." Some tumors are capable silver uptake but not reduction, and these may be demonstrated by the addition of an external reducing agent; these tumors are referred to as "argyrophilic." Carcinoid tumors of the midgut are typically argentaffin positive, while those in the hindgut are often mixed (6–70% argyrophilic and 8–16% argentaffin positive) [3]. Silver staining has been abandoned in favor of immunohistochemical staining for cytoplasmic proteins, including chromogranin, synaptophysin, and neuron-specific enolase [4].

Carcinoid tumors have been shown to produce at least 30 bioactive compounds [5]. These compounds include amines such as serotonin and histamine, proteins (including various hormones and kinins), and prostaglandins. Serotonin is derived from the amino acid tryptophan in a two-step process and is stored and transported in platelets. As tryptophan is an essential amino acid important in the production of proteins such as niacin (vitamin B_7) and nicotinamide (vitamin B_3), deficiencies of these vitamins may occur if large quantities of tryptophan are consumed in the production of serotonin by carcinoid tumors. Metabolism of serotonin occurs first in the liver (monoamine oxidase) and then in the kidney (aldehyde dehydrogenase) to produce 5-hydroxy-indole-acetic acid (5-HIAA), which is excreted in the urine.

Incidence and Distribution

Carcinoid tumors may originate in the foregut, midgut, or hindgut. Foregut tumors arise in the thymus, respiratory tract, stomach, duodenum, and pancreas. Midgut carcinoids originate in the jejunum, ileum, appendix, and proximal colon. Hindgut tumors arise in the distal colon and rectum. The distribution of carcinoids varies among reports. In a series of almost 3000 carcinoid tumors, Godwin [6] found that the most frequent site of origin was in the appendix (38%), followed by the ileum, rectum, and bronchus (23%, 13%, and 11.5%, respectively). Modlin and Sandor [7] combined Godwin's series with an additional 5000 carcinoid tumors and reported the most common site as the small bowel (28.7%) followed by the bronchus, appendix, and rectum (25.1%, 18.9%, and 12.6%, respectively). A recent report noted that since the implementation of screening colonoscopy in the United States, the incidence of rectal carcinoids has surpassed that of small bowel carcinoids [8]. Carcinoid tumors are associated with an increased risk of synchronous colorectal and small bowel tumors, as well as metachronous lung, prostate, and urinary tract neoplasms [9, 10]. The reason for this association is unknown; however, it has been theorized that the various peptides secreted by carcinoid tumors may have tumorigenic properties [9].

Clinical Presentation

Approximately half of all gastrointestinal carcinoids are diagnosed following appendectomy for suspected appendicitis. Carcinoids of the appendix are discussed in detail in Chap. 37. Colonic carcinoids most commonly occur in the seventh or eighth decade of life and are more common in women than in men [11]. They may present as a polyp or as a mass that is indistinguishable from a colon carcinoma, both grossly and on radiographic visualization. Many patients with colonic carcinoids are asymptomatic or have symptoms from another condition that prompt an investigation that leads to the diagnosis [12]. Those tumors that are symptomatic produce symptoms similar to colonic carcinomas (bleeding, abdominal pain, and change in bowel habits).

Carcinoids may arise throughout the colon; however, they are more commonly found in the cecum. Ballantyne and colleagues reported 48% of colonic carcinoids were found in the cecum, 16% in the ascending colon, 6% in the transverse colon, 11% in the descending colon, and 13% in the sigmoid colon [13]. Murray et al. reported similar results, with 73% of tumors found in the cecum, 7% in the ascending colon, and 20% in the sigmoid colon [14].

Symptoms of rectal carcinoids, when present, are typically rectal bleeding or change in bowel habits. Most rectal carcinoids, however, are asymptomatic and are found at the time of colorectal cancer screening. The incidence of rectal carcinoids in all patients undergoing sigmoidoscopy is estimated at 0.05% [15, 16]. These tumors typically appear as a solitary 1–1.5 cm mobile submucosal nodule with an intact overlying normal mucosa. Malignancy is frequently associated with carcinoids larger than 2 cm with invasion through the muscularis propria. These tumors often will appear ulcerated and present with rectal bleeding. Metastatic disease tends to occur less frequently in carcinoid tumors of the hindgut (rectum 18%) when compared with midgut carcinoids (small bowel 34%, colon 60%) and foregut tumors (stomach 23%, bronchopulmonary 21%) [6].

Carcinoid Syndrome

Systemic symptoms produced by carcinoid tumors are referred to as the carcinoid syndrome. Although classically described as the hallmark of carcinoid tumors, carcinoid syndrome occurs in only 10–18% of patients with carcinoids, and in only 50% of patients with advanced disease [3]. The symptoms include flushing of the skin, non-bloody diarrhea, and abdominal pain. The symptoms are often episodic and may be precipitated by stress or the ingestion of certain foods, caffeine, or alcohol. The flushing may involve the face or the entire body and may occur for a few minutes or last for several hours. Flushing may also be associated with excessive tearing, salivation, and bronchopulmonary spasm leading to wheezing. Flushing occurs in up to 85% of patients with the carcinoid syndrome, and it is believed that kallikrein secretion is responsible for these symptoms [17]. Abdominal symptoms such as cramping and watery diarrhea occur in 80% of patients with carcinoid syndrome, and are likely due to the secretion of serotonin. Intestinal obstruction may also develop secondary to mesenteric fibrosis, and fibrosis of the retroperitoneum may lead to ureteral obstruction. Treatment of symptoms of diarrhea includes loperamide, diphenoxylate/atropine, and other antidiarrheal medications. Antihistamines or H2 receptor antagonists may be helpful in reducing flushing symptoms.

Patients with carcinoid syndrome may also develop right-sided heart failure. Serotonin has an effect on myofibroblasts which results in fibroplasia, increased vascular tone, bronchoconstriction, and platelet aggregation. These effects may lead to pulmonary hypertension, tricuspid and pulmonary valve stenosis, and right ventricular hypertrophy and fibrosis [5]. Patients with higher levels of serotonin (higher urinary

5-HIAA levels) have been found to have increased valvular damage [3]. The left side of the heart is spared from the effects of carcinoid products as the lungs are capable of inactivating these substances. Surgical repair or replacement of the affected valves has been met with significant postoperative morbidity.

The liver is capable of metabolizing and inactivating most of the peptide hormones secreted by carcinoid tumors. It is for this reason that the carcinoid syndrome typically develops only after the tumor has developed metastases in the liver. Alternatively, primary carcinoid tumors located outside the portal venous system (bronchopulmonary) or gastrointestinal tumors that develop lymph node metastases or direct invasion into the retroperitoneum may also present with carcinoid syndrome [18].

Carcinoid syndrome occurs most frequently in patients with metastatic disease from a midgut carcinoid tumor. In fact, 90% of patients with carcinoid syndrome have midgut carcinoids, and 60% of patients with metastatic small bowel carcinoids will develop symptoms. This is likely due to the ability of midgut carcinoids to produce high levels of serotonin [19]. In contrast, foregut tumors typically lack the enzyme required to convert 5-hydroxytryptophan into serotonin, and hindgut carcinoids rarely produce serotonin. Therefore rectal carcinoids, even in the presence of metastatic disease in the liver, almost never result in the carcinoid syndrome.

Diagnostic Tests

The majority of carcinoid tumors of the colon and rectum are found during colonoscopy or are discovered during abdominal exploration for another condition. Full endoscopic evaluation of the colon and rectum should be performed to evaluate for synchronous malignancies. Endoscopic ultrasonography has been used in the evaluation of rectal carcinoids, and has been shown to have a 75% accuracy rate in determining the depth of invasion and presence of lymph node metastases [20]. This may be helpful in determining whether the carcinoid is amenable to endoscopic resection [21].

When endoscopic biopsy is not feasible, biochemical tests may help to make the diagnosis of carcinoid. Although carcinoid tumors may produce a variety of hormones, the most widely used tests are related to serotonin. The most useful biochemical test for diagnosing carcinoid in the symptomatic patient is the 24 h urine 5-HIAA assay. Normal excretion ranges from 2 to 8 mg/24 h, and a diagnosis of carcinoid syndrome in patients with excretion exceeding these levels has a sensitivity and specificity of 73% and 100%, respectively [22]. Certain medications including acetaminophen and salicylates, as well as serotonin-rich foods such as bananas, pineapples, nuts, and avocadoes may falsely elevate urinary 5-HIAA levels and should therefore be avoided during the test.

In addition to a CT scan of the chest, abdomen, and pelvis to evaluate for metastatic disease, somatostatin receptor scintigraphy (SRS) may be helpful in identifying occult metastases and to determine if the patient is likely to respond to treatment with octreotide. The majority of carcinoid tumors express receptors (SSTR 1–3) that have an affinity for somatostatin [23]. SRS therefore has a high sensitivity in detecting carcinoids; however, approximately 10% of tumors do not express the somatostatin receptor. Whole body positron emission tomography (PET) using ^{18}F-Dopa may also be useful in detecting carcinoid tumors. Hoegerle et al. compared the use of CT, SRS, and PET scans in the localization of primary and metastatic carcinoid tumors and found that PET imaging was more sensitive in localizing primary tumors and lymph node involvement, while CT was more sensitive in identifying distant disease [24]. Krausz et al. compared ^{18}F-Dopa PET/CT imaging with SRS and found that PET/CT demonstrated more true positive tumor foci and was better tolerated by patients [25]. The TNM staging of carcinoid tumors is similar to that of adenocarcinomas of the colon (Table 38-1).

Treatment

The treatment of carcinoid tumors is surgical resection. The type of surgery depends on a variety of factors, including whether the tumor is amenable to local or endoscopic resection and whether surgical debulking of tumor may help to reduce the symptoms of the carcinoid syndrome. The choice of the appropriate procedure is based on the location of the tumor, the likelihood of residual primary disease, and the presence of lymph node or metastatic disease. Guidelines for resection are summarized in Table 38-2.

Carcinoids of the small bowel are frequently multicentric and have a propensity for developing obstruction secondary to intussusception, mesenteric fibrosis, and kinking of the bowel (Figure 38-1a, b). Metastasis to regional lymph nodes approaches 50% [26], and tumors less than 1 cm in diameter are associated with a 20–30% incidence of lymph node involvement. Size of the tumor is a poor predictor of distant metastasis, as tumors less than 0.5 cm have been shown to metastasize to the liver. Surgical management should therefore include a formal small bowel resection with wide mesenteric excision of the associated lymph nodes. This should be performed even in the presence of metastatic disease to reduce the incidence of small bowel obstruction due to tumor or fibrosis of the mesentery. As one-third of carcinoids of the small bowel may be multicentric, it is important to examine the entire small intestine to evaluate for synchronous lesions [26].

Carcinoids arising in the colon are often asymptomatic until they develop into large tumors with lymph node metastases. Colonic resection similar to that performed for adenocarcinoma is therefore recommended, with the extent

TABLE 38-1. TNM staging of carcinoid tumors

Stage	Characteristics
Tumor	
T1	Tumor invades submucosa
T2	Tumor invades muscularis propria
T3	Tumor invades through muscularis propria into subserosa or nonperitonealized pericolic or perirectal tissues
T4	Tumor directly invades other organs or structures and/or perforates visceral peritoneum
Regional nodal metastases	
NX	Regional lymph nodes cannot be assessed
N0	No nodal metastasis
N1	Metastasis in 1–3 pericolic or perirectal nodes
N2	Metastasis in four to more pericolic or perirectal nodes
N3	Metastasis in any node along course of a named vascular trunk and/or metastasis to apical node
Distant metastasis	
MX	Presence of distant metastasis cannot be assessed
M0	No distant metastasis
M1	Distant metastasis

Adapted from the AJCC Cancer Staging Manuel, 7ed. (Edge, Byrd, Compton, Fritz, Green, Trotti, Eds.) Publ. Springer, NY. 2010

TABLE 38-2. Guidelines for resection

Primary tumor	Factor	Extent of resection
Small bowel	Locally limited disease	Resection of primary and metastatic tumors
	Extensive disease	Resection or bypass of primary tumor
		Debulking of metastasis
Colon		Colectomy
Rectum	<1 cm	Local excision
	1–1.9 cm	Local excision or proctectomy
	>2 cm	Proctectomy

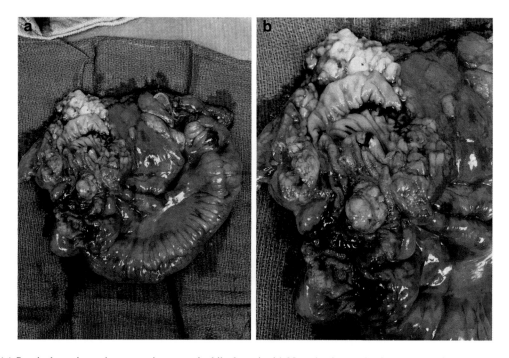

FIGURE 38-1. (**a**) Surgical specimen demonstrating a terminal ileal carcinoid. Note the desmoplastic response of the mesentery. (**b**) Close-up view of the lesion.

determined by the location of the disease [27]. Outcomes following colectomy for colonic carcinoids are varied. Welch and Donaldson [28] reported that 5-year survival was similar to that of survival in patients with carcinoma of the colon, while Berardi noted that the average survival following resection of colonic carcinoid was 26 months [29]. Location of the primary tumor may affect outcomes, as in one series cecal tumors were found to have an incidence of 71% metastases while tumors elsewhere in the colon had only a 33% incidence [30]. Spread and colleagues [31] noted that survival in patients with colonic carcinoids was significantly lower when compared with carcinoid tumors of the rectum or appendix, and was also significantly lower than survival in patients with adenocarcinoma. Al Natour and colleagues recently reviewed 929 patients with colonic carcinoids and found that those patients with intramucosal tumors less than 1 cm in diameter had only a 4% risk of lymph node metastasis [32]. They concluded that small tumors confined to the mucosa may be appropriately treated by endoscopic resection.

As carcinoid tumors of the rectum may be amenable to local excision, less invasive treatment may be an option in some patients. It is important to balance the benefits of a less morbid intervention with the risks of local recurrence and nodal involvement (and hence the risk of metastatic disease). Transanal or endoscopic excision is adequate for most tumors less than 1 cm in diameter. Formal transanal excision of the full thickness of the rectal wall allows for a precise assessment of the depth of penetration, and is more likely to result in negative margins of resection. However, this may not be necessary for many patients, as recurrence is rare even when there is an involved margin following endoscopic excision of tumors less than 1 cm in diameter. Invasion of the muscularis propria (T2) has been associated with lymph node metastases in up to 47% of patients [33]. In an analysis of 106 patients with rectal carcinoid, muscularis invasion was the only independent prognostic factor for predicting 5-year survival, and size of the tumor was significantly associated with muscular invasion [34].

In addition to muscularis propria invasion, rectal carcinoids whose size is greater than 2 cm in diameter are also at significant risk of lymph node metastases. Patients should therefore be considered for proctectomy with excision of the mesorectum to allow for assessment and clearance of the nodal basin. The treatment of rectal carcinoids measuring between 1 and 1.9 cm remains uncertain and must be individualized based on tumor features and the overall health of the patient. In a series of 62 patients, lymph node metastases were found in 69% of patients with tumors ranging 1.1–2 cm in diameter [35]. Shields and colleagues evaluated 202 patients with rectal carcinoids and found that tumor size greater than 1 cm and evidence of lymphovascular invasion were independent predictors of lymph node involvement [36]. Lymph node involvement was also associated with the development of distant metastasis and significant decrease in

survival. Perineural invasion has also been demonstrated as a poor prognostic factor [37]. These findings have led some authors to conclude that rectal carcinoids larger than 1 cm should routinely be treated with radical resection in suitable patients [35, 36].

Carcinoid tumors are typically slow-growing and patients often exhibit favorable 5- and 10-year survival rates despite the presence of extensive metastatic disease. Surgical treatment of metastatic carcinoid in the liver may be of benefit in improving survival and may help to provide long-term palliation of hormone-related symptoms in patients who are unable to tolerate or do not respond to medical treatment with somatostatin analogues. Various techniques have been employed, including hepatic resection, radiofrequency ablation, cryosurgery, and chemoembolization. Wedge resection or lobectomy of hepatic metastases not only improves symptoms associated with the carcinoid syndrome but also has been shown to prolong survival [38]. As metastatic carcinoid tumors derive the majority of their blood supply from the hepatic artery (while hepatocytes receive blood supply primarily from the portal venous system), chemoembolization may play an important role in patients who are unable to tolerate hepatic resection. Patients with large tumors or those who are refractory to somatostatin frequently experience significant short-term improvement in their symptoms [39]. Liver transplantation has also been employed in patients with metastatic carcinoid, with outcome similar to those seen in patients who undergo transplantation for hepatocellular carcinoma [40].

The efficacy of systemic chemotherapy in the treatment of metastatic carcinoid is limited. Various agents have been used, including 5-FU, streptozotocin, cisplatin, doxorubicin, etoposide, and dacarbazine, either as monotherapy or in combination. The largest study reported is a comparative trial of combination therapy with 5-FU and doxorubicin versus 5-FU and streptozotocin [41]. This study demonstrated an improvement in median survival in the streptozotocin arm (24.3 months vs. 15.7 months); however, there were no differences between the two treatments with regard to response rate (16% vs. 15.9%) or progression-free survival (5.3 months vs. 4.5 months). More aggressive carcinoids may respond well to combination therapy with cisplatin and etoposide [42]. The use of continuous infusion 5-FU combined with octreotide has also shown some promise, with reports of a 24% partial response rate and disease stabilization in 69% in a small series of patients [43].

More than 80% of carcinoid tumors express surface receptors for somatostatin (especially receptor subtype 2), and therapeutic strategies have therefore focused on the development of agents that target these receptors. Activation of these receptors results in reduced hormone synthesis and secretion, thereby leading to complete or partial relief of symptoms associated with the carcinoid syndrome in up to 90% of patients [44]. Somatostatin analogues that have been used in the treatment of carcinoid include octreotide and lanreotide.

Octreotide may be given as a subcutaneous, intramuscular, or long-acting depot injection. Lanreotide has a longer half-life than octreotide; however, its use is not currently approved for use in the United States. In addition to the ability to control symptoms, somatostatin analogues may also help to limit the progression of disease. In a placebo-controlled double-blind, randomized trial of 85 patients, octreotide was associated with a significantly better median time to tumor progression (14.3 months vs. 6 months) and stable disease at 6 months of treatment (66.7% vs. 37.2%), although the trial did not comment on overall survival [45]. Interferon-alpha has also been used to treat metastatic carcinoid tumors with some success. Di Bartolomeo and colleagues reported symptomatic control in 80% of patients and reduction of 5-HIAA levels in 58% of patients treated with daily intramuscular injections of interferon-alpha [46]. When combined with octreotide in a randomized trial, interferon-alpha was found to significantly reduce the risk of progression when compared with octreotide alone, although again no survival benefit was found [47]. Significant side effects of fever, fatigue, and weight loss often limit the routine use of interferon therapy.

GISTs

Gastrointestinal stromal tumors (GISTs) are the most common mesenchymal neoplasm of the gastrointestinal tract and account for approximately 0.1–3% of all intestinal cancers. GISTs were first described by Mazur and Clark, who used electron microscopy to differentiate these tumors from other soft tissue sarcomas [48]. Most tumors arising from mesenchymal elements of the gastrointestinal tract were considered leiomyomas, leiomyosarcomas, and leiomyoblastomas; however, it was discovered that GISTs lack features associated with smooth muscle cells. Instead, it is believed that GISTs arise from the interstitial cells of Cajal or other pluripotential mesenchymal stem cells. The interstitial cells of Cajal coordinate autonomic movements of the gastrointestinal tract and are located within muscle layer of the intestinal wall.

Histology

Histologically, gastrointestinal stromal tumors typically have a spindle cell appearance and stain positive for the CD117 antigen, a marker for the KIT tyrosine kinase oncoprotein. In addition, 60–70% of GISTs will stain positive for CD34, a hematopoietic progenitor cell antigen [49]. These features help to differentiate GISTs from other sarcomas; leiomyomas stain negative for KIT and CD34 but positive for desmin, smooth muscle actin, and S100 [50].

Incidence and Distribution

GISTs typically occur in the sixth to seventh decade of life and affect men and women equally. Most tumors are sporadic; however, several hereditary syndromes are associated with GISTs. Carney's triad consists of (1) synchronous or metachronous GISTs, (2) extra-adrenal paraganglionomas, and (3) pulmonary chondromas [51]. This is usually seen in women before age 30 and is not associated with a KIT mutation. Patients with neurofibromatosis type I are also more commonly affected with GISTs. Tumors in these patients are more likely to occur at a younger age and often present with multiple small intestinal GISTs [52].

Gastrointestinal stromal tumors are most commonly found in the stomach (approximately two-thirds of cases), followed by the small intestine (about one-quarter of cases). Esophageal GISTs are rare, but tumors may also arise in extra-GI locations, principally in the mesentery, omentum, and retroperitoneum. Tumors located in the colon and rectum account for only 10–20% of GISTs, and of those, the majority arise in the rectum.

Clinical Presentation

GISTs are usually slow-growing lesions, and are often discovered incidentally during endoscopy or in the treatment of other conditions. The most common clinical symptoms are rectal bleeding and abdominal or rectal pain. Advanced lesions may present with a palpable mass, obstruction, or perforation (Figure 38-2). Kingham et al. found that symptoms were more common in patients with larger tumors; the median size of tumors was 8.9 cm in symptomatic patients, compared to 2.7 cm in asymptomatic patients [51]. Metastatic disease most frequently occurs in the liver and peritoneum; metastatic disease in the lymph nodes is uncommon [52].

Diagnostic Tests

Evaluation of a patient with a suspected GIST includes colonoscopy as well as endoscopic ultrasound, if feasible. Lesions are usually submucosal; however, biopsy may be aided with the use of endoscopic ultrasound-guided fine needle aspiration. Care must be taken as these tumors are frequently associated with neovascularization, and biopsy may result in significant hemorrhage [53]. Percutaneous biopsy with fine or core needle aspiration is an option for tumors that cannot be reached endoscopically; however, concern over tumor rupture and spread has been reported [51]. CT and MRI may aid staging and determining whether surgical resection is feasible. GISTs typically involve the muscularis propria, and radiographically have a characteristic appearance of a

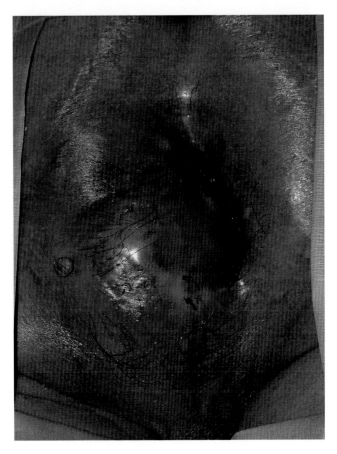

FIGURE 38-2. GIST of the rectum presenting as a perianal mass.

well-circumscribed intramural mass. Larger lesions may have evidence of central necrosis. PET scanning is not helpful in diagnosis, however may be of benefit in evaluating the response to treatment [54].

Treatment

Surgical resection of GISTs offers the best chance for cure and is therefore the treatment of choice. It is recommended that resection include the tumor en bloc with any associated contiguous tissues with margins of at least 1 cm [55]. As GISTs rarely metastasize to the lymphatic system, lymphadenectomy is not necessary [56]. Although many gastrointestinal stromal tumors may have a pseudocapsule, enucleation of the tumor without resection of the pseudocapsule should be avoided, as this has been associated with increased risk of tumor recurrence.

Resection of rectal GISTs may be accomplished by radical resection (low anterior resection or abdominoperineal resection) or local excision (transanal excision or transanal endoscopic microsurgery), provided that the tumor and pseudocapsule can be removed with adequate margins (Video 38.1). Liu et al. evaluated 21 patients with rectal GISTs and found that most patients with tumors located

within 5 cm of the anal verge were successfully treated with local excision; however, positive resection margin was associated with poorer disease-free survival [57]. Changchien et al. reported outcomes of 29 patients with rectal GISTs [58]. Higher local recurrence rates were seen in those patients who underwent wide local excision vs. those who underwent radical resection (77% vs. 31%), despite smaller mean tumor size in the local excision group (4.5% vs. 7.2%).

The development of imatinib has significantly impacted the treatment of gastrointestinal stromal tumors. As mentioned previously, the majority of GISTs have abnormal activation of the KIT oncoprotein which results in unregulated cellular proliferation. Imatinib is a selective tyrosine kinase inhibitor which blocks activation of the KIT oncoprotein. When used in adjuvant therapy, imatinib has been shown to significantly decrease the risk of recurrence. The American College of Surgeons Oncology Group (ACOSOG) conducted a prospective trial of 106 patients who had undergone complete gross tumor removal but were deemed to be high risk for recurrence [59]. Patients were given 400 mg of imatinib per day for 1 year and followed radiographically. The 5-year overall survival rate of those treated was 83%, significantly better than historical 5-year survival rates of 35%. Imatinib has also been used in patients where the tumor was felt to be too large to resect. In this situation, the use of imatinib has been shown to result in tumor shrinkage in more than 50% of patients [60, 61], thereby allowing surgical resection in selected patients.

Neoadjuvant imatinib therapy for rectal gastrointestinal stromal tumors has also been reported. Wang et al. reported three patients with GISTs in the distal rectum that would require abdominoperineal resection to achieve cure [62]. Following treatment with imatinib, all three patients had both significant shrinkage of the tumor and extension of the distance to the anal verge that allowed for sphincter-preserving procedures. Tielen et al. also found that patients treated with neoadjuvant imatinib had significant reduction in the size of their rectal GISTs; however, this did not lead to less extensive surgery when compared with patients who did not undergo neoadjuvant therapy [63].

The reported incidence of local recurrence and metastatic disease following complete surgical resection of GISTs varies, but approaches 50% in some series [56]. Yeh et al. reported outcomes of 40 patients who underwent resection of rectal GISTs and found that younger age (<50 years) and a high histologic grade of tumor were the two most significant prognostic factors for recurrence [64]. In the ACOSOG trial, the recurrence-free survival rate was found to be lower with increasing tumor size, high mitotic rate, and older age [59]. Patients with metastatic GISTs are typically treated with imatinib and evaluated radiographically. Approximately 45% of patients will demonstrate partial response and 30% will have stable disease; if response to therapy is seen, lifelong treatment can be used [65]. Overall survival is significantly better in patients with metastatic GISTs when treated with imatinib. Blanke et al. reported a median survival of 58 months, in contrast to a median of 15 months in historical controls treated with cytotoxic chemotherapy [66]. In patients whose tumors develop resistance to imatinib, sunitinib has been used as a second line treatment with some success [51]. Patients with unresectable hepatic metastases may also be candidates for radiofrequency ablation or hepatic artery embolization.

Lymphomas

The gastrointestinal tract is the most common site of extranodal lymphoma. While the majority of these lymphomas arise in the stomach (74.6%), small bowel and colonic lymphoma are less common, accounting for 8.6% and 7%, respectively [67]. In fact, in a recent review of the Surveillance, Epidemiology, and End Results (SEER) database, primary colonic lymphoma accounted for only 0.4% of all colonic malignancies, however the incidence more than doubled between 1973 and 2004 [68].

Histology

Most lymphomas of the gastrointestinal tract are non-Hodgkin's lymphoma. Diffuse large B-cell lymphoma is the most common histologic type seen in the colon [69]. Other pathologic types in the colon include MALT-associated low-grade b-cell lymphoma, mantle cell lymphoma, and T cell lymphoma [70, 71]. Correct determination of the subtype is important for optimal treatment and prognosis. It is believed that lymphomas begin in the submucosal lymphoid tissue and spread either by direct extension or through lymphatic channels. Dawson et al. established criteria for differentiating between primary gastrointestinal lymphoma and secondary involvement of the intestinal tract by systemic lymphoma [72]. The diagnosis of primary lymphoma can be made: (1) in the absence of enlarged superficial lymph nodes, (2) absence of enlarged mediastinal lymph nodes, (3) normal total and differential and white cell count, (4) at laparotomy, only regional lymph nodes have metastatic disease, and (5) the liver and spleen are unaffected.

Incidence and Distribution

Most colonic lymphomas arise in the cecum or ascending colon, likely due to the increased lymphoid tissue in this segment of the colon. In fact, 70% of lymphomas occur proximal to the hepatic flexure [73]. Patients are typically between the ages of 50 and 70; sex predominance varies among different reports. Prolonged steroid use, inflammatory bowel disease, HIV, and EBV have been postulated as possible risk factors for the development of colonic lymphoma [74]. Both a modified Ann Arbor staging system and the TNM system have been used to stage gastrointestinal lymphomas.

Clinical Presentation and Diagnostic Tests

The most common presenting symptom of lymphomas of the colon is abdominal pain. Other symptoms mimic those of adenocarcinoma and include weight loss, rectal bleeding, change in bowel habits, anemia, weakness, and possibly fever. Tender abdominal masses may be present in up to 80% of patients at the time of presentation [75]. Growth of the lesions leads to obstruction in 20–25% of cases; however, perforation is uncommon (Figure 38-3). Colonoscopy with biopsy should be performed; however, in some cases superficial biopsies may not be sufficient to confirm the diagnosis. CT scan of the chest, abdomen, and pelvis should be obtained to extraintestinal disease.

Treatment

In patients with lymphoma that is confined to the bowel, treatment is surgical excision or systemic chemotherapy. Historically, given that a sizeable fraction of patients presented with symptomatic disease that required semi-urgent operation or underwent operation to establish a diagnosis, surgical resection was most often employed as therapy. In patients with localized disease where the diagnosis can be made preoperatively, the rationale for surgical treatment is to remove tumor that has the potential to obstruct, perforate, or

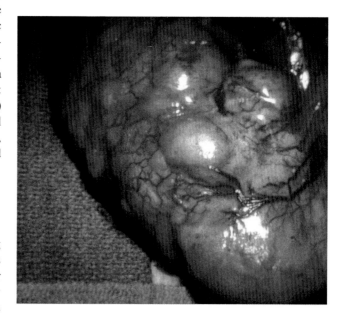

FIGURE 38-3. Lymphoma of the sigmoid colon invading the ileum (Courtesy of the ASCRS Image Library, Bruce Orkin, M.D.).

bleed, and potentially cure the patient if the tumor has not yet spread. Adjuvant chemotherapy, typically vincristine, cyclophosphamide, bleomycin, and doxorubicin, has been used to improve survival. Radiation therapy has also been advocated following resection of rectal lymphomas [76]. An alternative strategy is to treat with systemic chemotherapy and potentially avoid operation. One of the potential risks is perforation of the bowel if chemotherapy causes tumor necrosis. Given the low incidence of the disease, there are no randomized controlled trials to rely upon when making treatment decisions.

Aviles et al. treated 53 patients with B-cell lymphomas of the colon with surgery combined with chemotherapy and reported a 10-year survival of 83% [77]. Other authors, however, have reported far worse outcomes. Jinnai et al. reported results on a series of 130 patients who underwent surgical resection of colonic lymphomas [78]. Complete resection was possible in 55% of cases; however, 5-year survival was less than 40%. Prognosis was better in patients with tumors <5 cm in diameter and the absence of lymph node metastases. Lai et al. found that patients treated with surgery and chemotherapy had a 5-year survival of 62%, while 5-year survival in similar patients treated with surgery alone was only 14% [79]. Kim and colleagues compared response to treatment of 78 patients with B-cell lymphoma and 17 patients with T-cell lymphoma [80]. Those with T-cell lymphomas were younger, were more likely to present with perforation, and overall had a worse prognosis.

References

1. Oberndorfer S. Karzinoide tumoren des dunndarms. Frankf Z Pathol. 1907;1:7.
2. Kulke MH, Mayer RJ. Carcinoid tumors. N Engl J Med. 1999;340(11):858–68.
3. Ganim RB, Norton JA. Recent advances in carcinoid pathogenesis, diagnosis and management. Surg Oncol. 2000;9(4):173–9.
4. Eriksson B, Oberg K, Stridsberg M. Tumor markers in neuroendocrine tumors. Digestion. 2000;62 Suppl 1:33–8.
5. Lips CJ, Lentjes EG, Hoppener JW. The spectrum of carcinoid tumours and carcinoid syndromes. Ann Clin Biochem. 2003;40(Pt 6):612–27.
6. Godwin 2nd JD. Carcinoid tumors. An analysis of 2,837 cases. Cancer. 1975;36(2):560–9.
7. Modlin IM, Sandor A. An analysis of 8305 cases of carcinoid tumors. Cancer. 1997;79(4):813–29.
8. Taghavi S, Jayarajan SN, Powers BD, Davey A, Willis AI. Examining rectal carcinoids in the era of screening colonoscopy: a surveillance, epidemiology, and end results analysis. Dis Colon Rectum. 2013;56(8):952–9.
9. Habal N, Sims C, Bilchik AJ. Gastrointestinal carcinoid tumors and second primary malignancies. J Surg Oncol. 2000;75(4):310–6.
10. Tichansky DS, Cagir B, Borrazzo E, Topham A, Palazzo J, Weaver EJ, et al. Risk of second cancers in patients with colorectal carcinoids. Dis Colon Rectum. 2002;45(1):91–7.
11. Rosenberg JM, Welch JP. Carcinoid tumors of the colon. A study of 72 patients. Am J Surg. 1985;149(6):775–9.
12. Orloff MJ. Carcinoid tumors of the rectum. Cancer. 1971;28(1):175–80.
13. Ballantyne GH, Savoca PE, Flannery JT, Ahlman MH, Modlin IM. Incidence and mortality of carcinoids of the colon. Data from the Connecticut Tumor Registry. Cancer. 1992;69(10):2400–5.
14. Murray SE, Lloyd RV, Sippel RS, Chen H. Clinicopathologic characteristics of colonic carcinoid tumors. J Surg Res. 2013;184(1):183–8.
15. Matsui K, Iwase T, Kitagawa M. Small, polypoid-appearing carcinoid tumors of the rectum: clinicopathologic study of 16 cases and effectiveness of endoscopic treatment. Am J Gastroenterol. 1993;88(11):1949–53.
16. Pronay G, Nagy G, Ujszaszy L, Minik K. Carcinoid tumours of the rectum. Dtsch Z Verdau Stoffwechselkr. 1983;43(2):78–81.
17. Lucas KJ, Feldman JM. Flushing in the carcinoid syndrome and plasma kallikrein. Cancer. 1986;58(10):2290–3.
18. Schreurs AJ, Westermann CJ, van den Bosch JM, Vanderschueren RG, Brutel de la Riviere A, Knaepen PJ. A twenty-five-year follow-up of ninety-three resected typical carcinoid tumors of the lung. J Thorac Cardiovasc Surg. 1992;104(5):1470–5.
19. Barclay TH, Schapira DV. Malignant tumors of the small intestine. Cancer. 1983;51(5):878–81.
20. Yoshikane H, Tsukamoto Y, Niwa Y, Goto H, Hase S, Mizutani K, et al. Carcinoid tumors of the gastrointestinal tract: evaluation with endoscopic ultrasonography. Gastrointest Endosc. 1993;39(3):375–83.
21. Kobayashi K, Katsumata T, Yoshizawa S, Sada M, Igarashi M, Saigenji K, et al. Indications of endoscopic polypectomy for rectal carcinoid tumors and clinical usefulness of endoscopic ultrasonography. Dis Colon Rectum. 2005;48(2):285–91.
22. Feldman JM. Carcinoid tumors and syndrome. Semin Oncol. 1987;14(3):237–46.
23. Reubi JC, Laissue J, Waser B, Horisberger U, Schaer JC. Expression of somatostatin receptors in normal, inflamed, and neoplastic human gastrointestinal tissues. Ann N Y Acad Sci. 1994;733:122–37.
24. Hoegerle S, Altehoefer C, Ghanem N, Koehler G, Waller CF, Scheruebl H, et al. Whole-body 18F dopa PET for detection of gastrointestinal carcinoid tumors. Radiology. 2001;220(2):373–80.
25. Krausz Y, Freedman N, Rubinstein R, Lavie E, Orevi M, Tshori S, et al. 68Ga-DOTA-NOC PET/CT imaging of neuroendocrine tumors: comparison with (1)(1)(1)In-DTPA-octreotide (OctreoScan(R)). Mol Imaging Biol. 2011;13(3):583–93.
26. Stinner B, Kisker O, Zielke A, Rothmund M. Surgical management for carcinoid tumors of small bowel, appendix, colon, and rectum. World J Surg. 1996;20(2):183–8.
27. Memon MA, Nelson H. Gastrointestinal carcinoid tumors: current management strategies. Dis Colon Rectum. 1997;40(9):1101–18.
28. Welch JP, Donaldson GA. Recent experience in the management of cancer of the colon and rectum. Am J Surg. 1974;127(3):258–66.
29. Berardi RS. Carcinoid tumors of the colon (exclusive of the rectum): review of the literature. Dis Colon Rectum. 1972;15(5):383–91.

30. Sanders RJ, Axtell HK. Carcinoids of the gastrointestinal tract. Surg Gynecol Obstet. 1964;119:369–80.

31. Spread C, Berkel H, Jewell L, Jenkins H, Yakimets W. Colon carcinoid tumors. A population-based study. Dis Colon Rectum. 1994;37(5):482–91.

32. Al Natour RH, Saund MS, Sanchez VM, Whang EE, Sharma AM, Huang Q, et al. Tumor size and depth predict rate of lymph node metastasis in colon carcinoids and can be used to select patients for endoscopic resection. J Gastrointest Surg. 2012; 16(3):595–602.

33. Naunheim KS, Zeitels J, Kaplan EL, Sugimoto J, Shen KL, Lee CH, et al. Rectal carcinoid tumors—treatment and prognosis. Surgery. 1983;94(4):670–6.

34. Wang M, Peng J, Yang W, Chen W, Mo S, Cai S. Prognostic analysis for carcinoid tumours of the rectum: a single institutional analysis of 106 patients. Colorectal Dis. 2011;13(2): 150–3.

35. Wang YZ, Diebold A, Boudreaux P, Raines D, Campeau R, Anthony L, et al. Surgical treatment options for rectal carcinoid cancer: local versus low radical excision. Am Surg. 2014;80(1): 31–5.

36. Shields CJ, Tiret E, Winter DC, International Rectal Carcinoid Study Group. Carcinoid tumors of the rectum: a multi-institutional international collaboration. Ann Surg. 2010;252(5): 750–5.

37. Yoon SN, Yu CS, Shin US, Kim CW, Lim SB, Kim JC. Clinicopathological characteristics of rectal carcinoids. Int J Colorectal Dis. 2010;25(9):1087–92.

38. Sarmiento JM, Heywood G, Rubin J, Ilstrup DM, Nagorney DM, Que FG. Surgical treatment of neuroendocrine metastases to the liver: a plea for resection to increase survival. J Am Coll Surg. 2003;197(1):29–37.

39. Christante D, Pommier S, Givi B, Pommier R. Hepatic artery chemoinfusion with chemoembolization for neuroendocrine cancer with progressive hepatic metastases despite octreotide therapy. Surgery. 2008;144(6):885–93. discussion 93-4.

40. Gedaly R, Daily MF, Davenport D, McHugh PP, Koch A, Angulo P, et al. Liver transplantation for the treatment of liver metastases from neuroendocrine tumors: an analysis of the UNOS database. Arch Surg. 2011;146(8):953–8.

41. Sun W, Lipsitz S, Catalano P, Mailliard JA, Haller DG, Eastern Cooperative Oncology Group. Phase II/III study of doxorubicin with fluorouracil compared with streptozocin with fluorouracil or dacarbazine in the treatment of advanced carcinoid tumors: Eastern Cooperative Oncology Group Study E1281. J Clin Oncol. 2005;23(22):4897–904.

42. Moertel CG, Kvols LK, O'Connell MJ, Rubin J. Treatment of neuroendocrine carcinomas with combined etoposide and cisplatin. Evidence of major therapeutic activity in the anaplastic variants of these neoplasms. Cancer. 1991;68(2):227–32.

43. Brizzi MP, Berruti A, Ferrero A, Milanesi E, Volante M, Castiglione F, et al. Continuous 5-fluorouracil infusion plus long acting octreotide in advanced well-differentiated neuroendocrine carcinomas. A phase II trial of the Piemonte oncology network. BMC Cancer. 2009;9:388.

44. Modlin IM, Pavel M, Kidd M, Gustafsson BI. Review article: somatostatin analogues in the treatment of gastroenteropancreatic neuroendocrine (carcinoid) tumours. Aliment Pharmacol Ther. 2010;31(2):169–88.

45. Rinke A, Muller HH, Schade-Brittinger C, Klose KJ, Barth P, Wied M, et al. Placebo-controlled, double-blind, prospective, randomized study on the effect of octreotide LAR in the control of tumor growth in patients with metastatic neuroendocrine midgut tumors: a report from the PROMID Study Group. J Clin Oncol. 2009;27(28):4656–63.

46. Di Bartolomeo M, Bajetta E, Zilembo N, de Braud F, Di Leo A, Verusio C, et al. Treatment of carcinoid syndrome with recombinant interferon alpha-2a. Acta Oncol. 1993;32(2):235–8.

47. Kolby L, Persson G, Franzen S, Ahren B. Randomized clinical trial of the effect of interferon alpha on survival in patients with disseminated midgut carcinoid tumours. Br J Surg. 2003; 90(6):687–93.

48. Mazur MT, Clark HB. Gastric stromal tumors. Reappraisal of histogenesis. Am J Surg Pathol. 1983;7(6):507–19.

49. Davila RE, Faigel DO. GI stromal tumors. Gastrointest Endosc. 2003;58(1):80–8.

50. Steigen SE, Eide TJ. Gastrointestinal stromal tumors (GISTs): a review. APMIS. 2009;117(2):73–86.

51. Kingham TP, DeMatteo RP. Multidisciplinary treatment of gastrointestinal stromal tumors. Surg Clin North Am. 2009; 89(1):217–33. x.

52. Miettinen M, Fetsch JF, Sobin LH, Lasota J. Gastrointestinal stromal tumors in patients with neurofibromatosis 1: a clinicopathologic and molecular genetic study of 45 cases. Am J Surg Pathol. 2006;30(1):90–6.

53. Stelow EB, Stanley MW, Mallery S, Lai R, Linzie BM, Bardales RH. Endoscopic ultrasound-guided fine-needle aspiration findings of gastrointestinal leiomyomas and gastrointestinal stromal tumors. Am J Clin Pathol. 2003;119(5):703–8.

54. Goerres GW, Stupp R, Barghouth G, Hany TF, Pestalozzi B, Dizendorf E, et al. The value of PET, CT and in-line PET/CT in patients with gastrointestinal stromal tumours: long-term outcome of treatment with imatinib mesylate. Eur J Nucl Med Mol Imaging. 2005;32(2):153–62.

55. DeMatteo RP, Lewis JJ, Leung D, Mudan SS, Woodruff JM, Brennan MF. Two hundred gastrointestinal stromal tumors: recurrence patterns and prognostic factors for survival. Ann Surg. 2000;231(1):51–8.

56. Eisenberg BL, Judson I. Surgery and imatinib in the management of GIST: emerging approaches to adjuvant and neoadjuvant therapy. Ann Surg Oncol. 2004;11(5):465–75.

57. Liu H, Yan Z, Liao G, Yin H. Treatment strategy of rectal gastrointestinal stromal tumor (GIST). J Surg Oncol. 2014;109(7):708–13.

58. Changchien CR, Wu MC, Tasi WS, Tang R, Chiang JM, Chen JS, et al. Evaluation of prognosis for malignant rectal gastrointestinal stromal tumor by clinical parameters and immunohistochemical staining. Dis Colon Rectum. 2004;47(11):1922–9.

59. DeMatteo RP, Ballman KV, Antonescu CR, Corless C, Kolesnikova V, von Mehren M, et al. Long-term results of adjuvant imatinib mesylate in localized, high-risk, primary gastrointestinal stromal tumor: ACOSOG Z9000 (Alliance) intergroup phase 2 trial. Ann Surg. 2013;258(3):422–9.

60. Fernandes Gdos S, Blanke CD, Freitas D, Guedes R, Hoff PM. Perioperative treatment of gastrointestinal stromal tumors. Oncology. 2009;23(1):54–61.

61. Gold JS, Dematteo RP. Combined surgical and molecular therapy: the gastrointestinal stromal tumor model. Ann Surg. 2006;244(2):176–84.

62. Wang JP, Wang T, Huang MJ, Wang L, Kang L, Wu XJ. The role of neoadjuvant imatinib mesylate therapy in sphincter-preserving procedures for anorectal gastrointestinal stromal tumor. Am J Clin Oncol. 2011;34(3):314–6.

63. Tielen R, Verhoef C, van Coevorden F, Reyners AK, van der Graaf WT, Bonenkamp JJ, et al. Surgical management of rectal gastrointestinal stromal tumors. J Surg Oncol. 2013;107(4): 320–3.

64. Yeh CY, Chen HH, Tang R, Tasi WS, Lin PY, Wang JY. Surgical outcome after curative resection of rectal leiomyosarcoma. Dis Colon Rectum. 2000;43(11):1517–21.

65. Verweij J, Casali PG, Zalcberg J, LeCesne A, Reichardt P, Blay JY, et al. Progression-free survival in gastrointestinal stromal tumours with high-dose imatinib: randomised trial. Lancet. 2004;364(9440):1127–34.

66. Blanke CD, Rankin C, Demetri GD, Ryan CW, von Mehren M, Benjamin RS, et al. Phase III randomized, intergroup trial assessing imatinib mesylate at two dose levels in patients with unresectable or metastatic gastrointestinal stromal tumors expressing the kit receptor tyrosine kinase: S0033. J Clin Oncol. 2008;26(4):626–32.

67. Koch P, del Valle F, Berdel WE, Willich NA, Reers B, Hiddemann W, et al. Primary gastrointestinal non-Hodgkin's lymphoma: II. Combined surgical and conservative or conservative management only in localized gastric lymphoma—results of the prospective German Multicenter Study GIT NHL 01/92. J Clin Oncol. 2001;19(18):3874–83.

68. Gustafsson BI, Siddique L, Chan A, Dong M, Drozdov I, Kidd M, et al. Uncommon cancers of the small intestine, appendix and colon: an analysis of SEER 1973–2004, and current diagnosis and therapy. Int J Oncol. 2008;33(6):1121–31.

69. Myung SJ, Joo KR, Yang SK, Jung HY, Chang HS, Lee HJ, et al. Clinicopathologic features of ileocolonic malignant lymphoma: analysis according to colonoscopic classification. Gastrointest Endosc. 2003;57(3):343–7.

70. Howell JM, Auer-Grzesiak I, Zhang J, Andrews CN, Stewart D, Urbanski SJ. Increasing incidence rates, distribution and histological characteristics of primary gastrointestinal non-Hodgkin lymphoma in a North American population. Can J Gastroenterol. 2012;26(7):452–6.

71. Shaheen S, Guddati AK. Secondary mucosa-associated lymphoid tissue (MALT) lymphoma of the colon. Med Oncol. 2013;30(2):502.

72. Dawson IM, Cornes JS, Morson BC. Primary malignant lymphoid tumours of the intestinal tract. Report of 37 cases with a study of factors influencing prognosis. Br J Surg. 1961;49:80–9.

73. Fan CW, Changchien CR, Wang JY, Chen JS, Hsu KC, Tang R, et al. Primary colorectal lymphoma. Dis Colon Rectum. 2000;43(9):1277–82.

74. Dionigi G, Annoni M, Rovera F, Boni L, Villa F, Castano P, et al. Primary colorectal lymphomas: review of the literature. Surg Oncol. 2007;16 Suppl 1:S169–71.

75. Henry CA, Berry RE. Primary lymphoma of the large intestine. Am Surg. 1988;54(5):262–6.

76. Devine RM, Beart Jr RW, Wolff BG. Malignant lymphoma of the rectum. Dis Colon Rectum. 1986;29(12):821–4.

77. Aviles A, Neri N, Huerta-Guzman J. Large bowel lymphoma: an analysis of prognostic factors and therapy in 53 patients. J Surg Oncol. 2002;80(2):111–5.

78. Jinnai D, Iwasa Z, Watanuki T. Malignant lymphoma of the large intestine—operative results in Japan. Jpn J Surg. 1983; 13(4):331–6.

79. Lai YL, Lin JK, Liang WY, Huang YC, Chang SC. Surgical resection combined with chemotherapy can help achieve better outcomes in patients with primary colonic lymphoma. J Surg Oncol. 2011;104(3):265–8.

80. Kim YH, Lee JH, Yang SK, Kim TI, Kim JS, Kim HJ, et al. Primary colon lymphoma in Korea: a KASID (Korean Association for the Study of Intestinal Diseases) study. Dig Dis Sci. 2005;50(12):2243–7.

Index

soft-tissue reconstruction, 581–582
spinal reconstructive component, 581
transperineal portion, 578
urinary conduit, 578
vasiloops, 577
Restorative proctocolectomy (RPC), 269
Retroflexion, 66–67
Retroperitoneal metastases, 605
Retrorectal tumors
    classification, 374
    neoadjuvant therapy, 377
    posterior approach, 377–379
    preoperative planning, 377
    shelled out, 378
    skin incision, 378
    surgical approach, 377
    surgical treatment, 377–380
Rhomboid flap, 298, 300
Right colectomy
    anastomosis, 447–449
    caudad and cephalad aspects, 452
    cecum, 445
    duodenum, 451
    ileocolic pedicle, 446
    laparoscopic colectomy, 449, 450
    ligament of Treitz, 446
    medial-to-lateral approach, 450–451
    middle colic vessels, 452
    omental attachments, 447
    peritoneal cavity, 445
    retroperitoneum, 446
    transverse colon, 447
    Trendelenburg, 451
Right hemicolectomy, 626
Rigid proctoscopy, 48
Rigid proctosigmoioscope, 48
Robotic low anterior resection, 524–525
RPC. *See* Restorative proctocolectomy (RPC)
Rubber band ligation, 188–190
RUF. *See* Rectourethral fistula (RUF)

S
Sacrectomy
    anterior component, 579
    posterior component, 579–581
    spinal reconstructive component, 581
Sacropelvic resection
    advanced pelvic malignancies, 584
    long-term survivors, 584
    lumbosacral skeletal components, 583
    multivisceral and neuromusculoskeletal resection, 583
Scabies
    ivermectin, 339
    pruritic rash, 339
SCIP. *See* Surgical Care Improvement Project guidelines (SCIP)
Sclerotherapy, 191–192
Sedation, 60
Sedation complications, 67
Self-expanding metallic stents (SEMS), 167
SEMS. *See* Self-expanding metallic stents (SEMS)
Serrated polyposis syndrome (SPS), 387
    at-risk relatives, 398–399
    bleeding and diarrhea, 397
    cancer risk, 398
    clinical phenotypes, 397
    CRC risk, 398

diagnosis, 398
genetics, 398
screening, 398
treatment, 398
Sessile serrated adenomas (SSAs), 398
Setons
    anal fistulas, 231
    internal opening, 233
    non-cutting/draining, 233
    skin and anoderm, 232
Sexually transmitted diseases (STD), 312
Sexually transmitted infections (STIs)
    cervical cancer/anal cancer, 325
    chancroid, 333–334
    chlamydia, 329–331
    diarrhea and abdominal cramping, 327
    empiric therapy, 326
    genital lesions, 326
    gonorrhea, 327–329
    granuloma inguinale, 334
    herpes, 335
    high-risk sexual behavior, 325
    HIV and AIDS, 337–338
    HPV, 335, 337
    HSV-1 and HSV-2, 334–335
    lymphogranuloma venereum, 331 332
    molluscum contagiosum, 338
    MSM, 325
    proctitis, 326–327
    proctocolitis, 327
    pubic lice infestation, 338
    scabies, 339
    syphilis, 332–333
SGA. *See* Subjective global assessment (SGA)
Short chain fatty acids (SCFA), 31
Short *vs.* long course preoperative radiotherapy
    APR, 486
    chemoradiotherapy, systemic therapies, 486
    cytotoxic effect, 485
    cytotoxicity, 485
    disease-free survival, 485
    dose-fractionation schedule, 485
    long-term oncologic, 485
    MRI staging, 486
    neoadjuvant radiotherapy regimen, 486
    neoadjuvant treatment period, 485
    pelvic control, 485
    regimens, 485
    Trans Tasman Radiation Oncology Group, 485
Sigmoid colon, 62–63
Sigmoid-descending junction, 63
Sigmoidoscopic examination, 537
Sigmoidoscopy, 48
Simultaneous resection, 593, 597
Sister Mary Joseph node, 434
Skin preparation, 130
Slide-by technique, 53, 54
small (pediatric) Hirschmann anoscope, 48
Small bowel anastomoses, 144–145
Solitary fibrous tumor, 179
Spasm, 179
Sphincter reconstruction, 252–254, 260, 261
Sphincterotomy
    hypertrophied muscle segment, 209
    multimodal approach, 210
    topical agents, 210
    treatment failure, 209